EVIDENCE-BASED PRACTICE of CRITICAL CARE

EVIDENCE-BASED PRACTICE of CRITICAL CARE

third edition

Clifford S. Deutschman, MS, MD, FCCM

Vice Chair, Research
Department of Pediatrics
Steven and Alexandra Cohen Children's Medical Center
New Hyde Park, New York
Professor of Pediatrics and Molecular Medicine
Hofstra-Northwell School of Medicine
Hempstead, New York
Professor of Molecular Medicine, Feinstein Institute for Medical Research and
Professor, The Elmezzi Graduate School of Molecular Medicine
Manhasset, New York

Patrick J. Neligan, MA, MB, FCAI, FJFICMI

Consultant in Anaesthesia, Special Interest in Intensive Care
Medical Director, Critical Care
Galway University Hospitals
Honorary Professor of Anaesthesia and Intensive Care
National University of Ireland, Galway
Clincal Lead in Sepsis
Saolta Healthcare Group
Ireland

ELSEVIER

1600 John F. Kennedy Blvd.
Ste 1800
Philadelphia, PA 19103-2899

EVIDENCE-BASED PRACTICE OF CRITICAL CARE,
THIRD EDITION

ISBN: 978-0-323-64068-8

Notice

Practitioners and researchers must always rely on their own experience and knowledge in evaluating
and using any information, methods, compounds or experiments described herein. Because of rapid
advances in the medical sciences, in particular, independent verification of diagnoses and drug dosages
should be made. To the fullest extent of the law, no responsibility is assumed by Elsevier, authors, editors
or contributors for any injury and/or damage to persons or property as a matter of products liability,
negligence or otherwise, or from any use or operation of any methods, products, instructions, or ideas
contained in the material herein.

Library of Congress Control Number: 2019946281

Content Strategist: Nancy Anastasi Duffy
Senior Content Development Specialist: Rae L. Robertson
Publishing Services Manager: Deepthi Unni
Senior Project Manager: Manchu Mohan
Design Direction: Patrick Ferguson

Printed in the United States of America

Last digit is the print number: 9 8 7 6 5 4 3

Working together
to grow libraries in
developing countries

www.elsevier.com • www.bookaid.org

To my family:

Cate, Beth, and Nicki, who make us so proud, and Chris,
for truly being my better half for three and a half decades.

Clifford S. Deutschman, MS, MD

To Diane, David, Conor, and Kate and to
my parents, Maurice and Dympna Neligan,
for their continued support and wisdom.

Patrick J. Neligan, MA, MB, FCAI, FJFICIMI

In memory of Brian Kavanagh

friend and colleague, clinician and scientist
contributor to the first edition, mentor to many of the authors of this one
and, too sadly, not here to be embarrassed by this dedication.

Gareth L. Ackland, PhD, FRCA, FFICM
Reader in Perioperative Medicine
Translational Medicine & Therapeutics
William Harvey Research Institute
Barts and The London School of Medicine
and Dentistry, Queen Mary University of
London
London, United Kingdom

**Adeel Rafi Ahmed, MB BCh, BAO,
MRCPI, MRCP(UK), PGDip(ClinEd)**
Registrar/Fellow
Department of Nephrology
University Hospital Galway
Galway, Ireland

Djillali Annane, MD, PhD
Professor and Director, General Intensive
Care Unit
Hospital Raymond Poincaré, Assistance
Publique Hôpitaux de Paris
Dean, School of Medicine Simone Veil,
at University of Versailles Saint Quentin
en Yvelines
University Paris Saclay
Garches, France

Eman Ansari, MD, MPH
Faculty Physician
Department of Medicine
Boston Children's Hospital
Instructor of Pediatrics
Harvard Medical School
Boston, Massachusetts

Hubertus Axer, MD
Professor
Hans Berger Department of Neurology
Jena University Hospital
Jena, Germany

Jan Bakker, MD, PhD, FCCP, FCCM
Department of Pulmonology
and Critical Care
New York University and Columbia
University Medical Center
New York, New York
Intensive Care, Adults
Erasmus MC University Medical Center
Rotterdam, The Netherlands
Department of Intensive Care
Pontificia Universidad Católica de Chile
Santiago, Chile

Ian J. Barbash, MD, MS
Assistant Professor
Division of Pulmonary, Allergy & Critical
Care Medicine, Department of Medicine
University of Pittsburgh
Pittsburgh, Pennsylvania

**John James Bates, MB, BCh, BAO,
MRCPI, FCAI, FCICM, FJFICMI**
Consultant in Anaesthesia & Intensive Care
Galway University Hospitals
Honorary Professor of Anaesthesia and
Intensive Care
National University of Ireland, Galway
Clinical Lead for Critical Care
Saolta Healthcare Group
Ireland

Michael Bauer, MD
Director, Department of Anaesthesiology
and Intensive Care
Chief Executive Director, Center for Sepsis
Control & Care
Jena University Hospital
Jena, Germany

Amy L. Bellinghausen, MD
Fellow
Department of Pulmonary, Critical Care
and Sleep Medicine
University of California San Diego
San Diego, California

William S. Bender, MD, MPH
Assistant Professor
Division of Pulmonary, Allergy, Critical
Care and Sleep Medicine
Emory University School of Medicine
Atlanta, Georgia

Matthew R. Biery, DO
Attending Physician
Department of Critical Care and
Emergency Medicine
Jefferson Health System
Assistant Clinical Professor of Emergency
Medicine
Philadelphia College of Osteopathic
Medicine
Philadelphia, Pennsylvania

Alexandra Binnie, MD, DPhil
Associate Staff Physician
Department of Critical Care
William Osler Health System
Brampton, Canada

Thomas P. Bleck, MD, MCCM, FNCS
Professor of Neurology
Northwestern University Feinberg School
of Medicine
Emeritus Professor of Neurological
Sciences, Neurosurgery, Anesthesiology,
and Medicine
Rush Medical College
Chicago, Illinois

Christina Boncyk, MD
Assistant Professor
Department of Anesthesiology
Vanderbilt University Medical Center
Nashville, Tennessee

Jason C. Brainard, MD
Associate Professor
Department of Anesthesiology
University of Colorado School of Medicine
Aurora, Colorado

Scott C. Brakenridge, MD, FACS, MSCS
Assistant Professor of Surgery and
Anesthesiology
Department of Surgery, Division of Acute
Care Surgery
University of Florida
Gainesville, Florida

Frank Martin Brunkhorst, MD
Director, Center of Clinical Studies
Professor of Anaesthesiology and Intensive
Care Medicine
Jena University Hospital
Jena, Germany

Tara Cahill, BSc(Physio), MSc
Respiratory Physiotherapy
Galway University Hospital, Saolta
University Healthcare Group
National University of Ireland Galway
Galway, Ireland

**Christina Campbell, Mb BCh,
BAO, RCPI**
Respiratory Specialist Registrar
Galway University Hospital, Saolta
University Healthcare Group
National University of Ireland Galway
Galway, Ireland

Jonathan Dale Casey, MD, MSCI
Assistant Professor of Medicine
Division of Allergy, Pulmonary, and
Critical Care
Vanderbilt University Medical Center
Nashville, Tennessee

Jean-Marc Cavaillon, Dr.Sc
Professor
Experimental Neuropathology
Institut Pasteur
Paris, France

Maurizio Cereda, MD
Associate Professor
Department of Anesthesiology and Critical Care
Perelman School of Medicine at the University of Pennsylvania
Philadelphia, Pennsylvania

David J. Cooper, BMBS, MD
Professor of Intensive Care Medicine
Monash University
Melbourne, Australia

Craig M. Coopersmith, MD, FACS, FCCM
Professor
Department of Surgery
Emory Critical Care Center
Emory University
Atlanta, Georgia

Jennifer Cruz, DO
Cardiovascular Disease Fellow
Department of Cardiovascular Disease
Cooper University
Camden, New Jersey

Cheston B. Cunha, MD
Medical Director, Antimicrobial Stewardship
Infectious Disease Division
Alpert School of Medicine, Brown University
Providence, Rhode Island

Gerard F. Curley, MB, PhD, FCAI FJFICMI
Professor & Chair of Anaesthesiology & Critical Care
Royal College of Surgeons in Ireland
Consultant in Anaesthesia & Intensive Care
Beaumont Hospital
Dublin, Ireland

Allison Dalton, MD
Assistant Professor
Department of Anesthesia & Critical Care
University of Chicago
Chicago, Illinois

Daniel De Backer, MD, PhD
Professor
Intensive Care Department
CHIREC Hospitals, Université Libre de Bruxelles
Brussels, Belgium

Clifford S. Deutschman, MS, MD, MCCM
Vice Chair, Research
Department of Pediatrics
Steven and Alexandra Cohen Children's Medical Center
New Hyde Park, New York
Professor of Pediatrics and Molecular Medicine
Hofstra-Northwell School of Medicine
Hempstead, New York
Professor of Molecular Medicine, Feinstein Institute for Medical Research and Professor, The Elmezzi
Graduate School of Molecular Medicine
Manhasset, New York

David Devlin, FRCA, MRCPI
Clinical Fellow
Galway University Hospital
Galway, Ireland

Claudia C. Dos Santos, MSc, MD
Associate Professor of Medicine
Scientist, Institute of Medical Sciences
University of Toronto
Scientist, Keenan Research Centre for Biomedical Science
St. Michael's Hospital
Toronto, Canada

Tomas Drabek, MD, PhD, FASA
Associate Professor
Department of Anesthesiology and Perioperative Medicine
Scientist
Safar Center for Resuscitation Research
University of Pittsburgh
Pittsburgh, Pennsylvania

Laura Dragoi, MD
Fellow
Department of Critical Care Medicine
Sunnybrook Health Sciences Centre
Toronto, Canada

Martin Dres, MD, PhD
Sorbonne Université
Neurophysiologie Respiratoire Expérimentale et Clinique
Pneumologie, Médecine Intensive – Réanimation
La Pitié Salpêtrière Hospital
Paris, France

Anne M. Drewry, MD, MSCI
Associate Professor of Anesthesiology
Department of Anesthesiology
Washington University School of Medicine
St. Louis, Missouri

Stephen Duff, MD
School of Medicine
University College Dublin
Dublin, Ireland

Philip A. Efron, MD, FACS, FCCM
Professor of Surgery
Department of Surgery, Division of Acute Care Surgery
University of Florida
Gainesville, Florida

Sinéad Egan, MB, BCH, BAO, FCAI
Department of Anesthesia and Intensive Care
Beaumont Hospital
Dublin, Ireland

Ali A. El Solh, MD, MPH
Professor
Department of Medicine, Epidemiology, and Environmental Health
Jacobs School of Medicine and Biomedical Sciences and School of Public Health and Health Professions
University at Buffalo
Associate Chief of Staff for Research
VA Western New York Healthcare System
Buffalo, New York

E. Wesley Ely, MD, MPH
Grant Liddle Honorary Chair, Professor of Medicine
Critical Illness, Brain Dysfunction, and Survivorship (CIBS) Center
Assoc. Director of Aging Research, VA Tennessee Valley GRECC
Vanderbilt University Medical Center
Nashville, Tennessee

Laura Evans, MD, MSc
Associate Professor
Departments of Pulmonary, Critical Care, and Sleep Medicine
New York University School of Medicine
New York, New York

Jessica Falco-Walter, MD
Clinical Assistant Professor
Department of Neurology and Neurological Sciences
Stanford University
Palo Alto, California

Jonathan K. Frogel, MD
Senior Anesthestiologist
Sheba Medical Center
Department of Anesthesiology
Ramat Gan, Israel

Niall D. Ferguson, MD, MSc
Professor
Interdepartmental Division of Critical Care
Medicine
University of Toronto
Head, Critical Care Medicine
University Health Network and Sinai
Health System
Toronto, Ontario, Canada

Joseph S. Fernandez-Moure, MD, MS
Instructor
Department of Surgery
Division of Traumatology, Critical Care,
and Emergency Surgery
University of Pennsylvania
Philadelphia, Pennsylvania

Jakub Furmaga, MD
Assistant Professor of Emergency Medicine
University of Texas Southwestern Medical
Center
Dallas, Texas

David Foster Gaieski, MD
Professor
Department of Emergency Medicine
Sidney Kimmel Medical College
Thomas Jefferson University
Philadelphia, Pennsylvania

Ognjen Gajic, MD
Professor of Medicine
Division of Pulmonary and Critical Care
Mayo Clinic
Rochester, Minnesota

Alice Gallo De Moraes, MD, FACP
Assistant Professor of Medicine
Department of Medicine, Division of
Pulmonary and Critical Care
Mayo Clinic
Rochester, Minnesota

Kelly R. Genga, MD, PhD
Center for Heart Lung Innovation
University of British Columbia
Vancouver, British Columbia, Canada

Pierce Geoghegan, MB, BCh, BAO, BA
Specialist Registrar
Departments of Anaesthesia, Intensive Care
and Pain Medicine
St. Vincent's University Hospital
Dublin, Ireland

Evangelos J. Giamarellos-Bourboulis, MD, PhD
4th Department of Internal Medicine
National and Kapodistrian University of
Athens, Medical School
Athens, Greece

Rick Gill, MD
Assistant Professor
Department of Neurology
Loyola University Chicago
Chicago, Illinois

Ewan C. Goligher, MD, PhD
Department of Medicine, Division of
Respirology
University Health Network
Assistant Professor of Medicine
Interdepartmental Division of Critical Care
Medicine
University of Toronto
Scientist
Toronto General Hospital Research
Institute
Toronto, Canada

Emily K. Gordon, MD, MSEd
Associate Professor of Clinical
Anesthesiology and Critical Care
Department of Anesthesiology and
Critical Care
Perelman School of Medicine at the
University Hospital of Pennsylvania
Philadelphia, Pennsylvania

W. Robert Grabenkort, PA, MMSc, FCCM
Physician Assistant
Emory Healthcare
Atlanta, Georgia

Garima Gupta, DO, MPH
Clinical Fellow
Department of Critical Care Medicine
University of Pittsburgh Medical Center
Pittsburgh, Pennsylvania

Jacob T. Gutsche, MD
Associate Professor
Cardiothoracic and Vascular Section;
Anesthesiology and Critical Care
The Perelman School of Medicine at the
University of Pennsylvania
Philadelphia, Pennsylvania

Goksel Guven, MD
Department of Intensive Care
Erasmus Medical Center, Erasmus
University of Rotterdam
Rotterdam, The Netherlands
Department of Translational Physiology
Academic Medical Center, University of
Amsterdam
Amsterdam, The Netherlands

Paige Guyatt
Research Assistant
Department of Health Research Methods,
Evidence, and Impact
McMaster University
Hamilton, Canada

Nicholas Heming, MD
General Intensive Care Unit
Raymond Poincaré Hospital (AP-HP)
University of Versailles SQY
Laboratory of Inflammation and Infection
U1173 INSERM
Garches, France

Cheralyn J. Hendrix, MD
Resident
Department of Surgery
George Washington University Hospital
Washington, D.C.

McKenzie K. Hollen, BA
Department of Surgery, Division of Acute
Care Surgery
University of Florida
Gainesville, Florida

Steven M. Hollenberg, MD
Professor of Medicine
Hackensack Meridian Medical School at
Seton Hall
Associate Director, Cardiothoracic
Intensive Care Unit
Hackensack Meridian University Hospital
Hackensack, New Jersey

Vivien Hong Tuan Ha, MD
Assistant Specialist
Intensive Care
Raymond Poincaré University Hospital
Garches, France

Shahd Horie, BSc, MSc, PhD
Lung Biology Group
Regenerative Medicine Institute (REMEDI)
at CÚRAM Centre for Research in Medical
Devices
National University of Ireland Galway
Galway, Ireland

Catherine L. Hough, MD, MSc
Professor of Medicine
University of Washington
Seattle, Washington

Can Ince, PhD
Professor
Department of Intensive Care
Erasmus Medical Center
University Medical Center
Rotterdam, The Netherlands

Theodore J. Iwashyna, MD, PhD
Director of Health Services Research
Pulmonary and Critical Care Medicine
University of Michigan
Ann Arbor, Michigan

Judith Jacobi, PharmD, FCCP, MCCM, BCCCP
Critical Care Clinical Pharmacist
Indiana University Health Methodist Hospital
Indianapolis, Indiana

Marc Jeschke, MD, PhD, FACS, FCCM, FRCS(C)
Professor
Department of Surgery, Division of Plastic
Surgery, Department of Immunology
University of Toronto
Chair in Burn Research
Ross Tilley Burn Centre
Sunnybrook Health Sciences Centre
Senior Scientist
Sunnybrook Research Institute
Toronto, Canada

Nicholas J. Johnson, MD
Assistant Professor
Department of Emergency Medicine
Adjunct Assistant Professor
Division of Pulmonary, Critical Care, and
Sleep Medicine, Department of Medicine
University of Washington/Harborview
Medical Center
Seattle, Washington

Jeremy M. Kahn, MD, MS
Professor and Vice Chair
Department of Critical Care Medicine
University of Pittsburgh
Pittsburgh, Pennsylvania

Lewis J. Kaplan, MD, FACS, FCCM, FCCP
Professor of Surgery
Department of Surgery; Division of
Trauma, Surgical Critical Care and
Emergency Surgery
Perelman School of Medicine, University
of Pennsylvania
Section Chief, Surgical Critical Care
Department of Surgery
Corporal Michael J Crescenz VA Medical
Center
Philadelphia, Pennsylvania

Mark T. Keegan, MB, MRCPI, D.ABA, MSc, FCCM
Professor of Anesthesiology
Division of Critical Care, Department of
Anesthesiology and Perioperative Medicine
Mayo Clinic and Mayo Clinic College of
Medicine and Science
Rochester, Minnesota

Jordan Anthony Kempker, MD, MSc
Assisstant Professor
Department of Pulmonary, Allergy, Critical
Care and Sleep Medicine
Emory University
Atlanta, Georgia

Leo G. Kevin, MD, FCARCSI
Department of Intensive Care
University Hospital Galway
Galway, Ireland

Yasin A. Khan, MD
Clinical Fellow
Interdepartmental Division of Critical Care
University of Toronto
Toronto, Ontario, Canada

Ruth Kleinpell, PhD, RN, AG-ACNP, FCCM
Assistant Dean for Clinical Scholarship
Professor
Vanderbilt University School of Nursing
Nashville, Tennessee

Kurt Kleinschmidt, MD
Professor of Emergency Medicine
Division Chief, Medical Toxicology
University of Texas Southwestern Medical
Center
Dallas, Texas

Michael Klompas, MD, MPH
Professor of Population Medicine
Department of Population Medicine
Harvard Medical School and Harvard
Pilgrim Healthcare Institute
Hospital Epidemiologist
Brigham and Women's Hospital
Boston, Massachusetts

Patrick M. Kochanek, MD, MCCM
Ake N. Grenvik Professor in Critical Care
Medicine
Professor and Vice Chair, Critical Care
Medicine
Professor of Anesthesiology, Pediatrics,
Bioengineering, and Clinical and
Translational Science
Director, Safar Center for Resuscitation
Research
University of Pittsburgh School of
Medicine
Pittsburgh, Pennsylvania

W. Andrew Kofke, MD, MBA, FCCM, FNCS
Professor, Director of Neuroscience in
Anesthesiology and Critical Care Program
Co-Director, Neurocritical Care
Co-Director, Perioperative Medicine and
Pain Clinical Research Unit
Departments of Anesthesiology and
Critical Care and Neurosurgery
University of Pennsylvania
Philadelphia, Pennsylvania

Benjamin Kohl, MD, FCCM
Chief, Critical Care
Professor of Anesthesiology
Department of Anesthesiology
Thomas Jefferson University
Philadelphia, Pennsylvania

Andreas Kortgen, MD
Department of Anaesthesiology and
Critical Care Medicine
Center for Sepsis Control and Care
Jena University Hospital
Jena, Germany

David Kung, MD
Assistant Professor
Department of Neurosurgery
University of Pennsylvania
Philadelphia, Pennsylvania

John G. Laffey, MD, MA, FCAI, FJFICMI
Professor, Anaesthesia and Intensive Care
Medicine,
Vice-Dean Research, College of Medicine,
Nursing and Health Sciences
NUI Galway
Consultant, Anaesthesia and Intensive Care
Medicine
Galway University Hospitals
Galway, Ireland

Joel Lage, BS
Vila Real de Santo Antonio, Portugal

David William Lappin, MB, PhD, FRCPI
Consultant Nephrologist
Galway University Hospitals
Honorary Personal Professor of
Nephrology and Hypertension
Department of Medicine
National University of Ireland, Galway
Galway, Ireland

Francois Lamontagne, MD, MSc
Professor
Université de Sherbrooke
Scientist
Centre de Recherche du CHU de Sherbrooke
Intensivist
Centre Intégré Universitaire de Santé et de
Services Sociaux Sherbrooke
Sherbrooke, Quebec, Canada

Daniel E. Leisman, BS
Visting Scholar
Department of Pediatrics
Feinstein Institute for Medical Research
Manhasset, New York
Icahn School of Medicine at Mount Sinai
New York, New York

Ron Leong, MD
Fellow
Department of Anesthesiology
Hospital of the University of Pennsylvania
Philadelphia, Pennsylvania

Joshua M. Levine, MD
Associate Professor
Departments of Neurology, Neurosurgery,
and Anesthesiology & Critical Care
Chief, Division of Neurocritical Care
Department of Neurology
Perelman School of Medicine at the
University of Pennsylvania
Philadelphia, Pennsylvania

Andrew T. Levinson, MD, MPH
Assistant Professor of Medicine
Division of Pulmonary, Critical Care, and
Sleep Medicine
Warren Alpert School of Medicine, Brown
University
Providence, Rhode Island

Mitchell M. Levy, MD
Professor of Medicine
The Warren Alpert Medical School of
Brown University
Chief, Division of Pulmonary, Critical
Care, and Sleep Medicine
Director, Medical Intensive Care Unit
Rhode Island Hospital
Providence, Rhode Island

Ariane Lewis, MD
Associate Professor
Department of Neurology and
Neurosurgery
New York University Langone Medical
Center
New York, New York

Ariel Tamara Slavin, MD
Resident Physician
Department of Obstetrics & Gynecology
Drexel University
Philadelphia, Pennsylvania

Olivier Lheureux, MD
Department of Intensive Care
CUB Erasme Hospital
Brussels, Belgium

Vincent X. Liu, MD, MSc
Research Scientist
Division of Research
Kaiser Permanente
Oakland, California

Craig Lyons, MB, MCAI
Specialist Registrar in Anaesthesia
Department of Anaesthesia and Intensive
Care Medicine
Galway University Hospitals
Galway, Ireland

Jason H. Maley, MD
Fellow
Division of Pulmonary and Critical Care
Medicine
Massachusetts General Hospital
Division of Pulmonary, Critical Care, and
Sleep Medicine
Beth Israel Deaconess Medical Center
Boston, Massachusetts

Atul Malhotra, MD
Peter C. Farrell Presidential Chair in
Respiratory Medicine
Research Chief of Pulmonary, Critical Care
and Sleep Medicine
University of California, San Diego School
of Medicine
La Jolla, California

Joshua A. Marks, MD, FACS
Assistant Professor of Surgery
Program Director, Surgical Critical Care
Fellowship
Medical Director, Surgical Intensive Care
Unit
Sidney Kimmel Medical College at Thomas
Jefferson University
Philadelphia, Pennsylvania

Greg S. Martin, MD, MSc
Professor of Medicine
Executive Associate Division Director
Department of Pulmonary, Allergy, Critical
Care and Sleep Medicine
Emory University
Grady Memorial Hospital
Atlanta, Georgia

Niels D. Martin, MD, FACS, FCCM
Section Chief of Surgical Critical Care
Division of Traumatology, Surgical Critical
Care & Emergency Surgery
Department of Surgery
Perelman School of Medicine at the
University of Pennsylvania
Philadelphia, Pennsylvania

Claire Masterson, BSc, MSc, PhD
Post Doctoral Researcher, Lung Biology
Group
Regenerative Medicine Institute (REMEDI)
at CÚRAM Centre for Research in Medical
Devices
National University of Ireland Galway
Galway, Ireland

Yunis Mayasi, MD, MS
Division of Neurosciences Critical Care
Departments of Anesthesia and Critical
Care Medicine and Neurology
Johns Hopkins University
Baltimore, Maryland

Virginie Maxime, MD
Réanimation Médicale
Assistance Publique-Hôpitaux de Paris
Garches, Frances

**Bairbre Aine McNicholas, BSc, MB,
BCh, MRCPI, PhD, FJFICMI**
Department of Anaesthesia and Intensive
Care Medicine
Galway University Hospitals
Galway, Ireland

Jakob McSparron, MD
Assistant Professor of Medicine
Division of Pulmonary and Critical Care
Medicine
University of Michigan
Ann Arbor, Michigan

Maureen O. Meade, MD, MSc
Professor
Departments of Medicine and Health
Research Methods, Evidence and Impact
McMaster University
Hamilton, Ontario, Canada

Mark E. Mikkelsen, MD, MSCE
Associate Professor of Medicine
Pulmonary, Allergy, and Critical Care
Division
Perelman School of Medicine at the
University Hospital of Pennsylvania
Philadelphia, Pennsylvania

Alicia M. Mohr, MD, FACS, FCCM
Professor of Surgery
Department of Surgery, Division of Acute
Care Surgery
University of Florida
Gainesville, Florida

**Peter Moran, MB, BCh, BAO, MRCPI,
FCAI, FJFICMI, EDIC**
Specialist Registrar in Intensive Care Medicine
Intensive Care
University Hospital Galway
Galway, Ireland

Stephanie Royer Moss, MD
Associate Staff
Department of Hospital Medicine,
Medicine Institute
Department of Pediatric Hospital
Medicine, Pediatrics Institute
Cleveland Clinic Foundation
Cleveland, Ohio

**Patrick T. Murray, MD, FASN, FRCPI,
FJFICMI**
School of Medicine
University College Dublin
Dublin, Ireland

**Patrick J. Neligan, MA, MB, FCAI,
FJFICMI**
Consultant in Anaesthesia, Special Interest
in Intensive Care
Medical Director, Critical Care
Galway University Hospitals
Honorary Professor of Anaesthesia and
Intensive Care
National University of Ireland, Galway
Clincal Lead in Sepsis
Saolta Healthcare Group
Ireland

Larry X. Nguyen, DO, FACOI
Faculty Intensivist
Department of Critical Care Medicine
Jefferson Health Northeast
Philadelphia, Pennsylvania

**Alistair D. Nichol, MB BCh, BAO,
FCICM, FCARCSI, JFICMI, PhD**
Professor of Critical Care
University College Dublin, NUI
Consultant in Anaesthesia and Intensive
Care
St. Vincent's University Hospitals
Dublin, Ireland

Katherine Lyn Nugent, MD
Assistant Professor
Department of Emergency Medicine
Emory Critical Care Center
Emory University School of Medicine
Atlanta, Georgia

Mark E. Nunnally, MD, FCCM
Professor
Departments of Anesthesiology,
Perioperative Care & Pain Medicine,
Neurology, Surgery & Medicine
New York University Langone Health
New York, New York

Michael F. O'Connor, MD
Professor
Department of Anesthesia and Critical
Care, Department of Medicine
University of Chicago
Chicago, Illinois

Yewande Odeyemi, MBBS, MS
Senior Associate Consultant
Assistant Professor
Department of Pulmonary and Critical
Care Medicine
Mayo Clinic
Rochester, Minnesota

Steven M. Opal, MD
Clinical Professor of Medicine
Department of Medicine
The Alpert Medical School of Brown
University
Infectious Disease Division
Rhode Island Hospital
Providence, Rhode Island

Anthony O'Regan, MD, FRCPI
Professor
Department of Medicine
Consultant in Respiratory Medicine
Chief Academic Officer
Saolta University Health Care Group
Professor (personal) of Medicine
National University of Ireland Galway
Galway, Ireland

John O'Regan, MD
Nephrology Division
University Hospital Galway
Galway, Ireland

**Michelle O'Shaughnessy, MB, BCh,
MRCPI, MS, FASN**
Clinical Assistant Professor of Medicine
Division of Nephrology, Department of
Medicine
Stanford University School of Medicine
Palo Alto, California

Robert L. Owens, MD
Associate Professor of Medicine
Department of Pulmonary, Critical Care
and Sleep Medicine
University of California San Diego
La Jolla, California

Pratik Pandharipande, MD, MSCI
Department of Anesthesiology, Division of
Anesthesiology Critical Care Medicine
Critical Illness, Brain Dysfunction, and
Survivorship (CIBS) Center
Vanderbilt University
Nashville, Tennessee

Ithan D. Peltan, MD, MSc
Clinician Investigator
Division of Pulmonary and Critical Care
Medicine
Intermountain Medical Center
Murray, Utah
Adjunct Assistant Professor
Division of Pulmonary and Critical Care
Medicine
University of Utah School of Medicine
Salt Lake City, Utah

Anders Perner, MD, PhD
Professor
Department of Intensive Care
Rigshospitalet
Copenhagen, Denmark

**Michael R. Pinsky, MD, CM, Dr hc,
MCCM**
Professor of Critical Care Medicine
University of Pittsburgh
Pittsburgh, Pennsylvania

Greta Piper, MD
Assistant Professor of Surgery
Department of Surgery
New York University Langone Health
New York, New York

Lauren A. Plante, MD, MPH, FACOG
Professor
Departments of Obstetrics & Gynecology
and Anesthesiology
Drexel University College of Medicine
Philadelphia, Pennsylvania

Ariella Pratzer, MD
Department of Internal Medicine
New York University
New York, New York

Jean-Charles Preiser, MD, PhD
Professor
Intensive Care Unit
Erasme University Hospital
Université libre de Bruxelles
Brussels, Belgium

Hallie C. Prescott, MD, MSc
Assistant Professor of Internal Medicine
University of Michigan
Investigator, VA Center for Clinical
Management Research
VA Ann Arbor Healthcare System
Ann Arbor, Michigan

Megan T. Quintana, MD
Trauma and Critical Care
R. Adams Cowley Shock Trauma Center
University of Maryland Medical Center
Baltimore, Maryland

Lindsay Raab, MD
Resident Physician
Department of Neurology
Hospital of the University of Pennsylvania
Philadelphia, Pennsylvania

Jason S. Radowsky, MD
Trauma and Critical Care
R. Adams Cowley Shock Trauma Center
University of Maryland Medical Center
Baltimore, Maryland

Jesse M. Raiten, MD
Associate Professor
Anesthesiology and Critical Care
University of Pennsylvania Health System
Philadelphia, Pennsylvania

Bryan T. G. Reidy, MB, BAO, BCh, FCAI
Specialist Registrar Anaesthesia and Critical
Care Medicine
Department of Anaesthesia
University Hospital Galway
Galway, Ireland

Patrick M. Reilly, MD, FACS
Professor of Surgery
Department of Surgery
Perelman School of Medicine at the
University of Pennsylvania
Philadelphia, Pennsylvania

Kenneth E. Remy, MD, MHSc, MSCI
Assistant Professor of Pediatrics and
Internal Medicine
Washington University in St. Louis, School
of Medicine
Barnes-Jewish Hospital
St. Louis Children's Hospital
St. Louis, Missouri

Emanuele Rezoagli, MD
Lung Biology Group
Regenerative Medicine Institute (REMEDI)
at CÚRAM Centre for Research in Medical
Devices
National University of Ireland Galway
Department of Anesthesia and Intensive
Care Medicine
Galway University Hospitals
SAOLTA University Health Group
Galway, Ireland
Department of Medicine and Surgery
University of Milan-Bicocca
Monza, Italy

Zaccaria Ricci, MD
Department of Cardiology and Cardiac
Surgery
Pediatric Cardiac Intensive Care Unit
Bambino Gesù Children's Hospital
Rome, Italy

Lisbi Rivas, MD
Resident Physician
Department of Surgery
George Washington University
Washington, DC

Bram Rochwerg, MD, MSc, FRCPC
Assistant Professor
Department of Medicine
McMaster University
Hamilton, Ontario, Canada

Kristen Carey Rock, MD
Assistant Professor
Anesthesia and Critical Care Medicine
University of Pennsylvania
Philadelphia, Pennsylvania

Claudio Ronco, MD
Professor of Nephrology
Department of Medicine
Università degli Studi di Padova
Director, Department of Nephrology,
Dialysis and Transplantation
International Renal Research Institute
(IRRIV)
San Bortolo Hospital
Vicenza, Italy

James A. Russell, MD
Centre for Heart Lung Innovation
Division of Critical Care Medicine,
Department of Medicine
St. Paul's Hospital and University of British
Columbia
Vancouver, British Columbia, Canada

Danielle K. Sandsmark, MD, PhD
Assistant Professor
Departments of Neurology, Neurosurgery,
and Anesthesiology/Critical Care
Hospital of the University of Pennsylvania
Philadelphia, Pennsylvania

Joshua Iokepa Santos, MD
Anesthesiology Critical Care Fellow
Department of Anesthesiology & Critical
Care
University of Colorado School of Medicine
Aurora, Colorado

Babak Sarani, MD, FACS, FCCM
Professor of Surgery and Emergency
Medicine
Director, Center for Trauma and Critical
Care
Director, George Washington Patient
Logistics Center
George Washington University
Washington, DC

Damon C. Scales, MD, PhD
Professor
Interdepartmental Division of Critical Care
Medicine and Department of Medicine
University of Toronto
Staff Intensivist and Clinician Scientist
Department of Critical Care Medicine
Sunnybrook Health Sciences Centre and
Sunnybrook Research Institute
Toronto, Canada

Michael Scully, MB BCh, MD, FRCA, MRCPI, FCICM, FJFICMI
Senior Lecturer in Critical Care
National University of Ireland, Galway,
Consultant in Anaesthesia & Intensive Care
Galway University Hospitals
Galway, Ireland

Jon Sevransky, MD, MHS
Professor of Medicine
Emory University
Atlanta, Georgia

Sam D. Shemie, MD
Department of Pediatric Critical Care
Montreal Children's Hospital, McGill
University and Health Centre
Montreal, Canada

Carrie A. Sims, MD, PhD, FACS
Associate Professor of Surgery and Director
of Research
Section Chief, Geriatric Acute Care Surgery
Division of Trauma, Surgical Critical Care,
and Emergency Surgery
University of Pennsylvania
Philadelphia, Pennsylvania

Brian P. Smith, MD
Assistant Professor of Surgery
Department of Surgery
The Hospital of the University of
Pennsylvania
Philadelphia, Pennsylvania

Audrey E. Spelde, MD
Resident Physician
Department of Anesthesiology and Critical
Care
The University of Pennsylvania
Philadelphia, Pennsylvania

Robert David Stevens, MD, FCCM
Associate Professor
Department of Anesthesiology and Critical
Care Medicine, Neurology, Neurosurgery,
and Radiology
Johns Hopkins University School of
Medicine
Baltimore, Maryland

B. Taylor Thompson, MD
Division Pulmonary and Critical Care
Medicine
Massachusetts General Hospital
Professor of Medicine
Harvard Medical School
Boston, Massachusetts

**Samuel A. Tisherman, MD, FACS,
FCCM**
Professor
Department of Surgery and the Program in
Trauma
University of Maryland School of Medicine
Baltimore, Maryland

Mark Trinder, MSC
Centre for Heart Lung Innovation
Experimental Medicine Program
University of British Columbia
Vancouver, British Columbia, Canada

Isaiah R. Turnbull, MD, PhD
Assistant Professor
Department of Surgery
Washington University School of Medicine
St. Louis, Missouri

**Ida-Fong Ukor, MBBS, FCICM,
FANZCA, BMed Sci**
Centre for Heart Lung Innovation and
Division of Critical Care Medicine
University of British Columbia
Vancouver, British Columbia, Canada

Tom van der Poll, MD, PhD
Professor
Division of Infectious Diseases & Center of
Experimental and Molecular Medicine
Amsterdam UMC, Academic Medical
Center, University of Amsterdam
Amsterdam, The Netherlands

Tjitske S.R. van Engelen, MD, MSc
Center for Experimental Molecular
Medicine and Department of Internal
Medicine
Amsterdam University Medical Centers
University of Amsterdam
Amsterdam, The Netherlands

Charles R. Vasquez, MD
Surgical Resident
Division of Traumatology, Surgical Critical
Care & Emergency Surgery
Department of Surgery
Perelman School of Medicine at the
University of Pennsylvania
Philadelphia, Pennsylvania

Michael A. Vella, MD, MBA
Instructor in Surgery
Division of Traumatology, Surgical Critical
Care & Emergency Surgery
Perelman School of Medicine at the
University of Pennsylvania
Philadelphia, Pennsylvania

William J. Vernick, MD
Assistant Professor
Department of Anesthesiology and Critical
Care
The Perelman School of Medicine at the
University Hospital of Pennsylvania
Philadelphia, Pennsylvania

Gianluca Villa, MD
Department of Health Science, Section of
Anaesthesiology, Intensive Care and Pain
Medicine
University of Florence
Department of Anaesthesia and Intensive
Care, Section of Oncological Anaesthesia
and Intensive Care Unit
Azienda Ospedaliero Universitaria Careggi
Florence, Italy

Jean-Louis Vincent, MD, PhD
Professor of Intensive Care Medicine
Department of Intensive Care
Erasme Hospital, Université libre de
Bruxelles
Brussels, Belgium

Amy C. Walker, BSc, MD
Resident Physician
Department of Emergency Medicine
University of Washington
Seattle, Washington

Keith R. Walley, MD
Professor of Medicine
University of British Columbia
Vancouver, British Columbia, Canada

Lorraine B. Ware, MD
Professor of Medicine
Division of Allergy, Pulmonary and Critical
Care Medicine
Department of Medicine
Department of Pathology, Microbiology
and Immunology
Vanderbilt University School of Medicine
Nashville, Tennessee

Stuart J. Weiss, MD, PhD
Associate Professor
Chief, Division of Cardiac Anesthesiology
Department of Anesthesiology and Critical
Care
University of Pennsylvania
Philadelphia, Pennsylvania

Anna E. Garcia Whitlock, MD
Resident in General Surgery
University of Pennsylvania
Philadelphia, Pennsylvania

Pauline Whyte, MB BCh, FRCAI
Consultant in Anaesthesia & Intensive Care
Galway University Hospitals
Galway, Ireland

We are delighted to present this third edition of *Evidence-Based Practice of Critical Care*. Critical care is a fast moving field with an abundance of new publications that result in subtle but frequent changes in our thinking. To produce a state of the art book that covers the full spectrum of our specialty has required the participation of a large number of experts and their mentees. We are truly grateful for their participation. We would like to thank the many critical care practitioners who have purchased the prior editions of the book and complimented us on its value and content. This edition is not an updated facsimile of the second. We have significantly revised the content:

- Some of the basic principles we highlighted previously have stood the test of time—at least of the last few years. These successes reinforce our belief that care of the critically ill patient will continue to improve.
- Evidence continues to support the value of consistently applying proven interventions (Chapters 1, 2, 8, 38). However, while we may now have a better sense of which individual approaches carry the most profound benefit (Chapters 9, 16, 18, 24, 34), we are profoundly aware that many may not (Chapters 25, 48) and that, in most cases, the evidence remains equivocal (Chapters 7, 8, 18, 20, 26, 57, 73, 84).
- We have a better understanding of some aspects of the pathobiology of critical illness (Chapters 14, 17, 25, 29, 38, 40, 41, 62, 63, 69), but a great deal remains elusive (Chapters 5, 32, 33, 38, 69).
- The use of large datasets to identify disorders has increased (Chapters 1, 2, 3, 5, 13, 21, 31, 34, 37, 38), mostly to the benefit of critically ill patients. Data-based approaches have aided in the early identification of disorders of profound importance, for example, sepsis (Chapter 31). The impact of comorbidities as well as preexisting and predisposing conditions is now clearer (Chapters 5, 11, 15, 21,79), but controversy remains (Chapter 27).
- Critical illness does not end with discharge from the ICU; in fact, some unfortunate patients never fully recover (Chapters 3, 22, 40). A pathobiologic understanding is only just emerging (Chapters 3, 4, 12, 40, 41) and identification/validation of therapeutic approaches is limited (Chapter 4, 22).
- Definitions for sepsis, acute respiratory distress syndrome (ARDS), and ventilator-associated pneumonia have been revised (Chapters 13, 30, 47). It is now appreciated that a definition ("what a thing *is*") differs from the clinical criteria used to identify a disorder (Chapters 13, 30, 31, 47) because there are few gold standards that can be used to unequivocally identify most diagnoses that underlie critical illness. Critical criteria to identify patients with sepsis and

ARDS have been derived and validated using large datasets (Chapters 13, 31). There remains a pressing need to develop and validate evidence-driven consensus criteria for other disorders (e.g., brain death, Chapter 87).
- Many aspects of critical care practice remain poorly understood, controversial, or unproven (Chapters 25, 26, 32, 33, 39, 57, 68, 73). And while some of the things we do may be bad (Chapters 6, 10, 24, 60, 61), we continue to do them.
- Early identification of several disorders, especially those involving infection, trauma, or the vasculature, is of paramount importance (Chapters 34, 38, 46, 52, 53, 54, 64, 65, 66, 67, 74, 75, 77, 80).
- Determining if outcomes from critical illness have improved, or if interventions have been effective, remains problematic (Chapters 2, 5, 17, 18, 19, 20, 21, 22, 37, 38, 39, 47, 68, 73). And we continue to search for the elusive "better way" (Chapter 84).
- Critical care practice has long been recognized as a "team sport." We recognize that the critical care team is composed of diversely educated coequals; while each member may have a specific area of expertise, we also support and learn from each other (Chapters 85, 86).
- The results of many studies continue to be negative or equivocal. But we have increasingly come to recognize that this result is virtually unavoidable when we globally apply a specific therapy to all patients with a given disorder. A major challenge for future critical care practitioners will be to identify those specific patients in whom a therapeutic approach is most likely to work. Genetics or other aspects of the host response will be major determinants (Chapters 5, 32, 33, 40, 41, 46, 63), but so will the characteristics of the disorder, for example, the importance of the specific infecting agent that precipitates sepsis remains virtually unexplored (Chapter 43).
- Finally, critical care practice has become more patient-centric (Chapters 2, 3, 4, 5, 84, 86, 88), and this trend must continue.

Reading, writing, and editing the chapters in this book has been hugely enjoyable and thought provoking. In particular, we would like to commend the individuals who are contributing for the first time, having not participated in the first two editions. It is gratifying to recognize that their enthusiasm for critical care equals our own, and that their understanding of our field exceeds our own. These individuals represent the future of critical care—and the field is in good hands.

Clifford S. Deutschman
Patrick J. Neligan
March 2019

CONTENTS

EVIDENCE-BASED PRACTICE of CRITICAL CARE

1

Has Evidence-Based Medicine Changed the Practice of Critical Care?

Andrew T. Levinson and Mitchell M. Levy

The Evidence-Based Medicine movement, that originated in the mid-1990s, has resulted in monumental changes in critical care medicine. During that period, practice shifted from a reliance on expert opinion to a critical appraisal of the available literature to answer focused clinical questions.[1,2] Systematic examination of what works and what does not, while valuing clinical experience and patient preferences, has led to a surprising and thought-provoking journey that has resulted in dramatic improvements in the care of the critically ill patient. Many of the lessons learned during the evidence-based medicine era would have never been predicted two decades ago.

In this chapter, we describe five important lessons learned in intensive care during the evidence-based medicine era:
1. We need to look beyond single randomized clinical trials (RCTs).
2. It is the small things that make a difference.
3. Accountability is critically important.
4. We often need to do less to patients rather than more.
5. It is the multidisciplinary intensive care unit (ICU) team, not the individual provider, that is the most responsible for good clinical outcomes and high-quality critical care.

LOOKING BEYOND SINGLE RANDOMIZED CONTROLLED TRIALS

By critically appraising the entire body of literature on specific interventions and clinical outcomes, we have learned many lessons about what is most important in the delivery of critical care. However, we have learned that we must wait before we immediately embrace the results of a single RCT with very impressive results and instead base our clinical practices on more comprehensive, cautious, and critical appraisals of all of the available literature.

The decades of critical care research since the 1990s are filled with stories of impressive findings from single-center RCTs that could not be replicated in larger multicenter RCTs. Unfortunately, in many cases, the initial positive single-center results have been embraced by early adopters, only to have the

results refuted by subsequent follow-up trials. The story of tight glycemic control in critical illness is illustrative. A single-center study of the management of hyperglycemia in a population consisting primarily of postcardiac surgical patients found that intensive glucose management with insulin infusion with a target blood glucose of 80 to 110 mg/dL dramatically reduced mortality when compared with a more lenient target blood glucose of 160 to 200 mg/dL.[3] The results of this single-center study were embraced by many intensivists and rapidly generalized to a wide variety of critically ill patents. The factors behind this rapid adoption by the field are multiple, including ease of implementation and cost. Unfortunately, a subsequent similar study of medical patients showed no significant benefit of an intensive insulin therapy protocol in the critically ill medical patient.[4] Ultimately, the most comprehensive multicenter trial of medical and surgical critically ill patients found significantly increased mortality in the group randomized to a tight glycemic control protocol, compared with targeting a blood glucose level of less than 180 mg/dL. This excess mortality was likely due to the much higher rates of severe hypoglycemia.[5]

In 2001, the era of early goal-directed therapy (EGDT) was introduced through the publication of a single-center RCT. EGDT was widely adopted, and multiple subsequent published trials, all prospective cohort series, confirmed its benefit.[6] More recently, three large RCTs[7–9] failed to demonstrate a survival benefit when protocolized resuscitation was compared with "usual care." It is possible that these results, at least in part, reflect the effect of the original EGDT trial; the widespread adoption of aggressive, early resuscitation; and the broad-based implementation of the Surviving Sepsis Campaign Guidelines and bundles.[10] If this continues to define usual care, then perhaps it is no longer necessary to mandate specific protocols for resuscitation because it appears that standard sepsis management has evolved to be consistent with published protocols.

The evidence for the use of hydrocortisone in the treatment of septic shock is an example of a sepsis treatment in which the initial promising study was embraced quite early,[11] only to be questioned by subsequent conflicting evidence.[12] A multicenter placebo controlled trial of hydrocortisone in septic shock which enrolled 3800 patients, published in 2018, has only increased the ambiguity. It found a quicker resolution in shock but no mortality benefit.[13] After more than 15 years and multiple large studies we are still awaiting the final answer about the clinical administration of corticosteroids as an adjunctive therapy in septic shock.

Activated protein C is an example of how little we still currently know about the pathobiology of sepsis and the difficulty in developing targeted therapies. Activated protein C, used as an adjunct therapy for patients with sepsis, was initially thought to be quite promising,[14] but was ultimately abandoned after subsequent RCTs failed to duplicate the original results.[15] Newly adopted medications and interventions based on limited data may suffer the same fate.[16,17]

SMALL THINGS MAKE A BIG DIFFERENCE

The evidence-based era has taught us that small, often neglected or overlooked details of everyday bedside care can play a large role in determining whether our patients survive their ICU stay. Pneumonia that develops after the initiation of mechanic ventilation (ventilator-associated pneumonia [VAP]) is associated with high morbidity and mortality and significantly increased costs for critically ill patients. Several simple targeted interventions to address this problem have significantly reduced VAP rates. Simply keeping our intubated patients' heads elevated at least 30 degrees rather than leaving them supine (as was customary two decades ago) has resulted in major reductions in VAP.[18,19] In addition, a focus on better oral hygiene of mechanically ventilated patients via the administration of oral chlorhexidine has even further reduced the VAP rates.[20-23]

Another simple small intervention in the evidence-based era, the early mobilization of our critically ill patients, has also been found to significantly improve patient outcomes. Critically ill patients were kept immobilized for several weeks in the belief that this was necessary for their recovery. The result was very high rates of ICU-acquired weakness that required prolonged periods of rehabilitation in ICU survivors.[24] More recent studies have shown dramatic improvements in functional status and significantly decreased ICU length of stay (LOS) when critically ill patients are mobilized as soon and as much as possible.[25,26]

ACCOUNTABILITY IS IMPORTANT

Another important lesson learned during the evidence-based era is the importance of tracking clinical behavior through performance measures. Published reports have demonstrated a significant gap between intensivists' perceptions of their ability to adhere to current evidence-based medicine and actual practice.[27] This dichotomy has been noted in adherence to low tidal volume strategies in acute respiratory distress

syndrome and other common "best ICU practices." These findings have led to the development of checklists and performance metrics to foster clinician accountability that have provided tangible improvements in clinical care. Multifaceted interventions using checklists have dramatically reduced catheter-related blood stream infections[28] as well as complications from surgical procedures.[29]

In acute situations, checklists have also been shown to improve delivery of care.[30] Continuous measurement of individual performance in the evidence-based medicine era has allowed ongoing, real-time feedback to individual clinicians and groups of providers. Application of this approach to sepsis care has resulted in significant improvements in adherence to evidence-based guidelines and in patient outcomes.[31]

DO LESS, NOT MORE

The evidence-based era has also taught us that we often should do less, not more, to and for our critically ill patients. We have learned that interrupting sedation and awakening mechanically ventilated patients each day, and thus reducing the amount of medication administered, can reduce ICU LOS.[32,33] When coupled with a daily weaning trial, daily awaking of ICU patients reduced mortality.[34] There remains, however, some clinical equipoise regarding the additive effect of daily sedation interruption in addition to protocolized sedation.[35] It has also been learned that decreasing the need for mechanic ventilation by first using noninvasive strategies in specific groups of patients with acute respiratory distress may improve outcome.[36] In addition, use of smaller tidal volumes in mechanically ventilated patients has been shown to be lifesaving.[37] We have also learned that reducing the amount of blood given to patients who are critically ill, even in some situations where the patient is actively bleeding, can significantly improve outcomes.[38,39]

IT IS NOT JUST THE INTENSIVIST

Finally, it has been learned that it is not the physician, but rather the entire health-care team, that is responsible for the delivery of high-quality care in the ICU. In a large observational cohort study based on the Acute Physiology and Chronic Health Evaluation IV (APACHE IV) model for predicting ICU LOS, investigators found that the key factors for predicting ICU LOS were structural and administrative. Specific APACHE IV variables of importance include reduced nurse-to-patient ratios, specific discharge policies, and the utilization of protocols. Structural and administrative factors were significantly different in high-performing ICUs with decreased LOS when adjusting for patient variables.[40,41]

The use of weaning protocols managed by respiratory therapists has resulted in reductions in the duration of mechanic ventilation relative to the subjective individualized assessment of an ICU clinician.[42,43] In addition, a 2013 study revealed that staffing academic ICUs with intensivists overnight did not change clinical outcomes.[44] Finally, a landmark 2006 study found that empowering critical care nurses to intervene when they witnessed breaches in sterility was a key component in reducing catheter-related blood stream infections.[28] Taken together, these and other data strongly suggest that it is not solely the intensivist, but the entire critical care team, that is key to high-quality care.

SUMMARY

In summary, it seems that lessons offered by evidence-based medicine suggest that patience, keeping it simple, paying attention to detail, and working as a team are the key elements of good clinical care.

Key Points

1. Look beyond single randomized controlled trials.
2. Small things make a big difference.
3. Accountability is important.
4. Do less, not more.
5. It is not just the intensivist.

AUTHORS' RECOMMENDATIONS

- Single randomized controlled trials may be misleading, and the totality of evidence should be evaluated.
- Simple interventions such as head of bed elevation and early mobilization make a significant difference to outcomes.
- Measuring performance levels with checklists and audit improves outcomes. Accountability is important.
- Taking a conservative approach to interventions and therapies appears to confer patient benefit: "do less, not more."
- High-quality organized multidisciplinary intensive care improves outcomes: it is not just the intensivist.

REFERENCES

1. Smith R, Rennie D. Evidence-based medicine—an oral history. *JAMA*. 2014;311(4):365-367.
2. Evidence-Based Medicine Working Group. Evidence-based medicine. A new approach to teaching the practice of medicine. *JAMA*. 1992;268(17):2420-2425.
3. Van den Berghe G, Wouters P, Weekers F, et al. Intensive insulin therapy in critically ill patients. *N Engl J Med*. 2001;345(19):1359-1367.
4. Van den Berghe G, Wilmer A, Hermans G, et al. Intensive insulin therapy in the medical ICU. *N Engl J Med*. 2006;354(5):449-461.
5. NICE-SUGAR Study Investigators, Finfer S, Chittock DR, et al. Intensive versus conventional glucose control in critically ill patients. *N Engl J Med*. 2009;360(13):1283-1297.
6. Rivers E, Nguyen B, Havstad S, et al. Early goal-directed therapy in the treatment of severe sepsis and septic shock. *N Engl J Med*. 2001;345(19):1368-1377.
7. Angus DC, Yealy DM, Kellum JA, ProCESS Investigators. Protocol-based care for early septic shock. *N Engl J Med*. 2014;371(4):386.
8. ARISE Investigators; ANZICS Clinical Trials Group, Preake SL, et al. Goal-directed resuscitation for patients with early septic shock. *N Engl J Med*. 2014;371(16):1496-1506.
9. Mouncey PR, Osborn TM, Power GS, et al. Trial of early, goal-directed resuscitation for septic shock. *N Engl J Med*. 2015;372(14):1301-1311.
10. Rhodes A, Evans LE, Alhazzani W, et al. Surviving Sepsis Campaign: international guidelines for management of sepsis and septic shock, 2016. *Intensive Care Med*. 2017;43(3):304-377.
11. Annane D, Sébille V, Charpentier C, et al. Effect of treatment with low doses of hydrocortisone and fludrocortisone on mortality in patients with septic shock. *JAMA*. 2002;288(7):862-871.
12. Sprung CL, Annane D, Keh D, et al. Hydrocortisone therapy for patients with septic shock. *N Engl J Med*. 2008;358(2):111-124.
13. Venkatesh B, Finfer S, Cohen J, et al. Adjunctive glucocorticoid therapy in patients with septic shock. *N Engl J Med*. 2018;378(9):797-808.
14. Bernard GR, Vincent JL, Laterre PF, et al. Efficacy and safety of recombinant human activated protein C for severe sepsis. *N Engl J Med*. 2001;344(10):699-709.
15. Ranieri VM, Thompson BT, Barie PS, et al. Drotrecogin alfa (activated) in adults with septic shock. *N Engl J Med*. 2012;366(22):2055-2064.
16. Khanna A, English SW, Wang XS, et al. Angiotensin II for treatment of vasodilatory shock. *N Engl J Med*. 2017;377(5):419-430.
17. Marik PE, Khangoora V, Rivera R, Hooper MH, Catravas J. Hydrocortisone, vitamin C, and thiamine for the treatment of severe sepsis and septic shock. *Chest*. 2017;151(6):1229-1238.
18. Torres A, Serra-Batlles J, Ros E, et al. Pulmonary aspiration of gastric contents in patients receiving mechanical ventilation: the effect of body position. *Ann Intern Med*. 1992;116(7):540-543.
19. Orozco-Levi M, Torres A, Ferrer M, et al. Semirecumbent position protects from pulmonary aspiration but not completely from gastroesophageal reflux in mechanically ventilated patients. *Am J Respir Crit Care Med*. 1995;152(4 Pt 1):1387-1390.
20. Shi Z, Xie H, Wang P, et al. Oral hygiene care for critically ill patients to prevent ventilator-associated pneumonia. *Cochrane Database Syst Rev*. 2013;8:CD008367.
21. Chan EY, Ruest A, Meade MO, Cook DJ. Oral decontamination for prevention of pneumonia in mechanically ventilated adults: systematic review and meta-analysis. *BMJ*. 2007;334(7599):889.
22. Labeau SO, Van de Vyver K, Brusselaers N, Vogelaers D, Blot SI. Prevention of ventilator-associated pneumonia with oral antiseptics: a systematic review and meta-analysis. *Lancet Infect Dis*. 2011;11(11):845-854.
23. Price R, MacLennan G, Glen J, SuDDICU Collaboration. Selective digestive or oropharyngeal decontamination and topical oropharyngeal chlorhexidine for prevention of death in general intensive care: systematic review and network meta-analysis. *BMJ*. 2014;348:g2197.
24. Schweickert WD, Kress JP. Implementing early mobilization interventions in mechanically ventilated patients in the ICU. *Chest*. 2011;140(6):1612-1617.
25. Schweickert WD, Pohlman MC, Pohlman AS, et al. Early physical and occupational therapy in mechanically ventilated, critically ill patients: a randomised controlled trial. *Lancet*. 2009;373(9678):1874-1882.
26. Stiller K. Physiotherapy in intensive care: an updated systematic review. *Chest*. 2013;144(3):825-847.
27. Brunkhorst FM, Engel C, Ragaller M, et al. Practice and perception—a nationwide survey of therapy habits in sepsis. *Crit Care Med*. 2008;36(10):2719-2725.
28. Pronovost P, Needham D, Berenholtz S, et al. An intervention to decrease catheter-related bloodstream infections in the ICU. *N Engl J Med*. 2006;355(26):2725-2732.

29. de Vries EN, Prins HA, Crolla RM, et al. Effect of a comprehensive surgical safety system on patient outcomes. *N Engl J Med*. 2010; 363(20):1928-1937.

30. Arriaga AF, Bader AM, Wong JM, et al. Simulation-based trial of surgical-crisis checklists. *N Engl J Med*. 2013;368(3): 246-253.

31. Levy MM, Dellinger RP, Townsend SR, et al. The Surviving Sepsis Campaign: results of an international guideline-based performance improvement program targeting severe sepsis. *Crit Care Med*. 2010;38(2):367-374.

32. Kress JP, Pohlman AS, O'Connor MF, Hall JB. Daily interruption of sedative infusions in critically ill patients undergoing mechanical ventilation. *N Engl J Med*. 2000;342(20):1471-1477.

33. Hughes CG, McGrane S, Pandharipande PP. Sedation in the intensive care setting. *Clin Pharmacol*. 2012;4:53-63.

34. Girard TD, Kress JP, Fuchs BD, et al. Efficacy and safety of a paired sedation and ventilator weaning protocol for mechanically ventilated patients in intensive care (Awakening and Breathing Controlled trial): a randomised controlled trial. *Lancet*. 2008;371 (9607):126-134.

35. Mehta S, Burry L, Cook D, et al. Daily sedation interruption in mechanically ventilated critically ill patients cared for with a sedation protocol. *JAMA*. 2012;308(19):1985-1992.

36. Brochard L, Mancebo J, Wysocki M, et al. Noninvasive ventilation for acute exacerbations of chronic obstructive pulmonary disease. *N Engl J Med*. 1995;333(13):817-822.

37. Futier E, Constantin JM, Paugam-Burtz C, et al. A trial of intraoperative low-tidal-volume ventilation in abdominal surgery. *N Engl J Med*. 2013;369(5):428-437.

38. Villanueva C, Colomo A, Bosch A, et al. Transfusion strategies for acute upper gastrointestinal bleeding. *N Engl J Med*. 2013;368(1): 11-21.

39. Jairath V, Hearnshaw S, Brunskill SJ, et al. Red cell transfusion for the management of upper gastrointestinal haemorrhage. *Cochrane Database Syst Rev*. 2010;(9):CD006613.

40. Zimmerman JE, Kramer AA, McNair DS, Malila FM, Shaffer VL. Intensive care unit length of stay: benchmarking based on Acute Physiology and Chronic Health Evaluation (APACHE) IV. *Crit Care Med*. 2006;34(10):2517-2529.

41. Zimmerman JE, Alzola C, Von Rueden KT. The use of benchmarking to identify top performing critical care units: a preliminary assessment of their policies and practices. *J Crit Care*. 2003;18(2):76-86.

42. Ely EW, Baker AM, Dunagan DP, et al. Effect on the duration of mechanical ventilation of identifying patients capable of breathing spontaneously. *N Engl J Med*. 1996;335(25):1864-1869.

43. Blackwood B, Burns KE, Cardwell CR, O'Halloran P. Protocolized versus non-protocolized weaning for reducing the duration of mechanical ventilation in critically ill adult patients. *Cochrane Database Syst Rev*. 2014;(11):CD006904.

44. Kerlin MP, Halpern SD. Nighttime physician staffing in an intensive care unit. *N Engl J Med*. 2013;369(11):1075.

2

Do Protocols/Guidelines Actually Improve Outcomes?

Jon Sevransky, William S. Bender, and Bram Rochwerg

Critical illness and injury that results in intensive care unit (ICU) admission requires complex, coordinated, and often invasive treatment. The sheer number of clinicians, consultants, and caregivers coordinating the rapid delivery of life-saving therapy to patients with evolving physiology in a busy environment can make it challenging to ensure that all patients receive appropriate and evidence-based care. One way to increase the chance of receiving optimal care and to decrease the possibility of unnecessary variation in practice is to create protocols that explicitly delineate desired care pathways. Protocolization allows for consideration of specific pre-set treatment algorithms for patients who have life-threatening illness or injury. For example, it seems rational that a patient with sepsis admitted to the ICU on Tuesday morning would get similar and appropriate care as a patient with the same complaint admitted late Saturday evening. Thus, standardizing care through the use of protocols would ensure that patients receive similar and appropriate care at various times of the day and week with differing bedside clinicians.

Protocols may be based on local practice, derived from clinician's experiences and modified to suit specific patient phenotypes, or adapted from national or international clinical practice guidelines (CPGs) that provide direction for patients' treatment options. Whether the basis for a specific protocol is local or national, it is imperative that the standardization of clinical practice be modified based on the individual setting in order to fit the available resources and serve the local patient population in the best possible manner.

Over the past few years, guidelines have been established to help direct practitioners in the care of ICU patients with sepsis, acute respiratory failure, and delirium.[1-3] To be considered trustworthy, guidelines are best created using a platform that allows for:
- clear and reproducible documentation of how the guideline was created
- assessment and management of potential conflicts of interest in panel members
- involvement of all relevant stakeholders
- a clear linkage to the summary of the currently available evidence
- clear and actionable recommendations
- an assessment of the level of evidence supporting each recommendation within the guideline

This chapter will review the development and use of protocols and guidelines in critical illness as well as potential limitations and hazards in using such protocols and guidelines.

WHAT IS A PROTOCOL?

Protocols are locally produced care pathways that mandate a course of therapy or care. They are often codified into clinical order sets, serve as a template for the delivery of specific patient care.[4,5] Protocols are most often created with the aim of improving care for specific disorders and ensuring that appropriate, desired, and evidence-based care is delivered to patients who meet specific criteria.[4] Protocols can be produced and used by physicians, nurses, respiratory therapists, and often involve numerous providers allowing for coordinated and optimal clinical management. Protocol initiation may be triggered by admission to an ICU; more commonly, protocol initiation coincides with a specific level of care (e.g., a patient requiring intubation and delivery of invasive mechanical ventilation) or when a patient is diagnosed with a certain disorder (e.g., sepsis). While protocols are often developed from evidence summaries, others may be produced based on experiential practice with certain types of patients.[6]

WHAT IS A GUIDELINE?

Clinical Practice Guidelines (CPGs) are care pathways, constructed from expert opinion based on analysis of evidence, that suggest a course of therapy or care. CPGs are intended to provide contextualized guidance to bedside clinicians and ultimately inform the best care for patients. CPGs have evolved dramatically since the 1990s. This evolution culminated in the publication of the Institute of Medicine's monograph entitled "Clinical Practice Guidelines we can Trust" in 2011.[7] The Institute identified key tenets necessary for the production of trustworthy guidelines. These include:
- transparency
- identification and management of potential conflicts of interest
- comprehensive panel composition including all relevant stakeholders
- ensuring that all recommendations are informed by comprehensive systematic reviews of the relevant evidence

The Grading of Recommendations, Assessment, Development and Evaluation (GRADE) approach is a widely used guideline methodology that systematically includes these crucial components.[8] GRADE is used by many critical care societies in developing their CPGs.[1,3]

We will focus the discussion on GRADE methodology because, in our opinion, it offers distinct advantages over alternatives. These advantages include providing guidance on optimizing panel composition, managing potential conflicts of interest, prioritizing outcomes of interest, assessing the certainty of the evidence based on specific domains, and providing direction on how to move from evidence summary to recommendations.[9] Recommendations are directive and clear; "we recommend" is used for strong recommendations and "we suggest" for conditional or weak recommendations. Although the validity of evidence is crucial in deciding on the strength of recommendations, other concerns are considered when generating recommendations. These factors include cost, individual patient values and preferences, feasibility, and the balance of benefits and harms associated with specific interventions.[10] Most guidelines are reviewed and updated every few years as additional evidence is generated to inform clinical practice.[1,4,5]

HOW DOES A PROTOCOL DIFFER FROM A GUIDELINE?

Guidelines produced using a methodology such as GRADE embrace uncertainty. Strong recommendations, usually appropriate only in the setting of moderate or high certainty evidence, are relatively rare. Recommendations tend to be more nuanced and mandate shared decision-making between clinician, patients, and other stakeholders in order to make the best decision for each individual. Conditional recommendations (also known as weak recommendations) establish the course of action that is likely to be preferred by the majority of patients; however, they recognize that a large minority of patients may in fact choose the alternative. A transparent and comprehensive description of these considerations is provided following each actionable recommendation to better inform clinical decision-making.

Protocols may be derived from guidelines but tend to be created at a local level (hospital or health system). When adapting a guideline into a protocol, it is important to adapt the protocol to address the local patient population, ICU staffing models, available resources, and local practice patterns. While protocols may be equally informed by a summary of the best evidence, they tend to be more prescriptive in their direction. Clinical direction is often provided in an all-or-none sequential manner. This ensures standardization of care and that nothing is missed. An accompanying justification to inform the protocol's specific directions is only rarely provided; rather it is inherently assumed that the protocol was developed with best practices in mind. Given this, one might assume that only interventions with high certainty and clear beneficial effects are the ones that should be incorporated into protocols. We should note that sometimes protocols are developed in order to minimize unnecessary variation in practice even when the evidence supporting the protocol may be less than certain.

As illustrated, guidelines and protocols are not synonymous. Each has inherent strengths, limitations, and distinct settings where they should be used.

EPIDEMIOLOGY OF PROTOCOLS IN THE INTENSIVE CARE UNIT

Given the complex ICU environment, it is not surprising that most institutions have a number of clinical protocols. A survey of 69 United States ICUs demonstrated that the median number of protocols per ICU was 19.[6] Despite some concerns, it has been demonstrated that the presence of a protocol does not adversely affect trainee learning.[11] Importantly, the mere presence of a protocol does not ensure that the protocol will be followed or that patient outcomes will be better in an ICU with more protocols.[6] In fact, protocol uptake and efficacy seems better when implemented for a single illness or process of care than when introduced for all aspects of ICU care.[12–14] A careful attempt to introduce several protocols all at once into multiple Brazilian ICUs did not improve survival. It is possible that the team building necessary for successful implementation of protocols is augmented by focusing on a single process or illness (e.g., sepsis, prevention of catheter-associated bloodstream infections). This approach may be necessary to create changes in care that lead to improved outcomes.[13,14]

CHALLENGES FOR PROTOCOLS IN THE INTENSIVE CARE UNIT

As noted earlier, protocols are often developed to standardize care in a busy environment such as the ICU. The desired goal may be prevention of clinical omissions, especially during times of high acuity or other forms of clinical distraction.[15] The same situational factors that drive the potential benefit of protocols also serve as potential challenges. Patients who are critically ill tend to present with variable phenotypes, including different underlying disorders, different demographics with varying ages and ethnicities, and, at times, different types of acute illness. Developing a single protocol to meet the needs of all patients can be daunting. As discussed earlier, it is crucial that the needs of the patient primarily inform protocol development; however, the available resources of the hospital, including personnel, must be considered. More general protocols can and should be adapted to the environment in which they will be delivered. At times, a protocol may be used on a patient who does not meet the criteria for which the protocol was developed. It is especially important for protocol developers to consider this possibility because of the many syndromes prevalent in the ICU that lack a gold-standard diagnostic test.[1,16]

A more global challenge for protocol use in the critical care setting is to ensure that the clinicians charged with implementing them are willing to do so. One important way of accomplishing this goal is to assure that protocol development includes all relevant stakeholders (in particular the bedside providers who will be directly involved). This approach provides all parties with a stake in protocol ownership and will help in developing clinical champions for use. Variable compliance with protocols has even been observed even in hospitals where clinicians are invested in implementing standard types of care.[6,17,18] Providing a feedback loop tailored to the ICU and to involved clinicians is also essential so that they better reflect on their own compliance with the protocols.[14,19,20] Lastly, there is an opportunity cost to every protocol developed; time spent developing, championing, and evaluating the use of a protocol cannot be spent on competing tasks.

PROTOCOL-DRIVEN CARE VERSUS INDIVIDUALIZED CARE

Increasing evidence suggests that standardizing care is a useful tool for increasing compliance with a desired therapy and, consequently, for improving clinical outcomes. Protocols have been successfully used to:
- limit excessive exposure to sedation
- increase mobilization and early rehabilitation in the ICU
- deliver lung-protective invasive mechanical ventilation
- liberate patients from mechanical ventilation in a timely manner
- facilitate treatment of patients with sepsis[18,21–23]

In fact, protocols aimed at limiting sedation and liberating patients from invasive mechanical ventilation are found in many ICUs and have been used as platforms to extend additional treatments or to add on related protocols; e.g., increasing mobilization or augmenting the involvement of families and caregivers in ICU care.[2] Importantly, protocol use need not limit a clinician's ability to individualize care. For example, the presence of a protocol to assure the use of lung-protective ventilation, a need to correct severe respiratory acidosis, or to treat elevated intracranial pressure, can take precedence over the use of tidal volumes of 6 mL/kg. Similar flexibility can be applied to intravenous fluid resuscitation in sepsis.[24] A protocol in this situation might direct clinicians to administer fluid amounts based on a specific physiologic parameter or on a number of parameters, while ensuring adequate resuscitation.[1,25] It has been argued that protocolization will lead to misalignment of treatment patterns in which the encapsulated care within the protocol could be inappropriate.[26] We believe that one result of allowing individual providers to individualize care for every patient will be unnecessary variation in care. Simply put, for the majority of patients, attempts to individualize care most often reflects the usual practice arm of studies that have demonstrated this approach to be inferior to protocolized care.[21,27]

As future advances in ICU care develop, it may be possible to modify interventions based on individual patients' physiology. For example, assessment of lung compliance using esophageal balloons, currently the subject of a Phase II trial, may allow clinicians to titrate positive end expiratory pressure (PEEP) more precisely.[28] However, physiology-based or individualized care has not always led to improved clinical outcomes. Examples include titration of ventilator support to target higher partial pressures of oxygen, accomplished using higher tidal volumes, inhaled nitric oxide, or higher concentrations of supplemental oxygen,[18,29,30] or adding nonspecific nitric oxide synthase inhibitors to increase blood pressure.[31]

Alternatively, there are a number of instances in which individualized care does make sense—for example, limiting the use of steroids for shock in those at high risk for neuropsychiatric agitation or limiting the use of aggressive life-support modalities based on patients' values and preferences. It is always important to carefully consider the effect on a single patient when using a protocol.

PROTOCOLS AND GUIDELINES: SEPSIS AS A CASE STUDY

Sepsis and septic shock continue to be a frequent and often lethal cause of emergency department and ICU admissions. It is estimated that there are approximately 1.5 million ICU admissions and 300,000 deaths in the United States each year due to sepsis.[32] Because decreased time to appropriate therapy is associated with improved clinical outcomes, sepsis remains a common target for protocol and guideline creation.

The Surviving Sepsis Campaign (SSC), a combined effort of the European Society of Intensive Care Medicine and the Society of Critical Care Medicine (as well as other professional societies), was initiated in 2002. The approach used by the SSC was to increase awareness and improve care for patients with severe sepsis and septic shock.[33] Since inception and initial publication, the guidelines have been updated four times. Using formal guideline development methodology, the SSC created evidence-based guidelines for the management of patients with severe sepsis and septic shock with the aim of decreasing mortality and morbidity resulting from sepsis.[33] Using the evidence-based recommendations, the campaign created two bundles, which are in essence protocols, to standardize the treatment of sepsis and to assist with the translation of knowledge to bedside users (clinician and patient). The details[34] are reviewed in Chapter 38. However, two items about the first SSC guidelines should be highlighted. First, both in North America and Europe, implementation efforts across many hospitals led to uptake and improvements in compliance with these bundles, and use of these bundles was associated with decreased mortality after implementation.[35–37] Of note, despite low initial implementation in the United States, improvements over time were associated with an adjusted absolute decrease in sepsis mortality of 0.8% per quarter and an overall drop of 5.4% (95% confidence interval 2.5%–8.4%) over the subsequent 2 years.[34] Similarly, in Spain, an implementation effort (Edusepsis) led to an increase in sepsis bundle compliance which was associated with an improvement in sepsis survival nationwide.[35] Second, some of the items present in these initial bundles, such as early goal-directed therapy, use of tight glucose control, and administration of activated protein C, were later found to have no benefit, and in the case of tight glucose control, might potentially be harmful. These elements have been removed from the sepsis bundles.[38–40]

The changes in the SSC guidelines highlight the importance of updating both guidelines and protocols to reflect new study findings. With most guidelines, this occurs in cycles every few years.[1,4] There has been a recent push to move towards "living guidelines"; recommendations being constantly updated real-time in response to evolving evidence. However, the cost and human resource implications associated with operationalization is high. Compliance with the updated SSC bundles was noted to be associated with a 25% relative risk reduction in mortality over a period of 7.5 years when studied in nearly 30,000 patients across three continents.[37]

The New York State mandate (Rory's rules) serves as an additional example of how standardizing sepsis treatment can lead to improvements in patient outcomes. Rory Staunton was a young patient who died of septic shock after delayed recognition, and his death led New York State to develop a mandated sepsis treatment protocol. In early 2013 the state of New York began requiring hospitals to initiate evidence-based protocols for the early identification and treatment of severe sepsis and septic shock.[41] While the protocols could be tailored to specific hospitals, they required core measures similar to those included in the SSC bundles—administration of antibiotics within 3 hours of patient identification, drawing blood cultures before administering said antibiotics, and measuring serum lactate levels within 3 hours of hospital presentation. A 6-hour bundle consisted of administration of a 30 mL/kg bolus of intravenous fluid for patients with hypotension or serum lactate measuring ≥4 mmol/L, initiation of vasopressor therapy for refractory hypotension, and repeated measurement of lactate within 6 hours of bundle initiation. The implementation of compliance with this mandate was associated with shorter lengths of stay and lower risk and risk-adjusted mortality.[41] More recent evaluation of the effect of compliance with these bundles suggest that completion of most of the bundle elements was associated with decreased mortality.[42] However, while there is evidence that the implementation of the New York state mandated sepsis initiative has increased compliance with desired care and decreased mortality in patients with sepsis, a smaller study examining compliance and clinical outcomes could not demonstrate benefit with a different set of protocols (SEP-1) in patients with sepsis.[34] While the differences in outcomes between these two studies may be related to the power of the studies or differences between the study sites, this differential finding highlights the need to validate guidelines.

The examples highlighted earlier demonstrate some of the positive effects associated with both guidelines and protocols and how they can be used and adapted to optimize the management of sepsis and septic shock. The implementation of a protocol can create a standardized approach treating sepsis within an institution.[43] In the case of sepsis, synthesizing evidence-based guideline recommendations into a local protocol that fits a specific environment complete with its own particular practice patterns, staffing models, and resources is a challenging but necessary undertaking that requires engagement of a multiprofessional team.

HOW TO DEVELOP A PROTOCOL LOCALLY

It seems obvious but the major local decision to make is what illness or treatment pathway should be addressed with the protocol. As noted, it is best to target a single practice because wholescale adoption of many protocols has not improved outcomes in the critically ill.[12] Once consensus on the value the process has been achieved, a multiprofessional team with adequate representation of all of the involved disciplines should be constructed (Fig. 2.1). Each of the major stakeholders involved in protocol development and implementation should be comfortable communicating with each other as peers and a hierarchical framework should be avoided.

Over 2 years, our own institutions implemented a system-wide sepsis protocol to replace multiple departmental and hospital level protocol. We initiated monthly sepsis meetings that included ward, ICU, and emergency department nursing and physician leadership as well as representatives from our quality management team. These meetings, where everyone is seen as an equal partner in the implementation and continued improvement of our sepsis protocol, have allowed for robust buy-in across our system. Reviews of relative real-time adherence data and identification of opportunities for improvement are more easily accomplished in this collaborative environment as are the execution of projects designed to enhance protocol utilization and adherence. Continued maintenance of this synergistic environment is undoubtedly one of the most important elements for our institution and its delivery of sepsis care as we look to respond to external pressures, such as guideline and regulatory agency changes as well as changing patient demographics.

WHAT OUTCOMES SHOULD BE USED TO VALIDATE A PROTOCOL OR GUIDELINE?

Protocols and guidelines are time intensive to create and implement. For example, generation of the 2016 SSC guidelines involved more than 50 people performing more than 70 literature searches, systematic reviews, data abstractions, and meta-analyses to generate the evidence summary used to inform the guidelines.[1] In addition, creating a local protocol requires time

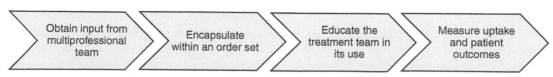

Fig. 2.1 Implementing and validating a local protocol locally.

and commitment from a multiprofessional team. As an example, at one of the author's institutions (JS), it took over a year to create a mobilization protocol, and 2 years to standardize sepsis treatment amongst all practitioners. Because this opportunity cost exists, it is important that we implement protocols that are both feasible to operationalize within an institution and that we meet the initially identified goals, which in general include decreasing practice variability or improved patient outcomes. Some protocols have not improved clinical outcomes, and others proven less beneficial in some hospitals.[44] Table 2.1 provides examples of the level of evidence needed to change clinician behavior. Box 2.1 presents a framework for creating and validating a treatment guideline.

TABLE 2.1 What Level of Evidence Should Change Practice?

Unit of Decision	Evidence Needed to Change Practice
Single Patient	Physicians knowledge and experience: patient preferences
Single Institution	Collective agreement of clinicians based on local implementation; experience with treatment at same institution, ideally backed up by data
Most Physicians	≥1 Randomized controlled trial in a similar patient population; in specific circumstances a strong observational trial may suffice
Treatment Guidelines	≥1 Randomized controlled trial in a similar patient population; review of evidence by multiprofessional including patients, and evaluation or risk benefit and costs of treatment

BOX 2.1 Suggestions for Implementing and Validating a Set of Guidelines Nationally.

1. Assemble a team of experts to review the evidence behind treatment of an illness.
2. Formally assess and manage potential conflicts of interest.
3. Establish questions and outcomes that the team should evaluate using both patient and clinician input. Consider importance from a patient outlook.
4. Perform systematic reviews of the literature for each question of interest and summarize evidence with meta-analysis and pooling of data where appropriate.
5. Use a validated methodology to establish the strength of the evidence.
6. Develop actionable recommendations considering the evidence and certainty (strength) but also the balance between benefits and harms, costs and resources, and patient values and preferences.
7. Disseminate the recommendations, including decision aids if possible.
8. Study the effect of implementing the guidelines on important patient outcomes.
9. Update the guidelines on a regular basis.

SUMMARY

Both protocols and guidelines can improve the care of critically ill and injured patients. Both can increase the likelihood that patients will get appropriate and desired care and can also empower all members of the multiprofessional team. While no one protocol or guideline will be appropriate for all patients, a well-developed protocol is a good starting point to deliver appropriate care for many patients with life-threatening illness and injury.

AUTHORS' RECOMMENDATIONS
- Guidelines are usually intended for wide distribution to hospitals and clinicians over a broad geographic area.
- Protocols tend to be derived from guidelines and are intended for a local hospital or health system.
- It is important that both guidelines and protocols be regularly reviewed and updated.[8]
- Guidelines and protocols should be based on the best available evidence.
- Stakeholders should strive to evaluate the impact of these documents, ensuring their use leads to improvement in patient care.

REFERENCES

1. Rhodes A, Evans LE, Alhazzani W, et al. Surviving Sepsis Campaign: international guidelines for management of sepsis and septic shock: 2016. *Intensive Care Med.* 2017;43(3):304-377.
2. Barnes-Daly MA, Pun BT, Harmon LA, et al. Improving health care for critically ill patients using an evidence-based collaborative approach to ABCDEF bundle dissemination and implementation. *Worldviews Evid Based Nurs.* 2018;15(3):206-216.
3. Fan E, Del Sorbo L, Goligher EC, et al. An official American Thoracic Society/European Society of Intensive Care Medicine/Society of Critical Care Medicine clinical practice guideline: mechanical ventilation in adult patients with acute respiratory distress syndrome. *Am J Respir Crit Care Med.* 2017;195(9):1253-1263.
4. Dellinger RP, Levy MM, Rhodes A, et al. Surviving sepsis campaign: international guidelines for management of severe sepsis and septic shock: 2012. *Crit Care Med.* 2013;41(2):580-637.
5. Guyatt GH, Norris SL, Schulman S, et al. Methodology for the development of antithrombotic therapy and prevention of thrombosis guidelines: Antithrombotic Therapy and Prevention of Thrombosis, 9th ed: American College of Chest Physicians Evidence-Based Clinical Practice Guidelines. *Chest.* 2012;141(suppl 2):53S-70S.
6. Sevransky JE, Checkley W, Herrera P, et al. Protocols and hospital mortality in critically ill patients: the United States Critical Illness and Injury Trials Group Critical Illness Outcomes Study. *Crit Care Med.* 2015;43(10):2076-2084.
7. Institute of Medicine (US) Committee on Standards for Developing Trustworthy Clinical Practice Guidelines, Graham R, Mancher M, Wolman DM, Greenfield S, Steinberg E, eds. *Clinical Practice Guidelines We Can Trust.* Washington, DC: National Academies Press; 2011.

8. Guyatt GH, Oxman AD, Vist GE, et al. GRADE: an emerging consensus on rating quality of evidence and strength of recommendations. *BMJ*. 2008;336(7650):924-926.

9. Guyatt GH, Oxman AD, Kunz R, et al. Going from evidence to recommendations. *BMJ*. 2008;336(7652):1049-1051.

10. Guyatt GH, Oxman AD, Kunz R, et al. Incorporating considerations of resources use into grading recommendations. *BMJ*. 2008;336(7654):1170-1173.

11. Prasad M, Holmboe ES, Lipner RS, et al. Clinical protocols and trainee knowledge about mechanical ventilation. *JAMA*. 2011; 306(9):935-941.

12. Writing Group for the CHECKLIST-ICU Investigators and the Brazilian Research in Intensive Care Network (BRICNet), Cavalcanti AB, Bozza FA, et al. Effect of a quality improvement intervention with daily round checklists, goal setting, and clinician prompting on mortality of critically ill patients: a randomized clinical trial. *JAMA*. 2016;315(14):1480-1490.

13. Pronovost P, Needham D, Berenholtz S, et al. An intervention to decrease catheter-related bloodstream infections in the ICU. *N Engl J Med*. 2006;355(26):2725-2732.

14. Miller RR III, Dong L, Nelson NC, et al. Multicenter implementation of a severe sepsis and septic shock treatment bundle. *Am J Respir Crit Care Med*. 2013;188(1):77-82.

15. Morris AH. Protocol management of adult respiratory distress syndrome. *New Horiz*. 1993;1(4):593-602.

16. ARDS Definition Task Force, Ranieri VM, Rubenfeld GD, et al. Acute respiratory distress syndrome: the Berlin definition. *JAMA*. 2012;307(23):2526-2533.

17. Umoh NJ, Fan E, Mendez-Tellez PA, et al. Patient and intensive care unit organizational factors associated with low tidal volume ventilation in acute lung injury. *Crit Care Med*. 2008; 36(5):1463-1468.

18. Acute Respiratory Distress Syndrome Network, Brower RG, Matthay MA, et al. Ventilation with lower tidal volumes as compared with traditional tidal volumes for acute lung injury and the acute respiratory distress syndrome. *N Engl J Med*. 2000;342(18):1301-1308.

19. Seitz KP, Sevransky JE, Martin GS, Roback JD, Murphy DJ. Evaluation of RBC transfusion practice in adult ICUs and the effect of restrictive transfusion protocols on routine care. *Crit Care Med*. 2017;45(2):271-281.

20. Murphy DJ, Lyu PF, Gregg SR, et al. Using incentives to improve resource utilization: a quasi-experimental evaluation of an ICU quality improvement program. *Crit Care Med*. 2016;44(1):162-170.

21. Ely EW, Baker AM, Dunagan DP, et al. Effect on the duration of mechanical ventilation of identifying patients capable of breathing spontaneously. *N Engl J Med*. 1996;335(25):1864-1869.

22. Girard TD, Kress JP, Fuchs BD, et al. Efficacy and safety of a paired sedation and ventilator weaning protocol for mechanically ventilated patients in intensive care (Awakening and Breathing Controlled trial): a randomised controlled trial. *Lancet*. 2008;371(9607):126-134.

23. Kress JP, Pohlman AS, O'Connor MF, Hall JB. Daily interruption of sedative infusions in critically ill patients undergoing mechanical ventilation. *N Engl J Med*. 2000;342(20):1471-1477.

24. Monnet X, Marik PE, Teboul JL. Prediction of fluid responsiveness: an update. *Ann Intensive Care*. 2016;6(1):111.

25. Sevransky JE. Dynamic measures to determine volume responsiveness: logical, biologically plausible, and unproven. *Crit Care Med*. 2016;44(10):1923-1926.

26. Deans KJ, Minneci PC, Danner RL, Eichacker PQ, Natanson C. Practice misalignments in randomized controlled trials: identification, impact, and potential solutions. *Anesth Analg*. 2010;111(2):444-450.

27. Checkley W, Martin GS, Brown SM, et al. Structure, process, and annual ICU mortality across 69 centers: United States Critical Illness and Injury Trials Group Critical Illness Outcomes Study. *Crit Care Med*. 2014;42(2):344-356.

28. Talmor D, Sarge T, Malhotra A, et al. Mechanical ventilation guided by esophageal pressure in acute lung injury. *N Engl J Med*. 2008;359(20):2095-2104.

29. Taylor RW, Zimmerman JL, Dellinger RP, et al. Low-dose inhaled nitric oxide in patients with acute lung injury: a randomized controlled trial. *JAMA*. 2004;291(13):1603-1609.

30. Chu DK, Kim LH, Young PJ, et al. Mortality and morbidity in acutely ill adults treated with liberal versus conservative oxygen therapy (IOTA): a systematic review and meta-analysis. *Lancet*. 2018;391(10131):1693-1705.

31. López A, Lorente JA, Steingrub J, et al. Multiple-center, randomized, placebo-controlled, double-blind study of the nitric oxide synthase inhibitor 546C88: effect on survival in patients with septic shock. *Crit Care Med*. 2004;32(1):21-30.

32. Gaieski DF, Edwards JM, Kallan MJ, Carr BG. Benchmarking the incidence and mortality of severe sepsis in the United States. *Crit Care Med*. 2013;41(5):1167-1174.

33. Dellinger RP, Carlet JM, Masur H, et al. Surviving Sepsis Campaign guidelines for management of severe sepsis and septic shock. *Crit Care Med*. 2004;32(3):858-873.

34. Levy MM, Dellinger RP, Townsend SR, et al. The Surviving Sepsis Campaign: results of an international guideline-based performance improvement program targeting severe sepsis. *Crit Care Med*. 2010;38(2):367-374.

35. Ferrer R, Artigas A, Levy MM, et al. Improvement in process of care and outcome after a multicenter severe sepsis educational program in Spain. *JAMA*. 2008;299(19):2294-2303.

36. Levy MM, Pronovost PJ, Dellinger RP, et al. Sepsis change bundles: converting guidelines into meaningful change in behavior and clinical outcome. *Crit Care Med*. 2004;32(suppl 11):S595-S597.

37. Levy MM, Rhodes A, Phillips GS, et al. Surviving Sepsis Campaign: association between performance metrics and outcomes in a 7.5-year study. *Crit Care Med*. 2015;43(1):3-12.

38. Abraham E, Laterre PF, Garg R, et al. Drotrecogin alfa (activated) for adults with severe sepsis and a low risk of death. *N Engl J Med*. 2005;353(13):1332-1341.

39. NICE-SUGAR Study Investigators, Finfer S, Chittock DR, et al. Intensive versus conventional glucose control in critically ill patients. *N Engl J Med*. 2009;360(13):1283-1297.

40. PRISM Investigators, Rowan KM, Angus DC, et al. Early, goal-directed therapy for septic shock - a patient-level meta-analysis. *N Engl J Med*. 2017;376(23):2223-2234.

41. Seymour CW, Gesten F, Prescott HC, et al. Time to treatment and mortality during mandated emergency care for sepsis. *N Engl J Med*. 2017;376(23):2235-2244.

42. Levy MM, Gesten FC, Phillips GS, et al. Mortality changes associated with mandated public reporting for sepsis: the results of the New York State initiative. *Am J Respir Crit Care Med*. 2018. doi:10.1164/rccm.201712-2545OC. [Epub ahead of print].

43. Prasad M, Christie JD, Bellamy SL, Rubenfeld GD, Kahn JM. The availability of clinical protocols in US teaching intensive care units. *J Crit Care*. 2010;25(4):610-619.

44. Rhee C, Filbin MR, Massaro AF, et al. Compliance with the national SEP-1 quality measure and association with sepsis outcomes: a multicenter retrospective cohort study. *Crit Care Med*. 2018;46(10):1585-1591.

3

What Happens to Critically Ill Patients After They Leave the ICU?

Jason H. Maley and Mark E. Mikkelsen

Each year over 5.7 million patients are admitted to intensive care units (ICUs) in the United States; worldwide, millions more are admitted.[1] Over the past several decades, improvements in critical care delivery have resulted in significantly reduced mortality, leading to a growing number of ICU survivors.[2] In fact, the majority of patients cared for in an ICU will survive to leave the hospital.

The path from survival to recovery after critical illness is marked with numerous obstacles, beginning in the ICU and continuing long after hospital discharge. Many survivors of critical illness experience post-intensive care syndrome (PICS), defined as new or progressive difficulties in cognition, mental and/or physical health that linger after critical illness. In this chapter, we explore the experience of patients after they survive critical illness, including the epidemiology of ICU survivorship, the challenges faced, and the opportunities to improve the recovery and lives of this growing population of patients.

LOOKING BACK TO FORWARD

Prior to understanding "what happens to ICU survivors after they leave the ICU," we must begin by examining the lives of patients before critical illness. Increasingly, studies of health-related quality of life, mortality, and health-care resource utilization following critical illness have revealed that post-ICU outcomes may have as much to do with a patient's health prior to the ICU as they do with critical illness itself.[3,4]

Critical illness may come as an "asteroid strike" (e.g., the young, previously healthy patient who incurs sepsis or trauma). However, for most, critical illness arrives on the heels of gradual health deterioration.[5] From this trajectory perspective, new insights have emerged. For example, pre-ICU hearing and vision impairment have been strongly associated with poor functional recovery in the 6 months following critical illness.[6] Furthermore, a higher burden of medical (e.g., chronic obstructive pulmonary disease, congestive heart failure, diabetes) and behavioral health comorbidities (e.g., anxiety, depression) prior to an ICU stay are independently associated with worse appetite, fatigue, pain, joint stiffness, and breathlessness at 12 months post-ICU discharge.[7]

Remarkably, in a large matched cohort of ICU survivors within the Scottish ICU registry, factors relating to the severity of acute illness had little or no influence on post-ICU health-care resource use. In contrast, pre-illness factors, including prior hospital resource use and preexisting comorbidities had the strongest association with subsequent health-care resource use.[4] Similarly, in a large prospective study of health-related quality of life following ICU survival in Sweden, investigators surveyed survivors over a 36-month period. The authors found that the majority of the reduction in health-related quality of life after critical illness was related to preexisting conditions rather than the critical illness itself.[8] In understanding the epidemiology of critical illness at various steps along the health-care continuum, these pre-illness factors serve as a critical starting point to the story of ICU survivorship.

WITHIN THE INTENSIVE CARE UNIT

Opportunities to improve ICU survivorship begin in the ICU, as a patient begins to improve from an episode of shock, respiratory failure, or other critical illness. At these early stages, survivors and their loved ones crave information.[9] Unfortunately, issues of survivorship are rarely addressed during an ICU stay.[10]

Fortunately, ICU clinicians are well positioned to begin the process of patient and family education. To close the gap between what survivors need and what they receive at this critical juncture, we recommend the following steps:
1. Inform the patient and family of what has transpired in words that they can understand, including their diagnosis (e.g., "sepsis, caused by a pneumonia") and prognosis.
   - When discussing prognosis, we recommend providing anticipatory guidance for what to expect in the short and longer term.
   - As most patients will have some degree of cognitive impairment at the time of ICU discharge, and as a strategy to reduce long-term psychological stress amongst survivors and their caregivers, we recommend the use of an ICU diary to facilitate meeting this first aim.[11–14] The diary, which includes entries by staff and family, can be reviewed during the hospitalization and thereafter, to reorient the patient to what they experienced and how far they have come in their recovery.
2. Given the prevalence of functional impairment after critical illness, engage physical and occupational therapists and

social work colleagues early to ensure that appropriate therapies are continued and postdischarge services are arranged.

3. In partnership with providers on the medical or surgical ward who will be discharging the patient, ensure that the discharge summary includes pertinent details of the ICU stay and highlights that the patient is at high risk for developing PICS.
4. For those who develop PICS, provide patients with information about regional support groups and post-ICU clinics to connect patients and families with other survivors and centers with experience and expertise in ICU survivorship.[15]

Though further evidence is needed to optimally guide these novel interventions, the potential exists to meaningfully impact the recovery of ICU survivors and their families.[16,17]

ON THE MEDICAL WARDS

At the time of discharge from the ICU, patients commonly transfer to a medical or surgical inpatient ward. Alternatively, select patients leave the hospital directly from the ICU to recover at a long-term acute care hospital (LTACH) or, occasionally and in select cases, directly home.[18] This period of transition from the ICU presents a number of challenges to patients and families.

In an ICU setting, patients and families find comfort in close monitoring and 1:1 or 1:2 nurse-to-patient ratios, as well as frequent contact with ICU physicians. When moved to a medical ward, a change in these factors may result in physical and psychological disturbances known as relocation stress.[19,20]

On the ward, patients and families experience less frequent contact with nurses, physical therapists, and physicians and advanced practice professionals. Patients who have suffered loss of physical function as a result of their ICU stay, and are dependent on assistance from others, may have the most difficulty with this transition. Those patients who functioned independently prior to their critical illness frequently have a new need for assistance with eating, bathing, toileting, and other activities of daily living. With more patients for a given nurse and less frequent monitoring, patients may experience isolation, fear, anxiety, and depression.[21,22]

Following transition to the ward, given the potential for acute deterioration amongst this vulnerable patient population, readmission to the ICU prior to leaving the hospital is a known, albeit rare, risk. In a retrospective cohort study of 196,202 patients from 156 medical and surgical ICUs within 106 community and academic hospitals, Brown and colleagues[23] found that approximately 2% of ICU survivors experienced ICU readmission from the ward within 48 hours, and 4% within 120 hours. The most common reasons for readmission in this cohort were respiratory failure, respiratory arrest, heart failure, and cardiac arrest.

Readmitted patients had a significantly higher mortality (20.7%) than first-time ICU admissions (3.7%), consistent with international epidemiological studies.[24] While some patients were readmitted due to inadequate resolution of the primary problem, many readmissions were due to a new problem such as aspiration, venous thromboembolism, or new infection.

While an ICU readmission is an important, potentially pivotal, event in a patient's health trajectory, evidence suggests that readmissions are not preventable.[25] Furthermore, while organizational factors, such as being discharged at night or when experiencing ICU strain, are associated with ICU readmission, ICU readmissions are not causally linked to in-hospital mortality.[26–28] As an event that (1) reflects a state of frailty, (2) is rarely preventable, and (3) is not causally linked to outcome, its consideration as a measure of ICU quality has been undermined.

POST-ACUTE CARE

Given functional impairments, patients frequently require post-acute care services or placement following an ICU stay. Post-acute care includes home health services, skilled nursing facility, or long-term acute care hospital placement. Less frequently, given national policy restricting access to patients with 1 of 13 qualifying conditions, survivors of critical illness in the United States are admitted to acute rehabilitation.[29] However, as a qualifying condition, patients who survive a stroke are more often discharged to acute rehabilitation.

The transition to post-acute care marks another potential period of relocation stress. To date, little is known about post-acute care use after critical illness: for example, whether outcomes differ across post-acute care options is unknown. What is known is that post-acute care use is costly, albeit variably so, ranging from an average of US$2720 for a home health-care episode, to US$11,357 for placement in a skilled care facility, to US$15,000 for acute rehabilitation.[29]

LTACHs, a costly post-acute care option (e.g., standard prolonged mechanical ventilation LTACH payment is $79,128), provide an opportunity for chronically critically ill patients to leave the ICU, serving a "step-down" purpose to facilitate the lengthy recovery process of such patients.[29]

While LTACH utilization has increased, long-term outcomes remain poor. Between 1997 and 2006, LTACH admissions increased from 13,732 to 40,353. At 1 year, more than half of these patients had died, with a 1-year mortality rate of 50.7% for LTACH admissions for the period 1997–2000 and 52.2% for those admitted for the period 2004–2006.[30] Further, in the year following an LTACH admission, transitions in care were the norm, with a median of four transitions of care and two of three patients being rehospitalized at least once.[31]

To better understand the experience of the chronically critically ill while in an LTACH, Lamas and colleagues conducted a mixed-methods study examining health-related quality-of-life, expectations for the future, and planning for setbacks among patients and families.[32] These investigators conducted semistructured interviews with a total of 50 subjects (30 patients and 20 surrogates), and performed thematic analysis of recorded conversations. Patients reported their quality of life to be poor, and surrogates reported stress and anxiety. Patients and families revealed optimistic health expectations, yet there was poor planning for medical setbacks, coupled with disruptive care transitions. While nearly four of five patients and their families identified going home as a goal, only 38% were at home at 1 year following admission. The average stay was 48 days (range, 8 to 203 days), with the most common discharge destination being a skilled nursing facility. For patients scheduled for discharge from the ICU to an LTACH, to bridge the gap between expectations and outcomes, we recommend an ICU communication strategy that encourages the patient and family to hope for the best, while preparing for the worst.

REHOSPITALIZATION

Readmission to the hospital following an episode of critical illness is common and serves as a significant obstacle to recovery after critical illness. In addition to the new health challenges that a hospital readmission brings, readmission to the hospital may exacerbate symptoms of PICS, including posttraumatic stress disorder (PTSD), depression, anxiety, and physical impairment.

Through examination of the New York Statewide Planning and Research Cooperative System, an administrative database of all hospital discharges in New York State, Hua and colleagues described the epidemiology of readmissions from a cohort of nearly 500,000 ICU survivors over 3 years.[33] Readmission within 30 days occurred in 16% of patients, with over one-quarter (28.6%) of these patients requiring care in an ICU during their readmission. Most often, early readmissions following critical illness were due to a new episode of sepsis or congestive heart failure. Hospital mortality in this cohort was 7.6% for all rehospitalizations and 15.7% for patients who received ICU care during the readmission. A longer index hospitalization was the factor most strongly associated with early rehospitalization. Other factors associated with early hospital readmission were initial discharge to a skilled nursing facility, dialysis, and an index hospitalization diagnosis of sepsis.

Sepsis survivors, in particular, are at high risk for hospital readmission, as nearly one out of four survivors are rehospitalized within 30 days.[34] Liu and colleagues[35] examined 6344 sepsis patients in an integrated health system and found that the need for intensive care during an initial sepsis admission was predictive of the need for early readmission following sepsis, compared with sepsis admissions that did not require ICU admission. After a sepsis hospitalization, healthcare utilization increased nearly threefold compared with presepsis levels.

LONG-TERM SURVIVAL

Survivors of critical illness may remain at higher risk of death for years following critical illness, and particularly in the first few months after their hospitalization. While partially attributable to preexisting medical conditions, the association between critical illness and an increased risk of subsequent mortality has been identified consistently across continents.

As shown in Table 3.1, survivors of critical illness experience a higher mortality rate compared with hospital or general population controls in multiple large retrospective studies across several countries. This increased mortality has been observed up to 5 years from the time of discharge from the hospital. A variety of patient and disease-specific factors may play a role in these findings. In a Dutch cohort of over 91,000 ICU patients who survived to hospital discharge, patients admitted to medical intensive care units and those with cancer had significantly worse outcomes over the 3-year study period compared with elective surgery and cardiac surgery patients who required intensive care.[36] In a matched, retrospective cohort study of United States Medicare beneficiaries, ICU survivors had a higher 3-year mortality compared with hospitalized controls, a difference largely driven by ICU survivors

TABLE 3.1 Long-Term Mortality Risk After Critical Illness.

Author	Period of Study	Country	Design	Study Population	Control	ICU Survivor Mortality	Adjusted Hazard Ratio for Mortality
Brinkman et al.[36]	2007–2010	Netherlands	Retrospective cohort study	91,203 medical and surgical ICU patients	General population data from national registry	Mortality at 1, 2, and 3 years: 12.5%, 19.3%, and 27.5%, respectively	1-year mortality: medical patients HR 1.41 ($P < .05$) compared with general ICU population
Lone et al.[4]	2005–2010	Scotland	Matched retrospective cohort using the Scottish ICU registry	7656 medical and surgical ICU patients	Hospital controls from Scottish registry of acute hospital admissions	Mortality at 1 and 5 years: 10.9% and 32.3%, respectively	5-year mortality: 1.33 ($P < .001$) compared with hospital controls
Wunsch et al.[37]	2003–2006	United States	Matched retrospective cohort of Medicare beneficiaries	35,308, medical and surgical ICU patients	Hospitalized and non-hospitalized Medicare beneficiaries	Mortality at 6 months and 3 years: 14.1% and 39.5%, respectively	3-year mortality: 1.07 ($P < .001$) compared with hospital controls; 2.39 ($P < .001$) compared with general population

who received mechanical ventilation.[37] These patients had markedly higher mortality (57.6% vs. 32.8% hospital controls), compared with ICU survivors who did not receive mechanical ventilation (38.3% vs. 34.6% hospital controls). The difference in mortality largely occurred during the first 6 months after discharge; in this period, mortality was 30.1% for those receiving mechanical ventilation, compared with 9.6% for matched hospital controls. Discharge to a skilled nursing facility, relative to discharge home, was identified as an additional risk factor for higher 6-month mortality.

In a cohort study of 5259 Scottish ICU survivors matched with hospital controls, examined over a 5-year period, Lone and colleagues found that ICU survivors had higher mortality (32.3% vs. 22.7%) and greater resource utilization (mean hospital admission rate, 4.8 vs. 3.3/person/5 years) at a higher cost ($25,608 vs. $16,913/patient).[4]

Given increased mortality and resource utilization among critical care survivors, an important consideration after an ICU admission (or an ICU readmission during the same hospitalization) is whether aggressive care is consistent with the patient's goals and preferences. Through deliberate and empathic communication, when discussing an individual's diagnosis and prognosis, an important goal should be to elicit patient's values and preferences. Clinicians should engage the expertise of palliative care colleagues, as necessary, in these important discussions. With a shared understanding of what is valued and important to the patient, it should be anticipated that some patients will opt for comfort measures and/or hospice care at the time of hospital discharge.

LONG-TERM FUNCTIONAL OUTCOMES

Patients and families commonly experience long-term impairments in health-related quality of life following critical illness. Physical, psychiatric, and cognitive impairments that follow an episode of critical illness can be severe and enduring. New or worsened impairment in one or more of these domains is common following an episode of critical illness and defines PICS.[38]

Patients who have experienced severe and prolonged critical illness, particularly due to septic shock and respiratory failure, are at greatest risk for development of PICS. Additional risk factors associated with long-term physical and/or neuropsychological impairment include prolonged mechanical ventilation, deep sedation, multisystem organ failure, prolonged ICU length of stay, duration of delirium, glucose dysregulation, and the use of corticosteroids.[39–43]

Physical impairment is common following critical illness, occurring in over half of ICU survivors.[44] New or progressive cognitive impairment is an important and underrecognized consequence of critical illness.[45] In a prospective study of survivors of shock and respiratory failure, Pandharipande and colleagues performed neurocognitive testing on survivors of critical illness.[42] Patients had a median age of 61 years and only 6% had cognitive impairment at baseline. The authors reported that 40% of survivors performed neurocognitive testing at a level consistent with moderate traumatic brain injury

3 months following their illness, 26% performed at a level consistent with mild Alzheimer disease, and these impairments frequently persisted. Psychiatric illness seen in PICS manifests as symptoms of anxiety, depression, or PTSD. This commonly affects both patients and their family members.

Further impairments to quality of life may occur in the form of financial challenges due to medical bills and job loss (i.e., financial shock), and interpersonal challenges resulting from a change in family dynamics and family members serving as caregivers. Joblessness is common after critical illness. In a study of acute respiratory distress syndrome (ARDS) survivors conducted by Kamdar and colleagues,[46] joblessness and lost earnings were assessed 12 months after an ICU stay. They found that 1 year following hospitalization for ARDS, 44% of previously employed survivors, with a mean age of 45 years, were unemployed. They calculated that 71% of nonretired survivors accrued lost earnings averaging nearly US$27,000. Survivors displayed a shift towards government-funded health care, with a 14% absolute decrease in private health insurance (from 44% pre-ARDS) and a 16% absolute increase in Medicare and Medicaid use (from 33%).

RESILIENCE AND POSTTRAUMATIC GROWTH

Resilience is a potentially modifiable trait that relates to one's ability to overcome setbacks and obstacles in life. In a study of ICU survivors from two medical intensive care units within a single institution, survivors were surveyed 6 to 12 months after ICU discharge for symptoms of PICS, to assess resilience, and to understand barriers to and facilitators of recovery. Resilience, normal or high in 63% and 9% of survivors, respectively, was inversely correlated with self-reported executive dysfunction, symptoms of anxiety, depression, and PTSD, difficulty with self-care, and pain ($P < .05$).[44]

Beyond resilience, the concept of posttraumatic growth describes positive change and personal growth following a traumatic experience. This has been described in the pediatric literature, related to parents of intensive care patients.[47] Though data in adult ICU populations are lacking, we believe that posttraumatic growth and resilience can be fostered through the implementation of a longitudinal care delivery pathway that spans the ICU to outpatient practice and is designed to mitigate PICS and educate, empower, and support the patient and family through recovery.

CONCLUSION

Survivors of critical illness commonly suffer long-term impairments that impact upon health-related quality of life. Furthermore, survivors often experience medical setbacks, manifested as increased health-care utilization, and their survival is threatened. To combat these losses and threats, survivors (patients and families) need to be educated and empowered, beginning with a simple conversation between ICU clinicians and patients and families prior to discharge from the ICU. This early intervention can set the stage for further education about PICS and arrangement of services to manage and rehabilitate cognitive, psychiatric, and physical impairments. While the optimal postdischarge care pathway remains unclear, novel strategies are being implemented to meet the needs of survivors more effectively.

AUTHORS' RECOMMENDATIONS

- Post-intensive care syndrome, defined as new or progressive difficulties in cognition, mental health, and/or physical health after critical illness, is common.
- Health-related quality of life after critical illness is low; however, preexisting conditions contribute substantially to the reduced quality of life.
- Transition to the floor can be challenging.
- Relocation stress, manifest as isolation, fear, anxiety, and depression and exacerbated by dependence on others for activities of daily living, is common.
- ICU readmissions are uncommon and are often not preventable.
- Post-acute care use, given survivors' functional impairments, is common and costly, and includes home health services and placement in skilled care facilities and long-term acute care hospitals.
- In the United States, despite functional impairments, discharge to acute rehabilitation is uncommon for many survivors of critical illness given national policy; however, certain patients (e.g., stroke) are more likely to receive this type of post-acute care as 1 of the 13 preferred, qualifying conditions.
- Nearly one out of five survivors of critical illness will be rehospitalized within 30 days; more than one out of four of these rehospitalizations will require care in an ICU again.
- Survivors of critical illness incur a long-term mortality risk.
- Despite these losses and impairments, resilience amongst survivors of critical illness is the norm, and the potential for posttraumatic growth exists.
- To promote a culture of resilience amongst survivors, providers need to educate, empower, and prepare patients and caregivers for life after critical illness; these efforts should begin in the ICU.

REFERENCES

1. Society of Critical Care Medicine. *Critical Care Statistics*. https://www.sccm.org/Communications/Critical-Care-Statistics.
2. Zimmerman JE, Kramer AA, Knaus WA. Changes in hospital mortality for United States intensive care unit admissions from 1988 to 2012. *Crit Care*. 2013;17(2):R81.
3. Prescott HC, Sjoding MW, Langa KM, et al. Late mortality after acute hypoxic respiratory failure. *Thorax*. 2018;73:618-625.
4. Lone NI, Gillies MA, Haddow C, et al. Five-year mortality and hospital costs associated with surviving intensive care. *Am J Respir Crit Care Med*. 2016;194(2):198-208.
5. Iwashyna TJ, Prescott HC. When is critical illness not like an asteroid strike? *Am J Respir Crit Care Med*. 2013;188(5):525-527.
6. Ferrante LE, Pisani MA, Murphy TE, et al. Factors associated with functional recovery among older intensive care unit survivors. *Am J Respir Crit Care Med*. 2016;194(3):299-307.
7. Griffith DM, Salisbury LG, Lee RJ, et al. Determinants of health-related quality of life after ICU: importance of patient demographics, previous comorbidity, and severity of illness. *Crit Care Med*. 2018;46(4):594-601.
8. Orwelius L, Nordlund A, Nordlund P, et al. Pre-existing disease: the most important factor for health related quality of life long-term after critical illness: a prospective, longitudinal, multicentre trial. *Crit Care*. 2010;14(2):R67.
9. Lee CM, Herridge MS, Matte A, Cameron JI. Education and support needs during recovery in acute respiratory distress syndrome survivors. *Crit Care*. 2009;13(5):R153.
10. Govindan S, Iwashyna TJ, Watson SR, et al. Issues of survivorship are rarely addressed during intensive care unit stays. Baseline results from a statewide quality improvement collaborative. *Ann Am Thorac Soc*. 2014;11(4):587-591.
11. Kamdar BB, King LM, Collop NA, et al. The effect of a quality improvement intervention on perceived sleep quality and cognition in a medical ICU. *Crit Care Med*. 2013;41(3):800-809.
12. Jones C, Bäckman C, Capuzzo M, et al. Intensive care diaries reduce new onset post traumatic stress disorder following critical illness: a randomised, controlled trial. *Crit Care*. 2010;14(5):R168.
13. Jones C, Bäckman C, Griffiths RD. Intensive care diaries and relatives' symptoms of posttraumatic stress disorder after critical illness: a pilot study. *Am J Crit Care*. 2012;21(3):172-176.
14. Garrouste-Orgeas M, Coquet I, Périer A, et al. Impact of an intensive care unit diary on psychological distress in patients and relatives. *Crit Care Med*. 2012;40(7):2033-2040.
15. Society of Critical Care Medicine. https://www.sccm.org/Research/Quality/THRIVE. Accessed August 31, 2018.
16. Mikkelsen ME, Jackson JC, Hopkins RO, et al. Peer support as a novel strategy to mitigate post-intensive care syndrome. *AACN Adv Crit Care*. 2016;27(2):221-229.
17. Haines KJ, Beesley SJ, Hopkins RO, et al. Peer support in critical care: a systematic review. *Crit Care Med*. 2018;46(9):1522-1531.
18. Stelfox HT, Soo A, Niven DJ, et al. Assessment of the safety of discharging select patients directly home from the intensive care unit: a multicenter population-based cohort study. *JAMA Intern Med*. 2018;178(10):1390-1399.
19. Carpentino L. *Nursing Diagnosis: Application to Clinical Practice*. 12th ed. Philadelphia: Lippincott,Williams & Wilkins; 2007.
20. Beard H. Does intermediate care minimize relocation stress for patients leaving the ICU? *Nurs Crit Care*. 2005;10(6):272-278.
21. McKinney AA, Melby V. Relocation stress in critical care: a review of the literature. *J Clin Nurs*. 2002;11(2):149-157.
22. Field K, Prinjha S, Rowan K. 'One patient amongst many': a qualitative analysis of intensive care unit patients' experiences of transferring to the general ward. *Crit Care*. 2008;12(1):R21.
23. Brown SE, Ratcliffe SJ, Kahn JM, Halpern SD. The epidemiology of intensive care unit readmissions in the United States. *Am J Respir Crit Care Med*. 2012;185(9):955-964.
24. Chen LM, Martin CM, Keenan SP, Sibbald WJ. Patients readmitted to the intensive care unit during the same hospitalization: clinical features and outcomes. *Crit Care Med*. 1998;26(11):1834-1841.
25. Al-Jaghbeer MJ, Tekwani SS, Gunn SR, Kahn JM. Incidence and etiology of potentially preventable ICU readmissions. *Crit Care Med*. 2016;44(9):1704-1709.
26. Renton J, Pilcher DV, Santamaria JD, et al. Factors associated with increased risk of readmission to intensive care in Australia. *Intensive Care Med*. 2011;37(11):1800-1808.

27. Wagner J, Gabler NB, Ratcliffe SJ, et al. Outcomes among patients discharged from busy intensive care units. *Ann Intern Med.* 2013;159(7):447-455.

28. Brown SES, Ratcliffe SJ, Halpern SD. Assessing the utility of ICU readmissions as a quality metric: an analysis of changes mediated by residency work-hour reforms. *Chest.* 2015; 147(3):626-636.

29. Medicare Payment Advisory Commission. Chapter 10: inpatient rehabilitation facility services. In: *Report to the Congress: Medicare Payment Policy.* 2018. Available at: http://www.medpac. gov/-documents-/reports. Accessed August 10, 2018.

30. Kahn JM, Benson NM, Appleby D, et al. Long-term acute care hospital utilization after critical illness. *JAMA.* 2010; 303(22):2253-2259.

31. Unroe M, Kahn JM, Carson SS, et al. One-year trajectories of care and resource utilization for recipients of prolonged mechanical ventilation: a cohort study. *Ann Intern Med.* 2010;153(3):167-175.

32. Lamas DJ, Owens RL, Nace RN, et al. Opening the door: the experience of chronic critical illness in a long-term acute care hospital. *Crit Care Med.* 2017;45(4):e357-e362.

33. Hua M, Gong MN, Brady J, Wunsch H. Early and late unplanned rehospitalizations for survivors of critical illness. *Crit Care Med.* 2015;43(2):430-438.

34. Maley JH, Mikkelsen ME. Short-term gains with long-term consequences: the evolving story of sepsis survivorship. *Clin Chest Med.* 2016;37(2):367-380.

35. Liu V, Lei X, Prescott HC, et al. Hospital readmission and healthcare utilization following sepsis in community settings. *J Hosp Med.* 2014;9(8):502-507.

36. Brinkman S, de Jonge E, Abu-Hanna A, et al. Mortality after hospital discharge in ICU patients. *Crit Care Med.* 2013;41(5): 1229-1236.

37. Wunsch H, Guerra C, Barnato AE, et al. Three-year outcomes for Medicare beneficiaries who survive intensive care. *JAMA.* 2010;303(9):849-856.

38. Needham DM, Davidson J, Cohen H, et al. Improving long-term outcomes after discharge from intensive care unit: report from a stakeholders' conference. *Crit Care Med.* 2012;40(2): 502-509.

39. Iwashyna TJ, Ely EW, Smith DM, Langa KM. Long-term cognitive impairment and functional disability among survivors of severe sepsis. *JAMA.* 2010;304(16):1787-1794.

40. Mikkelsen ME, Christie JD, Lanken PN, et al. The adult respiratory distress syndrome cognitive outcomes study: long-term neuropsychological function in survivors of acute lung injury. *Am J Respir Crit Care Med.* 2012;185(12):1307-1315.

41. Hopkins RO, Weaver LK, Collingridge D, et al. Two-year cognitive, emotional, and quality-of-life outcomes in acute respiratory distress syndrome. *Am J Respir Crit Care Med.* 2005;171(4):340-347.

42. Pandharipande PP, Girard TD, Jackson JC, et al. Long-term cognitive impairment after critical illness. *N Engl J Med.* 2013;369(14):1306-1316.

43. Saczynski JS, Marcantonio ER, Quach L, et al. Cognitive trajectories after postoperative delirium. *N Engl J Med.* 2012;367(1):30-39.

44. Maley JH, Brewster I, Mayoral I, et al. Resilience in survivors of critical illness in the context of the survivors' experience and recovery. *Ann Am Thorac Soc.* 2016;13(8):1351-1360.

45. Marra A, Pandharipande PP, Girard TD, et al. Co-occurrence of post-intensive care syndrome problems among 406 survivors of critical illness. *Crit Care Med.* 2018;46(9):1393-1401.

46. Kamdar BB, Huang M, Dinglas VD, et al. Joblessness and lost earnings after acute respiratory distress syndrome in a 1-year national multicenter study. *Am J Respir Crit Care Med.* 2017;196(8):1012-1020.

47. Aftyka A, Rozalska-Walaszek I, Rosa W, et al. Post-traumatic growth in parents after infants' neonatal intensive care unit hospitalisation. *J Clin Nurs.* 2017;26(5-6):727-734.

4

What Can Be Done to Enhance Recognition of the Post-ICU Syndrome (PICS)? What Can Be Done to Prevent It? What Can Be Done to Treat It?

Jakob I. McSparron and Theodore J. Iwashyna

This topic covers an area of rapidly evolving research; an exhaustive approach is guaranteed to quickly become outdated. Therefore this chapter seeks to provide an approach to the problems faced by survivors of critical illness with a focus on patients surviving acute respiratory distress syndrome (ARDS) and severe sepsis.

WHAT PROBLEMS ARE PREVALENT AMONG SURVIVORS OF CRITICAL ILLNESS?

Survivors of critical illness must deal with many problems. Indeed, compared with an age-matched population, survivors of critical illness face nearly every medical complication imaginable. As is discussed in the next section, some of these issues reflect preexisting illnesses, some of which may even have led to the development of critical illness. However, regardless of when they developed, the long-term problems prevalent among critical illness survivors have significant consequences for survivors, their families, and their clinicians. A magisterial summary of the literature on issues plaguing patients surviving severe sepsis has been provided by Prescott and Angus.[1]

Following discharge from the hospital, some survivors of critical illness face a substantially elevated mortality. This problem is best documented for sepsis. For example, Quartin et al.[2] compared patients with severe sepsis in the 1980s to matched non-septic patients hospitalized during the same time period. Among patients who had lived for at least 180 days after their illness, patients with sepsis were 3.4 times more likely to die in the subsequent 6 months (that is, days 181–365 after hospitalization) than controls (95% confidence interval: 2.3, 4.2) . Indeed, among those who lived at least 2 full years, survivors of sepsis were still 2.2 times as likely as controls to die by year 5. Yende et al.[3] and Prescott et al.[4] have shown similar rates of excess post-discharge mortality among sepsis survivors. In contrast, Wunsch et al.[5] looked at intensive care unit (ICU) patients who did or did not require mechanical ventilation and compared them with the general population and with hospitalized controls; these authors suggested that mechanical ventilation is associated with a substantial excess mortality. However, this excess mortality occurred largely in the first 6 months post-discharge. Prescott et al.[6] similarly found that excess mortality in patients with hypoxic respiratory failure occurred well before that observed in patients hospitalized with similar conditions who did not develop frank respiratory failure.

The term *post-intensive care syndrome* (PICS) was coined to provide an intellectual framework for organizing the problems prevalent among those who survive this excess mortality.[7,8] A working description of PICS was developed over several years and involved extensive contributions from stakeholders—including patients, families, caregivers, administrators, and others—within critical care and throughout the broader medical and rehabilitation communities. Within PICS, it is valuable to consider three broad domains specific to the patient: physical health, cognitive impairment, and mental health. The notion of PICS-F (Family) recognizes that family members of the adult critically ill are also deeply affected, while the PICS-P (Pediatrics) framework generalizes these issues for the developmental needs of children during ICU recovery.[9]

Most work after critical illness has focused on the presence and persistence of neuromuscular weakness. In our opinion, enduring weakness, which can be profound and disabling, is the central patient-centered physical problem facing the population of survivors as a whole. Abnormalities of motor function, united under the useful umbrella of "ICU-acquired weakness," include myopathies and polyneuropathies.[10] The biology of this syndrome remains an area of active research, but there is little evidence that the origin (nerve or muscle) of the underlying defect affects either prognosis or specific treatment. Physical and occupational therapies are the mainstay of recovery.[11] These preventive strategies are probably most effective if initiated early in the ICU stay[12]; little work has been done on optimal strategies for promoting recovery among those with established deficits post-ICU.

Other physical problems are common but less well-studied. Transient and enduring renal failure has been noted.[13] High rates of cardiovascular disease are reported.[14] Dyspnea and low exercise tolerance, even in the face of seemingly normal or near-normal pulmonary function tests, are ubiquitous after severe ARDS.[15,16] Other survivors report subglottic stenosis and profound cosmetic changes.[14] High rates of cachexia, injurious falls, incontinence, and impaired hearing and vision have all been reported.[17]

A spectrum of cognitive impairment is also common after critical illness. Abnormalities range from dysfunction in specific tasks (defects in executive function are particularly common) to frank cognitive impairment. The prevalence seems to be high, although there is disagreement about how severe an abnormality must be to be "bad enough to be counted."[18-23] Patients who experience severe delirium in the ICU may be at risk for loss of cognitive function at a later time,[24] but the duration of the ICU-acquired cognitive dysfunction is probably months to years; therefore it is unlikely to be a simple extension of ICU- or hospital-acquired delirium.

There is also evidence that ICU survivors experience high degrees of depression, anxiety, and posttraumatic stress disorder (PTSD). Assessments of depression with the Hospital Anxiety and Depression Scale (HADS) have tended to emphasize the PTSD finding.[25-27] In contrast, Jackson and colleagues[28] suggested that the HADS may be insufficiently sensitive to somatic symptoms of depression and that symptoms attributed to PTSD were not tied to the critical illness experience. Although these issues are being addressed, it is clear that many patients have significant emotional disorders.[29,30]

In summary, survivors of critical illness face a wide array of problems. Only some of these have been adequately studied, and there are specific interventions for even fewer. These problems lead to high rates of ongoing health-care resource use and frequent rehospitalization.[4,31,32] There is growing recognition that the consequences of critical illness also place substantial strain on families of ICU survivors, who often bear the brunt of high levels of ongoing informal care.[33-41]

In the face of such high prevalence, it is understandable that critical care practitioners may develop a certain nihilism or sense of hopelessness. Obviously, this is an issue that must be addressed by each individual involved. However, it seems important to stress that the inability to save everyone does not mean that many are not saved. The newly appreciated prevalence of PICS represents a problem to be tackled and eventually solved, not an inevitable fate to which all ICU patients are doomed. Indeed, as Cuthbertson and colleagues noted in their longitudinal cohort of Scottish sepsis survivors, "At five years all patients stated they would be willing to be treated in an ICU again if they become critically ill... [and] 80% were either very happy or mostly happy with their current QOL [quality of life]."[42]

WHICH OF THE PROBLEMS FACED BY SURVIVORS ARE CONSEQUENCES OF CRITICAL ILLNESS?

It is sometimes rhetorically useful to frame studies of long-term consequences as extremes on a spectrum, as if all problems of ICU survivors must be caused by critical illness. One unfortunate consequence of such a dichotomy is the development of a false sense of hierarchy—asking, "Which is more important?" It is rather more valuable to examine the extent to which acute changes and preexisting conditions contribute in any given patient.

Perhaps the best research on this particular problem lies in the domain of cognitive impairment after critical illness. A large group of investigators followed 5888 older Americans in the Cardiovascular Health Study, a population-based observational cohort.[23] Patients were examined every year with the Teng Modified Mini-Mental Status examination. Shah et al.[23] noted that patients who went on to have pneumonia were more likely to have relatively low premorbid cognitive scores and/or scores that had been declining before the development of pneumonia. However, irrespective of baseline trajectory, patients who contracted pneumonia had an increasingly rapid transition to dementia. Iwashyna et al.[22] found similar results with sepsis, and Ehlenbach et al.[43] noted this finding in a group of critically ill patients.

In other cases, findings have been less consistent. Wunsch et al.[29] used elegantly detailed Danish records to show that depression and other mental health disorders were diagnosed much more commonly in patients after critical illness with mechanical ventilation than in the years before the critical illness. However, Davydow et al.[30] showed that US survivors of sepsis did not exhibit a change in the (already very high) level of depressive symptoms present before or after their critical illness. It is possible to reconcile these findings by attributing them to the known low sensitivity of general medical practice for the detection of depression and an increased level of surveillance in the years following a critical illness. The Davydow findings might also be explained by an insufficiently responsive scale for symptoms; the Wunsch finding might reflect high levels of persistent or restarted antipsychotics and anxiolytics after ICU care.

In some cases it appears that the prevalent problems after critical illness are primarily the result of preexisting morbidity. Further complicating work suggesting this to be the case due to the fact that older Americans are at increasing risk for both critical illness and potential complications. Thus, work in the Health and Retirement Study showed dramatic increases in rates of injurious falls and incontinence in survivors of sepsis relative to both the general population of older adults and even compared with the same patients when measured presepsis.[17] However, any apparent effect of sepsis disappeared when the "morbidity growth curve" of older Americans was controlled (i.e., their presepsis trajectory of increasing development of morbidity).

In summary, patients with critical illness typically had both a level of functionality that was worse than the general population before the development of their critical illness and were on trajectories of more rapid decline before their critical illness. However, it is common for function to decline more rapidly following critical illness. This finding is not universal: for example, exacerbations after critical illness were not detectable for geriatric conditions such as injurious falls.

It may also not be true for impaired quality of life, particularly because people may be able to adapt to their new post-critical illness deficits.

WHY DOES IT MATTER WHETHER THE PROBLEM PRECEDES CRITICAL ILLNESS OR IS A CONSEQUENCE OF CRITICAL ILLNESS?

Having established that there are substantial problems that are highly prevalent among survivors of critical illness, it is important to ask what can be done to make things better. The next section discusses specific strategies. However, in general, three approaches have been used: (1) in-ICU prevention, (2) treatment and remediation, and (3) triage. In-ICU prevention strategies are only effective for problems that develop over the course of critical illness; while it may be possible to prevent acceleration of development, it is impossible to prevent a problem that already exists. Therefore it is important to identify those conditions that are specific to each individual patient, as opposed to the population of survivors as a whole, and which did or did not precede the development of critical illness.

When newly acquired diagnoses are evaluated, it is essential to distinguish the degree of morbidity that is caused by critical illness from complications that arise from interventions to treat and/or support the patient. For example, ICU-acquired weakness is common in survivors of critical illness. However, it is difficult to determine to what extent this disability results from the critical illness itself as opposed to the treatment modalities, including prolonged bed rest, use of neuromuscular blocking agents, antibiotics, or other drugs, decreased respiratory muscle activity resulting from mechanical ventilation, and inadequate metabolic/nutritional support. Indeed, PICS is an acronym for "post-intensive care syndrome," not "postcritical illness syndrome," but health-care providers should not let this untested assertion provide false assurances as to where the problems may lie. Attribution to the management of problems that are really a consequence of critical illness itself could lead to faulty triage decisions, in which patients with a critical illness are kept out of the ICU to spare them the perceived risk of exposure to ICU-associated risk. However, such triage would also preclude these patients from receiving improvements in care that can only be delivered in an ICU.[44] However, ICU care may be of lower marginal value and prone to excess interventions, invasive monitoring, and bed rest. In that case, the decision to avoid ICU care would be fully appropriate. Conversely, an incorrect belief that a complication is a component of the underlying disorder may lead to overuse of therapy; for example, it appears that less sedation reduces the psychological sequelae of critical care rather than providing the preventive amnesia that some once hoped it would. There is an urgent need for objective data to inform this debate; in particular, data should not merely catalog the problems in one place but also catalog comparative effectiveness in research on care in alternative settings.

GIVEN THE ABSENCE OF PROVEN THERAPIES, WHAT CAN BE DONE TO ENHANCE PREVENTION, RECOGNITION, AND TREATMENT OF PICS?

Patients surviving critical illness labor under a complex burden of problems—some newly developed as a consequence of the acute episode, some present before critical illness but exacerbated by the episode to the point of decompensation, and some preexisting in occult form that are unmasked critical illness. There are no proven therapies specifically remediating long-term problems after the ICU. There are several potentially promising approaches or interventions that could be initiated in the ICU. A pragmatic approach, which is based on the work of Lachman and Agrigoroaei in a different setting,[45] that the authors have found to be clinically valuable involves six steps detailed here:

1. *Prevention*: There is frustratingly little to prove that excellent in-ICU care prevents post-ICU problems. However, the physiologic rationale that minimizing the extent of critical illness is an essential step to improving the lives of patients who survive the ICU is compelling. It is our practice to emphasize aggressive sepsis detection and resuscitation, low tidal volume ventilation, sedation minimization, and early mobilization of mechanically ventilated patients. We feel that the ABCDE bundle is one standardized method that plays a major role in the prevention of the development of PICS.[46] In the 90-days after an ICU stay—particularly for sepsis—rehospitalizations are concentrated in a handful of diagnoses that might be avoided by better outpatient care, more careful discharge practices, and more careful anticipatory counseling (Fig. 4.1).

2. *Protection*: ICU patients frequently experience discontinuities of care after transfer out of the ICU.[47] Essential home medications often are not restarted. Antipsychotics intended only for short-term delirium management may be continued for prolonged periods.[48,49] The receiving team may not be made aware of the appearance of new radiographic findings, and follow-up does not occur.[50] Potentially, ambulatory care-sensitive conditions may go untreated and blossom into rehospitalizations.[51] There are multiple process-of-care efforts to prevent such discontinuities. While the evidence is inconsistent, we feel that minimizing sedation and initiating early physical therapy will improve physical functioning in ICU survivors and should thus be standard of care in critical care units.[52] There appears to be a role for diaries in the ICU; these have been shown to decrease post-hospitalization PTSD symptoms.[53] Finally, we are confident there are other as-of-yet unproven therapies that will prevent ICU patients from having new neuromuscular and emotional deficits in the first place.

3. *Treatment*: Previously unrecognized or undiagnosed problems are often uncovered in the ICU. In some cases (e.g., the patient whose diabetes first presents as diabetic ketoacidosis), there are well-established procedures not only to correct the acute problem but also to ensure appropriate follow-up, including education and communication with

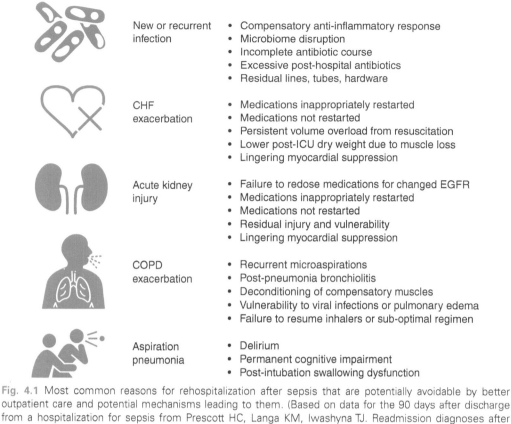

New or recurrent infection
- Compensatory anti-inflammatory response
- Microbiome disruption
- Incomplete antibiotic course
- Excessive post-hospital antibiotics
- Residual lines, tubes, hardware

CHF exacerbation
- Medications inappropriately restarted
- Medications not restarted
- Persistent volume overload from resuscitation
- Lower post-ICU dry weight due to muscle loss
- Lingering myocardial suppression

Acute kidney injury
- Failure to redose medications for changed EGFR
- Medications inappropriately restarted
- Medications not restarted
- Residual injury and vulnerability
- Lingering myocardial suppression

COPD exacerbation
- Recurrent microaspirations
- Post-pneumonia bronchiolitis
- Deconditioning of compensatory muscles
- Vulnerability to viral infections or pulmonary edema
- Failure to resume inhalers or sub-optimal regimen

Aspiration pneumonia
- Delirium
- Permanent cognitive impairment
- Post-intubation swallowing dysfunction

Fig. 4.1 Most common reasons for rehospitalization after sepsis that are potentially avoidable by better outpatient care and potential mechanisms leading to them. (Based on data for the 90 days after discharge from a hospitalization for sepsis from Prescott HC, Langa KM, Iwashyna TJ. Readmission diagnoses after hospitalization for severe sepsis and other acute medical conditions. *JAMA.* 2015;313[10]:1055-1057.)

primary care providers. However, other conditions, in particular depression and mental health issues, are often neglected. A balanced approach to improving life after the ICU must ensure appropriate follow-up for all new problems diagnosed or likely to be exacerbated in the ICU. A proven approach to specifically ensure appropriate follow-up after the ICU is lacking, but work on transitions of care for geriatric patients may provide promising models. Multidisciplinary ICU follow-up clinics have been developed in order to address the complex needs of ICU survivors and family members.[54] Various models exist; there is limited and conflicting evidence about the benefits of these efforts.[53,55, 56] There is evidence to suggest that critical care pharmacists play a key role in these clinics, with one center reporting a median of four pharmacy interventions per patient.[57] In particular, pharmacists are able to identify and prevent adverse drug events in this susceptible population.

4. *Remediation*: The evidence increasingly suggests that disability after critical illness is rooted in muscle weakness, cognitive impairment, and lack of social support. Many practitioners strongly recommend early and ongoing physiotherapy for all patients in the ICU, with follow-up as an outpatient when appropriate. However, the appropriate approach to physiotherapy should be one of preventing any loss of functioning while in the ICU as opposed to only treating those with demonstrable weakness. Moreover, work by Hopkins and others[58] has shown that physical therapy in the ICU may also have important cognitive and psychiatric

benefits. It is essential that a patient's family or other support group be intimately involved in the process of providing ICU care. The work of Netzer and Sullivan,[40] who defined a "family ICU syndrome," demonstrates the incredible toll that ICUs take on families. However, if patients are especially vulnerable in the period immediately after discharge, family participation may be an essential and underused determinant of whether the patients have a trajectory of recovery or a trajectory of disability.

5. *Compensation*: Even with the best medical care and physical therapy, some patients will have new problems after the ICU. There is an ongoing struggle to find a systematic approach to evaluating their needs. The model of a comprehensive geriatrics assessment may hold great promise, but it needs to be customized to the ICU.[59] In this approach, there is a structured questionnaire tied to initial interventions to assess a range of potential needs. The sort of pragmatic assistance that geriatricians routinely provide to allow weak, older patients to stay in their homes may be of great value to ICU patients in their recovery.

6. *Enhancement*: The next frontier of recovery from critical illness will be finding ways to empower survivors to help each other by developing innovative peer support models.[60,61] This approach allows patients to become partners in discovering new approaches to facilitate recovery. Such groups have fundamentally transformed recovery from cancer, stroke, Alzheimer disease, and other disabling conditions. This powerful tool holds enormous promise for improving outcomes after the ICU.

CONCLUSION

Many, but not all, patients have a range of physical, cognitive, and emotional challenges after critical illness. There is a limited number of validated tools to identify patients at risk for PICS, and thus a large number of patients must be assumed to be vulnerable.[18] Likewise, neither critical care nor primary care professionals have developed specific, validated therapies to prevent or treat these multifactorial problems. Primary care services often do not exist or are inadequate for many populations of critically ill patients. However, simply hoping that the patient's own primary care will sort out all their post-ICU needs is an untenable approach. There is reason to believe that post-ICU services can be of benefit for navigating the complex sets of problems faced by these patients; preventing iatrogenic injury from disruptions in medications and other aspects of health care, catching and treating early new "second-hit" illnesses that would otherwise derail recovery, and helping patients and family develop a path to recovery and posttraumatic growth.

AUTHORS' RECOMMENDATIONS

- A significant proportion of patients have a range of physical, cognitive, and emotional challenges after critical illness; this is known as PICS (post-intensive care syndrome).
- Critical illness also places substantial strain on families of ICU survivors, who often bear the brunt of high levels of ongoing informal care as well as financial toxicities.
- There are few validated tools to identify patients at risk for PICS; the risk of PICS does not correlate well with severity of illness in the ICU.
- Patients likely to have complex post-ICU courses may benefit from targeted post-ICU help in the form of peer support, a post-ICU clinic, and/or a revisit with a clinician familiar with their course.
- Existing primary care practices do not reliably provide adequate access and services for medically complex patients in the post-ICU period, and cannot be assumed to be able to sort out all post-ICU issues given the rapid pace of change of ICU technology and the frequent inadequacies of post-ICU hand-offs.

REFERENCES

1. Prescott HC, Angus DC. Enhancing recovery from sepsis: a review. *JAMA*. 2018;319(1):62-75.
2. Quartin AA, Schein RMH, Kett DH, Peduzzi PN. Magnitude and duration of the effect of sepsis on survival. *JAMA*. 1997;277:1058-1063.
3. Yende S, Linde-Zwirble W, Mayr F, Weissfeld LA, Reis S, Angus DC. Risk of cardiovascular events in survivors of severe sepsis. *Am J Respir Crit Care Med*. 2014;189:1065-1074.
4. Prescott HC, Langa KM, Liu V, Escobar GJ, Iwashyna TJ. Increased 1-year healthcare use in survivors of severe sepsis. *Am J Respir Crit Care Med*. 2014;190:62-69.
5. Wunsch H, Guerra C, Barnato AE, Angus DC, Li G, Linde-Zwirble WT. Three-year outcomes for Medicare beneficiaries who survive intensive care. *JAMA*. 2010;303:849-856.
6. Prescott HC, Sjoding MW, Langa KM, Iwashyna TJ, McAuley DF. Late mortality after acute hypoxic respiratory failure. *Thorax*. 2017;73(7).
7. Needham DM, Davidson J, Cohen H, et al. Improving long-term outcomes after discharge from intensive care unit: report from a stakeholders' conference. *Crit Care Med*. 2012;40;502-509.
8. Elliott D, Davidson JE, Harvey MA, et al. Exploring the scope of post-intensive care syndrome therapy and care: engagement of non-critical care providers and survivors in a second stakeholders meeting. *Crit Care Med*. 2014;42:2518-2526.
9. Manning JC, Pinto NP, Rennick JE, Colville G, Curley MAQ. Conceptualizing post intensive care syndrome in children—the PICS-p framework. *Pediatr Crit Care Med*. 2018;19(4): 298-300.
10. Schweickert WD, Hall J. ICU-acquired weakness. *Chest*. 2007;131: 1541-1549.
11. Schweickert WD, Pohlman MC, Pohlman AS, et al. Early physical and occupational therapy in mechanically ventilated, critically ill patients: a randomised controlled trial. *Lancet*. 2009;373 (9678):1874-1882.
12. Hodgson CL, Iwashyna TJ, Schweickert WD. All that work and no gain: what should we do to restore physical function in our survivors? *Am J Respir Crit Care Med*. 2016;193(10):1071-1072.
13. Mehta RL, Pascual MT, Soroko S, et al. Spectrum of acute renal failure in the intensive care unit: the PICARD experience. *Kidney Int*. 2004;66:1613-1621.
14. Griffiths RD, Jones C. Recovery from intensive care. *BMJ*. 1999;319:427-429.
15. Herridge MS, Cheung AM, Tansey CM, et al. One-year outcomes in survivors of the acute respiratory distress syndrome. *N Engl J Med*. 2003;348:683-693.
16. Herridge MS, Tansey CM, Matté A, et al. Functional disability 5 years after acute respiratory distress syndrome. *N Engl J Med*. 2011;364:1293-1304.
17. Iwashyna TJ, Netzer G, Langa KM, Cigolle C. Spurious inferences about long-term outcomes: the case of severe sepsis and geriatric conditions. *Am J Respir Crit Care Med*. 2012;185:835-841.
18. Woon FL, Dunn C, Hopkins RO. Predicting cognitive sequelae in survivors of critical illness with cognitive screening tests. *Am J Respir Crit Care Med*. 2012;186:333-340.
19. Hopkins RO, Weaver LK, Pope D, Orme JF, Bigler ED, Larson-LOHR V. Neuropsychological sequelae and impaired health status in survivors of severe acute respiratory distress syndrome. *Am J Respir Crit Care Med*. 1999;160:50-56.
20. Hopkins RO, Weaver LK, Collingridge D, Parkinson RB, Chan KJ, Orme Jr JF. Two-year cognitive, emotional, and quality-of-life outcomes in acute respiratory distress syndrome. *Am J Respir Crit Care Med*. 2005;171:340-347.
21. Wilcox ME, Brummel NE, Archer K, Ely EW, Jackson JC, Hopkins RO. Cognitive dysfunction in ICU patients: risk factors, predictors, and rehabilitation interventions. *Crit Care Med*. 2013; 41:S81-S98.
22. Iwashyna TJ, Ely EW, Smith DM, Langa KM. Long-term cognitive impairment and functional disability among survivors of severe sepsis. *JAMA*. 2010;304:1787-1794.
23. Shah F, Pike F, Alvarez K, et al. Bidirectional relationship between cognitive function and pneumonia. *Am J Respir Crit Care Med*. 2013;188:586-592.
24. Pandharipande PP, Girard TD, Jackson JC, et al. Long-term cognitive impairment after critical illness. *N Engl J Med*. 2013;369:1306-1316.
25. Davydow DS, Gifford JM, Desai SV, Bienvenu OJ, Needham DM. Depression in general intensive care unit survivors: a systematic review. *Intensive Care Med*. 2009;35:796-809.

26. Davydow DS, Gifford JM, Desai SV, Needham DM, Bienvenu OJ. Posttraumatic stress disorder in general intensive care unit survivors: a systematic review. *Gen Hosp Psychiatry*. 2008;30:421-434.

27. Davydow DS, Desai SV, Needham DM, Bienvenu OJ. Psychiatric morbidity in survivors of the acute respiratory distress syndrome: a systematic review. *Psychosom Med*. 2008;70:512-519.

28. Jackson JC, Pandharipande PP, Girard TD, et al., Bringing to light the Risk Factors and Incidence of Neuropsychological dysfunction in ICU survivors (BRAIN-ICU) study investigators. Depression, post-traumatic stress disorder, and functional disability in survivors of critical illness in the brain-ICU study: a longitudinal cohort study. *Lancet Respir Med*. 2014;2:369-379.

29. Wunsch H, Christiansen CF, Johansen MB, et al. Psychiatric diagnoses and psychoactive medication use among nonsurgical critically ill patients receiving mechanical ventilation. *JAMA*. 2014;311:1133-1142.

30. Davydow DS, Hough CL, Langa KM, Iwashyna TJ. Symptoms of depression in survivors of severe sepsis: a prospective cohort study of older Americans. *Am J Geriatr Psychiatry*. 2013;21:887-897.

31. Weycker D, Akhras KS, Edelsberg J, Angus DC, Oster G. Long-term mortality and medical care charges in patients with severe sepsis. *Crit Care Med*. 2003;31:2316-2323.

32. Coopersmith CM, Wunsch H, Fink MP, et al. A comparison of critical care research funding and the financial burden of critical illness in the United States. *Crit Care Med*. 2012;40:1072-1079.

33. Cameron JI, Herridge MS, Tansey CM, McAndrews MP, Cheung AM. Well-being in informal caregivers of survivors of acute respiratory distress syndrome. *Crit Care Med*. 2006;34:81-86.

34. Chelluri L, Im KA, Belle SH, et al. Long-term mortality and quality of life after prolonged mechanical ventilation. *Crit Care Med*. 2004;32:61-69.

35. Azoulay E, Pochard F, Kentish-Barnes N, et al. Risk of post-traumatic stress symptoms in family members of intensive care unit patients. *Am J Respir Crit Care Med*. 2005;171:987-994.

36. Davidson JE, Jones C, Bienvenu OJ. Family response to critical illness: postintensive care syndrome-family. *Crit Care Med*. 2012;40:618-624.

37. Davidson JE, Daly BJ, Agan D, Brady NR, Higgins PA. Facilitated sensemaking: a feasibility study for the provision of a family support program in the intensive care unit. *Crit Care Nurs Q*. 2010;33:177-189.

38. Verceles AC, Corwin DS, Afshar M, et al. Half of the family members of critically ill patients experience excessive daytime sleepiness. *Intensive Care Med*. 2014;40:1124-1131.

39. Sullivan DR, Liu X, Corwin DS, et al. Learned helplessness among families and surrogate decision-makers of patients admitted to medical, surgical, and trauma ICUs. *Chest*. 2012;142:1440-1446.

40. Netzer G, Sullivan DR. Recognizing, naming, and measuring a family intensive care unit syndrome. *Ann Am Thorac Soc*. 2014;11:435-441.

41. Davydow DS, Hough CL, Langa KM, Iwashyna TJ. Depressive symptoms in spouses of older patients with severe sepsis. *Crit Care Med*. 2012;40:2335-2341.

42. Cuthbertson BH, Elders A, Hall S, et al. Mortality and quality of life in the five years after severe sepsis. *Crit Care*. 2013;17:R70.

43. Ehlenbach WJ, Hough CL, Crane PK, et al. Association between acute care and critical illness hospitalization and cognitive function in older adults. *JAMA*. 2010;303:763-770.

44. Valley TS, Sjoding MW, Ryan AM, Iwashyna TJ, Cooke CR. Association of intensive care unit admission with mortality among older patients with pneumonia. *JAMA*. 2015;314(12):1272-1279.

45. Lachman ME, Agrigoroaei S. Promoting functional health in midlife and old age: long-term protective effects of control beliefs, social support, and physical exercise. *PLoS One*. 2010;5(10):e13297.

46. Pandharipande P, Banerjee A, McGrane S, Ely EW. Liberation and animation for ventilated ICU patients: the ABCDE bundle for the back-end of critical care. *Crit Care*. 2010;14(3):157.

47. Bell CM, Brener SS, Gunraj N, et al. Association of ICU or hospital admission with unintentional discontinuation of medications for chronic diseases. *JAMA*. 2011;306:840-847.

48. Morandi A, Vasilevskis E, Pandharipande PP, et al. Inappropriate medication prescriptions in elderly adults surviving an intensive care unit hospitalization. *J Am Geriatr Soc*. 2013;61:1128-1134.

49. Morandi A, Vasilevskis EE, Pandharipande PP, et al. Inappropriate medications in elderly ICU survivors: where to intervene? *Arch Intern Med*. 2011;171:1032-1034.

50. Gandhi TK. Fumbled handoffs: one dropped ball after another. *Ann Intern Med*. 2005;142:352-358.

51. Prescott HC, Langa KM, Iwashyna TJ. Readmission diagnoses after hospitalization for severe sepsis and other acute medical conditions. *JAMA*. 2015;313(10):1055-1057.

52. Calvo-Ayala E, Khan BA, Farber MO, Ely EW, Boustani MA. Interventions to improve the physical function of ICU survivors: a systematic review. *Chest*. 2013;144(5):1469-1480.

53. Mehlhorn J, Freytag A, Schmidt K, et al. Rehabilitation interventions for postintensive care syndrome: a systematic review. *Crit Care Med*. 2014;42(5):1263-1271.

54. Sevin CM, Bloom SL, Jackson JC, Wang L, Ely EW, Stollings JL. Comprehensive care of ICU survivors: Development and implementation of an ICU recovery center. *J Crit Care*. 2018;46:141-148.

55. Schmidt K, Worrack S, Von Korff M, et al. Effect of a primary care management intervention on mental health-related quality of life among survivors of sepsis: a randomized clinical trial. *JAMA*. 2016;315(24):2703-2711.

56. McPeake J, Iwashyna TJ, Devine H, MacTavish P, Quasim T. Peer support to improve recovery following critical care discharge: a case-based discussion. *Thorax*. 2017;72(9):856-858.

57. Stollings JL, Bloom SL, Wang L, Ely EW, Jackson JC, Sevin CM. Critical care pharmacists and medication management in an ICU recovery center. *Ann Pharmacother*. 2018;52(8):713-723.

58. Hopkins RO, Suchyta MR, Farrer TJ, Needham D. Improving post-intensive care unit neuropsychiatric outcomes: understanding cognitive effects of physical activity. *Am J Respir Crit Care Med*. 2012;186:1220-1228.

59. Stuck AE, Siu AL, Wieland GD, Adams J, Rubenstein LZ. Comprehensive geriatric assessment: a meta-analysis of controlled trials. *Lancet*. 1993;342:1032-1036.

60. Mikkelsen ME, Jackson JC, Hopkins RO, et al. Peer support as a novel strategy to mitigate post-intensive care syndrome. *AACN Adv Crit Care*. 2016;27(2):221-229.

61. Haines KJ, Beesley SJ, Hopkins RO, et al. Peer support in critical care: a systematic review. *Crit Care Med*. 2018;46(9):1522-1531.

5

How Have Genomics Informed Our Understanding of Critical Illness?

Kelly R. Genga, Mark Trinder, and James A. Russell

INTRODUCTION

Per the Biomarkers Definitions Working Group, a biomarker is a characteristic that is objectively measured and evaluated as an indicator of normal biological processes, pathogenic processes, or pharmacologic responses to a therapeutic intervention.[1] In many areas of clinical medicine (e.g., cancer and heart disease), genomic biomarkers are routinely used for diagnosis, prognosis, and prediction. In cancer care, genomic biomarkers are used to identify responders to specific chemotherapies and to guide and select treatment regardless of anatomic or cellular origin. The clinical laboratory assays (or kits) are usually either based on variations in genomic DNA, most commonly either single nucleotide polymorphisms (SNPs) or copy number variants (CNVs), or use RNA to identify specific patterns of gene expression in either tissue or in circulating peripheral blood monocytes (PBMCs).

The story is different in critical care. Despite years of intense research and investigation into more than 200 distinct biological molecules that fulfill some validation criteria,[2] no clinically viable genomic biomarkers in sepsis, acute respiratory distress syndrome (ARDS), acute kidney injury (AKI), or trauma have emerged. Indeed, the international Surviving Sepsis Campaign (SSC) Guidelines did not review or recommend a single genomic biomarker in sepsis.[3] However, recent advances and approaches suggest that some biomarkers are close to clinical utility in critical illness.

We use the convention that genes are denoted in italics (e.g., interleukin-1β gene [*IL-1β*]) while proteins and transcripts are not italicized (e.g., IL-1-β). We mainly discuss SNPs, insertion/deletion variants (indels), CNVs, and rare mutations (<1%). Polymorphisms that are inherited together because they are linked along the genome are said to be in linkage disequilibrium. This is relevant because we do not usually measure every SNP or CNV, but rather measure tag SNPs that mark a genomic region (in or between genes), that may not have a known function, but that may mark a known functional variant.

Most genomics studies of critical illness are population based. The characteristics of strong population genomics studies include appropriate controls in case-control studies, adequate sample size and power, correction for multiple comparisons (and there are many comparisons in most population genomics studies), control for ethnicity, confirmation

that the genomic variant has a known function, and, eventually, evidence that the variant has high clinical utility, i.e., a clinician would use a kit to detect the variant and a payer would pay for it because results of the genomic variant test add useful information that complements other assessments. We now briefly review genomics discovery methods.

GENOMICS DISCOVERY METHODS—BRIEFLY

Functional genomics can:

- focus on a single gene and how the alteration of the gene sequence changes gene expression
- focus on a small number of candidate genes
- use genome-wide association studies (GWAS) that canvass specific variants (SNPs) across the whole genome or
- even measure (by sequencing) the whole exon or the whole genome.

Functional genomics methods include SNP analysis, genetic interaction mapping, mutagenesis, RNA interference (RNAi), and genome annotation. GWAS has been successful in identifying genetic variants associated with many common diseases (e.g., type 2 diabetes, cystic fibrosis, asthma, and neurofibromatosis).

Transcriptomics (also known as expression profiling) measures RNA transcript abundance in tissues and/or blood cells in cases (disease of interest) and controls. Challenges involved in the study of critical illnesses include which tissue to sample, the rapid disease process (leading to lead time bias in clinical studies), and accurately establishing the diagnosis of sepsis, ARDS, trauma, and other critical illnesses.[4]

GENOMIC DIAGNOSTIC AND PROGNOSTIC BIOMARKERS IN SEPSIS

The gold standard for diagnosing bacteremia remains the traditional microbiology laboratory broth blood culture followed by identification and susceptibility testing. Novel molecular techniques that use genetic analysis for molecular organism detection including hybridization (fluorescence in situ hybridization [FISH], arrays), amplification (polymerase chain reaction [PCR], multiplex PCR), post-amplification detection (PCR + hybridization/MALDI-TOF mass spectrometry [MS]), and non-nucleic acid-based strategies (proteomics, spectrometry) are rapidly gaining ground.[5] PCR and multiplex post-amplification techniques accelerate the diagnosis of bacteremia and detection of the most common resistant genotypes. However, the majority of molecular tests require a positive blood culture before widespread clinical application. The main benefits of pathogen detection by PCR, multiplex PCR, and MS is the possibility of having results reported as soon as 6 hours after sampling. To our knowledge, there has been no large, multicenter, multinational randomized controlled trial (RCT) comparing conventional blood culture to a strategy of blood culture plus molecular organism detection in sepsis.

Barriers to the universal approval of PCR detection of pathogens include limited sensitivity of the test (i.e., statistical sensitivity), discordance between molecular results and blood cultures (i.e., specificity), and a poor ability to detect *Streptococcus pneumoniae* bacteremia (i.e., sensitivity).[6] Several molecular strategies allow molecular detection of pathogens: pathogen-specific assays targeting species- or genus- specific genes; assays targeting conserved sequences in the bacterial or fungal genome (panbacterial 16S, 5S, or 23S rRNA genes or panfungal 18S, 5.8S, and 28S rDNAs), and multiplex assays allowing parallel detection of different pathogens.[7]

Microarray techniques have been applied to the diagnosis of sepsis but are still limited to the detection of *Staphylococcus aureus*, *Pseudomonas aeruginosa*, and *Escherichia coli* in positive blood cultures.[8] In a study of neonatal sepsis ($n = 172$ clinical cases), 10% tested positive by PCR and nearly 5% by blood culture.[9]

The most used molecular pathogen detection test is the SeptiFast test (Roche Diagnostics), a multiplex real-time PCR-based assay that detects 25 pathogens with modest sensitivity for detection of bacteremia. However, SeptiFast had variable pathogen detection compared with traditional blood culture testing.[6,10,11] In a prospective severe sepsis study, PCR positivity even with a negative blood culture was associated with higher sequential organ failure assessment (SOFA) scores and a trend towards higher mortality.[12]

The only molecular direct pathogen detection test approved by the Food and Drug Administration (FDA) is the Cepheid Xpert that yields rapid detection of *Neisseria gonorrhoeae/Chlamydia*, *Mycobacterium tuberculosis* (MTB) complex, MTB specimens with rifampin-resistance (*rpoB* gene) and MRSA. Other pathogen detection tests in variable stages of development include the SepsiTest (Molyzm, Germany), Magicplex (Seegene, Korea), and VYOO (SIRSLab, Germany). These tests are in their infancy with limited or no observational studies to date.[13]

EFFECTS OF SEPSIS ON GENE EXPRESSION

Host gene expression changes could be used to diagnose sepsis. Human leukocyte response to endotoxin challenge[14-17] demonstrated that the greatest change in mononuclear cell gene expression occurred at 6 hours post-endotoxin with increased expression (induction) of 439 and decreased expression (repression) of 428 genes and return to baseline by 24 hours. The upregulated genes included genes associated with pathogen recognition molecules and signaling cascades linked to receptors associated with cell mobility and activation as well as cytokines, chemokines, and their respective receptors, acute-phase transcription factors, proteases, arachidonate metabolites, and oxidases. Repressed genes included defense response genes such as those associated with co-stimulatory molecules, T and cytotoxic lymphocytes, natural killer (NK) cells, and protein synthesis.

A recent study identified a novel gene expression profile in blood that defined early sepsis.[18] The genes are involved in the development of endotoxin tolerance: a second exposure to endotoxin elicits a less profound inflammatory and immune response than the first endotoxin exposure. Several other groups have evaluated whole blood or specific leukocyte gene expression as a diagnostic for sepsis.[17,19]

Transcriptomics provides another novel approach to sepsis diagnosis (Table 5.1). Gene expression in sepsis was highly homogeneous, with 70% of genes differentially expressed between septic and controls.[20] Tang et al.[21] measured gene expression in peripheral whole-blood samples and compared septic and nonseptic critically ill patients and gram-positive vs. gram-negative sepsis and found no major differences. These findings suggest that gram-positive and gram-negative infections share a common host response.[22]

TABLE 5.1   Transcriptomic Expression Profiles Showing Upregulated and Downregulated Genes In Studies of Human Sepsis.

Pathway	Upregulated	Downregulated
Inflammatory	TLR1 and 2[20]	TNF[20]
	CD14[20]	TNF receptor 1b[21]
	FPRL1[20]	
	Properdin P factor	Prokineticin 2[21]
	C1q receptor	LPS-induced
	C3a receptor 1	TNF factor[21]
	S100A8, S100A12[20]	Raf-1[21]
	PF4[20]	BMP5[20]
	Matrix metallopeptidase-8 (MMP-8)[23]	
Immune regulatory	Fc-γ receptor I and II	IL-8[21]
	LILRA3, LILRB2, LILRB3 and LILRB4	IL-8RA[20]
	Protein kinase C	Chemokine Ligand 4[21]
	MAPK14[20] or p38, PAK2	Chitinase-3[21]
	PI3K	
	Src, JAK, Ras, Rho	
	15-Hydroxy-PG DH[21]	
	LAIR 1[21]	
	NFKBIA[21]	
	IL-11, 18[20]	

Septic shock subclass stratification by Wong et al.[19] is based on whole-blood RNA from 98 children and identified 6934 differentially regulated genes. These genes generated 10 regulated gene cluster pathways and they stratified patients into three subclasses corresponding to phenotypic outcomes.

Several examples of gene association studies in sepsis are shown in Table 5.2. We have evaluated and found associations of SNPs of inflammatory, coagulation, innate immunity, and endotoxin clearance-regulating genes with altered outcomes in sepsis.[24–34] If validated, several of these discoveries could guide the use of vasopressors.[27,35–37]

In contrast to candidate gene association studies, GWAS is a nonbiased approach to evaluate genetic variants across the human genome and gives insights into the breadth of genomic risks for sepsis. Many novel pathways—including pathways that were never suspected in sepsis—are important in sepsis. To date, there have been few published GWAS studies in sepsis.[52]

TABLE 5.2 Genetic Association Studies in Human Sepsis.

Pathway	Genes	Comment
Pattern recognition receptors	CD14	GG of rs2569190 with increased risk of severe sepsis[38]
	TLR2	rs3804099 associated with neonatal sepsis and gram-positive infections[39]
	TLR4	Asp299Gly/Thr39
		9Ile—more severe sepsis and gram-negative infections[40]
	TLR5	rs5744105 associated with neonatal sepsis[39]
Intracellular signaling proteins	IRAK1	
Proinflammatory	IL-1α	rs1800587 associated with sepsis susceptibility
	IL-1β	CT and TT of rs1143643 with increased risk of sepsis[38]
		rs143634 TT genotype associated with decreased risk of sepsis[41]
	IL-6	G-174C—possible association of GG genotype with improved survival[42]
	Lymphotoxin-alpha (LTA)	rs1800629-AG associated with susceptibility to sepsis[43]
	CD86	rs17281995G/C associated with pneumonia induced sepsis[44]
	TNF-α	TNF-30—TNF2 allele associated with increased susceptibility and mortality[45]
	TNF-β	TNF Ncol—TNFB2 allele associated with susceptibility to sepsis and poor outcome[46]
	FcγR	FcRIIa-R131, FcRIIIa-F158, FcRIIIb-NA2—deficient phenotype associated with increased susceptibility and mortality[47]
Anti-inflammatory	IL-10	rs1800896 associated with neonatal sepsis and gram-negative infections[39]
	IL-1 receptor antagonist (IL-RA)	VNTR polymorphism with increased sepsis susceptibility[41]
Chemokines	IL-8 CXCL10	AT of rs4073 with increased risk of severe sepsis[38]
Endothelial	PAI-1	4G/5G—strong association of PAI-1 4G allele with poor outcome from sepsis[48]
	ACE	I/D—DD genotype is associated with higher mortality[49]
Others	Bactericidal-permeability increasing protein (BPI)	rs4358188-AG associated with reduced susceptibility to sepsis[38]
		Taq GG and 216 AG or GG associated with gram-negative sepsis and death[50]
	Mannose-binding lectin (MBL)	Exon1 (AB/BB) associated with the risk of sepsis in neonates[51]
	Matrix metalloproteinase-16 (MMP-16)	GG of rs2664349GG with increased risk of sepsis[38]
	Serpine1	
	Heat shock protein12A	
	Ring finger protein 175	
	Phospholipase A2, Group IIA (PLA2G2A)	rs1891320 associated with sepsis in neonates and gram-positive infections[39]

GENOMIC PREDICTIVE BIOMARKERS IN SEPSIS AND SEPTIC SHOCK

Predictive biomarkers define the response to a drug or device and seek to identify and validate genomic biomarkers to stratify patients so that one can define which patients respond well—or not—to a particular drug. There are many predictive biomarkers for drugs used in fields such as cancer or cardiovascular disease that identify those patients who will respond to a drug (efficacy predictive biomarker) or who will have an adverse event (safety predictive biomarker). There are no approved or clinically used predictive genomic biomarkers for use of drugs in sepsis but potential biomarkers have been proposed. To discuss these, we first need to review some sepsis prognostic genomic biomarkers (i.e., to estimate prognosis).

Sepsis is a very heterogeneous condition and there have been no drugs approved for its treatment. One approach to increase the efficacy of drugs in sepsis and septic shock is to discover and validate (genomic) predictive biomarker(s) that predict responses to drugs. To date, there have been efforts but no successes in getting a predictive biomarker into clinical use in sepsis and septic shock. However, there are possibilities. For example, if sepsis represents the imbalance between pro- and anti-inflammatory biomarkers, then SNPs within genes of cytokines such as tumor necrosis factor alpha (TNF-α) could be strong candidate predictive biomarkers in sepsis for drugs that alter TNF-α (e.g., anti-TNFα). Elevated serum TNF-α is associated with poor outcomes in sepsis[53,54] and TNF-α SNPs may be associated with the altered TNF-α production. The TNF-α promoter region SNP at position 308 confers either high (A) or low (G) gene transcription.[55] The -308 A allele is associated with increased susceptibility to and mortality from septic shock. TNF-α 308 G/A SNP could be used as a predictive biomarker to define responders to anti-TNF-α antibodies or soluble TNF-α receptors.[56–58]

Activated protein C (APC)—drotrecogin alfa (activated)—was at one time approved for the treatment of sepsis but was removed from the market after the negative PROWESS SHOCK trial.[59] Nonetheless, it provided an opportunity to examine a set of predictive biomarkers. In a novel propensity matched case-control trial of patients who were randomized in the APC clinical trial,[60] patients with severe sepsis at high risk of death (with DNA available for analysis) were matched to controls adjusting for age, APACHE II or SAPS II, organ dysfunction, ventilation, medical/surgical status, infection site, and propensity score (probability that a patient would have received APC given their baseline characteristics). Independent genotyping and two-phase data transfer mitigated bias; 692 patients treated with DrotAA were successfully matched to 1935 patients not treated with DrotAA. There was no significant genotype by treatment interaction for mortality or several secondary endpoints. The study was "negative" but highlighted a method that could be used to discover and develop predictive biomarker(s) for drugs in critical illness.[61]

Similar methods have been used to discover a panel of cytokine biomarkers that predict response to corticosteroids in septic shock[62] and an SNP variant of vasopressinase that predicts response to vasopressin in septic shock.[36] SNPs of the thrombomodulin gene[63] could predict response to treatment with recombinant thrombomodulin.[64]

GENOMIC DIAGNOSTIC AND PROGNOSTIC BIOMARKERS IN ACUTE RESPIRATORY DISTRESS SYNDROME

ARDS may complicate sepsis, trauma, and other critical illnesses. Like sepsis, ARDS is highly heterogeneous regarding the underlying clinical risk factor and timing of presentation, and, to date, there is no robust biomarker for risk assessment, diagnosis, prognosis, or prediction of response to therapy for ARDS. Despite the Berlin Definition, the limited accuracy of chest radiographs and the clinical heterogeneity of ARDS often lead to misdiagnosis.[65,66] As with sepsis, no pharmacologic intervention has been proven to decrease duration of mechanical ventilation,[67] reduce mortality rates,[68,69] or improve oxygenation in ARDS.[70]

ARDS is a polygenic disorder related to multiple genetic variants, each one contributing only with a limited effect,[71] and environmental risks, a classic gene–environment interaction. Not all patients who are exposed to equivalent risk factors for ARDS actually develop it. Accordingly, patients who develop similar "ARDS phenotypes" have distinctively different outcomes: that is, some patients die due to refractory respiratory dysfunction, despite initiation of therapy, while some recover lung function. It is likely that genetics play a role in the individual predisposition and mortality associated with ARDS.[66] Gene–environment interaction is central to risk prediction in ARDS pathobiology and mortality.[66,72]

Several biomarkers have been studied to predict ARDS risk,[73] organ dysfunction in ARDS,[63] response to therapy,[74] and prognosis[75] (Table 5.3). However, no biomarker is currently used in clinical practice because of limited accuracy and lack of robust validation in large, adequately powered studies. However, genomic biomarker studies add insights about ARDS pathophysiology and the roles of genomic variation in ARDS risk and outcome.[76,77]

To date, there are no reports of ARDS affecting multiple members of the same family, distinct from diseases with well-known heritability. Genomics research in ARDS is therefore most often based on nested case-control studies comparing genetic variations at specific genomic regions, particularly using the candidate gene approach. Several genomic discovery studies using GWAS, whole exome sequencing (WES), and whole genome sequencing (WGS) have been done in ARDS but have not identified clinical biomarkers.[84,88,89] GWAS studies require large cohorts in order to have adequate power to detect common genetic variants that have small-to-moderate effect sizes[90] and must achieve strict P values corrected for multiple comparisons (e.g., $P < 10^{-8}$ to 10^{-10}) to be statistically significant. Thus, rare variants and true associations of SNPs with small effect size may not be

TABLE 5.3   Genomic Biomarkers in ARDS.

Author (Year)	Type of Study	Gene(s)	Patients	Findings
Meyer et al. (2011)[78]	Two-stage genetic association study using SNP genotyping array method	ANGPT2	Stage I: African American critically ill subjects with trauma. Stage II: European American patients with trauma-related ARDS	Increased risk of ARDS in patients carrying the two ANGPT2 SNPs rs1868554 and rs2442598
Bajwa et al. (2011)[79]	Candidate gene association case-control study	NFKB1 promoter polymorphism (rs28362491): a four base pair insertion/deletion (−94ins/delATTG)	ICU-admitted patients at risk for ARDS vs. ARDS patients	Patients under 70 carrying the variant (del/del) had increased OR for ARDS; among ARDS patients, this variant was also associated with increased 60-day mortality in comparison to WT and heterozygous patients
Dahmer et al. (2011)[80]	Prospective cohort genetic association study	SFTPB	African American children with community-acquired pneumonia	Greater need for mechanical ventilation in patients with ARDS induced by pneumonia in children carrying the variants rs1130866 or +1580 C/T, and rs3024793
Acosta-Herrera et al. (2015)[81]	Candidate gene association case-control study	NFE2L2	Patients with ARDS secondary to sepsis	ARDS susceptibility was associated with 10 noncoding NFE2L2 SNPs that were in tight linkage disequilibrium
Meyer et al. (2013)[82]	Multistage genetic association study using SNP genotyping array method	IL-1RN	Three critically ill populations. Stage I: patients with trauma-associated ARDS. Stage II: trauma control patients. Stage III: nested case-control population of mixed subjects	The C allele of rs315952 reduced the risk of ARDS in around 20% and was associated with increased levels of IL-1RA
O'Mahony et al. (2012)[83]	Candidate gene association nested case-control study	IL-6	Caucasians patients with SIRS diagnosis	IL-6 SNP rs2069832 was associated with increased risk for ARDS
Bime et al. (2018)[84]	GWAS	SELPLG	African American patients	Identification of the SELPLG variant rs2228315 and ARDS
Morrell et al. (2018)[85]	Two-stage gene association study (candidate gene association)	MAP3K1	Stage I: patients with ARDS from the ARDSNet FACTT. Stage II: patients with ARDS from a different center in the United States	A genetic variant rs832582 was associated with decreased ventilator-free days in ARDS patients
Kangelaris et al. (2015)[86]	Case-control study using WGE analysis (whole blood)	OLFM4, CD24, LCN2, BPI	Critically ill patients with sepsis	OLFM4, CD24, LCN2, BPI (mediators of the initial neutrophil response to infection) were upregulated in patients with sepsis and ARDS vs. patients with sepsis alone

Continued

TABLE 5.3	Genomic Biomarkers In ARDS.—cont'd			
Author (Year)	Type of Study	Gene(s)	Patients	Findings
Kovach et al. (2015)[87]	Case-control study using microarray analysis (alveolar macrophages and circulating leukocytes)	*S100A12* and *IL-1R2*	Patients with ARDS that were enrolled in the Acute Lung Injury	Upregulation of S100A12 and the anti-inflammatory IL-1 decoy receptor IL-1R2 in ARDS vs. control group; increased levels of IL-1R2 in plasma found in nonsurvivors compared with survivors at later stages of ARDS
Grigoryev et al. (2015)[88]	eGWAS of combined 8 ARDS models (case-control study)	Several	Analysis of more than 120 publicly available microarray samples of ARDS in the ARDS datasets were collected from GEO	Identification of 42 ARDS candidate genes, two-thirds of which was previously linked to lung injury. The top 5 genes were *IL-1R2, IL-1B, CLC4D, CLC4E, CD300LF*

revealed.[91] There are also concerns about what population represents the appropriate control group for patients with ARDS. Control subjects should be exposed to similar risk factors for ARDS but should not develop ARDS. The use of healthy individuals as controls mitigates the relevance and even the significance of any associations.[72] Genome- or exome-wide sequencing studies are alternatives to GWAS studies but require careful quality assurance and interpretation to discriminate which variants are truly meaningful.[91]

Candidate genes are selected based on previous knowledge of ARDS biology and pathogenesis[72] and, as such, are driven by a priori hypotheses. The effectiveness of candidate gene studies can be increased by the use of multiplex candidate genes. The disadvantages of these designs include potential inaccuracy when selecting genes and/or gene variants and limitations regarding the number of gene/variants analyzed.[91]

Another option for genomic research in ARDS is the study of intermediate traits involved in ARDS pathogenesis. The intermediate trait can be a plasma biomarker or an mRNA transcript that can then be used in combination with Mendelian randomization analysis. Mendelian randomization analysis takes the assumption that genetic variants —like an intervention in an RCT—are randomly assigned to offspring from each of the two parents. Mendelian randomization analysis can yield inferences about causality between genetic variants, intermediate traits, and ARDS (e.g., genetic variants of and increased levels of IL-1β and/or angiotensin-2 vs. risk of ARDS).[66,90]

Gene expression studies (e.g., mRNA microarray methods) of circulating cells (such as monocytes) identify genes associated with ARDS by comparing levels of transcript abundance between control and ARDS. Gene expression (mRNA) is linked with gene pathway analysis, and can include quantification of gene expression over time. This approach led to the discovery of a possible protective role of the elafin (*PI3*) gene in ARDS.[92] This is an hypothesis-generating discovery with limitations, such as definition of "normal" expression.[72] The use of circulating cells may be problematic because gene expression does not necessarily mirror the transcription changes in the lung epithelial or endothelial cells (key cells in the ARDS pathophysiology).[90] However, lung biopsies are not commonly performed in ARDS and bronchoalveolar lavage (BAL)-derived cells have been exposed to non-ARDS conditions that alter gene expression (e.g., smoking, air pollution).[93]

MicroRNA (miRNA) and epigenetic studies have been performed in ARDS. miRNAs are noncoding RNAs that control the activity of a large fraction of the protein-coding genes in mammals.[94] Several miRNAs have been associated with initiation, maintenance, and resolution of ARDS in human cells because of their regulatory effects on ARDS-related gene expression. Examples include *MYLK* (miR-374a, miR-374b, miR-520c-3p, and miR-1290),[95] *PBEF/NAMPT* (miR-374a and miR-568),[96] and *SERT* (miR-16).[97] Recently, two epigenetic variants within the *MYLK* gene (an ARDS candidate gene associated with vascular barrier regulatory functions) were associated with ARDS, suggesting that epigenetics contributes to the expression of ARDS-related genes.[98]

Expression quantitative trait loci (eQTL) studies combine gene expression and gene association analysis, providing data about genetic variants that are associated with changes in transcript abundance.[91] One exome-wide case-control study in ARDS validated a platelet-associated locus (among 5 loci),[99] based on the hypothesis that platelets might be a causal mediator of the genetic effects on ARDS development.[89]

In future studies, the integration of different genomic methods and/or the use of a multiple 'omics approach (e.g., genomics, proteomics, metabolomics, transcriptomics, and epigenomics) could lead to discovery and validation of accurate biomarkers that may predict risk, response to therapy, mortality, and even novel drugs for ARDS.[66,100,101]

DIAGNOSTIC AND PROGNOSTIC BIOMARKERS IN ARDS

Since early reports evaluated polymorphisms in surfactant genes (SP-A, SP-B, and SP-D), more than 40 ARDS-related candidate genes have been described.[102] These possibilities included genes encoding cytokines (IL-8, IL-10, MIF, PBEF1, TNF, VEGF), blood pressure regulators (ACE), proteins involved in endothelial barrier function (MYLK), antioxidant enzymes (SOD-3, NQO1), coagulation factors (PLAU, F5, thrombomodulin [REFS]), regulators of iron homeostasis (FTL, HMOX2), and immune response-related proteins (MBL2, IL-1β). More recent discoveries are related predominantly to genes associated with lung permeability, alveolar function, endothelial activation, and inflammation.

In two separate cohorts, two SNPs in the angiopoietin 2 gene (*ANGPT2*) (rs1868554 and rs2442598) were associated with increased risk of trauma-related ARDS.[78] These findings are interesting because the *ANGPT2* gene has previously been associated with increased pulmonary vascular leak in models of lung injury.[103] Other variants of genes that regulate vascular permeability (*MYLK*, *PBEF1*, and *VEGFA*) have also been associated with risk of ARDS.[103–105]

NFKB1, a transcription factor that regulates many proinflammatory genes, was previously associated with ARDS severity.[106] The presence of the *NFKB1* promoter polymorphism (rs28362491)—a four-base pair insertion/deletion (-94ins/delATTG) genotype—was independently associated with greater risk of ARDS in patients under 70 years old and with mortality in a case-control study comparing at-risk vs. ARDS patients.[79]

Surfactant protein B (SP-B) (gene *SFTPB)* maintains alveolar surface tension.[80] SP-B concentration is low in BAL fluid obtained from patients with ARDS. Polymorphisms in *SFTPB* are associated with increased risk of ARDS.[107,108] In African American children with community-acquired pneumonia, two specific *SFTPB* variants (rs1130866 or +1580 C/T, and rs3024793) were associated with greater need for mechanical ventilation in patients with ARDS induced by pneumonia.[80]

ARDS pathogenesis involves oxidative stress.[109] Nuclear factor erythroid 2-like 2 (*NFE2L2*) is a transcription factor that controls the expression of antioxidant genes. Common variants in *NFE2L2* were evaluated in a case-control study in subjects with ARDS secondary to sepsis.[81] ARDS susceptibility was associated with 10 noncoding SNPs that were in tight linkage disequilibrium. Interestingly, one of the identified SNPs (rs672961) was formerly shown to alter the promoter activity of the *NFE2L2* gene,[110] leading to reduction in the antioxidative response induced by this gene.

A genetic variant in the *IL1RN* gene (rs315952), which encodes IL-1 receptor antagonist protein (IL-1RA), was identified as protective from ARDS in a multistage genetic association study, in two cohorts of trauma patients and one cohort of patients admitted to a mixed intensive care unit. The C allele of rs315952 reduced the risk of ARDS by 20% and was associated with increased levels of IL-1RA.[82] This finding supports previous animal studies that demonstrated that IL-1RA mitigates the increased lung permeability induced by IL-1β.[111]

A nested case-control study investigated common variants in genes related to inflammation, innate immunity, epithelial cell function, and angiogenesis in Caucasian patients with

systemic inflammatory response syndrome (SIRS). An *IL-6* SNP (rs2069832) showed significant associations with risk for ARDS,[83] corroborating the key role of IL-6 in ARDS pathophysiology and replicating previous studies.[112,113]

Recently, a novel gene associated with increased ARDS susceptibility in African American patients was discovered in a GWAS studies in ARDS. A nonsynonymous coding SNP (rs2228315) in the *SELPLG* gene encodes P-selectin glycoprotein ligand 1, a protein involved in the endothelium activation in sepsis was associated with ARDS.[84]

A variant of the mitogen-activated protein (MAP) kinase 1 gene (*MAP3K1*) rs832582 was associated with decreased ventilator-free days in ARDS.[85] MAP kinase 1 modulates inflammation, apoptosis, and cytoskeletal dysfunction.[114]

To briefly summarize, although genomic studies in ARDS have expanded in recent years, many gaps in the understanding of genomics of ARDS remain. Furthermore, several inherent limiting characteristics (e.g., phenotype heterogeneity, limited sample size and statistical power, mixing of risk factors, misdiagnosis of included cases) generate ongoing difficulties in design and interpretation. There are no clinically approved genomic diagnostic, prognostic, or predictive biomarkers for ARDS (and there are no approved drugs for ARDS).

GENOMIC BIOMARKERS IN OTHER CRITICAL ILLNESSES

In addition to sepsis and ARDS, use of genetic biomarkers for critical illnesses such as AKI, trauma, and traumatic brain injury (TBI) holds promise.

Genomic studies provide novel information on risk factors, etiology, prognosis, and pathogenesis of AKI. The discovery that hypovolemic AKI and ischemic reperfusion AKI have profoundly different genomic transcriptional responses has led to the identification of subtype-specific biomarkers of AKI in human urine.[115] This is important because identification of AKI by conventional plasma creatinine measurement fails to identify AKI in a large proportion of critically ill patients with low urine output. Genetic differences are also risk factors for AKI development. Septic shock patients with the minor alleles of SNPs rs2093266 and rs1955656 that occur in apoptosis-related genes (*SERPINA4* and *SERPINA5*, respectively) have a reduced risk of developing AKI.[116] In contrast, Caucasian patients suffering AKI with either rs1050851 or rs2233417 minor alleles in the *NFKBIA* gene have a significantly increased risk of developing AKI.[117] The performance of large unbiased investigations using an exploratory approach (e.g., GWAS, RNA sequencing)[118] requires further exploration, as do approaches using in vitro and in vivo basic science studies to confirm the biological plausibility and to identify mechanisms.

Studies of trauma patients by the Inflammation and the Host Response to Injury Collaborative Research Program (Glue Grant investigators) have provided important information regarding the near-universal presence of SIRS and subsequent compensatory anti-inflammatory response syndrome (CARS).[119] The profound longitudinal "genomic storm" in leukocytes after trauma includes rapid (within hours following injury) upregulation of innate immune genes and repression of genes involved in adaptive immunity. Observed changes are more pronounced and prolonged in patients who have complicated outcomes.[120–122] These studies generated prognostic biomarkers and identified potential drug targets.[122]

A 63 gene set expression signature in leukocytes at 12–24 hours following trauma yields more accurate prediction of post-trauma complications than the APACHE II or new injury score severity clinical assessments in a retrospective cohort of 167 traumatized patients.[120,121] Additional analysis of a small patient subgroup who developed gram-negative bacteremia revealed suppression of leukocyte genes related to innate and adaptive immunity at 96 hours.[123] These gene expression signatures could guide initiation of immune-stimulating therapies (e.g., interferon-gamma) to mitigate the risk of bacteremia. Furthermore, the genomic signature of trauma is similar to severe burns, despite differences in tissue response acuity and mechanism of injury.[122] Stimulation of healthy human whole blood ex vivo with lipopolysaccharide also recapitulates many of the gene signature features attributed to polytrauma.[120] These findings highlight remarkable similarities in the immunologic changes that occur in humans following trauma, severe burns, and sepsis.[120,122,123]

Genomics studies also address inter-individual variability in TBI and could provide accurate prognosis of long-term functional outcomes.[124–126] Genetics influence both the injury (e.g., pro- and anti-inflammatory cytokines) and repair (e.g., neurotrophic genes) phases following TBI. Specifically, several minor alleles of SNPs within inflammatory cytokine genes such as *TNF-α* (rs1800629), *IL-1α* (rs1800587), and *IL-1β* (rs1143634) are associated with unfavorable TBI outcomes.[125] *Apolipoprotein E* genotype (*APOE4*), best-known for its association with Alzheimer disease, may be an important marker in TBI as well. Meta-analyses indicate that the *APOE4* genotype was associated with poor prognoses in a severity- and ethnicity-dependent manner.[127,128] *APOE* genotyping is currently available as a clinical test to assist in the diagnosis of late-onset Alzheimer disease or to confirm the diagnosis of type III hyperlipoproteinemia (dysbetalipoproteinemia). *APOE4* genotype may also increase risk of chronic traumatic encephalopathy in athletes, but the utility of prophylactic testing is deterred by ethical conundrums.[129]

Unfortunately, there are no genomics tests that are suitable for clinical practice in critical illness at this time. However, growing efforts could increase chances of success because of (1) increased sample size of cohorts through collaborations, (2) decreased cost of exon and gene sequencing, and (3) combined use of multi- 'omics (genomics, proteomics, metabolomics, and lipidomics).

GENOMICS FOR DRUG DISCOVERY

We have proposed a novel drug discovery strategy that incorporates (1) a focus on the early infectious stage of sepsis,

(2) multiple 'omics (multi- 'omics), and (3) an inverted drug discovery sequence. All these factors increase the chances of discovering effective sepsis drugs. We focus on early sepsis because antibiotics are recommended within 1 hour of presentation and each 1-hour delay is associated with a 4–6% decrease in survival.[130,131] A limitation of antibiotics is that they do not directly remove bacterial endotoxins (such as lipopolysaccharide [LPS] and lipotechoic acid [LTA], components of gram-negative and gram-positive bacteria, respectively). Almost all recently successful drugs were developed based on an initial understanding and targeting of a relevant mechanistic pathway. An 'omics association is typically an unbiased discovery that points to a possible mechanistic pathway. Multi 'omics confirmation (genetics, genomics, proteomics, lipidomics, and metabolomics) validates the discovery and refines mechanistic understanding so that high-probability drug targets can be identified.

Surprisingly, death from infection is more heritable than death from cancer or heart disease.[132] Thus, evaluating the associations of genetic variations with impaired endotoxin clearance, organ dysfunction, and decreased survival could facilitate discovery of new drugs.

We used a candidate gene approach and discovered that inhibition of proprotein convertase subtilisin/kexin type 9 (PCSK9) increased survival in sepsis.[31–33,133] Briefly, loss-of-function SNPs of PCSK9 were consistently associated with increased survival in sepsis, and PCSK9 knock-out as well as PCSK9 inhibitor treatment after induction of sepsis increased survival from sepsis.[34]

There are no approved drugs for the treatment of sepsis. To address this huge barrier to the development of new drugs, we suggested inversion (as shown by our PCSK9 discovery) of the generally accepted standard drug discovery sequence (Fig. 5.1). We propose starting with human 'omics for drug candidate discovery (instead of animal models), confirming mechanisms in human cell and clinically relevant animal models, and only then making a go/no-go decision for clinical development. For example, we could extend our PCSK9 inhibition genomics-based approach by adding multi- 'omics to discover and develop other novel candidate sepsis targets. The specific approach would include:

1. Sequencing genes of a relevant pathway—such as the 32 genes of the endotoxin clearance cascade—in well-powered cohorts.
2. Identifying associations of genetic variants with 28-day survival.
3. Measuring plasma proteins, lipids, and metabolites in the same sepsis cohorts.
4. Determining associations of genetic variants with plasma proteins, lipids, and metabolites in those cohorts.
5. Examining associations of gene variants with plasma proteins, lipids, and metabolites in a cohort of human volunteers administered low-dose lipopolysaccharide.
6. Selecting candidate targets that have
    a. variants significantly associated with decreased survival
    b. at least one significantly different level of plasma proteins, lipids, and/or metabolites in sepsis and

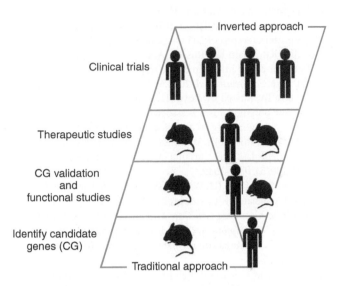

Inverted approach

Clinical trials

Therapeutic studies

CG validation
and
functional studies

Identify candidate
genes (CG)

Traditional approach

Fig. 5.1 An Inverted Drug Discovery Sequence for Sepsis and Septic Shock. We have proposed a novel drug discovery strategy that incorporates (1) a focus on the early infectious stage of sepsis, (2) multiple 'omics' (multiomics), and (3) an inverted drug discovery sequence: all to increase the chances of discovering effective sepsis drugs. We would start with human 'omics' for drug candidate discovery (instead of animal models), confirm mechanisms in human cell and clinically relevant sepsis models, and only then make go/no-go decisions for potential validated targets for clinical development.

c. at least one significantly different level of plasma proteins, lipids, and/or metabolites in the human LPS infusion cohort.

7. Evaluating these selected candidate targets for potential mechanisms of action in

   a. a human hepatocyte (because the liver clears endotoxins) model and

   b. murine gene knock-out septic shock models (e.g., peritonitis).

8. Selecting candidate targets with a significant mechanism of action for subsequent drug synthesis using both antibody and small molecule methods.

We have a done a small feasibility study of genomics, proteomics, lipidomics, and metabolomics in 24 septic shock patients and 99 heathy controls (AJRCCM abstract citation) and found dramatic differences in proteomics, lipidomics, and metabolomics. The septic shock group had significantly lower levels of discriminant proteins, lipids, and metabolites than healthy controls. We used the *PCSK9* gene to illustrate linking genomics with proteomics, lipidomics, and metabolomics and found significant differences in key proteins, lipids, and metabolites between PCSK9 loss-of-function and wild-type patients

In summary, by focusing on early sepsis, harnessing the power of multiomics, and inverting the drug discovery sequence, this novel strategy could enhance drug discovery in sepsis and septic shock that could benefit patients by improving survival and quality of life.

REFERENCES

1. Biomarkers Definitions Working Group. Biomarkers and surrogate endpoints: preferred definitions and conceptual framework. *Clin Pharmacol Ther.* 2001;69(3):89-95.
2. Douglas JJ, Roussel JA. The role of genomics to identify biomarkers and signaling molecules during severe sepsis. *Minerva Anestesiol.* 2016;82(3):343-358.
3. Rhodes A, Evans LE, Alhazzani W, et al. Surviving Sepsis Campaign: International Guidelines for Management of Sepsis and Septic Shock: 2016. *Crit Care Med.* 2017;45(3):486-552.
4. Maslove DM, Wong HR. Gene expression profiling in sepsis: timing, tissue, and translational considerations. *Trends Mol Med.* 2014;20(4):204-213.
5. Liesenfeld O, Lehman L, Hunfeld KP, Kost G. Molecular diagnosis of sepsis: new aspects and recent developments. *Eur J Microbiol Immunol (Bp).* 2014;4(1):1-25.
6. Josefson P, Strålin K, Ohlin A, et al. Evaluation of a commercial multiplex PCR test (SeptiFast) in the etiological diagnosis of community-onset bloodstream infections. *Eur J Clin Microbiol Infect Dis.* 2011;30(9):1127-1134.
7. Mancini N, Carletti S, Ghidoli N, Cichero P, Burioni R, Clementi M. The era of molecular and other non-culture-based methods in diagnosis of sepsis. *Clin Microbiol Rev.* 2010;23(1):235-251.
8. Cleven BE, Palka-Santini M, Gielen J, Meembor S, Krönke M, Krut O. Identification and characterization of bacterial pathogens causing bloodstream infections by DNA microarray. *J Clin Microbiol.* 2006;44(7):2389-2397.
9. Shang S, Chen G, Wu Y, Du L, Zhao Z. Rapid diagnosis of bacterial sepsis with PCR amplification and microarray hybridization in 16S rRNA gene. *Pediatr Res.* 2005;58(1):143-148.
10. Lehmann LE, Hunfeld KP, Steinbrucker M, et al. Improved detection of blood stream pathogens by real-time PCR in severe sepsis. *Intensive Care Med.* 2010;36(1):49-56.
11. Herne V, Nelovkov A, Kütt M, Ivanova M. Diagnostic performance and therapeutic impact of LightCycler SeptiFast assay in patients with suspected sepsis. *Eur J Microbiol Immunol (Bp).* 2013;3(1):68-76.
12. Bloos F, Hinder F, Becker K, et al. A multicenter trial to compare blood culture with polymerase chain reaction in severe human sepsis. *Intensive Care Med.* 2010;36(2):241-247.
13. Jacob D, Sauer U, Housley R, et al. Rapid and high-throughput detection of highly pathogenic bacteria by Ibis PLEX-ID technology. *PLoS One.* 2012;7(6):e39928.
14. Talwar S, Munson PJ, Barb J, et al. Gene expression profiles of peripheral blood leukocytes after endotoxin challenge in humans. *Physiol Genomics.* 2006;25(2):203-215.
15. Boyd JH, Russell JA, Fjell CD. The meta-genome of sepsis: host genetics, pathogens and the acute immune response. *J Innate Immun.* 2014;6(3):272-283.

16. Fjell CD, Russell JA. Could altered leukocyte gene expression profile in trauma patients guide immune interventions to prevent gram-negative bacteremia? *Crit Care Med.* 2014;42(6):1550-1551.

17. Thair SA, Russell JA. Sepsis in transit: from clinical to molecular classification. *Crit Care.* 2012;16(6):173.

18. Pena OM, Hancock DG, Lyle NH, et al. An endotoxin tolerance signature predicts sepsis and organ failure at first clinical presentation. *EBioMedicine.* 2014;1(1):64-71.

19. Wong HR, Cvijanovich N, Allen GL, et al. Genomic expression profiling across the pediatric systemic inflammatory response syndrome, sepsis, and septic shock spectrum. *Crit Care Med.* 2009;37(5):1558-1566.

20. Prucha M, Ruryk A, Boriss H, et al. Expression profiling: toward an application in sepsis diagnostics. *Shock.* 2004; 22(1):29-33.

21. Tang BM, McLean AS, Dawes IW, Huang SJ, Lin RC. The use of gene-expression profiling to identify candidate genes in human sepsis. *Am J Respir Crit Care Med.* 2007;176(7): 676-684.

22. Tang BM, McLean AS, Dawes IW, Huang SJ, Cowley MJ, Lin RC. Gene-expression profiling of gram-positive and gram-negative sepsis in critically ill patients. *Crit Care Med.* 2008;36(4):1125-1128.

23. Solan PD, Dunsmore KE, Denenberg AG, Odoms K, Zingarelli B, Wong HR. A novel role for matrix metalloproteinase-8 in sepsis. *Crit Care Med.* 2012;40(2):379-387.

24. Wacharasint P, Nakada TA, Boyd JH, Russell JA, Walley KR. AA genotype of IL-8 -251A/T is associated with low PaO(2)/FiO(2) in critically ill patients and with increased IL-8 expression. *Respirology.* 2012;17(8):1253-1260.

25. Thain KR, Nakada TA, Boyd JH, Russell JA, Walley KR. A common polymorphism in the 5′ region of the human protein c gene binds USF1. *Thromb Res.* 2012;130(3):451-457.

26. Nakada TA, Russell JA, Boyd JH, Walley KR. IL17A genetic variation is associated with altered susceptibility to Gram-positive infection and mortality of severe sepsis. *Crit Care.* 2011;15(5):R254.

27. Nakada TA, Russell JA, Boyd JH, et al. Association of angiotensin II type 1 receptor-associated protein gene polymorphism with increased mortality in septic shock. *Crit Care Med.* 2011;39(7):1641-1648.

28. Sutherland AM, Walley KR, Nakada TA, Sham AH, Wurfel MM, Russell JA. A nonsynonymous polymorphism of IRAK4 associated with increased prevalence of gram-positive infection and decreased response to toll-like receptor ligands. *J Innate Immun.* 2011;3(5):447-458.

29. Thair SA, Walley KR, Nakada TA, et al. A single nucleotide polymorphism in NF-kappaB inducing kinase is associated with mortality in septic shock. *J Immunol.* 2011;186(4): 2321-2328.

30. Wurfel MM, Gordon AC, Holden TD, et al. Toll-like receptor 1 polymorphisms affect innate immune responses and outcomes in sepsis. *Am J Respir Crit Care Med.* 2008; 178(7):710-720.

31. Nakada TA, Wacharasint P, Russell JA, et al. The IL20 genetic polymorphism is associated with altered clinical outcome in septic shock. *J Innate Immun.* 2018;10(3):181-188.

32. Boyd JH, Fjell CD, Russell JA, Sirounis D, Cirstea MS, Walley KR. Increased plasma PCSK9 levels are associated with reduced endotoxin clearance and the development of acute organ failures during sepsis. *J Innate Immun.* 2016;8(2):211-220.

33. Topchiy E, Cirstea M, Kong HJ, et al. Lipopolysaccharide is cleared from the circulation by hepatocytes via the low density lipoprotein receptor. *PLoS One.* 2016;11(5):e0155030.

34. Walley KR, Thain KR, Russell JA, et al. PCSK9 is a critical regulator of the innate immune response and septic shock outcome. *Sci Transl Med.* 2014;6(258):258ra143.

35. Nakada TA, Russell JA, Boyd JH, et al. beta2-Adrenergic receptor gene polymorphism is associated with mortality in septic shock. *Am J Respir Crit Care Med.* 2010;181(2):143-149.

36. Nakada TA, Russell JA, Wellman H, et al. Leucyl/cystinyl aminopeptidase gene variants in septic shock. *Chest.* 2011;139(5):1042-1049.

37. Anantasit N, Boyd JH, Walley KR, Russell JA. Serious adverse events associated with vasopressin and norepinephrine infusion in septic shock. *Crit Care Med.* 2014;42(8):1812-1820.

38. Esposito S, Zampiero A, Pugni L, et al. Genetic polymorphisms and sepsis in premature neonates. *PLoS One.* 2014; 9(7):e101248.

39. Abu-Maziad A, Schaa K, Bell EF, et al. Role of polymorphic variants as genetic modulators of infection in neonatal sepsis. *Pediatr Res.* 2010;68(4):323-329.

40. Lorenz E, Mira JP, Frees KL, Schwartz DA. Relevance of mutations in the TLR4 receptor in patients with gram-negative septic shock. *Arch Intern Med.* 2002;162(9):1028-1032.

41. Zhang AQ, Pan W, Gao JW, et al. Associations between interleukin-1 gene polymorphisms and sepsis risk: a meta-analysis. *BMC Med Genet.* 2014;15:8.

42. Schlüter B, Raufhake C, Erren M, et al. Effect of the interleukin-6 promoter polymorphism (-174 G/C) on the incidence and outcome of sepsis. *Crit Care Med.* 2002; 30(1):32-37.

43. Watanabe E, Buchman TG, Hirasawa H, Zehnbauer BA. Association between lymphotoxin-alpha (tumor necrosis factor-beta) intron polymorphism and predisposition to severe sepsis is modified by gender and age. *Crit Care Med.* 2010;38(1):181-193.

44. Song H, Tang L, Xu M, et al. CD86 polymorphism affects pneumonia-induced sepsis by decreasing gene expression in monocytes. *Inflammation.* 2015;38(2):879-885.

45. Tang GJ, Huang SL, Yien HW, et al. Tumor necrosis factor gene polymorphism and septic shock in surgical infection. *Crit Care Med.* 2000;28(8):2733-2736.

46. Stüber F, Petersen M, Bokelmann F, Schade U. A genomic polymorphism within the tumor necrosis factor locus influences plasma tumor necrosis factor-alpha concentrations and outcome of patients with severe sepsis. *Crit Care Med.* 1996;24(3):381-384.

47. Platonov AE, Shipulin GA, Vershinina IV, Dankert J, van de Winkel JG, Kuijper EJ. Association of human Fc gamma RIIa (CD32) polymorphism with susceptibility to and severity of meningococcal disease. *Clin Infect Dis.* 1998;27(4):746-750.

48. Westendorp RG, Hottenga JJ, Slagboom PE. Variation in plasminogen-activator-inhibitor-1 gene and risk of meningococcal septic shock. *Lancet.* 1999;354(9178):561-563.

49. Marshall RP, Webb S, Bellingan GJ, et al. Angiotensin converting enzyme insertion/deletion polymorphism is associated with susceptibility and outcome in acute respiratory distress syndrome. *Am J Respir Crit Care Med;* 2002;166(5): 646-650.

50. Michalek J, Svetlikova P, Fedora M, et al. Bactericidal permeability increasing protein gene variants in children with sepsis. *Intensive Care Med.* 2007;33(12):2158-2164.

51. Luo J, Xu F, Lu GJ, Lin HC, Feng ZC. Low mannose-binding lectin (MBL) levels and MBL genetic polymorphisms associated with the risk of neonatal sepsis: an updated meta-analysis. *Early Hum Dev.* 2014;90(10):557-564.

52. Man M, Close SL, Shaw AD, et al. Beyond single-marker analyses: mining whole genome scans for insights into treatment responses in severe sepsis. *Pharmacogenomics J.* 2013;13(3):218-226.

53. Debets JM, Kampmeijer R, van der Linden MP, Buurman WA, van der Linden CJ. Plasma tumor necrosis factor and mortality in critically ill septic patients. *Crit Care Med.* 1989;17(6):489-494.

54. Girardin EP, Berner ME, Grau GE, Suter S, Lacourt G, Paunier L. Serum tumour necrosis factor in newborns at risk for infections. *Eur J Pediatr.* 1990;149(9):645-647.

55. Kroeger KM, Carville KS, Abraham LJ. The -308 tumor necrosis factor-alpha promoter polymorphism effects transcription. *Mol Immunol.* 1997;34(5):391-399.

56. Parsons PE, Matthay MA, Ware LB, Eisner MD. Elevated plasma levels of soluble TNF receptors are associated with morbidity and mortality in patients with acute lung injury. *Am J Physiol Lung Cell Mol Physiol.* 2005;288(3):L426-L431.

57. Abraham E, Wunderink R, Silverman H, et al. Efficacy and safety of monoclonal antibody to human tumor necrosis factor alpha in patients with sepsis syndrome. A randomized, controlled, double-blind, multicenter clinical trial. TNF-alpha MAb Sepsis Study Group. *JAMA.* 1995;273(12):934-941.

58. Abraham E, Laterre PF, Garbino J, et al. Lenercept (p55 tumor necrosis factor receptor fusion protein) in severe sepsis and early septic shock: a randomized, double-blind, placebo-controlled, multicenter phase III trial with 1,342 patients. *Crit Care Med.* 2001;29(3):503-510.

59. Ranieri VM, Thompson BT, Barie PS, et al. Drotrecogin alfa (activated) in adults with septic shock. *N Engl J Med.* 2012;366(22):2055-2064.

60. Annane D, Mira JP, Ware LB, et al. Design, conduct, and analysis of a multicenter, pharmacogenomic, biomarker study in matched patients with severe sepsis treated with or without drotrecogin Alfa (activated). *Ann Intensive Care.* 2012;2(1):15.

61. Annane D, Mira JP, Ware LB, et al. Pharmacogenomic biomarkers do not predict response to drotrecogin alfa in patients with severe sepsis. *Ann Intensive Care.* 2018;8(1):16.

62. Bentzer P, Fjell C, Walley KR, Boyd J, Russell JA. Plasma cytokine levels predict response to corticosteroids in septic shock. *Intensive Care Med.* 2016;42(12):1970-1979.

63. Sapru A, Liu KD, Wiemels J, et al. Association of common genetic variation in the protein C pathway genes with clinical outcomes in acute respiratory distress syndrome. *Crit Care.* 2016;20(1):151.

64. Vincent JL, Ramesh MK, Ernest D, et al. A randomized, double-blind, placebo-controlled, Phase 2b study to evaluate the safety and efficacy of recombinant human soluble thrombomodulin, ART-123, in patients with sepsis and suspected disseminated intravascular coagulation. *Crit Care Med.* 2013;41(9):2069-2079.

65. Fan E, Brodie D, Slutsky AS. Acute respiratory distress syndrome: advances in diagnosis and treatment. *JAMA.* 2018;319(7):698-710.

66. Reilly JP, Christie JD, Meyer NJ. Fifty years of research in ARDS. Genomic contributions and opportunities. *Am J Respir Crit Care Med.* 2017;196(9):1113-1121.

67. McAuley DF, Laffey JG, O'Kane CM, et al. Simvastatin in the acute respiratory distress syndrome. *N Engl J Med.* 2014;371(18):1695-1703.

68. Gao Smith F, Perkins GD, Gates S, et al. Effect of intravenous beta-2 agonist treatment on clinical outcomes in acute respiratory distress syndrome (BALTI-2): a multicentre, randomised controlled trial. *Lancet.* 2012;379(9812):229-235.

69. National Heart, Lung, and Blood Institute ARDS Clinical Trials Network; Truwit JD, Bernard GR, et al. Rosuvastatin for sepsis-associated acute respiratory distress syndrome. *N Engl J Med.* 2014;370(23):2191-2200.

70. McAuley DF, Cross LM, Hamid U, et al. Keratinocyte growth factor for the treatment of the acute respiratory distress syndrome (KARE): a randomised, double-blind, placebo-controlled phase 2 trial. *Lancet Respir Med.* 2017;5(6):484-491.

71. Flores C, Pino-Yanes MM, Casula M, Villar J. Genetics of acute lung injury: past, present and future. *Minerva Anestesiol.* 2010;76(10):860-864.

72. Gao L, Barnes KC. Recent advances in genetic predisposition to clinical acute lung injury. *Am J Physiol Lung Cell Mol Physiol.* 2009;296(5):L713-L725.

73. Greene KE, Ye S, Mason RJ, Parsons PE. Serum surfactant protein-A levels predict development of ARDS in at-risk patients. *Chest.* 1999;116(suppl 1):90S-91S.

74. Calfee CS, Delucchi K, Parsons PE, et al. Subphenotypes in acute respiratory distress syndrome: latent class analysis of data from two randomised controlled trials. *Lancet Respir Med.* 2014;2(8):611-620.

75. McClintock D, Zhuo H, Wickersham N, Matthay MA, Ware LB. Biomarkers of inflammation, coagulation and fibrinolysis predict mortality in acute lung injury. *Crit Care.* 2008;12(2):R41.

76. Bhargava M, Wendt CH. Biomarkers in acute lung injury. *Transl Res.* 2012;159(4):205-217.

77. Sweeney RM, McAuley DF. Acute respiratory distress syndrome. *Lancet.* 2016;388(10058):2416-2430.

78. Meyer NJ, Li M, Feng R, et al. ANGPT2 genetic variant is associated with trauma-associated acute lung injury and altered plasma angiopoietin-2 isoform ratio. *Am J Respir Crit Care Med.* 2011;183(10):1344-1353.

79. Bajwa EK, Cremer PC, Gong MN, et al. An NFKB1 promoter insertion/deletion polymorphism influences risk and outcome in acute respiratory distress syndrome among Caucasians. *PLoS One.* 2011;6(5):e19469.

80. Dahmer MK, O'Cain P, Patwari PP, et al. The influence of genetic variation in surfactant protein B on severe lung injury in African American children. *Crit Care Med.* 2011;39(5):1138-1144.

81. Acosta-Herrera M, Pino-Yanes M, Blanco J, et al. Common variants of NFE2L2 gene predisposes to acute respiratory distress syndrome in patients with severe sepsis. *Crit Care.* 2015;19:256.

82. Meyer NJ, Feng R, Li M, et al. IL1RN coding variant is associated with lower risk of acute respiratory distress syndrome and increased plasma IL-1 receptor antagonist. *Am J Respir Crit Care Med.* 2013;187(9):950-959.

83. O'Mahony DS, Glavan BJ, Holden TD, et al. Inflammation and immune-related candidate gene associations with acute lung injury susceptibility and severity: a validation study. *PLoS One.* 2012;7(12):e51104.

84. Bime C, Pouladi N, Sammani S, et al. Genome-wide association study in African Americans with acute respiratory distress syndrome identifies the selectin P ligand gene as a risk factor. *Am J Respir Crit Care Med.* 2018;197(11):1421-1432.

85. Morrell ED, O'Mahony DS, Glavan BJ, et al. Genetic variation in MAP3K1 associates with ventilator-free days in acute respiratory distress syndrome. *Am J Respir Cell Mol Biol.* 2018;58(1):117-125.

86. Kangelaris KN, Prakash A, Liu KD, et al. Increased expression of neutrophil-related genes in patients with early sepsis-induced ARDS. *Am J Physiol Lung Cell Mol Physiol.* 2015;308(11):L1102-L1113.

87. Kovach MA, Stringer KA, Bunting R, et al. Microarray analysis identifies IL-1 receptor type 2 as a novel candidate biomarker in patients with acute respiratory distress syndrome. *Respir Res.* 2015;16:29.

88. Grigoryev DN, Cheranova DI, Chaudhary S, Heruth DP, Zhang LQ, Ye SQ. Identification of new biomarkers for acute respiratory distress syndrome by expression-based genome-wide association study. *BMC Pulm Med.* 2015;15:95.

89. Wei Y, Wang Z, Su L, et al. Platelet count mediates the contribution of a genetic variant in LRRC16A to ARDS risk. *Chest.* 2015;147(3):607-617.

90. Meyer NJ. Beyond single-nucleotide polymorphisms: genetics, genomics, and other 'omic approaches to acute respiratory distress syndrome. *Clin Chest Med.* 2014;35(4):673-684.

91. Meyer NJ, Christie JD. Genetic heterogeneity and risk of acute respiratory distress syndrome. *Semin Respir Crit Care Med.* 2013;34(4):459-474.

92. Wang Z, Beach D, Su L, Zhai R, Christiani DC. A genome-wide expression analysis in blood identifies pre-elafin as a biomarker in ARDS. *Am J Respir Cell Mol Biol.* 2008;38(6):724-732.

93. Rush B, McDermid RC, Celi LA, Walley KR, Russell JA, Boyd JH. Association between chronic exposure to air pollution and mortality in the acute respiratory distress syndrome. *Environ Pollut.* 2017;224:352-356.

94. Ambros V. MicroRNA pathways in flies and worms: growth, death, fat, stress, and timing. *Cell.* 2003;113(6):673-676.

95. Adyshev DM, Moldobaeva N, Mapes B, Elangovan V, Garcia JG. MicroRNA regulation of nonmuscle myosin light chain kinase expression in human lung endothelium. *Am J Respir Cell Mol Biol.* 2013;49(1):58-66.

96. Adyshev DM, Elangovan VR, Moldobaeva N, Mapes B, Sun X, Garcia JG. Mechanical stress induces pre-B-cell colony-enhancing factor/NAMPT expression via epigenetic regulation by miR-374a and miR-568 in human lung endothelium. *Am J Respir Cell Mol Biol.* 2014;50(2):409-418.

97. Tamarapu Parthasarathy P, Galam L, Huynh B, et al. MicroRNA 16 modulates epithelial sodium channel in human alveolar epithelial cells. *Biochem Biophys Res Commun.* 2012;426(2):203-208.

98. Szilágyi KL, Liu C, Zhang X, et al. Epigenetic contribution of the myosin light chain kinase gene to the risk for acute respiratory distress syndrome. *Transl Res.* 2017;180:12-21.

99. Qayyum R, Snively BM, Ziv E, et al. A meta-analysis and genome-wide association study of platelet count and mean platelet volume in African Americans. *PLoS Genet.* 2012;8(3):e1002491.

100. Kan M, Shumyatcher M, Himes BE. Using omics approaches to understand pulmonary diseases. *Respir Res.* 2017;18(1):149.

101. Russell JA, Spronk P, Walley KR. Using multiple 'omics strategies for novel therapies in sepsis. *Intensive Care Med.* 2018;44(4):509-511.

102. Lin Z, Pearson C, Chinchilli V, et al. Polymorphisms of human SP-A, SP-B, and SP-D genes: association of SP-B Thr131Ile with ARDS. *Clin Genet.* 2000;58(3):181-191.

103. Parikh SM, Mammoto T, Schultz A, et al. Excess circulating angiopoietin-2 may contribute to pulmonary vascular leak in sepsis in humans. *PLoS Med.* 2006;3(3):e46.

104. Christie JD, Ma SF, Aplenc R, et al. Variation in the myosin light chain kinase gene is associated with development of acute lung injury after major trauma. *Crit Care Med.* 2008;36(10):2794-2800.

105. Zhai R, Gong MN, Zhou W, et al. Genotypes and haplotypes of the VEGF gene are associated with higher mortality and lower VEGF plasma levels in patients with ARDS. *Thorax.* 2007;62(8):718-722.

106. Adamzik M, Frey UH, Rieman K, et al. Insertion/deletion polymorphism in the promoter of NFKB1 influences severity but not mortality of acute respiratory distress syndrome. *Intensive Care Med.* 2007;33(7):1199-1203.

107. Gong MN, Wei Z, Xu LL, Miller DP, Thompson BT, Christiani DC. Polymorphism in the surfactant protein-B gene, gender, and the risk of direct pulmonary injury and ARDS. *Chest.* 2004;125(1):203-211.

108. Quasney MW, Waterer GW, Dahmer MK, et al. Association between surfactant protein B + 1580 polymorphism and the risk of respiratory failure in adults with community-acquired pneumonia. *Crit Care Med.* 2004;32(5):1115-1119.

109. Abilés J, de la Cruz AP, Castaño J, et al. Oxidative stress is increased in critically ill patients according to antioxidant vitamins intake, independent of severity: a cohort study. *Crit Care.* 2006;10(5):R146.

110. Cho HY, Reddy SP, Kleeberger SR. Nrf2 defends the lung from oxidative stress. *Antioxid Redox Signal.* 2006;8(1-2):76-87.

111. Herold S, Tabar TS, Janssen H, et al. Exudate macrophages attenuate lung injury by the release of IL-1 receptor antagonist in gram-negative pneumonia. *Am J Respir Crit Care Med.* 2011;183(10):1380-1390.

112. Flores C, Ma SF, Maresso K, Wade MS, Villar J, Garcia JG. IL6 gene-wide haplotype is associated with susceptibility to acute lung injury. *Transl Res.* 2008;152(1):11-17.

113. Sutherland AM, Walley KR, Manocha S, Russell JA. The association of interleukin 6 haplotype clades with mortality in critically ill adults. *Arch Intern Med.* 2005;165(1):75-82.

114. Tricker E, Arvand A, Kwan R, Chen GY, Gallagher E, Cheng G. Apoptosis induced by cytoskeletal disruption requires distinct domains of MEKK1. *PLoS One.* 2011;6(2):e17310.

115. Xu K, Rosenstiel P, Paragas N, et al. Unique transcriptional programs identify subtypes of AKI. *J Am Soc Nephrol.* 2017;28(6):1729-1740.

116. Vilander LM, Kaunisto MA, Vaara ST, Pettilä V; FINNAKI study group. Genetic variants in SERPINA4 and SERPINA5, but not BCL2 and SIK3 are associated with acute kidney injury in critically ill patients with septic shock. *Crit Care.* 2017;21(1):47.

117. Bhatraju P, Hsu C, Mukherjee P, et al. Associations between single nucleotide polymorphisms in the FAS pathway and acute kidney injury. *Crit Care.* 2015;19:368.

118. Larach DB, Engoren MC, Schmidt EM, Heung M. Genetic variants and acute kidney injury: a review of the literature. *J Crit Care.* 2018;44:203-211.

119. Tompkins RG. Genomics of injury: the Glue Grant experience. *J Trauma Acute Care Surg.* 2015;78(4):671-686.

120. Cuenca AG, Gentile LF, Lopez MC, et al. Development of a genomic metric that can be rapidly used to predict clinical outcome in severely injured trauma patients. *Crit Care Med.* 2013;41(5):1175-1185.

121. Warren HS, Elson CM, Hayden DL, et al. A genomic score prognostic of outcome in trauma patients. *Mol Med.* 2009;15(7-8):220-227.

122. Xiao W, Mindrinos MN, Seok J, et al. A genomic storm in critically injured humans. *J Exp Med.* 2011;208(13):2581-2590.

123. Thompson CM, Park CH, Maier RV, O'Keefe GE. Traumatic injury, early gene expression, and gram-negative bacteremia. *Crit Care Med.* 2014;42(6):1397-1405.

124. Weaver SM, Portelli JN, Chau A, Cristofori I, Moretti L, Grafman J. Genetic polymorphisms and traumatic brain injury: the contribution of individual differences to recovery. *Brain Imaging Behav.* 2014;8(3):420-434.

125. Waters RJ, Murray GD, Teasdale GM, et al. Cytokine gene polymorphisms and outcome after traumatic brain injury. *J Neurotrauma.* 2013;30(20):1710-1716.

126. Wilson M, Montgomery H. Impact of genetic factors on outcome from brain injury. *Br J Anaesth.* 2007;99(1):43-48.

127. Zhou W, Xu D, Peng X, Zhang Q, Jia J, Crutcher KA. Meta-analysis of APOE4 allele and outcome after traumatic brain injury. *J Neurotrauma.* 2008;25(4):279-290.

128. Zeng S, Jiang JX, Xu MH, et al. Prognostic value of apolipoprotein E epsilon4 allele in patients with traumatic brain injury: a meta-analysis and meta-regression. *Genet Test Mol Biomarkers.* 2014;18(3):202-210.

129. Katsnelson A. Gene tests for brain injury still far from the football field. *Nat Med.* 2011;17(6):638.

130. Liu VX, Fielding-Singh V, Greene JD, et al. The timing of early antibiotics and hospital mortality in sepsis. *Am J Respir Crit Care Med.* 2017;196(7):856-863.

131. Seymour CW, Gesten F, Prescott HC, et al. Time to treatment and mortality during mandated emergency care for sepsis. *N Engl J Med.* 2017;376(23):2235-2244.

132. Sørensen TI, Nielsen GG, Andersen PK, Teasdale TW. Genetic and environmental influences on premature death in adult adoptees. *N Engl J Med.* 1988;318(12):727-732.

133. Walley KR, Francis GA, Opal SM, Stein EA, Russell JA, Boyd JH. The central role of proprotein convertase subtilisin/kexin type 9 in septic pathogen lipid transport and clearance. *Am J Respir Crit Care Med.* 2015;192(11):1275-1286.

6

Is Oxygen Toxic?

Bryan T.G. Reidy, Pauline Whyte, and Patrick J. Neligan

INTRODUCTION

Supplementary oxygen is the most frequently used therapeutic intervention in clinical medicine. Oxygen is administered to treat hypoxia in acute and chronic respiratory failure, often in high inspired concentrations. Varying amounts are given in the perioperative period. Hyperbaric oxygen therapy (HBOT), in which oxygen is administered in a high-pressure chamber, is used to treat decompression illness and carbon monoxide poisoning, enhance wound healing, and kill anaerobic bacteria. Since the late 19th century, the toxic effects of hyperbaric oxygen have been known. Since the 1960s, it has been believed that high concentrations of normobaric oxygen may be toxic, in particular to lung tissue.[1]

This chapter aims to unravel the published data on oxygen toxicity, from both the normobaric and hyperbaric literature.[2] These data are of varying quality, often conflicting in their conclusions and rarely involve critically ill patients. Finally, we conclude with the question: Is oxygen beneficial?

MECHANISMS OF TOXICITY—REACTIVE OXYGEN SPECIES

Oxygen is a highly reactive element, a property that leads to its toxic potential. The oxygen molecule, an electron acceptor, is nontoxic, and normal mitochondrial function reduces most molecular oxygen to water through the sequential donation of four electrons. At mitochondrial level, less than 5% of oxygen molecules convert to the reactive oxygen species (ROS) that contribute extensively to oxidative damage.[3] The term *reactive oxygen species* encompasses both free radicals and chemicals that take part in radical-type reactions (gain or loss of electrons); the latter do not contain unpaired electrons and therefore are not true radicals in themselves. The most common ROS include the superoxide anion (O_2^-), hydrogen peroxide (H_2O_2), hydroxyl radicals (OH^-), singlet oxygen (O^-), the hypochlorous anion ($HOCl^-$), and ozone (O_3).[4] Cellular sources of ROS include the mitochondrial electron transport chain, oxidant enzymes such as xanthine oxidase, phagocytic cells through NADPH oxidase, cyclooxygenase during arachidonic acid metabolism, cellular auto-oxidation of Fe^{2+} and epinephrine, and metabolic enzymes such as the cytochrome P-450 family and the nitric oxide synthetases when inadequate substrate is available.[5]

ROS cause structural injury to lipid membranes, proteins, and nucleic acids. These structural changes lead to disruptions in normal intracellular signaling, protein transcription, and enzyme function. Actively dividing cells are particularly vulnerable to oxidative damage due to exposure of rapidly replicating DNA. Effective protection in this setting may be achieved by cells entering a transient growth-arrested state.[6] Therefore, oxygen can lead to a wide spectrum of damage, from disordered gene expression to disrupted growth and even necrosis.

Oxidative stress occurring as a result of ROS production is thought to be an ongoing process at physiologic levels of oxygen. When the balance between ROS and scavenging systems is altered, free radicals may contribute to the normal aging process, development of cancers, heart failure, and diabetic vascular and cerebrovascular disease.

The effects of oxidative stress are potentially increased during normobaric administration of oxygen at high concentrations and are accentuated further under hyperbaric conditions. Endogenous scavenging systems include superoxide dismutases, a group of metalloproteins, catalase, and components of the glutathione redox cycle including glutathione peroxidase and glutathione reductase. Nonenzyme antioxidants, including vitamins C and E, beta-carotene and uric acid, also reduce ROS to less harmful molecules. However, in the presence of hyperoxia, these may become overwhelmed, giving rise to injury.[4]

In summary, high levels of oxygen at the cellular level result in the formation of ROS. ROS cause lipid peroxidation, oxidative injury to nucleic acid chains, and oxidative protein damage.

THE EVIDENCE FOR TOXICITY—FROM BENCH TO BEDSIDE

Hyperoxia is toxic in a variety of animal models, but data demonstrating similar effects in humans are scant. Thus, while lung injury from elevated levels of administered oxygen is frequently invoked in critical care, actual damage is difficult to substantiate. The bulk of the literature describing pulmonary oxygen toxicity was written in the 1950s to 1970s.[2] However, inspired fractions of oxygen (FiO_2) between 50% and 60% are well tolerated for prolonged periods.[2] At higher levels the potential for toxicity exists. The development of toxicity depends not only on the partial pressure of oxygen but also on the duration of exposure and there is likely to be significant inter-individual variation.[7] In addition, animals who survive exposure to high concentrations may acclimate and adapt.[2]

Pathologic examination of animal lungs exposed to high concentrations of oxygen identifies distinctive features at both macroscopic and microscopic levels. Gross examination reveals lungs and respiratory mucosa that are inflamed, atelectatic, with areas of consolidation and fluid in the pleural space. Microscopic changes include pulmonary edema with diffuse alveolar membrane damage.[7] The clinical progression of diffuse alveolar damage (DAD) mirrors that of the acute respiratory distress syndrome (ARDS). An initial exudative phase, characterized by increasing dyspnea, bilateral crackles, frothy and bloody sputum, and widespread infiltrates on chest radiograph, may evolve into a fibrotic phase. While some studies have attempted to define the impact of oxygen toxicity on acute lung injury in a critical care setting, the large number of confounding variables and conditions—ventilator-associated pneumonia, ventilator-related barotrauma, and volutrauma (ventilator-induced lung injury [VILI]), and the underlying disease processes—makes interpretation of the findings difficult.

Many of the oft-cited studies were carried out in otherwise healthy volunteers, which limits generalizability to patients with comorbidities.[8–10] Available evidence reinforces results from animal studies that demonstrate early dyspnea, cough, and chest pain. Absorption atelectasis leads to reduced lung volumes with spirometric evidence of falling vital capacity.[11] Application of findings from an oft-quoted 1967 study is limited because strategies for mechanical ventilation so profoundly differ from those currently used.[12] Thus, damage from oxygen cannot be separated from that of VILI.

OXYGEN TOXICITY IN PRACTICE—FROM THE CRADLE TO THE GRAVE

Neonates

Newborn infants, particularly those born prematurely, are at particular risk for oxygen toxicity. Therefore, systematic reviews and meta-analyses have led to reduction in the use of high FiO_2 for both neonatal resuscitation and respiratory dysfunction.[13] Traditionally, both adult and neonatal resuscitation were performed with 100% oxygen. High-quality data now demonstrate that substitution of air (FiO_2 0.21) is associated with a survival benefit of up to 30%.[14] Lower oxygen concentrations during resuscitation are also associated with a decrease in the overall duration of oxygen support, development of chronic lung disease, and markers of oxidative injury.[15]

Data from the BOOST and SUPPORT studies revealed the association between higher oxygenation targets and the retinopathy of prematurity. However, both data from studies also suggested that lower O_2 targets (ratio of oxygen saturation by pulse oximetry [SpO_2] 85–89%) were associated with higher mortality (relative risk [RR] 1.45, 95% confidence interval [CI] 1.15–1.84). Importantly, the higher saturation targets of 91–95% would be considered conservative in an adult population.[16,17]

Adults

While there is compelling evidence for pulmonary oxygen toxicity or hyperoxic lung injury in both animals and neonates, the evidence in adults is less clear. Problems start with the use of nomenclature that is confused. While the term 'hyperoxia' is used ubiquitously, there is a difference between hyperoxia (a high inspired concentration of oxygen) and hyperoxemia (a high partial pressure of oxygen in blood), usually denoted by a PaO_2 between 120 and 200 mm Hg, with a PaO_2 >200 mm Hg characterizing severe hyperoxemia. Interestingly, one study identified a linear relationship between time spent in hyperoxemia and mortality.[18]

The majority of human studies were performed in healthy volunteers, and involved small sample sizes. Thus, relevance to clinical practice, particularly in the critically ill, is uncertain. Identified clinical features include early retrosternal discomfort, pleuritic chest pain, cough, and dyspnea.[19] Inflammatory change became visible on bronchoscopic examination after 6 hours of breathing oxygen at >90%.[20] Resolution of symptoms usually occurred over a number of days. In a small retrospective study, Elliot and colleagues attempted to define predictors for lung function in survivors of ARDS and found that duration of administration FiO_2 >0.6 was the only variable related to reduced diffusion capacity at 1 year.[21] A larger retrospective study that corrected for severity of illness uncovered an independent association between mean FiO_2 during intensive care unit (ICU) stay and in-hospital mortality.[22] The effects of hyperoxia on respiratory measurements are unclear[23,24] and the pathologic substrate remain unknown.

The contribution of oxygen toxicity to morbidity and mortality in the critically ill is difficult to identify, at least in part because of the confounding effects of mechanical ventilation. Much of the early literature was reported before the advent of lung protective ventilation and, as such, further trials are required to elicit the contribution of oxygen to VILI. A single-center study by Giradis et al.[25] demonstrated an association between conservative (SpO_2 94–98% vs. 97–100%) oxygen management and demonstrated an absolute risk reduction of 8.6% (95% CI 1.7–15%, $P = .01$) in ICU mortality. A trial of hyperoxia in patients with septic shock was stopped early due to an excess of adverse events in the hyperoxia group.[26] In a large systematic review and meta-analysis of 16,037 acutely unwell patients, oxygen strategies where the mean FiO_2 was 0.52 (range 0.28–1.0) were associated with increased 30-day and last follow-up hospital mortality. Indeed, for every 1% increase in SpO_2 the relative risk of in-hospital mortality increased by 25%.[27] A Dutch study revealed hyperoxemia ($PaO_2 > 100$ mm Hg (13 kPa)) in >40% of 126,778 arterial blood gases (ABG) obtained from mechanically ventilated ICU patients.[28] Finally, hyperoxemia (PaO_2 101–300 mm Hg) during extracorporeal membrane oxygenation (ECMO) in patients with cardiac and respiratory failure was associated with increased mortality.[29,30]

In summary, hyperoxic lung injury in healthy volunteers is associated with a syndrome analogous to ARDS, starting with an inflammatory phase and followed by a fibroproliferative phase. In critically ill patients, hyperoxia and hyperoxemia appear to be harmful and FiO_2 should be tailored to the individual patient's needs, with the lowest safe level that is compatible with life.

HYPEROXIA AND CARBON DIOXIDE

For many years it has been accepted that hyperoxia leads to a reduction in ventilatory drive in patients with hypercapneic respiratory failure. Aubier et al.[31] described a transient, self-limiting reduction in minute ventilation in subjects exposed to hyperoxia that did not correlate with the subsequent degree of hypercapnea. The development of hypercapnea is more likely explained by increases in V/Q mismatch and dead space secondary to the reversal of hypoxic pulmonary vasoconstriction (HPV) and the Haldane effect (the reduced ability of oxyhemoglobin to bind carbon dioxide).

HYPEROXIA IN CARDIAC ARREST, TRAUMATIC BRAIN INJURY, AND STROKE

Hyperoxia impairs endothelial-mediated vasodilatation in the peripheral, coronary, and cerebral vasculature, an effect that is mediated through inhibition of nitric oxide synthesis.[32] These findings bely the routine practice of administering oxygen to patients with acute coronary and intracerebral events. Recent studies on patients with acute myocardial infarction indicated that oxygen administration increased infarct size and recurrent myocardial ischemia.[33,34]

Registry data from the United States demonstrated that postcardiac arrest exposure to $PaO_2 > 300$ mm Hg was associated with mortality in excess of that observed in either normoxia or hypoxia. In a secondary analysis, this mortality difference was even more pronounced in patients with $PaO_2 > 400$ mm Hg. Functional status was also significantly worse in the group exposed to hyperoxia.[35]

The impact of hyperoxia on outcome in traumatic brain injury (TBI) is unclear and, because hypoxia is unequivocally detrimental, high FiO_2 is frequently administered to increase brain oxygen tension. Most studies involve retrospective analyses of datasets and results are inconsistent. A retrospective

analysis of 1547 consecutive patients with severe TBI who survived past 12 hours found that patients with PaO_2 levels >200 mm Hg had significantly higher mortality and lower discharge Glasgow Coma Scale (GCS) scores than patients with PaO_2 between 100 and 200 mm Hg. This difference persisted even after controlling for age, sex, injury severity score, mechanism of injury, and admission GCS. Patients with high PaO_2 levels (>200 mm Hg) had significantly higher mortality and lower discharge GCS scores than patients with a normal PaO_2 (100–200 mm Hg) ($P < .05$).[36] Conversely, an analysis of 24,148 patients with TBI in 129 ICUs was unable to identify an association between hyperoxia ($PaO_2 > 300$ mm Hg during the first 24 hours) and mortality in adjusted analysis.[37] These contrasting studies illustrate why the use of hyperoxia following traumatic brain injury is difficult to justify.

Hyperoxemia may be harmful in stroke. Rincon and colleagues[38] looked at 554 patients over 5 years who were mechanically ventilated with acute ischemic stroke (19%), subarachnoid hemorrhage (32%), and intracerebral hemorrhage (49%). Patients were divided into three exposure groups: hyperoxia ($PaO_2 \geq 300$ mm Hg [40 kPa]), normoxia, and hypoxia ($PaO_2 < 60$ mm Hg). Hyperoxia was associated with higher in-hospital mortality. These data may reflect the increase in risk of hyperoxia associated with mechanical ventilation, rather than brain injury, as reported by Page and colleagues[39] in a study of mechanically ventilated emergency room patients.

THERAPEUTIC HYPEROXIA

Surgical Site Infection

Perioperative use of therapeutic hyperoxia has been touted as an approach to reducing the risk of surgical site infections (SSIs). There are theoretical underpinnings to support this contention: oxidative killing by neutrophils, an important defense against surgical pathogens, is dependent on free radicals, which are generated from the oxygen not used for oxidative phosphorylation.

An initial noninterventional, prospective study of subcutaneous wound oxygen tension ($PsqO_2$) in 230 patients revealed an inverse relationship between wound oxygen tension and the risk for developing SSIs.[40] The authors suggested that manipulating FiO_2 may increase PsqO and reduce SSIs. Several subsequent studies supported this hypothesis.[41,42] An unblinded study randomized 500 patients undergoing colorectal resection to 80% or 30% inspired oxygen during the surgery and for 2 hours postoperatively. Higher FiO_2 was associated with a 55% relative and 6% absolute reduction in SSIs (5.2% vs. 11.2%). These data were replicated in a smaller study from Spain.[42] A study of 2050 patients randomized FiO_2 values of either 80% or 30%, plus 70% nitrous oxide; the higher FiO_2 was associated with significantly lower rates of major complications and severe nausea and vomiting.[43] However, the study was designed to assess this impact of nitrous oxide, not oxygen. The study was subsequently included in meta-analyses despite the authors protesting that SSI detection was not a purpose of the study.[44]

In contrast to previously described studies, an investigation randomizing 165 patients undergoing general surgery to 80% oxygen in the operating room and for 2 hours postoperatively found that the higher FiO$_2$ was associated with an increased risk of surgical site complications (25.0% vs. 11.3%; $P = .02$).[45] However, a number of concerns were raised, the most important of these being that wound infection was identified by retrospective chart review. In addition, patients receiving 80% oxygen were more likely to be obese, had longer operations, and lost more blood. Along these lines, a trial of 400 bariatric surgery patients, randomized to 80% vs. 30% oxygen intraoperatively and until the first postoperative morning also was unable to a benefit from hyperoxia.[46] The PROXI trial, which randomized 1400 patients undergoing laparotomy to an FiO$_2$ of either 80% or 30% oxygen, failed to show any differences in SSI, mortality, length of stay, or pulmonary complications.[47] A similar inability to identify benefits from hyperoxia was noted following colorectal surgery patients.[48] A 2018 meta-analysis of available studies concluded that higher FiO$_2$ was associated with a reduced risk of SSI—but only in high-quality studies.[49] Concerns with all the studies and the meta-analysis include the wide interstudy range in the incidence of SSI and significant heterogeneity of other data. Indeed, SSI rates—timing of antibiotics, body temperature, blood glucose, body mass index, fluid resuscitation, and skin preparation—affect many different factors, most of which are standardized across studies. In addition, examination of a database of almost 80,000 patients found a dose-dependent relationship between intraoperative FiO$_2$ and a composite of respiratory complications (reintubation, respiratory failure, pulmonary edema, and pneumonia) within 7 days after surgery.[50] Despite these concerns, the World Health Organization[51] has recommended the use of high FiO$_2$ during general anesthesia and tracheal intubation, but we and others believe this to be misguided.[44]

A major additional issue, however, has been uncovered in patients who had long-term follow-up. It appears that hyperoxia is associated with an untoward effect on cancer recurrence. A 4-year follow-up of the PROXI trial found that the cancer-free survival interval was significantly shorter in the 80% oxygen group.[52]

These findings and the associated concerns, especially those regarding long-term complications, lead us to conclude that the use of intraoperative hyperoxia to prevent SSIs cannot be recommended at this time.

MANAGEMENT AND PREVENTION OF OXYGEN TOXICITY

Concerns that oxygen therapy may be associated with toxicity has prompted updated guidance from both the British and the Australian/New Zealand Thoracic Societies. Recommended target oxygen saturations are within a range of 92–96% (Au/NZ) and 94–98% (British) for those not at risk of hypercapneic respiratory failure. Both advocate a saturation target of 88–92% for those with chronic hypercapnea.[53,54]

A target PaO$_2$ of 55–80 mm Hg (7.4–10.7 kPa) has been recommended by the ARDSnet group.[55]

Hyperoxic lung injury may play a role in the development of VILI. The use of several forms nonoxygen therapies to achieve improved oxygenation (positive end-expiratory pressure [PEEP] titration,[56] lung protective ventilation[55]) in critically ill patients. Other approaches (conservative fluid therapy,[57] prone positioning,[58] ECMO[59]) may be appropriate under specific conditions but should not be universally applied. Importantly, it may be impossible to avoid use of elevated FiO$_2$ levels in critically ill patients; the need to achieve adequate oxygen delivery often outweighs concerns regarding oxygen toxicity. Decisions are best made on a case-by-case basis.

In summary, while a growing body of evidence suggests that there is an association between administration of supplemental oxygen and organ toxicity in the critically ill, consensus on the maximum safe concentration and duration of oxygen therapy is lacking. It seems reasonable to limit FiO$_2$ to <60% and PaO$_2$ to <100 mm Hg (13.3 kPa), but these targets are not evidence based.

HYPERBARIC OXYGEN THERAPY AND OXYGEN TOXICITY

Patients have been treated with HBOT for almost two centuries, principally to aid wound healing. More recently, HBOT has been used to treat carbon monoxide poisoning, gas embolism, anaerobic infections, and diabetic vascular insufficiency/foot ulcers (Box 6.1). However, HBOT requires careful organization and risk assessment and is associated with various complications (Table 6.1). Most have been identified in recreational divers. In 2017, the European Committee for Hyperbaric Medicine published consensus guidelines on indications for hyperbaric oxygen treatment, including a review of the evidence supporting each treatment indication.[60] While high-level evidence for any indication is lacking, there is moderate evidence and strong agreement between the authors for eight indications. An additional five indications

BOX 6.1 Indications for Hyperbaric Oxygen Therapy

Carbon monoxide poisoning
Open fractures with crush injury
Prevention of osteoradionecrosis after dental extraction
Osteoradionecrosis (mandible)
Soft tissue radionecrosis (cystitis proctitis)
Decompression illness
Gas embolism
Anaerobic or mixed bacterial infections
Sudden deafness
Diabetic foot lesions
Femoral head necrosis
Compromised skin grafts and musculocutaneous flaps
Central retinal artery occlusion

TABLE 6.1 Oxygen Toxicity Associated With Hyperbaric Oxygen Use.

Symptoms	No. of cases	Percentage
Convulsions	46	9.2
Twitching lips	303	60.6
Vertigo	44	8.8
Nausea	43	8.6
Respiratory disturbance	19	3.8
Dyspnea	8	
Cough	6	
Other	5	
Twitching, other than lips	16	3.2
Sensation of abnormality	16	3.2
Visual disturbance[61–64]	5	1
Acoustic hallucinations	3	0.6
Paresthesia	2	0.4

Modified from Fock A, Millar I. Oxygen toxicity in recreational and technical diving. *Diving Hyperb Med.* 2008:38(2):86-90.

had strong agreement between the authors, but lower levels of evidence.

AUTHORS' RECOMMENDATIONS

- Hyperoxia leads to development of reactive oxygen species. These ROS can cause oxidative damage to lipids, nucleic acids, and proteins that has been linked to cellular injury and inflammation.
- Hyperoxia-induced lung injury probably contributes to the morbidity and mortality of ventilator-induced lung injury.
- There is good-quality evidence linking hyperoxia and mortality. However, what level of FiO_2 or PaO_2 constitutes "hyperoxia" is unknown.
- While not supported by evidence, recent recommendations support avoidance, whenever possible, of FiO_2 >0.6. There is insufficient evidence to support withholding higher FiO_2 levels if required to maintain "safe" arterial oxygen tension levels.
- While not supported by direct evidence, it is reasonable to limit exposure to hyperoxia, and more importantly hyperoxemia, by choosing conservative oxygen targets of 92–96% in most patients, and 88–92% in those at risk for respiratory failure.
- Data supporting the use of hyperoxia to prevent surgical site infections is equivocal, and is countered by studies suggesting the potential for long-term harm.
- While no consensus definition for hyperoxemia exists, most studies have used a threshold of PaO_2 >100 mm Hg/13.3 kPa. It seems reasonable to aim to reduce FiO_2 in response to a PaO_2 >100 mm Hg.

REFERENCES

1. van der Walt J. Oxygen: elixir of life or Trojan horse? Part 1: oxygen and neonatal resuscitation. *Paediatr Anaesth.* 2006;16(11):1107-1111.
2. Kallet RH, Matthay MA. Hyperoxic acute lung injury. *Respir Care.* 2013;58(1):123-141.
3. Turrens JF. Mitochondrial formation of reactive oxygen species. *J Physiol.* 2003;552(Pt 2):335-344.
4. Jackson RM. Pulmonary oxygen toxicity. *Chest.* 1985;88(6):900-905.
5. Magder S. Reactive oxygen species: toxic molecules or spark of life? *Crit Care.* 2006;10(1):208.
6. Davies KJ. Oxidative stress, antioxidant defenses, and damage removal, repair, and replacement systems. *IUBMB Life.* 2000;50(4-5):279-289.
7. Weir FW, Bath DW, Yevich P, Oberst FW. Study of effects of continuous inhalation of high concentrations of oxygen at ambient pressure and temperature. *J Occup Med.* 1965;7(9):486.
8. Clark JM, Lambertsen CJ. Rate of development of pulmonary O_2 toxicity in man during O_2 breathing at 2.0 Ata. *J Appl Physiol.* 1971;30(5):739-752.
9. Clark JM, Jackson RM, Lambertsen CJ, Gelfand R, Hiller WD, Unger M. Pulmonary function in men after oxygen breathing at 3.0 ATA for 3.5 h. *J Appl Physiol (1985).* 1991;71(3):878-885.
10. Clark JM, Lambertsen CJ, Gelfand R, et al. Effects of prolonged oxygen exposure at 1.5, 2.0, or 2.5 ATA on pulmonary function in men (predictive studies V). *J Appl Physiol (1985).* 1999;86(1):243-259.
11. Magnusson L, Spahn DR. New concepts of atelectasis during general anaesthesia. *Br J Anaesth.* 2003;91(1):61-72.
12. Nash G, Blennerhassett JB, Pontoppidan H. Pulmonary lesions associated with oxygen therapy and artificial ventilation. *N Engl J Med.* 1967;276(7):368-374.
13. Manley BJ, Owen LS, Hooper SB, et al. Towards evidence-based resuscitation of the newborn infant. *Lancet.* 2017;389(10079):1639-1648.
14. Saugstad OD, Vento M, Ramji S, Howard D, Soll RF. Neurodevelopmental outcome of infants resuscitated with air or 100% oxygen: a systematic review and meta-analysis. *Neonatology.* 2012;102(2):98-103.
15. Vento M, Moro M, Escrig R, et al. Preterm resuscitation with low oxygen causes less oxidative stress, inflammation, and chronic lung disease. *Pediatrics.* 2009;124(3):e439-e449.
16. SUPPORT Study Group of the Eunice Kennedy Shriver NICHD Neonatal Research Network; Carlo WA, Finer NN, et al. Target ranges of oxygen saturation in extremely preterm infants. *N Engl J Med.* 2010;362(21):1959-1969.
17. BOOST II United Kingdom Collaborative Group; BOOST II Australia Collaborative Group; BOOST II New Zealand Collaborative Group, et al. Oxygen saturation and outcomes in preterm infants. *N Engl J Med.* 2013;368(22):2094-2104.
18. Helmerhorst HJ, Arts DL, Schultz MJ, et al. Metrics of arterial hyperoxia and associated outcomes in critical care. *Crit Care Med.* 2017;45(2):187-195.
19. Montgomery AB, Luce JM, Murray JF. Retrosternal pain is an early indicator of oxygen toxicity. *Am Rev Respir Dis.* 1989;139(6):1548-1550.
20. Sackner MA, Landa J, Hirsch J, Zapata A. Pulmonary effects of oxygen breathing. A 6-hour study in normal men. *Ann Intern Med.* 1975;82(1):40-43.
21. Elliott CG, Rasmusson BY, Crapo RO, Morris AH, Jensen RL. Prediction of pulmonary function abnormalities after adult respiratory distress syndrome (ARDS). *Am Rev Respir Dis.* 1987;135(3):634–638.

22. de Jonge E, Peelen L, Keijzers PJ, et al. Association between administered oxygen, arterial partial oxygen pressure and mortality in mechanically ventilated intensive care unit patients. *Crit Care.* 2008;12(6):R156.

23. Singer MM, Wright F, Stanley LK, Roe BB, Hamilton WK. Oxygen toxicity in man: a prospective study in patients after open-heart surgery. *N Engl J Med.* 1970;283(27):1473-1478.

24. Barber RE, Hamilton WK. Oxygen toxicity in man. A prospective study in patients with irreversible brain damage. *N Engl J Med.* 1970;283(27):1478-1484.

25. Girardis M, Busani S, Damiani E, et al. Effect of conservative vs conventional oxygen therapy on mortality among patients in an intensive care unit: the oxygen-ICU randomized clinical trial. *JAMA.* 2016;316(15):1583-1589.

26. Asfar P, Schortgen F, Boisramé-Helms J, et al. Hyperoxia and hypertonic saline in patients with septic shock (HYPERS2S): a two-by-two factorial, multicenter, randomised, clinical trial. *Lancet Respir Med.* 2017;5(3):180-190.

27. Chu DK, Kim LH, Young PJ, et al. Mortality and morbidity in acutely ill adults treated with liberal versus conservative oxygen therapy (IOTA): a systematic review and meta-analysis. *Lancet.* 2018;391(10131):1693-1705.

28. de Graaff AE, Dongelmans DA, Binnekade JM, de Jonge E. Clinicians' response to hyperoxia in ventilated patients in a Dutch ICU depends on the level of FiO_2. *Intensive Care Med.* 2011;37(1):46-51.

29. Thiagarajan RR, Barbaro RP, Rycus PT, et al. Extracorporeal Life Support Organization Registry International Report 2016. *ASAIO J.* 2017;63(1):60-67.

30. Munshi L, Kiss A, Cypel M, Keshavjee S, Ferguson ND, Fan E. Oxygen thresholds and mortality during extracorporeal life support in adult patients. *Crit Care Med.* 2017;45(12):1997-2005.

31. Aubier M, Murciano D, Milic-Emili J, et al. Effects of the administration of O_2 on ventilation and blood gases in patients with chronic obstructive pulmonary disease during acute respiratory failure. *Am Rev Respir Dis.* 1980;122(5):747-754.

32. Cornet AD, Kooter AJ, Peters MJ, Smulders YM. The potential harm of oxygen therapy in medical emergencies. *Crit Care.* 2013;17(2):313.

33. Stub D, Smith K, Bernard S, et al. Air versus oxygen in ST-segment elevation myocardial infarction. *Circulation.* 2015;131(24):2143-2150.

34. Hofmann R, James SK, Jernberg T, et al. Oxygen therapy in suspected acute myocardial infarction. *N Engl J Med.* 2017;377(13):1240-1249.

35. Roberts BW, Kilgannon JH, Hunter BR, et al. Association between early hyperoxia exposure after resuscitation from cardiac arrest and neurological disability: a prospective multicenter protocol-directed cohort study. *Circulation.* 2018;137(20):2114-2124.

36. Brenner M, Stein D, Hu P, Kufera J, Wooford M, Scalea T. Association between early hyperoxia and worse outcomes after traumatic brain injury. *Arch Surg.* 2012;147(11):1042-1046.

37. Ó Briain D, Nickson C, Pilcher DV, Udy AA. Early hyperoxia in patients with traumatic brain injury admitted to intensive care in Australia and New Zealand: a retrospective multicenter cohort study. *Neurocrit Care.* 2018;29(3):443-451.

38. Rincon F, Kang J, Maltenfort M, et al. Association between hyperoxia and mortality after stroke: a multicenter cohort study. *Crit Care Med.* 2014;42(2):387-396.

39. Page D, Ablordeppey E, Wessman BT, et al. Emergency department hyperoxia is associated with increased mortality in mechanically ventilated patients: a cohort study. *Crit Care.* 2018;22(1):9.

40. Hopf HW, Hunt TK, West JM, et al. Wound tissue oxygen tension predicts the risk of wound infection in surgical patients. *Arch Surg.* 1997;132(9):997-1004; discussion 1005.

41. Greif R, Akça O, Horn EP, Kurz A, Sessler DI; Outcomes Research Group. Supplemental perioperative oxygen to reduce the incidence of surgical-wound infection. *N Engl J Med.* 2000;342(3):161-167.

42. Belda FJ, Aguilera L, García de la Asunción J, et al. Supplemental perioperative oxygen and the risk of surgical wound infection: a randomized controlled trial. *JAMA.* 2005;294(16):2035-2042.

43. Leslie K, Myles PS, Chan MT, et al. Nitrous oxide and long-term morbidity and mortality in the ENIGMA trial. *Anesth Analg.* 2011;112(2):387-393.

44. Myles PS, Kurz A. Supplemental oxygen and surgical site infection: getting to the truth. *Br J Anaesth.* 2017;119(1):13-15.

45. Pryor KO, Fahey TJ 3rd, Lien CA, Goldstein PA. Surgical site infection and the routine use of perioperative hyperoxia in a general surgical population: a randomized controlled trial. *JAMA.* 2004;291(1):79-87.

46. Wadhwa A, Kabon B, Fleischmann E, Kurz A, Sessler DI. Supplemental postoperative oxygen does not reduce surgical site infection and major healing-related complications from bariatric surgery in morbidly obese patients: a randomized, blinded trial. *Anesth Analg.* 2014;119(2):357-365.

47. Meyhoff CS, Wetterslev J, Jorgensen LN, et al. Effect of high perioperative oxygen fraction on surgical site infection and pulmonary complications after abdominal surgery: the PROXI randomized clinical trial. *JAMA.* 2009;302(14):1543-1550.

48. Kurz A, Fleischmann E, Sessler DI, et al. Effects of supplemental oxygen and dexamethasone on surgical site infection: a factorial randomized trial. *Br J Anaesth.* 2015;115(3):434-443.

49. Cohen B, Schacham YN, Ruetzler K, et al. Effect of intraoperative hyperoxia on the incidence of surgical site infections: a meta-analysis. *Br J Anaesth.* 2018;120(6):1176-1186.

50. Staehr-Rye AK, Meyhoff CS, Scheffenbichler FT, et al. High intraoperative inspiratory oxygen fraction and risk of major respiratory complications. *Br J Anaesth.* 2017;119(1):140-149.

51. Allegranzi B, Zayed B, Bischoff P, et al. New WHO recommendations on intraoperative and postoperative measures for surgical site infection prevention: an evidence-based global perspective. *Lancet Infect Dis.* 2016;16(12):e288-e303.

52. Meyhoff CS, Jorgensen LN, Wetterslev J, Siersma VD, Rasmussen LS; PROXI Trial Group. Risk of new or recurrent cancer after a high perioperative inspiratory oxygen fraction during abdominal surgery. *Br J Anaesth.* 2014;113(suppl 1):i74-i81.

53. Beasley R, Chien J, Douglas J, et al. Thoracic Society of Australia and New Zealand oxygen guidelines for acute oxygen use in adults: 'Swimming between the flags'. *Respirology.* 2015;20(8):1182-1191.

54. O'Driscoll B, Howard L, Earis J, Mak V; British Thoracic Society Emergency Oxygen Guideline Group; BTS Emergency Oxygen Guideline Development Group. BTS guideline for oxygen use in adults in healthcare and emergency settings. *Thorax.* 2017;72(suppl 1):ii1-ii90.

55. Acute Respiratory Distress Syndrome Network; Brower RG, Matthay MA, et al. Ventilation with lower tidal volumes as compared with traditional tidal volumes for acute lung injury

and the acute respiratory distress syndrome. *N Engl J Med.* 2000;342(18):1301-1308.

56. Brower RG, Lanken PN, MacIntyre N, et al. Higher versus lower positive end-expiratory pressures in patients with the acute respiratory distress syndrome. *N Engl J Med.* 2004;351(4):327-336.

57. National Heart, Lung, and Blood Institute Acute Respiratory Distress Syndrome (ARDS) Clinical Trials Network; Wiedemann HP, Wheeler AP, et al. Comparison of two fluid-management strategies in acute lung injury. *N Engl J Med.* 2006;354(24):2564-2575.

58. Guerin C, Reignier J, Richard JC, et al. Prone positioning in severe acute respiratory distress syndrome. *N Engl J Med.* 2013;368(23):2159-2168.

59. Abrams D, Brodie D. Extracorporeal membrane oxygenation for adult respiratory failure: 2017 update. *Chest.* 2017;152(3):639-649.

60. Mathieu D, Marroni A, Kot J. Tenth European Consensus Conference on Hyperbaric Medicine: recommendations for accepted and non-accepted clinical indications and practice of hyperbaric oxygen treatment. *Diving Hyperb Med.* 2017;47(1):24-32.

61. Palmquist BM, Philipson B, Barr PO. Nuclear cataract and myopia during hyperbaric oxygen therapy. *Br J Ophthalmol.* 1984;68(2):113-117.

62. Fledelius HC, Jansen EC, Thorn J. Refractive change during hyperbaric oxygen therapy. A clinical trial including ultrasound oculometry. *Acta Ophthalmol Scand.* 2002;80(2): 188-190.

63. Onoo A, Kiyosawa M, Takase H, Mano Y. Development of myopia as a hazard for workers in pneumatic caissons. *Br J Ophthalmol.* 2002;86(11):1274-1277.

64. Gesell LB, Trott A. De novo cataract development following a standard course of hyperbaric oxygen therapy. *Undersea Hyperb Med.* 2007;34(6):389-392.

7

What Is the Role of Noninvasive Respiratory Support and High-Flow Nasal Cannula in the Intensive Care Client?

Joshua Iokepa Santos and Jason C. Brainard

INTRODUCTION

Noninvasive respiratory support (NIRS) involves the application of positive pressure to the airway through an interface that does not require instrumentation of the larynx—such as a face mask, nasal mask, helmet, or high-flow nasal device. Noninvasive (positive pressure) ventilation (NIV) is a long established therapy for respiratory failure due to chronic obstructive pulmonary disease (COPD) (Box 7.1). Continuous positive airway pressure (CPAP), which does not include additional flow in inspiration, is used to treat obstructive sleep apnea, postoperative hypoxemia, and acute cardiogenic pulmonary edema.[1,2] High-flow nasal cannulas (HFNCs), which apply high-flow oxygen to the nasal cavity and oropharynx, improving oxygenation—partially due to low levels of CPAP, and ventilation, due to washout of dead space—are now widely used to treat moderate levels of hypoxemia and hypercarbia.

DELIVERY OF MECHANICAL NONINVASIVE RESPIRATORY SUPPORT

There are two main approaches to mechanical NIRS: CPAP and NIV. The latter usually involves some form of pressure-limited support in inspiration, such as pressure support ventilation, but may involve assist-control, synchronized intermittent mandatory ventilation or any other mode, volume or pressure targeted, that can be delivered noninvasively. "BiPAP", a proprietary term, is often used incorrectly and interchangeably with NIV, but in fact refers to a single mode on a Respironics/Philips noninvasive ventilator.

CPAP is continuous airway pressure delivered to the patient during both inhalation and exhalation, usually through a tight-fitting face mask or helmet. It functions principally to stent the upper airways and alveoli open, prevent cyclic derecruitment, and improve oxygenation. There is no additional flow in inspiration, but baseline flow is high and this may reduce the work of breathing. CPAP is used chronically to treat obstructive sleep apnea and acutely to treat postoperative hypoxemia (reversing atelectasis) and in the management of acute left ventricular failure.

NIV is used in a medley of clinical situations, most frequently in acute exacerbations of COPD. The most commonly used mode of NIV is analogous to pressure support ventilation. For example, in bilevel positive airway pressure (BiPAP), the ventilator cycles from expiratory positive airway pressure (EPAP) to inspiratory positive airway pressure (IPAP), which is pressure targeted and flow cycled. IPAP may be delivered without EPAP, particularly in patients with significant bullous lung disease. All modern noninvasive ventilators can deliver mandatory and assisted breaths, analogous to volume or pressure assist-control ventilation. This is widely used for patients with late-stage neuromuscular diseases such as motor neuron disease (amyotrophic lateral sclerosis), myotonic dystrophy, and multiple sclerosis—situations where the patient may be unable to trigger the ventilator.

SELECTING PATIENTS FOR NONINVASIVE RESPIRATORY SUPPORT

The first question that should be addressed when selecting patients for NIRS is whether the patient needs ventilatory support. Such patients usually have moderate-to-severe respiratory distress, signs of increased work of breathing, such as tachypnea, increased use of accessory muscles, or abdominal paradox. Arterial blood gases (ABG) should be obtained before starting NIV to assess the severity of the gas exchange derangement, particularly partial pressure of arterial carbon dioxide ($PaCO_2$), and to establish a baseline for comparison after the first 1–2 hours. The response at the 1–2-hour time point is highly predictive of subsequent outcome; patients improving at this point are likely to succeed, but those without improvement are likely to fail and require intubation and invasive ventilation or palliative care. Risk factors for failure after 2 hours of NIV are listed in Box 7.2.[1–3]

CONTRAINDICATIONS TO NONINVASIVE RESPIRATORY SUPPORT

When the need for ventilatory assistance is established, candidates for NIRS should be screened for possible contraindications. In general, if patients are unable to protect their airway due to sedation, coma, or slowly reversible impairment of consciousness, they are poor candidates. Large amounts of upper airway secretions, gastrointestinal hemorrhage, impaired swallowing, and frequent vomiting are risk factors for aspiration and identify poor candidates. Uncooperative and agitated patients and those with severe claustrophobia are unlikely to tolerate the mask. Patients in respiratory distress with cardiovascular instability and cardiogenic shock are probably unsuitable.[3] Upper airway obstruction due to epiglottitis or angioedema is best treated with intubation to avoid progression to complete airway obstruction and the need for emergent cricothyrotomy. This differs from upper airway obstruction due to glottic edema after extubation which may respond well to NIRS.[4] However, carbon dioxide narcosis associated with COPD exacerbations should not be considered a contraindication, and one trial has shown good outcomes with NIV use in these patients (Box 7.3).[5]

APPLICATIONS OF NONINVASIVE RESPIRATORY SUPPORT IN THE INTENSIVE CARE UNIT

NIRS has been trialed for many types of acute respiratory failure in the intensive care unit (ICU) and the evidence to support these applications varies depending on the specific diagnosis. In the following sections, we discuss the evidence supporting the various applications in more detail, starting with those supported by the strongest evidence.

BEST EVIDENCE/FIRST-LINE THERAPY

Chronic Obstructive Pulmonary Disease

Acute Exacerbation

Multiple randomized controlled trials (RCTs), meta-analyses, and comparative effectiveness analyses have shown decreased intubation and improved mortality rates with NIV compared with standard medical therapy in patients with exacerbations of COPD.[1,2,6–10] Thus NIV should be considered the standard of care in patients with COPD exacerbations requiring ventilatory support in the absence of contraindications. The physiologic rationale in these patients is that inspiratory pressure unloads the inspiratory muscles and increases tidal volume, decreases the dead space-to-tidal volume ratio, lowers respiratory rate, and improves alveolar ventilation.[6] The addition of positive end-expiratory pressure (PEEP) decreases the work of breathing by decreasing the inspiratory threshold load imposed by auto-PEEP that is frequently present in these patients.[11]

Extubating COPD Patients

Extubation of COPD patients who have failed spontaneous breathing trials to NIV reduces hospital mortality and duration of mechanical ventilation.[12,13] However, this approach is limited by whether the patient is hemodynamically stable, cooperative, has a strong cough, manageable secretions, and is not a difficult reintubation. The pressure support limit should not exceed 15 cm H_2O.

Acute Cardiogenic Pulmonary Edema

Multiple RCTs and meta-analyses have shown that CPAP lowers intubation rates and mortality when compared with conventional medical therapy in patients with cardiogenic pulmonary edema.[14–25] Higher intrathoracic pressure increases functional residual capacity (FRC), recruiting flooded alveoli, improving gas exchange, and improving lung compliance. An increase in intrathoracic pressure also reduces cardiac preload and afterload.[26,27] Longer-term use of CPAP in stable congestive heart failure patients improves left ventricular ejection fraction, decreases mitral regurgitation, and decreases atrial natriuretic peptide levels compared with controls.[28]

MODERATE EVIDENCE FOR USE

Asthma

CPAP stents open smaller airways, preventing dynamic airway collapse and reducing the transpulmonary pressure required to move gas into the lungs. This decreases the work of breathing. A small ($n = 53$) single-center RCT found that patients with acute severe asthma treated with NIV compared with conventional therapy had significantly decreased ICU and hospital length of stay (38 vs. 54 hours and 24 vs. 101 hours, respectively).[29] Murase et al.[30] demonstrated a significant decrease in the need for endotracheal intubation when comparing NIV with conventional therapy (3.5% vs. 18%). These data probably reflect selection and publication bias. However, it may be reasonable to cautiously trial NIV in patients with severe asthma exacerbations who fail to respond to initial bronchodilator therapy and have persistently increased work of breathing.

Pneumonia

Remarkably few studies have evaluated the use of NIV in pneumonia/hypoxic respiratory failure. Ferrer et al.[31] demonstrated decreased ICU mortality rates (18% vs. 39%) and intubation rates (25% vs. 52%) among younger patients receiving NIV compared with standard oxygen therapy for acute hypoxemic respiratory failure due to pneumonia. A retrospective study by Stefan et al.[32] demonstrated a mortality benefit in patients with pneumonia and concomitant heart failure or COPD. Failure rates have exceeded 60% in some studies.[33] Indeed, in patients with PaO_2/FiO_2 (ratio of partial pressure of arterial oxygen to the fraction of inspired oxygen) <150, NIV was associated with increased mortality, probably due to "self-induced lung injury"/volutrauma.[34] Acute respiratory distress syndrome (ARDS) is a progressive, multisystem disease that evolves over days and is associated with high PEEP and driving pressure requirements; it requires careful tidal volume management. If a trial of CPAP/NIV is undertaken, a strict time limit, such as 12 hours, should be set before the process is abandoned in favor of invasive mechanical ventilation.

Immunocompromised States

Several very small randomized trials from the 1990s demonstrated decreased mortality with NIV compared with oxygen therapy alone in immunocompromised patients with hypoxemic respiratory failure.[35,36] The mechanism of this improvement is believed to reflect a reduction in infectious complications.[37] However, overall outcomes in this patient cohort have improved over the past two decades. Lemiale and colleagues[38] randomized 374 patients to NIV vs. oxygen therapy in France and Belgium. There was no mortality difference between the groups. The lower-than-expected mortality rate resulted in the study being underpowered, and the use of HFNC may have been a confounder, although this appears to have been refuted.[39]

It is reasonable to consider instituting this NIRS early when there is a window of opportunity to avoid the progression to overt respiratory failure and the need for intubation. Once intubated, mortality rates among the immunocompromised remain high.[37,40]

Preoxygenation for Intubation

NIV can be an effective way of preoxygenating critically ill patients with hypoxemic respiratory failure for intubation.[41] In one randomized trial, patients managed with NIV in preparation for intubation had improved oxygen saturation and a decreased incidence of clinically significant desaturation during intubation.[41]

Postoperative Respiratory Failure

A systematic review by Ferreyra et al.[42] found a decreased intubation rate, atelectasis, and pneumonia with the use of CPAP compared with oxygen supplementation alone in patients who underwent abdominal surgery. Zhu et al.[43] systematically reviewed 14 RCTs and 1740 patients that examined NIV after cardiac surgery. There was a significant improvement in oxygen saturation and decrease in intubation rate and no significant increase in cardiopulmonary complications.[43] Squadrone and colleagues[44] reported significantly reduced reintubation rates in post abdominal surgery patients, treated with NIV via a helmet device.

Obesity Hypoventilation Syndrome

Acute hypercapnic respiratory failure related to obesity hypoventilation (OHS) is becoming more prevalent given the obesity epidemic in the general population. When used for acute hypercapnic respiratory failure in the ICU, NIV for OHS patients has similar efficacy and better outcomes than for COPD patients.[45]

Neuromuscular Disease

NIV is widely used at home in patients with progressive neuromuscular disorders such as myopathies, muscular dystrophies, spinal muscular atrophy, scoliosis, and amyotrophic lateral sclerosis (motor neuron disease).[46–49] NIV reverses hypoventilation, stabilizes the upper airway, and improves obstructive sleep apnea. Hospital admission is usually due to respiratory infection and sputum retention and aggressive respiratory and physical therapy is warranted to avoid intubation.[50]

A retrospective observational study in patients with myasthenic crises showed that early use of NIV reduced the need for intubation and prolonged mechanical ventilation.[51] Conversely, NIV is not an appropriate therapy for rapidly progressive neuromuscular disorders, such as Guillain–Barré syndrome, or tetanus, that involves "bulbar" muscles—impairing swallowing and the ability to mobilize secretions.

Palliative Care

NIV has a potential role in the treatment of patients with do-not-resuscitate/do-not-intubate (DNR/DNI) orders and end-of-life care. A study of NIV use in patients with heterogeneous respiratory failure and DNR/DNI status showed favorable outcomes in those with the types of respiratory failure expected to respond to NIV, including COPD and cardiogenic pulmonary edema.[52] NIV can also be used for palliation of dyspnea as part of a multidisciplinary multi-modal approach to end-of-life cases, in select circumstances.

Interstitial Lung Disease

Patients with respiratory failure secondary to fibrotic or interstitial lung disease do poorly in an ICU, particularly if they are intubated and ventilated.[53] There are no RCTs of NIV vs. invasive ventilation in this setting, and studies published demonstrating improved outcomes from NIV have issues with selection bias.[53,54]

CONFLICTING EVIDENCE/ DELETERIOUS EFFECT

Acute Lung Injury and Acute Respiratory Distress Syndrome

Few data support the use of NIV in ARDS.[55] However, frequently, the diagnosis of ARDS is one of exclusion—for example of atelectasis, pneumonia, transfusion-related acute lung injury, fluid overload, or left ventricular failure. In those settings CPAP or alternative oxygen therapies such as HFNC may be administered while a reversible component is sought. This approach may prevent endotracheal intubation and shorten hospital stay.

When used as first-line therapy for "ARDS patients" admitted to an ICU, NIV appeared to prevent subsequent intubation in 54% of patients.[56] It is likely that ARDS was overdiagnosed in this study in view of the extraordinary difference in mortality between patients who required intubation and those who did not (53% vs. 6%; $P < .001$).

Postextubation Respiratory Failure

Patients who develop postextubation respiratory failure do poorly when "rescued" with NIV.[57] Mortality appears to increase due to delayed reintubation. However, it may be reasonable to extubate specific cohorts of patients, such as those with COPD[58,59] or morbid obesity, to NIV as a prophylactic measure to prevent lung derecruitment.[60]

High-Flow Nasal Cannula Oxygen Therapy

HNFC oxygen therapy can reliably deliver up to 60 L/min of oxygen via nasal cannula; it is a component of modern NIRS. HFNC has multiple benefits to traditional high-flow systems (e.g., nonrebreather face mask, Venturi mask): (1) allows for heating and humidification of inspired oxygen, which decreases desiccation-associated mucosal injury and increases the water content of mucous secretions, thereby allowing for easier clearance of secretions; (2) high flow rates create a CPAP effect (approximately 0.5 cm H_2O for every 10 L/min); (3) less entrainment of room air and washout of oropharyngeal dead space; and (4) improved comfort with pliable nasal prongs.[61]

Many patients who are intolerant of tight-fitting CPAP or NIV face masks will manage well with HFNC that allow the patient to eat, speak, and sleep comfortably.

Increasing use of HFNC has resulted in academic interest in these devices in preventing intubation, preventing reintubation

and for airway surgery, apneic oxygenation, and difficult airway management.

High-Flow Nasal Cannula in Acute Hypoxemic Respiratory Failure

HFNC improve oxygenation and reduce respiratory rate compared with conventional oxygen therapy.[62–64] Frat et al.[65] randomized patients with acute hypoxemic respiratory failure (AHRF) to HFNC, NIV, or conventional oxygen therapy. While HFNC did not appear to reduce the need for intubation, patients spent fewer days on the ventilator compared with the other groups and had lower 90-day mortality compared with NIV and standard oxygen therapy. This suggests that NIV may be harmful in this patient population. These data support the use of HFNC in patients with acute hypoxemia during the time window that reversible causes are being treated, prior to intubation, but care should be taken to avoid delayed intubation.[66,67]

In immunocompromised patients with hypoxemia, HFNC was not superior to conventional oxygen therapy.[39]

Prevention of Postextubation Respiratory Failure

HFNC therapy reduced the reintubation rate in selected high-risk hypoxic patients in ICUs (4% vs. 21%).[68] However, it is unclear whether or not HFNC prevents reintubation in a heterogeneous group of patients extubated in an ICU.[69] Studies in the postoperative population of HFNC have, thus far, been disappointing.[70,71] It is unclear what specific questions these studies were addressing and whether or not the studies were adequately powered to detect postoperative pulmonary complications.

Apneic Oxygenation During Intubation

Many studies have demonstrated that the use of low-flow nasal cannula oxygen applied prior to and during intubation to provide apneic oxygenation significantly prolongs time to desaturation and decreases lowest oxygen saturations during intubation in the operating room.[72] However, to date, studies of HFNC vs. standard therapy for intubation in the ICU have been underwhelming.[73,74]

AUTHORS' RECOMMENDATIONS

- Noninvasive respiratory support includes CPAP, NIV (or pressure support ventilation), and HFNC oxygen therapy.
- NIV is associated with better outcomes than endotracheal intubation and mechanical ventilation in exacerbations of COPD.
- CPAP is effective in treating cardiogenic pulmonary edema, postoperative atelectasis, and obstructive sleep apnea.
- NIV may also be used in asthma, pneumonia, immunocompromised states, preoxygenation, postoperative respiratory failure, obesity hypoventilation syndrome, neuromuscular disease, and palliative care.
- NIV has no role in the management of the patient with ARDS and may be associated with worse outcomes when used in acute hypoxemic respiratory failure.
- HFNC is an effective therapy for acute respiratory failure as it increases nonhypoxic apneic duration and may be used to prevent reintubation.

REFERENCES

1. Lightowler JV, Wedzicha JA, Elliott MW, Ram FS. Non-invasive positive pressure ventilation to treat respiratory failure resulting from exacerbations of chronic obstructive pulmonary disease: Cochrane systematic review and meta-analysis. *BMJ*. 2003;326(7382):185.
2. Keenan SP, Sinuff T, Cook DJ, Hill NS. Which patients with acute exacerbation of chronic obstructive pulmonary disease benefit from noninvasive positive pressure ventilation? A systematic review of the literature. *Ann Intern Med*. 2003;138(11):861-870.
3. Gray AJ, Goodacre S, Newby DE, et al. A multicentre randomised controlled trial of the use of continuous positive airway pressure and non-invasive positive pressure ventilation in the early treatment of patients presenting to the emergency department with severe acute cardiogenic pulmonary oedema: the 3CPO trial. *Health Technol Assess*. 2009;13(33):1-106.
4. Nava S, Gregoretti C, Fanfulla F, et al. Noninvasive ventilation to prevent respiratory failure after extubation in high-risk patients. *Crit Care Med*. 2005;33(11):2465-2470.
5. Díaz G, Alcaraz AC, Talavera JC, et al. Noninvasive positive-pressure ventilation to treat hypercapnic coma secondary to respiratory failure. *Chest*. 2005;127(3):952-960.
6. Brochard L, Isabey D, Piquet J, et al. Reversal of acute exacerbations of chronic obstructive lung disease by inspiratory assistance with a face mask. *N Engl J Med*. 1990;323(22):1523-1530.
7. Bott J, Carroll MP, Conway JH, et al. Randomised controlled trial of nasal ventilation in acute ventilatory failure due to chronic obstructive airways disease. *Lancet*. 1993;341(8860):1555–1557.
8. Kramer N, Meyer TJ, Meharg J, Cece RD, Hill NS. Randomized, prospective trial of noninvasive positive pressure ventilation in acute respiratory failure. *Am J Respir Crit Care Med*. 1995;151(6):1799-1806.
9. Plant PK, Owen JL, Elliott MW. Early use of non-invasive ventilation for acute exacerbations of chronic obstructive pulmonary disease on general respiratory wards: a multicentre randomised controlled trial. *Lancet*. 2000;355(9219):1931-1935.
10. Lindenauer PK, Stefan MS, Shieh MS, Pekow PS, Rothberg MB, Hill NS. Outcomes associated with invasive and noninvasive ventilation among patients hospitalized with exacerbations of chronic obstructive pulmonary disease. *JAMA Intern Med*. 2014;174(12):1982-1993.
11. Appendini L, Patessio A, Zanaboni S, et al. Physiologic effects of positive end-expiratory pressure and mask pressure support during exacerbations of chronic obstructive pulmonary disease. *Am J Respir Crit Care Med*. 1994;149(5):1069-1076.
12. Ferrer M, Esquinas A, Arancibia F, et al. Noninvasive ventilation during persistent weaning failure: a randomized controlled trial. *Am J Respir Crit Care Med*. 2003;168(1):70-76.
13. Nava S, Ambrosino N, Clini E, et al. Noninvasive mechanical ventilation in the weaning of patients with respiratory failure due to chronic obstructive pulmonary disease. A randomized, controlled trial. *Ann Intern Med*. 1998;128(9):721-728.
14. Bersten AD, Holt AW, Vedig AE, Skowronski GA, Baggoley CJ. Treatment of severe cardiogenic pulmonary edema with continuous positive airway pressure delivered by face mask. *N Engl J Med*. 1991;325(26):1825-1830.
15. Lin M, Yang YF, Chiang HT, Chang MS, Chiang BN, Cheitlin MD. Reappraisal of continuous positive airway pressure therapy in acute cardiogenic pulmonary edema. Short-term results and long-term follow-up. *Chest*. 1995;107(5):1379-1386.
16. Nava S, Carbone G, DiBattista N, et al. Noninvasive ventilation in cardiogenic pulmonary edema: a multicenter randomized trial. *Am J Respir Crit Care Med*. 2003;168(12):1432-1437.
17. Crane SD, Elliott MW, Gilligan P, Richards K, Gray AJ. Randomised controlled comparison of continuous positive airways pressure, bilevel non-invasive ventilation, and standard treatment in emergency department patients with acute cardiogenic pulmonary oedema. *Emerg Med J*. 2004;21(2):155-161.
18. Pang D, Keenan SP, Cook DJ, Sibbald WJ. The effect of positive airway pressure on mortality and the need for intubation in cardiogenic pulmonary edema. *Chest*. 1998;114(4):1185-1192.
19. Räsänen J, Heikkilä J, Downs J, Nikki P, Väisänen I, Viitanen A. Continuous positive airway pressure by face mask in acute cardiogenic pulmonary edema. *Am J Cardiol*. 1985;55(4):296-300.
20. Lin M, Chiang HT. The efficacy of early continuous positive airway pressure therapy in patients with acute cardiogenic pulmonary edema. *J Formos Med Assoc*. 1991;90(8):736-743.
21. Masip J, Roque M, Sánchez B, Fernández R, Subirana M, Expósito JA. Noninvasive ventilation in acute cardiogenic pulmonary edema: systematic review and meta-analysis. *JAMA*. 2005;294(24):3124-3130.
22. Ho KM, Wong K. A comparison of continuous and bi-level positive airway pressure non-invasive ventilation in patients with acute cardiogenic pulmonary oedema: a meta-analysis. *Crit Care*. 2006;10(2):R49.
23. Mehta S, Jay GD, Woolard RH, et al. Randomized, prospective trial of bilevel versus continuous positive airway pressure in acute pulmonary edema. *Crit Care Med*. 1997;25(4):620-628.
24. Winck JC, Azevedo LF, Costa-Pereira A, Antonelli M, Wyatt JC. Efficacy and safety of non-invasive ventilation in the treatment of acute cardiogenic pulmonary edema—a systematic review and meta-analysis. *Crit Care*. 2006;10(2):R69.
25. Weng CL, Zhao YT, Liu QH, et al. Meta-analysis: noninvasive ventilation in acute cardiogenic pulmonary edema. *Ann Intern Med*. 2010;152(9):590-600.
26. Naughton MT, Rahman MA, Hara K, Floras JS, Bradley TD. Effect of continuous positive airway pressure on intrathoracic and left ventricular transmural pressures in patients with congestive heart failure. *Circulation*. 1995;91(6):1725-1731.
27. Tkacova R, Rankin F, Fitzgerald FS, Floras JS, Bradley TD. Effects of continuous positive airway pressure on obstructive sleep apnea and left ventricular afterload in patients with heart failure. *Circulation*. 1998;98(21):2269-2275.
28. Tkacova R, Liu PP, Naughton MT, Bradley TD. Effect of continuous positive airway pressure on mitral regurgitant fraction and atrial natriuretic peptide in patients with heart failure. *J Am Coll Cardiol*. 1997;30(3):739-745.
29. Gupta D, Nath A, Agarwal R, Behera D. A prospective randomized controlled trial on the efficacy of noninvasive ventilation in severe acute asthma. *Respir Care*. 2010;55(5):536-543.
30. Murase K, Tomii K, Chin K, et al. The use of non-invasive ventilation for life-threatening asthma attacks: changes in the need for intubation. *Respirology*. 2010;15(4):714-720.
31. Ferrer M, Esquinas A, Leon M, Gonzalez G, Alarcon A, Torres A. Noninvasive ventilation in severe hypoxemic respiratory failure: a randomized clinical trial. *Am J Respir Crit Care Med*. 2003;168(12):1438-1444.

32. Stefan MS, Priya A, Pekow PS, et al. The comparative effectiveness of noninvasive and invasive ventilation in patients with pneumonia. *J Crit Care*. 2018;43:190-196.

33. Jolliet P, Abajo B, Pasquina P, Chevrolet JC. Non-invasive pressure support ventilation in severe community-acquired pneumonia. *Intensive Care Med*. 2001;27(5):812-821.

34. Bellani G, Laffey JG, Pham T, et al. Noninvasive ventilation of patients with acute respiratory distress syndrome. Insights from the LUNG SAFE study. *Am J Respir Crit Care Med*. 2017;195(1):67-77.

35. Hilbert G, Gruson D, Vargas F, et al. Noninvasive ventilation in immunosuppressed patients with pulmonary infiltrates, fever, and acute respiratory failure. *N Engl J Med*. 2001;344(7):481-487.

36. Antonelli M, Conti G, Bufi M, et al. Noninvasive ventilation for treatment of acute respiratory failure in patients undergoing solid organ transplantation: a randomized trial. *JAMA*. 2000;283(2):235-241.

37. Hauringa AJ, Leyva FJ, Girault SA, et al. Outcome of bone marrow transplantation patients requiring mechanical ventilation. *Crit Care Med*. 2000;28(4):1014-1017.

38. Lemiale V, Mokart D, Resche-Rigon M, et al. Effect of noninvasive ventilation vs oxygen therapy on mortality among immunocompromised patients with acute respiratory failure: a randomized clinical trial. *JAMA*. 2015;314(16):1711-1719.

39. Azoulay E, Lemiale V, Mokart D, et al. Effect of high-flow nasal oxygen vs standard oxygen on 28-day mortality in immunocompromised patients with acute respiratory failure: the HIGH randomized clinical trial. *JAMA*. 2018;320(20):2099-2107.

40. Azoulay E, Lemiale V, Mokart D, et al. Acute respiratory distress syndrome in patients with malignancies. *Intensive Care Med*. 2014;40(8):1106-1114.

41. Baillard C, Fosse JP, Sebbane M, et al. Noninvasive ventilation improves preoxygenation before intubation in hypoxic patients. *Am J Respir Crit Care Med*. 2006;174(2):171-177.

42. Ferreyra GP, Baussano I, Squadrone V, et al. Continuous positive airway pressure for treatment of respiratory complications after abdominal surgery: a systematic review and meta-analysis. *Ann Surg*. 2008;247(4):617-626.

43. Zhu G, Huang Y, Wei D, Shi Y. Efficacy and safety of noninvasive ventilation in patients after cardiothoracic surgery. A PRISMA-compliant systematic review and meta-analysis. *Medicine (Baltimore)*. 2016;95(38):e4734.

44. Squadrone V, Coha M, Cerutti E, et al. Continuous positive airway pressure for treatment of postoperative hypoxemia: a randomized controlled trial. *JAMA*. 2005;293(5):589-595.

45. Carrillo A, Ferrer M, Gonzalez-Diaz G, et al. Noninvasive ventilation in acute hypercapnic respiratory failure caused by obesity hypoventilation syndrome and chronic obstructive pulmonary disease. *Am J Respir Crit Care Med*. 2012;186(12):1279-1285.

46. Simonds AK, Muntoni F, Heather S, Fielding S. Impact of nasal ventilation on survival in hypercapnic Duchenne muscular dystrophy. *Thorax*. 1998;53(11):949-952.

47. Young HK, Lowe A, Fitzgerald DA, et al. Outcome of noninvasive ventilation in children with neuromuscular disease. *Neurology*. 2007;68(3):198-201.

48. Bach JR, Saltstein K, Sinquee D, Weaver B, Komaroff E. Long-term survival in Werdnig-Hoffmann disease. *Am J Phys Med Rehabil*. 2007;86(5):339-345.

49. Simonds AK, Elliott MW. Outcome of domiciliary nasal intermittent positive pressure ventilation in restrictive and obstructive disorders. *Thorax*. 1995;50(6):604-609.

50. Tzeng AC, Bach JR. Prevention of pulmonary morbidity for patients with neuromuscular disease. *Chest*. 2000;118(5):1390-1396.

51. Seneviratne J, Mandrekar J, Wijdicks EF, Rabinstein AA. Noninvasive ventilation in myasthenic crisis. *Arch Neurol*. 2008;65(1):54-58.

52. Levy MM, Tanios MA, Nelson D, et al. Outcomes of patients with do-not-intubate orders treated with noninvasive ventilation. *Crit Care Med*. 2004;32(10):2002-2007.

53. Vianello A, Arcaro G, Battistella L, et al. Noninvasive ventilation in the event of acute respiratory failure in patients with idiopathic pulmonary fibrosis. *J Crit Care*. 2014;29(4):562-567.

54. Güngör G, Tatar D, Saltürk C, et al. Why do patients with interstitial lung disease fail in the ICU? A 2-center cohort study. *Respir Care*. 2013;58(3):525-531.

55. Rana S, Jenad H, Gay PC, Buck CF, Hubmayr RD, Gajic O. Failure of non-invasive ventilation in patients with acute lung injury: observational cohort study. *Crit Care*. 2006;10(3):R79.

56. Antonelli M, Conti G, Esquinas A, et al. A multiple-center survey on the use in clinical practice of noninvasive ventilation as a first-line intervention for acute respiratory distress syndrome. *Crit Care Med*. 2007;35(1):18-25.

57. Esteban A, Frutos-Vivar F, Ferguson ND, et al. Noninvasive positive-pressure ventilation for respiratory failure after extubation. *N Engl J Med*. 2004;350(24):2452-2460.

58. Krishna B, Sampath S, Moran JL. The role of non-invasive positive pressure ventilation in post-extubation respiratory failure: an evaluation using meta-analytic techniques. *Indian J Crit Care Med*. 2013;17(4):253-261.

59. Lin C, Yu H, Fan H, Li Z. The efficacy of noninvasive ventilation in managing postextubation respiratory failure: a meta-analysis. *Heart Lung*. 2014;43(2):99-104.

60. El-Solh AA, Aquilina A, Pineda L, Dhanvantri V, Grant B, Bouquin P. Noninvasive ventilation for prevention of post-extubation respiratory failure in obese patients. *Eur Respir J*. 2006;28(3):588-595.

61. Hyzy R. Heated and humidified high-flow nasal oxygen in adults: practical considerations and potential applications. UpToDate. 2018. Available at https://www.uptodate.com/contents/heated-and-humidified-high-flow-nasal-oxygen-in-adults-practical-considerations-and-potential-applications. Accessed January 9, 2019.

62. Roca O, Riera J, Torres F, Masclans JR. High-flow oxygen therapy in acute respiratory failure. *Respir Care*. 2010;55(4):408-413.

63. Sztrymf B, Messika J, Bertrand F, et al. Beneficial effects of humidified high flow nasal oxygen in critical care patients: a prospective pilot study. *Intensive Care Med*. 2011;37(11):1780-1786.

64. Roca O, de Acilu MG, Caralt B, Sacanell J, Masclans JR; ICU collaborators. Humidified high flow nasal cannula supportive therapy improves outcomes in lung transplant recipients readmitted to the intensive care unit because of acute respiratory failure. *Transplantation*. 2015;99(5):1092-1098.

65. Frat JP, Thille AW, Mercat A, et al. High-flow oxygen through nasal cannula in acute hypoxemic respiratory failure. *N Engl J Med*. 2015;372(23):2185-2196.

66. Helviz Y, Einav S. A systematic review of the high-flow nasal cannula for adult patients. *Crit Care*. 2018;22(1):71-79.

67. Kang BJ, Koh Y, Lim CM, et al. Failure of high-flow nasal cannula therapy may delay intubation and increase mortality. *Intensive Care Med*. 2015;41(4):623-632.

68. Maggiore SM, Idone FA, Vaschetto R, et al. Nasal high-flow versus Venturi mask oxygen therapy after extubation. Effects on oxygenation, comfort, and clinical outcome. *Am J Respir Crit Care Med*. 2014;190(3):282-288.

69. Hernández G, Vaquero C, González P, et al. Effect of postextubation high-flow nasal cannula vs conventional oxygen therapy on reintubation in low-risk patients. *JAMA*. 2016;315(13):1354-1361.

70. Zhu Y, Yin H, Zhang R, Wei J. High-flow nasal cannula oxygen therapy vs conventional oxygen therapy in cardiac surgical patients: a meta-analysis. *J Crit Care*. 2017;38:123-128.

71. Futier E, Paugam-Burtz C, Godet T, et al. Effect of early postextubation high-flow nasal cannula vs conventional oxygen therapy on hypoxaemia in patients after major abdominal surgery: a French multicentre randomised controlled trial (OPERA). *Intensive Care Med*. 2016;42(12):1888–1898.

72. Gleason JM, Christian BR, Barton ED. Nasal cannula apneic oxygenation prevents desaturation during endotracheal intubation: an integrative literature review. *West J Emerg Med*. 2018;19(2):403-411.

73. Jaber S, Monnin M, Girard M, et al. Apnoeic oxygenation via high-flow nasal cannula oxygen combined with non-invasive ventilation preoxygenation for intubation in hypoxaemic patients in the intensive care unit: the single-centre, blinded, randomised controlled OPTINIV trial. *Intensive Care Med*. 2016;42(12):1877-1887.

74. Simon M, Wachs C, Braune S, de Heer G, Frings D, Kluge S. High-flow nasal cannula versus bag-valve-mask for preoxygenation before intubation in subjects with hypoxemic respiratory failure. *Respir Care*. 2016;61(9):1160-1167.

8

What Is the Role of PEEP and Recruitment Maneuvers in ARDS?

Sinead Egan and Gerard F. Curley

INTRODUCTION

Positive end-expiratory pressure (PEEP) has been used in the management of patients with acute respiratory distress syndrome (ARDS) since the initial description of ARDS by Ashbaugh and colleagues in 1967.[1] Adjusting PEEP levels improves gas exchange by preventing alveolar derecruitment and reducing intrapulmonary shunt.[2] PEEP also mitigates ventilator-induced lung injury (VILI), by reducing atelectrauma, and pulmonary edema formation.[3–5] Thus, PEEP is not only a means to improve oxygenation but also a tool to protect the lung.

PEEP, however, increases mean airway pressure, leading to overdistension of less-diseased lung units and increased alveolar dead space. PEEP also increases pulmonary vascular resistance, reduces right atrial filling and right ventricular stroke volume, resulting in hypotension.[6,7] Moreover, excessive PEEP may damage the lungs and worsen oxygenation by compressing already recruited lung units.

Lung recruitment maneuvers (RMs) are used to reopen collapsed lung units to make them available for gas exchange. In theory, this should improve oxygenation and reduce driving pressure. Conversely, when applied inappropriately, RMs may damage the lung due to volutrauma and barotrauma, and cause cardiovascular instability.

This chapter explores the theoretical and practical basis behind the use of PEEP and the continued challenge to find the ideal PEEP for individual patients. We examine the "open lung" approach to ARDS and address the current role of RMs in mechanical ventilation.

VENTILATOR-INDUCED LUNG INJURY

Mechanical ventilation damages the lungs by a variety of mechanisms. In the 1970s Webb and Tierney[3] demonstrated that pulmonary edema and alveolar flooding developed within 13–35 minutes in rats ventilated with 45 cm H_2O peak airway pressure. This process, a stretch injury, is now known as volutrauma. Crucially, Webb and Tierney showed that edema was reduced when 10 cm H_2O PEEP was applied, even with a peak inspiratory pressure of 45 cm H_2O.[3] Thus, PEEP appears to be lung protective. Later studies demonstrated less epithelial injury in lungs ventilated with higher PEEP levels compared with zero end-expiratory pressure (ZEEP).[8] PEEP prevented phasic atelectasis, thus mitigating injury due to repetitive opening and closing of terminal units—a mechanism of injury termed atelectrauma.[9]

Injured lungs are particularly susceptible to volutrauma and atelectrauma because the number of aerated and recruitable alveoli is reduced.[10] Within the "baby lung," both fully aerated and nonaerated, but recruitable, respiratory units exist in close proximity.[11] The preferential distribution of ventilation to the less-injured units, as well as the heterogeneities at the interfaces between aerated and atelectatic regions, places these units at a high risk for injury.[12]

That mechanical ventilation damages the lungs is now universally accepted.[13] Ventilation strategies that reduce lung stretch save lives.[14,15] In 2000, "ARMA," a landmark randomized controlled trial (RCT), demonstrated a 9% absolute mortality reduction using a strategy of low tidal volume (V_t) (6 mL/kg predicted body weight [PBW]), and limitation of plateau pressure (30 cm H_2O) compared with a high-stretch approach.[14] A statistically significant decrease in nonpulmonary organ failure days (15 vs. 12) was also observed. In addition, the lower tidal volume strategy led to lower levels of plasma interleukins IL-6 and IL-8 and tumor necrosis factor receptor 1 (TNFR1) over the first 1–3 days,[16] suggesting the potential contribution of reduced "biotrauma" to decreased mortality.

THE OPEN LUNG VENTILATION APPROACH

PEEP prevents end-expiratory collapse of unstable lung units, and should lessen atelectrauma. In addition, PEEP appeared to restore the pulmonary compartmentalization of proinflammatory cytokines in preclinical studies.[17,18] In theory, once the lung has been reopened (i.e., collapsed lung units reinflated or "recruited" using RMs), adequate PEEP or mean airway pressure sufficient to keep the lung "open," when applied, should improve oxygenation and reduce driving and plateau pressures. The application of this theory is known as "open lung ventilation" (OLV) or the "open lung approach" (OLA). This may include the use of long inspiratory times to increase mean airway pressure; tidal volumes (TV) are usually limited to <6 mL/kg of PBW.

The scientific basis of this approach evolved in the late 1980s when computed tomography (CT) revealed that some lung regions in ARDS appear, radiographically, to be relatively normal, whereas other areas are partially or completely collapsed and unable to participate in gas exchange.[19] However, some collapsed or atelectatic areas of the lung can be re-expanded by the application of a brief period of high transpulmonary pressure (RM), followed by the application of adequate levels of PEEP to keep the newly aerated regions open.[20] While RMs can open the lung, the primary factor for the sustained improved oxygenation is the level of PEEP after the RM. Because PEEP is an expiratory setting, its level should be tailored after having recruited the lung: that is, identifying the lowest PEEP level that keeps the recruited lung open.

The OLV approach should result in reduced volutrauma, atelectrauma, and biotrauma.[8,21] However, clinical trials, to date, have failed to confirm or disconfirm its utility.[22] In the next section we carefully deconstruct the high vs. low PEEP trials and then address RMs.

CLINICAL TRIALS OF PEEP STRATEGIES

Although PEEP is a standard of care for the management of the patient with hypoxic respiratory failure, there is controversy regarding the amount of PEEP required, how that is determined, and whether the goal of PEEP should be improved oxygenation or improved lung mechanics.

Following an initial study of the OLA by Amato and colleagues[15] which suggested that a low-stretch mechanical ventilation strategy plus relatively high levels of PEEP improved patient outcomes, three large studies were funded to address high vs. low PEEP in low-stretch mechanical ventilation in ARDS. These were the Assessment of Low Tidal Volume and Elevated End-Expiratory Volume to Obviate Lung Injury (ALVEOLI) trial, published in 2004[16]; the Lung Open Ventilation Study (LOVS) in 2008[23]; and the ExPress trial, also in 2008.[24] These trials all used the intervention approach from the ARMA trial as their control (i.e., TV < 6 mL/kg PBW and P_{plat} <30 cm H_2O) and used higher PEEP levels on the intervention side.

- The ALVEOLI trial[16] used a PEEP table to adjust PEEP according to FiO_2: between 4 and 6 cm H_2O above the comparable PEEP level in the control group. There was no process in place to determine whether or not the patient was PEEP responsive, in terms of compliance or oxygenation. The ratios of partial pressure of arterial oxygen to the fraction of inspired oxygen (PaO_2/FiO_2 or PF ratios) in the control group at the time of recruitment were 165 vs. 151 in the higher PEEP group ($P = 0.003$) (Table 8.1). RMs were used in the first 80 patients in the higher PEEP group, then quietly abandoned as there was a belief that RMs were ineffective. The primary endpoint was unusual for this type of study: the proportion of patients who died before they were discharged home, while breathing without assistance. The mortality rates in both groups were lower than expected—24.9% (low PEEP), 27.5% high PEEP ($P = 0.48$). The slightly higher mortality in the intervention group was not significant, although patients in this group were sicker and more hypoxemic.

- The LOVS trial, from Canada,[23] used an open lung strategy of pressure-controlled ventilation (PCV), higher PEEP, and RM after ventilator disconnections. Again, PEEP was adjusted according to an FiO_2 table, derived semiarbitrarily. The PF ratio in the control group was 144.6 vs. 144.8 in the intervention group; approximately 15% of patients in each group had PF ratios >200. The outcome measure was "all-cause hospital mortality"—which was 36.4% in the high PEEP group and 40.4% in the control group ($P = 0.49$): 28-day mortality was 28.4% vs. 32.3% (control). The control group received more rescue therapy, such as inhaled nitric oxide, high frequency ventilation, prone positioning, and extracorporeal membrane oxygenation (ECMO).

- In the ExPress trial,[24] which was a French multicenter study, the control group was limited to a PEEP level of between 5 and 9 cm H_2O, irrespective of the PF ratio, and the intervention group PEEP was adjusted to be kept as high as possible, but P_{plat} could not exceed 30 cm H_2O. RMs were permitted but not encouraged. The PF ratios were 143 in the control group and 144 in the high PEEP group. The intervention group received, on average, 7 cm H_2O more PEEP over the first few days, compared with controls, and this translated to improved compliance, improved oxygenation (lower FiO_2) but similar partial pressure of arterial carbon dioxide ($PaCO_2$) levels. The main outcome measure was 28-day mortality, which was 31.2% in the control group and 27.8% in the high PEEP group ($P = 0.31$). Almost twice as many patients in the control group required rescue therapy—such as prone positioning and inhaled nitric oxide. There were more ventilator-free days in the high PEEP group.

- A Spanish trial ARIES,[25] that included 103 patients, was published in 2006. This study used similar methodology to that of Amato et al.,[15] and set the PEEP in the intervention group above the lower inflection point of the volume–pressure curve. The authors reported a statistically significant mortality benefit in the open lung group: 32% (ICU mortality) vs. 53.3%; $P = 0.4$. Note, though, that tidal volumes were relatively high in both groups (almost 10 mL/kg) and that 8 patients were removed from the study due to protocol violations.

- An individual patient-level meta-analysis was published by Briel et al.[28] in 2010 combining ALVOLI, LOVS, and ExPress trials ($n = 2299$). The investigators found a correlation between the severity of lung injury and the likelihood of benefit for high PEEP. For example, for patients with a PF ratio of <200 (ARDS by all definitions [$n = 1892$]), higher PEEP/OLV was associated with a 5% absolute reduction in the risk of death (34.1 vs. 39.1%; $P < 0.05$). The implication of this meta-analysis was that patients with less extensive severe lung disease were unlikely to benefit from higher levels of PEEP. Conversely, with worsening ARDS, higher levels of PEEP/OLV appeared to confer a mortality benefit. Two subsequent meta-analyses, which used essentially the same data,[29,30] failed to demonstrate a mortality benefit from higher

TABLE 8.1   Select Studies of Acute Respiratory Distress Syndrome.

Study	No. of Patients	Control Group	Inx Group	Outcome Variable	PaO$_2$/FiO$_2$ Intervention/Control Group	Control Mortality (%)	Inx Mortality (%)	P Value
Amato 1998[15]	53	10–12 mL	6 mL/kg P$_{plat}$ < 40 PEEP > LIP	28-day mortality	112 / 134	71	38	<.001*
ARMA 2000[14]	861	10–12 mL P$_{plat}$ >45	<6 mL P$_{plat}$ < 30	28-day mortality	138 / 134	39.8	31	<.05*
ALVEOLI 2004[16]	549	<6 mL/kg Low PEEP (8)	<6 mL/kg High PEEP (13)	Hospital mortality	151 / 165	24.9	27.5	.48
Aries 2006[25]	103	9–11 mL/kg Low PEEP (5)	5–8 PEEP > LIP	Hospital mortality	109 (median) / 110 (median)	55.5	34	.04
ExPress 2008[24]	226	<6 mL/kg Low PEEP	<6 mL/kg High PEEP	28-day mortality	143 / 144	31.2	27.8	.31
LOVS 2008[23]	933	<6 mL/kg P$_{plat}$ < 30	<6 mL/kg P$_{plat}$ < 30 High PEEP RM	Hospital mortality	144.6 / 144.8	40.4	36.4	.19
PROSEVA 2013[26]	466	<6 mL/kg P$_{plat}$ < 30	<6 mL/kg P$_{plat}$ < 30 Prone positioning 16 hours/day	28-day mortality	100 / 100	32.8	16	<.001*
OSCILLATE 2013[27]	548	<6 mL/kg	HFOV P$_{plat}$ < 30	In-hospital mortality	121 / 114	35	47	<.001*
ART 2017[22]	1010	<6 mL/kg P$_{plat}$ <30 Low PEEP (ARDSnet)	<6 mL/kg P$_{plat}$ < 30 RM—PCV 15 + PEEP up to 45* *Reduced due to cardiac arrests	28-day mortality	119 / 117	49.3	55.3	.04*

*Outcome was statistically significant.
HFOV, High frequency oscillation ventilation; *Inx,* investigation group; *LIP,* lower inflection point (of the volume pressure curve); *PCV,* pressure controlled ventilation; *PEEP,* positive end expiratory pressure; *Pplat,* plateau pressure; *RM,* recruitment maneuvers.

PEEP, but probably disregarded the signal identified by Briel for patients with worse lung injuries. Nevertheless, the issue of high vs. low PEEP remains unresolved and will require further research, probably to include individualized PEEP settings for patients recruited.

CLINICAL TRIALS OF RECRUITMENT MANEUVERS

A lung RM is commonly utilized as part of the open lung protective ventilation strategy, and has been widely used in anesthesia and intensive care. Opening collapsed lung tissue requires pressures adequate to overcome the sum of defined counterforces: (a) compressive forces due to the increased lung weight; (b) the surface tension forces due to the moving of air/liquid interface from the small airway to the alveolar space; and (c) the pressure needed to lift up the chest wall.[31]

Cardiovascular compromise, manifest by a fall in the blood pressure, is often encountered during RMs, but is usually self-limiting. Increased airway pressure decreases right atrial preload and increases right ventricular afterload, leading to underfilling of the left ventricle and reduced cardiac output. Barotrauma is also a concern, although the incidence of RM-induced pneumothorax appears low.[32]

A Cochrane review[33] in 2016 looked at 10 trials of RMs in ARDS. The analysis was problematic due to the heterogeneity of the data and the contamination of most of the trials by confounders such as other aspects of the OLA. Although the analysis concluded that, while RMs decrease critical care mortality, they had no effect on 28-day or hospital mortality; the primary data was low in quality.

Kacmarek and colleagues[34] conducted an RCT in 200 ARDS patients with persistent hypoxemia comparing the ARDSnet protocol with an OLA. This involved RMs and a decremental PEEP trial identifying the PEEP level associated with the maximum dynamic compliance. OLA improved oxygenation and respiratory system mechanics; there was no difference in 60-day mortality, ventilator-free days, or barotrauma. This trial identified the need for a larger RCT using RMs in association with PEEP titrated by compliance of the respiratory system to test whether this approach is able to increase survival in patients with persistent ARDS.

The efficacy of the OLA was evaluated in the Alveolar Recruitment for Acute Respiratory Distress Syndrome Trial (ART). Patients were randomized to an OLA or a conventional low tidal volume and PEEP strategy as per the protocol from the ARMA trial. The OLA strategy involved an initial RM with the application of increasing levels of PEEP (25, 35, and 45 cm H_2O) with a driving pressure of 15 cm H_2O to achieve maximal P_{plat} of 60 cm H_2O. While the OLA arm showed an improvement in hypoxemia, it resulted in higher mortality (55.3% vs. 49.3%; $P = 0.041$) and also more hypotension and barotrauma. A small but statistically significant difference in ventilator-free days favored the control group (5.3 days in the OLA group vs. 6.4 days in the control group). Patients in the OLA group required more vasopressors within 1 hour of beginning the protocol, and three patients experienced cardiac arrests (resulting in a late change to the protocol).

A similar trial of RMs in ARDS, PHARLAP (Permissive Hypercapnia, Alveolar Recruitment and Low Airway Pressure)[35] halted patient recruitment after the publication of the ART study; the outcomes data have yet to be published.

Does the ART trial signal the "end for the OLA approach"? We think not. It is worth noting that the 28-day mortality rate in both arms of the study were very high (49.3% in the control group, 55.3% in the intervention group), with approximately 60% mortality at 6 months in both groups. For comparison, the PROSEVA trial,[26] in which patients were randomized to standard care vs. 16 hours per day of prone positioning, had 28-day mortality rates of 32.8% (controls) vs. 16% (proned); the control group mortality rate was 41% at 90 days—significantly lower than either group in the ARM trial (see Table 8.1). It could also be argued that prone positioning—in and of itself—represents a form or RM. Only 10% of each group of the ART trial was turned prone. Moreover, all intensivists are aware that a cohort of patients have lung injuries that are nonresponsive to PEEP, RM, and prone positioning.[36] Application of OLV to these patients has no apparent benefit and a high likelihood of harm. Villar and colleagues[37] have raised a number of other critiques of this study, questioning the quality control of a complex intervention in a 120-center study, the absence of comorbidity exclusion criteria, the low reported rate of protocol violations, 24-minute recruitment process (compared with 10–12 minutes in the Kacmarek trial) and the likelihood of the mechanical ventilation strategy increasing the risk of VILI.

INDIVIDUALIZED PEEP TITRATION AT THE BEDSIDE

Although the protective role of PEEP in ARDS is widely acknowledged,[38] there remains no ideal method of setting optimal PEEP at the bedside. Clinical trials have tended to use charts to set the PEEP according to FiO_2 and PF ratio.[16,24] However, individualized PEEP titration (IPT) is more likely to result in a safer profile, both in terms of oxygenation and in terms of VILI, and further trials of OLV will probably include some form of IPT.[34] Different techniques of IPT have been proposed: multiple pressure–volume curves, measurement of lung volume, use of esophageal pressure (P_{es}) and transpulmonary pressure, use of lung ultrasound, and CT.

IMAGING

Repeated CT scanning is a costly and resource-intensive way of assessing recruitment that may only be suitable in the research and nonclinical setting. Cressoni et al.[31] looked at 33 patients with mild, moderate, and severe ARDS and measured lung recruitment, atelectrauma, and lung ventilation inhomogeneities using two low-dose end-expiratory CT scans at PEEP 5 and 15 cm H_2O and four end-inspiratory CT scans (from 19 to 40 cm H_2O). The fraction of tissue that regained lung inflation was defined as recruitment. Intratidal tissue collapse at 5 and 15 cm H_2O PEEP was used as a measure of atelectrauma. The ratio of inflation between neighboring lung units was used to estimate lung ventilation inhomogeneities. In patients with early ARDS at 30 cm H_2O airway pressure, a generally accepted threshold of safety for mechanical ventilation, 10–30% of the potentially recruitable lung tissue remained closed in patients with moderate and severe ARDS. A tidal volume of 6–8 mL/kg and 15 cm H_2O of PEEP was insufficient to prevent cyclic lung tissue opening and closing. Finally, increasing PEEP decreased inhomogeneity by 3–4% of the total lung volume in mild and moderate ARDS, while in the severe ARDS groups it was unmodified.

Lung ultrasound (LUS) has been suggested as a practical, cost-effective approach to assess lung recruitment in response to PEEP. Xirouchaki et al.[39] demonstrated that LUS had better diagnostic yield than a chest radiograph for pleural effusions, pneumothorax, and alveolar consolidation. LUS has been shown to accurately reflect PEEP-induced lung recruitment,[40] but not hyperinflation.

OXYGENATION RESPONSE TO PEEP

Clinical trials have used an oxygenation table to titrate PEEP. This has many drawbacks, including the possible presence of intracardiac shunt, the influence of hemodynamics, and relatively poor correlation between recruitment and oxygenation.[41] The large RCTs evaluating PEEP did not attempt to offer high PEEP to responders and low PEEP to nonresponders.[16] A recent post hoc analysis of those trials suggested that, among patients in whom PEEP was increased after randomization, the higher the increase in oxygenation after PEEP the greater the reduction in mortality associated with PEEP.[42]

ESOPHAGEAL PRESSURE

Transpulmonary pressure is defined as the pressure difference between the pleural space and the alveolar space.[43] Conditions that decrease chest wall compliance, such as kyphoscoliosis, can increase airway pressure and lead to a false impression that lung stress is also increased. Measuring transpulmonary pressures can more accurately reflect the stress on lung parenchyma, as the measurement is independent of chest wall compliance. If transpulmonary pressure remains within normal limits, then it may be appropriate to ventilate above the accepted airway plateau pressures.

Esophageal pressure can be measured by positioning an air- or liquid-filled catheter (manometer) in the lower-third of the esophagus, and this can be used to estimate pleural pressure. Accuracy is variable due to patient positioning, the presence or absence of lung disease, and the position of the diaphragm.[38] Talmor and colleagues have suggested correcting the esophageal pressure by –5 cm H_2O mid-lung height, to estimate the true pleural pressure.[44,45]

In a single-center RCT (EPVent study), Talmor et al.[46] compared mechanical ventilation guided by P_{es} measurements (experimental arm) with ventilation based on the ARMA trial protocol (control arm). Patients who had PEEP titrated to ensure a positive end-expiratory transpulmonary pressure experienced a higher PaO_2/FiO_2, better respiratory system compliance as a possible consequence of improved recruitment, but no difference in 28-day mortality. Limitations to the measurement include the fact that a single measurement of esophageal pressure is unlikely to accurately reflect pleural pressure throughout the lung. It is also a resource-intensive measurement requiring two to three operators.

COMPLIANCE CURVES

Amato et al.[15,47] used quasistatic pressure–volume curves to set PEEP in their open lung studies. A lower inflection point (P_{flex}) was identified, above which PEEP was set. Although mortality was reduced in this setting, their results were confounded by the simultaneous use of a low tidal volume mechanical ventilation strategy in the intervention group.

ELECTRICAL IMPEDANCE TOMOGRAPHY

Electrical impedance tomography (EIT) has emerged as a noninvasive, bedside monitoring technique that provides semicontinuous, real-time information about the regional distribution of changes in the electrical resistivity of lung tissue due to variations in ventilation (or blood flow/perfusion) in relation to a reference state.[48]

EIT has been used to assess ventilation distribution and guide PEEP titration.[49] To date, EIT has not been used in a large RCT, and data are limited to its efficacy. For example, Franchineau and colleagues[50] looked at a cohort of 15 patients with severe ARDS treated with extracorporeal support. They utilized EIT to monitor a PEEP to determine the ideal point between recruitment and overdistension. A broad variability in optimal PEEP was observed.

CONCLUSION AND FUTURE DIRECTIONS

Despite extensive evidence in experimental models that PEEP and RMs can reduce VILI, large randomized clinical trials of higher PEEP and RMs have now failed to demonstrate improved clinical outcomes for the average patient, while one trial (using ART) suggested harm. However, only approximately 50% of all patients with ARDS responded to higher airway pressures by recruiting previously atelectatic or flooded alveoli,[36,51] and a reanalysis of PEEP studies provides a rationale for titrating PEEP to improvements in oxygenation.[42] Therefore, an OLV approach is more likely to be beneficial in patients with recruitable lungs. The best method for setting PEEP levels has still not been established. Further refinements in the OLV strategy with less aggressive attempts at lung recruitment and a focus on identifying patients who recruit in response to PEEP may lead to more favorable results.

REFERENCES

1. Ashbaugh DG, Bigelow DB, Petty TL, Levine BE. Acute respiratory distress in adults. *Lancet*. 1967;2(7511):319-323.
2. Falke KJ, Pontoppidan H, Kumar A, Leith DE, Geffin B, Laver MB. Ventilation with end-expiratory pressure in acute lung disease. *J Clin Invest*.1972;51(9):2315-2323.
3. Webb HH, Tierney DF. Experimental pulmonary edema due to intermittent positive pressure ventilation with high inflation pressures. Protection by positive end-expiratory pressure. *Am Rev Respir Dis*. 1974;110(5):556-565.
4. Tremblay L, Valenza F, Ribeiro SP, Li J, Slutsky AS. Injurious ventilatory strategies increase cytokines and c-fos m-RNA expression in an isolated rat lung model. *J Clin Invest*. 1997;99(5):944-952.
5. Ranieri VM, Suter PM, Tortorella C, et al. Effect of mechanical ventilation on inflammatory mediators in patients with acute respiratory distress syndrome: a randomized controlled trial. *JAMA*. 1999;282(1):54-61.
6. Suter PM, Fairley B, Isenberg MD. Optimum end-expiratory airway pressure in patients with acute pulmonary failure. *N Engl J Med*. 1975;292(6):284-289.
7. Kirby RR, Downs JB, Civetta JM, et al. High level positive end expiratory pressure (PEEP) in acute respiratory insufficiency. *Chest*. 1975;67(2):156-163.
8. Muscedere JG, Mullen JB, Gan K, Slutsky AS. Tidal ventilation at low airway pressures can augment lung injury. *Am J Respir Crit Care Med*. 1994;149(5):1327-1334.
9. Slutsky AS. Lung injury caused by mechanical ventilation. *Chest*. 1999;116(suppl 1):9S-15S.
10. Gattinoni L, Marini JJ, Pesenti A, Quintel M, Mancebo J, Brochard L. The "baby lung" became an adult. *Intensive Care Med*. 2016;42(5):663-673.
11. Maunder RJ, Shuman WP, McHugh JW, Marglin SI, Butler J. Preservation of normal lung regions in the adult respiratory distress syndrome. Analysis by computed tomography. *JAMA*. 1986;255(18):2463-2465.
12. Mead J, Takishima T, Leith D. Stress distribution in lungs: a model of pulmonary elasticity. *J Appl Physiol*. 1970;28(5):596-608.
13. Petrucci N, De Feo C. Lung protective ventilation strategy for the acute respiratory distress syndrome. *Cochrane Database Syst Rev*. 2013;2:CD003844.
14. Acute Respiratory Distress Syndrome Network; Brower RG, Matthay MA, et al. Ventilation with lower tidal volumes as compared with traditional tidal volumes for acute lung injury and the acute respiratory distress syndrome. *N Engl J Med*. 2000;342(18):1301-1308.
15. Amato MB, Barbas CS, Medeiros DM, et al. Effect of a protective-ventilation strategy on mortality in the acute respiratory distress syndrome. *N Engl J Med*. 1998;338(6):347-354.
16. Brower RG, Lanken PN, MacIntyre N, et al. Higher versus lower positive end-expiratory pressures in patients with the acute respiratory distress syndrome. *N Engl J Med*. 2004;351(4):327-336.
17. Haitsma JJ, Uhlig S, Göggel R, Verbrugge SJ, Lachmann U, Lachmann B. Ventilator-induced lung injury leads to loss of alveolar and systemic compartmentalization of tumor necrosis factor-alpha. *Intensive Care Med*. 2000;26(10):1515-1522.
18. Herrera MT, Toledo C, Valladares F, et al. Positive end-expiratory pressure modulates local and systemic inflammatory responses in a sepsis-induced lung injury model. *Intensive Care Med*. 2003;29(8):1345-1353.
19. Gattinoni L, Pesenti A. The concept of "baby lung." *Intensive Care Med*. 2005;31(6):776-784.
20. Girgis K, Hamed H, Khater Y, Kacmarek RM. A decremental PEEP trial identifies the PEEP level that maintains oxygenation after lung recruitment. *Respir Care*. 2006;51(10):1132-1139.
21. Suarez-Sipmann F, Böhm SH, Tusman G, et al. Use of dynamic compliance for open lung positive end-expiratory pressure titration in an experimental study. *Crit Care Med*. 2007; 35(1):214-221.
22. Writing Group for the Alveolar Recruitment for Acute Respiratory Distress Syndrome Trial (ART) Investigators; Cavalcanti AB, Suzumura ÉA, et al. Effect of lung recruitment and titrated positive end-expiratory pressure (PEEP) vs low PEEP on mortality in patients with acute respiratory distress syndrome: a randomized clinical trial. *JAMA*. 2017;318(14):1335-1345.
23. Meade MO, Cook DJ, Guyatt GH, et al. Ventilation strategy using low tidal volumes, recruitment maneuvers, and high positive end-expiratory pressure for acute lung injury and acute respiratory distress syndrome: a randomized controlled trial. *JAMA*. 2008;299(6):637-645.
24. Mercat A, Richard JC, Vielle B, et al. Positive end-expiratory pressure setting in adults with acute lung injury and acute respiratory distress syndrome: a randomized controlled trial. *JAMA*. 2008;299(6):646-655.
25. Villar J, Kacmarek RM, Pérez-Méndez L, Aguirre-Jaime A. A high positive end-expiratory pressure, low tidal volume ventilatory strategy improves outcome in persistent acute respiratory distress syndrome: a randomized, controlled trial. *Crit Care Med*. 2006;34(5):1311-1318.
26. Guérin C, Reignier J, Richard JC, et al. Prone positioning in severe acute respiratory distress syndrome. *N Engl J Med*. 2013;368(23):2159-2168.

27. Ferguson ND, Cook DJ, Guyatt GH, et al. High-frequency oscillation in early acute respiratory distress syndrome. *N Engl J Med*. 2013;368(9):795-805.
28. Briel M, Meade M, Mercat A, et al. Higher vs lower positive end-expiratory pressure in patients with acute lung injury and acute respiratory distress syndrome: systematic review and meta-analysis. *JAMA*. 2010;303(9):865-873.
29. Walkey AJ, Del Sorbo L, Hodgson CL, et al. Higher PEEP versus lower PEEP strategies for patients with acute respiratory distress syndrome. A systematic review and meta-analysis. *Ann Am Thorac Soc*. 2017;14(suppl 4):S297-S303.
30. Santa Cruz R, Rojas JI, Nervi R, Heredia R, Ciapponi A. High versus low positive end-expiratory pressure (PEEP) levels for mechanically ventilated adult patients with acute lung injury and acute respiratory distress syndrome. *Cochrane Database Syst Rev*. 2013;(6):CD009098.
31. Cressoni M, Chiumello D, Algieri I, et al. Opening pressures and atelectrauma in acute respiratory distress syndrome. *Intensive Care Med*. 2017;43(5):603-611.
32. Hodgson CL, Tuxen DV, Davies AR, et al. A randomised controlled trial of an open lung strategy with staircase recruitment, titrated PEEP and targeted low airway pressures in patients with acute respiratory distress syndrome. *Crit Care*. 2011;15(3):R133.
33. Hodgson C, Goligher EC, Young ME, et al. Recruitment manoeuvers for adults with acute respiratory distress syndrome receiving mechanical ventilation. *Cochrane Database Syst Rev*. 2016;11:CD006667.
34. Kacmarek RM, Villar J, Sulemanji D, et al. Open lung approach for the acute respiratory distress syndrome: a pilot, randomized controlled trial. *Crit Care Med*. 2016;44(1):32-42.
35. Hodgson C, Cooper DJ, Arabi Y, et al. Permissive Hypercapnia, Alveolar Recruitment and Low Airway Pressure (PHARLAP): a protocol for a phase 2 trial in patients with acute respiratory distress syndrome. *Crit Care Resusc*. 2018;20(2):139-149.
36. Gattinoni L, Caironi P, Cressoni M, et al. Lung recruitment in patients with the acute respiratory distress syndrome. *N Engl J Med*. 2006;354(17):1775-1786.
37. Villar J, Suárez-Sipmann F, Kacmarek RM. Should the ART trial change our practice? *J Thorac Dis*. 2017;9(12):4871-4877.
38. Sahetya SK, Goligher EC, Brower RG. Fifty years of research in ARDS. Setting positive end-expiratory pressure in acute respiratory distress syndrome. *Am J Respir Crit Care Med*. 2017;195(11):1429-1438.
39. Xirouchaki N, Magkanas E, Vaporidi K, et al. Lung ultrasound in critically ill patients: comparison with bedside chest radiography. *Intensive Care Med*. 2011;37(9):1488-1493.
40. Bouhemad B, Brisson H, Le-Guen M, Arbelot C, Lu Q, Rouby JJ. Bedside ultrasound assessment of positive end-expiratory pressure-induced lung recruitment. *Am J Respir Crit Care Med*. 2011;183(3):341-347.
41. Maggiore SM, Jonson B, Richard JC, Jaber S, Lemaire F, Brochard L. Alveolar derecruitment at decremental positive end-expiratory pressure levels in acute lung injury: comparison with the lower inflection point, oxygenation, and compliance. *Am J Respir Crit Care Med*. 2001;164(5):795-801.
42. Goligher EC, Kavanagh BP, Rubenfeld GD, et al. Oxygenation response to positive end-expiratory pressure predicts mortality in acute respiratory distress syndrome. A secondary analysis of the LOVS and ExPress trials. *Am J Respir Crit Care Med*. 2014;190(1):70-76.
43. Loring SH, Topulos GP, Hubmayr RD. Transpulmonary pressure: the importance of precise definitions and limiting assumptions. *Am J Respir Crit Care Med*. 2016;194(12):1452-1457.
44. Talmor D, Sarge T, O'Donnell CR, et al. Esophageal and transpulmonary pressures in acute respiratory failure. *Crit Care Med*. 2006;34(5):1389-1394.
45. Washko GR, O'Donnell CR, Loring SH. Volume-related and volume-independent effects of posture on esophageal and transpulmonary pressures in healthy subjects. *J Appl Physiol (1985)*. 2006;100(3):753-758.
46. Talmor D, Sarge T, Malhotra A, et al. Mechanical ventilation guided by esophageal pressure in acute lung injury. *N Engl J Med*. 2008;359(20):2095-2104.
47. Amato MB, Barbas CS, Medeiros DM, et al. Beneficial effects of the "open lung approach" with low distending pressures in acute respiratory distress syndrome. A prospective randomized study on mechanical ventilation. *Am J Respir Crit Care Med*. 1995;152(6 Pt 1):1835-1846.
48. Bodenstein M, David M, Markstaller K. Principles of electrical impedance tomography and its clinical application. *Crit Care Med*. 2009;37(2):713-724.
49. Kobylianskii J, Murray A, Brace D, Goligher E, Fan E. Electrical impedance tomography in adult patients undergoing mechanical ventilation: a systematic review. *J Crit Care*. 2016;35:33-50.
50. Franchineau G, Bréchot N, Lebreton G, et al. Bedside contribution of electrical impedance tomography to setting positive end-expiratory pressure for extracorporeal membrane oxygenation-treated patients with severe acute respiratory distress syndrome. *Am J Respir Crit Care Med*. 2017;196(4):447-457.
51. Grasso S, Fanelli V, Cafarelli A, et al. Effects of high versus low positive end-expiratory pressures in acute respiratory distress syndrome. *Am J Respir Crit Care Med*. 2005;171(9):1002-1008.

9

What Is the Best Way to Wean and Liberate Patients from Mechanical Ventilation?

Alistair Nichol, Pierce Geoghegan, Stephen Duff, David Devlin, and David J. Cooper

INTRODUCTION

"Weaning" refers to the transition from full mechanical ventilatory support to spontaneous ventilation with minimal support. "Liberation" refers to the discontinuation of mechanical ventilation.[1] This chapter focuses on the clinical assessment of readiness to wean, the technique for conducting a spontaneous breathing trial (SBT), and the assessment of readiness for extubation. In addition, we review the evidence supporting various ventilator strategies in the difficult-to-wean patient.

Mechanically ventilated intensive care patients may be classified as simple to wean, difficult to wean, or prolonged weaning.[2] Simple-to-wean patients are extubated on the first attempt, make up the vast majority of the patients in the intensive care unit (ICU; ~69%), and have a low mortality rate (~5%).[3,4] The remaining cohort of difficult-to-wean (requiring up to three attempts or up to 7 days from the onset of weaning) or prolonged-wean (over three attempts or greater than 7 days from the onset of weaning) patients require greater effort to successfully liberate from mechanical ventilation. These difficult-to-wean and prolonged-wean patients have an associated higher mortality rate (~25%).[3,4]

Prolonged mechanical ventilation is associated with increased mortality[5] and costs (mechanical ventilation costs > US$2000/day).[6] It has been estimated that the 6% of patients who require prolonged mechanical ventilation consume 37% of ICU resources,[7] and 40–50% of the time spent undergoing mechanical ventilation occurs after this weaning process has started.[3,5,8] In part, the reason is that more severely ill patients usually require longer periods of mechanical ventilation. Prolonged weaning may result, however, from an excessive use of sedatives, the absence of weaning–liberation protocols, and the myriad of organizational and cultural factors that fail to optimize weaning conditions. In general, the duration of mechanical ventilation should be minimized, and liberation from mechanical ventilation should be considered as soon as possible.

Expert consensus[2] has proposed that the weaning process be considered in the following six steps:

1. Treatment of acute respiratory failure
2. Clinical judgment that weaning may be possible
3. Assessment of the readiness to wean
4. An SBT
5. Extubation
6. Possibly reintubation

Depending on the mechanism of acute respiratory failure—whether it is a problem of oxygenation, ventilation, or airway (or a combination)—most critically ill patients require a period in which they will require full ventilatory support after intubation. Consideration of the weaning process should begin very soon after intubation. Weaning involves several discrete logical and sequential steps. If patients fail to make sufficient progress, then a contingency plan is required. Failure to wean/liberate involves either (1) the failure of an SBT or (2) the need for reintubation/ventilation or death within 48 hours of extubation.[2]

CLINICAL SUSPICION THAT WEANING MAY BE POSSIBLE

Because of the significant morbidity and mortality associated with prolonged mechanical ventilation, it is generally accepted that all ventilated ICU patients should be assessed for their readiness to wean at least on a daily basis. The importance of this "readiness" assessment has been highlighted by several trials that have demonstrated that weaning can be achieved in most patients after the first formal assessment of readiness[9,10] and the finding that nearly 50% of unexpected self-extubations during the weaning process did not require reintubation.[11,12] The benefit of early weaning should be balanced against the significant morbidity and mortality associated with failed extubation. Two large prospective observational studies found a fivefold to tenfold increased mortality in patients requiring reintubation.[12,13] Though it is unclear how much of this effect is confounded by population and disease severity differences.[13]

ASSESSMENT OF READINESS TO WEAN

The clinical assessment of readiness to wean is a two-step process that is based on (1) the assessment of predictors of weaning and (2) the successful completion of an SBT. Both of these steps require a reliable and reproducible institutional sedation strategy that maximizes the patient's capability of being assessed and undergoing SBTs. Ventilator liberation protocols should be developed locally and in concert with analgesia protocols.[14,15]

The concept of nocturnal rest, in conjunction with daytime respiratory muscle training, is an important one for those patients whose weaning is more difficult and prolonged.

Predictors of Successful Weaning

The initial screening evaluation of readiness to wean is composed of a clinical examination and an assessment of several objective criteria (respiratory, cardiovascular, and neurologic) that aim to predict the likelihood of successfully weaning[3,4,8–10,16,17] (Table 9.1). Individually, these predictors are neither highly sensitive nor specific, but together with the clinical examination, they allow the clinician to identify patients who will clearly not be suitable for weaning and who may have detrimental effects from an aggressive reduction in ventilatory support. All other patients should undergo a SBT. This is an important point because (1) many patients who meet some but not all of the criteria for weaning will still successfully wean and (2) clinicians frequently underestimate the ability of patients to wean.

General Limitations of the Readiness-to-Wean Predictors

It is important to be aware of the general limitations of prediction criteria in assessing readiness to wean. The most significant difficulty is that in most studies failing an SBT (arguably a surrogate outcome) and reintubation after extubation (a patient important outcome) are treated as equivalent under a term such as "failure to wean." Confidence in the validity of this equivalence is undermined by the observation that a high percentage of patients ($> 50\%$) who experience unplanned extubation, and were presumably therefore judged not suitable for extubation, do not require reintubation.[18] An argument has been made that this equivalence therefore results in the conflation of "failure to extubate," a decision not to extubate, with "failed extubation" for an indeterminately large proportion of patients.[19] This means that the performance characteristics (e.g., negative predictive value) of a predictive weaning test in relation to the patient important outcome of extubation without reintubation is unknown in general. To accurately determine such performance characteristics would require extubation of all patients, including those failing the predictive test, and this seems unlikely to happen because of the ethical challenges involved in extubating a patient who has failed a predictive test. In the meantime, we are stuck, at least partly, predicting the results of SBTs. Fortunately, SBTs can be performed very easily and there is no evidence that a failed SBT harms the patient.

Individual Limitations of the Readiness-to-Wean Predictors

General limitations aside, it is additionally important to be aware of the individual limitations of the various prediction criteria because many have been examined only retrospectively, and of those which have been studied prospectively, many have demonstrated high false-positive and false-negative rates.

TABLE 9.1	**Clinical and Objective Measures of Readiness to Wean.**
Clinical Assessment	Resolution of Acute Process Requiring: Intubation/ventilation
	Patient awake and cooperative
	Chest wall pain controlled
	Adequate cough
	Absence of excessive tracheobronchial secretions
	Absence of
	Nasal flaring
	Suprasternal and intercostal recession
	Paradoxical movement of the rib cage or abdomen
Objective Measures	Respiratory Stability: Oxygenation
	$Sao_2 > 90\%$ on $Fio_2 \leq 0.4$
	$Pao_2 \geq 50\text{–}60$ mm Hg on $Fio_2 \leq 0.5$
	Alveolar-arterial Po_2 gradient < 350 mm Hg (Fio_2 1.0)
	$Pao_2/Fio_2 \geq 150$
	Respiratory Stability: Function
	Respiratory rate ≤ 35 breath/min
	Maximal inspiratory pressure ≤ -20 to -25 cm H_2O
	Tidal volume > 5 mL/kg
	Minute ventilation <10 L/min
	No significant respiratory acidosis
	Respiratory rate/tidal volume < 105 breaths/min/L[a]
	CROP index > 13 mL/breath/min[b]
	Integrative index of Jabour < 4 per minute[c]
	IWI of ≥ 25 mL/cm H_2O breaths/min/L[d]
	Cardiovascular Stability
	Heart rate <140 beats/min
	Systolic blood pressure > 90 and < 160 mm Hg
	Minimal inotropic/vasopressor support
	Neurologic Function
	Including normal mentation on sedation

[a]The respiratory rate/tidal volume ratio is also known as the RSBI.
[b]CROP index = [compliance (dynamic) × maximum inspiratory pressure × (arterial partial pressure of oxygen/alveolar partial pressure of oxygen)]/respiratory rate.
[c]Integrative index of Jabour = pressure time product × (minute ventilation to bring the $Paco_2$ to 40 mm Hg/tidal volume during spontaneous breathing).
[d]IWI = (compliance (static) × arterial oxygen saturation/(respiratory rate/tidal volume during spontaneous breathing).
CROP, Compliance, Respiratory rate, arterial Oxygenation and maximal inspiratory Pressure; *Fio₂*, fraction of inspired oxygen; *IWI*, integrative weaning index; *Pao₂*, partial pressure of arterial oxygen; *Po₂*, partial pressure of oxygen; *RSBI*, rapid shallow breathing index; *Sao₂*, arterial oxygen saturation.

A *minute ventilation* less than 10 L/min is only associated with a positive predictive value of 50% and a negative predictive value of 40%.[20] The *maximal inspiratory pressure*, a measure of respiratory muscle strength, was initially suggested to be a good indicator of weaning success.[21] These findings were not replicated in subsequent trials.

Static compliance (i.e., tidal volume/plateau pressure–positive end expiratory pressure) has a low positive predictive value (60%) and negative predictive value (53%).[20] *Occlusion pressure* (P0.1) is the airway pressure 0.1 second after the initiation of a spontaneous breath in a measure of respiratory drive. The results from studies determining the utility of this index have been conflicting to date.[22–24]

A reduction in central venous saturation of more than 4.5% at the 13th minute of an SBT in patients who had failed their first T-tube SBT was an independent predictor of reintubation, with a sensitivity of 88% and a specificity of 95%.[25] A previous study showed that on discontinuation of the ventilator, mixed venous oxygen saturation fell progressively in the failure group ($P = .01$), whereas it did not change in the success group.[26]

A low left ventricular ejection fraction (LVEF) (36% [27–55] vs. 51% [43–55], $P = .04$), shortened deceleration time of E wave (DTE), and increased Doppler E velocity to tissue Doppler E′ velocity ratio (E/E′) assessed by transesophageal echocardiography with an experienced operator were predictive of extubation failure in a prospective observational study.[27] This is obviously a test that is not routinely available at the bedside in most ICUs, and carries some additional risk, such as esophageal perforation.

B-type natriuretic peptide (BNP) and N-terminal pro-BNP levels either at baseline[28] or the relative change during an SBT[29–31] have been associated with extubation failure due to heart failure. There was significant heterogeneity, though, between results, which may be explained by the different populations studied, fluid balance, the use of cardioactive drugs, and underlying cardiovascular or renal dysfunction.

The rapid shallow breathing index (RSBI) (respiratory rate/tidal volume) measured over 1 minute in the spontaneously breathing patient has demonstrated a high sensitivity (97%) and a moderate specificity (65%) for predicting patients who will subsequently successfully pass an SBT compared with the other predictors.[20] The measurement of RSBI value may be affected by the airway pressure protocol. In prospective studies, RSBI values were significantly lower in patients while they were on a continuous positive airway pressure (CPAP) of 5 cm H_2O compared with T-piece (median 71 vs. 90 breaths/L/min)[32] or a spontaneously breathing room air trial without ventilator support (median 36 vs. 71 breaths/L/min).[33]

The trend rather than an individual value of RSBI may be a better predictor of weaning success. RSBI remained unchanged or decreased in successful extubation; in contrast, RSBI tended to increase in those who failed extubation in three prospective observational studies.[32,34–36] Although many clinicians use RSBI in their clinical practice, there is some controversy as to its utility: one small randomized controlled trial (RCT) reported that the use of this measure prolonged weaning time and did not reduce the incidence of extubation failure or tracheostomy.[37] This trial was small, though, and there was a high likelihood of selection bias and crossover in the non-RSBI utilization arm. Results from another RCT suggested that the predictive value of RSBI may be increased using automatic tube compensation (ATC).[38]

Overall, individual "predictor" criteria should not be considered as reliable indicators to predict successful weaning. However, it has been argued that combined with clinical examination they may assist the clinician in identifying patients who will clearly *not* be suitable for weaning and who may have detrimental effects from an unnecessary SBT. Empirical support for this philosophy requires further development and should not be considered as dogma.

The failure of individual indices to predict successful weaning prompted various investigators to combine several individual indices in an attempt to increase specificity and sensitivity. However, these predictors (see Table 9.1) are more complex and are more commonly used in clinical trials than in routine clinical practice.

A Compliance, Respiratory rate, arterial Oxygenation and maximal inspiratory Pressure (CROP) index (see Table 9.1) of more than 13 mL/breath/min has prospectively determined a positive predictive value of 71% and a negative predictive value of 70% to predict weaning success.[20] A *Jabour pressure time product* (see Table 9.1) of less than 4 per minute has been shown in a retrospective study to have a positive predictive value of 96% and a negative predictive value of 95%.[39]

An *integrative weaning index (IWI)* (see Table 9.1) of 25 mL/cm H_2O breaths/min/L or more has been shown in a prospective study to have a positive predictive value of 0.99 and a negative predictive value of 0.86 to predict weaning success ($n = 216$ in the prospective-validation group).[40] Future research is required to identify simple predictors that are sufficiently sensitive and specific to predict successful weaning. In the absence of such measures, the clinician should have a low threshold for conducting a daily SBT.

Spontaneous Breathing Trial

The initiation of the weaning process is defined as the commencement of the first SBT. There are several techniques that can be used to conduct an SBT. These include techniques such as (1) T-tube/T-piece, (2) PSV, or (3) ATC, all of which may be used with or without CPAP. Failure of an SBT is defined as the development of respiratory (function or oxygenation), cardiovascular, or neurologic instability and is determined by clinical assessment and objective testing during the trial (Table 9.2).[1] There appears to be little predictive advantage by increasing the duration of the SBT assessment to greater than 20–30 minutes.[4,41] Prospective studies have demonstrated that most patients successfully pass their first SBTs and more than 60% of patients successfully wean[2] (Table 9.3). Interestingly, to date, trials have not demonstrated that any one of these techniques is superior in its ability to predict weaning success (see Table 9.3). Recent guidelines have advocated the use of inspiratory pressure augmentation (5–8 cm H_2O) rather than without (T-piece or CPAP).[42] Nevertheless, clinicians still need to be aware of the relative advantages and disadvantages of each technique.

T-Tube/T-piece: This well-established method involves attaching the end of the endotracheal tube to a short piece of tubing that acts as a reservoir and a connection to the humidified fresh gas flow. There were initial concerns that

TABLE 9.2   Clinical and Objective Determinants of Failure of an SBT.

Clinical Assessment	Agitation and anxiety
	Reduced level of consciousness
	Significant sweating
	Cyanosis
	Evidence of increased respiratory muscle effort
	Increased accessory muscle usage
	Facial signs of distress
	Dyspnea
Objective Measures	Respiratory Stability: Oxygenation
	$PaO_2 \leq 50–60$ mm Hg on $FiO_2 \geq 0.5$ or $SaO_2 < 90\%$
	Respiratory Stability: Function
	$PaCO_2 > 50$ mm Hg or an increase in $PaCO_2 > 8$ mm Hg
	pH < 7.32 or a decrease of pH ≥ 0.07 pH units
	Respiratory rate/tidal volume >105 breaths/min/L[a]
	Respiratory rate > 35 breaths/min or increase $\geq 50\%$
	Cardiovascular Stability
	Heart rate > 140 beats/min (or increase $\geq 20\%$)
	Systolic blood pressure >180 mm Hg (or increase $\geq 20\%$)
	Systolic blood pressure < 90 mm Hg
	Significant cardiac arrhythmias
	Neurologic function
	Reduced level of consciousness

[a]The respiratory rate/tidal volume is also known as the RSBI.
FiO₂, fraction of inspired oxygen; *PaCO₂*, partial pressure of arterial carbon dioxide; *PaO₂*, partial pressure of arterial oxygen; *RSBI*, rapid shallow breathing index; *SaO₂*, arterial oxygen saturation; *SBT*, spontaneous breathing trial.

the increased resistance to airflow and the increased work of breathing induced by the endotracheal tube resulted in a workload in excess of that required when the tube was removed. These studies, however did not account for the airway inflammation and edema that frequently accompany extubation, which results in little difference between the preextubation and postextubation workload.[43,44] Therefore many clinicians use this method because it is simple, well tested, and imposes a pulmonary workload that is comparable to that encountered after extubation.

Pressure support ventilation: PSV is the most frequently used method for conducting the SBT and recent guidelines have endorsed defaulting to use of PSV during SBTs.[42] Despite the theoretical concerns that (1) the use of PSV may not mimic the "true" postextubation workload and (2) there is difficulty in predicting the level of PSV necessary to completely compensate for the resistive load,[45] this does not appear problematic in practice.[8,46,47] Pressure support is typically reduced to relatively low levels (≤ 10 cm H_2O) so that most of its impact is dissipated because of tube resistance and the patient

experiences no elevation in inspiratory pressure at the end of the endotracheal tube.[8,46–48] The major advantage of this technique over the T-piece is that it does not require disconnection from the ventilator, and apnea alarms and pressure monitors remain in place. Recent meta-analysis of RCTs relevant to the question of superiority of PSV in this context demonstrated that conducting the SBT with pressure augmentation was more likely to be successful (84.6% vs. 76.7%; risk ratio [RR] 1.11, 95% confidence interval [CI] 1.02–1.18); resulted in a higher rate of extubation success (75.4% vs. 68.9%; RR 1.09, 95% CI 1.02–1.18); and was associated with a trend towards lower ICU mortality (8.6% vs. 11.6%; RR 0.74, 95% CI 0.45–1.24).[42] It therefore seems likely that PSV will continue to be popular during SBTs.

Automatic tube compensation: ATC is an automatic method by which the ventilator compensates for the degree of resistance provided by the endotracheal tube that is increasingly found on modern ventilators. Because tube resistance varies with length, girth, and secretions, this is theoretically advantageous, but literature is limited. Haberthür and colleagues reported that ATC was as effective as PSV or T-piece weaning.[46] This result was subsequently confirmed by a larger RCT comparing PSV with ATC in 190 patients.[38] Figueroa-Casas and colleagues compared ATC with CPAP during SBT.[49] There was no difference in duration of weaning, rate of unsuccessful extubation, or duration of mechanical ventilation. A bench study showed that ATC may not sufficiently compensate for the pressure–time product increase caused by tracheal secretions and higher tidal volume.[50] Because low-level PSV achieves the same goals and because most weaning patients receive some PSV either alone or in conjunction with another ventilatory mode, the potential for ATC to add any clinically relevant benefit during weaning is questionable.

Continuous positive airway pressure: Proponents of CPAP argue that it increases functional residual capacity, maintains small airway patency, may be beneficial on left ventricular dysfunction, and has minimal harmful effects.[51] Despite the potential risk that a patient may pass the SBT but experience cardiac failure on extubation, most clinicians are comfortable using low levels of CPAP (<5 cm H_2O) in combination with the techniques mentioned earlier.

Automated weaning: Systems aim to reduce the requirement for clinician input in the weaning process and improve outcomes. The most commonly studied systems are SmartCare (Dräger Ventilators) and Adaptive Support Ventilation (ASV).[52] ASV can automatically switch from controlled to spontaneous ventilation, while SmartCare requires clinician input to initiate this. However, SmartCare can automatically reduce pressure support based on patient demographic and ventilator feedback parameters. It will provide the patient with SBT and recommend consideration of extubation when it considers an SBT successful.

A Cochrane meta-analysis compared automated weaning with usual care and found that pooled data from 16 trials

TABLE 9.3   Success of SBT and Success in Weaning from Mechanical Ventilation.

Author	Year	Number	Passed Initial SBT	Extubated at 48 h (From All Extubated)	Method
Trials Describing Success Rate of Initial SBT and Extubation					
Brochard[9]	1994	456	347 (76%)	330 (95%)	T-piece
Esteban[10]	1995	546	416 (76%)	358 (86%)	T-piece
Vallverdu[16]	1998	217	148 (68%)	125 (84%)	T-piece
Esteban[4]	1999	526	416 (79%)	346 (82%)	T-piece
Trials Describing Success Rate of Initial SBT and Extubation With Differing Techniques					
Esteban[95]	1997	484	397 (82%)	323 (81%)	PSV/T-piece
Subgroup		236	205 (86%)	167 (81%)	PSV 7 cm H_2O
Subgroup		246	192 (78%)	156 (81%)	T-piece
Farias[48]	2001	257	201 (78%)	173 (86%)	PSV/T-piece
Subgroup		125	99 (79%)	79 (80%)	PSV 10 cm H_2O
Subgroup		132	102 (77%)	89 (87%)	T-piece
Haberthur[a,46]	2002	90	78 (87%)	62 (79%)	ATC/PSV/T-piece
Subgroup		30	29 (96%)	25 (86%)	ATC
Subgroup		30	23 (77%)	18 (78%)	PSV 5 cm H_2O
Subgroup		30	24 (80%)	19 (79%)	T-piece
Matić[47]	2004	260	200 (77%)	Not specified	PSV/T-piece
Subgroup		110	80 (73%)	Not specified	T-piece
Subgroup		150	120 (80%)	Not specified	PSV
Cohen	2006	99	90 (91%)	73 (74%)	ATC/CPAP
Subgroup		51	49 (96%)	42 (82%)	ATC
Subgroup		48	41 (85%)	31 (65%)	CPAP
Cohen[38]	2009	190	161 (85%)	139 (86%)	ATC/PSV
Subgroup		87	81 (93%)	71 (88%)	ATC
Subgroup		93	80 (86%)	68 (85%)	PSV
Figueroa-Casas[49]	2010	118	108 (92%)	115 (97%)	ATC/CPAP
Subgroup		58	56 (97%)	57 (99%)	ATC
Subgroup		60	52 (87%)	58 (97%)	CPAP

[a]Some patients initially randomized to the T-piece/PSV groups who failed an SBT were subsequently extubated after an ATC trial.
ATC, automatic tube compensation; *CPAP,* continuous positive airway pressure; *PSV,* pressure support ventilation; *SBT,* spontaneous breathing trial.

indicated that automated systems reduced mean weaning duration by 30% (95% CI 13–45%), though with substantial heterogeneity.[53] The authors concluded that automated systems may reduce weaning and ventilation duration and ICU stay but cautioned that due to substantial trial heterogeneity, an adequately powered, high-quality, multi-center RCT is needed to demonstrate this definitively. Consequently, routine use of automated weaning systems cannot be recommended at present outside of a research setting.

SUITABILITY FOR EXTUBATION

Extubation is the final stage in successful liberation of a patient from the mechanical ventilator, but it would be unwise to extubate any patient before assessing the ability of the patient to protect and maintain a patent airway. This clinical assessment involves (1) testing for an adequate level of consciousness, (2) cough strength, (3) frequency of secretions, and (4) airway patency. The likelihood of undergoing a successful extubation is significantly higher if the Glasgow Coma Score is 8 or greater.[54] In addition, although there are several objective measures of cough strength (e.g., card moistening[55] and spirometry[56]), most clinicians subjectively determine the presence of a moderate to strong cough before extubation. The presence of a weak cough, measured as a cough peak flow of 60 L/min or less, is a strong independent risk factor for extubation failure.[56–58] It is important to evaluate the volume and thickness of secretions because the likelihood of weaning success diminishes with increased secretions and reduced suctioning intervals.[17,55] Poor cough strength and greater secretions may have synergistic effects, reducing the chances of extubation success in burn and medical ICU patients.[57]

The most common test for airway patency is determination of a "cuff leak," which is neither sensitive nor specific. The presence of a "leak" after deflation of the endotracheal tube cuff is reassuring; however, the absence of a leak does not predict extubation failure.[59,60] In a recent systematic review,[61] the pooled likelihood ratio in published studies (three in total) for reintubation after failing a cuff leak test was 4.04 (95% CI 2.21–7.40) and after passing a cuff leak test was 0.46 (95% CI 0.26–0.82). Another meta-analysis, which included 16 studies, demonstrated that the area under the receiver operating curve (AUC) for laryngeal edema and reintubation was 0.89 and 0.82, respectively.[62] These performance characteristics have led to recent recommendations to restrict use of the cuff leak test to those at high risk of post stridor.[63] What should be done when a cuff leak is absent? Specifically, should corticosteroids be administered prior to any subsequent extubation attempt? In a recent guideline, the effect of systemic steroid therapy in patients who failed a cuff leak test was evaluated by pooling the estimates from three randomized trials.[63] Systemic steroid therapy reduced both the reintubation rate (5.8 vs. 17.0%; RR 0.32, 95% CI 0.14–0.76) and postextubation stridor rate (10.8 vs. 31.9%; RR 0.35, 95% CI 0.20–0.63) in patients who had failed a cuff leak test. A double-blind multicenter trial of 761 adults considered at high risk for postextubation laryngeal edema (ventilated > 36 hours) were pretreated and posttreated with methylprednisolone 12 hours before and every 4 hours after planned extubation, without regard to cuff leak testing.[64] Corticosteroid therapy reduced the incidence of reintubation by 4% and laryngeal edema by 11%. These data led to a consensus recommendation that patients who fail a cuff leak test but are otherwise ready for extubation receive systemic steroids for at least 4 hours before extubation.[63]

A recent multicenter RCT suggests one further step in patients who pass the SBT—reconnection to mechanical ventilation for 1 hour following a successful SBT.[65] In this study of 470 patients, the intervention group were reconnected to the ventilator at prior settings for 1 hour after successfully passing an SBT, whereas the control group were immediately extubated. The intervention was successful in reducing 48-hour reintubation rates (primary outcome 5% vs. 14%; odds ratio [OR] 0.33, 95% CI 0.16–0.65). The SBT and physiotherapy protocols were different from hospital to hospital and large numbers of potentially recruitable patients were excluded from the study. There were no differences in ICU length of stay, or mortality. Nevertheless, consideration should be made to integrating this into practice on the basis that it is cheap, simple, and carries little risk of harm.

Prior to extubation, consideration should also be given to the use of noninvasive ventilation (NIV) or high-flow nasal oxygen (HFNO) after extubation to reduce the risk of reintubation. NIV has been shown in some studies to reduce the risk of reintubation, particularly in patients with chronic lung disease.[66] The picture is complicated by notable failures to replicate such observations, particularly in patients without chronic lung disease.[67,68] Nevertheless, the use of NIV after extubation is gaining in popularity[69] and its use

in high-risk patients has been endorsed by recent consensus guidelines.[42] However, increasingly HFNO is being considered as an alternative strategy to reduce reintubation risk.[70] Hernández and colleagues undertook a multicenter RCT of critically ill patients at low risk of failed extubation.[71] They demonstrated that reintubation within 72 hours was lower in those randomized to HFNO postextubation compared to facemask oxygen therapy (absolute risk reduction 7.2%; 95% CI 2.5–12.2%). In a separate open-label, noninferiority, multicenter RCT, HFNO was noninferior to NIV in preventing reintubation in patients at high risk of failed extubation. After exclusion of nonrespiratory related reintubations, reintubation rate was 15.9% in the NIV group, and 16.9% in the HFNO group (absolute difference 1%; 95% CI −4.9%–6.9%). Therefore a growing body of evidence suggests that HFNO may be helpful in the prevention of postextubation respiratory failure and extubation failure in both high- and low-risk populations.[70]

VENTILATOR MANAGEMENT OF THE DIFFICULT-TO-WEAN PATIENT

The difficult-to-wean patient has already failed at least one SBT or required reintubation within 48 hours of extubation. The failure of an SBT may be accompanied by significantly increased inspiratory effort,[72] which translates to increased respiratory muscle workload.[73] This extra burden does not appear to cause long-lasting (low-frequency) fatigue, but it is uncertain whether it may induce short-lasting (high-frequency) fatigue.[72] Therefore after the failure of either an SBT or trial of extubation, the clinician must (1) determine the presence of exacerbating factors that reduced the success of weaning[2,74] (Table 9.4) and (2) provide ventilatory management to balance the need for adequate ventilator support (minimizing respiratory fatigue) against the need to minimize support (increase patient respiratory autonomy) to improve the chances of subsequent successful weaning.

The clinician should conduct a careful physical examination and review the patient's diagnostic tests to uncover and treat any reversible contributory factors (see Table 9.4). In the absence of any obvious remedial conditions or while such conditions are being treated, the patient should "rest" on the ventilator. The most commonly used modes of ventilation are assist-control mechanical ventilation (ACV), synchronized intermittent mechanical ventilation (SIMV), and PSV.

Assist-control mechanical ventilation: ACV is widely used to rest the respiratory muscles after the increased pulmonary workload during a failed weaning attempt. The diaphragm, in failure-to-wean patients, though, does not demonstrate that low-frequency muscle fatigue[75] and even short periods of ACV may induce diaphragm dysfunction and injury.[76] Weaning techniques that include respiratory muscle exercise are required to minimize respiratory muscle atrophy and dysfunction.

Synchronized intermittent mechanical ventilation: The use of SIMV as a weaning tool involves a progressive reduction of the mechanical ventilator respiratory rate in steps of

TABLE 9.4 Assessment of Factors that Reduce the Success of Weaning.

Respiratory	Increased restrictive load: broncho-spasm, tube kinking, tube obstruction Increased chest wall elastic load: pleural effusion, pneumothorax, abdominal distension Increase lung elastic load: infection, edema, hyperinflation
Cardiovascular	Cardiac dysfunction either long standing or secondary to increased load
Neuromuscular	Depressed central drive: metabolic alkalosis, sedatives, analgesics Neural transmission: spinal cord injury, Guillain–Bárre syndrome, myasthenia gravis, phrenic nerve injury Peripheral dysfunction: critical illness neuropathy and myopathy
Neurophysiologic	Delirium Depression Anxiety
Metabolic	Hypophosphatemia Hypomagnesemia Hypokalemia Hyperglycemia Steroid use—controversial
Nutrition	Obesity Malnutrition Overfeeding
Anemia	Hemoglobin 7.0–10.0 g/dL

1–3 breaths/min, and 30–60 minutes later, the patient is assessed for signs of failure to adapt to the increased patient load (similar to failure of breathing trial criteria; see Table 9.2). Accumulated evidence suggests that SIMV is a suboptimal weaning mode.

SIMV involves three different types of breath: a volume- or pressure-controlled breath, a volume- or pressure-assisted breath, and a spontaneous breath that is usually pressure supported. SIMV may contribute to respiratory muscle fatigue or prevent recovery from fatigue[10] secondary to an increased work of breathing associated with patient–ventilator dyssynchrony, increased effort to activate the SIMV demand valve, inadequate gas flow,[77,78] or the inability of the respiratory center to coordinate with the intermittent nature of the support and different types of breath.[73]

A 457-patient RCT demonstrated that SIMV (with T-piece SBTs) resulted in a slightly longer duration of mechanical ventilation (9.9 ± 8.2 days) compared with a PSV strategy (9.7 ± 3.7 days).[9] This trial also found that SIMV had higher rates of weaning failure (SIMV 42%, PSV 23%, T-piece 43%). Esteban and colleagues looked at four different weaning approaches involving 546 patients and reported that an SIMV-based weaning strategy resulted in longer duration of mechanical ventilation (5 days) compared with a PSV-based strategy (4 days) and T-piece ventilation (3 days).[10]

Pressure support ventilation: PSV allows the patient to determine the depth, length, flow, and rate of breathing.[79] PSV can be used for SBTs (typically ≤ 10 cm H_2O) or, less effectively, as a weaning tool involving the gradual reduction of pressure support by 2–4 cm H_2O once or twice a day as tolerated. This method results in a progressive reduction in ventilatory support over hours to days. Two large RCTs have demonstrated that PSV is superior to SIMV in reducing the duration of mechanical ventilation of difficult-to-wean patients.[9,10] Although one of these trials demonstrated that PSV weaning was more efficient than T-piece weaning,[9] the other trial demonstrated T-piece trials to be superior.[10] However, these potentially contradictory results may be accounted for by differences in the trial weaning protocols. One small, prospective RCT has suggested that pressure support weaning is superior to T-piece weaning in patients with chronic obstructive pulmonary disease (COPD).[80] Overall, progressive decrements in pressure support, as part of a challenge-to-wean protocol, should be limited to patients who fail spontaneous weaning trials.

T-piece trials: This method is the oldest ventilator weaning technique and involves sequentially increasing the amount of time the patient spends on the T-piece.[9,10] Traditionally, many units repeatedly placed patients on T-tubes for a short period multiple times each day. The demonstration that single daily T-tube trials were as efficient, though, has significantly reduced the clinical use of this more labor-intensive practice.[10] T-piece trials are limited by the absence of apnea and volume alarms in this setting.

Noninvasive ventilation: The increasing clinical use and familiarity with NIV in the critical care setting makes it an attractive tool in the difficult-to-wean patient. The potential advantages of NIV are to avoid the complications of intubation and sedation and reduce the total time of invasive mechanical ventilation. The use of NIV in weaning can be separated into (1) preventing extubation failure in selected patients, (2) being used as a rescue therapy for postextubation respiratory distress, and (3) permitting early extubation in patients who fail to meet standard extubation criteria.

1. ***Preventing extubation failure in selected patients (prophylactic therapy):*** Prophylactic NIV has the potential to prevent hypoxia, hypercapnia, and atelectasis and reduce the work of breathing, thereby reducing the rate of respiratory complications. RCTs have demonstrated that in high-risk postoperative patients (vascular, abdominal, and thoracicoabdominal surgery), NIV results in trends toward improved oxygenation and reduced infection rate, reintubation rate, length of hospital stay, and mortality.[81–83] This has resulted in a strong recommendation in recent guidelines that patients who are at high risk for extubation failure and who have passed a spontaneous breathing trial be extubated to preventive NIV.

2. ***Rescue therapy to avoid reintubation for postextubation respiratory distress (rescue therapy):*** NIV for patients

with acute postextubation respiratory failure (in the ICU) is ineffective.[66] A meta-analysis of two RCTs that compared NIV with the standard medical therapy in patients ($n = 302$) with postextubation respiratory failure did not demonstrate a reduction in the reintubation rate (RR 1.03, 95% CI 0.84–1.25) or ICU mortality (RR 1.14, 95% CI 0.43–3.0) in the NIV group.[84]

3. *Permitting early extubation in patients who fail to meet standard extubation criteria (facilitation therapy):* Interest has emerged in using NIV in highly selected patients to facilitate earlier removal of the endotracheal tube while still allowing a progressive stepwise reduction of ventilator support. This strategy involves extubating the patient who has failed an SBT directly on to NIV (PSV + CPAP) compared with standard therapy (invasive mechanical ventilation). Clearly, this approach can only be successful for patients who have good airway protection, a strong cough, and minimal secretions; therefore they are likely to be conscious, alert patients with slowly resolving lung injury but who retain good respiratory neuromuscular function. In the existing literature, these patients frequently have COPD. A meta-analysis of 16 trials involving 994 participants, most of whom had COPD, estimated that compared with continued invasive weaning, noninvasive weaning significantly reduced mortality (RR 0.53, 95% CI 0.36–0.80) without increasing the risk of weaning failure or reintubation.[85] However, invasive ventilation of patients with COPD has become less common, limiting the generalizability of these findings to modern ICU practice. Therefore, this paradigm has been significantly informed by a large, recent trial in a more heterogeneous cohort, the vast majority of whom did not have COPD (Breathe Trial).[86,87] The authors compared early extubation using protocolized noninvasive weaning with protocolized weaning with invasive ventilation in intubated patients who had failed their first spontaneous breathing trial. The primary outcome, time from randomization to liberation from both forms of ventilation, was not significantly different between the two groups, though patients in the noninvasive group did receive less invasive ventilation. In this way, the authors demonstrated that patients who failed a spontaneous breathing trial could be extubated to noninvasive ventilation, thereby shortening the period of invasive ventilation, but this change in the mode of ventilatory support did not appear to change the overall duration of ventilation of any form. Furthermore, there were no differences between groups across a series of prespecified secondary outcomes and important subgroup analyses, including rates of reintubation, tracheostomy, mortality at 30 and 180 days, and long-term health-related quality of life. In post hoc analyses, patients in the noninvasive ventilation group had fewer days with sedation and a shorter length of ICU stay. Following this study, clinicians might reasonably conclude that, for patients in whom a spontaneous breathing trial fails, ventilation is still required, although not necessarily via the endotracheal

route.[87] NIV may offer advantages such as the ability to speak, and perhaps reduced need for sedation and intensive care nursing and resources. In deciding between invasive and noninvasive weaning, clinicians may wish to take into account the relative advantages of each and their value to individual patients.

Role of Tracheostomy in Weaning

The insertion of a tracheostomy tube (whether surgical or percutaneous) is an important tool in the difficult-to-wean patient. Tracheostomy is usually far less irritating to the patient than an endotracheal tube, and the decreased sedation requirements usually enable weaning strategies that would otherwise not be possible. Tracheostomy also provides a more secure airway,[88] reduces vocal cord damage, reduces the work of breathing, and facilitates airway toilet.[89,90] A meta-analysis of RCTs comparing early with late or no tracheostomy concluded that the accumulated evidence suggested that early tracheostomy was not associated with lower mortality but may reduce the incidence of pneumonia in the ICU.[91]

Consideration of Weaning Protocols

Several studies have reported that either lack of attention to screening for the ability to progress or the unnecessary delay in progression through the weaning steps is associated with increased morbidity and mortality[3,17,92] and that weaning protocols have resulted in reduced ventilator-associated pneumonia, self-extubation rates, tracheostomy rates, and cost.[3,8] A Cochrane review suggested that a protocolized weaning strategy may result in a shorter duration of weaning and ICU stay.[93] Reductions were most likely to occur in medical, surgical, and mixed ICUs, but not in neurosurgical ICUs. However, significant heterogeneity among studies means caution should be exercised in generalizing results. Some authors of the included studies suggested that organizational context may influence outcomes; however, these factors were not considered in all included studies and could not be evaluated on review. The use of such protocols therefore remains controversial, with some suggesting that informed clinical judgment is superior. In an Italian multicenter study, higher levels of physician-to-patient ratios resulted in shorter weaning duration, suggesting that physician input is important to earlier weaning.[94]

AUTHORS' RECOMMENDATIONS
- Assessment of readiness to wean and reduction in sedative infusions should be considered early and frequently in critically ill patients receiving mechanical ventilation.
- Unless contraindicated, clinicians should commence weaning as early as possible following intubation.
- Once the acute insult has resolved, clinicians should have a low threshold for conducting an SBT in all critically ill patients.
- The SBT should last more than 30 minutes and may use the following:
  - A T-piece/T-tube
  - PSV (≤ 10 cm H_2O)

- ATC
- ± CPAP (≤ 5 cm H_2O)
- Current data support PSV as being the simplest and most effective technique.
- If the patient fails an SBT, then the clinician should do the following:
  - Address all contributory causes of failure to wean
  - Not perform a repeat SBT for 24 hours
  - Support the patient with a nonfatiguing mode of ventilation (most commonly PSV)
  - Consider tracheostomy.
- Consideration should be given to liberation to noninvasive ventilation or high-flow nasal cannulae in high-risk patients.
- Weaning, challenge to wean, and liberation protocols should be considered in ICUs.

REFERENCES

1. Slutsky AS. Mechanical ventilation. American College of Chest Physicians' Consensus Conference. *Chest.* 1993;104(6):1833-1859.
2. Boles JM, Bion J, Connors A, et al. Weaning from mechanical ventilation. *Eur Respir J.* 2007;29(5):1033-1056.
3. Ely EW, Baker AM, Dunagan DP, et al. Effect on the duration of mechanical ventilation of identifying patients capable of breathing spontaneously. *N Engl J Med.* 1996;335(25):1864-1869.
4. Esteban A, Alía I, Tobin MJ, et al. Effect of spontaneous breathing trial duration on outcome of attempts to discontinue mechanical ventilation. *Am J Respir Crit Care Med.* 1999;159(2):512-518.
5. Esteban A, Anzueto A, Frutos F, et al. Characteristics and outcomes in adult patients receiving mechanical ventilation: a 28-day international study. *JAMA.* 2002;287(3):345-355.
6. Cooper LM, Linde-Zwirble WT. Medicare intensive care unit use: analysis of incidence, cost, and payment. *Crit Care Med.* 2004;32(11):2247-2253.
7. Wagner DP. Economics of prolonged mechanical ventilation. *Am Rev Respir Dis.* 1989;140(2 Pt 2):S14-S18.
8. Kollef MH, Shapiro SD, Silver P, et al. A randomized, controlled trial of protocol-directed versus physician-directed weaning from mechanical ventilation. *Crit Care Med.* 1997;25(4):567-574.
9. Brochard L, Rauss A, Benito S, et al. Comparison of three methods of gradual withdrawal from ventilatory support during weaning from mechanical ventilation. *Am J Respir Crit Care Med.* 1994;150(4):896-903.
10. Esteban A, Frutos F, Tobin MJ, et al. A comparison of four methods of weaning patients from mechanical ventilation. Spanish Lung Failure Collaborative Group. *N Engl J Med.* 1995;332(6):345-350.
11. Epstein SK, Nevins ML, Chung J. Effect of unplanned extubation on outcome of mechanical ventilation. *Am J Respir Crit Care Med.* 2000;161(6):1912-1916.
12. Thille AW, Harrois A, Schortgen F, Brun-Buisson C, Brochard L. Outcomes of extubation failure in medical intensive care unit patients. *Crit Care Med.* 2011;39(12):2612-2618.
13. Menon N, Joffe AM, Deem S, et al. Occurrence and complications of tracheal reintubation in critically ill adults. *Respir Care.* 2012; 57(10):1555-1563.
14. Kress JP, Pohlman AS, O'Connor MF, Hall JB. Daily interruption of sedative infusions in critically ill patients undergoing mechanical ventilation. *N Engl J Med.* 2000;342(20):1471-1477.
15. Kress JP, Gehlbach B, Lacy M, Pliskin N, Pohlman AS, Hall JB. The long-term psychological effects of daily sedative interruption on critically ill patients. *Am J Respir Crit Care Med.* 2003;168(12):1457-1461.
16. Vallverdú I, Calaf N, Subirana M, Net A, Benito S, Mancebo J. Clinical characteristics, respiratory functional parameters, and outcome of a two-hour T-piece trial in patients weaning from mechanical ventilation. *Am J Respir Crit Care Med.* 1998;158(6): 1855-1862.
17. Coplin WM, Pierson DJ, Cooley KD, Newell DW, Rubenfeld GD. Implications of extubation delay in brain-injured patients meeting standard weaning criteria. *Am J Respir Crit Care Med.* 2000;161(5):1530-1536.
18. Chao CM, Sung MI, Cheng KC, et al. Prognostic factors and outcomes of unplanned extubation. *Sci Rep.* 2017;7(1):8636.
19. Aberegg SK. *Medical evidence blog*: bite the bullet and pull it: the NIKE approach to extubation. Medical Evidence Blog. 2012. Available at: http://www.medicalevidenceblog. com/2012/12/just-do-it-nike-approach-to-extubation.html. Accessed October 13, 2018.
20. Yang KL, Tobin MJ. A prospective study of indexes predicting the outcome of trials of weaning from mechanical ventilation. *N Engl J Med.* 1991;324(21):1445-1450.
21. Sahn SA, Lakshminarayan S. Bedside criteria for discontinuation of mechanical ventilation. *Chest.* 1973;63(6):1002-1005.
22. Herrera M, Blasco J, Venegas J, Barba R, Doblas A, Marquez E. Mouth occlusion pressure (P0.1) in acute respiratory failure. *Intensive Care Med.* 1985;11(3):134-139.
23. Capdevila XJ, Perrigault PF, Perey PJ, Roustan JP, d'Athis F. Occlusion pressure and its ratio to maximum inspiratory pressure are useful predictors for successful extubation following T-piece weaning trial. *Chest.* 1995;108(2):482-489.
24. Montgomery AB, Holle RH, Neagley SR, Pierson DJ, Schoene RB. Prediction of successful ventilator weaning using airway occlusion pressure and hypercapnic challenge. *Chest.* 1987;91(4):496-499.
25. Teixeira C, da Silva NB, Savi A, et al. Central venous saturation is a predictor of reintubation in difficult-to-wean patients. *Crit Care Med.* 2010;38(2):491-496.
26. Jubran A, Mathru M, Dries D, Tobin MJ. Continuous recordings of mixed venous oxygen saturation during weaning from mechanical ventilation and the ramifications thereof. *Am J Respir Crit Care Med.* 1998;158(6):1763-1769.
27. Caille V, Amiel JB, Charron C, Belliard G, Vieillard-Baron A, Vignon P. Echocardiography: a help in the weaning process. *Crit Care.* 2010;14(3):R120.
28. Mekontso-Dessap A, de Prost N, Girou E, et al. B-type natriuretic peptide and weaning from mechanical ventilation. *Intensive Care Med.* 2006;32(10):1529-1536.
29. Chien JY, Lin MS, Huang YC, Chien YF, Yu CJ, Yang PC. Changes in B-type natriuretic peptide improve weaning outcome predicted by spontaneous breathing trial. *Crit Care Med.* 2008; 36(5):1421-1426.
30. Grasso S, Leone A, De Michele M, et al. Use of N-terminal pro-brain natriuretic peptide to detect acute cardiac dysfunction during weaning failure in difficult-to-wean patients with chronic obstructive pulmonary disease. *Crit Care Med.* 2007;35(1):96-105.
31. Zapata L, Vera P, Roglan A, Gich I, Ordonez-Llanos J, Betbesé AJ. B-type natriuretic peptides for prediction and diagnosis of weaning failure from cardiac origin. *Intensive Care Med.* 2011;37(3):477-485.

32. Patel KN, Ganatra KD, Bates JH, Young MP. Variation in the rapid shallow breathing index associated with common measurement techniques and conditions. *Respir Care*. 2009; 54(11):1462-1466.

33. El-Khatib MF, Jamaleddine GW, Khoury AR, Obeid MY. Effect of continuous positive airway pressure on the rapid shallow breathing index in patients following cardiac surgery. *Chest*. 2002;121(2):475-479.

34. Verceles AC, Diaz-Abad M, Geiger-Brown J, Scharf SM. Testing the prognostic value of the rapid shallow breathing index in predicting successful weaning in patients requiring prolonged mechanical ventilation. *Heart Lung*. 2012;41(6):546-552.

35. Adams RC, Gunter OL, Wisler JR, et al. Dynamic changes in respiratory frequency/tidal volume may predict failures of ventilatory liberation in patients on prolonged mechanical ventilation and normal preliberation respiratory frequency/tidal volume values. *Am Surg*. 2012;78(1):69-73.

36. Segal LN, Oei E, Oppenheimer BW, et al. Evolution of pattern of breathing during a spontaneous breathing trial predicts successful extubation. *Intensive Care Med*. 2010;36(3):487-495.

37. Tanios MA, Nevins ML, Hendra KP, et al. A randomized, controlled trial of the role of weaning predictors in clinical decision making. *Crit Care Med*. 2006;34(10):2530-2535.

38. Cohen J, Shapiro M, Grozovski E, Fox B, Lev S, Singer P. Prediction of extubation outcome: a randomised, controlled trial with automatic tube compensation vs. pressure support ventilation. *Crit Care*. 2009;13(1):R21.

39. Jabour ER, Rabil DM, Truwit JD, Rochester DF. Evaluation of a new weaning index based on ventilatory endurance and the efficiency of gas exchange. *Am Rev Respir Dis*. 1991;144(3 Pt 1):531-537.

40. Nemer SN, Barbas CS, Caldeira JB, et al. A new integrative weaning index of discontinuation from mechanical ventilation. *Crit Care*. 2009;13(5):R152.

41. Perren A, Domenighetti G, Mauri S, Genini F, Vizzardi N. Protocol-directed weaning from mechanical ventilation: clinical outcome in patients randomized for a 30-min or 120-min trial with pressure support ventilation. *Intensive Care Med*. 2002;28(8):1058-1063.

42. Ouellette DR, Patel S, Girard TD, et al. Liberation from mechanical ventilation in critically ill adults: an official American College of Chest Physicians/American Thoracic Society clinical practice guideline: inspiratory pressure augmentation during spontaneous breathing trials, protocols minimizing sedation, and noninvasive ventilation immediately after extubation. *Chest*. 2017;151(1):166-180.

43. Straus C, Louis B, Isabey D, Lemaire F, Harf A, Brochard L. Contribution of the endotracheal tube and the upper airway to breathing workload. *Am J Respir Crit Care Med*. 1998;157(1):23-30.

44. Mehta S, Nelson DL, Klinger JR, Buczko GB, Levy MM. Prediction of post-extubation work of breathing. *Crit Care Med*. 2000;28(5):1341-1346.

45. Nathan SD, Ishaaya AM, Koerner SK, Belman MJ. Prediction of minimal pressure support during weaning from mechanical ventilation. *Chest*. 1993;103(4):1215-1219.

46. Haberthür C, Mols G, Elsasser S, Bingisser R, Stocker R, Guttmann J. Extubation after breathing trials with automatic tube compensation, T-tube, or pressure support ventilation. *Acta Anaesthesiol Scand*. 2002;46(8):973-979.

47. Matić I, Majerić-Kogler V. Comparison of pressure support and T-tube weaning from mechanical ventilation: randomized prospective study. *Croat Med J*. 2004;45(2):162-166.

48. Farias JA, Retta A, Alía I, et al. A comparison of two methods to perform a breathing trial before extubation in pediatric intensive care patients. *Intensive Care Med*. 2001;27(10):1649-1654.

49. Figueroa-Casas JB, Montoya R, Arzabala A, Connery SM. Comparison between automatic tube compensation and continuous positive airway pressure during spontaneous breathing trials. *Respir Care*. 2010;55(5):549-554.

50. Oto J, Imanaka H, Nakataki E, Ono R, Nishimura M. Potential inadequacy of automatic tube compensation to decrease inspiratory work load after at least 48 hours of endotracheal tube use in the clinical setting. *Respir Care*. 2012;57(5):697-703.

51. Hess D. Ventilator modes used in weaning. *Chest*. 2001;120 (6 suppl):474S-476S.

52. Rose L, Schultz MJ, Cardwell CR, Jouvet P, McAuley DF, Blackwood B. Automated versus non-automated weaning for reducing the duration of mechanical ventilation for critically ill adults and children: a cochrane systematic review and meta-analysis. *Crit Care*. 2015;19(1):48.

53. Burns KE, Lellouche F, Lessard MR, Friedrich JO. Automated weaning and spontaneous breathing trial systems versus non-automated weaning strategies for discontinuation time in invasively ventilated postoperative adults. *Cochrane Database Syst Rev*. 2014;(2):CD008639.

54. Namen AM, Ely EW, Tatter SB, et al. Predictors of successful extubation in neurosurgical patients. *Am J Respir Crit Care Med*. 2001;163(3 Pt 1):658-664.

55. Khamiees M, Raju P, DeGirolamo A, Amoateng-Adjepong Y, Manthous CA. Predictors of extubation outcome in patients who have successfully completed a spontaneous breathing trial. *Chest*. 2001;120(4):1262-1270.

56. Smina M, Salam A, Khamiees M, Gada P, Amoateng-Adjepong Y, Manthous CA. Cough peak flows and extubation outcomes. *Chest*. 2003;124(1):262-268.

57. Salam A, Tilluckdharry L, Amoateng-Adjepong Y, Manthous CA. Neurologic status, cough, secretions and extubation outcomes. *Intensive Care Med*. 2004;30(7):1334-1339.

58. Smailes ST, McVicar AJ, Martin R. Cough strength, secretions and extubation outcome in burn patients who have passed a spontaneous breathing trial. *Burns*. 2013;39(2):236-242.

59. Fisher MM, Raper RF. The 'cuff-leak' test for extubation. *Anaesthesia*. 1992;47(1):10-12.

60. Maury E, Guglielminotti J, Alzieu M, Qureshi T, Guidet B, Offenstadt G. How to identify patients with no risk for postextubation stridor? *J Crit Care*. 2004;19(1):23-28.

61. Ochoa ME, Marín Mdel C, Frutos-Vivar F, et al. Cuff-leak test for the diagnosis of upper airway obstruction in adults: a systematic review and meta-analysis. *Intensive Care Med*. 2009; 35(7):1171-1179.

62. Zhou T, Zhang HP, Chen WW, et al. Cuff-leak test for predicting postextubation airway complications: a systematic review. *J Evid Based Med*. 2011;4(4):242-254.

63. Girard TD, Alhazzani W, Kress JP, et al. An Official American Thoracic Society/American College of Chest Physicians clinical practice guideline: liberation from mechanical ventilation in critically ill adults. Rehabilitation protocols, ventilator liberation protocols, and cuff leak tests. *Am J Respir Crit Care Med*. 2017; 195(1):120-133.

64. François B, Bellissant E, Gissot V, et al. 12-h pretreatment with methylprednisolone versus placebo for prevention of postextubation laryngeal oedema: a randomised double-blind trial. *Lancet*. 2007;369(9567):1083-1089.

65. Fernandez MM, González-Castro A, Magret M, et al. Reconnection to mechanical ventilation for 1 h after a successful spontaneous breathing trial reduces reintubation in critically ill patients: a multicenter randomized controlled trial. *Intensive Care Med.* 2017;43(11):1660-1667.

66. Glossop AJ, Shephard N, Bryden DC, Mills GH. Non-invasive ventilation for weaning, avoiding reintubation after extubation and in the postoperative period: a meta-analysis. *Br J Anaesth.* 2012;109(3):305-314.

67. Girault C, Bubenheim M, Abroug F, et al. Noninvasive ventilation and weaning in patients with chronic hypercapnic respiratory failure: a randomized multicenter trial. *Am J Respir Crit Care Med.* 2011;184(6):672-679.

68. Su CL, Chiang LL, Yang SH, et al. Preventive use of noninvasive ventilation after extubation: a prospective, multicenter randomized controlled trial. *Respir Care.* 2011;57(2):204-210.

69. Demoule A, Chevret S, Carlucci A, et al. Changing use of noninvasive ventilation in critically ill patients: trends over 15 years in francophone countries. *Intensive Care Med.* 2016;42(1):82-92.

70. McGuigan P, Nutt C, Gowers C, Trainor D, MacSweeney R. *Critical Care Reviews Book 2018* (website). 2018. Available at: https://www.criticalcarereviews.com/index.php/2014-07-17-22-24-12/ccr16-book. Accessed October 14, 2018.

71. Hernández G, Vaquero C, González P, et al. Effect of postextubation high-flow nasal cannula vs conventional oxygen therapy on reintubation in low-risk patients: a randomized clinical trial. *JAMA.* 2016;315(13):1354.

72. Jubran A, Tobin MJ. Pathophysiologic basis of acute respiratory distress in patients who fail a trial of weaning from mechanical ventilation. *Am J Respir Crit Care Med.* 1997;155(3):906-915.

73. Imsand C, Feihl F, Perret C, Fitting JW. Regulation of inspiratory neuromuscular output during synchronized intermittent mechanical ventilation. *Anesthesiology.* 1994;80(1):13-22.

74. Alía I, Esteban A. Weaning from mechanical ventilation. *Crit Care.* 2000;4(2):72.

75. Laghi F, Cattapan SE, Jubran A, et al. Is weaning failure caused by low-frequency fatigue of the diaphragm? *Am J Respir Crit Care Med.* 2003;167(2):120-127.

76. Vassilakopoulos T, Petrof BJ. Ventilator-induced diaphragmatic dysfunction. *Am J Respir Crit Care Med.* 2004;169(3):336-341.

77. Gherini S, Peters RM, Virgilio RW. Mechanical work on the lungs and work of breathing with positive end-expiratory pressure and continuous positive airway pressure. *Chest.* 1979;76(3):251-256.

78. Gibney RT, Wilson RS, Pontoppidan H. Comparison of work of breathing on high gas flow and demand valve continuous positive airway pressure systems. *Chest.* 1982;82(6):692-695.

79. MacIntyre NR. Respiratory function during pressure support ventilation. *Chest.* 1986;89(5):677-683.

80. Matić I, Danić D, Majerić-Kogler V, Jurjević M, Mirković I, Mrzljak Vucinić N. Chronic obstructive pulmonary disease and weaning of difficult-to-wean patients from mechanical ventilation: randomized prospective study. *Croat Med J.* 2007;48(1):51-58.

81. Böhner H, Kindgen-Milles D, Grust A, et al. Prophylactic nasal continuous positive airway pressure after major vascular surgery: results of a prospective randomized trial. *Langenbecks Arch Surg.* 2002;387(1):21-26.

82. Squadrone V, Coha M, Cerutti E, et al. Continuous positive airway pressure for treatment of postoperative hypoxemia: a randomized controlled trial. *JAMA.* 2005;293(5):589.

83. Kindgen-Milles D, Müller E, Buhl R, et al. Nasal-continuous positive airway pressure reduces pulmonary morbidity and length of hospital stay following thoracoabdominal aortic surgery. *Chest.* 2005;128(2):821-828.

84. Agarwal R, Aggarwal AN, Gupta D, Jindal SK. Role of noninvasive positive-pressure ventilation in postextubation respiratory failure: a meta-analysis. *Respir Care.* 2007;52(11):1472-1479.

85. Burns KE, Meade MO, Premji A, Adhikari NK. Noninvasive ventilation as a weaning strategy for mechanical ventilation in adults with respiratory failure: a Cochrane systematic review. *CMAJ.* 2014;186(3):E112-E122.

86. Perkins GD, Mistry D, Gates S, et al; Breathe Collaborators. Effect of protocolized weaning with early extubation to noninvasive ventilation vs invasive weaning on time to liberation from mechanical ventilation among patients with respiratory failure: the Breathe Randomized Clinical Trial. *JAMA.* 2018;320(18):1881-1888.

87. Munshi L, Ferguson ND. Weaning from mechanical ventilation: what should be done when a patient's spontaneous breathing trial fails? *JAMA.* 2018;320(18):1865-1867.

88. Stauffer JL, Olson DE, Petty TL. Complications and consequences of endotracheal intubation and tracheotomy. A prospective study of 150 critically ill adult patients. *Am J Med.* 1981;70(1):65-76.

89. Diehl JL, El Atrous S, Touchard D, Lemaire F, Brochard L. Changes in the work of breathing induced by tracheotomy in ventilator-dependent patients. *Am J Respir Crit Care Med.* 1999;159(2):383-388.w

90. Davis Jr K, Campbell RS, Johannigman JA, Valente JF, Branson RD. Changes in respiratory mechanics after tracheostomy. *Arch Surg.* 1999;134(1):59-62.

91. Siempos II, Ntaidou TK, Filippidis FT, Choi AMK. Effect of early versus late or no tracheostomy on mortality and pneumonia of critically ill patients receiving mechanical ventilation: a systematic review and meta-analysis. *Lancet Respir Med.* 2015;3(2):150-158.

92. Ely EW, Baker AM, Evans GW, Haponik EF. The prognostic significance of passing a daily screen of weaning parameters. *Intensive Care Med.* 1999;25(6):581-587.

93. Blackwood B, Burns KE, Cardwell CR, O'Halloran P. Protocolized versus non-protocolized weaning for reducing the duration of mechanical ventilation in critically ill adult patients. *Cochrane Database Syst Rev.* 2014;(11):CD006904.

94. Polverino E, Nava S, Ferrer M, et al. Patients' characterization, hospital course and clinical outcomes in five Italian respiratory intensive care units. *Intensive Care Med.* 2010;36(1):137-142.

95. Esteban A, Alía I, Gordo F, et al. Extubation outcome after spontaneous breathing trials with T-tube or pressure support ventilation. The Spanish Lung Failure Collaborative Group. *Am J Respir Crit Care Med.* 1997;156(2 Pt 1):459-465.

10

How Does Mechanical Ventilation Damage Lungs? What Can Be Done to Prevent It?

Ron Leong, Joshua A. Marks, and Maurizio Cereda

INTRODUCTION AND DEFINITIONS

In order to address the question of how mechanical ventilation damages lungs, one must first understand several commonly utilized related terms:

Ventilator-induced lung injury (VILI) is the term used to denote acute lung damage that develops during mechanical ventilation. Alveolar overdistension, lung strain, and atelectasis are the key inciting and defining features of VILI. Overdistension or lung stress reflects the presence of an elevated transpulmonary pressure—the difference between the airway pressure and the pleural pressure—at the end of inspiration. Strain is the ratio of the volume of gas delivered during a tidal breath to the amount of aerated lung receiving that breath: larger strain is matched by a higher mechanical stress on alveolar structures.[1] In animal models, VILI is characterized by inflammatory cell infiltrates, hyaline membranes, alveolar hemorrhage, increased vascular permeability, pulmonary edema, loss of functional surfactant, and ultimately alveolar collapse. In patients, the clinical presentation of VILI is largely indistinguishable from ARDS. Nevertheless, ventilator strategies designed to reduce VILI have improved outcomes among patients with acute respiratory distress syndrome (ARDS) and in the perioperative setting, highlighting the clinical importance of VILI.

The *"baby lung"* concept explains how larger tidal volumes (V_T) worsen ARDS. In previously healthy animal lungs, very large (not used clinically) V_T is necessary to cause VILI.[1] However, early studies using computed tomography (CT) in supine ARDS patients[2] showed heterogeneous consolidation and atelectasis in dorsal lung regions. Therefore, inspired gas is concentrated in a smaller, yet otherwise functional fraction of ventilated parenchyma in the ventral lung. This gas maldistribution causes regional overdistension and excessive strain from a clinically 'acceptable' V_T.[2] Conceptually, this is akin to delivering an "adult" V_T to a "baby lung." Later studies using metabolic imaging confirmed that tissue in the "baby lung" is inflamed in proportion to regional strain.[3]

Atelectrauma occurs with the repetitive, cyclic, opening and closing of airways and lung units during inspiration and expiration, respectively. The stretching or shear forces between aerated and atelectatic alveoli cause epithelial and endothelial cell injury and regional inflammation. Furthermore, air fluid levels cause epithelial shear and cell damage in the conducting small airways.[4]

Stress amplification occurs in areas where collapsed and ventilated airspaces are intermingled. High-resolution imaging shows that the ARDS lung is heterogeneous at a very small scale. Mechanical stress is then focally amplified at the interfaces between ventilated and nonventilated tissue,[5] and in areas where lung inflation is reduced due to microscopic atelectasis.[6] In these regions, large tidal changes in aeration ("unstable inflation") were associated with worse progression of injury (in animal models) and with mortality in human ARDS.[7]

Barotrauma is the result of ventilating at high lung volumes, which can lead to alveolar rupture, air leaks or even pneumothoraces, pneumomediastinum and subcutaneous emphysema. The critical component remains regional lung overdistension, however, and not necessarily high airway pressure. *Volutrauma* refers to the concept that volume, or rather lung stretching and not airway pressures, is the determinant of injury.

Biotrauma results from the physical forces of atelectrauma, barotrauma, and volutrauma that cause the release of intracellular mediators. Cells are either directly injured by these mediators or indirectly injured through the activation of cell-signaling pathways in epithelial, endothelial, or inflammatory cells. The translocation of these mediators or bacteria from the airspaces into the systemic circulation through areas of increased alveolar-capillary permeability—as is classically seen in ARDS or which may be a result of volutrauma —may lead to multiorgan dysfunction and death.[8]

Patient self-inflicted lung injury (P-SILI) refers to an injurious pattern of spontaneous breathing that worsens the initial injury when respiratory drive if strong. There are multiple proposed mechanisms through which spontaneous breathing during mechanical ventilation can worsen lung injury. These include large transpulmonary pressure and V_T, dorsal lung stretch due to vigorous diaphragmatic contractions,[9] exaggerated pulmonary blood flow,[10] and patient–ventilator dyssynchrony.[11]

HOW DO VENTILATORS DAMAGE THE LUNGS IN PATIENTS?

VILI is typically considered a form of secondary injury, and it is clearly an essential contributor to the evolution of ARDS.

It is also likely that mechanical ventilation influences the earliest stages of lung injury, before ARDS is established. However, how this happens is less clear.

Moderate V_T (i.e., 12 mL/kg) worsens survival of preexisting ARDS.[12] In an effort to reduce inspiratory strain, clinicians prescribe lower V_T (i.e., 6 mL/kg) according to patient's predicted body weight,[12] but there are two corollaries to the "baby lung" model that have relevant implications on clinical management.

First, the capacity and the strain of the ventilated lung are variable in patients, depending on the severity of injury. Indeed, patients with small lung capacity may undergo unacceptable stretch even with a low V_T.[13] Since it is hard to quantify overdistension and strain at the bedside—inspiratory airway pressures are notoriously inaccurate and a safe threshold is unknown—it is much more difficult to identify those subjects at increased risk of VILI who might benefit from an even further reduction in V_T.

The second corollary of the "baby lung" model is that there are some data that suggest that mechanical ventilation, associated with larger tidal volumes and low positive end-expiratory pressure (PEEP), may increase pulmonary complications in non-ARDS patients,[14] including intraoperative subjects.[15] Animal studies showed that the presence of systemic inflammation, as in sepsis, may raise the sensitivity to mechanical stress in lung tissue—less deformation is required to cause injury.[16] However, low V_T did not prevent lung injury after prolonged ventilation in a large animal model of sepsis.[17]

Atelectasis could contribute to generating injury in ARDS and in non-ARDS patients by increasing susceptibility to V_T dimensions. According to accepted paradigms of VILI, atelectrauma occurs in injured, collapsible regions,[18] but recent evidence showed that atelectasis modifies the distribution of mechanical stress and, consequently, of inflammation, in the lungs.[19] Poorly recruited lung units may render lungs more vulnerable to moderate V_T by reciprocally increasing stretch in ventilated airspaces.[19,20] Such mechanical stress is locally amplified where inflation is reduced or discontinuous.

Despite this compelling experimental evidence on the role of atelectasis in VILI, clinical trials showed only marginal effects of lung recruitment and high PEEP in established ARDS.[21–23] This could be due to the frequent ineffectiveness of study recruitment. A key characteristic of ARDS is the inflammatory changes that are heterogeneously distributed throughout the lung parenchyma,[3] an aspect ignored by consensus definitions of ARDS[24] and by most study enrollment criteria. This spatial variation may explain the inconsistent findings of many human trials. While a specific treatment such as high PEEP may very well improve one area of lung (e.g., by recruiting atelectasis), it may simultaneously worsen another (by stretching the "baby lung").[25]

Understanding spontaneous breathing during mechanical ventilation can help minimize P-SILI. Spontaneous breathing can be beneficial, as it preserves diaphragmatic muscle integrity and improves ventilation/perfusion matching in the dependent lung.[26] However, in a classic animal experiment, induced spontaneous hyperventilation led to an injury pattern similar to VILI.[27] The biological effects of spontaneous breathing superimposed on mechanical ventilation may depend on the degree of the preexisting lung injury: it could be helpful in mild—and harmful in severe—injury.[28] Supporting this concept, the early use of neuromuscular blockers increased the survival of severe ARDS.[29] Spontaneous breathing may be more harmful when inflammation and aeration are heterogeneously distributed, leading to a disproportionate level of lung strain.[3] In this setting, the negative pleural pressure that is generated is no longer distributed evenly across the lung surface. Instead, the inhomogeneity of aeration causes regional differences in pleural pressure, which is more negative in the dependent lung near the diaphragm.[9] The distending pressure gradient between the nondependent and dependent lung leads to pendelluft (intrapulmonary gas transfer), tidal recruitment, and local overstretch of the dependent lung. Furthermore, an unintended, augmented V_T and transpulmonary pressure can occur with a spontaneous breath due to a more negative pleural pressure during a ventilator-delivered breath. A high respiratory drive can lead to patient–ventilator dyssynchrony and is most commonly seen as "double triggering," the occurrence of two delivered ventilator breaths with a single patient-triggered effort, resulting in double the V_T.[30]

The interaction between the heart, pulmonary vasculature and lungs may also provide further insight into other mechanisms of VILI. During a spontaneous breath, the negative pleural pressure increases the pulmonary transvascular pressure—the difference between pulmonary capillary hydrostatic pressure and pleural pressure—leading to pulmonary edema in the presence of increased alveolar-capillary permeability.[9] Additionally, positive pressure ventilation will present varying loading conditions to the left and right side of the heart and, in certain situations, cause a harmful surge in pulmonary blood flow. A recent study showed that high volume inflation, potentiated by negative pleural pressure swings, can lead to fluctuating right ventricular output, cyclic disruption with amplified pulmonary blood flow, and ultimately pulmonary microvascular injury.[10] Interestingly, higher PEEP can potentially reduce the injurious breathing pattern by reducing the amplitude of negative pleural pressure swings, pendelluft, regional rapid inflation–deflation, cyclic interruption, and exaggeration of pulmonary blood flow.[9,10,31,32]

Recent interest in lung deflation-mediated injury may also provide further insight into VILI and is worth considering. While most attention is paid to the damage done by lung inflation, a "deflation injury" can also occur after sustained lung inflation with sudden deflation. Looking specifically at this ventilatory pattern in rats, a 2018 study showed compelling evidence for lung injury caused by increased pulmonary hydrostatic pressures from transient left ventricular strain (increased preload with sustained afterload).[32] Furthermore, expiratory kinetics may also play a role in VILI as stored elastic energy during lung inflation is preferentially distributed to the lung parenchyma during sudden deflation.[33]

Goebel and colleagues have demonstrated attenuation in stress amplification by decreasing the peak expiratory flow rate, thus preventing sudden lung deflation.[34]

HOW TO MINIMIZE LUNG DAMAGE

Ventilation with 6 mL/kg V_T rather than 12 mL/kg V_T improves ARDS outcomes[12] and is currently the accepted standard of care in established ARDS. An observational study confirmed a dose–response relationship between V_T size and ARDS mortality.[35] This study also showed that the effects of V_T selection during the ICU course extend into the long term.

The current clinical approach is to set the ventilator index V_T to predicted body weight (PBW) as a surrogate of lung size.[12] V_T is set to 4–6 mL/kg ideal body weight (IBW), assuring that the plateau pressure is less than 30 cm H_2O and accepting high $PaCO_2$ (partial pressure of arterial carbon dioxide). There is no universally accepted method of setting PEEP, but it may be adjusted according to ARDSnet protocols to maintain a goal PaO_2 (partial pressure of arterial oxygen) of 55–80 mm Hg and a SpO_2 (oxygen saturation by pulse oximetry) of 88–95%. Hypercapnia is tolerated, although the limits of acceptable pH and the effectiveness of metabolic correction remain unclear. While this strategy decreases mortality, it represents "a one size fits all model" that does not account for individual patient characteristics, such as lung capacity, recruitable atelectasis, and chest wall mechanics. As a consequence, weight-based V_T settings may leave a proportion of severely ill patients underprotected, while others may be treated with unnecessary aggressiveness (i.e., obese patients with low chest wall compliance). It is not clear how to personalize treatment. While bedside measurements of lung capacity and strain remain experimental, a promising approach seems to be titration to transpulmonary pressure measured via esophageal manometry.[36] This methodology allows to correct airway pressure for the effect of chest wall mechanics and to personalize both PEEP and V_T settings, aiming to minimize peak pulmonary distension while maintaining recruitment.[37]

The introduction of "driving pressure," measured as the difference between plateau pressure and PEEP, provides a more elegant way of titrating V_T to the patient's respiratory compliance (as a surrogate for lung capacity). The driving pressure represents the cyclical strain that is imposed on the ventilated lung parenchyma. Large meta-analyses in patients with ARDS and in patients undergoing general anesthesia have shown a correlation between higher driving pressure and increased mortality and pulmonary complications.[38,39] Although the available evidence on the use of driving pressure is promising, and it provides a valuable, complementary tool to identify patients at higher risk of death and VILI, we are still awaiting large clinical trials to fully validate its use.

For patients with the highest severity illness, it is possible that even the most aggressive V_T reduction does not achieve sufficient lung protection. The use of extracorporeal lung assist methods has been hypothesized and

implemented in select situations,[40] but a single, design-limited randomized trial is the only evidence of outcome benefit.[41] The EOLIA trial of 249 patients with severe ARDS demonstrated a 9% absolute mortality difference at 60 days with extracorporeal membrane oxygenation (ECMO), versus conventional mechanical ventilation (with crossover), but this was not statistically significant (relative risk 0.76, 95% confidence interval [CI] 0.55–1.04; $P = .09$).[42] This study appears underpowered, as mortality was significantly lower than anticipated in both groups. In addition, there was a high rate of crosssover (rescue ECMO was given to 28% of patients), which probably diluted any potential benefit from ECMO. An ongoing trial is investigating the efficacy of extracorporeal CO_2 removal with ultraprotective ventilation (4 mL/kg PBW) in ARDS patients.[43] High-frequency oscillatory ventilation (HFOV), an appealing technique for extreme V_T reduction and aggressive recruitment, was shown to increase mortality in a high-quality randomized controlled trial (RCT).[44]

Based on the existing evidence, ventilator management targeted to recruitment with high PEEP ("open lung ventilation") cannot be recommended as the standard of care in all ventilated patients.[21–23] A meta-analysis showed some benefit in ARDS patients with more severe hypoxemia.[45] In an effort to personalize PEEP settings, a recent trial[46] randomized ARDS patients to conventional lower PEEP vs. a more aggressive recruitment strategy targeting lower driving pressure. The study treatment was associated with worse mortality than the control group, which may be due to nonselective patient enrollment, aggressive recruitment maneuvers, and limited efficacy in driving pressure reduction.

The role of lung recruitment during general anesthesia is also undefined. The application of higher PEEP vs. lower PEEP was not beneficial in patients who were ventilated with low V_T during major abdominal surgery.[47] Furthermore, a recent trial tested driving-pressure guided management of intraoperative PEEP but found no decrease in postoperative complications (the primary outcome). However, the post hoc analysis detected some improvements in pulmonary and infections complications as well as a shorter ICU length of stay.[48] Future studies may provide more support for a personalized approach, possibly utilizing better instruments to stratify patients and monitor effectiveness, such as physiologic responses,[49] CT imaging,[50,51] esophageal manometry,[37] or bedside imaging tools such as electrical impedance tomography. In the meantime, the benefits of the "open lung" approach should be weighed in each patient against its tangible adverse effects. Similar caution should be applied to alternative ventilator modalities that augment mean airway pressures with the goal of maximizing recruitment, where published data, to date, exhibit high potential for bias.[52] Careful patient selection and monitoring of the effects of higher airway pressure on lung overdistension, pulmonary and systemic circulation,[53] and alveolar dead space should be used to avoid undesired responses.

The ACURASYS trial suggested that the outcomes of severe ARDS can be improved with the early adoption of a course of muscle relaxation.[29] It is likely that, by maintaining tight control of inspired strain and avoiding asynchronies in the early stage of severe ARDS, muscle paralysis optimizes protection from VILI or P-SILI. However, the design of this particular study did not clarify the impact of patient inspiratory effort nor the optimal or maximal duration of neuromuscular blockade. An ongoing trial is currently reassessing the impact of muscle relaxation in a larger population of patients.[54]

Managing patients in the prone position had dramatic positive effects on outcomes of severe ARDS.[55] In the PROS-EVA trial, prone positioning was used for longer periods of time (16 hours) and in more severely ill patients than in previous studies that had more ambiguous results. This favorable outcome was probably due to better lung protection from VILI rather than to gas exchange improvement. In fact, placing patients prone reopens collapsed dorsal lung regions without causing overdistension, a frequent side effect of PEEP.[56] Furthermore, experimental studies have shown that prone position attenuates the progression of mild lung injury, an effect that was related to decreased local stress in the dorsal lung vs. The supine position.[17,57] Therefore, prone positioning seems to have an effect of injury control and should be considered as a first-line adjunct to lung protective strategies in high-risk patients.

Approximately 67% of ARDS cases arise after hospital admission,[58] which provides ample opportunity for preventive interventions. It is thus likely that ventilator management has a role in generating new lung injury and worsening preexisting pulmonary lesions. However, predicting which patients are at risk for developing lung injury and ARDS as well as the potential severity of illness remains challenging. Scoring systems have been developed to identify patients at risk but are inconsistent in their application and ability to connect specific treatments with disease prevention.[59]

A meta-analysis showed beneficial outcome effects from the use of lower versus higher V_T in heterogeneous populations of non-ARDS patients in the ICU and in the operating room.[14] Based on this evidence, the use of low V_T seems logical in ventilated patients at risk of progression to ARDS. However, a word of caution is warranted. Many studies in non-ARDS groups have shown outcome differences when comparing largely different V_T values. Whether smaller differences in V_T would have shown similar effects is unclear, but many practitioners have already abandoned such large V_T (i.e., >10 mL/kg) in non-ARDS. To address this point, an ongoing international trial (PRotective VENTilation in patients without ARDS (PReVENT-NL, NCT02153294) is testing the effects of V_T 4–6 mL/kg vs. 9–10 mL/kg PBW in a population of ventilated non-ARDS patients.[60]

Use of surrogate outcomes such as onset of ARDS to gauge the effectiveness of preventive strategies does not guarantee success in improving end result: death or long-term functional impairment.[61] In the case of low V_T ventilation, its success in a population at high risk for mortality due to ARDS does not necessarily translate into benefits in patients

who are at much lower risk, such as those ventilated in the operating room. Contrarily, undesired effects—often undetected by underpowered clinical trials—may affect more patients than the beneficial ones.[62] For example, decreasing V_T in a patient without ARDS may worsen atelectasis, leading to possible increased lung damage and hypoxemia. Although studies so far have not reported an increased requirement for sedation when lower vs. higher V_T is used,[63] sedation practices and goals are known to be variable between centers. If minimal sedation and spontaneous breathing modes—as opposed to deeper sedation and controlled ventilation—are the usual practice, reducing V_T may have more relevant consequences on P-SILI, patient discomfort, ventilator dyssynchrony, and eventually on sedation usage, with all of the resultant sequelae.

CONCLUSIONS

Our knowledge of alveolar mechanics and ventilator-induced lung injury is improving. The outcomes of ARDS can be improved by implementation of existing evidence and better pathophysiologic knowledge. Ventilator settings should be dynamically adapted to individual subjects' characteristics rather than to body weight alone. Regional force distribution and inflation heterogeneity are major players in determining the response of lung tissue to ventilator settings and possibly other therapies, such as prone positioning.

AUTHORS' RECOMMENDATIONS
- Ventilator-induced lung injury (VILI) is caused by stretch injury (volutrauma—"baby lung"), atelectrauma, stress amplification, barotrauma, biotrauma, and patient self-inflicted lung injury (P-SILI).
- Large tidal volumes (>12 mL/kg of predicted body weight) damage the lungs in acute respiratory distress syndrome (ARDS), when "baby lung" is present.
- Significant lung injury probably also occurs due to inflation and deflation of injured or atelectatic lung tissue.
- Large, swinging, transpulmonary pressures may also lead to maldistribution of pulmonary capillary blood flow, worsening capillary leak, and increasing extravascular lung water.
- Strong data support limiting tidal volumes and plateau pressures in patients with ARDS. Weak evidence supports extending this approach to all mechanically ventilated patients.
- High driving pressures are associated with worse outcomes in ARDS.
- There is no best method of setting positive end expiratory pressure (PEEP), and current evidence does not support the "open lung approach" of high PEEP and recruitment maneuvers.
- Neuromuscular blockade may reduce VILI by limiting transpulmonary pressures.
- Prone positioning likely improves outcomes in ARDS by attenuating VILI
- Extracorporeal membrane oxygenation (ECMO) is used as a rescue therapy in ARDS, but remains controversial.

REFERENCES

1. Protti A, Cressoni M, Santini A, et al. Lung stress and strain during mechanical ventilation: Any safe threshold? *Am J Respir Crit Care Med.* 2011;183(10):1354-1362.
2. Gattinoni L, Pesenti A, Avalli L, et al. Pressure-volume curve of total respiratory system in acute respiratory failure. Computed tomographic scan study. *Am Rev Respir Dis.* 1987;136(3):730-736.
3. Bellani G, Guerra L, Musch G, et al. Lung regional metabolic activity and gas volume changes induced by tidal ventilation in patients with acute lung injury. *Am J Respir Crit Care Med.* 2011;183(9):1193-1199.
4. Bilek AM, Dee KC, Gaver DP 3rd. Mechanisms of surface-tension-induced epithelial cell damage in a model of pulmonary airway reopening. *J Appl Physiol.* 2003;94(2):770-783.
5. Cressoni M, Cadringher P, Chiurazzi C, et al. Lung inhomogeneity in patients with acute respiratory distress syndrome. *Am J Respir Crit Care Med.* 2014;189(2):149-158.
6. Borges JB, Costa EL, Bergquist M, et al. Lung inflammation persists after 27 hours of protective Acute Respiratory Distress Syndrome Network Strategy and is concentrated in the nondependent lung. *Crit Care Med.* 2015;43:e123-e132.
7. Cereda M, Xin Y, Hamedani H, et al. Tidal changes on CT and progression of ARDS. *Thorax.* 2017;72: 981-989.
8. Imai Y, Parodo J, Kajikawa O, et al. Injurious mechanical ventilation and end-organ epithelial cell apoptosis and organ dysfunction in an experimental model of acute respiratory distress syndrome. *JAMA.* 2003;289:2104-2112.
9. Yoshida T, Torsani V, Gomes S, et al. Spontaneous effort causes occult pendelluft during mechanical ventilation. *Am J Respir Crit Care Med.* 2013;188:1420-1427.
10. Katira BH, Giesinger RE, Engelberts D, et al. Adverse heart–lung interactions in ventilator-induced lung injury. *Am J Respir Crit Care Med.* 2017;196:1411-1421.
11. Pohlman MC, McCallister KE, Schweickert WD, et al. Excessive tidal volume from breath stacking during lung-protective ventilation for acute lung injury. *Crit Care Med.* 2008;36:3019-3023.
12. Acute Respiratory Distress Syndrome Network, Brower RG, Matthay MA, et al. Ventilation with lower tidal volumes as compared with traditional tidal volumes for acute lung injury and the acute respiratory distress syndrome. *N Engl J Med.* 2000;342(18):1301-1308.
13. Terragni PP, Rosboch G, Tealdi A, et al. Tidal hyperinflation during low tidal volume ventilation in acute respiratory distress syndrome. *Am J Respir Crit Care Med.* 2007;175(2):160-166.
14. Serpa Neto A, Cardoso SO, Manetta JA, et al. Association between use of lung-protective ventilation with lower tidal volumes and clinical outcomes among patients without acute respiratory distress syndrome: a meta-analysis. *JAMA.* 2012;308(16):1651-1659.
15. Futier E, Constantin JM, Paugam-Burtz C, et al. A trial of intraoperative low-tidal-volume ventilation in abdominal surgery. *N Engl J Med.* 2013;369(5):428-437.
16. Levine GK, Deutschman CS, Helfaer MA, Margulies SS. Sepsis-induced lung injury in rats increases alveolar epithelial vulnerability to stretch. *Crit Care Med.* 2006;34(6):1746-1751.
17. Motta-Ribeiro G, Hashimoto S, Winkler T, et al. Deterioration of regional lung strain and inflammation during early lung injury. *Am J Respir Crit Care Med.* 2018;198(7):891-902.
18. Tremblay L, Valenza F, Ribeiro SP, et al. Injurious ventilatory strategies increase cytokines and c-fos m-RNA expression in an isolated rat lung model. *J Clin Invest.* 1997;99(5):944-952.
19. Tsuchida S, Engelberts D, Peltekova V, et al. Atelectasis causes alveolar injury in nonatelectatic lung regions. *Am J Respir Crit Care Med.* 2006;174(3):279-289.
20. Cereda M, Emami K, Xin Y, et al. Imaging the interaction of atelectasis and overdistension in surfactant-depleted lungs. *Crit Care Med.* 2013;41(2):527-535.
21. Meade MO, Cook DJ, Guyatt GH, et al. Ventilation strategy using low tidal volumes, recruitment maneuvers, and high positive end-expiratory pressure for acute lung injury and acute respiratory distress syndrome: a randomized controlled trial. *JAMA.* 2008;299(6):637-645.
22. Mercat A, Richard JC, Vielle B, et al. Positive end-expiratory pressure setting in adults with acute lung injury and acute respiratory distress syndrome: a randomized controlled trial. *JAMA.* 2008;299(6):646-655.
23. Brower RG, Lanken PN, MacIntyre N, et al. Higher versus lower positive end-expiratory pressures in patients with the acute respiratory distress syndrome. *N Engl J Med.* 2004; 351(4):327-336.
24. Force ADT, Ranieri VM, Rubenfeld GD, et al. Acute respiratory distress syndrome: the Berlin Definition. *JAMA.* 2012;307(23): 2526-2533.
25. Vieira SR, Puybasset L, Richecoeur J, et al. A lung computed tomographic assessment of positive end-expiratory pressure-induced lung overdistension. *Am J Respir Crit Care Med.* 1998; 158(5 Pt 1):1571-1577.
26. Neumann P, Wrigge H, Zinserling J, et al. Spontaneous breathing affects the spatial ventilation and perfusion distribution during mechanical ventilatory support. *Crit Care Med.* 2005;33: 1090-1095.
27. Mascheroni D, Kolobow T, Fumagalli R, et al. Acute respiratory failure following pharmacologically induced hyperventilation: an experimental animal study. *Intensive Care Med.* 1988;15:8-14.
28. Yoshida T, Uchiyama A, Matsuura N, et al. The comparison of spontaneous breathing and muscle paralysis in two different severities of experimental lung injury. *Crit Care Med.* 2013;41: 536-545.
29. Papazian L, Forel JM, Gacouin A, et al. Neuromuscular blockers in early acute respiratory distress syndrome. *N Engl J Med.* 2010;363(12):1107-1116.
30. Gilstrap D, MacIntyre N. Patient–ventilator interactions. Implications for clinical management. *Am J Respir Crit Care Med.* 2013;188:1058-1068.
31. Yoshida T, Roldan R, Beraldo MA, et al. Spontaneous effort during mechanical ventilation: maximal injury with less positive end-expiratory pressure. *Crit Care Med.* 2016;44: e678-e688.
32. Katira BH, Engelberts D, Otulakowski G, et al. Abrupt deflation after sustained inflation causes lung injury. *Am J Respir Crit Care Med.* 2018;198(9):1165-1176.
33. Pelosi P, Rocco PR. Effects of mechanical ventilation on the extracellular matrix. *Intensive Care Med.* 2008;34:631-639.
34. Goebel U, Haberstroh J, Foerster K, et al. Flow-controlled expiration: a novel ventilation mode to attenuate experimental porcine lung injury. *Br J Anaesth.* 2014;113(3):474-483.
35. Needham DM, Colantuoni E, Mendez-Tellez PA, et al. Lung protective mechanical ventilation and two year survival in patients with acute lung injury: prospective cohort study. *BMJ.* 2012;344:e2124.
36. Yoshida T, Amato MBP, Grieco DL, et al. Esophageal manometry and regional transpulmonary pressure in lung injury. *Am J Respir Crit Care Med.* 2018;197(8):1018-1026.

37. Talmor D, Sarge T, Malhotra A, et al. Mechanical ventilation guided by esophageal pressure in acute lung injury. *N Engl J Med*. 2008;359(20):2095-2104.
38. Amato MBP, Meade MO, Slutsky AS, et al. Driving pressure and survival in the acute respiratory distress syndrome. *N Engl J Med*. 2015;372:747-755.
39. Neto AS, Hemmes SNT, Barbas CSV, et al. Association between driving pressure and development of postoperative pulmonary complications in patients undergoing mechanical ventilation for general anaesthesia: a meta-analysis of individual patient data. *Lancet Respir Med*. 2016;4:272-280.
40. Terragni PP, Del Sorbo L, Mascia L, et al. Tidal volume lower than 6 ml/kg enhances lung protection: role of extracorporeal carbon dioxide removal. *Anesthesiology*. 2009;111(4):826-835.
41. Peek GJ, Mugford M, Tiruvoipati R, et al. Efficacy and economic assessment of conventional ventilatory support versus extracorporeal membrane oxygenation for severe adult respiratory failure (CESAR): a multicentre randomised controlled trial. *Lancet*. 2009;374(9698):1351-1363.
42. Combes A, Hajage D, Capellier G, et al. Extracorporeal membrane oxygenation for severe acute respiratory distress syndrome. *N Engl J Med*. 2018;378:1965-1975.
43. Allardet-Servent J, et al. Enhanced lung protective ventilation with ECCO2R during ARDS (PROVE). ClinicalTrials.gov. Identifier: NCT03525691.
44. Ferguson ND, Slutsky AS, Meade MO. High-frequency oscillation for ARDS. *N Engl J Med*. 2013;368(23):2233-2234.
45. Briel M, Meade M, Mercat A, et al. Higher vs lower positive end-expiratory pressure in patients with acute lung injury and acute respiratory distress syndrome: systematic review and meta-analysis. *JAMA*. 2010;303(9):865-873.
46. Writing Group for the Alveolar Recruitment for Acute Respiratory Distress Syndrome Trial (ART) Investigators, Cavalcanti AB, Suzumura ÉA, et al. Effect of lung recruitment and titrated positive end-expiratory pressure (PEEP) vs low PEEP on mortality in patients with acute respiratory distress syndrome. A randomized clinical trial. *JAMA*. 2017;318(14):1335-1345.
47. PROVE Network Investigators for the Clinical Trial Network of the European Society of Anaesthesiology, Hemmes SN, Gama de Abreu M, et al. High versus low positive end-expiratory pressure during general anaesthesia for open abdominal surgery (PROVHILO trial): a multicentre randomised controlled trial. *Lancet*. 2014;384(9942):495-503.
48. Ferrando C, Soro M, Unzueta C, et al. Individualised perioperative open-lung approach versus standard protective ventilation in abdominal surgery (iPROVE): a randomised controlled trial. *Lancet Respir Med*. 2018;6(3):193-203.
49. Goligher EC, Kavanagh BP, Rubenfeld GD, et al. Oxygenation response to positive end-expiratory pressure predicts mortality in acute respiratory distress syndrome. A secondary analysis of the LOVS and ExPress trials. *Am J Respir Crit Care Med*. 2014;190(1):70-76.
50. Gattinoni L, Caironi P, Cressoni M, et al. Lung recruitment in patients with the acute respiratory distress syndrome. *N Engl J Med*. 2006;354(17):1775-1786.
51. Jabaudon M, Godet T, Futier E, et al. Rationale, study design and analysis plan of the lung imaging morphology for ventilator settings in acute respiratory distress syndrome study (LIVE study): study protocol for a randomised controlled trial. *Anaesth Crit Care Pain Med*. 2017;36(5):301-306.
52. Andrews PL, Shiber JR, Jaruga-Killeen E, et al. Early application of airway pressure release ventilation may reduce mortality in high-risk trauma patients: a systematic review of observational trauma ARDS literature. *J Trauma Acute Care Surg*. 2013;75(4):635-641.
53. Jardin F, Vieillard-Baron A. Right ventricular function and positive pressure ventilation in clinical practice: from hemodynamic subsets to respirator settings. *Intensive Care Med*. 2003;29(9):1426-1434.
54. Huang DT, Angus DC, Moss M, et al. Design and rationale of the reevaluation of systemic early neuromuscular blockade trial for acute respiratory distress syndrome. *Ann Am Thorac Soc*. 2017;14(1):124-133.
55. Guérin C, Reignier J, Richard JC, et al. Prone positioning in severe acute respiratory distress syndrome. *N Engl J Med*. 2013;368(23):2159-2168.
56. Cornejo RA, Diaz JC, Tobar EA, et al. Effects of prone positioning on lung protection in patients with acute respiratory distress syndrome. *Am J Respir Crit Care Med*. 2013;188:440-448.
57. Xin Y, Cereda M, Hamedani H, et al. Unstable inflation causing injury. Insight from prone position and paired computed tomography scans. *Am J Respir Crit Care Med*. 2018;198(2):197-207.
58. Shari G, Kojicic M, Li G, et al. Timing of the onset of acute respiratory distress syndrome: a population-based study. *Respir Care*. 2011;56(5):576-582.
59. Gajic O, Dabbagh O, Park PK, et al. Early identification of patients at risk of acute lung injury: evaluation of lung injury prediction score in a multicenter cohort study. *Am J Respir Crit Care Med*. 2011;183(4):462-470.
60. Simonis FD, Binnekade JM, Braber A, et al. PReVENT—protective ventilation in patients without ARDS at start of ventilation: study protocol for a randomized controlled trial. *Trials*. 2015;16(1):226.
61. Rubenfeld GD. Who cares about preventing ARDS? *Am J Respir Crit Care Med*. 2015;191(3):255-260.
62. Goldenberg NM, Steinberg BE, Lee WL, et al. Lung-protective ventilation in the operating room: time to implement? *Anesthesiology*. 2014;121(1):184-188.
63. Determann RM, Royakkers A, Wolthuis EK, et al. Ventilation with lower tidal volumes as compared with conventional tidal volumes for patients without acute lung injury: a preventive randomized controlled trial. *Crit Care*. 2010;14(1):R1.

11

How Should Exacerbations of COPD Be Managed in the Intensive Care Unit?

Christina Campbell, Tara Cahill, and Anthony O'Regan

PREVALENCE OF COPD

The Global Burden of Disease (GBD) project ranked chronic obstructive pulmonary disease (COPD) 8th of the 315 causes of the Global Burden of Disease in 2015.[1] It estimated 3.2 million people died from COPD worldwide in 2015; this is an increase of 11% from 1990, despite a decrease in the overall age-standardized death rate of 42%. The prevalence of COPD increased by 44% in the same period. Worldwide, COPD affects 105 million males and 70 million females, with an age-standardized prevalence of 3% in males and 2% in females. However, age-standardized disability-adjusted life years (DALYs) rates in males are almost double the rates in females, which reflects a higher male-to-female ratio for mortality than prevalence.[1]

Smoking and exposure to ambient particulate matter are the main risk factors for development of COPD, followed by household air pollution, occupational exposures, ozone, and environmental tobacco smoke.[1] In countries with a higher sociodemographic index (SDI), smoking contributes to 69% of COPD burden, whereas environmental risks are more prevalent in lower SDI countries, contributing to 58% of COPD cases.[1] A significant proportion of COPD remains unexplained. The GBD group plan to expand their data to include a personal history of pulmonary tuberculosis as a risk factor, given the emergence of evidence for a causal relationship.[1–3]

A 2011 French study had demonstrated that exacerbations of COPD contribute to 1.6–2.6% of all medical admissions.[4] Of these admissions, in-hospital mortality were 6–8%, with the mortality rates in males being significantly higher than in females (6–9% vs. 5–7%, respectively). The rates of COPD admission increased by 38% from 1998 to 2007, despite a drop in inpatient lethality from 7.6% to 6%.[5] The US National Hospital Discharge Survey reported an increase in admissions between 1990 and 1999.[5] Data from Italy, Australia, and Canada show similar trends.[5–7] This may reflect improving care, leading to longer life expectancy and thus more admissions.

As expected, admission rates increase with age, particularly over 45 years and show a definite seasonal pattern, related to the peaks of prevalence of influenza-like illnesses.[4]

Acute episodes of respiratory failure in patients with COPD are estimated to account for between 5% and 10% of acute emergency hospital medical admissions. Failure of first-line medical treatment is a common source of intensive care unit (ICU) referrals, accounting for 2–3% of non-surgical ICU admissions.[8] In a cohort of 1016 patients who were hospitalized for acute exacerbations, half of whom required intensive care, the in-hospital mortality rate was 11%.[9] The 6-month and 1-year mortality rates were 33% and 43%, respectively. Those who survived the first hospitalization had a 50% rate of rehospitalization within 6 months after discharge.

RESPIRATORY FAILURE

The pathophysiology of acute respiratory failure in COPD is not completely understood but may be precipitated by any condition that increases the work of breathing. Respiratory failure may be predominantly hypoxic (type 1) or hypercapnic (type 2). The mechanism of hypercapnea in COPD is not clear, but it is no longer believed to reflect problems with respiratory drive as suggested by the concept of "pink puffers and blue bloaters." Gas exchange abnormalities appear to predominantly reflect ventilation–perfusion mismatching due to airflow limitation, and progressive respiratory failure reflects a combination of severe airflow obstruction, hyperinflation, and respiratory muscle fatigue. Regardless of the pathophysiology, the presence of hypercapnea and the need for assisted ventilation identify patients that have high initial (up to 27%) and 12-month mortality (up to 50%).[10]

CLINICAL PRECIPITANTS OF RESPIRATORY FAILURE

It has been shown that viral and bacterial infections account for between 50% and 70% of acute exacerbations and the majority of cases of acute respiratory failure in COPD.[11,12] Numerous viral and bacterial agents have been implicated, but rhinoviruses, respiratory syncytial virus, *Haemophilus influenzae*, *Moraxella catarrhalis*, and *Streptococcus pneumoniae* are the most common pathogens.[12–15] *Pseudomonas aeruginosa*, Enterobacteriaceae, and *Stenotrophomonas* spp. are also frequently isolated, particularly from patients with severe COPD and those requiring mechanical ventilation.[16] Therefore, although still uncommon, clinicians should consider more resistant gram-negative organisms in patients requiring ICU care with COPD exacerbations. The prevalence of atypical organisms such as *Mycoplasma* and *Chlamydia* is less well defined.

Up to 10% of COPD flares are caused by environmental pollution and airway irritants such as smoke or fumes. There is growing body of evidence that gastroesophageal reflux disease contributes to acute exacerbations in the COPD population,[17] particularly those not on acid suppressive therapies.[18] For many other cases the etiology of acute exacerbations is not clear.

Medical conditions can mimic or cause COPD exacerbations, and patients with COPD have higher rates of comorbid illnesses, in part reflecting exposure to cigarette smoke. This is supported by results from the Towards a Revolution in COPD Health (TORCH) trial; only 35% of deaths were adjudicated as due to pulmonary causes, with cardiovascular disease being the other major cause of death at 27% and cancer third at 21%. A further study has demonstrated patients are at a higher risk of myocardial infarction or stroke following an exacerbation of COPD, possibly due to higher rates of systemic inflammation following exacerbations of COPD.[19] Pulmonary embolism (PE) can be an occult cause of acute respiratory failure in COPD. A systematic review found that 16% of patients with an exacerbation of COPD had a PE, but other studies report a lower incidence at presentation to hospital.[20] Signs of infection were seen less commonly with PE, with pleuritic chest pain and cardiac failure being more common.[20]

PROGNOSTIC INDICATORS IN PATIENTS WITH ACUTE EXACERBATIONS OF COPD

There are several potential prognostic indicators that should be considered when admitting a patient to ICU with an acute exacerbation of COPD. The DECAF score has been developed to predict mortality. It is based on the five strongest predictors of mortality in a study from the UK in 2012: dyspnea, eosinophilia, consolidation, acidemia, and atrial fibrillation.[21] As a combined score, this has been shown to be a stronger predictor of mortality than the CURB-65 score in patients with COPD and pneumonia, and as such, is a useful triage tool. Other factors commonly cited in literature include patients' age, their forced expiratory volume in 1 second (FEV$_1$), the degree of hypoxemia or hypercapnea, the presence of other comorbidities, such as cardiovascular disease, or a history of prior or frequent exacerbations. Frequent exacerbations accelerate disease progression and

mortality, leading to a faster decline in lung function and quality of life.[22] The 2-year mortality after a COPD exacerbation is approximately 50%. Finally, a patient who has failed adequate treatment for a COPD exacerbation over 48 hours ("late failure") has a very poor prognosis in the setting of escalation to invasive mechanical ventilation.[23]

Patients with chronic hypercapnic respiratory failure are particularly high risk, and, as a result, noninvasive ventilation (NIV) at home is being increasingly used. Base excess, which represents a metabolic response to chronic hypercapnia (increased bicarbonate, reduced chloride), was found to be one of the strongest prognostic indicators in this setting, as reported in a study published in 2007 by Budweiser and colleagues.[24] They also found that in a cohort of COPD patients sent home from hospital on NIV, the 5-year survival rate was 26.4%, with deaths predominantly from respiratory causes (73.8%). A recent study demonstrated that domiciliary NIV following an exacerbation prolongs time to next admission if patients are selected for persistent hypercapnia at 4 weeks post discharge and NIV is titrated to normalize pCO$_2$.[25]

MANAGEMENT OF COPD

The treatment guidelines for management of acute exacerbation of COPD requiring admission to ICU are broadly similar to those principles employed in patients without respiratory failure, although significantly more attention must be paid to safe and appropriate gas exchange. Addressing the issue of poor respiratory mechanics due to dynamic hyperinflation, loss of alveolar volume and impaired ventilation is fundamental to COPD management. Compensated chronic respiratory failure can rapidly decompensate due to poor chest wall mechanics, suboptimal respiratory muscle function, malnutrition, obesity, and myopathy. Reducing the work of breathing using NIV to improve oxygenation, rest muscles, and manage hyperinflation has become key in the management of COPD.

Indications for referral to ICU include dyspnea that does not respond to emergency treatment, changes in mental status (confusion, drowsiness, or coma), persistent or worsening hypoxemia, and/or severe or worsening hypercapnia, acidosis, or hemodynamic instability.[26]

Corticosteroids

A number of randomized controlled trials (RCTs) have shown that for patients hospitalized with acute exacerbations of COPD, systemic corticosteroids administered for up to 2 weeks are helpful.[27] Treatment of an exacerbation of COPD with oral or parenteral corticosteroids increases the rate of improvement in lung function and dyspnea over the first 72 hours.[28] Corticosteroids also reduce the duration of hospital stay.[29] The optimal dose and need for tapering, route of administration, and length of treatment are uncertain.

Most recent guidelines suggest intravenous corticosteroids should be given to patients who present with a severe exacerbation, including all those requiring ICU admission, or those who may have impaired absorption due to decreased splanchnic perfusion (e.g., patients in shock or congestive heart failure). Nonetheless, if tolerated, oral corticosteroid administration is equally effective as intravenous.[30] There appears to be no benefit to prolonged treatment beyond 2 weeks.[31] There is a significant side-effect profile, the most common side effect being hyperglycemia occurring in approximately 15%.[31]

Studies have shown that nebulized steroid therapy is superior to placebo but not better than parenteral therapy.[32]

Bronchodilators

Inhaled short-acting beta-adrenergic agonists are the mainstay of therapy for an acute exacerbation of COPD because of their rapid onset of action and efficacy in producing bronchodilation. RCTs have consistently demonstrated their efficacy.[27] Parenteral or subcutaneous injection of short-acting beta-adrenergic agonists is reserved for situations in which inhaled administration is not possible. Parenteral use of these agents results in greater inotropic and chronotropic effects, which may cause arrhythmias or myocardial ischemia in susceptible individuals and is not generally recommended. These medications may be administered via a nebulizer or a metered dose inhaler (MDI) with a spacer device; however, despite evidence that neither method has been shown to be superior, physicians tend to favor the nebulized route, due to the ease of administration. Patients should revert to appropriate inhaled preparations as soon as possible.

Anticholinergic bronchodilators, such as ipratropium, are equally efficacious,[33] and some studies have found that combination therapy with inhaled beta-agonists provides better bronchodilation than either alone.[34] The array of inhalers available for use in stable COPD patients is widening, and newer combination inhalers include a long-acting beta-agonist with a long-acting anticholinergic. These dual bronchodilators have been shown to improve symptoms and lung function in COPD patients where single bronchodilators may be insufficient,[35] but there is no proven efficacy for their use in acute exacerbations.

Methylxanthines have a long history in the treatment of COPD; however, despite widespread clinical use, their role in the acute setting is controversial. Current guidelines based on meta-analysis of four RCTs recommend that theophylline should not be used in the acute setting, as efficacy beyond that induced by inhaled bronchodilator and glucocorticoid therapy has not been demonstrated. In addition to lack of efficacy, methylxanthines have caused significantly more nausea and vomiting than placebo and trended toward more frequent tremor, palpitations, and arrhythmias.[36]

Antibiotics

In patients with severe exacerbations requiring mechanical ventilation, antibiotic therapy is beneficial and has been shown to significantly decrease mortality (4% vs. 22%), the need for additional courses of antibiotics, the duration of mechanical ventilation, and the duration of hospital stay.[37] Other studies show inconsistent benefit from antibiotics, but the decision to withhold antimicrobials is difficult and potentially risky in severe exacerbations. Unfortunately, early investigations using inflammatory markers such as procalcitonin have not shown a reduction in antibiotic use.[38]

Current guidelines suggest the use of antimicrobials with a spectrum of activity to cover beta-lactamase-producing organisms. While choice is somewhat dependent on the local streptococcal resistance patterns, amoxicillin–clavulanic acid, second-generation cephalosporin, or macrolides are all acceptable. A treatment of 3–7 days is recommended (GOLD).[39] Wider-spectrum antibiotics such as fluoroquinolones or beta-lactam with antipseudomonal activity should be used in those at risk of resistant gram-negative infections (i.e., recent hospitalization, previous colonization, previous severe exacerbation or <4 exacerbations per year) or prior culture for pseudomonas.

Oxygen Therapy

Adequate oxygenation can be achieved in most patients with acute exacerbations of COPD. Ventilation–perfusion mismatch is usually improved by 24–28% oxygen. There appears to be a tendency to develop CO_2 retention at $FiO_2 > 30\%$. The mechanism is more likely to reflect a combination of ventilation–perfusion mismatching and the Haldane effect rather than any effect on hypoxic drive for ventilation. Controlled or titrated oxygen therapy has been shown to significantly reduce hypercapnia, acidosis, and mortality.[40] In critical care, the use of high-flow facemasks or nasal devices provides better titration of oxygen therapy compared to simple facemasks or nasal cannulae, Venturi masks or other variable performance devices.

Assisted Ventilation

Recognition of need for assisted ventilation is essential and should be considered in any patient with type 2 or hypercapnic respiratory failure. NIV is definitely indicated if the pH remains <7.32 and probably indicated if the pH remains <7.36. Studies have shown that pH and degree of hypercapnia are better predictors of need for mechanical ventilation than hypoxia.[41] There are a number of absolute and relative contraindications to NIV:

- Respiratory arrest
- Impaired level of consciousness
- Cardiovascular collapse
- Profound hypoxemia (ARDS)
- Vomiting or very high aspiration risk due to excessive secretions
- Uncooperative patient
- Extreme obesity
- Recent facial surgery
- Burns

A number of RTCs have validated the use of NIV in the setting of acute hypercapnic respiratory failure in COPD[42] and indeed several studies have demonstrated the superiority of NIV over tracheal intubation and mechanical ventilation. NIV reduces intubation by up to 42%[42] and appears to reduce nosocomial complications and mortality.[42,43] Some studies have also found that patients with COPD who were randomly assigned to NIV had a shorter stay in the ICU. The use of

NIV has certainly improved care for many COPD sufferers and allowed some to undergo a more intense level of treatment than perhaps may have been previously available to them.

NIV on respiratory care wards and intermediate care settings is highly efficacious, with a reported failure rate of 5–20%. Studies have shown that staff training and experience are more important than location in regards to NIV, and can be given effectively outside of the ICU.[44] However, when patients are admitted to intensive care, presumably in worse clinical condition, the failure rate is up to 60%.[43,45] This is particularly problematic in patients who present late with advanced respiratory failure, and mortality is higher compared with patients who receive NIV at an earlier stage.[10] There are many reasons for failing NIV, including patient intolerance, inadequate augmentation of tidal volume, and problems with triggering.

The response to NIV treatment needs to be closely monitored using arterial blood gases, respiratory rate, hemodynamics, and overall degree of respiratory distress. Patients who respond within 1–4 hours are consistently shown to have better outcomes.[46] An initial reduction in respiratory rate is generally a good indicator of a positive response to NIV. Failure of or contraindications to NIV, or imminent cardiorespiratory arrest, should prompt endotracheal intubation and mechanical ventilation. Ideally this should be performed in the controlled setting of ICU, as intubation can precipitate a cardiovascular collapse in the setting of significant air trapping.[8]

Once intubation has been performed, hypoxemia can be corrected, usually with modest FiO_2. Subsequently, respiratory acidosis is corrected slowly using low rates and tidal volumes guided by air pressures and expiratory phase. This approach is to limit auto-PEEP from air trapping, which can result in significant hemodynamic compromise and can be difficult to detect.[47]

In the first 12–24 hours, paralysis may be required to prevent ventilator dyssynchrony, which can increase airway resistance and decrease alveolar ventilation. Airway resistance and hyperinflation can both contribute to the need for high inflation pressures to achieve tidal volume. High mean airway pressures may lead to a number of serious problems, including circulatory collapse, pneumothorax, or barotrauma. It is unclear whether pressure-controlled or pressure-limited ventilation is safer than volume control. Nevertheless, efforts should be made to minimize auto-PEEP and end inspiratory stretch.[47]

Weaning can pose problems in ventilated COPD patients, with 20–30% of those patients meeting the traditional extubation criteria failing trial of weaning.[8] Failure to wean raises the risks of the complications associated with prolonged ventilation. There is some evidence that expiratory flow limitation may predict successful extubation.[32] Nava and colleagues randomly assigned patients with COPD who were intubated for 48 hours to extubation and NIV or to continued invasive ventilation and conventional liberation, after an unsuccessful initial spontaneous breathing trial.[48] The study demonstrated improved outcomes in the noninvasive group, as measured by the percentage of patients in whom assisted ventilation could be discontinued, the duration of assisted ventilation, survival, the length of stay in the ICU, and the incidence of ventilator-associated pneumonia. Ornico and colleagues demonstrated a significant reduction of reintubation rates and in-hospital mortality when nasal NIV was commenced after planned extubation, as compared with continuous oxygen therapy.[49] Risk factors for postextubation respiratory failure includes an age over 65 years, cardiac failure as a cause for respiratory distress, an APACHE score of 12 or greater at the time of extubation, the diagnosis of an acute exacerbation of COPD, or the presence of chronic respiratory disease with over 48 hours of mechanical ventilation and hypercapnea during a spontaneous breathing trial. If patients do develop postextubation respiratory distress, they should be reintubated, as persisting with NIV in this setting may worsen outcomes.[50] High-flow nasal cannula (HFNC) oxygen therapy was recently been shown to be at least as effective as NIV in reducing reintubation rates (see below).

HFNC Oxygen Therapy

HFNC oxygen therapy is now widely used for the treatment of both hypoxic and hypercapnic respiratory failure in COPD. HFNC delivers humidified and heated air at flows up to 60 L/min and FiO_2 from 21% to 100%. HFNC is postulated to reduce anatomical dead space and provide 4–5 cm H_2O of positive end-expiratory pressure (PEEP).[51] HFNC has been shown to significantly decrease dyspnea in patients with acute respiratory failure, when compared with conventional therapy.[52] In the FLORALI trial, HFNC was noninferior to NIV in preventing intubation of patients with hypoxic respiratory failure, but patients that were intubated spent less time on mechanical ventilation and had significantly reduced 90-day mortality.[53] HFNC has also been shown to reduce the rates of reintubation, when compared with conventional therapy and NIV.[54,55]

The use of HFNC in hypercapnic respiratory failure is expanding. Kim and colleagues[51] retrospectively examined a small cohort of patients who presented principally with pneumonia, hypercarbia, and hypoxemia over a 2-year period. Compared with conventional oxygen therapy, which increased $PaCO_2$, HFNC was associated with a reduction in $PaCO_2$ by 4.2 ± 5.5 and 3.7 ± 10.8 mm Hg at 1 and 24 hours, respectively.[51] Lee and colleagues compared HFNC oxygen therapy to NIV in hypercapnic respiratory failure in 92 patients. They found no difference in 30-day mortality or intubation rates between both groups,[56] nor in pH, PaO_2 or $PaCO_2$ after 24 hours. Jeong et al. showed that HFNC reduced hypercapnia but did not prevent progression to NIV or invasive ventilation.[57] Finally, a study of 604 patients found that HFNC was not inferior to NIV for preventing postextubating respiratory failure.[55] Although these are small studies, HFNC could be used as an adjunct in patients with respiratory failure, particularly as an alternative to conventional oxygen therapy, particularly those failing NIV and after extubation. It is worth noting that many of these trials are not specific to COPD and further research is required.

PROGNOSIS AND OUTCOMES

Despite reasonable survival to hospital discharge, the decision to admit to the ICU in advanced cases is difficult and there is no consensus. One has to take into account expected prognosis, comorbidities and estimate likely quality of life assuming survival to hospital discharge. Factors affecting the decision to mechanically ventilate include cultural attitudes towards disability, perceived impact of treatment, financial resources, the availability of ICU and long-term ventilator beds, local medical practice, and patient wishes.

Past perception has been that survival following ICU admission was poor, especially in those deemed to have severe or end-stage disease. However, short-term survival following invasive mechanical ventilation ranges from 63% to 86%, more than would be expected in unplanned medical admissions.[58] In addition, survival following mechanical ventilation has been shown to be better in the absence of a major precipitating cause for acute deterioration, perhaps as shorter periods of assisted ventilation are required and thus length of ICU stay and associated complications are lessened.[59]

However, a difficulty still remains in identifying those patients most likely to derive benefit from aggressive management. Long-term survival rates are not quite as encouraging as survival to discharge figures. Rates of 52%, 42%, and 37% at 1, 2, and 3 years, respectively, were reported in one UK study[60] and similar numbers have been reported from other centers.

Poor prognostic indicators include:
- Increased age; presence of severe respiratory disease
- Increased length of stay in hospital before ICU admission
- Cardiopulmonary resuscitation within 24 hours before admission
- Low Pao_2/FiO_2 gradient
- Hypercapnea
- Low serum albumin
- Low body mass index (BMI)
- Cardiovascular organ failure; neurologic organ failure; and renal organ failure

While all of these factors have been associated with increased in-hospital mortality,[61] there is currently no reliable or definitive method for identifying patients at high risk of inpatient or 6-month mortality. Therefore, these parameters should not influence decisions about instituting, continuing, or withdrawing life-sustaining treatment.

A small 2001 study of 166 COPD patients requiring mechanical ventilation found that absence of comorbid condition more than halved in-hospital mortality rates (28% vs. 12%).[62] A higher mortality rate among those patients who required >72 hours of mechanical ventilation (37% vs. 16%), those without previous episodes of mechanical ventilation (33% vs. 11%), and those with a failed extubation attempt (36% vs. 11%) was also noted. Further larger studies would be helpful to assist in decision making.

While the above material can guide treatment decisions, patient preference represents an essential component of our assessment. A prospective cohort study carried out in 92 ICUs and 3 respiratory high dependency units in the UK examined outcomes in patients with COPD admitted to the ICU for decompensated hypercarbic respiratory failure, including survival and quality of life at 180 days.[63] Of the survivors, 73% considered their quality of life to be the same as or better than it had been in the stable period before they were admitted, and 96% would choose similar treatment again.

The GOLD guidelines state that acute mortality among COPD patients is lower than patients ventilated for non-COPD causes. However, there is evidence that patients are denied admission to intensive care for intubation due to excessive prognostic pessimism.[64] Taking all of this into account, current treatment guidelines suggest that failure of NIV in most cases should be followed by a short trial of invasive mechanical ventilation. Early reevaluation is then recommended. Patient wishes play an important role in this decision and advances directives based on discussion, ideally occurring during a medically stable period, regarding risks and complications of invasive ventilation are advocated.

END-OF-LIFE DECISIONS IN SEVERE COPD

In the severe and end-stage COPD patient population, decisions regarding end-of-life care and palliation should be addressed. Factors that may lead to an end-of-life discussion include[65]:
- FEV_1 below 30% predicted
- Oxygen dependence
- Requirement of domiciliary NIPPV (noninvasive positive pressure ventilation)
- One or more hospital admissions in the past year with an acute exacerbation of COPD
- Weight loss or cachexia
- Decreased functional status/decreased independence
- Age over 70 years
- On maximal medical management

A retrospective study performed in the Mayo Clinic,[66] involving 591 patients admitted to ICU with an acute exacerbation of COPD, found that the factors most associated with a poor 1-year mortality were age and length of hospital stay. These patients may benefit from early communication regarding end of life and palliation, prior to their next hospital admission.

As COPD is a chronic progressive disease, there is opportunity to have the discussion early, with the knowledge that in severe and end-stage COPD patients, they will likely require more aggressive care (e.g., mechanical ventilation), with a possibly fatal outcome in an unpredictably acute setting. Given the opportunity, three primary end-of-life topics can be discussed[32]:
- Their disease course and likely prognosis
- Establishing a ceiling of care
- Symptom management and control

Knowing their own disease course allows patients to participate in their management strategy and provides context for the acute decisions made during an exacerbation. When discussed early in the course of the disease, it may improve compliance with therapy, and towards more end-stage disease, it allows patients to know what to expect and make informed end-of-life decisions, including establishing the ceiling of care and whether or not to be admitted to intensive care for ventilation. In a French study regarding patients with COPD admitted to intensive care, only 56% of patients had discussed intensive care as a possibility with their physician.[67]

A ceiling of care can be established by considering the patient's comorbidities and prognosis, but it is also important to consider the patient's quality of life, the functionality of activities of daily living, and their wishes with regards to their treatment. In particular, deciding whether the patient should be for mechanical ventilation in an ICU or for a trial of noninvasive ventilation should be established if possible. The SUPPORT trial published in 2000 compared patients with stage III and IV lung cancer with severe COPD, and found that 60% of patients in each group wanted comfort-focused care.[68]

AUTHORS' RECOMMENDATIONS

- COPD accounts for a large proportion of medical ICU admissions; 25% of COPD patients will require ICU at some stage in their disease. Half of those will not survive 1 year.
- The majority of acute exacerbations of COPD are associated with viral or bacterial infection.
- The DECAF (Dyspnea, Eosinophilia, Consolidation, Acidemia, and Atrial Fibrillation) score may be used to predict mortality.
- Oxygen therapy, corticosteroids, beta-adrenoceptor agonists and anticholinergic agents continue to be the mainstay of therapy. Methylxanthines are probably ineffective.
- Noninvasive ventilation (NIV) is effective and economical in moderate to severe cases and is associated with reduced mortality, reduced invasive ventilation, and nosocomial complications.
- In severe cases intubation is necessary, and extreme care is required to control dyssynchrony, auto-PEEP, and end-inspiratory lung stretch.
- Weaning and liberation can be difficult. Extubation to NIV may shorted duration of ICU and hospital stay.
- High-flow nasal cannula oxygen therapy may be a useful adjuvant for patients with hypoxic or hypercapnic respiratory failure, failing NIV or postintubation.
- Advanced age, low body weight, cardiovascular disease, and multiple previous ICU admissions predict poor outcomes in COPD, although no specific scoring system exists. Advanced directives and treatment limitation planning should be undertaken.

REFERENCES

1. GBD 2015 Chronic Respiratory Disease Collaborators. Global, regional, and national deaths, prevalence, disability-adjusted life years, and years lived with disability for chronic obstructive pulmonary disease and asthma, 1990-2015: a systematic analysis for the Global Burden of Disease Study 2015. *Lancet Respir Med.* 2017;5(9):691-706.
2. Buist AS, McBurnie MA, Vollmer WM, et al. International variation in the prevalence of COPD (the BOLD Study): a population-based prevalence study. *Lancet.* 2007;370(9589):741-750.
3. Lee CH, Lee MC, Lin HH, et al. Pulmonary tuberculosis and delay in anti-tuberculous treatment are important risk factors for chronic obstructive pulmonary disease. *PLoS One.* 2012;7(5):e37978.
4. Fuhrman C, Roche N, Vergnenègre A, Zureik M, Chouaid C, Delmas MC. Hospital admissions related to acute exacerbations of chronic obstructive pulmonary disease in France, 1998-2007. *Respir Med.* 2011;105(4):595-601.
5. Public Health Agency of Canada. Life and breath: respiratory disease in Canada. 2007. Available at http://publications.gc.ca/pub?id=9.690355&sl=0. Accessed October 10, 2018.
6. Trerotoli P, Bartolomeo N, Moretti AM, Serio G. Hospitalisation for COPD in Puglia: the role of hospital discharge database to estimate prevalence and incidence. *Monaldi Arch Chest Dis.* 2008;69(3):94-106.
7. Wilson DH, Tucker G, Frith P, Appleton S, Ruffin RE, Adams RJ. Trends in hospital admissions and mortality from asthma and chronic obstructive pulmonary disease in Australia, 1993-2003. *Med J Aust.* 2007;186(8):408-411.
8. Global Initiative for Chronic Obstructive Lung Disease. Global strategy for the diagnosis, management, and prevention of chronic obstructive pulmonary disease (Gold Report). 2018. Available at http://www.goldcopd.com. Accessed October 10, 2018.
9. Davidson AC. The pulmonary physician in critical care: 11: critical care management of respiratory failure resulting from COPD. *Thorax.* 2002;57(12):1079-1084.
10. Chandra D, Stamm JA, Taylor B, et al. Outcomes of noninvasive ventilation for acute exacerbations of chronic obstructive pulmonary disease in the United States, 1998-2008. *Am J Respir Crit Care Med.* 2012;185(2):152-159.
11. Papi A, Bellettato CM, Braccioni F, et al. Infections and airway inflammation in chronic obstructive pulmonary disease severe exacerbations. *Am J Respir Crit Care Med.* 2006;173(10):1114-1121.
12. Soler N, Torres A, Ewig S, et al. Bronchial microbial patterns in severe exacerbations of chronic obstructive pulmonary disease (COPD) requiring mechanical ventilation. *Am J Respir Crit Care Med.* 1998;157(5 Pt 1):1498-1505.
13. Monsó E, Ruiz J, Rosell A, et al. Bacterial infection in chronic obstructive pulmonary disease: a study of stable and exacerbated outpatients using the protected specimen brush. *Am J Respir Crit Care Med.* 1995;152(4 Pt 1):1316-1320.
14. Rutschmann OT, Cornuz J, Poletti PA, et al. Should pulmonary embolism be suspected in exacerbation of chronic obstructive pulmonary disease? *Thorax.* 2007;62(2):121-125.
15. Snow V, Lascher S, Mottur-Pilson C, et al. Evidence base for management of acute exacerbations of chronic obstructive pulmonary disease. *Ann Intern Med.* 2001;134(7):595-599.
16. Wood-Baker RR, Gibson PG, Hannay M, Walters EH, Walters JA. Systemic corticosteroids for acute exacerbations of chronic obstructive airway disease. *Cochrane Database Syst Rev.* 2005;(1):CD001288.
17. Bigatao AM, Herbella FAM, Del Grande LM, Nascimento OA, Jardim JR, Patti MG. Chronic obstructive pulmonary disease exacerbations are influenced by gastroesophageal reflux disease. *Am Surg.* 2018;84(1):51-55.
18. Ingebrigtsen TS, Marott JL, Vestbo J, Nordestgaard BG, Hallas J, Lange P. Gastro-esophageal reflux disease and exacerbations in chronic obstructive pulmonary disease. *Respirology.* 2015;20(1):101-107.
19. Donaldson GC, Hurst JR, Smith CJ, Hubbard RB, Wedzicha JA. Increased risk of myocardial infarction and stroke following exacerbation of COPD. *Chest.* 2010;137(5):1091-1097.

20. Aleva FE, Voets LWLM, Simons SO, de Mast Q, van der Ven AJAM, Heijdra YF. Prevalence and localization of pulmonary embolism in unexplained acute exacerbations of COPD: a systematic review and meta-analysis. *Chest*. 2017;151(3):544-554.

21. Steer J, Gibson J, Bourke SC. The DECAF Score: predicting hospital mortality in exacerbations of chronic obstructive pulmonary disease. *Thorax*. 2012;67(11):970-976.

22. Anzueto A. Impact of exacerbations on COPD. *Eur Respir Rev*. 2010;19(116):113-118.

23. Lightowler JV, Elliott MW. Predicting the outcome from NIV for acute exacerbations of COPD. *Thorax*. 2000;55(10):815-816.

24. Budweiser S, Jörres RA, Riedl T, et al. Predictors of survival in COPD patients with chronic hypercapnic respiratory failure receiving noninvasive home ventilation. *Chest*. 2007;131(6):1650-1658.

25. Murphy PB, Rehal S, Arbane G, et al. Effect of home noninvasive ventilation with oxygen therapy vs oxygen therapy alone on hospital readmission or death after an acute COPD exacerbation: a randomized clinical trial. *JAMA*. 2017;317(21):2177-2186.

26. Tillie-Leblond I, Marquette CH, Perez T, et al. Pulmonary embolism in patients with unexplained exacerbation of chronic obstructive pulmonary disease: prevalence and risk factors. *Ann Intern Med*. 2006;144(6):390-396.

27. de Jong YP, Uil SM, Grotjohan HP, Postma DS, Kerstjens HA, van den Berg JW. Oral or IV prednisolone in the treatment of COPD exacerbations: a randomized, controlled, double-blind study. *Chest*. 2007;132(6):1741-1747.

28. Nouira S, Marghli S, Belghith M, Besbes L, Elatrous S, Abroug F. Once daily oral ofloxacin in chronic obstructive pulmonary disease exacerbation requiring mechanical ventilation: a randomized placebo-controlled trial. *Lancet*. 2001;358(9298):2020-2025.

29. O'Driscoll BR, Taylor RJ, Horsley MG, Chambers DK, Bernstein A. Nebulised salbutamol with and without ipratropium bromide in acute airflow obstruction. *Lancet*. 1989;1(8652):1418-1420.

30. Barr RG, Rowe BH, Camargo Jr CA. Methylxanthines for exacerbations of chronic obstructive pulmonary disease: meta-analysis of randomized trials. *BMJ*. 2003;327(7416):643.

31. Falagas ME, Avgeri SG, Matthaiou DK, Dimopoulos G, Siempos II. Short- versus long-duration antimicrobial treatment for exacerbations of chronic bronchitis: a meta-analysis. *J Antimicrob Chemother*. 2008;62(3):442-450.

32. Dean MM. End-of-life care for COPD patients. *Prim Care Respir J*. 2008;17(1):46-50.

33. Karpel JP. Bronchodilator responses to anticholinergic and beta-adrenergic agents in acute and stable COPD. *Chest*. 1991;99(4):871-876.

34. Maltais F, Ostinelli J, Bourbeau J, et al. Comparison of nebulised budesonide and oral prednisolone with placebo in the treatment of acute exacerbation of COPD: a randomized control trial. *Am J Respir Crit Care Med*. 2002;165(5):698-703.

35. Bateman ED, Ferguson GT, Barnes N, et al. Dual bronchodilation with QVA149 versus single bronchodilator therapy: the SHINE study. *Eur Respir J*. 2013;42(6):1484-1494.

36. In chronic obstructive pulmonary disease, a combination of ipratropium and albuterol is more effective than either agent alone: an 85-day multicenter trial. COMBIVENT Inhalation Aerosol Study Group. *Chest*. 1994;105(5):1411-1419.

37. Vollenweider DJ, Frei A, Steurer-Stey CA, et al. Antibiotics for exacerbations of chronic obstructive pulmonary disease. *Cochrane Database Syst Rev*. 2018;29;10:CD010257.

38. Huang DT, Yealy DM, Filbin MR, et al. Procalcitonin-guided use of antibiotics for lower respiratory tract infection. *N Engl J Med*. 2018;379(3):236-249.

39. Global Initiative for Chronic Obstructive Lung Disease (2019 report). Available at https://goldcopd.org/wp-content/uploads/2018/11/GOLD-2019-v1.7-FINAL.

40. Austin MA, Wills KE, Blizzard L, Walters EH, Wood-Baker R. Effect of high flow oxygen on mortality in chronic obstructive pulmonary disease patients in prehospital setting: randomised controlled trial. *BMJ*. 2010;341:c5462.

41. Antonelli M, Conti G, Rocco M, et al. A comparison of noninvasive positive-pressure ventilation and conventional mechanical ventilation in patients with acute respiratory failure. *N Engl J Med*. 1998;339(7):429-435.

42. Brochard L, Mancebo J, Wysocki M, et al. Noninvasive ventilation for acute exacerbations of chronic obstructive pulmonary disease. *N Engl J Med*. 1995;333(13):817-822.

43. Moretti M, Cilione C, Tampieri A, Fracchia C, Marchioni A, Nava S. Incidence and causes of non-invasive mechanical ventilation failure after initial success. *Thorax*. 2000;55(10):819-825.

44. Elliott MW, Confalonieri M, Nava S. Where to perform noninvasive ventilation? *Eur Respir J*. 2002;19(6):1159-1166.

45. Alvesi V, Romanello A, Badet M, Gaillard S, Philit F, Guérin C. Time course of expiratory flow limitation in COPD patients during acute respiratory failure requiring mechanical ventilation. *Chest*. 2003;123(5):1625-1632.

46. Nevins ML, Epstein SK. Predictors of outcome for patients with COPD requiring invasive mechanical ventilation. *Chest*. 2001;119(6):1840-1849.

47. Plant PK, Elliott MW. Chronic obstructive pulmonary disease. 9. Management of ventilatory failure in COPD. *Thorax*. 2003;58(6):537-542.

48. Nava S, Ambrosino N, Clini E, et al. Noninvasive mechanical ventilation in the weaning of patients with respiratory failure due to chronic obstructive pulmonary disease. A randomized, controlled trial. *Ann Intern Med*. 1998;128(9):721-728.

49. Ornico SR, Lobo SM, Sanches HS, et al. Noninvasive ventilation immediately after extubation improves weaning outcome after acute respiratory failure: a randomized controlled trial. *Crit Care*. 2013;17(2):R39.

50. Esteban A, Frutos-Vivar F, Ferguson ND, et al. Noninvasive positive-pressure ventilation for respiratory failure after extubation. *N Engl J Med*. 2004;350(24):2452-2460.

51. Kim ES, Lee H, Kim SJ, et al. Effectiveness of high-flow nasal cannula oxygen therapy for acute respiratory failure with hypercapnia. *J Thorac Dis*. 2018;10(2):882-888.

52. Lenglet H, Sztrymf B, Leroy C, Brun P, Dreyfuss D, Ricard JD. Humidified high flow nasal oxygen during respiratory failure in the emergency department: feasibility and efficacy. *Respir Care*. 2012;57(11):1873-1878.

53. Frat JP, Thille AW, Mercat A, et al. High-flow oxygen through nasal cannula in acute hypoxemic respiratory failure. *N Engl J Med*. 2015;372(23):2185-2196.

54. Hernández G, Vaquero C, González P, et al. Effect of postextubation high-flow nasal cannula vs conventional oxygen therapy on reintubation in low-risk patients: a randomized clinical trial. *JAMA*. 2016;315(13):1354-1361.

55. Hernández G, Vaquero C, Colinas L, et al. Effect of postextubation high-flow nasal cannula vs noninvasive ventilation on reintubation and postextubation respiratory failure in high-risk patients: a randomized clinical trial. *JAMA*. 2016;316(15):1565-1574.

56. Lee MK, Choi J, Park B, et al. High flow nasal cannulae oxygen therapy in acute-moderate hypercapnic respiratory failure. *Clin Respir J.* 2018;12(6):2046-2056.

57. Jeong JH, Kim DH, Kim SC, et al. Changes in arterial blood gases after use of high-flow nasal cannula therapy in the ED. *Am J Emerg Med.* 2015;33(10):1344-1349.

58. Seneff MG, Wagner DP, Wagner RP, Zimmerman JE, Knaus WA. Hospital and 1-year survival of patients admitted to intensive care units with acute exacerbation of chronic obstructive pulmonary disease. *JAMA.* 1995;274(23):1852-1857.

59. Breen D, Churches T, Hawker F, Torzillo PJ. Acute respiratory failure secondary to chronic obstructive pulmonary disease treated in the intensive care unit: a long term follow up study. *Thorax.* 2002;57(1):29-33.

60. Sapey E, Stockley RA. COPD exacerbations. 2: aetiology. *Thorax.* 2006;61(3):250-258.

61. Wildman MJ, Harrison DA, Brady AR, Rowan K. Case mix and outcomes for admissions to UK adult, general critical care units with chronic obstructive pulmonary disease: a secondary analysis of the ICNARC Case Mix Programme Database. *Crit Care.* 2005;9(suppl 3):S38-S48.

62. Nevins ML, Epstein SK. Predictors of outcome for patients with COPD requiring invasive mechanical ventilation. *Chest.* 2001;119(6):1840-1849.

63. Wildman MJ, Sanderson CF, Groves J, et al. Survival and quality of life for patients with COPD or asthma admitted to intensive care in a UK multicentre cohort: the COPD and Asthma Outcome Study (CAOS). *Thorax.* 2009;64(2):128-132.

64. Wildman MJ, Sanderson C, Groves J, et al. Implications of prognostic pessimism in patients with chronic obstructive pulmonary disease (COPD) or asthma admitted to intensive care in the UK within the COPD and asthma outcome study (CAOS): multicentre observational cohort study. *BMJ.* 2007;335(7630):1132.

65. Patel K, Janssen DJ, Curtis JR. Advance care planning in COPD. *Respirology.* 2012;17(1):72-78.

66. Batzlaff CM, Karpman C, Afessa B, Benzo RP. Predicting 1-year mortality rate for patients admitted with an acute exacerbation of chronic obstructive pulmonary disease to an intensive care unit: an opportunity for palliative care. *Mayo Clin Proc.* 2014;89(5):638-643.

67. Schmidt M, Demoule A, Deslandes-Boutmy E, et al. Intensive care unit admission in chronic obstructive pulmonary disease: patient information and the physician's decision-making process. *Crit Care.* 2014;18(3):R115

68. Claessens MT, Lynn J, Zhong Z, et al. Dying with lung cancer or chronic obstructive pulmonary disease: insights from SUPPORT. Study to understand prognoses and preferences for outcomes and risks of treatments. *J Am Geriatr Soc.* 2000;48(suppl 5):S146-S153.

12

Is Diaphragmatic Dysfunction a Major Problem Following Mechanical Ventilation?

Ewan C. Goligher and Martin Dres

INTRODUCTION

Critically ill patients are at high risk of developing acute generalized muscle injury and weakness. Injury and dysfunction of the respiratory muscles, especially the diaphragm, is of particular concern in mechanically ventilated patients because of the crucial role played by these muscles in enabling a patient to be liberated from mechanical ventilation. Mounting evidence suggests that diaphragmatic dysfunction developing during critical illness presents a serious obstacle to recovery. As yet there are no proven therapies for diaphragmatic dysfunction, but the field is evolving rapidly with a number of potential approaches to prevention and treatment on the horizon.

DEFINITION AND EPIDEMIOLOGY

The diaphragm is a thin, dome-shaped muscular structure separating the thoracic and abdominal cavities. Under normal conditions, the diaphragm acts like a piston within a syringe, generating flow as its dome descends, enabling tidal breathing.[1] The pressure generated across the dome between the thoracic and abdominal cavities is called the transdiaphragmatic pressure and is proportional to the tension developed within the muscle fibers.

Diagnostic Criteria

Diaphragmatic dysfunction can be defined as a reduction in the force-generating capacity of the diaphragm. Several methods are available to detect the presence of diaphragmatic dysfunction in critically ill patients. Bilateral anterior magnetic phrenic stimulation (BAMPS) is regarded as the reference technique because it generates a consistent level of diaphragm activation independent of volitional effort.[2,3] BAMPS elicits an isolated contraction (twitch) of the diaphragm to measure the change in transdiaphragmatic pressure or airway pressure.[4] Using this method, diaphragmatic dysfunction is defined by a decrease in its capacity to generate a negative intrathoracic pressure, usually below 11 cm H_2O.[2] While BAMPS provides a rigorous assessment of the diaphragm function, it is only available in expert centers and requires costly equipment, which precludes its widespread use.

An alternative means of evaluating diaphragmatic function in the intensive care unit (ICU) is ultrasound. When the diaphragm contracts, it thickens, and this thickening can be quantified by directly visualizing the muscle on ultrasound.[5] the motion (excursion) of the dome of the diaphragm during inspiration can also be visualized.[6] To assess thickening, the diaphragm is examined on its zone of apposition to the rib cage. In this location, ultrasound can measure end-expiratory and peak-inspiratory diaphragm thickness. Diaphragm-thickening fraction is computed as the fractional increase in diaphragm thickness during inspiration. Thickening fraction is tightly correlated with transdiaphragmatic pressure.[7,8] Thickening fraction is also correlated with the twitch pressure generated by BAMPS ($r = 0.87$), provided that patients trigger the ventilator. A thickening fraction below 30% is diagnostic for diaphragmatic dysfunction.[9]

Diaphragm excursion can be used to assess diaphragm function but only during nonassisted breathing; otherwise the downward displacement of the diaphragm may reflect passive insufflation of the chest by the ventilator. Diaphragm excursion ≤1 cm during resting unsupported breathing is diagnostic for diaphragmatic dysfunction.[6]

Respiratory muscle function can also be assessed by airway pressures generated during maximal inspiratory efforts against an occluded airway.[10] Transient airway occlusion for up to 20 seconds can be used to enhance respiratory drive and ensure maximal volition in mechanically ventilated patients.[11] Using this technique, respiratory muscle weakness is defined as maximal inspiratory pressure below 30–40 cm H_2O, although expected values vary somewhat with age.[10]

Epidemiology

Diaphragm weakness is strikingly common in mechanically ventilated patients. Diaphragmatic dysfunction is present in up to 63% of patients within 24 hours of ICU admission and intubation.[12] Since the initial severity of diaphragm weakness upon ICU admission is associated with the number and magnitude of organ failures, this early diaphragm weakness might simply be a form of organ failure associated with critical illness.[12]

At the time of weaning, diaphragmatic dysfunction is present in between 63% and 80% of patients.[13,14] Using diaphragm ultrasound, Kim et al. identified diaphragmatic dysfunction in 24/82 medical ICU patients (29%) undergoing a first spontaneous breathing trial.[15] Using BAMPs at time of weaning, diaphragmatic dysfunction was present in 63% of nonselected ICU patients[13] and in 80% of patients with critical illness polyneuropathy and polyneuropathy.[14]

Later in the course of ventilation, diaphragm weakness is nearly universal in mechanically ventilated patients. The severity of diaphragm weakness is directly correlated with the duration of ventilation.[16,17] In several studies, average twitch transdiaphragmatic pressures ranged between 7 and 10 cm H_2O, well below the lower limit of normal values in healthy subjects (28–30 cm H_2O).[4,18,19] In one study, 30% of patients had twitch transdiaphragmatic pressure below 5 cm H_2O, consistent with nearly complete muscle paralysis.[18]

The very high prevalence of profound diaphragm weakness is particularly striking when one considers that these studies generally excluded patients with any antecedent history of neuromuscular disease. Within a given patient, diaphragmatic function varies considerably through time. A recent cohort study found that many patients with profound diaphragm weakness on admission exhibited substantial recovery, while others without diaphragm weakness at baseline developed significant weakness.[20] The time-dependent variation in diaphragmatic function reflects the complex interplay of various waxing and waning pathophysiologic insults responsible for the development of muscle injury at weakness throughout the course of critical illness.

PATHOGENESIS

A variety of factors contribute to the high prevalence of diaphragmatic dysfunction among mechanically ventilated patients (Fig. 12.1).

Sepsis

Sepsis acutely impairs muscle function by several mechanisms. It interferes with systemic oxygen delivery and oxygen utilization (septic shock). Circulating inflammatory mediators directly impair the function of contractile proteins involved in the myofilament's force-generating mechanism.[21] Inflammatory cytokines also amplify nitric oxide production within muscle tissue by upregulating inducible nitric oxide synthase expression in specific tissues, including the diaphragm, leading to rapid impairment in muscle force generation.[22] As sepsis resolves, diaphragmatic function may rapidly improve.[20]

Metabolic Factors

Many metabolic derangements commonly associated with critical illness contribute to diaphragm weakness, including hypercapnia,[23,24] hypokalemia, hypophosphatemia, malnutrition, and hypoxemia.[25] Shock states also induce acute diaphragm weakness and fatigue by impairing oxygen delivery to the strenuously active respiratory muscles,[26,27] despite the redirection of oxygen delivery away from vital organs to the diaphragm.[28]

Pharmacologic Exposures

Sedative agents may directly injure the diaphragm or impair muscle function apart from causing muscle disuse (see below). For example, propofol causes acute diaphragm weakness in healthy subjects undergoing anesthesia[29] and activates muscle proteolysis in experimental models.[30] Corticosteroids are well-known to cause atrophy and myopathy with long-term administration by activating muscle proteolytic pathways.[31] Their impact on the development of ICU-acquired weakness and diaphragmatic dysfunction is less

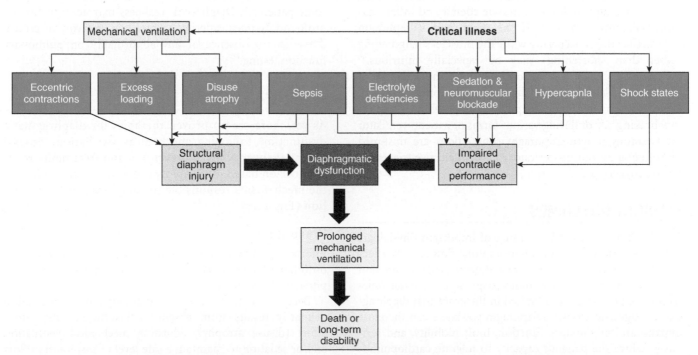

Fig. 12.1 Mechanisms of diaphragm injury and diaphragmatic dysfunction during critical illness.

certain, as recent studies do not bear out an association between corticosteroid exposure and ICU-acquired weakness[32] or diaphragm atrophy.[33]

Mechanical Ventilation

By suppressing respiratory muscle effort, mechanical ventilation can induce a remarkably rapid disuse atrophy of the diaphragm. This phenomenon has been demonstrated repeatedly in a range of experimental models.[34–37] Histologic studies in brain-dead organ donors and living mechanically ventilated patients have documented significant reductions in diaphragm myofiber cross-sectional area compared with that of other axial skeletal muscles.[16,38–40] Using bedside ultrasound, several clinical studies have documented widespread progressive thinning of the diaphragm over several days of mechanical ventilation.[33,41–43] The rate of thinning is directly related to the level of diaphragm contractile activity: patients with low or absent diaphragm contractility during mechanical ventilation exhibit significantly faster atrophy.[33] On the other hand, changes in diaphragm thickness were minimal when diaphragm thickening fraction (a sonographic marker for contractile effort) was similar to that of healthy subjects breathing at rest.

Diaphragm injury and diaphragmatic dysfunction may also result from insufficient ventilatory assistance. The work of breathing is often excessive in ventilated patients because of elevated respiratory load (compromised respiratory mechanics) and significantly increased respiratory drive (owing to a variety of chemoreceptive, mechanoreceptive, and cortical stimuli).[44] If the respiratory muscles are not adequately unloaded by mechanical ventilation, acute diaphragm injury can result. Sepsis and systemic inflammation render the myofiber cell membrane (sarcolemma) more fragile and susceptible to injury from mechanical stress; sarcolemma rupture leads to muscle edema and inflammation.[45] Eccentric loading of the diaphragm (diaphragm contractile efforts occurring while the muscle is lengthening rather than shortening) may be especially injurious.[46] Eccentric diaphragm contractions may occur in the context of significant atelectasis, where the diaphragm contracts during expiration to maintain end-expiratory lung volume ("expiratory braking"),[47] or during various forms of patient–ventilator dyssynchrony, where diaphragm contractions are mistimed and often occur during expiratory flow (ineffective triggering, reverse triggering).[48,49]

CLINICAL OUTCOMES

The diaphragm muscle has a range of important physiologic functions—the generation of inspiratory flow, cough effectiveness, posture, and maintenance of hemodynamic function in the face of intravascular volume depletion.[50–53] Axial skeletal muscle performance is limited in the event that diaphragmatic fatigue develops.[54] Diaphragm weakness can therefore impair cardiopulmonary function, limit mobility, and seriously reduce the patient's capacity to tolerate cardiopulmonary insults. In ventilated patients, diaphragmatic function is

a crucial determinant of weaning success.[55] Diaphragmatic dysfunction is associated with a substantial increase in the risk of weaning failure.[13,15,56] Patients with diaphragm weakness also require a significantly greater duration of weaning from mechanical ventilation and a prolonged ICU stay, and are at higher risk of death in the ICU or in hospital.[13,15] Of note, at the time of the first trial of spontaneous breathing, diaphragm muscle weakness has a much greater impact on prognosis than limb muscle weakness (Fig. 12.2).[13]

Similarly, the development of diaphragm atrophy during mechanical ventilation portends a much greater risk of reintubation, tracheostomy, and prolonged ventilation (Fig. 12.3).[57] This finding is important because it suggests that a potentially avoidable mechanism of injury, disuse atrophy from ventilator overassistance or oversedation, is responsible for prolonged ventilation and poor outcomes. Avoiding diaphragm atrophy may therefore prevent diaphragm weakness and the attendant poor outcomes.

The impact of diaphragm weakness after critical illness extends beyond the initial period of respiratory failure. The risk of readmission to ICU or hospital is substantially increased in patients with diaphragm weakness, persisting 7 days after ICU discharge.[58] Long-term outcomes are also probably significantly affected: patients with diaphragm weakness at ICU discharge are at significantly greater risk of death at 1 year after ICU discharge.[59] Given that diaphragm weakness prolongs ICU admission, and ICU admission in turn consistently predicts long-term functional disability in ICU survivors, the development of diaphragm weakness probably contributes to poor long-term functional status and quality of life. Although diaphragmatic dysfunction and poor long-term outcomes have not yet been directly linked, available data suggest that impaired respiratory muscle strength may persist for months and years after ICU admission in some patients.[32] Diaphragm weakness may account for the profound dyspnea experienced by some survivors of critical illness in the absence of any abnormality on pulmonary function testing.[60]

POTENTIAL THERAPIES

As yet, there are no proven therapies for diaphragmatic dysfunction following mechanical ventilation. Several potential approaches to prevention and treatment are on the horizon based on a rapidly evolving understanding of the mechanisms responsible for diaphragmatic dysfunction (Fig. 12.4).

Prevention

Efforts to prevent diaphragm weakness are primarily focused on different mechanistic aspects of ventilator-induced diaphragmatic dysfunction.

Because ventilator-induced diaphragmatic dysfunction primarily results from absent or insufficient inspiratory effort (disuse atrophy), adjusting mechanical ventilation and/or sedation to maintain a safe level of inspiratory effort may prevent disuse atrophy and diaphragm weakness. This

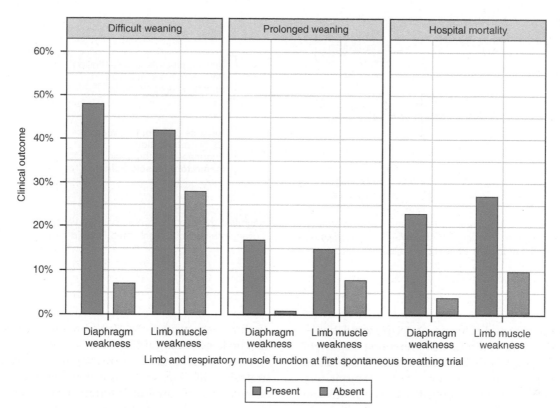

Fig. 12.2 Diaphragm weakness is more strongly associated with prognosis than limb muscle weakness at the time of the first trial of spontaneous breathing. (From Schreiber A, Bertoni M, Goligher EC. Avoiding respiratory and peripheral muscle injury during mechanical ventilation: diaphragm-protective ventilation and early mobilization. *Crit Care Clin.* 2018;34[3]:357-381. Based on data from Dres M, Dubé B-P, Mayaux J, et al. Coexistence and impact of limb muscle and diaphragm weakness at time of liberation from mechanical ventilation in medical intensive care unit patients. *Am J Respir Crit Care Med.* 2017;195[1]:57-66.)

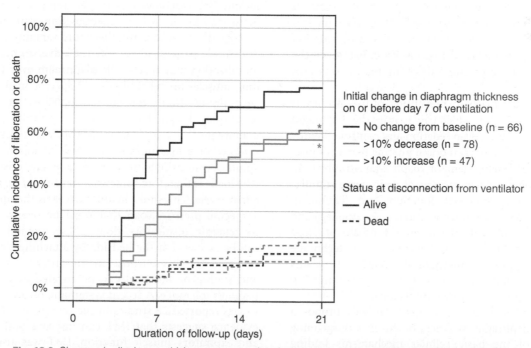

Fig. 12.3 Changes in diaphragm thickness are associated with delayed liberation from mechanical ventilation. In patients with early decreases or increases in thickness, the risk of remaining on mechanical ventilation at day 21 is approximately doubled. (From Goligher EC, Dres M, Fan E, et al. Mechanical ventilation-induced diaphragm atrophy strongly impacts clinical outcomes. *Am J Respir Crit Care Med.* 2018;197[2]:204-213.)

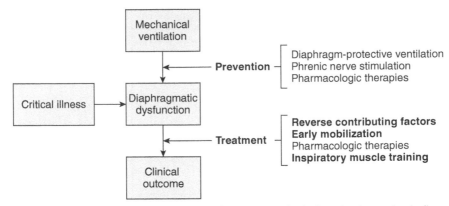

Fig. 12.4 Approach to prevention and treatment of diaphragmatic dysfunction in mechanically ventilated patients. The benefits of preventive strategies remain unproven. Interventions highlighted in **bold** have at least moderate evidence in support of clinical benefit.

approach—referred to as diaphragm-protective ventilation—offers a promising potential means of preventing diaphragm weakness.[61] In support of this concept, a recent study found that both insufficient and excessive levels of inspiratory effort were associated with prolonged ventilation, while an intermediate level of effort (similar to that of healthy subjects breathing at rest) was associated with a relatively shorter duration of ventilation.[57] These data provide a potential therapeutic target. However, in view of competing concerns such as the need to prevent ventilator-induced lung injury by maintaining a protective tidal volume and the need to ensure that patients are adequately sedated to be calm and comfortable, it is unclear whether the benefits of diaphragm protection outweigh the potential harms of maintaining spontaneous breathing.[62] It is also unclear whether it is possible to titrate ventilation and/or sedation to achieve the desired level of inspiratory effort, given the very high levels of respiratory drive in many conscious critically ill patients.

An alternative approach to preventing disuse atrophy is phrenic nerve stimulation, which can activate the diaphragm while permitting ongoing deep sedation and controlled ventilation as indicated. In animal models, phrenic nerve stimulation prevents the development of diaphragm atrophy.[63] In patients undergoing cardiac surgery, phrenic nerve stimulation maintains mitochondrial function and diaphragm muscle fiber force generation while mitigating autophagy and oxidative stress,[64–66] all cardinal features of ventilator-induced diaphragmatic dysfunction. The benefits of this technique have yet to be explored in mechanically ventilated patients with respiratory failure; patient selection and stimulation dosing remain important areas of uncertainty.

A variety of pharmacologic agents have been proposed for preventing diaphragm weakness based on a burgeoning understanding of the basic cellular mechanisms leading to diaphragmatic dysfunction. For example, a number of antioxidant agents or antiproteolytic agents have shown promise in preventing cellular derangements associated with diaphragm inactivity.[67–69,70] However, none of these therapies have undergone clinical testing.

While awaiting the confirmation of effective preventive strategies, clinicians can reasonably aim to ensure a comfortable and safe level of inspiratory effort in their ventilated patients by attending to patient effort levels and minimizing exposure to unnecessary sedation or neuromuscular blockade.

Treatment

Diaphragmatic function will improve as the factors that contribute to muscle weakness are addressed. Effective treatment of sepsis and avoidance of immobility are paramount. Pharmacologic agents, including levosimendan and methylxanthines such as theophylline, can improve diaphragmatic function but their role remains undefined in critically ill patients given potential adverse effects.[71,72] Early mobilization may recruit the diaphragm even as it recruits limb muscles for rehabilitation.[73] Specific inspiratory muscle training (IMT) can be accomplished by a variety of techniques designed to load the inspiratory muscles and diaphragm.[74] Two basic forms of IMT may be distinguished: flow-resistive loading and threshold loading. The former applies a resistance to inspiratory flow; the resistive pressure (the load) is therefore somewhat dependent on the patient's effort levels. Threshold loading involves the application of a specific pressure load that must be overcome in order to generate inspiratory flow. These methods of loading can be achieved at the bedside by attaching simple devices designed for this purpose to the airway. The magnitude and timing of the load can be titrated according to the patient's tolerance. A recent systematic review of IMT techniques reported 28 studies in the literature.[75] The available evidence suggests that IMT can improve both inspiratory and expiratory muscle function. IMT was also associated with a shorter duration of ventilation and ICU stay, but further trials are awaited to definitively confirm this finding.

AUTHORS' RECOMMENDATIONS

- Diaphragmatic dysfunction (DD) is extremely common in mechanically ventilated patients, occurring in two-thirds of patients within 24 hours, and directly contributes to poor clinical outcomes in critical illness.
- DD can be defined as a reduction in the force-generating capacity of the diaphragm: a decrease in its capacity to generate a negative intrathoracic pressure, usually below 11 cm H_2O.
- DD can be diagnosed using ultrasound at the level of the rib cage—to assess diaphragmatic thickness on inspiration and expiration. A thickening fraction below 30% is diagnostic.
- Epidemiologic factors for DD include sepsis, metabolic derangements, drugs (sedatives, neuromuscular blockers and, possibly, corticosteroids), mechanical ventilation, and inadequate ventilatory support.
- DD significantly contributes to weaning failure, prolonged mechanical ventilation, and readmission to ICU, and is associated with increased 1-year mortality.
- Preventive strategies for DD include avoidance of critical illness, by treating and source controlling sepsis early, avoidance of oversedation, "diaphragm-protective ventilation," phrenic nerve stimulation, and metabolic support.
- Therapeutic approaches to DD include early mobilization and inspiratory muscle training (flow resistive and threshold loading).

REFERENCES

1. Gauthier AP, Verbanck S, Estenne M, Segebarth C, Macklem PT, Paiva M. Three-dimensional reconstruction of the in vivo human diaphragm shape at different lung volumes. *J Appl Physiol.* 1994; 76(2):495-506.
2. American Thoracic Society/European Respiratory Society. ATS/ERS statement on respiratory muscle testing. *Am J Respir Crit Care Med.* 2002;166(4):518-624.
3. Moxham J, Goldstone J. Assessment of respiratory muscle strength in the intensive care unit. *Eur Respir J.* 1994;7(11):2057-2061.
4. Watson AC, Hughes PD, Louise Harris M, et al. Measurement of twitch transdiaphragmatic, esophageal, and endotracheal tube pressure with bilateral anterolateral magnetic phrenic nerve stimulation in patients in the intensive care unit. *Crit Care Med.* 2001;29(7):1325-1331.
5. Matamis D, Soilemezi E, Tsagourias M, et al. Sonographic evaluation of the diaphragm in critically ill patients. Technique and clinical applications. *Intensive Care Med.* 2013;39(5):801-810.
6. Boussuges A, Gole Y, Blanc P. Diaphragmatic motion studied by M-mode ultrasonography: methods, reproducibility, and normal values. *Chest.* 2009;135(2):391-400.
7. Vivier E, Mekontso Dessap A, Dimassi S, et al. Diaphragm ultrasonography to estimate the work of breathing during non-invasive ventilation. *Intensive Care Med.* 2012;38(5):796-803.
8. Goligher EC, Laghi F, Detsky ME, et al. Measuring diaphragm thickness with ultrasound in mechanically ventilated patients: feasibility, reproducibility and validity. *Intensive Care Med.* 2015;41(4):734.
9. Dubé BP, Dres M, Mayaux J, Demiri S, Similowski T, Demoule A. Ultrasound evaluation of diaphragm function in mechanically ventilated patients: comparison to phrenic stimulation and prognostic implications. *Thorax.* 2017;72(9):811-818.
10. Evans JA, Whitelaw WA. The assessment of maximal respiratory mouth pressures in adults. *Respir Care.* 2009;54(10):1348-1359.
11. Truwit JD, Marini JJ. Validation of a technique to assess maximal inspiratory pressure in poorly cooperative patients. *Chest.* 1992; 102(4):1216-1219.
12. Demoule A, Jung B, Prodanovic H, et al. Diaphragm dysfunction on admission to the intensive care unit. Prevalence, risk factors, and prognostic impact—a prospective study. *Am J Respir Crit Care Med.* 2013;188(2):213-219.
13. Dres M, Dubé BP, Mayaux J, et al. Coexistence and impact of limb muscle and diaphragm weakness at time of liberation from mechanical ventilation in medical intensive care unit patients. *Am J Respir Crit Care Med.* 2017;195(1):57-66.
14. Jung B, Moury PH, Mahul M, et al. Diaphragmatic dysfunction in patients with ICU-acquired weakness and its impact on extubation failure. *Intensive Care Med.* 2016;42(5):853-861.
15. Kim WY, Suh HJ, Hong SB, Koh Y, Lim CM. Diaphragm dysfunction assessed by ultrasonography: influence on weaning from mechanical ventilation. *Crit Care Med.* 2011;39(12):2627-2630.
16. Jaber S, Petrof BJ, Jung B, et al. Rapidly progressive diaphragmatic weakness and injury during mechanical ventilation in humans. *Am J Respir Crit Care Med.* 2011;183(3):364-371.
17. Hermans G, Agten A, Testelmans D, Decramer M, Gayan-Ramirez G. Increased duration of mechanical ventilation is associated with decreased diaphragmatic force: a prospective observational study. *Crit Care.* 2010;14(4):R127.
18. Supinski GS, Callahan LA. Diaphragm weakness in mechanically ventilated critically ill patients. *Crit Care.* 2013;17(3):R120.
19. Cattapan SE, Laghi F, Tobin MJ. Can diaphragmatic contractility be assessed by airway twitch pressure in mechanically ventilated patients? *Thorax.* 2003;58(1):58-62.
20. Demoule A, Molinari N, Jung B, et al. Patterns of diaphragm function in critically ill patients receiving prolonged mechanical ventilation: a prospective longitudinal study. *Ann Intensive Care.* 2016;6(1):75.
21. Shindoh C, Hida W, Ohkawara Y, et al. TNF-alpha mRNA expression in diaphragm muscle after endotoxin administration. *Am J Respir Crit Care Med.* 1995;152(5 Pt 1):1690-1696.
22. Boczkowski J, Lanone S, Ungureanu-Longrois D, Danialou G, Fournier T, Aubier M. Induction of diaphragmatic nitric oxide synthase after endotoxin administration in rats: role on diaphragmatic contractile dysfunction. *J Clin Invest.* 1996;98(7):1550-1559.
23. Juan G, Calverley P, Talamo C, Schnader J, Roussos C. Effect of carbon dioxide on diaphragmatic function in human beings. *N Engl J Med.* 1984;310(14):874-879.
24. Michelet P, Carreira S, Demoule A, et al. Effects of acute respiratory and metabolic acidosis on diaphragm muscle obtained from rats. *Anesthesiology.* 2015;122(4):876-883.
25. Laghi F, Tobin MJ. Disorders of the respiratory muscles. *Am J Respir Crit Care Med.* 2003;168(1):10-48.
26. Aubier M, Trippenbach T, Roussos C. Respiratory muscle fatigue during cardiogenic shock. *J Appl Physiol Respir Environ Exerc Physiol.* 1981;51(2):499-508.
27. Rutledge FS, Hussain SN, Roussos C, Magder S. Diaphragmatic energetics and blood flow during pulmonary edema and hypotension. *J Appl Physiol.* 1988;64(5):1908-1915.
28. Hussain SN, Roussos C. Distribution of respiratory muscle and organ blood flow during endotoxic shock in dogs. *J Appl Physiol.* 1985;59(6):1802-1808.
29. Shaw IC, Mills GH, Turnbull D. The effect of propofol on airway pressures generated by magnetic stimulation of the phrenic nerves. *Intensive Care Med.* 2002;28(7):891-897.

30. Bruells CS, Maes K, Rossaint R, et al. Sedation using propofol induces similar diaphragm dysfunction and atrophy during spontaneous breathing and mechanical ventilation in rats. *Anesthesiology*. 2014;120(3):665-672.
31. Sassoon CS, Caiozzo VJ. Bench-to-bedside review: diaphragm muscle function in disuse and acute high-dose corticosteroid treatment. *Crit Care*. 2009;13(5):221.
32. Fan E, Dowdy DW, Colantuoni E, et al. Physical complications in acute lung injury survivors: a two-year longitudinal prospective study. *Crit Care Med*. 2014;42(4):849-859.
33. Goligher EC, Fan E, Herridge MS, et al. Evolution of diaphragm thickness during mechanical ventilation. Impact of inspiratory effort. *Am J Respir Crit Care Med*. 2015;192(9):1080-1088.
34. Powers SK, Shanely RA, Coombes JS, et al. Mechanical ventilation results in progressive contractile dysfunction in the diaphragm. *J Appl Physiol*. 2002;92(5):1851-1858.
35. Sassoon CS, Caiozzo VJ, Manka A, Sieck GC. Altered diaphragm contractile properties with controlled mechanical ventilation. *J Appl Physiol*. 2002;92(6):2585-2595.
36. Anzueto A, Peters JI, Tobin MJ, et al. Effects of prolonged controlled mechanical ventilation on diaphragmatic function in healthy adult baboons. *Crit Care Med*. 1997;25(7):1187-1190.
37. Yang L, Luo J, Bourdon J, Lin MC, Gottfried SB, Petrof BJ. Controlled mechanical ventilation leads to remodeling of the rat diaphragm. *Am J Respir Crit Care Med*. 2002;166(8):1135-1140.
38. Levine S, Nguyen T, Taylor N, et al. Rapid disuse atrophy of diaphragm fibers in mechanically ventilated humans. *N Engl J Med*. 2008;358(13):1327-1335.
39. Hooijman PE, Beishuizen A, Witt CC, et al. Diaphragm muscle fiber weakness and ubiquitin-proteasome activation in critically ill patients. *Am J Respir Crit Care Med*. 2015;191(10):1126-1138.
40. Hussain SN, Cornachione AS, Guichon C, et al. Prolonged controlled mechanical ventilation in humans triggers myofibrillar contractile dysfunction and myofilament protein loss in the diaphragm. *Thorax*. 2016;71(5):436-445.
41. Grosu HB, Lee YI, Lee J, Eden E, Eikermann M, Rose KM. Diaphragm muscle thinning in patients who are mechanically ventilated. *Chest*. 2012;142(6):1455-1460.
42. Schepens T, Verbrugghe W, Dams K, Corthouts B, Parizel PM, Jorens PG. The course of diaphragm atrophy in ventilated patients assessed with ultrasound: a longitudinal cohort study. *Crit Care*. 2015;19(1):422.
43. Zambon M, Beccaria P, Matsuno J, et al. Mechanical ventilation and diaphragmatic atrophy in critically ill patients: an ultrasound study. *Crit Care Med*. 2016;44(7):1347-1352.
44. Marini JJ, Rodriguez RM, Lamb V. The inspiratory workload of patient-initiated mechanical ventilation. *Am Rev Respir Dis*. 1986;134(5):902-909.
45. Lin MC, Ebihara S, El Dwairi Q, et al. Diaphragm sarcolemmal injury is induced by sepsis and alleviated by nitric oxide synthase inhibition. *Am J Respir Crit Care Med*. 1998;158(5 Pt 1):1656-1663.
46. Gea J, Zhu E, Gáldiz JB, et al. [Functional consequences of eccentric contractions of the diaphragm]. *Arch Bronconeumol*. 2009;45(2):68-74. [in Spanish]
47. Pellegrini M, Hedenstierna G, Roneus A, Segelsjö M, Larsson A, Perchiazzi G. The diaphragm acts as a brake during expiration to prevent lung collapse. *Am J Respir Crit Care Med*. 2016;195(12):1608-1616.
48. Akoumianaki E, Lyazidi A, Rey N, et al. Mechanical ventilation-induced reverse-triggered breaths: a frequently unrecognized form of neuromechanical coupling. *Chest*. 2013;143(4):927-938.
49. Chao DC, Scheinhorn DJ, Stearn-Hassenpflug M. Patient-ventilator trigger asynchrony in prolonged mechanical ventilation. *Chest*. 1997;112(6):1592-1599.
50. Troyer A, Loring SH. Action of the respiratory muscles. *Compr Physiol*. 2011;(suppl 12):443-461.
51. Irwin RS, Rosen MJ, Braman SS. Cough. A comprehensive review. *Arch Intern Med*. 1977;137(9):1186-1191.
52. Hodges PW, Butler JE, McKenzie DK, Gandevia SC. Contraction of the human diaphragm during rapid postural adjustments. *J Physiol*. 1997;505(Pt 2):539-548.
53. Skytioti M, Søvik S, Elstad M. Respiratory pump maintains cardiac stroke volume during hypovolemia in young, healthy volunteers. *J Appl Physiol*. 2018;124(5):1319-1325.
54. Sheel AW, Derchak PA, Morgan BJ, Pegelow DF, Jacques AJ, Dempsey JA. Fatiguing inspiratory muscle work causes reflex reduction in resting leg blood flow in humans. *J Physiol*. 2001;537(Pt 1):277-289.
55. Vassilakopoulos T, Zakynthinos S, Roussos C. The tension–time index and the frequency/tidal volume ratio are the major pathophysiologic determinants of weaning failure and success. *Am J Respir Crit Care Med*. 1998;158(2):378-385.
56. DiNino E, Gartman EJ, Sethi JM, McCool FD. Diaphragm ultrasound as a predictor of successful extubation from mechanical ventilation. *Thorax*. 2014;69(5):423-427.
57. Goligher EC, Dres M, Fan E, et al. Mechanical ventilation-induced diaphragm atrophy strongly impacts clinical outcomes. *Am J Respir Crit Care Med*. 2018;197(2):204-213.
58. Adler D, Dupuis-Lozeron E, Richard JC, Janssens JP, Brochard L. Does inspiratory muscle dysfunction predict readmission after intensive care unit discharge? *Am J Respir Crit Care Med*. 2014;190(3):347-350.
59. Medrinal C, Prieur G, Frenoy É, et al. Respiratory weakness after mechanical ventilation is associated with one-year mortality—a prospective study. *Crit Care*. 2016;20(1):231.
60. Wilcox ME, Patsios D, Murphy G, et al. Radiologic outcomes at 5 years after severe ARDS. *Chest*. 2013;143(4):920-926.
61. Heunks L, Ottenheijm C. Diaphragm-protective mechanical ventilation to improve outcomes in ICU patients? *Am J Respir Crit Care Med*. 2018;197(2):150-152.
62. Yoshida T, Fujino Y, Amato MB, Kavanagh BP. Fifty years of research in ARDS. Spontaneous breathing during mechanical ventilation. Risks, mechanisms, and management. *Am J Respir Crit Care Med*. 2017;195(8):985-992.
63. Reynolds SC, Meyyappan R, Thakkar V, et al. Mitigation of ventilator-induced diaphragm atrophy by transvenous phrenic nerve stimulation. *Am J Respir Crit Care Med*. 2017;195(3):339-348.
64. Martin AD, Joseph AM, Beaver TM, et al. Effect of intermittent phrenic nerve stimulation during cardiothoracic surgery on mitochondrial respiration in the human diaphragm. *Crit Care Med*. 2014;42(2):e152-e156.
65. Ahn B, Beaver T, Martin T, et al. Phrenic nerve stimulation increases human diaphragm fiber force after cardiothoracic surgery. *Am J Respir Crit Care Med*. 2014;190(7):837-839.
66. Mankowski RT, Ahmed S, Beaver T, et al. Intraoperative hemidiaphragm electrical stimulation reduces oxidative stress and upregulates autophagy in surgery patients undergoing mechanical ventilation: exploratory study. *J Transl Med*. 2016;14(1):305.
67. Powers SK, Hudson MB, Nelson WB, et al. Mitochondria-targeted antioxidants protect against mechanical ventilation-induced diaphragm weakness. *Crit Care Med*. 2011;39(7):1749-1759.

68. Supinski GS, Callahan LA. β-hydroxy-β-methylbutyrate (HMB) prevents sepsis-induced diaphragm dysfunction in mice. *Respir Physiol Neurobiol.* 2014;196:63-68.

69. Agten A, Maes K, Thomas D, et al. Bortezomib partially protects the rat diaphragm from ventilator-induced diaphragm dysfunction. *Crit Care Med.* 2012;40(8):2449-2455.

70. Agten A, Maes K, Smuder A, Powers SK, Decramer M, Gayan-Ramirez G. N-Acetylcysteine protects the rat diaphragm from the decreased contractility associated with controlled mechanical ventilation. *Crit Care Med.* 2011; 39(4):777-782.

71. Doorduin J, Sinderby CA, Beck J, et al. The calcium sensitizer levosimendan improves human diaphragm function. *Am J Respir Crit Care Med.* 2012;185(1):90-95.

72. Aubier M, Roussos C. Effect of theophylline on respiratory muscle function. *Chest.* 1985;88(suppl 2):91S-97S.

73. Dantas CM, Silva PF, Siqueira FH, et al. Influence of early mobilization on respiratory and peripheral muscle strength in critically ill patients. *Rev Bras Ter Intensiva.* 2012;24(2): 173-178.

74. Bissett B, Leditschke IA, Green M, Marzano V, Collins S, Van Haren F. Inspiratory muscle training for intensive care patients: a multidisciplinary practical guide for clinicians. *Aust Crit Care.* 2018. doi:10.1016/j.aucc.2018.06.001. [Epub ahead of print].

75. Vorona S, Sabatini U, Al-Maqbali S, et al. Inspiratory muscle rehabilitation in critically ill adults. A systematic review and meta-analysis. *Ann Am Thorac Soc.* 2018;15(6):735-744.

13

ARDS: Are the Current Definitions Useful?

Jason H. Maley and B. Taylor Thompson

INTRODUCTION

Following the initial 1967 description of the acute respiratory distress syndrome (ARDS) in a case series of 12 patients, numerous efforts have sought to define ARDS in a manner meaningful to clinicians and researchers.[1–3] in this initial description, ARDS was noted to be acute in onset and accompanied by hypoxemia, tachypnea, and decreased respiratory system compliance. Despite multiple iterative changes to the definition of ARDS since that time, the defining characteristics set forth in 1967 remain essential features. The current definition of ARDS, known as the "Berlin definition," emerged from an international expert panel convened in Berlin, Germany in 2011 to review and update the 1994 American–European Consensus Conference (AECC) definition.[3,4] in this chapter, we explore the development of the Berlin definition, discuss the definition's impact on the diagnosis and management of patients with ARDS, and describe limitations to the definition's use in both clinical and research settings.

CREATING THE BERLIN DEFINITION—AN EVIDENCE-BASED CONSENSUS

In updating the AECC definition, the Berlin panel reviewed epidemiologic and clinical trials data to create a definition based on feasibility, reliability, and validity.[4] Feasibility was an essential aim as this describes a definition's ability to identify the condition using readily available testing (e.g., chest radiographs) in a timely manner to facilitate rapid identification of cases for both guiding clinical care and facilitating clinical trial enrollment. Reliable definitions allow consistent identification of patients across studies (e.g., accurate interpretation of chest radiographs for qualifying opacities) and allow clinicians to apply study results to patients. With regards to validity, both face and predictive validity were examined.[5] the panel took a novel approach of utilizing a patient-level meta-analysis of existing epidemiologic and trials data to refine the definition with regards to predictive (or prognostic) validity for mortality.[6] the core aspects of previous definitions of

ARDS, including acute onset, bilateral radiographic opacities, and severe hypoxemia, were incorporated into the definition, as discussed in the following section. The initial Berlin draft also incorporated three grades of severity of hypoxemia, and four ancillary variables for severe ARDS. These ancillary variables were radiographic severity, respiratory system compliance (≤ 40 mL/cm H_2O), positive end-expiratory pressure (PEEP) (≥ 10 cm H_2O), and corrected (for partial pressure of arterial carbon dioxide [$PaCO_2$]) minute ventilation (≥ 10 L/min). Surprisingly, the addition of these severity criteria identified subgroups with a similar mortality to the larger subgroup identified with a much simpler severity metric, a PaO_2/FiO_2 <100 on 5 cm H_2O or more of PEEP. Thus, the four ancillary variables for severe ARDS added only complexity to the definition and were abandoned.

THE BERLIN DEFINITION

The Berlin panel's final product was a definition of ARDS that incorporates readily accessible clinical, radiographic, and laboratory data (Table 13.1). Based on a patient's history, the definition requires that the onset of symptoms occurred within 1 week of presentation or known clinical insult. As ARDS is an acute process, this distinguishes the entity from inflammatory lung diseases such as cryptogenic organizing pneumonia, which can follow a more indolent course, though might otherwise meet criteria for ARDS. Chest imaging was expanded to include either a chest radiograph or a chest computed tomography (CT) scan, and must either demonstrate bilateral opacities not fully explained by effusions, lobar/lung collapse, or nodules. The addition of CT scan to the criteria, and an emphasis on exclusion of alternative explanations for imaging findings (such as a mass, atelectasis, or a pleural effusion), aimed to increase the specificity of the definition and facilitate reliable interpretation. Additionally, the edema seen on imaging must not be fully explained by cardiac failure or fluid overload based on a clinician's judgment. If a clear risk factor for ARDS, such as sepsis, is not present, then clinicians should take further steps to exclude

TABLE 13.1   The Berlin Definition of ARDS.

Timing	Within 1 week of a known clinical insult or new/worsening respiratory symptoms		
Chest imaging	Bilateral opacities—not fully explained by effusions, lobar/lung collapse, or nodules		
Origin of edema	Respiratory failure not fully explained by cardiac failure or fluid overload; need objective assessment (e.g., echocardiography) to exclude hydrostatic edema if no risk factor present		
	Mild	**Moderate**	**Severe**
Severity of hypoxemia	$200 < PaO_2{:}FiO_2 \leq 300$ with PEEP or CPAP 5 cm H_2O	$100 < PaO_2{:}FiO_2 \leq 200$ with PEEP 5 cm H_2O	$PaO_2{:}FiO_2 \leq 100$ with PEEP 5 cm H_2O

hydrostatic edema, typically with transthoracic echocardiography. Patients must be receiving PEEP (or continuous positive airway pressure [CPAP] if mild severity) of at least 5 cm H_2O prior to assessing the degree of hypoxemia. Finally, severity of ARDS is graded in the Berlin definition based on the degree of arterial hypoxemia using the ratio of partial pressure of arterial oxygen to the fraction of inspired oxygen (PaO_2/FiO_2). ARDS is considered mild if $200 < PaO_2/FiO_2 \leq 300$, moderate if $100 < PaO_2/FiO_2 \leq 200$, and, as noted above, severe if $PaO_2/FiO_2 \leq 100$.

COMPARING THE BERLIN AND AECC DEFINITIONS

Several important changes distinguish the Berlin definition from the previous AECC definition. These changes are a result of evidence, accumulated over the nearly 20 years since the AECC definition, which informed the feasibility, reliability, and validity of the Berlin definition. The first major change relates to the distinction between hydrostatic edema and ARDS. The AECC definition stated that if a pulmonary artery catheter was present, the pulmonary artery occlusion pressure (PAOP) should be less than 18 mm Hg to exclude left atrial hypertension as the cause of pulmonary edema. In contrast, the Berlin definition makes no mention of the use of pulmonary capillary wedge pressure for the diagnosis of ARDS. The Berlin panel also removed the previous AECC definition statement that clinicians should determine that there was "no evidence of left atrial hypertension" if a PAOP measurement was not available. Both these modifications acknowledged growing evidence that ARDS and cardiogenic edema may coexist. This coexistence of ARDS and hydrostatic edema has, in fact, been demonstrated in multiple studies, including a randomized trial of pulmonary artery catheter vs. central venous catheter-guided fluid management in 1000 patients with ARDS.[6,7,8,9] Wheeler and colleagues reported that 29% of the patients enrolled, all of whom were deemed to have ARDS "without evidence of left atrial hypertension," were found upon insertion of a pulmonary artery catheter to have a PAOP exceeding the AECC upper-allowable limit of 18 mm Hg. Accordingly, the Berlin definition changes the emphasis away from prior definitions, including the AECC, which insisted that ARDS could only be diagnosed in the absence of left atrial hypertension, to stating that in patients with both conditions, the respiratory failure should not be fully explained by cardiac failure or fluid overload. Clinical vignettes were provided to help clinicians make this distinction as no biomarker, including brain natriuretic peptide (BNP), can reliably do so.

Compared with the AECC definition, the Berlin definition newly required 5 cm H_2O of PEEP (or CPAP in mild ARDS) to diagnose and grade the severity of ARDS. Following application of PEEP, a proportion of patients may have improved oxygenation and no longer meet diagnostic criteria for ARDS. This requirement may, therefore, exclude a proportion of patients who are unlikely to have pathologic diffuse alveolar damage and reduce the heterogeneity of populations enrolled in clinical studies. Notably, patients with severe ARDS, in the data examined by the Berlin authors, did not have a significant change in mortality when defined with this additional PEEP requirement. This is probably because severely hypoxemic patients are already managed with greater levels of PEEP based on current standard practices.

The stratification of patients by degree of hypoxemia, as assessed by PaO_2/FiO_2, was a significant change to the AECC definition. In the patient-level data analyzed by the Berlin panel, mortality in patients with mild, moderate, and severe ARDS was 27%, 32%, and 45% respectively. Median duration of mechanical ventilation was 5 days for mild ARDS, 7 days for moderate, and 9 days for severe ARDS. Overall, the area under the receiver operating characteristic (ROC) curve for mortality was 0.577 for the Berlin definition vs. 0.536 for AECC.[4]

The Berlin definition authors attempted to bolster reliability through supplemental material containing chest radiographs interpreted by the authors. This supplement demonstrates examples of opacities consistent with edema, those not consistent with edema, and radiographs where the distinction cannot be made. As discussed later in the chapter, despite these attempts, radiographic interpretation may remain a barrier to the accurate and reliable diagnosis of ARDS.

COMPARING THE BERLIN DEFINITION TO LUNG PATHOLOGY

Diffuse alveolar damage (DAD) has been considered the gold standard pathologic finding for ARDS on postmortem examination and lung biopsy since the original description of ARDS in 1967. Autopsy studies, however, have demonstrated that clinical criteria for ARDS do not always identify patients with pathologic DAD. In an autopsy series of 712 patient deaths within a single intensive care unit (ICU) over a 20-year period, Thille and colleagues described a subset of 356 patients who met the Berlin definition for ARDS. The authors aimed to better understand the relationship between clinical ARDS and pathologic findings. Within the cohort, 14% had mild, 40% moderate, and 46% severe ARDS by the Berlin definition. The authors reported that only 45% of the total 356 patients who met the Berlin definition had DAD on pathologic specimens. The proportion of patients with DAD was greatest in the group with severe ARDS, where 58% of the patients had DAD, compared with 40% in the moderate ARDS group, and 12% in the mild ARDS group. When either DAD, pneumonia, or both were considered as the reference standard for pathologic ARDS, the sensitivity of the Berlin definition increased to 88%, while the specificity remained low at 37%. In this study, the origin of ARDS did not influence the likelihood of DAD on pathology. DAD was present in 49% of patients with a primary pulmonary process (e.g., pneumonia) causing ARDS and in 42% of patients with extrapulmonary (e.g., pancreatitis, sepsis) ARDS. Normal lung pathology was found in approximately one in every eight patients with ARDS.[10]

Importantly, Thille and colleagues reported that a lower proportion of DAD were found in patients with ARDS over the latter decade of study (2001–2010) when compared with patients from the period 1991–2000. For the 2001–2010 period, patients were also ventilated with lower average tidal volumes than patients in the 1991–2000 cohort, probably as a result of the landmark ARDS network trial supporting the use of lower tidal volume targets.[11] This observation supports experimental evidence that DAD is, to some degree, the histologic finding of ventilator-induced lung injury.

In 2004, Esteban and colleagues examined autopsy findings within the same series of patients to understand the relationship between lung pathology and the AECC criteria[12]: 127 patients met the AECC definition for ARDS and 112 of these patients (88%) had diffuse alveolar damage on autopsy. The overall sensitivity of the clinical definition was 75% and the specificity was 84%. The lack of specificity of the Berlin definition for DAD, as compared with AECC, probably results from the addition of a mild ARDS category ($200 < PaO_2:FiO_2 \le 300$). Patients with mild ARDS were previously considered non-ARDS acute lung injury in the AECC definition. Given the low prevalence of DAD in mild ARDS, the inclusion of these patients will decrease the specificity of the Berlin definition for DAD within this subset of ARDS.

Taken together, autopsy data from patients meeting clinical criteria for ARDS suggest that clinical trials for ARDS most likely enroll a significant proportion of patients who do not have pathologic diffuse alveolar damage. Furthermore, the inclusion of pneumonia and other findings of lung edema and hemorrhage on pathologic specimens, with DAD, may better link pulmonary pathologic changes to clinical ARDS.[10,11,13] The imperfect correlation between clinical criteria for ARDS and pathologic DAD underscores the importance of developing more advanced methods of identifying ARDS beyond clinical criteria. These methods may include molecular phenotyping (i.e., biomarkers) to support characterization of patients by biologic criteria in addition to clinical criteria. These biomarkers are essential for drug-discovery and interventional trials, as the study of therapies for the underlying pathology of ARDS will depend on accurately enrolling patients with that specific pathology.

LIMITATIONS OF THE BERLIN DEFINITION FOR RECOGNITION AND MANAGEMENT OF ARDS

Despite the Berlin definition's improved feasibility, reliability, and validity, limitations to its application remain. These limitations affect both research and clinical work, and arise from numerous factors, including the potential for misinterpretation of radiographic criteria, lack of specific biomarkers, heterogeneity of the ARDS population, and absence of objective noninvasive assessment of causes of edema.

The Large observational study to UNderstand the Global impact of Severe Acute respiratory FailurE (LUNG SAFE) examined a cohort of over 29,000 ICU patients, over 3000 of whom had ARDS.[14] the LUNG SAFE investigators identified patients fulfilling the Berlin definition of ARDS and examined the incidence and outcomes of ARDS, as well as clinician recognition, ventilator management, and use of adjunct treatments for ARDS. Over a 4-week study period in the winter of 2014, the prevalence of mild, moderate, and severe ARDS was 30%, 46.6%, and 23.4%, respectively.

Clinician recognition of ARDS was assessed at the time of screening for the study and at the study conclusion with a simple questionnaire. Clinicians were asked at study enrollment the cause of their patient's hypoxemia and were asked at the conclusion if ARDS was present at any time during the ICU stay. The percentage of patients correctly identified as having ARDS ranged from 78.5% for severe ARDS to 51.3% for mild ARDS. When ARDS was recognized, this was associated with utilization of a higher level of PEEP, greater use of neuromuscular blockade, and use of prone positioning.

Tidal volumes used for ventilation in patients with ARDS were, on average, 7.5–7.8 mL/kg predicted body weight, with no significant difference across degrees of severity. While it is encouraging to see an increased use of adjunctive therapies in moderate and severe ARDS as compared with mild ARDS, these treatments were still employed in a minority of patients. Neuromuscular blockade was used in 37.8% of patients with severe ARDS, while these patients were managed with prone positioning only 16% of the time. When stratified by severity, the in-hospital mortality for these patients was 34.9% for mild ARDS, 40.3% for moderate ARDS, and 46.1% for those with severe ARDS. Similarly, ICU mortality and 28-day mortality were significantly different between grades of severity, all supporting the prognostic value of the Berlin PaO_2/FiO_2 thresholds.

While the Berlin panel included sample radiographs to assist clinicians and researchers in the radiographic assessment of ARDS, radiographic interpretation may be an ongoing limitation to the recognition of ARDS. To better understand this limitation, Goddard and colleagues conducted a randomized trial of an educational intervention to improve the accuracy and reliability of the radiographic diagnosis of ARDS. Prior to a test module, they randomized a total of 463 LUNG SAFE study coordinators to either an educational intervention consisting of clinical vignettes and radiographic examples or to a control arm with no education prior to the module. Out of 11 total radiographs in the test module, the participants identified 6.43 (intervention) and 6.18 (control) cases correctly, with no significant difference between groups. Overall, the accuracy and reliability for the diagnosis of ARDS by LUNG SAFE coordinators were poor and were not improved by an educational intervention. If study investigators and coordinators have difficulty identifying ARDS accurately, clinicians as a whole may be similarly challenged. Additionally, this limitation may lead to significant heterogeneity of patients enrolled in clinical studies, thus impacting the effects of interventions and interpretation of trial results.[15]

In resource-limited settings, strict use of the Berlin definition may fail to identify patients with ARDS. In a prospective observational cohort of patients hospitalized at the University Teaching Hospital of Kigali, Rwanda, Riviello and colleagues examined the utility of the Berlin definition and a modification termed the Kigali modification of the Berlin definition for identifying patients with ARDS.[16] the Kigali modification used the ratio of oxygen saturation by pulse oximetry to the fraction of inspired oxygen (SpO_2:FiO_2) rather than PaO_2:FiO_2, removed the PEEP requirement, and allowed for chest radiograph or ultrasound imaging to be used for the diagnosis of bilateral pulmonary opacities. Of 1046 adult patients admitted to the hospital over the 6-week study period, 42 patients were diagnosed with ARDS by Kigali modification while no patients met the traditional Berlin definition of ARDS. The mortality of ARDS by Kigali modification of the Berlin definition was 50% in this cohort. The limitation of the Berlin definition was primarily due to the inability to measure PaO_2 in this setting and the limited utilization of PEEP due to reduced availability of mechanical ventilators. Appropriate modifications to ARDS criteria, such as those by Riviello and colleagues, are essential for expanding both research and clinical care in resource-limited settings.

CONCLUSION

In 2011, the Berlin panel convened with the aim of improving the feasibility, reliability, and validity of the definition of ARDS. The new definition was successful in many of these respects, allowing clinicians to identify patients with ARDS using readily available diagnostic information and clinical judgment. By stratifying patients based on severity of hypoxemia, the Berlin definition more tightly linked physiology to outcomes. Despite these advancements, ARDS remains underrecognized, thereby limiting the appropriate use of evidence-based adjunctive therapies, some with very strong evidence to support their use (e.g., prone ventilation in severe ARDS). Further complicating the process of defining ARDS is the fact that the pathologic gold standard of ARDS, diffuse alveolar damage, is frequently not present in patients meeting the clinical definition of ARDS and may be even less common in the low tidal volume era. The limitations of the Berlin definition are illustrative of the broader challenge of using clinical criteria rather than specific biomarkers to define a pathologic process. Future work must therefore focus on identifying and incorporating biomarkers for ARDS into a clinical definition, in the hope of improving clinician identification of patients with ARDS and advancing the study of specific targeted therapies in clinical trials.

AUTHORS' RECOMMENDATIONS

- The current consensus definitions for ARDS were derived from a meeting in Berlin in 2011 and are colloquially known as the "Berlin definition."
- The definition eliminated the term "acute lung injury" and stratified ARDS into mild, moderate, and severe, related to the PaO_2/FiO_2 (PF) ratio: this more tightly linked physiology to outcomes.
- The addition of a minimal PEEP or CPAP level (5 cm H_2O), probably removed many patients that had hypoxemia and patchy infiltrates on chest X-ray but not ARDS.
- ARDS remains underrecognized—as demonstrated by the LUNG SAFE trial.
- This results in patients not receiving evidence-based adjunctive therapies—such as neuromuscular blockade and prone positioning.
- The pathologic gold standard of ARDS, diffuse alveolar damage (DAD), is frequently not present in patients meeting the clinical definition of ARDS and may be even less common in the low tidal volume era.
- The limitations of the Berlin definition are illustrative of the broader challenge of using clinical criteria rather than specific biomarkers to define a pathologic process.

REFERENCES

1. Ashbaugh DG, Bigelow DB, Petty TL, Levine BE. Acute respiratory distress in adults. *Lancet*. 1967;2(7511):319-323.
2. Murray JF, Matthay MA, Luce JM, Flick MR. An expanded definition of the adult respiratory distress syndrome. *Am Rev Respir Dis*. 1988;138(3):720-723.
3. Bernard GR, Artigas A, Brigham KL, et al. The American-European Consensus Conference on ARDS. Definitions, mechanisms, relevant outcomes, and clinical trial coordination. *Am J Respir Crit Care Med*. 1994;149(3 Pt 1):818-824.
4. Ranieri VM, Rubenfeld GD, Thompson BT, et al. Acute respiratory distress syndrome: the Berlin Definition. *JAMA*. 2012;307(23):2526-2533.
5. Thompson BT, Moss M. A new definition for the acute respiratory distress syndrome. *Semin Respir Crit Care Med*. 2013;34(4):441-447.
6. Ferguson ND, Fan E, Camporota L, et al. The Berlin definition of ARDS: an expanded rationale, justification, and supplementary material. *Intensive Care Med*. 2012;38(10):1573-1582.
7. Harvey S, Harrison DA, Singer M, et al. Assessment of the clinical effectiveness of pulmonary artery catheters in management of patients in intensive care (PAC-Man): a randomised controlled trial. *Lancet*. 2005;366(9484):472-477.

8. Wheeler AP, Bernard GR, Thompson BT, et al. Pulmonary-artery versus central venous catheter to guide treatment of acute lung injury. *N Engl J Med*. 2006;354(21):2213-2224.

9. Ferguson ND, Meade MO, Hallett DC, Stewart TE. High values of the pulmonary artery wedge pressure in patients with acute lung injury and acute respiratory distress syndrome. *Intensive Care Med*. 2002;28(8):1073-1077.

10. Thille AW, Esteban A, Fernández-Segoviano P, et al. Comparison of the Berlin definition for acute respiratory distress syndrome with autopsy. *Am J Respir Crit Care Med*. 2013;187(7):761-767.

11. Brower RG, Matthay MA, Morris A, et al. Ventilation with lower tidal volumes as compared with traditional tidal volumes for acute lung injury and the acute respiratory distress syndrome. *N Engl J Med*. 2000;342(18):1301-1308.

12. Esteban A, Fernández-Segoviano P, Frutos-Vivar F, et al. Comparison of clinical criteria for the acute respiratory distress syndrome with autopsy findings. *Ann Intern Med*. 2004;141(6):440-445.

13. Thompson BT, Matthay MA. The Berlin definition of ARDS versus pathological evidence of diffuse alveolar damage. *Am J Respir Crit Care Med*. 2013;187(7):675-677.

14. Bellani G, Laffey JG, Pham T, et al. Epidemiology, patterns of care, and mortality for patients with acute respiratory distress syndrome in intensive care units in 50 countries. *JAMA*. 2016;315(8):788-800.

15. Goddard SL, Rubenfeld GD, Manoharan V, et al. The randomized educational acute respiratory distress syndrome diagnosis study: a trial to improve the radiographic diagnosis of acute respiratory distress syndrome. *Crit Care Med*. 2018;46(5):743-748.

16. Riviello ED, Kiviri W, Twagirumugabe T, et al. Hospital incidence and outcomes of the acute respiratory distress syndrome using the Kigali Modification of the Berlin Definition. *Am J Respir Crit Care Med*. 2016;193(1):52-59.

14

What Are the Pathologic and Pathophysiologic Changes That Accompany ARDS?

Jonathan Dale Casey and Lorraine B. Ware

INTRODUCTION

Despite substantial progress since the initial description of acute respiratory distress syndrome (ARDS) by Ashbaugh and colleagues in 1967, the pathophysiology of ARDS remains incompletely understood.[1] the condition develops after an injury to the lung that can be direct (pneumonia, aspiration of gastric contents, pulmonary contusion, inhalation injury near-drowning, or fat, amniotic fluid embolism) or indirect (sepsis from a nonpulmonary source, multiple trauma, cardiopulmonary bypass, drug overdose, acute pancreatitis, transfusion of blood products).[2–7] Pneumonia, aspiration, and sepsis are the most common causes of ARDS, and were identified as the inciting event in 85% of the patients enrolled in recent clinical trials of ARDS patients.[8] There have been significant efforts in recent years to elucidate better ways to differentiate patients within the broader clinical syndrome of ARDS, beyond the mechanism of injury.[9–11] Regardless of the cause, the central tenets of ARDS pathophysiology are accumulation and activation of immune cells and platelets, dysregulation of inflammation, increased permeability of the alveolar-capillary barrier, and activation of coagulation pathways.[2,4,12,13] The pathophysiologic changes evolve over the course of the disease as the lung injury progresses through three phases: an exudative phase, a proliferative phase, and a fibrotic phase.[8] Previously, it was believed that these phases were distinct, with a predictable time course of progression, but it is now recognized that there is significant temporal and spatial heterogeneity in ARDS, such that different regions of the lung may be in different phases of ARDS.[14]

PATHOGENESIS

The Exudative Phase

Activation of the Innate Immune System and Platelets

The exudative phase is the lung's initial response to injury, which begins within 24 hours of the insult (Fig. 14.1).[8] It is characterized by activation of the innate immune system, damage to both the alveolar epithelial and endothelial barriers, increased permeability of the alveolar-capillary barrier, and influx of protein-rich edema fluid into the interstitium and alveolar space.[15] An early event in the development of ARDS is the activation of alveolar macrophages by exposure to microbial components of pathogenic organisms (pathogen-associated molecular patterns [PAMPs]) or damage-associated molecular patterns (DAMPs) released from injured cells such as HMGB1 (high mobility group box 1) and mitochondrial DNA.[4,16–18] Resident macrophages then activate the complement system and release proinflammatory cytokines (such as tumor necrosis factor alpha [TNF-α] and interleukins IL-6 and IL-17) and chemokines (such as IL-8, CCL2, CCL7, CXCL8, and CXCL10) which recruit neutrophils and monocytes or macrophages to the site of insult.[19,20] The resultant endothelial damage leads to the breakdown in the capillary wall, to which platelets adhere. There has been an increasing recognition of the role that platelets play in ARDS as platelet-derived thromboxane A2 (TXA2) and P-selectin activate neutrophils, further exacerbating cytokine release.[21–23] Activated platelets induce expression of ICAM-1 on endothelial cells and secrete platelet-derived chemokines CCL5 and CXCL4, both of which promote further neutrophil adhesion and migration.[22,24]

While ARDS can develop in the absence of neutrophils and has been well documented in neutropenic patients, neutrophils play a significant role in amplifying inflammation and tissue damage in most patients with ARDS.[25] Biopsy and bronchoalveolar lavage (BAL) fluid studies show a significant increase in the number of neutrophils, and labeled neutrophils transfused into ARDS patients show a predilection for the lung.[26,27] Neutrophils in the lungs of ARDS patients are phenotypically distinct from blood neutrophils, displaying delayed apoptosis but preserved oxidative burst and phagocytosis, and BAL fluid from patients with ARDS has been shown to inhibit neutrophil apoptosis ex vivo.[28–30] Clinical studies have shown an association between the number of neutrophils in the lung and disease severity.[31] Once activated in the lungs of ARDS patients, neutrophils contribute to lung damage by releasing proteases, various cytokines, leukotrienes, and cytotoxic reactive oxygen species (ROS). Neutrophils also release neutrophil extracellular traps (NETs), extracellular strands of decondensed DNA in complex with histones, and neutrophil granule proteins that capture pathogens but are also proinflammatory and can cause endothelial injury and contribute to thrombosis.[32]

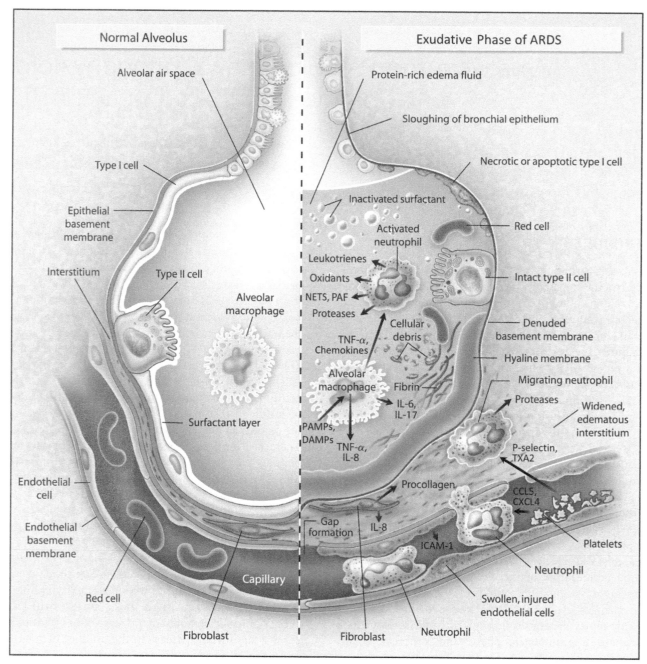

Normal Alveolus

- Alveolar air space
- Type I cell
- Epithelial basement membrane
- Interstitium
- Type II cell
- Alveolar macrophage
- Surfactant layer
- Endothelial cell
- Endothelial basement membrane
- Red cell
- Capillary
- Fibroblast

Exudative Phase of ARDS

- Protein-rich edema fluid
- Sloughing of bronchial epithelium
- Necrotic or apoptotic type I cell
- Inactivated surfactant
- Activated neutrophil
- Red cell
- Leukotrienes
- Oxidants
- NETS, PAF
- Proteases
- Intact type II cell
- Cellular debris
- TNF-α, Chemokines
- Denuded basement membrane
- Hyaline membrane
- Alveolar macrophage
- Fibrin
- Migrating neutrophil
- IL-6, IL-17
- Proteases
- PAMPs, DAMPs
- Widened, edematous interstitium
- TNF-α, IL-8
- P-selectin, TXA2
- Procollagen
- CCL5, CXCL4
- Gap formation
- IL-8
- Platelets
- ICAM-1
- Neutrophil
- Swollen, injured endothelial cells
- Fibroblast
- Neutrophil

Fig. 14.1 The normal alveolus is shown on the left, and the exudative phase of ARDS is shown on the right. Following the initial injury of ARDS (direct or indirect), alveolar macrophages are activated by exposure to molecular components of pathogenic organisms (PAMPs) or products released from injured cells (DAMPs) such as HMGB1 and mitochondrial DNA. The activated alveolar macrophages release proinflammatory cytokines (TNF-α, IL-6, and IL-17) and chemokines (IL-8, CCL2, CCL7, CXCL8, and CXCL10) which recruit neutrophils and monocytes or macrophages. Once activated in the lungs of ARDS patients, neutrophils release leukotrienes, cytotoxic reactive oxygen species, NETs, platelet-activating factor, and proteases, which cause necrosis and sloughing of the bronchial and alveolar epithelial cells, denuding of the basement membrane, and formation of hyaline membranes. Breakdown of the alveolar-capillary barrier leads to flooding of the alveolar and interstitial space with protein-rich edema fluid. Surfactant is inactivated and fibrin deposition occurs. TNF-α-induced upregulation of tissue factor leads to dysregulated intravascular and intra-alveolar coagulation and platelet aggregation causing microthrombi and macrothrombi. Activated platelets secrete the chemokines CCL5 and CXCL4 and induce the expression of ICAM-1 on endothelial cells, all of which promote further neutrophil adhesion and migration. Activated platelets also release P-selectin and thromboxane A2, which activate neutrophils and cause further release of proinflammatory cytokines. *CCL,* C-C motif chemokine; *CXCL,* C-X-C motif chemokine; *DAMP,* damage-associated molecular pattern; *HMGB1,* high mobility group box 1; *ICAM-1,* intercellular adhesion molecule 1; *IL,* interleukin; *NET,* neutrophil extracellular trap; *PAF,* platelet-activating factor; *PAMP,* pathogen-associated molecular pattern; *TNF,* tumor necrosis factor; *TXA2,* thromboxane A2. (From Ware LB, Matthay MA. The acute respiratory distress syndrome. *N Engl J Med.* 2000;342:1334–1349. Copyright 2000, Massachusetts Medical Society. All rights reserved.)

Alveolar-Capillary Barrier Dysfunction and Permeability Pulmonary Edema

Activation of the innate immune system with neutrophil recruitment and activation results in injury to the alveolar epithelium and the capillary endothelium. Injury to both of these structures is required to increase the permeability of the alveolar-capillary barrier and cause alveolar accumulation of protein-rich edema fluid, the defining pathophysiologic feature of ARDS.[21,26]

The alveolar epithelium is composed of flat type I cells and cuboidal type II cells. The type I cells make up 96% of the alveolar surface area and facilitate gas exchange. Type II cells are present in similar numbers to type I cells but make up only 4% of the alveolar surface area.[33] Type II cells produce surfactant, participate in ion transport, and differentiate to repopulate type I cells after injury. In a healthy lung (see Fig. 14.1), type I cells are connected by tight junctions that form a barrier regulating the passage of molecules between the alveolar space and the interstitium. The epithelial barrier is much less permeable than the endothelial barrier, and the movement of fluid from the alveolar space into the lung interstitium is controlled by channels and ion pumps on the surface of lung epithelial cells.[33,34] Neutrophils cause bystander damage to host cells by releasing ROS, NETs, and proteinases such as neutrophil elastase and matrix metalloproteinases that directly degrade the extracellular matrix and components of the paracellular space, disrupting tight junctions and accelerating apoptosis of both type 1 and type 2 cells.[19,21,35] The migration of neutrophils across the endothelium and epithelium also causes structural deformations that augment tissue damage.[19]

Epithelial injury leads to loss of alveolar ion pumps, impairing the generation of osmotic forces required for alveolar fluid clearance and further contributing to sustained flooding of the alveolar space. Faster rates of alveolar fluid clearance are associated with better clinical outcomes in patients with ARDS, probably as a reflection of the extent of lung epithelial injury.[36,37] The extent of lung epithelial injury can also be assessed by plasma levels of the receptor for advanced glycation end-products (RAGE), a membrane receptor that is expressed in type I cells and is released in the setting of alveolar epithelial injury, particularly in patients receiving higher tidal volumes.[38,39] Damage to type II cells also reduces surfactant production, increasing surface tension and promoting alveolar collapse.[40]

Endothelial injury and activation during the exudative phase contribute to the dysfunction of the alveolar-capillary barrier, by increasing vascular permeability and flooding the interstitial space (see Fig. 14.1). Many of the proinflammatory and injurious mediators of the exudative process, including TNF-α, IL-6, lipopolysaccharide (LPS), ROS, and histamine, have been shown also to cause endothelial activation, adhesion molecule expression, and microvascular injury.[8] IL-6 induces inflammatory signaling in pulmonary endothelium and increases vascular permeability by a mechanism that is potentiated by mechanical stretch, suggesting one possible pathway through which ventilator-induced lung injury (VILI) leads to microvascular injury.[41] There has been significant interest in identifying the molecules that modulate endothelial permeability, including pathways modulated by ligation of the vascular endothelial growth factor (VEGF) and Tie2 receptors. Angiopoietin-2, a partial agonist of Tie2, has been shown to increase endothelial cell permeability and is a well-validated marker of endothelial injury in ARDS that correlates with pulmonary leak and mortality.[42–44] Endothelial injury is particularly important in cases of ARDS, due to an indirect injury, and elevated levels of biomarkers of endothelial activation and injury (von Willebrand factor [VWF], sFlt-1, and Ang-2) can identify which patients with nonpulmonary sepsis will develop ARDS.[45] Furthermore, a two-biomarker panel consisting of Ang-2 and RAGE performed well across multiple patient cohorts and outperformed clinical providers for diagnosing ARDS in severe trauma.[46]

Activation of the Coagulation Cascade

Under normal conditions, the systemic circulation is in a state of homeostasis with a balance between thrombotic and anticoagulant/profibrinolytic processes. This homeostasis is disturbed in ARDS with the activation of coagulation pathways and the inhibition of fibrinolysis, leading to fibrin formation and accumulation in the alveolar space.[47,48] TNF-α has been shown to upregulate tissue factor (TF), a major initiator of the extrinsic coagulation cascade, in the injured lung, and TF is found in the alveolar space and in alveolar macrophages of patients with ARDS.[49,50] The expression of TF leads to dysregulated intravascular and intra-alveolar coagulation and platelet aggregation.[8] Both microthrombi and macrothrombi are common during ARDS and have been reported to be present in 95% and 86%, respectively, of lung specimens collected at autopsy.[51]

Proliferative Phase

The proliferative phase of ARDS represents the lung's attempt to restore homeostasis by reestablishing epithelial integrity, absorbing alveolar edema, and developing a scaffold for repair of the alveolar architecture. This phase is marked by a transient expansion of resident fibroblasts and the formation of a provisional fibrin/fibronectin-rich matrix along injured basement membranes.[8] Type II cells and airway progenitor cells (endogenous stem cells) proliferate, migrate and differentiate into type I pulmonary epithelial cells to reepithelialize the injured basement membrane.[52,53] Once the alveolar-capillary barrier is reestablished, alveolar ion channels are reexpressed in alveolar epithelial cells, facilitating alveolar edema fluid resorption.[37,54] During this phase, tissue neutrophils undergo apoptosis and are cleared by reparative or M2-like alveolar macrophages, which release proresolving lipids such as resolvins and lipoxins to promote repair.[8,55] Regulatory T lymphocytes also have an important role in the resolution of lung injury via effects on alveolar macrophages and epithelial regeneration, in a process that is modulated by DNA methylation and transforming growth factor beta (TGF-β).[4,56,57] Interestingly, apoptotic neutrophils may produce mediators that suppress inflammation and promote the proliferation of type II cells.[58]

Fibrotic Phase

Many patients transition from the proliferative phase into a period of resolution during which the fibrin/fibronectin-rich matrix is removed and normal lung architecture is reestablished. For reasons that remain unclear, some patients do not transition to a normal repair process, instead progressing to a fibrotic phase of ARDS. While the risk factors for and mechanism of progression into the fibrotic phase have not been fully elucidated, the extent of damage to the basement membrane seems to be an important predictor.[59] In the fibrotic phase, profibrotic mediators, particularly TGF-β_1, are released and lead to filling of the alveolar space with mesenchymal cells and new blood vessels.[60] Recent studies have demonstrated that, in some patients, the fibrosis process starts shortly after injury; the presence of any fibrosing alveolitis on biopsy specimens in ARDS is associated with prolonged mechanical ventilation and increased mortality.[61] Studies that collected BAL fluid of patients early in their course of ARDS demonstrated that the level of procollagen III peptide, a precursor of collagen synthesis, is associated with the risk of death.[62,63] Despite the prognostic significance of fibrosis during the acute illness of ARDS, studies of survivors have shown that the fibrosis resolves in the vast majority of patients and does not seem to be a significant contributor to the ongoing dyspnea that many of these patients experience.[64] Many experts believe that the fibrotic phase of ARDS is driven primarily by VILI and may be decreasing with improvements in ARDS care such as lung protective ventilation and protocols to shorten the duration of mechanical ventilation.[65–67]

IATROGENIC LUNG INJURY

In ARDS, positive pressure mechanical ventilation is almost universally employed. Although lifesaving and necessary, positive pressure ventilation can worsen preexisting lung injury and cause new injury in healthy lungs.[68] The concept of VILI has existed for many years, but it has received considerable attention since the publication of a seminal clinical trial from the NHLBI ARDS Clinical Trials Network in 2000, which demonstrated that a ventilation strategy which deemphasized the correction of respiratory acidosis in favor of a "lung protective" strategy of low tidal volumes and low plateau pressures significantly improved mortality of ARDS patients.[65]

VILI can occur through several mechanisms. Overdistention of alveoli leads to damage in a process known as volutrauma. Although volutrauma is correlated with high peak airway pressures, experimental data suggest that the critical variable mediating damage is lung stretching.[69] Atelectrauma is the term for the deleterious repeated opening of collapsed alveoli, which occurs during ventilation with low lung volumes and/or low positive end-expiratory pressure (PEEP). Volutrauma and atelectrauma activate the inflammatory cascade in a way that is similar to that seen with any other form of direct lung insult. Implicated mediators include neutrophils, IL-6 and IL-8, and TNF-α.[68,70] In addition, the damage to the epithelial wall seen in VILI may facilitate bacterial translocation into the capillary space and from there into the circulation.[71,72] Pathologically,

this process leads to epithelial sloughing, hyaline membrane formation, and pulmonary edema.[68,73] Atelectrauma has also been shown to contribute to the diminution in surfactant that occurs during ARDS.[74,75] Injury from positive pressure ventilation is potentiated by the fact that lung aeration is heterogeneous during ARDS. Some alveoli are collapsed and do not participate in air exchange, whereas other segments are patent and receive more volume than intended.[68] The extent of lung inhomogeneity correlates with the severity of ARDS and mortality.[76] Increasing PEEP decreases inhomogeneity, but many patients with ARDS will experience regional volutrauma and atelectrauma concurrently, regardless of the chosen ventilation strategy.[76] The risk of VILI may, in part, explain the robust mortality benefit observed in clinical trials that successfully shortened the duration of mechanical ventilation with daily awakening and breathing trials.[66]

The lung injury processes that characterize VILI may not be unique to positive pressure ventilation. In animal models, increasing minute ventilation to supernormal levels by manipulating the central drive to breath causes acute lung injury similar to that seen in patients on positive pressure ventilation.[77] Nonventilated patients with acute hypoxic respiratory failure similarly breathe with large tidal volumes and high minute ventilation, and the regional forces generated by the respiratory muscles may lead to injurious effects on the lung at a regional level, a process that has been termed patient self-inflicted lung injury (P-SILI).[78] These findings raise important questions that remain to be answered, including

- Should we avoid noninvasive ventilation for acute hypoxemic respiratory failure (which has been shown to increase tidal volumes)?
- Should we "prophylactically" intubate and sedate spontaneously breathing patients who are able to sufficiently oxygenate and ventilate but do so at the cost of large tidal volumes and high minute ventilation?[78]

PHYSIOLOGIC CONSEQUENCES

The primary clinical manifestations of ARDS are hypoxemia, increased work of breathing and respiratory acidosis which are consequences of impaired gas exchange, decreased lung compliance, and increased dead space. It is also important to recognize the nonpulmonary complications of ARDS, as multiorgan dysfunction frequently occurs. The most common causes of death in ARDS patients are sepsis and malignancy, while death from refractory respiratory failure is uncommon.[79,80]

Impaired Gas Exchange

The hypoxemia that characterizes ARDS results from several important physiologic derangements: ventilation–perfusion mismatch, shunt, and diffusion impairment. Alveoli in some parts of the lung are filled with exudative edema fluid and/or are atelectatic. The inflammatory mediators present in the exudative phase of ARDS can disrupt hypoxic vasoconstriction in these areas, leading to ventilation–perfusion mismatch in hypoxic, poorly ventilated areas of the lung. Severely affected areas may have perfusion but no ventilation (right-to-left shunt). Oxygenation can be further impaired by areas that are both ventilated and perfused as the edema fluid increases the distance through which oxygen must diffuse.

Low Compliance

The dysfunction of the alveolar-capillary barrier and subsequent flooding of the interstitium and alveolar space with permeability pulmonary edema lead to severely reduced pulmonary compliance. In spontaneously breathing patients, significantly labored breathing is required to maintain an adequate minute ventilation. For mechanically ventilated patients, high peak and plateau pressures may be required to deliver sufficient tidal volumes to poorly compliant lungs. As ARDS progresses, areas of fibrotic lung may develop that remain stiff and poorly compliant, even after the inflammation resolves and the edema fluid is resorbed. High-resolution computed tomography (CT) scans in ARDS have shown that the amount of radiographic reticulation and bronchiectasis is inversely correlated with lung compliance.[81]

Increased Dead Space

Patients with ARDS generally require a significantly elevated minute ventilation to maintain a normal arterial partial pressure of CO_2, even in the setting of normal CO_2 production. This is due to an increase in dead space (regions of the lung with ventilation but no or minimal perfusion), caused by microthrombi, vascular remodeling, and pathologic hypoxic vasoconstriction.[8] Positive pressure mechanical ventilation with high inspiratory pressures can also contribute to dead space by raising intra-alveolar pressures to levels that exceed perfusion pressures. The need for a high minute ventilation contributes to the marked increased in work of breathing in ARDS, and failure to maintain adequate minute ventilation results in respiratory acidosis. The amount of dead space in early ARDS (the dead-space fraction) is independently associated with the risk of death.[82]

Pulmonary Hypertension

The vascular processes that contribute to increased dead space in ARDS also lead to pulmonary hypertension and acute cor pulmonale (ACP). In one study, ACP was present in 22% of patients with moderate-to-severe ARDS. The clinical significance of ACP in ARDS is unclear, as hospital mortality did not differ between patients with and without ACP. Severe ACP, however, did appear to be an independent risk factor for mortality in ARDS, even after adjustment for other risk factors.[83]

PATHOLOGIC FINDINGS

"Diffuse alveolar damage" (DAD) is considered to be the pathognomonic histologic finding of ARDS. It is characterized by neutrophilic inflammation, hyaline membranes, intra-alveolar edema, alveolar type II proliferation covering denuded alveolar-capillary membrane, interstitial proliferation of fibroblasts and myofibroblasts, and organizing interstitial fibrosis. However, autopsy studies and studies of open lung biopsy in nonresolving

ARDS have demonstrated that DAD is only present in 45–66% of patients meeting clinical criteria for ARDS.[84–88] Common findings in patients who met clinical criteria for ARDS but did not have DAD were pneumonia, pulmonary edema, alveolar hemorrhage, and malignancy, but up to 15% of patients had no identifiable pulmonary lesions.[85,88] Although these studies have limitations related to patient selection, they do raise important questions regarding the prevalence of DAD in ARDS. A recent study demonstrated that patients with ARDS and DAD at postmortem had worse oxygenation and compliance, and higher SOFA (sequential organ failure assessment) and INR (international normalized ratio) scores than patients with ARDS and other histologic findings. Patients with DAD on biopsy were also more likely to die from hypoxemia and less likely to die from septic shock.[88] There is ongoing debate regarding whether DAD represents (1) a common but non-uniform finding of the larger syndrome of ARDS, (2) a defining feature of a specific subphenotype of ARDS, or (3) a response to VILI that is not directly related to the pathogenesis of ARDS.[8,88] Many experts believe that the failure to find effective biomarkers or treatments of ARDS is related to the "lumping" of heterogeneous, mechanistically distinct illnesses within this clinical syndrome and predict that improvements in subphenotyping in ARDS will enrich future clinical trials with patients likely to respond to specific therapies.

AUTHORS' RECOMMENDATIONS

- Acute respiratory distress syndrome (ARDS) is caused by activation of the innate immune system and platelets, dysregulated inflammation, altered permeability of the alveolar-capillary barrier, and activation of coagulation pathways.
- Although there is spatial and temporal heterogeneity in ARDS, the pattern of lung injury in ARDS progresses through three identifiable phases: an exudative phase, a proliferative phase, and finally either recovery or progression to fibrotic lung disease
- Volutrauma and atelectrauma are drivers of iatrogenic lung injury in ARDS patients (VILI), which may also occur in spontaneously breathing patients (P-SILI).
- The primary clinical manifestations of ARDS are hypoxemia (caused by ventilation–perfusion mismatch, shunt, and impaired diffusion), increased work of breathing, respiratory acidosis (caused by increased dead space), and decreased lung compliance.
- The classic pathologic characteristic of clinical ARDS, diffuse alveolar damage, is only present in approximately 50% of patients meeting clinical criteria for ARDS.

REFERENCES

1. Ashbaugh DG, Bigelow DB, Petty TL Levine BE. Acute respiratory distress in adults. *Lancet*. 1967;290(7511):319-323.
2. Ware LB, Matthay MA. The acute respiratory distress syndrome. *N Engl J Med*. 2000;342(18):1334-1349.
3. Hudson LD, Milberg JA, Anardi D, Maunder RJ. Clinical risks for development of the acute respiratory distress syndrome. *Am J Respir Crit Care Med*. 1995;151(2 Pt 1):293-301.

4. Matthay MA, Ware LB, Zimmerman GA. The acute respiratory distress syndrome. *J Clin Invest*. 2012;122(8):2731-2740.

5. Pepe PE, Potkin RT, Reus DH, Hudson LD, Carrico CJ. Clinical predictors of the adult respiratory distress syndrome. *Am J Surg*. 1982;144(1):124-130.

6. Ferguson ND, Frutos-Vivar F, Esteban A, et al. Clinical risk conditions for acute lung injury in the intensive care unit and hospital ward: a prospective observational study. *Crit Care*. 2007;11:R96.

7. Ware LB, Bastarache JA, Bernard GR. Acute respiratory distress syndrome. In: Vincent JL, Abraham E, Moore FA, Kochanek PM, Fink MP, eds. *Textbook of Critical Care*. 7th ed. Philadelphia: Elsevier; 2017:413-424.

8. Thompson BT, Chambers RC, Liu KD. Acute respiratory distress syndrome. *N Engl J Med*. 2017;377(6):562-572.

9. Calfee CS, Janz DR, Bernard GR, et al. Distinct molecular phenotypes of direct vs. indirect ARDS in single-center and multicenter studies. *Chest*. 2015;147(6):1539-1548.

10. Calfee CS, Delucchi K, Parsons PE, et al. Subphenotypes in acute respiratory distress syndrome: latent class analysis of data from two randomised controlled trials. *Lancet Respir Med*. 2014;2(8):611-620.

11. Famous KR, Delucchi K, Ware LB, et al. Acute respiratory distress syndrome subphenotypes respond differently to randomized fluid management strategy. *Am J Respir Crit Care Med*. 2017; 195(3):331-338.

12. Matthay MA, Zimmerman GA. Acute lung injury and the acute respiratory distress syndrome: four decades of inquiry into pathogenesis and rational management. *Am J Respir Cell Mol Biol*. 2005;33(4):319-327.

13. Matthay MA, Zimmerman GA, Esmon C, et al. Future research directions in acute lung injury: summary of a National Heart, Lung, and Blood Institute working group. *Am J Respir Crit Care Med*. 2003;167(7):1027-1035.

14. Otto CM, Markstaller K, Kajikawa O, et al. Spatial and temporal heterogeneity of ventilator-associated lung injury after surfactant depletion. *J Appl Physiol (1985)*. 2008;104(5):1485-1494.

15. Pugin J, Verghese G, Widmer MC, Matthay MA. The alveolar space is the site of intense inflammatory and profibrotic reactions in the early phase of acute respiratory distress syndrome. *Crit Care Med*. 1999;27(2):304-312.

16. Opitz B, van Laak V, Eitel J, Suttorp N. Innate immune recognition in infectious and noninfectious diseases of the lung. *Am J Respir Crit Care Med*. 2010;181(12):1294-1309.

17. Aggarwal NR, King LS, D'Alessio FR. Diverse macrophage populations mediate acute lung inflammation and resolution. *Am J Physiol Lung Cell Mol Physiol*. 2014;306(8):L709-L725.

18. Zhang Q, Raoof M, Chen Y, et al. Circulating mitochondrial DAMPs cause inflammatory responses to injury. *Nature*. 2010;464(7285):104-107.

19. Williams AE, Chambers RC. The mercurial nature of neutrophils: still an enigma in ARDS? *Am J Physiol Lung Cell Mol Physiol*. 2013; 306(3):L217-L230.

20. Williams AE, José RJ, Mercer PF, et al. Evidence for chemokine synergy during neutrophil migration in ARDS. *Thorax*. 2017;72(1):66-73.

21. Matthay MA, Zemans RL. The acute respiratory distress syndrome: pathogenesis and treatment. *Annu Rev Pathol*. 2011; 6:147-163.

22. Yadav H, Kor DJ. Platelets in the pathogenesis of acute respiratory distress syndrome. *Am J Physiol Lung Cell Mol Physiol*. 2015;309(9):L915-L923.

23. Zarbock A, Singbartl K, Ley K. Complete reversal of acid-induced acute lung injury by blocking of platelet-neutrophil aggregation. *J Clin Invest*. 2006;116(2):3211-3219.

24. Grommes J, Alard JE, Drechsler M, et al. Disruption of platelet-derived chemokine heteromers prevents neutrophil extravasation in acute lung injury. *Am J Respir Crit Care Med*. 2012;185(6): 628-636.

25. Vansteenkiste JF, Boogaerts MA. Adult respiratory distress syndrome in neutropenic leukemia patients. *Blut*. 1989;58(6): 287-290.

26. Ware LB. Pathophysiology of acute lung injury and the acute respiratory distress syndrome. *Semin Respir Crit Care Med*. 2006;27(4):337-349.

27. Pittet JF, Mackersie RC, Martin TR, Matthay MA. Biological markers of acute lung injury: prognostic and pathogenetic significance. *Am J Respir Crit Care Med*. 1997;155(4):1187-1205.

28. Matute-Bello G, Liles WC, Radella F, et al. Neutrophil apoptosis in the acute respiratory distress syndrome. *Am J Respir Crit Care Med*. 1997;156(6):1969-1977.

29. Lesur O, Kokis A, Hermans C, Fülöp T, Bernard A, Lane D. Interleukin-2 involvement in early acute respiratory distress syndrome: relationship with polymorphonuclear neutrophil apoptosis and patient survival. *Crit Care Med*. 2000;28(12): 3814-3822.

30. Juss JK, House D, Amour A, et al. Acute respiratory distress syndrome neutrophils have a distinct phenotype and are resistant to phosphoinositide 3-kinase inhibition. *Am J Respir Crit Care Med*. 2016;194(8):961-973.

31. Weiland JE, Davis WB, Holter JF, Mohammed JR, Dorinsky PM, Gadek J. Lung neutrophils in the adult respiratory distress syndrome. Clinical and pathophysiologic significance. *Am Rev Respir Dis*. 1986;133(2):218-225.

32. Sørensen OE, Borregaard N. Neutrophil extracellular traps—the dark side of neutrophils. *J Clin Invest*. 2016;126(5):1612-1620.

33. Guillot L, Nathan N, Tabary O, et al. Alveolar epithelial cells: master regulators of lung homeostasis. *Int J Biochem Cell Biol*. 2013;45(11):2568-2573.

34. Wiener-Kronish JP, Albertine KH, Matthay MA. Differential responses of the endothelial and epithelial barriers of the lung in sheep to *Escherichia coli* endotoxin. *J Clin Invest*. 1991;88(3):864-875.

35. Albertine KH, Soulier MF, Wang Z, et al. Fas and fas ligand are up-regulated in pulmonary edema fluid and lung tissue of patients with acute lung injury and the acute respiratory distress syndrome. *Am J Pathol*. 2002;161(5):1783-1796.

36. Ware LB, Matthay MA. Alveolar fluid clearance is impaired in the majority of patients with acute lung injury and the acute respiratory distress syndrome. *Am J Respir Crit Care Med*. 2001; 163(6):1376-1383.

37. Huppert LA, Matthay MA. Alveolar fluid clearance in pathologically relevant conditions: in vitro and in vivo models of acute respiratory distress syndrome. *Front Immunol*. 2017;8:371.

38. Uchida T, Shirasawa M, Ware LB, et al. Receptor for advanced glycation end-products is a marker of type I cell injury in acute lung injury. *Am J Respir Crit Care Med*. 2006;173(9):1008-1015.

39. Calfee CS, Ware LB, Eisner MD, et al. Plasma receptor for advanced glycation end products and clinical outcomes in acute lung injury. *Thorax*. 2008;63(12):1083-1089.

40. Greene KE, Wright JR, Steinberg KP, et al. Serial changes in surfactant-associated proteins in lung and serum before and after onset of ARDS. *Am J Respir Crit Care Med*. 1999;160(6):1843-1850.

41. Birukova AA, Tian Y, Meliton A, Leff A, Wu T, Birukov KG. Stimulation of Rho signaling by pathologic mechanical stretch is a "second hit" to Rho-independent lung injury induced by IL-6. *Am J Physiol-Lung Cell Mol Physiol.* 2012;302(9):L965-L975.

42. Calfee CS, Gallagher D, Abbott J, Thompson BT, Matthay MA; NHLBI ARDS Network. Plasma angiopoietin-2 in clinical acute lung injury: prognostic and pathogenetic significance. *Crit Care Med.* 2012;40(6):1731-1737.

43. Agrawal A, Matthay MA, Kangelaris KN, et al. Plasma angiopoietin-2 predicts the onset of acute lung injury in critically ill patients. *Am J Respir Crit Care Med.* 2013;187(7):736-742.

44. Zinter MS, Spicer A, Orwoll BO, et al. Plasma angiopoietin-2 outperforms other markers of endothelial injury in prognosticating pediatric ARDS mortality. *Am J Physiol Lung Cell Mol Physiol.* 2016;310(3):L224-L231.

45. Hendrickson CM, Matthay MA. Endothelial biomarkers in human sepsis: pathogenesis and prognosis for ARDS. *Pulm Circ.* 2018;8(2):2045894018769876.

46. Ware LB, Zhao Z, Koyama T, et al. Derivation and validation of a two-biomarker panel for diagnosis of ARDS in patients with severe traumatic injuries. *Trauma Surg Acute Care Open.* 2017; 2(1):e000121.

47. Ware LB, Bastarache JA, Wang L. Coagulation and fibrinolysis in human acute lung injury—new therapeutic targets? *Keio J Med.* 2005;54(3):142-149.

48. Abraham E. Coagulation abnormalities in acute lung injury and sepsis. *Am J Respir Cell Mol Biol.* 2000;22(4):401-404.

49. Sebag SC, Bastarache JA, Ware LB. Therapeutic modulation of coagulation and fibrinolysis in acute lung injury and the acute respiratory distress syndrome. *Curr Pharm Biotechnol.* 2011; 12(9):1481-1496.

50. Bastarache JA, Wang L, Geiser T, et al. The alveolar epithelium can initiate the extrinsic coagulation cascade through expression of tissue factor. *Thorax.* 2007;62(7):608-616.

51. Tomashefski Jr JF. Pulmonary pathology of acute respiratory distress syndrome. *Clin Chest Med.* 2000;21(3):435-466.

52. Vaughan AE, Brumwell AN, Xi Y, et al. Lineage-negative progenitors mobilize to regenerate lung epithelium after major injury. *Nature.* 2015;517(7536):621-625.

53. Chapman HA, Li X, Alexander JP, et al. Integrin α6β4 identifies an adult distal lung epithelial population with regenerative potential in mice. *J Clin Invest.* 2011;121(7):2855-2862.

54. Millar FR, Summers C, Griffiths MJ, Toshner MR, Proudfoot AG. The pulmonary endothelium in acute respiratory distress syndrome: insights and therapeutic opportunities. *Thorax.* 2016;71(5):462-473.

55. Levy BD, Serhan CN. Resolution of acute inflammation in the lung. *Annu Rev Physiol.* 2014;76:467-492.

56. Singer BD, Mock JR, Aggarwal NR, et al. Regulatory T cell DNA methyltransferase inhibition accelerates resolution of lung inflammation. *Am J Respir Cell Mol Biol.* 2015;52(5):641-652.

57. D'Alessio FR, Tsushima K, Aggarwal NR, et al. CD4+CD25+Foxp3+ Tregs resolve experimental lung injury in mice and are present in humans with acute lung injury. *J Clin Invest.* 2009;119(10):2898-2913.

58. Paris AJ, Liu Y, Mei J, et al. Neutrophils promote alveolar epithelial regeneration by enhancing type II pneumocyte proliferation in a model of acid-induced acute lung injury. *Am J Physiol Lung Cell Mol Physiol.* 2016;311(6):L1062-L1075.

59. Matthay MA, Wiener-Kronish JP. Intact epithelial barrier function is critical for the resolution of alveolar edema in humans. *Am Rev Respir Dis.* 1990;142(6 Pt 1):1250-1257.

60. Fukuda Y, Ishizaki M, Masuda Y, Kimura G, Kawanami O, Masugi Y. The role of intraalveolar fibrosis in the process of pulmonary structural remodeling in patients with diffuse alveolar damage. *Am J Pathol.* 1987;126(1):171-182.

61. Martin C, Papazian L, Payan MJ, Saux P, Gouin F. Pulmonary fibrosis correlates with outcome in adult respiratory distress syndrome. A study in mechanically ventilated patients. *Chest.* 1995;107(1):196-200.

62. Chesnutt AN, Matthay MA, Tibayan FA, Clark JG. Early detection of type III procollagen peptide in acute lung injury. Pathogenetic and prognostic significance. *Am J Respir Crit Care Med.* 1997;156(3 Pt 1):840-845.

63. Clark JG, Milberg JA, Steinberg KP, Hudson LD. Type III procollagen peptide in the adult respiratory distress syndrome. Association of increased peptide levels in bronchoalveolar lavage fluid with increased risk for death. *Ann Intern Med.* 1995;122(1):17-23.

64. Wilcox ME, Patsios D, Murphy G, et al. Radiologic outcomes at 5 years after severe ARDS. *Chest.* 2013;143(4):920-926.

65. Acute Respiratory Distress Syndrome Network; Brower RG, Matthay MA, et al. Ventilation with lower tidal volumes as compared with traditional tidal volumes for acute lung injury and the acute respiratory distress syndrome. *N Engl J Med.* 2000;342(18):1301-1308.

66. Girard TD, Kress JP, Fuchs BD, et al. Efficacy and safety of a paired sedation and ventilator weaning protocol for mechanically ventilated patients in intensive care (Awakening and Breathing Controlled trial): a randomised controlled trial. *Lancet.* 2008;371(9607):126-134.

67. Cabrera-Benitez NE, Laffey JG, Parotto M, et al. Mechanical ventilation-associated lung fibrosis in acute respiratory distress syndrome: a significant contributor to poor outcome. *Anesthesiology.* 2014;121(1):189-198.

68. Slutsky AS, Ranieri VM. Ventilator-induced lung injury. *N Engl J Med.* 2013;369(22):2126-2136.

69. Dreyfuss D, Soler P, Basset G, Saumon G. High inflation pressure pulmonary edema. Respective effects of high airway pressure, high tidal volume, and positive end-expiratory pressure. *Am Rev Respir Dis.* 1988;137(5):1159-1164.

70. Slutsky AS, Tremblay LN. Multiple system organ failure. Is mechanical ventilation a contributing factor? *Am J Respir Crit Care Med.* 1998;157(6 Pt 1):1721-1725.

71. Nahum A, Hoyt J, Schmitz L, et al. Effect of mechanical ventilation strategy on dissemination of intratracheally instilled *Escherichia coli* in dogs. *Crit Care Med.* 1997;25(10):1733-1743.

72. Murphy DB, Cregg N, Tremblay L, et al. Adverse ventilatory strategy causes pulmonary-to-systemic translocation of endotoxin. *Am J Respir Crit Care Med.* 2000;162(1):27-33.

73. Tremblay L, Valenza F, Ribeiro SP, Li J, Slutsky AS. Injurious ventilatory strategies increase cytokines and c-fos m-RNA expression in an isolated rat lung model. *J Clin Invest.* 1997; 99(5):944-952.

74. Albert RK. The role of ventilation-induced surfactant dysfunction and atelectasis in causing acute respiratory distress syndrome. *Am J Respir Crit Care Med.* 2012;185(7):702-708.

75. Maruscak AA, Vockeroth DW, Girardi B, et al. Alterations to surfactant precede physiological deterioration during high tidal volume ventilation. *Am J Physiol Lung Cell Mol Physiol.* 2008;294(5):L974-L983.

76. Cressoni M, Cadringher P, Chiurazzi C, et al. Lung inhomogeneity in patients with acute respiratory distress syndrome. *Am J Respir Crit Care Med.* 2014;189(2):149-158.

77. Mascheroni D, Kolobow T, Fumagalli R, Moretti MP, Chen V, Buckhold D. Acute respiratory failure following pharmacologically induced hyperventilation: an experimental animal study. *Intensive Care Med*. 1988;15(1):8-14.

78. Brochard L, Slutsky A, Pesenti A. Mechanical ventilation to minimize progression of lung injury in acute respiratory failure. *Am J Respir Crit Care Med*. 2017;195(4):438-442.

79. Stapleton RD, Wang BM, Hudson LD, Rubenfeld GD, Caldwell ES, Steinberg KP. Causes and timing of death in patients with ARDS. *Chest*. 2005;128(2):525-532.

80. Wang CY, Calfee CS, Paul DW, et al. One-year mortality and predictors of death among hospital survivors of acute respiratory distress syndrome. *Intensive Care Med*. 2014;40(3):388-396.

81. Burnham EL, Hyzy RC, Paine R, et al. Detection of fibroproliferation by chest high-resolution CT scan in resolving ARDS. *Chest*. 2014;146(5):1196-1204.

82. Nuckton TJ, Alonso JA, Kallet RH, et al. Pulmonary dead-space fraction as a risk factor for death in the acute respiratory distress syndrome. *N Engl J Med*. 2002;346(17):1281-1286.

83. Mekontso Dessap A, Boissier F, Charron C, et al. Acute cor pulmonale during protective ventilation for acute respiratory distress syndrome: prevalence, predictors, and clinical impact. *Intensive Care Med*. 2016;42(5):862-870.

84. Esteban A, Fernández-Segoviano P, Frutos-Vivar F, et al. Comparison of clinical criteria for the acute respiratory distress syndrome with autopsy findings. *Ann Intern Med*. 2004;141(6):440-445.

85. Thille AW, Esteban A, Fernández-Segoviano P, et al. Comparison of the Berlin definition for acute respiratory distress syndrome with autopsy. *Am J Respir Crit Care Med*. 2013;187(7):761-767.

86. Guerin C, Bayle F, Leray V, et al. Open lung biopsy in nonresolving ARDS frequently identifies diffuse alveolar damage regardless of the severity stage and may have implications for patient management. *Intensive Care Med*. 2015;41(2):222-230.

87. Kao KC, Hu HC, Chang CH, et al. Diffuse alveolar damage associated mortality in selected acute respiratory distress syndrome patients with open lung biopsy. *Crit Care*. 2015;19:228.

88. Lorente JA, Cardinal-Fernández P, Muñoz D, et al. Acute respiratory distress syndrome in patients with and without diffuse alveolar damage: an autopsy study. *Intensive Care Med*. 2015;41(11):1921-1930.

15

What Factors Predispose Patients to Acute Respiratory Distress Syndrome?

Yewande Odeyemi, Alice Gallo De Moraes, and Ognjen Gajic

Acute respiratory distress syndrome (ARDS) is a common complication of critical illness or injury associated with significant morbidity and mortality. The pathogenesis of ARDS involves mechanical and inflammatory injury to the lungs that causes marked derangement in alveolar-capillary permeability and the passage of protein-rich edema fluid into the air spaces.[1,2] ARDS usually occurs in a context of uncontrolled response to local or systemic inflammation and most recently two endotypes of ARDS—namely, hyperinflammatory and hypoinflammatory—have been identified with different therapeutic responses and prognoses.[3,4] The clinical pathogenesis is often multifactorial, with complex interaction of risk factors and risk modifiers (Fig. 15.1).

PREDISPOSING CONDITIONS

Sepsis, pneumonia, and shock are the most common conditions predisposing to ARDS.[5,6] However, only a minority of these patients with these disorders actually have ARDS (Fig. 15.2). Other typical predisposing conditions include gastropulmonary aspiration, trauma, and massive blood product transfusion.[7,8] Atypical respiratory infections, including viral (*influenza*) and fungal (*Pneumocystis jiroveci*, *Histoplasma* spp., *Blastomyces* spp.) infections, are unusual but important causes of ARDS, especially in patients with compromised immune systems. Several pathogens, such as severe acute respiratory syndrome (SARS), Middle East respiratory syndrome-coronavirus, and epidemic H1N1 influenza, have attracted widespread attention, and confer increased risk for ARDS.[9] Additional patient risk factors include gastroesophageal reflux disease, chronic silent aspiration, and drug exposures.[5,10]

Observational studies and clinical trials have noted a distinct subtype of ARDS without known risk factors.[11] Of note, these patients may have better prognoses.[12]

Certain host genetic variants have been associated with development of sepsis and ARDS,[13] including mutations in the surfactant protein B.[14] Recently, a genome-wide association study comparing 232 African-American patients with ARDS and 162 at-risk control subjects identified selectin P ligand gene (*SELPLG*) as a novel ARDS susceptibility gene.[15] Genetic associations have been generally difficult to replicate, and the role of genetic predisposition in development of ARDS is presently unclear.[14]

RISK MODIFIERS

Sepsis in alcoholics is associated with a distinctly high risk of ARDS. Chronic alcohol use carries a twofold to threefold increase in ARDS development.[16,17] The exact mechanism of this association remains unknown, but it may be related to a reduction in the antioxidant capacity of the lung.[17] In addition, acute and chronic consumption of alcohol cause an increase in the systemic levels of adenosine[18,19] and a dose-dependent reduction in alveolar fluid clearance through stimulation of the adenosine type 1 receptor, adding to the lung injury.[20,21] A 2014 study in trauma patients demonstrated that the risk of ARDS increased in direct proportion to the blood alcohol content.[22]

A history of tobacco exposure (including second-hand smoking) has been associated with an increased risk of ARDS in trauma patients.[23] Another study found an independent dose–response association between current cigarette smoking and subsequent development of ARDS.[24]

Hypoalbuminemia is a well-known marker of acute or chronic illness or malnutrition and poor surgical outcomes.[25,26] It was also found to be an independent risk factor for ARDS.[27] This appears to be mediated by decreases in plasma oncotic pressure with increased pulmonary permeability in the critically ill, independent of underlying cause and fluid status.[28]

Hypercapnic acidosis protects against ventilator-induced lung injury in several animal models of ARDS.[29,30] However, low pH and, in particular, metabolic acidosis have been associated with increased risk of ARDS.[31,32]

Obesity is also an independent risk factor for the development of ARDS.[33] Although the effects of body position and compression atelectasis may in part explain the observed association,[2] additional mechanisms have been proposed. These include an imbalance between proinflammatory and anti-inflammatory cytokines, which increases lung inflammation and injury through the tumor necrosis factor-α and interleukin-6 pathways.[34–37]

Diabetes mellitus seems to be associated with a lower risk of ARDS in septic shock.[38] Indeed, a meta-analysis that included a total of 12,794 adult patients suggested that diabetes protected against ARDS.[39] Although the exact mechanism is not known, one possible explanation is that diabetic patients

ARDS pathogens: "Multiple hit" hypothesis

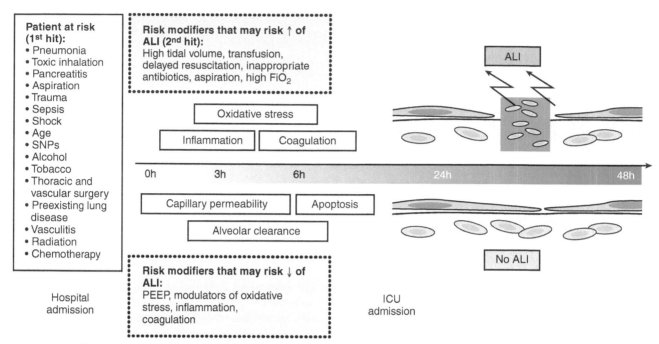

Patient at risk (1st hit):
- Pneumonia
- Toxic inhalation
- Pancreatitis
- Aspiration
- Trauma
- Sepsis
- Shock
- Age
- SNPs
- Alcohol
- Tobacco
- Thoracic and vascular surgery
- Preexisting lung disease
- Vasculitis
- Radiation
- Chemotherapy

Hospital admission

Risk modifiers that may risk ↑ of ALI (2nd hit): High tidal volume, transfusion, delayed resuscitation, inappropriate antibiotics, aspiration, high FiO₂

Oxidative stress

Inflammation   Coagulation

0h   3h   6h   24h   48h

Capillary permeability   Apoptosis

Alveolar clearance

Risk modifiers that may risk ↓ of ALI: PEEP, modulators of oxidative stress, inflammation, coagulation

ICU admission

ALI

No ALI

Fig. 15.1 Illustration of Interaction between Risk factors and Risk Modifiers in the Development of Acute respiratory Distress Syndrome. *ALI,* acute lung injury; *FiO₂,* fraction of inspired oxygen; *ICU,* intensive care unit; *PEEP,* positive end-expiratory pressure; *SNP,* single nucleotide polymorphism.

% ALI development according to predisposing conditions

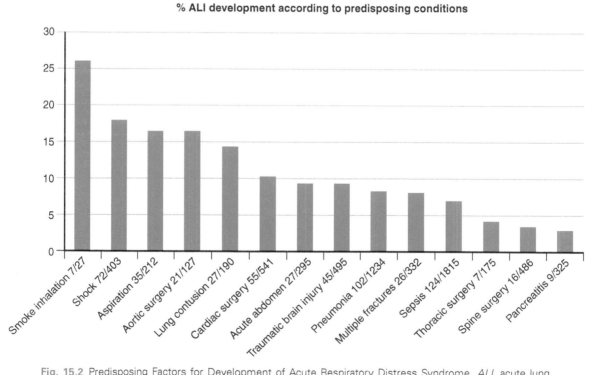

Fig. 15.2 Predisposing Factors for Development of Acute Respiratory Distress Syndrome. *ALI,* acute lung injury. (From Gajic et al.[31].)

have impaired activation of the inflammatory cascade in the lungs.[40]

An alternative hypothesis for ARDS pathogenesis has been proposed, suggesting that surfactant dysfunction may be a critical step in ARDS progression.[41] Both spontaneous and mechanical hyperventilation can induce surfactant dysfunction, leading to higher surface tension and atelectasis. This injury is augmented by supine position and sedation, and this effect can be particularly pronounced in obese patients.[2] However, trials administering surfactant in ARDS patients did not show an outcome benefit.[42]

RISK PREDICTION MODELS

The Lung Injury Prediction Score (LIPS) was created in 2011 with the intent to facilitate the design and conduct of ARDS prevention studies.[43] The model includes risk factors and risk modifiers present at the time of hospital admission, before ARDS occurs. It was later validated[31] and refined (Table 15.1). A simplified model, the Early Acute Lung Injury Score, predicts ARDS on the basis of oxygen requirement, respiratory rate, and presence of immunosuppression in patients with bilateral infiltrates on chest imaging.[44]

HOSPITAL-ACQUIRED EXPOSURES

Hospitalized patients are frequently exposed to various potentially harmful factors that may modify their risk of ARDS development. Compared with patients who died of other causes, ARDS decedents have a markedly higher incidence of potentially preventable adverse events (medical or surgical misadventures).[45] High tidal volume ventilation,[46–48] high oxygen concentration,[49] and plasma transfusion from multiparous female donors[50] each have been implicated as iatrogenic contributors to ARDS. In septic patients, delays in fluid resuscitation and in the initiation of antimicrobial treatment have also been associated with ARDS.[51] Although lung-protective mechanical ventilation is considered a standard of care for patients with established ARDS, a series of studies suggest that its application to all mechanically ventilated patients may be safe and beneficial.[46–48]

A large case-control study found iatrogenic risk factors to be significantly greater in patients with ARDS than in matched controls and deemed most of these factors to be preventable.[52] Multiple potential strategies directed at preventing ARDS have been proposed. These include early identification of "at-risk" patients, standardization of clinical

TABLE 15.1 LIPS Calculation Table.

	LIPS Points	Examples
Predisposing Conditions		(1) Patient with history of alcohol abuse with septic shock
Shock	2	from pneumonia requiring $FiO_2 > 0.35$ in the emergency
Aspiration	2	room: sepsis + shock + pneumonia + alcohol abuse +
Sepsis	1	$FiO_2 > 0.35$
Pneumonia	1.5	$1 + 2 + 1.5 + 1 + 2 = 7.5$
High-Risk Surgery[a]		
Orthopedic spine	1	
Acute abdomen	2	
Cardiac	2.5	
Aortic vascular	3.5	
High-Risk Trauma		(2) Motor vehicle accident with traumatic brain injury, lung
Traumatic brain injury	2	contusion, and shock requiring $FiO_2 > 0.35$
Smoke inhalation	2	Traumatic brain injury + lung contusion + shock +
Near drowning	2	$FiO_2 > 0.35$
Lung contusion	1.5	$2 + 1.5 + 2 + 2 = 7.5$
Multiple fractures	1.5	
Risk Modifiers		(3) Patient with history of diabetes mellitus and urosepsis
Alcohol abuse	1	with shock
Obesity (BMI > 30)	1	$1 + 2 - 1 = 2$
Hypoalbuminemia	1	
Chemotherapy	1	
$FiO_2 > 0.35$ (> 4 L/min)	2	
Tachypnea (RR > 30)	1.5	
$SpO_2 < 95\%$	1	
Acidosis (pH < 7.35)	1.5	
Diabetes mellitus[b]	−1	

[a]Add 1.5 points if emergency surgery.
[b]Only if sepsis.
BMI, body mass index; FiO_2, fraction of inspired oxygen; LIPS, Lung Injury Prediction Score; RR, respiratory rate; SpO_2, oxygen saturation by pulse oximetry.
From Gajic et al.[31]

practice to prevent iatrogenic injury, and early treatment of predisposing conditions.[52,53] The Checklist for Lung Injury Prevention (CLIP) has been developed to ensure compliance with evidence-based practice that may affect ARDS occurrence and is currently used in clinical trials of ARDS prevention.[54] CLIP items include lung-protective mechanical ventilation, aspiration precautions, early adequate antimicrobial therapy, restrictive fluid and transfusion management, and early assessment for extubation with daily awakening and breathing trials.

A population-based cohort study conducted in Olmsted County, Minnesota, reported a decrease in the incidence of ARDS from 82.4 cases per 100,000 person-years in 2001 to 38.9 cases per 100,000 person-years in 2008.[55] This decrease in ARDS incidence was observed despite a stable incidence of community-acquired ARDS and an increase in the population's severity of illness, comorbidity burden, and predisposing conditions for ARDS over the same time period. This decrease was attributed to the prevention strategies described above, including lung-protective ventilation strategies in all mechanically ventilated patients, restrictive transfusion practice, male-donor-predominant plasma, improved sepsis treatment, and more conservative fluid management.[50,55,56]

Although several potential pharmacologic therapies have emerged to target specific components of the underlying pathogenic pathway of ARDS, to date, none has been proven to be effective in the prevention of ARDS.

Most recently, a phase IIa double-blind multicenter randomized controlled trial (RCT) studying the feasibility of the combination of an inhaled corticosteroid and inhaled long-acting beta-adrenergic agonist in patients at an increased risk of ARDS (LIPS score > 4) showed an improvement in oxygenation when compared with placebo and, although not intended to study the effect on prevention of ARDS, there was a lower incidence of ARDS in the treatment group that became nonsignificant after adjustment for shock. Although this was only a pilot study and limited by sample size, this trial will help to inform future studies.[57]

The use of inhaled beta-adrenergic agonists only have also been formally evaluated in a phase II RCT. In 362 patients undergoing esophagectomy, intraoperative administration of inhaled salmeterol reduced several biomarkers of alveolar inflammation and injury and was associated with a decreased incidence of postoperative adverse events (predominantly pneumonia); however, the incidence of ARDS did not differ between the groups.[58]

The administration of aspirin was thought to be protective in earlier observational studies;[59,60] however, in a phase II RCT comparing aspirin and placebo in patients at an increased risk of ARDS (LIPS score >4), there was no difference in the incidence of ARDS or other important outcomes.[61] However, an ancillary mechanistic study demonstrated the important role of biomarkers for intravascular monocyte activation and a potential preventive effect of aspirin on ARDS development in per-protocol analysis.[62]

Animal studies had suggested that statins may be beneficial in modulating hyperinflammatory ARDS. However, the HARP-2 clinical trial of 540 patients failed to demonstrate benefit.[63] A systematic review of observational studies and other RCTs have shown no beneficial effect for statins in the prevention of ARDS in high-risk patients.[64,65]

Several other pharmacologic therapies for prevention of ARDS in patients at risk are being evaluated in clinical studies. These include[58] inhaled heparin,[66] inhaled steroids,[67] peroxisome proliferator receptor antagonist, angiotensin inhibitors, curcumin, and vitamin D.[68,69]

In conclusion, although sepsis, pneumonia, and shock commonly predispose patients to ARDS, many risk factors are potentially modifiable and early identification of those at risk is important. Ongoing clinical studies are evaluating various promising preventive strategies. Meanwhile, attention to best practices and avoidance of iatrogenic exposures is a simple and powerful strategy for reducing the burden of this important complication of critical illness.

AUTHORS' RECOMMENDATIONS

- Sepsis, pneumonia, and shock are the most common conditions predisposing to ARDS.
- Certain host genetic variants have been associated with development of sepsis and ARDS.
- Abuse of alcohol and tobacco predispose to ARDS, as does malnutrition and obesity.
- The LIPS and the simplified Early Acute Lung Injury Score predict ARDS based on clinical and investigational criteria.
- Hospital-acquired ARDS may result from a medley factors, of which high tidal volume ventilation, high oxygen concentration, and plasma transfusion are most commonly implicated.
- The Checklist for Lung Injury Prevention (CLIP) has been developed to ensure compliance with evidence-based practice that may affect ARDS occurrence.
- To date, no pharmacologic intervention has been shown to prevent ARDS.

REFERENCES

1. Matthay MA, Zemans RL. The acute respiratory distress syndrome: pathogenesis and treatment. *Annu Rev Pathol.* 2011;6:147-163.
2. Albert RK. The role of ventilation-induced surfactant dysfunction and atelectasis in causing acute respiratory distress syndrome. *Am J Respir Crit Care Med.* 2012;185(7):702-708.
3. Calfee CS, Delucchi K, Parsons PE, Thompson BT, Ware LB, Matthay MA. Subphenotypes in acute respiratory distress syndrome: latent class analysis of data from two randomised controlled trials. *Lancet Respir Med.* 2014;2(8):611-620.
4. Calfee CS, Delucchi KR, Matthay MA, et al. Consistent ARDS endotypes are identified using minimal data from a United Kingdom clinical trial. C96. Critical Care: New Discoveries In ARDS. American Thoracic Society; 2017.
5. Bice T, Li G, Malinchoc M, Lee AS, Gajic O. Incidence and risk factors of recurrent acute lung injury. *Crit Care Med.* 2011;39(5):1069-1073.
6. Wind J, Versteegt J, Twisk J, et al. Epidemiology of acute lung injury and acute respiratory distress syndrome in The Netherlands: a survey. *Respir Med.* 2007;101(10):2091-2098.

7. Wallis JP. Transfusion-related acute lung injury (TRALI): presentation, epidemiology and treatment. *Intensive Care Med.* 2007;33(suppl 1):S12-S16.

8. Khan H, Belsher J, Yilmaz M, et al. Fresh-frozen plasma and platelet transfusions are associated with development of acute lung injury in critically ill medical patients. *Chest.* 2007;131(5):1308-1314.

9. Kojicic M, Li G, Hanson AC, et al. Risk factors for the development of acute lung injury in patients with infectious pneumonia. *Crit Care.* 2012;16(2):R46.

10. Dhokarh R, Li G, Schmickl CN, et al. Drug-associated acute lung injury: a population-based cohort study. *Chest J.* 2012;142(4):845-850.

11. de Prost N, Pham T, Carteaux G, et al. Etiologies, diagnostic work-up and outcomes of acute respiratory distress syndrome with no common risk factor: a prospective multicenter study. *Ann Intensive Care.* 2017;7(1):69.

12. Harrington JS, Schenck EJ, Oromendia C, Choi AMK, Siempos II. Acute respiratory distress syndrome without identifiable risk factors: a secondary analysis of the ARDS network trials. *J Crit Care.* 2018;47:49-54.

13. Marshall RP, Webb S, Hill MR, Humphries SE, Laurent GJ. Genetic polymorphisms associated with susceptibility and outcome in ARDS. *Chest.* 2002;121(suppl 3):68S-69S.

14. Gong MN, Wei Z, Xu LL, Miller DP, Thompson BT, Christiani DC. Polymorphism in the surfactant protein-B gene, gender, and the risk of direct pulmonary injury and ARDS. *Chest.* 2004;125(1):203-211.

15. Bime C, Pouladi N, Sammani S, et al. Genome-wide association study in African Americans with acute respiratory distress syndrome identifies the selectin P ligand gene as a risk factor. *Am J Respir Crit Care Med.* 2018;197(11):1421-1432.

16. Moss M, Burnham EL. Chronic alcohol abuse, acute respiratory distress syndrome, and multiple organ dysfunction. *Crit Care Med.* 2003;31(suppl 4):S207-S212.

17. Moss M, Parsons PE, Steinberg KP, et al. Chronic alcohol abuse is associated with an increased incidence of acute respiratory distress syndrome and severity of multiple organ dysfunction in patients with septic shock. *Crit Care Med.* 2003;31(3):869-877.

18. Dohrman DP, Diamond I, Gordon AS. The role of the neuromodulator adenosine in alcohol's actions. *Alcohol Health Res World.* 1997;21(2):136-143.

19. Nagy LE, Diamond I, Collier K, Lopez L, Ullman B, Gordon AS. Adenosine is required for ethanol-induced heterologous desensitization. *Mol Pharmacol.* 1989;36(5):744-748.

20. Dada L, Gonzalez AR, Urich D, et al. Alcohol worsens acute lung injury by inhibiting alveolar sodium transport through the adenosine A1 receptor. *PLoS One.* 2012;7(1):e30448.

21. Factor P, Mutlu GM, Chen L, et al. Adenosine regulation of alveolar fluid clearance. *Proc Natl Acad Sci U S A.* 2007;104(10):4083-4088.

22. Afshar M, Smith GS, Terrin ML, et al. Blood alcohol content, injury severity, and adult respiratory distress syndrome. *J Trauma Acute Care Surg.* 2014;76(6):1447-1455.

23. Calfee CS, Matthay MA, Eisner MD, et al. Active and passive cigarette smoking and acute lung injury after severe blunt trauma. *Am J Respir Crit Care Med.* 2011;183(12):1660-1665.

24. Iribarren C, Jacobs Jr DR, Sidney S, Gross MD, Eisner MD. Cigarette smoking, alcohol consumption, and risk of ARDS: a 15-year cohort study in a managed care setting. *Chest.* 2000;117(1):163-168.

25. Buzby GP, Mullen JL, Matthews DC, Hobbs CL, Rosato EF. Prognostic nutritional index in gastrointestinal surgery. *Am J Surg.* 1980;139(1):160-167.

26. Dempsey DT, Mullen JL. Prognostic value of nutritional indices. *JPEN J Parenter Enteral Nutr.* 1987;11(suppl 5):109S-114S.

27. Mangialardi RJ, Martin GS, Bernard GR, et al. Hypoproteinemia predicts acute respiratory distress syndrome development, weight gain, and death in patients with sepsis. *Crit Care Med.* 2000;28(9):3137-3145.

28. Aman J, van der Heijden M, van Lingen A, et al. Plasma protein levels are markers of pulmonary vascular permeability and degree of lung injury in critically ill patients with or at risk for acute lung injury/acute respiratory distress syndrome. *Crit Care Med.* 2011;39(1):89-97.

29. Ijland MM, Heunks LM, van der Hoeven JG. Bench-to-bedside review: hypercapnic acidosis in lung injury–from 'permissive' to 'therapeutic'. *Crit Care.* 2010;14(6):237.

30. Wu SY, Wu CP, Kang BH, Li MH, Chu SJ, Huang KL. Hypercapnic acidosis attenuates reperfusion injury in isolated and perfused rat lungs. *Crit Care Med.* 2012;40(2):553- 559.

31. Gajic O, Dabbagh O, Park PK, et al. Early identification of patients at risk of acute lung injury: evaluation of lung injury prediction score in a multicenter cohort study. *Am J Respir Crit Care Med.* 2011;183(4):462-470.

32. Gong MN, Thompson BT, Williams P, Pothier L, Boyce PD, Christiani DC. Clinical predictors of and mortality in acute respiratory distress syndrome: potential role of red cell transfusion. *Crit Care Med.* 2005;33(6):1191-1198.

33. Karnatovskaia LV, Lee AS, Bender SP, et al. Obstructive sleep apnea, obesity, and the development of acute respiratory distress syndrome. *J Clin Sleep Med.* 2014;10(6):657-662.

34. Wang C. Obesity, inflammation, and lung injury (OILI): the good. *Mediators Inflamm.* 2014;2014:978463.

35. Leal Vde O, Mafra D. Adipokines in obesity. *Clin Chim Acta.* 2013;419:87-94.

36. Mancuso P. Obesity and lung inflammation. *J Appl Physiol (1985).* 2010;108(3):722-728.

37. Simpson SQ, Casey LC. Role of tumor necrosis factor in sepsis and acute lung injury. *Crit Care Clin.* 1989;5(1):27-47.

38. Moss M, Guidot DM, Steinberg KP, et al. Diabetic patients have a decreased incidence of acute respiratory distress syndrome. *Crit Care Med.* 2000;28(7):2187-2192.

39. Gu WJ, Wan YD, Tie HT, Kan QC, Sun TW. Risk of acute lung injury/acute respiratory distress syndrome in critically ill adult patients with pre-existing diabetes: a meta-analysis. *PLoS One.* 2014;9(2):e90426.

40. Filgueiras LR Jr, Martins JO, Serezani CH, Capelozzi VL, Montes MB, Jancar S. Sepsis-induced acute lung injury (ALI) is milder in diabetic rats and correlates with impaired NFκB activation. *PLoS One.* 2012;7(9):e44987.

41. Petty TL, Silvers GW, Paul GW, Stanford RE. Abnormalities in lung elastic properties and surfactant function in adult respiratory distress syndrome. *Chest.* 1979;75(5):571-574.

42. Kesecioglu J, Beale R, Stewart TE, et al. Exogenous natural surfactant for treatment of acute lung injury and the acute respiratory distress syndrome. *Am J Respir Crit Care Med.* 2009;180(10):989-994.

43. Trillo-Alvarez C, Cartin-Ceba R, Kor DJ, et al. Acute lung injury prediction score: derivation and validation in a population-based sample. *Eur Respir J.* 2011;37(3):604-609.

44. Levitt JE, Calfee CS, Goldstein BA, Vojnik R, Matthay MA. Early acute lung injury: criteria for identifying lung injury prior to the need for positive pressure ventilation. *Crit Care Med*. 2013;41(8):1929-1937.

45. TenHoor T, Mannino DM, Moss M. Risk factors for ARDS in the United States: analysis of the 1993 National Mortality Followback Study. *Chest*. 2001;119(4):1179-1184.

46. Serpa Neto A, Simonis FD, Barbas CS, et al. Association between tidal volume size, duration of ventilation, and sedation needs in patients without acute respiratory distress syndrome: an individual patient data meta-analysis. *Intensive Care Med*. 2014;40(7):950-957.

47. Gajic O, Dara SI, Mendez JL, et al. Ventilator-associated lung injury in patients without acute lung injury at the onset of mechanical ventilation. *Crit Care Med*. 2004;32(9): 1817-1824.

48. Serpa Neto A, Cardoso SO, Manetta JA, et al. Association between use of lung-protective ventilation with lower tidal volumes and clinical outcomes among patients without acute respiratory distress syndrome: a meta-analysis. *JAMA*. 2012;308(16):1651-1659.

49. Rachmale S, Li G, Wilson G, Malinchoc M, Gajic O. Practice of excessive FiO_2 and effect on pulmonary outcomes in mechanically ventilated patients with acute lung injury. *Respir Care*. 2012;57(11):1887-1893.

50. Toy P, Gajic O, Bacchetti P, et al. Transfusion-related acute lung injury: incidence and risk factors. *Blood*. 2012;119(7): 1757-1767.

51. Iscimen R, Cartin-Ceba R, Yilmaz M, et al. Risk factors for the development of acute lung injury in patients with septic shock: an observational cohort study. *Crit Care Med*. 2008; 36(5):1518-1522.

52. Ahmed AH, Litell JM, Malinchoc M, et al. The role of potentially preventable hospital exposures in the development of acute respiratory distress syndrome: a population-based study. *Crit Care Med*. 2014;42(1):31-39.

53. Litell JM, Gong MN, Talmor D, Gajic O. Acute lung injury: prevention may be the best medicine. *Respir Care*. 2011; 56(10):1546-1554.

54. Kor DJ, Talmor DS, Banner-Goodspeed VM, et al. Lung Injury Prevention with Aspirin (LIPS-A): a protocol for a multicentre randomised clinical trial in medical patients at high risk of acute lung injury. *BMJ Open*. 2012;2(5):e001606.

55. Li G, Malinchoc M, Cartin-Ceba R, et al. Eight-year trend of acute respiratory distress syndrome: a population-based study in Olmsted County, Minnesota. *Am J Respir Crit Care Med*. 2011;183(1):59-66.

56. National Heart, Lung, and Blood Institute Acute Respiratory Distress Syndrome (ARDS) Clinical Trials Network; Wiedemann H, Wheeler A, et al. Comparison of two fluid-management strategies in acute lung injury. *N Engl J Med*. 2006;354(24):2564-2575.

57. Festic E, Carr GE, Cartin-Ceba R, et al. Randomized clinical trial of a combination of an inhaled corticosteroid and beta agonist in patients at risk of developing the acute respiratory distress syndrome. *Crit Care Med*. 2017;45(5):798-805.

58. Perkins GD, McAuley DF, Thickett DR, Gao F. The beta-agonist lung injury trial (BALTI) a randomized placebo-controlled clinical trial. *Am J Respir Crit Care Med*. 2006; 173(3):281-287.

59. Erlich JM, Talmor DS, Cartin-Ceba R, Gajic O, Kor DJ. Prehospitalization antiplatelet therapy is associated with a reduced incidence of acute lung injury: a population-based cohort study. *Chest*. 2011;139(2):289-295.

60. Kor DJ, Erlich J, Gong MN, et al. Association of prehospitalization aspirin therapy and acute lung injury: results of a multicenter international observational study of at-risk patients. *Crit Care Med*. 2011;39(11):2393-2400.

61. Kor DJ, Carter RE, Park PK, et al. Effect of aspirin on development of ARDS in at-risk patients presenting to the emergency department: the LIPS-A randomized clinical trial. *JAMA*. 2016;315(22):2406-2414.

62. Abdulnour RE, Gunderson T, Barkas I, et al. Early intravascular events are associated with development of acute respiratory distress syndrome. a substudy of the LIPS-A clinical trial. *Am J Respir Crit Care Med*. 2018;197(12):1575-1585.

63. McAuley DF, Laffey JG, O'Kane CM, et al. Simvastatin in the acute respiratory distress syndrome. *N Engl J Med*. 2014; 371(18):1695-1703.

64. O'Neal HR Jr, Koyama T, Koehler EA, et al. Prehospital statin and aspirin use and the prevalence of severe sepsis and acute lung injury/acute respiratory distress syndrome. *Crit Care Med*. 2011;39(6):1343-1350.

65. Yadav H, Lingineni RK, Slivinski EJ, et al. Preoperative statin administration does not protect against early postoperative acute respiratory distress syndrome: a retrospective cohort study. *Anesth Analg*. 2014;119(4):891-898.

66. Dixon B, Schultz MJ, Smith R, Fink JB, Santamaria JD, Campbell DJ. Nebulized heparin is associated with fewer days of mechanical ventilation in critically ill patients: a randomized controlled trial. *Crit Care*. 2010;14(5):R180.

67. Karnatovskaia LV, Lee AS, Gajic O, Festic E; U.S. Critical Illness and Injury Trials Group: Lung Injury Prevention Study Investigators (USCITG-LIPS). The influence of prehospital systemic corticosteroid use on development of acute respiratory distress syndrome and hospital outcomes. *Crit Care Med*. 2013;41(7):1679-1685.

68. Jeng L, Yamshchikov AV, Judd SE, et al. Alterations in vitamin D status and anti-microbial peptide levels in patients in the intensive care unit with sepsis. *J Transl Med*. 2009;7:28.

69. Festic E, Kor DJ, Gajic O. Prevention of acute respiratory distress syndrome. *Curr Opin Crit Care*. 2015;21(1): 82-90.

16

What is the Best Mechanical Ventilation Strategy in ARDS?

Yasin A. Khan and Niall D. Ferguson

INTRODUCTION

Acute respiratory distress syndrome (ARDS) is the rapid and catastrophic response of the lung to an injury that results in severe, hypoxemic respiratory failure. The current Berlin definition defines ARDS as a process that occurs within 7 days of a known clinical insult, presents with bilateral opacities on chest imaging, and manifests with hypoxemia with a ratio of partial pressure of arterial oxygen (PaO_2) to fraction of inspired oxygen (FiO_2) ≤ 300 mm Hg. The definition further classifies the severity of ARDS based upon PaO_2/FiO_2 ratios.[1,2] Patients with ARDS account for 10% of intensive care unit (ICU) admissions, nearly 25% of patients undergoing mechanical ventilation, and have a mortality rate of 40%.[3] Mechanical ventilation is an essential tool in the management of ARDS, and in this chapter we review the evidence surrounding mechanical ventilation strategies and adjunctive therapies for ARDS.

VENTILATOR-INDUCED LUNG INJURY

In ARDS, mechanical ventilation supports gas exchange and allows the respiratory system to rest while the lung recovers from injury. However, inappropriate application of mechanical ventilation can worsen injury.[4] Before discussing the clinical evidence for mechanical ventilation in ARDS, we review the mechanisms by which ventilator-induced lung injury (VILI) can develop.

Volutrauma

During mechanical ventilation, injury can occur due to cyclic alveolar overdistension (volutrauma) with elevated inflation pressures. Dreyfuss et al.[5] found that high volume ventilation led to more lung injury when compared with lower volume and high airway pressure strategies, suggesting the injury in this model was due to lung stretching. Webb and Tierney[6] showed that ventilation with very high peak inflation pressures also caused injury due to overdistension. However, it is not absolute airway pressure, but transpulmonary pressure (alveolar pressure minus pleural pressure) that is the true distending pressure of the lung and the one that produces injury.[7–11] In ARDS, the lung is composed of areas that appear normally aerated, poorly aerated, overinflated, and nonaerated.[12,13] Although the normally aerated component, or *baby lung*, is still inflamed, it is functional, recruitable, and has near-normal compliance; its size is inversely correlated with the degree of ARDS (Fig. 16.1).[14] This small component bears the stress and strain during mechanical ventilation, explaining why elevated pressures and high volumes can cause VILI.[15,16]

Atelectrauma

Atelectasis is a common pathologic feature in ARDS and can contribute to another form of VILI, termed atelectrauma.[17] During tidal ventilation, repeated opening and closing of these atelectatic airways requires high forces and the resulting shear stress can lead to injury.[7] Furthermore, as atelectasis decreases the size of the baby lung, it also potentiates the effect of volutrauma (Fig. 16.2).[18–20]

Patient Self-Inflicted Lung Injury

Patient self-inflicted lung injury (P-SILI) is a form of VILI driven by a patient's own spontaneous respirations.[21] As mentioned earlier, transpulmonary pressure is the true distending pressure of the lung. When combined with a positive pressure breath, spontaneous breaths will decrease the pleural pressure, increasing transpulmonary pressure.[22] Spontaneous breathing can also cause ventilator dyssynchrony, which can lead to larger tidal volume delivery and higher transpulmonary pressures.[23] P-SILI can also be driven by a phenomenon called *pendelluft*, or "swinging air." In healthy lungs, flow through the airways and lungs is uniform, the changes in pleural pressure are equally distributed, and ventilation is homogeneous. In ARDS the lungs are heterogeneous, and so is the flow through the airways. When spontaneous breaths are present, changes in pleural pressure are not uniformly transmitted through the lung, leading to differential inflation of lung regions where air flows from one region to another (i.e., pendelluft) and the regional overdistension can cause injury.[23–25]

LUNG-PROTECTIVE VENTILATION

The term lung-protective ventilation refers to lower tidal volume (LTV) ventilation and limited inspiratory pressures.[26] In the seminal study of lung protective ventilation, the LTV

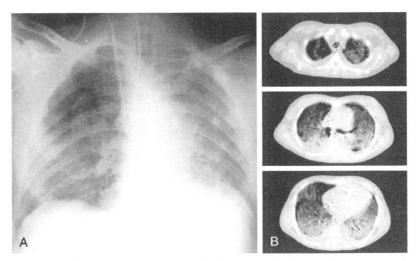

Fig. 16.1 A chest x-ray (A) and computed tomography (CT) scans (B) showing heterogeneous lung changes in a patient with acute respiratory distress syndrome (ARDS). (From Gattinoni L, Caironi P, Pelosi P, Goodman LR. What has computed tomography taught us about the acute respiratory distress syndrome? *Am J Respir Crit Care Med.* 2001;164[9]:1701-1711.)

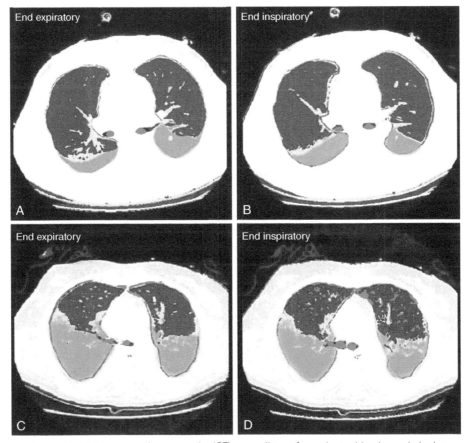

Fig. 16.2 Representative computed tomography (CT) scan slices of a patient with a larger baby lung component at end expiration (A) and after tidal inflation at end inspiration (B). A patient with a smaller baby lung component at end expiration (C) with hyperinflation of the previously normally aerated lung component after tidal inflation with lower tidal volume delivery (D) is shown. (Modified from Terragni PP, Rosboch G, Tealdi A, et al. Tidal hyperinflation during low tidal volume ventilation in acute respiratory distress syndrome. *Am J Respir Crit Care Med.* 2007;175[2]:160-166.)

group was ventilated with targeted tidal volumes of 6 mL/kg (ranging from 4 to 8 mL/kg) while maintaining a plateau pressure (P_{plat}) less than 30 cm H_2O; the traditional tidal volume group was ventilated with tidal volumes of 12 mL/kg PBW (predicted body weight) and P_{plat} <50 cm H_2O.[27]

Positive end-expiratory pressure (PEEP) and FiO_2 in both groups were titrated according to the same stepped protocol. The mean ± standard deviation (SD) tidal volumes for days 1–3 of the study were 6.2 ± 0.8 mL/kg PBW and 11.8 ± 0.8 mL/kg PBW in the LTV and traditional groups, respectively.

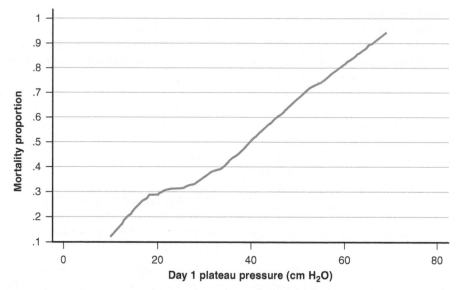

Fig. 16.3 A plot showing decreasing mortality associated with lower plateau pressure (P_{plat}) levels at day 1 in patients with acute respiratory distress syndrome (ARDS); no identifiable safe P_{plat} threshold is apparent. (From Hager DN, Krishnan JA, Hayden DL, Brower RG, Network ACT. Tidal volume reduction in patients with acute lung injury when plateau pressures are not high. *Am J Respir Crit Care Med.* 2005; 172[10]:1241-1245.).

The mean ± SD P_{plat} were 25 ± 6 and 33 ± 8 cm H_2O in the LTV and traditional groups, respectively. The study was stopped early after 861 patients were randomized because the LTV group had a mortality of 31.0% compared with 39.8% in the traditional tidal volume group, with an absolute risk reduction of 8.8% and number needed to treat (NNT) of 11 ($P < .05$).

Secondary analyses of the ARMA trial suggested that there was a benefit associated with tidal volume reduction, even when P_{plat} was relatively low and showed that P_{plat} independently predicted mortality when tidal volumes were held constant (Fig. 16.3).[28,29]

VILI can still occur, despite strict adherence to lung-protective, and further reductions in tidal volume could potentially be beneficial,[4,20,30] but very low tidal volumes can lead to respiratory acidosis.[31] Extracorporeal carbon dioxide removal (ECCO₂-R) has been suggested as a possible adjunct to lung-protective ventilation with ultra-low tidal volumes (<4 mL/kg PBW).[32–35] Early clinical studies have shown some promise, but the evidence is not yet adequate for widespread adoption.[36,37] Fortunately, The Protective Ventilation With Veno-Venous Lung Assist in Respiratory Failure (REST) trial (Clinicaltrials.gov Identifier: NCT02654327) and the Strategy of Ultraprotective Lung Ventilation With Extracorporeal CO₂ Removal for New-Onset Moderate to Severe ARDS (SUPERNOVA) trial (Clinicaltrials.gov Identifier: NCT02282657) are currently underway.

PEEP OPTIMIZATION AND RECRUITMENT MANEUVERS

An open lung approach includes higher levels of PEEP and recruitment maneuvers (RM) and can improve gas exchange by increasing end-expiratory lung volumes, reduce lung stress and strain, and minimize the effect of atelectrauma.[26,38–40]

Amato et al.[41] and Villar et al.[42] showed that ventilation strategies with higher PEEP levels were associated with reduced mortality when compared with strategies with lower PEEP levels. However, these findings were confounded by the concurrent use of higher tidal volumes in the lower PEEP groups.

The Assessment of Low Tidal Volume and Elevated End-Expiratory Pressure to Obviate Lung Injury trial (ALVEOLI) compared high-PEEP/FiO₂ and low-PEEP/FiO₂ titration strategies.[43] All study participants were also ventilated with LTV. This study was stopped early for futility and revealed no difference in in-hospital mortality between the lower-PEEP and higher-PEEP groups.

The Expiratory Pressure Study (ExPress) compared a minimal distension strategy to an increased recruitment strategy.[44] This trial was also stopped early and showed no difference in 28-day mortality between the groups. However, the increased recruitment group did have more ventilator-free days: 7 (interquartile range [IQR] 0–19) vs. 3 (IQR 0–17); $P = .004$.

In the Lung Open Ventilation Study (LOVS), a conventional ventilation protocol with lower PEEP was compared with an open lung protocol that included higher PEEP values and RM and there was no statistically significant difference in mortality between the groups.[45]

A meta-analysis of individual patient data from the ALVEOLI, ExPress, and LOVS trials showed that in patients with moderate-to-severe ARDS (with a threshold PaO₂/FiO₂ ratio of 200 mm Hg), the higher PEEP strategies were associated with lower mortality (34.1 vs. 39.1%; relative risk [RR] 0.90; 95% confidence interval [CI] 0.81–1.00; $P = .49$).[46] Another secondary analysis of the ExPress and LOVS trials showed that patients who responded to increased PEEP with improved oxygenation had lower mortality, and this association was stronger among patients with severe ARDS, with PaO₂/FiO₂ ≤150 mm Hg.[47]

RM involve a transient increase in transpulmonary pressure to levels higher than those achieved during tidal ventilation and can confer the same physiologic benefit as higher PEEP.[16,48–50] Several clinical studies of RM have been performed, and two secondary analyses of these studies suggested that RM were associated with significant mortality reduction (RR 0.81; 95% CI 0.69–0.95; $I^2 = 6\%$).[26,51]

The multicenter, randomized Alveolar Recruitment in ARDS Trial (ART) compared a protocol of RM and PEEP titration to a lower PEEP protocol.[52] It showed that RM with PEEP titration led to increased 28-day mortality (55.3 vs. 49.3%; $P = .041$), increased 60-day mortality (65.3 vs. 59.9%; $P = 0.04$), and fewer ventilator-free days (5.3 vs. 6.4%; $P = .03$).

Unlike some of the other clinical studies, RM in the ART trial led to only modest improvements in lung compliance and a reduction of driving pressure.[52–54] Furthermore, the ART trial did not include an assessment of baseline responsiveness to PEEP. This is important, because recruitability in patients with ARDS is variable and may be influenced by severity of disease and the oxygenation response to increased PEEP.[16,46,47,55]

In addition, patients with different inflammatory subphenotypes of ARDS can have different clinical manifestations in response to higher PEEP levels. In a secondary analysis of the AVEOLI trial participants, Calfee et al.[56] showed that patients with a more inflammatory phenotype of ARDS responded to higher PEEP with lower mortality and more ventilator-free and organ failure-free days than the phenotype with less inflammation.

A detailed summary of the aforementioned trials of the open lung approach in ARDS is presented in Table 16.1.

DRIVING PRESSURE

In ARDS, the concept of the baby lung provides a rationale for the mortality benefit associated with LTV ventilation.[14,27,41] Nearly all the studies of LTV delivered volumes based on PBW, which is calculated based on height. This approach assumes that the residual lung is a function of height, but it may be more appropriate to deliver a volume that corresponds to the residual functional lung, or baby lung component.[60] The compliance of the respiratory system is calculated as the tidal volume divided by the change in pressure (P_{plat} minus PEEP). In ARDS, the compliance of the respiratory system correlates with the amount of the functional lung: thus, compliance estimates the size of the baby lung.[61] Driving pressure can be understood as the tidal volume normalized to respiratory system compliance (i.e., baby lung) and can be calculated clinically as P_{plat} minus PEEP.[60] When the lung is recruitable, increased PEEP should decrease driving pressure, but when the lung is not recruitable, increased PEEP will lead to overdistension and will increase driving pressure.[16]

In a study of individual patient data from nine ARDS trials, Amato et al.[60] showed that higher driving pressures were associated with increased mortality. However, this relationship was tested only in patients who were receiving LTV and were breathing passively during the measurement of P_{plat} used to calculate driving pressure. Guérin et al.[62] showed a similar relationship between driving pressure and mortality of two other trials. Schmidt et al.[63] confirmed these findings again in a retrospective study of patients who were not enrolled in any trials. It is important to note that all these studies were observational and no interventional trials of ventilation adjusted to driving pressure have yet been performed.

MODES OF VENTILATION

Volume-Targeted vs. Pressure-Targeted Ventilation

In volume-targeted modes, the tidal volume and peak inspiratory flow are set by the clinician, and the airway pressure and driving pressure can vary with changes in lung compliance.[64,65] However, increased patient effort and breath-stacking dyssynchrony can lead to the delivery of tidal volumes above the set value.[66,67] In pressure-targeted modes, the clinician sets the driving pressure; the tidal volume and flow vary with changes in compliance and patient effort.[68,69]

Two systematic reviews and meta-analyses of 34 studies and 3 trials that compared volume-targeted and pressure-targeted modes of ventilation found no association between ventilator mode and clinical outcomes.[22,70]

Considering the available evidence, it is unclear if either volume-targeted or pressure-targeted modes are superior for ventilation of patients with ARDS. Regardless of the chosen mode, it is vital to understand how changes in severity of ARDS and lung compliance can influence the dependent variable in each mode. When using volume-targeted modes it is important to measure P_{plat} regularly, and when using pressure-targeted modes the tidal volumes should be monitored closely to ensure that these values remain within the limits of lung-protective ventilation.

Spontaneous Breathing

In some cases, controlled ventilation may be associated with increased risk of harm and this may be mitigated by the use of assisted spontaneous breathing. In the absence of any spontaneous respirations, diaphragmatic inactivity can cause disuse atrophy and can lead to prolonged weaning from ventilatory support.[71–74] Spontaneous respirations can also improve ventilation–perfusion matching through lung recruitment.[75] Controlled positive pressure ventilation preferentially ventilates the anterior and apical segments of the lung, leaving the poorly ventilated dependent regions prone to even more atelectasis,[17,76–78] whereas diaphragmatic contraction during spontaneous ventilation improves aeration in the usually well-perfused dependent segments of the lung, decreasing intrapulmonary shunting and improving oxygenation.[79,80]

In an observational study of 48 patients undergoing controlled ventilation, Cereda et al.[81] found that 79% of patients tolerated switching to pressure support ventilation (PSV) with no difference in oxygenation or mortality between the patients who tolerated PSV and those who required return to controlled ventilation. In a trial of 30 patients at risk for developing ARDS, Putensen et al.[82] showed that patients allowed to breath spontaneously with airway pressure release ventilation (APRV) had more ventilator-free days and shorter ICU stays compared with patients undergoing pressure control ventilation with neuromuscular blockade.

In a trial of 138 patients with ARDS ventilated with either APRV of volume assist-control ventilation, Zhou et al. showed that APRV led to more ventilator-free days (19 [IQR 8–22] vs. 2 [IQR 8–22]; $P < .001$), shorter ICU stays, required fewer RM, and patients underwent prone positioning less frequently.[83] However, patients ventilated with volume assist-control had more pneumonia and other comorbidities, including chronic obstructive pulmonary disease, and also had more shock that required vasopressors.[84]

Patients enrolled in these studies had mild-to-moderate ARDS. As discussed earlier, in severe ARDS spontaneous breathing can lead to pendelluft, which can cause VILI.[23–25] Therefore, the advantages associated with assisted spontaneous breathing are likely to be limited to patients with mild-to-moderate disease, and may actually be harmful in severe ARDS.[73]

The evidence available to date is not adequate to make definitive recommendations for or against the use of assisted spontaneous breathing in mild-to-moderate ARDS. However, the Early Spontaneous Breathing in ARDS (BiRDS) trial (Clinicaltrials.gov Identifier: NCT01862016), comparing spontaneous breathing with APRV to controlled volume-targeted ventilation, is ongoing and may provide more insight about the role for assisted spontaneous ventilation in ARDS ventilation.

High-Frequency Oscillatory Ventilation

During high-frequency oscillatory ventilation (HFOV), a high mean airway pressure is applied to the lungs and very small tidal volumes, typically 1–3 mL/kg, are delivered by an oscillating diaphragm at rates of 3–15 Hz, or 180–900 breaths per minute.[85–88] Theoretically, this should be an ideal approach to minimize VILI in ARDS. The small tidal volumes can prevent volutrauma, the high mean airway pressure can recruit collapsed lung and prevent atelectrauma, and the avoidance of high inspiratory pressure swings can prevent barotrauma.[40,89]

Two early trials of patients with ARDS with PaO_2/FiO_2 ratio ≤ mm Hg showed that there was no difference in mortality of ventilator-free days when HFOV was compared with pressure-controlled ventilation, suggesting HFOV was safe to use in ARDS.[90,91] However, the control groups in these trials did not receive LTV ventilation.

In 2013, Ferguson et al.[92] reported the results of the Oscillation for ARDS Treated Early (OSCILLATE) trial that compared HFOV with lung-protective ventilation with 6 mL/kg PBW tidal volumes, P_{plat} ≤35 cm H_2O, and high PEEP in patients with ARDS with PaO_2/FiO_2 ratio ≤200 mm Hg. The

trial was stopped after 548 of the planned 1200 patients had been randomized due to a signal of harm in the HFOV group. In-hospital mortality was 47% in the HFOV group and 35% in the control group (absolute risk 12%; RR 1.33, 95% CI 1.12–1.79; $P = .004$).

At the same time, Young et al.[93] reported the results of their large multicenter Oscillation in ARDS (OSCAR) trial that compared HFOV and conventional lung-protective ventilation in patients with ARDS with PaO_2/FiO_2 ratio ≤200 mm Hg. The trial included 789 patients and found no difference in 30-day mortality (41.7 vs. 41.1%; $P = .85$).

In the OSCILLATE trial, the conventional ventilation strategy was strictly protocolized, whereas patients in the conventional arm of the OSCAR trial were managed according to local practice. As a result, tidal volumes in the control group of the OSCILLATE trial were smaller than those in the OSCAR trial (6.1 ± 1.3 mL/kg PBW vs. 8.3 ± 2.9 mL/kg PBW) and PEEP levels were higher in the OSCILLATE trial (18 ± 3.2 cm H_2O vs. 11.4 ± 3.6 cm H_2O).[94]

Two meta-analyses of trials examining HFOV suggested that there is no benefit to using HFOV over conventional lung-protective ventilation and suggested that HFOV may actually cause harm.[26,95] A recent individual patient data meta-analysis, however, showed significant heterogeneity of treatment effect with HFOV vs. conventional ventilation, with baseline PaO_2/FiO_2 ratio being an important effect modifier.[96] Patients with severe hypoxemia appeared to benefit from HFOV, while those with moderate ARDS may have been harmed.

NEUROMUSCULAR BLOCKING AGENTS

Spontaneous breathing in ARDS can be associated with increased transpulmonary pressures, regional overdistension due to pendelluft, and above-target tidal volume delivery due to increased patient effort and ventilator dyssynchrony.[23–25,66,73] Neuromuscular blocking agents (NMBAs) have been used for decades for refractory hypoxemia, ventilator dyssynchrony, and decreased respiratory system compliance.[97,98]

Early trials of NMBAs showed that a 48-hour infusion of cisatracurium led to increased oxygenation in patients with ARDS with PaO_2/FiO_2 ratio ≤150 mm Hg ($P = .021$)[99] and with PaO_2/FiO_2 ratio ≤200 mm Hg ($P < .001$).[100] However, these studies were not powered to detect clinical outcomes.

The largest trial published to date on the use of NMBA in ARDS is the ARDS et Curarisation Systematique (ACURASYS) trial of 340 patients with ARDS with PaO_2/FiO_2 ratio ≤150 mm Hg within 48 hours of onset of disease.[101] All patients were deeply sedated and received lung-protective ventilation.[27] Patients in the NMBA group received cisatracurium as a 15 mg bolus followed by 37.5 mg/h continuous infusion for 48 hours. Patients in the control group received a bolus and continuous infusion of an identical-appearing placebo. Though there was no difference in overall 90-day mortality between NMBA and placebo (40.7 vs. 48.8%; $P = .08$), NMBA reduced 90-day mortality when adjusted for PaO_2/FiO_2 ratio, P_{plat}, and severity of illness

TABLE 16.1 Summary of Randomized Trials of Open Lung Strategies (High PEEP and/or Recruitment Maneuvers).

Study Name, First Author, Year, Reference	SUBJECTS Treatment	SUBJECTS Control	Inclusion Criteria	TARGET / MEASURED TIDAL VOLUMES Treatment	TARGET / MEASURED TIDAL VOLUMES Control	PEEP TITRATION STRATEGY / ACTUAL PEEP LEVELS Treatment	PEEP TITRATION STRATEGY / ACTUAL PEEP LEVELS Control	RECRUITMENT MANEUVER STRATEGY Treatment	RECRUITMENT MANEUVER STRATEGY Control	MORTALITY, TIME, RESULTS Treatment	MORTALITY, TIME, RESULTS Control
Amato et al., 1998[41]	29	24	ARDS, LIS ≥2.5; ventilation <1 week	<6 mL/kg; 348 ± 6 mL[a]	Target 12 mL/kg; 768 ± 13 mL[a]	PEEP set to P_{flex} + 2 cm H_2O; 16.4 ± 0.4 cm H_2O[a]	PEEP titrated to keep PaO_2 >60 mm Hg, FiO_2 <0.6; 8.7 ± 0.4 cm H_2O[a]	CPAP of 35–40 cm H_2O for 40 seconds	None	28-day mortality 11/29 (38%)	17/24 (71%); $P < .001$
ALVEOLI, Brower et al., 2004[43]	276	273	ARDS, PaO_2/FiO_2 ratio <300 mm Hg; <36 hours	Lower tidal volume according to ARMA; goal 6 mL/kg PBW; 6.0 ± 0.9 mL/kg PBW[b]	Lower tidal volume according to ARMA; goal 6 mL/kg PBW; 6.1 ± 0.8 mL/kg PBW[b]	Higher PEEP/FiO_2 table; 14.7 ± 3.5 cm H_2O[b]	Lower PEEP according to ARMA trial PEEP/FiO_2 table; 8.9 ± 3.5 cm H_2O[b]	CPAP of 35–40 cm H_2O for 30 seconds; in first 80 patients	None	Hospital mortality 68/273 (24.9%)	76/276 (27.5%); $P = .48$
Villar et al., 2006[42]	50 (45 included in analysis)	53 (50 included in analysis)	ARDS, PaO_2/FiO_2 ratio ≤250 mm Hg; acute onset	5–8 mL/kg PBW; Unavailable	9–11 mL/kg PBW; Unavailable	PEEP set to P_{flex} + 2 cm H_2O; Unavailable	PEEP ≥5 cm H_2O to maintain oxygenation goal; Unavailable	None	None	ICU mortality 16/50 (32%)	24/45 (53.3%); $P = .40$
LOVS, Meade et al., 2008[45]	475	508	ARDS, PaO_2/FiO_2 ratio <250 mm Hg; <48 hours	6 mL/kg PBW; allowance of 4–8 mL/kg PBW; P_{plat} <40 cm H_2O; 6.8 ± 1.4 mL/kg PBW[b]	Lower tidal volume according to ARMA; goal 6 mL/kg PBW; 6.8 ± 1.3 mL/kg PBW[b]	Higher PEEP/FiO_2 table; 15.6 ± 3.9 cm H_2O[b]	Lower PEEP according to ARMA trial PEEP/FiO_2 table; 10.1 ± 3.0 cm H_2O[b]	CPAP of 40 cm H_2O for 40 seconds	None	Hospital mortality 173/475 (36.4%)	205/508 (40.4%); RR, 0.90; 95% CI, 0.77–1.05; $P = .19$
ExPress, Mercat et al., 2008[44]	385	382	ARDS, PaO_2/FiO_2 ratio <300 mm Hg; <48 hours	6 mL/kg PBW; 6.1 ± 0.3 mL/kg PBW[b]	6 mL/kg PBW; 6.1 ± 0.4 mL/kg PBW[b]	PEEP set to maximal level to keep P_{plat} 38–30 cm H_2O; 14.6 ± 3.2 cm H_2O[b]	PEEP 5–9 cm H_2O; set to lowest level to maintain oxygenation target; 7.1 ± 1.8 cm H_2O[b]	None	None	28-day mortality 107/385 (27.8%)	28-day 119/382 (31.2%); RR, 1.12; 95% CI, 0.90–1.40; $P = .31$
Talmor et al., 2008[10]	30	31	ARDS, PaO_2/FiO_2 ratio <300 mm Hg; acute onset	6 mL/kg PBW; Unavailable	Lower tidal volume according to ARMA; goal 6 mL/kg PBW; Unavailable	PEEP titrated to keep end-expiratory TPP 0–10 cm H_2O; Unavailable	Lower PEEP according to ARMA trial PEEP/FiO_2 table; Unavailable	PIP increased to 40 cm H_2O for 30 seconds once before group allocation	PIP increased to 40 cm H_2O for 30 seconds once before group allocation	28-day mortality 5/30 (17%)	12/31 (39%); $P = .055$

Study	No. (Intervention)	No. (Control)	ARDS Definition	Intervention Tidal Volume (goal)	Intervention Measured Tidal Volume	Control Tidal Volume (goal)	Control Measured Tidal Volume	Intervention PEEP Strategy	Intervention Measured PEEP	Control PEEP Strategy	Control Measured PEEP	Recruitment Maneuver	Co-intervention	Mortality
Huh et al., 2009[57]	30	27	ARDS, PaO_2/FiO_2 ratio <200 mm Hg; <48 hours	Lower tidal volume according to ARMA; goal 6 mL/kg PBW	Unavailable	Lower tidal volume according to ARMA; goal 6 mL/kg PBW	Unavailable	PEEP level associated with first desaturation + 2 cm H_2O	Unavailable	Lower PEEP according to ARMA trial PEEP/FiO_2 table	7.0 ± 3.7	25% decrease in tidal volume, incremental PEEP to 25 cm H_2O; maximal PIP <55 cm H_2O	None	28-day mortality 12/30 (40%); 9/27 (33.3%); P = .784
Xi et al., 2010[58]	55	55	ARDS, PaO_2/FiO_2 ratio ≤200 mm Hg; duration not specified	6–8 mL/kg PBW	6.4 ± 0.6 mL/kg PBW[b]	6–8 mL/kg PBW	6.3 ± 0.7 mL/kg PBW[b]	PEEP titrated to maintain PaO_2 60–80 mm Hg with FiO_2 ≤0.6	10.5 ± 3.2 cm H_2O[b]	PEEP titrated to maintain PaO_2 60–80 mm Hg with FiO_2 ≤0.6	9.8 ± 2.3 cm H_2O[b]	CPAP of 40 cm H_2O applied for 40 seconds	None	Hospital mortality 23/55 (41.8%); 31/55 (56.4%); RR, 0.74; 95% CI, 0.50–1.10; P = .13
Hodgson et al., 2011[59]	10	10	ARDS, PaO_2/FiO_2 ratio <200 mm Hg; <72 hours	<6 mL/kg PBW	463 ± 42 mL[b]	<6 mL/kg PBW	563 ± 65 mL[b]	PEEP level associated with first desaturation + 2.5 cm H_2O	15 ± 1 cm H_2O[b]	Lower PEEP according to ARMA trial PEEP/FiO_2 table	10 ± 0.5 cm H_2O[b]	Incremental PEEP levels to 40 cm H_2O then decremental PEEP to point of desaturation	None	Hospital mortality 3/10 (30%); 2/10 (20%); P = .61
Kacmarek et al., 2016	101	99	ARDS, PaO_2/FiO_2 ratio <200 mm Hg; <48 hours	Lower tidal volume according to ARMA; goal 6 mL/kg PBW	5.6 ± 1.1 mL/kg PBW[b]	Lower tidal volume according to ARMA; goal 6 mL/kg PBW	6.2 ± 0.7 mL/kg PBW[b]	PEEP associated with highest compliance + 3 cm H_2O	15.8 ± 3.8 cm H_2O[b]	Lower PEEP according to ARMA trial PEEP/FiO_2 table	11.6 ± 2.5 cm H_2O[b]	Incremental PEEP levels to 35–45 cm H_2O to achieve PIP of 50–60 cm H_2O then decremental PEEP to best dynamic compliance	None	60-day mortality 33/101 (33%); 28/99 (29%); P = .18
ART, Cavalcanti et al., 2017[52]	501	509	ARDS, PaO_2/FiO_2 ratio ≤200 mm Hg; <72 hours	Lower tidal volume according to ARMA; goal 6 mL/kg PBW	5.6 (5.5–5.7) mL/kg PBW[b]	Lower tidal volume according to ARMA; goal 6 mL/kg PBW	5.7 (5.7–5.8) mL/kg PBW[b]	PEEP associated with highest compliance + 2 cm H_2O	16.2 (15.9–16.6) cm H_2O[b]	Lower PEEP according to ARMA trial PEEP/FiO_2 table	12.0 (11.7–12.3) cm H_2O[b]	Incremental PEEP levels up to 45 cm H_2O then decremental PEEP to best respiratory system compliance	None	28-day mortality 277/501 (55.3%); 251/509 (49.3%); HR 1.20; 95% CI, 1.01–1.42; P = .041

[a]Measured on day 3.
[b]Measured on day 1.

ARDS, acute respiratory distress syndrome; CI, confidence interval; CPAP, continuous positive airway pressure; HR, hazard ratio; ICU, intensive care unit; PBW, predicted body weight; PEEP, positive end-expiratory pressure; P_{plat}, plateau pressure; PIP, peak inspiratory pressure; P_{flex}, lower inflection point on the pressure–volume curve; RR, relative risk; TPP, transpulmonary pressure.

score (adjusted hazard ratio [HR] for death 0.68; 95% CI 0.48–0.98; $P = .04$). The NMBA group also had more ventilator-free days at day 28 ($P = .03$) and day 90 ($P = .04$). They also showed no difference in ICU-acquired paresis as defined by the Medical Research Council scale.

A systematic review and meta-analysis of these three trials found that NMBA with cisatracurium was associated with a lower risk of mortality at 28 days (RR 0.66; 95% CI 0.50–0.87; $P = .003$; $I^2 = 0$; NNT = 7).[102]

The patients in the control group of the ACURASYS trial were also deeply sedated, and this is not representative of usual practice and may have confounded the results of the trial.[103,104] The level of sedation in the control group was one of the factors that is evaluated in the open label Re-evaluation of Systemic Early Neuromuscular Blockade (ROSE) trial.[105] This trial included patients with ARDS with PaO_2/FiO_2 ratio <150 mm Hg (or a corresponding peripheral artery capillary oxygen saturation [SpO_2] to FiO_2 ratio). Patients in the treatment arm were deeply sedated and received NMBA as a bolus and then 48 hours infusion, whereas patients in the control arm were lightly sedated with no NMBA. This trial stopped early after 1006 patients were randomized; 28 day mortality was higher than in the Acurysys study, despite similar severity of illness. At 90 days, there was no mortality difference between the NMB group vs. the control group (42.5% vs. 42.8% 95% confidence interval, −6.4 to 5.9; P = 0.93). These data suggest that early adoption of NMB in moderate to severe ARDS may not be beneficial.

PRONE POSITIONING

In a supine patient, positive pressure from the ventilator lifts the ventral chest wall, but has minimal effect on the dorsal chest wall.[106] When in prone position, the positive pressure lifts the dorsal chest wall, but as the dorsal chest wall is less compliant, there is overall decreased chest wall compliance, leading to more diaphragmatic excursion.[107] Because the dorsal lung is larger than the ventral lung, dorsal recruitment exceeds ventral derecruitment, improving overall aeration and increasing lung compliance.[108,109] In addition to the effects of chest wall mechanics, gravity also causes dorsal lung compression when a patient is supine.[110] The heart combined with the heavy edematous lungs in ARDS, increase the ventral–dorsal pleural pressure gradient and cause dorsal lung collapse, which can be reduced by prone positioning.[107,111–113] As pulmonary blood flow is largely unchanged in the prone position, improved dorsal lung aeration also improves ventilation–perfusion matching.[114,115]

Early clinical trials found that prone positioning for 6, 8, and 20 hours in patients with ARDS and PaO_2/FiO_2 ratios <300 mm Hg, <150 mm Hg, and ≤200 mm Hg, respectively, improved oxygenation, but did not have any significant mortality benefit.[116–118]

Subsequently, Guérin et al.[119] published the results of the large Effect of Prone Positioning on Mortality in Patients with Severe Acute Respiratory Distress Syndrome (PROSEVA) trial. The trial included 466 patients with severe ARDS with PaO_2/FiO_2 ratio <100 mm Hg (mean PaO_2/FiO_2 ratio 100 ± 300 mm Hg in prone group and 100 ± 20 mm Hg in supine group). Prone positioning lasted at least 16 hours per day (mean 17.0 ± 3 hours) and could be applied daily for up to 28 days (mean 4.0 ± 4 sessions per patient). All patients received lung-protective ventilation with target tidal volumes of 6 mL/kg PBW. They found that prone positioning decreased 28-day mortality (16.0 vs. 32.8%; $P < .001$; HR 0.39; 95% CI 0.25–0.63; NNT = 6) and 90-day mortality (23.6 vs. 41.0%; $P < .001$; HR 0.44; 95% CI 0.29–0.67).

Two recent meta-analyses of prone positioning trials found no overall mortality benefit associated with prone positioning but did report that the intervention is associated with lower mortality when applied for more than 12 hours per day in patients with moderate-to-severe ARDS with PaO_2/FiO_2 ratio <200 mm Hg.[26,120]

Interestingly, the improved oxygenation seen with prone positioning in the PROSEVA trial participants was not predictive of survival, suggesting that the reduction in mortality was not solely due to improved oxygenation, but more likely due to decreased VILI.[119,121] Improved aeration during prone positioning leads to more uniform distribution of tidal volumes, more even transpulmonary pressures, and can facilitate sustained recruitment with the application of PEEP.[122,123] The more homogeneous aeration also reduces regional hyperinflation and reduces the area of interface between open and closed lung units, collectively decreasing barotrauma and atelectrauma.[106,109,124]

AUTHORS' RECOMMENDATIONS

- Patients with ARDS should be ventilated with low tidal volumes targeting 6 mL/kg PBW (range 4–8 mL/kg PBW) and P_{plat} should be maintained less than 30 cm H_2O.
- We recommend higher PEEP strategies in patients with moderate-to-severe ARDS. Recruitment maneuvers can be used with caution in patients with ARDS but should be limited to patients who have more recruitable lungs.
- We recommend targeting a driving pressure of less than 15 cm H_2O, though lower values may be associated with further reduction in mortality. Targeting driving pressure should be used in conjunction to proven lung-protective ventilation strategies proven to improve outcomes, and should not replace them.
- There is insufficient evidence to suggest superiority of either volume-targeted or pressure-targeted modes of ventilation. Regardless of the mode selected, tidal volumes and P_{plat} should be monitored closely to ensure they remain within lung-protective limits. There is inadequate evidence to recommend for or against assisted spontaneous ventilation in ARDS.
- We recommend that patients with ARDS with PaO_2/FiO_2 ≤ 150 mm Hg undergo neuromuscular blockade, which should be started within 48 hours of disease onset.
- We recommend that patients with ARDS with PaO_2/FiO_2 ratio <150 mm Hg receive prone positioning for more than 12 hours per day.

REFERENCES

1. Ranieri VM, Rubenfeld GD, Thompson BT, et al. Acute respiratory distress syndrome: the Berlin Definition. *JAMA*. 2012;307(23):2526-2533.
2. Ferguson ND, Fan E, Camporota L, et al. The Berlin definition of ARDS: an expanded rationale, justification, and supplementary material. *Intensive Care Med*. 2012;38(10):1573-1582.
3. Bellani G, Laffey JG, Pham T, et al. Epidemiology, patterns of care, and mortality for patients with acute respiratory distress syndrome in intensive care units in 50 countries. *JAMA*. 2016;315(8):788-800.
4. Slutsky AS, Ranieri VM. Ventilator-induced lung injury. *N Engl J Med*. 2013;369(22):2126-2136.
5. Dreyfuss D, Soler P, Basset G, Saumon G. High inflation pressure pulmonary edema. Respective effects of high airway pressure, high tidal volume, and positive end-expiratory pressure. *Am Rev Respir Dis*. 1988;137(5):1159-1164.
6. Webb HH, Tierney DF. Experimental pulmonary edema due to intermittent positive pressure ventilation with high inflation pressures. Protection by positive end-expiratory pressure. *Am Rev Respir Dis*. 1974;110(5):556-565.
7. Slutsky AS. Lung injury caused by mechanical ventilation. *Chest*. 1999;116(suppl 1):9S-15S.
8. Beitler JR, Malhotra A, Thompson BT. Ventilator-induced lung injury. *Clin Chest Med*. 2016;37(4):633-646.
9. Sajjad H, Schmidt GA, Brower RG, Eberlein M. Can the plateau be higher than the peak pressure? *Ann Am Thorac Soc*. 2018;15(6):754-759.
10. Talmor D, Sarge T, Malhotra A, et al. Mechanical ventilation guided by esophageal pressure in acute lung injury. *N Engl J Med*. 2008;359(20):2095-2104.
11. Mauri T, Yoshida T, Bellani G, et al. Esophageal and transpulmonary pressure in the clinical setting: meaning, usefulness and perspectives. *Intensive Care Med*. 2016;42(9):1360-1373.
12. Gattinoni L, Pesenti A. ARDS: the non-homogeneous lung; facts and hypothesis. *Intensive Crit Care Dig*. 1987;6:1-4.
13. Gattinoni L, Caironi P, Pelosi P, Goodman LR. What has computed tomography taught us about the acute respiratory distress syndrome? *Am J Respir Crit Care Med*. 2001;164(9):1701-1711.
14. Gattinoni L, Pesenti A. The concept of "baby lung". *Intensive Care Med*. 2005;31(6):776-784.
15. Gattinoni L, Marini JJ, Pesenti A, Quintel M, Mancebo J, Brochard L. The "baby lung" became an adult. *Intensive Care Med*. 2016;42(5):663-673.
16. Gattinoni L, Caironi P, Cressoni M, et al. Lung recruitment in patients with the acute respiratory distress syndrome. *N Engl J Med*. 2006;354(17):1775-1786.
17. Albert RK. The role of ventilation-induced surfactant dysfunction and atelectasis in causing acute respiratory distress syndrome. *Am J Respir Crit Care Med*. 2012;185(7):702-708.
18. Cereda M, Emami K, Xin Y, et al. Imaging the interaction of atelectasis and overdistension in surfactant-depleted lungs. *Crit Care Med*. 2013;41(2):527-535.
19. Tsuchida S, Engelberts D, Peltekova V, et al. Atelectasis causes alveolar injury in nonatelectatic lung regions. *Am J Respir Crit Care Med*. 2006;174(3):279-289.
20. Terragni PP, Rosboch G, Tealdi A, et al. Tidal hyperinflation during low tidal volume ventilation in acute respiratory distress syndrome. *Am J Respir Crit Care Med*. 2007;175(2):160-166.

21. Brochard L, Slutsky A, Pesenti A. Mechanical ventilation to minimize progression of lung injury in acute respiratory failure. *Am J Respir Crit Care Med*. 2017;195(4):438-442.
22. Rittayamai N, Katsios CM, Beloncle F, Friedrich JO, Mancebo J, Brochard L. Pressure-controlled vs. volume-controlled ventilation in acute respiratory failure: a physiology-based narrative and systematic review. *Chest*. 2015;148(2):340-355.
23. Yoshida T, Nakahashi S, Nakamura MAM, et al. Volume-controlled ventilation does not prevent injurious inflation during spontaneous effort. *Am J Respir Crit Care Med*. 2017;196(5):590-601.
24. Yoshida T, Torsani V, Gomes S, et al. Spontaneous effort causes occult pendelluft during mechanical ventilation. *Am J Respir Crit Care Med*. 2013;188(12):1420-1427.
25. Yoshida T, Uchiyama A, Matsuura N, Mashimo T, Fujino Y. Spontaneous breathing during lung-protective ventilation in an experimental acute lung injury model: high transpulmonary pressure associated with strong spontaneous breathing effort may worsen lung injury. *Crit Care Med*. 2012;40(5):1578-1585.
26. Fan E, Del Sorbo L, Goligher EC, et al. An official American Thoracic Society/European Society of Intensive Care Medicine/Society of Critical Care Medicine clinical practice guideline: mechanical ventilation in adult patients with acute respiratory distress syndrome. *Am J Respir Crit Care Med*. 2017;195(9):1253-1263.
27. Brower RG, Matthay MA, Morris A, et al. Ventilation with lower tidal volumes as compared with traditional tidal volumes for acute lung injury and the acute respiratory distress syndrome. *N Engl J Med*. 2000;342(18):1301-1308.
28. Hager DN, Krishnan JA, Hayden DL, Brower RG, Network ACT. Tidal volume reduction in patients with acute lung injury when plateau pressures are not high. *Am J Respir Crit Care Med*. 2005;172(10):1241-1245.
29. Brower RG, Matthay M, Schoenfeld D. Meta-analysis of acute lung injury and acute respiratory distress syndrome trials. *Am J Respir Crit Care Med*. 2002;166(11):1515-1517.
30. Morelli A, Del Sorbo L, Pesenti A, Ranieri VM, Fan E. Extracorporeal carbon dioxide removal (ECCO$_2$R) in patients with acute respiratory failure. *Intensive Care Med*. 2017;43(4):519-530.
31. Costa EL, Amato MB. Ultra-protective tidal volume: how low should we go? *Crit Care*. 2013;17(2):127.
32. Cove ME, MacLaren G, Federspiel WJ, Kellum JA. Bench to bedside review: Extracorporeal carbon dioxide removal, past, present and future. *Crit Care*. 2012;16(5):232.
33. Batchinsky AI, Jordan BS, Regn D, et al. Respiratory dialysis: reduction in dependence on mechanical ventilation by venovenous extracorporeal CO$_2$ removal. *Crit Care Med*. 2011;39(6):1382-1387.
34. Brodie D, Bacchetta M. Extracorporeal membrane oxygenation for ARDS in adults. *N Engl J Med*. 2011;365(20):1905-1914.
35. Del Sorbo L, Cypel M, Fan E. Extracorporeal life support for adults with severe acute respiratory failure. *Lancet Respir Med*. 2014;2(2):154-164.
36. Bein T, Weber-Carstens S, Goldmann A, et al. Lower tidal volume strategy ($\approx$ 3 ml/kg) combined with extracorporeal CO$_2$ removal versus 'conventional' protective ventilation (6 ml/kg) in severe ARDS: the prospective randomized Xtravent-study. *Intensive Care Med*. 2013;39(5):847-856.
37. Winiszewski H, Aptel F, Belon F, et al. Daily use of extracorporeal CO$_2$ removal in a critical care unit: indications and results. *J Intensive Care*. 2018;6:36.

38. Suter PM, Fairley B, Isenberg MD. Optimum end-expiratory airway pressure in patients with acute pulmonary failure. *N Engl J Med.* 1975;292(6):284-289.

39. Caironi P, Cressoni M, Chiumello D, et al. Lung opening and closing during ventilation of acute respiratory distress syndrome. *Am J Respir Crit Care Med.* 2010;181(6):578-586.

40. Lachmann B. Open up the lung and keep the lung open. *Intensive Care Med.* 1992;18(6):319-321.

41. Amato MB, Barbas CS, Medeiros DM, et al. Effect of a protective-ventilation strategy on mortality in the acute respiratory distress syndrome. *N Engl J Med.* 1998;338(6):347-354.

42. Villar J, Kacmarek RM, Pérez-Méndez L, Aguirre-Jaime A. A high positive end-expiratory pressure, low tidal volume ventilatory strategy improves outcome in persistent acute respiratory distress syndrome: a randomized, controlled trial. *Crit Care Med.* 2006;34(5):1311-1318.

43. Brower RG, Lanken PN, MacIntyre N, et al. Higher versus lower positive end-expiratory pressures in patients with the acute respiratory distress syndrome. *N Engl J Med.* 2004;351(4):327-336.

44. Mercat A, Richard JC, Vielle B, et al. Positive end-expiratory pressure setting in adults with acute lung injury and acute respiratory distress syndrome: a randomized controlled trial. *JAMA.* 2008;299(6):646-655.

45. Meade MO, Cook DJ, Guyatt GH, et al. Ventilation strategy using low tidal volumes, recruitment maneuvers, and high positive end-expiratory pressure for acute lung injury and acute respiratory distress syndrome: a randomized controlled trial. *JAMA.* 2008;299(6):637-645.

46. Briel M, Meade M, Mercat A, et al. Higher vs lower positive end-expiratory pressure in patients with acute lung injury and acute respiratory distress syndrome: systematic review and meta-analysis. *JAMA.* 2010;303(9):865-873.

47. Goligher EC, Kavanagh BP, Rubenfeld GD, et al. Oxygenation response to positive end-expiratory pressure predicts mortality in acute respiratory distress syndrome. A secondary analysis of the LOVS and ExPress trials. *Am J Respir Crit Care Med.* 2014;190(1):70-76.

48. Lapinsky SE, Aubin M, Mehta S, Boiteau P, Slutsky AS. Safety and efficacy of a sustained inflation for alveolar recruitment in adults with respiratory failure. *Intensive Care Med.* 1999;25(11):1297-1301.

49. Rimensberger PC, Cox PN, Frndova H, Bryan AC. The open lung during small tidal volume ventilation: concepts of recruitment and "optimal" positive end-expiratory pressure. *Crit Care Med.* 1999;27(9):1946-1952.

50. Crotti S, Mascheroni D, Caironi P, et al. Recruitment and derecruitment during acute respiratory failure: a clinical study. *Am J Respir Crit Care Med.* 2001;164(1):131-140.

51. Goligher EC, Hodgson CL, Adhikari NKJ, et al. Lung recruitment maneuvers for adult patients with acute respiratory distress syndrome. A systematic review and meta-analysis. *Ann Am Thorac Soc.* 2017;14(Suppl. 4):S304-S311.

52. Cavalcanti AB, Suzumura ÉA, Laranjeira LN, et al. Effect of lung recruitment and titrated positive end-expiratory pressure (PEEP) vs. low PEEP on mortality in patients with acute respiratory distress syndrome: a randomized clinical trial. *JAMA.* 2017;318(14):1335-1345.

53. Borges JB, Okamoto VN, Matos GF, et al. Reversibility of lung collapse and hypoxemia in early acute respiratory distress syndrome. *Am J Respir Crit Care Med.* 2006;174(3):268-278.

54. de Matos GF, Stanzani F, Passos RH, et al. How large is the lung recruitability in early acute respiratory distress syndrome: a prospective case series of patients monitored by computed tomography. *Crit Care.* 2012;16(1):R4.

55. Rubenfeld GD. How much PEEP in acute lung injury. *JAMA.* 2010;303(9):883-884.

56. Calfee CS, Delucchi K, Parsons PE, et al. Subphenotypes in acute respiratory distress syndrome: latent class analysis of data from two randomised controlled trials. *Lancet Respir Med.* 2014;2(8):611-620.

57. Huh JW, Jung H, Choi HS, Hong SB, Lim CM, Koh Y. Efficacy of positive end-expiratory pressure titration after the alveolar recruitment manoeuvre in patients with acute respiratory distress syndrome. *Crit Care.* 2009;13(1):R22. doi: 10.1186/cc7725.

58. Xi XM, Jiang L, Zhu B, RM group. Clinical efficacy and safety of recruitment maneuver in patients with acute respiratory distress syndrome using low tidal volume ventilation: a multi-center randomized controlled clinical trial. *Chin Med J (Engl).* 2010;123(21):3100-3105.

59. Hodgson CL, Tuxen DV, Davies AR, et al. A randomised controlled trial of an open lung strategy with staircase recruitment, titrated PEEP and targeted low airway pressures in patients with acute respiratory distress syndrome. *Crit Care.* 2011;15(3):R133. doi: 10.1186/cc10249

60. Amato MB, Meade MO, Slutsky AS, et al. Driving pressure and survival in the acute respiratory distress syndrome. *N Engl J Med.* 2015;372(8):747-755.

61. Gattinoni L, Pesenti A, Baglioni S, Vitale G, Rivolta M, Pelosi P. Inflammatory pulmonary edema and positive end-expiratory pressure: correlations between imaging and physiologic studies. *J Thorac Imaging.* 1988;3(3):59-64.

62. Guérin C, Papazian L, Reignier J, et al. Effect of driving pressure on mortality in ARDS patients during lung protective mechanical ventilation in two randomized controlled trials. *Crit Care.* 2016;20(1):384.

63. Schmidt MFS, Amaral ACKB, Fan E, Rubenfeld GD. Driving pressure and hospital mortality in patients without ARDS: a cohort study. *Chest.* 2018;153(1):46-54.

64. Chiumello D, Pelosi P, Calvi E, Bigatello LM, Gattinoni L. Different modes of assisted ventilation in patients with acute respiratory failure. *Eur Respir J.* 2002;20(4):925-933.

65. Marini JJ. Point: Is pressure assist-control preferred over volume assist-control mode for lung protective ventilation in patients with ARDS? Yes. *Chest.* 2011;140(2):286-290.

66. Beitler JR, Sands SA, Loring SH, et al. Quantifying unintended exposure to high tidal volumes from breath stacking dyssynchrony in ARDS: the BREATHE criteria. *Intensive Care Med.* 2016;42(9):1427-1436.

67. Kallet RH, Campbell AR, Dicker RA, Katz JA, Mackersie RC. Work of breathing during lung-protective ventilation in patients with acute lung injury and acute respiratory distress syndrome: a comparison between volume and pressure regulated breathing modes. *Respir Care.* 2005;50(12):1623-1631.

68. MacIntyre N. Counterpoint: Is pressure assist-control preferred over volume assist-control mode for lung protective ventilation in patients with ARDS? No. *Chest.* 2011;140(2):290-292.

69. Nichols D, Haranath S. Pressure control ventilation. *Crit Care Clin.* 2007;23(2):183-199, viii-ix.

70. Chacko B, Peter JV, Tharyan P, John G, Jeyaseelan L. Pressure-controlled versus volume-controlled ventilation for acute respiratory failure due to acute lung injury (ALI) or acute

respiratory distress syndrome (ARDS). *Cochrane Database Syst Rev.* 2015;1:CD008807.

71. Jaber S, Petrof BJ, Jung B, et al. Rapidly progressive diaphragmatic weakness and injury during mechanical ventilation in humans. *Am J Respir Crit Care Med.* 2011;183(3):364-371.

72. Levine S, Nguyen T, Taylor N, et al. Rapid disuse atrophy of diaphragm fibers in mechanically ventilated humans. *N Engl J Med.* 2008;358(13):1327-1335.

73. Rittayamai N, Brochard L. Recent advances in mechanical ventilation in patients with acute respiratory distress syndrome. *Eur Respir Rev.* 2015;24(135):132-140.

74. Goligher EC, Dres M, Fan E, et al. Mechanical ventilation-induced diaphragm atrophy strongly impacts clinical outcomes. *Am J Respir Crit Care Med.* 2018;197(2):204-213.

75. Marini JJ. Spontaneously regulated vs. controlled ventilation of acute lung injury/acute respiratory distress syndrome. *Curr Opin Crit Care.* 2011;17(1):24-29.

76. Katzenstein AL, Bloor CM, Leibow AA. Diffuse alveolar damage—the role of oxygen, shock, and related factors. A review. *Am J Pathol.* 1976;85(1):209-228.

77. Taskar V, John J, Evander E, Robertson B, Jonson B. Surfactant dysfunction makes lungs vulnerable to repetitive collapse and reexpansion. *Am J Respir Crit Care Med.* 1997;155(1):313-320.

78. Neumann P, Wrigge H, Zinserling J, et al. Spontaneous breathing affects the spatial ventilation and perfusion distribution during mechanical ventilatory support. *Crit Care Med.* 2005;33(5):1090-1095.

79. Wrigge H, Zinserling J, Neumann P, et al. Spontaneous breathing improves lung aeration in oleic acid-induced lung injury. *Anesthesiology.* 2003;99(2):376-384.

80. Froese AB, Bryan AC. Effects of anesthesia and paralysis on diaphragmatic mechanics in man. *Anesthesiology.* 1974;41(3):242-255.

81. Cereda M, Foti G, Marcora B, et al. Pressure support ventilation in patients with acute lung injury. *Crit Care Med.* 2000;28(5):1269-1275.

82. Putensen C, Zech S, Wrigge H, et al. Long-term effects of spontaneous breathing during ventilatory support in patients with acute lung injury. *Am J Respir Crit Care Med.* 2001;164(1):43-49.

83. Zhou Y, Jin X, Lv Y, et al. Early application of airway pressure release ventilation may reduce the duration of mechanical ventilation in acute respiratory distress syndrome. *Intensive Care Med.* 2017;43(11):1648-1659.

84. Mireles-Cabodevila E, Dugar S, Chatburn RL. APRV for ARDS: the complexities of a mode and how it affects even the best trials. *J Thorac Dis.* 2018;10(Suppl. 9):S1058-S1063.

85. Hickling KG, Henderson SJ, Jackson R. Low mortality associated with low volume pressure limited ventilation with permissive hypercapnia in severe adult respiratory distress syndrome. *Intensive Care Med.* 1990;16(6):372-377.

86. Ferguson ND, Villar J, Slutsky AS. Understanding high-frequency oscillation: lessons from the animal kingdom. *Intensive Care Med.* 2007;33(8):1316-1318.

87. Slutsky AS, Drazen JM. Ventilation with small tidal volumes. *N Engl J Med.* 2002;347(9):630-631.

88. Hager DN, Fessler HE, Kaczka DW, et al. Tidal volume delivery during high-frequency oscillatory ventilation in adults with acute respiratory distress syndrome. *Crit Care Med.* 2007;35(6):1522-1529.

89. Fessler HE, Derdak S, Ferguson ND, et al. A protocol for high-frequency oscillatory ventilation in adults: results from a roundtable discussion. *Crit Care Med.* 2007;35(7):1649-1654.

90. Derdak S, Mehta S, Stewart TE, et al. High-frequency oscillatory ventilation for acute respiratory distress syndrome in adults: a randomized, controlled trial. *Am J Respir Crit Care Med.* 2002;166(6):801-808.

91. Bollen CW, van Well GT, Sherry T, et al. High frequency oscillatory ventilation compared with conventional mechanical ventilation in adult respiratory distress syndrome: a randomized controlled trial [ISRCTN24242669]. *Crit Care.* 2005;9(4):R430-439.

92. Ferguson ND, Cook DJ, Guyatt GH, et al. High-frequency oscillation in early acute respiratory distress syndrome. *N Engl J Med.* 2013;368(9):795-805.

93. Young D, Lamb SE, Shah S, et al. High-frequency oscillation for acute respiratory distress syndrome. *N Engl J Med.* 2013;368(9):806-813.

94. Goffi A, Ferguson ND. High-frequency oscillatory ventilation for early acute respiratory distress syndrome in adults. *Curr Opin Crit Care.* 2014;20(1):77-85.

95. Goligher EC, Munshi L, Adhikari NKJ, et al. High-frequency oscillation for adult patients with acute respiratory distress syndrome. a systematic review and meta-analysis. *Ann Am Thorac Soc.* 2017;14(Suppl. 4):S289-S296.

96. Meade MO, Young D, Hanna S, et al. Severity of hypoxemia and effect of high-frequency oscillatory ventilation in acute respiratory distress syndrome. *Am J Respir Crit Care Med.* 2017;196(6):727-733.

97. Hansen-Flaschen JH, Brazinsky S, Basile C, Lanken PN. Use of sedating drugs and neuromuscular blocking agents in patients requiring mechanical ventilation for respiratory failure. A national survey. *JAMA.* 1991;266(20):2870-2875.

98. Mehta S, Burry L, Fischer S, et al. Canadian survey of the use of sedatives, analgesics, and neuromuscular blocking agents in critically ill patients. *Crit Care Med.* 2006;34(2):374-380.

99. Gainnier M, Roch A, Forel JM, et al. Effect of neuromuscular blocking agents on gas exchange in patients presenting with acute respiratory distress syndrome. *Crit Care Med.* 2004;32(1):113-119.

100. Forel JM, Roch A, Marin V, et al. Neuromuscular blocking agents decrease inflammatory response in patients presenting with acute respiratory distress syndrome. *Crit Care Med.* 2006;34(11):2749-2757.

101. Papazian L, Forel JM, Gacouin A, et al. Neuromuscular blockers in early acute respiratory distress syndrome. *N Engl J Med.* 2010;363(12):1107-1116.

102. Alhazzani W, Alshahrani M, Jaeschke R, et al. Neuromuscular blocking agents in acute respiratory distress syndrome: a systematic review and meta-analysis of randomized controlled trials. *Crit Care.* 2013;17(2):R43.

103. Barr J, Fraser GL, Puntillo K, et al. Clinical practice guidelines for the management of pain, agitation, and delirium in adult patients in the intensive care unit. *Crit Care Med.* 2013;41(1):263-306.

104. Reade MC, Finfer S. Sedation and delirium in the intensive care unit. *N Engl J Med.* 2014;370(5):444-454.

105. Huang DT, Angus DC, Moss M, et al. Design and rationale of the reevaluation of systemic early neuromuscular blockade trial for acute respiratory distress syndrome. *Ann Am Thorac Soc.* 2017;14(1):124-133.

106. Gattinoni L, Taccone P, Carlesso E, Marini JJ. Prone position in acute respiratory distress syndrome. Rationale, indications, and limits. *Am J Respir Crit Care Med.* 2013;188(11):1286-1293.

107. Pelosi P, D'Andrea L, Vitale G, Pesenti A, Gattinoni L. Vertical gradient of regional lung inflation in adult respiratory distress syndrome. *Am J Respir Crit Care Med.* 1994;149(1):8-13.

108. Gattinoni L, Pelosi P, Vitale G, Pesenti A, D'Andrea L, Mascheroni D. Body position changes redistribute lung computed-tomographic density in patients with acute respiratory failure. *Anesthesiology.* 1991;74(1):15-23.

109. Cornejo RA, Díaz JC, Tobar EA, et al. Effects of prone positioning on lung protection in patients with acute respiratory distress syndrome. *Am J Respir Crit Care Med.* 2013;188(4):440-448.

110. Lai-Fook SJ, Rodarte JR. Pleural pressure distribution and its relationship to lung volume and interstitial pressure. *J Appl Physiol.* 1991;70(3):967-978.

111. Malbouisson LM, Busch CJ, Puybasset L, Lu Q, Cluzel P, Rouby JJ. Role of the heart in the loss of aeration characterizing lower lobes in acute respiratory distress syndrome. CT Scan ARDS Study Group. *Am J Respir Crit Care Med.* 2000;161(6):2005-2012.

112. Puybasset L, Cluzel P, Chao N, Slutsky AS, Coriat P, Rouby JJ. A computed tomography scan assessment of regional lung volume in acute lung injury. The CT Scan ARDS Study Group. *Am J Respir Crit Care Med.* 1998;158(5 Pt 1):1644-1655.

113. Scholten EL, Beitler JR, Prisk GK, Malhotra A. Treatment of ARDS with prone positioning. *Chest.* 2017;151(1):215-224.

114. Prisk GK, Yamada K, Henderson AC, et al. Pulmonary perfusion in the prone and supine postures in the normal human lung. *J Appl Physiol (1985).* 2007;103(3):883-894.

115. Glenny RW, Lamm WJ, Albert RK, Robertson HT. Gravity is a minor determinant of pulmonary blood flow distribution. *J Appl Physiol (1985).* 1991;71(2):620-629.

116. Gattinoni L, Tognoni G, Pesenti A, et al. Effect of prone positioning on the survival of patients with acute respiratory failure. *N Engl J Med.* 2001;345(8):568-573.

117. Guerin C, Gaillard S, Lemasson S, et al. Effects of systematic prone positioning in hypoxemic acute respiratory failure: a randomized controlled trial. *JAMA.* 2004;292(19):2379-2387.

118. Taccone P, Pesenti A, Latini R, et al. Prone positioning in patients with moderate and severe acute respiratory distress syndrome: a randomized controlled trial. *JAMA.* 2009;302(18):1977-1984.

119. Guérin C, Reignier J, Richard JC, et al. Prone positioning in severe acute respiratory distress syndrome. *N Engl J Med.* 2013;368(23):2159-2168.

120. Munshi L, Del Sorbo L, Adhikari NKJ, et al. Prone position for acute respiratory distress syndrome. a systematic review and meta-analysis. *Ann Am Thorac Soc.* 2017;14(Suppl. 4):S280-S288.

121. Albert RK, Keniston A, Baboi L, Ayzac L, Guérin C; Proseva Investigators. Prone position-induced improvement in gas exchange does not predict improved survival in the acute respiratory distress syndrome. *Am J Respir Crit Care Med.* 2014;189(4):494-496.

122. Gattinoni L, Pesenti A, Carlesso E. Body position changes redistribute lung computed-tomographic density in patients with acute respiratory failure: impact and clinical fallout through the following 20 years. *Intensive Care Med.* 2013;39(11):1909-1915.

123. Cakar N, der Kloot TV, Youngblood M, Adams A, Nahum A. Oxygenation response to a recruitment maneuver during supine and prone positions in an oleic acid-induced lung injury model. *Am J Respir Crit Care Med.* 2000;161(6):1949-1956.

124. Galiatsou E, Kostanti E, Svarna E, et al. Prone position augments recruitment and prevents alveolar overinflation in acute lung injury. *Am J Respir Crit Care Med.* 2006;174(2):187-197.

17

Is Carbon Dioxide Harmful or Helpful in ARDS?

Claire Masterson, Shahd Horie, Emanuele Rezoagli, and John G. Laffey

INTRODUCTION

Arterial CO_2 tension ($PaCO_2$) represents a balance between CO_2 production and elimination via the lungs, and in health is maintained within a tight range (35–40 mm Hg). Traditional approaches to the CO_2 management of adults with acute respiratory failure, which focused on the potential for hypercapnia (HC) to exert deleterious effects, advocated increases in tidal and minute ventilation to minimize the risks of HC. However, in critically ill patients with acute respiratory failure, decrements in alveolar ventilation render maintenance of normocapnia challenging. The potential for high lung stretch to directly injure the lungs—termed ventilation-induced lung injury (VILI)—is now well recognized,[1–3] mandating the use of more protective ventilatory strategies that reduce lung stretch. These approaches improve survival in patients with acute respiratory distress syndrome (ARDS).[4,5]

Consequently, HC—and its associated hypercapnic acidosis (HCA)—is prevalent in the critically ill, permitted in order to realize the benefits of lower lung stretch. The increased frequency of ventilator strategies incorporating "permissive hypercapnia" in critically ill patients has generated significant experimental and clinical investigations designed to better understand the effects of HC. These studies reveal HC to be a potent biologic agent, with the potential to exert both beneficial and potentially harmful[6,7] effects. In recent years, advances in extracorporeal technologies have made possible the direct removal of CO_2 while maintaining[8,9] lung protective ventilation. Consequently, it is important to understand the biology of HC, in order to best determine when it should be encouraged, tolerated, or avoided in the critically ill.

PHYSIOLOGIC EFFECTS OF HYPERCAPNIA

The Respiratory System

Control of Breathing

The regulation and control of breathing in healthy individuals is governed by $PaCO_2$ levels, which are sensed by carotid chemoreceptors that rapidly respond to fluctuations,[10] and central chemoreceptive neurons which have a slower but more pronounced effect on ventilation in response to HC.[11] Questions remain as to whether ventilatory changes occur solely in response to HC or to the associated acidosis that occurs, given that both chemoreceptors respond to changes in both CO_2 and H^+[11,12]; however, it has been demonstrated that the ventilatory response to metabolic acidosis is more gradual than responses to elevated $PaCO_2$.[13,14] More recently, experiments have demonstrated that the loss of individual acid-sensing ion channel subunits does not alter ventilator responses to HC or hypoxia.[15] In response to HC, caudal medullary brainstem astrocytes in murine models release D-serine, which binds the NMDA receptor, resulting in an increased respiratory rate, which gives further insight to the central chemoreceptor response to HC.[16]

Pulmonary Vasculature

HC can improve arterial oxygenation by enhancing ventilation–perfusion matching by augmenting hypoxia-induced pulmonary arteriolar vasoconstriction.[17] This effect of hypercapnia can increase pulmonary vascular resistance,[18] increasing pulmonary vascular pressures and potentially worsen pulmonary hypertension. While this may increase fluid filtration and increase pulmonary edema development, HCA directly inhibits the increase in the whole lung filtration coefficient caused by increased vascular pressures by reducing mechanotransduction in the lung vasculature.[19] HCA also directly inhibits the increase in pulmonary endothelial permeability caused by ischemia–reperfusion induced lung injury,[20,21] and free-radical injury.[21]

Airways

In the airways, hypercapnia directly dilates small airways[22] but indirectly constricts larger airways via vagal stimulation,[23] which may contribute to ventilation–perfusion matching.

Lung Tissue

In experimental models, induced hypercapnia acidosis—termed therapeutic hypercapnia—has been demonstrated to directly attenuate lung injury induced by high lung stretch,[24,25] ischemia–reperfusion injury, endotoxin,[26] pulmonary bacterial infection,[27] and systemic polymicrobial sepsis.[28] In terms of dose–response, moderate HCA ($PaCO_2$ of 80–100 mm Hg) appears to be more effective than severe HCA ($PaCO_2 > 100$ mm Hg) in experimental ventilation induced injury,[29] and ischemia—reperfusion injury.[30] In experimental models of lung transplantation, lung function improved, lung injury was lowered, and the rate of cellular rejection after lung allograft was reduced when inspired CO_2 (8%) was applied.[31] A comparison of the relative effects of therapeutic vs. permissive HC in surfactant-depleted rabbits found that both reduced lung injury, with greater protection seen with reduced tidal volume (V_t).[32]

Alveolar fluid clearance, a critical step in the resolution of ARDS, can be affected by HC. In vitro moderate HC reduces cAMP-stimulated fluid secretion in human airway epithelial cells[33]; however, it has also been reported that HC impairs alveolar fluid clearance via downregulation of Na^+, K^+-ATPase.[34,35]

Respiratory Muscles

Postcritical illness weakness of skeletal[36,37] and respiratory muscles[37] is a critical factor in functional outcome in patients with ARDS.[37] ARDS survivors present diminished exercise capabilities, decreased muscle strength, a lower maximal inspiratory pressure, and a reduced quality of life.[37] The effect of HC on diaphragmatic function is as yet unclear. In spontaneously breathing patients, HCA impairs diaphragmatic contractility and increases diaphragmatic fatigue[38,39]; however, HC can restore diaphragmatic function due to prolonged mechanical ventilation where the minute ventilation is controlled.[40] The resulting myosin loss and inflammation resulting from prolonged ventilation can also be prevented by HC in experimental models.[41] In a small sample of critically ill patients receiving mechanical ventilation, HC did not influence muscle wasting as determined by diaphragm thickness and peripheral skeletal muscle cross-sectional area.[42]

The Cardiovascular System

Cardiac output (CO) and pulmonary vascular resistance can both be increased via HC-induced sympathetic activation, which increases myocardial contractility and decreases afterload, leading to a net increase in CO.[17,43] This counteracts the direct reduction of cardiac[44] and vascular smooth muscle[17] contractility by HCA. The net effect is that carbon dioxide increases cardiac index by 10–15% by each 10 mm Hg of $PaCO_2$ increase.[45,46]

Limiting peak inspiratory pressure in porcine models of ARDS leads to respiratory acidosis and HC that is associated with increased CO and regional blood flow in areas such as the myocardium, brain, and spinal cord, among others.[47] In preclinical polymicrobial sepsis models, HC improves tissue oxygenation and reduces lung edema formation, with hemodynamic effects comparable to dobutamine therapy.[48]

HC also directly protects the myocardium, limiting myocardial stunning in experimental models of ischemia–reperfusion injury.[49] Increases in $PaCO_2$ result in vasodilation to levels similar to that seen with a standard dose of adenosine, providing an alternative to pharmacologic vasodilators to ascertain myocardial blood flow during cardiac stress testing.[50]

Tissue Oxygenation Supply vs. Demand Balance

The effects of HC on cardiovascular hemodynamics and on pulmonary ventilation–perfusion (V/Q) matching increases arterial oxygenation and oxygen delivery to the tissues. HC and acidosis shift the hemoglobin–oxygen dissociation curve rightward, reducing the oxygen affinity of hemoglobin and may cause an elevation in hematocrit level,[51] further increasing tissue oxygen delivery. Concurrent reduced cellular respiration and oxygen consumption observed during acidosis may further improve oxygen supply–demand balance, particularly in the setting of compromised supply.[52]

Peripheral tissue oxygenation is linearly increased by mild intraoperative HC in healthy anesthetized subjects.[45] Improved tissue oxygenation reduces the risk of surgical site infection (SSI).[53] In normal weight,[54] and morbidly obese surgical patients (at high risk of SSI),[55] HC improved tissue oxygenation. However, a large trial of mild HC use in patients undergoing colon resection determined that there was little to no effect of HC on the development of SSI.[56]

The Central Nervous System

Both cerebral blood flow (CBF) and cerebral oxygen delivery are augmented by HC[57] via dilation of precapillary cerebral arterioles, which is attributed to acidosis rather than the increased $PaCO_2$,[58] and by increases in arterial oxygen tension (PaO_2).

The direct effects of HC in the injured brain are unclear. In rodents exposed to experimental hypoxia and cerebral stroke, HC reduced the size of cerebral infarcts,[59] and upregulated the synthetic and proliferative activity of nerve cells.[60] In contrast, in a hypoxia model in rats, activation of NLRP3 inflammasome release of IL-1β from activated microglia was enhanced by HC, increasing neuronal death and contributing to cognitive impairment.[61]

In healthy subjects, significant heterogeneity is seen in regional cerebral perfusion in response to HC.[62] Indeed, cerebral vascular reactivity to CO_2 measured by transcranial Doppler may be used as a risk predictor for ischemic stroke.[63]

Clear concerns exist regarding the potential for HC-induced increases in CBF, in the setting of reduced intracranial compliance, to critically elevate intracranial pressure.[64]

INTRACELLULAR MECHANISMS OF ACTION OF CO_2

The molecular effects of HC—both beneficial and harmful—are increasingly well understood (Fig. 17.1). HC inhibits key aspects of the innate immune response. The expression of interleukin-6 (IL-6) and tumor necrosis factor alpha (TNF-α) in alveolar macrophages is inhibited by HC and phagocytosis is decreased, indicating a reduction in innate immunity.[65] Recently, HC has been demonstrated to inhibit bacterial killing and autophagy in alveolar macrophages via a BCL-2– and BCL-XL–dependent mechanism.[66] These results and others suggest that hypercapnia may be deleterious in prolonged untreated bacterial infection.[67]

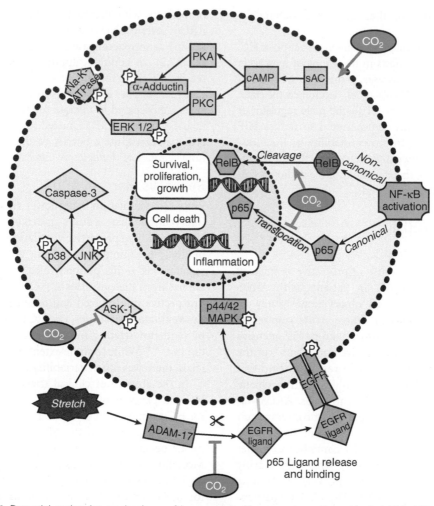

Fig. 17.1 Potential molecular mechanisms of hypercapnia. Hypercapnia and/or acidosis inhibit NF-κB signal transduction pathways at multiple levels. Hypercapnia prevents p65 translocation to the nucleus (canonical pathway) and reduces inflammatory gene expressions, while promotion of RelB activation (noncanonical pathway) influences gene expressions responsible for survival, proliferation, and cell growth. CO_2 activates soluble adenylate cyclase *(sAC)* and increases intracellular cAMP levels, which in turn activates protein kinases *(PKA/PKC)*. Phosphorylation of α-adductin and ERK1/2 by PKA/PKC initiates the endocytosis of Na^+/K^+-ATP-ase, leading to reduced alveolar fluid transport. Mechanical stretch-induced inflammatory response and apoptosis are also inhibited by hypercapnia. Hypercapnia prevents "shedding" of EGFR Ligand by inhibiting metalloproteases (ADAM-17). This in turn leads to reduced activation of the p44/42 mitogen-activated protein kinase *(MAPK)* pathway dependent inflammatory gene expression. Hypercapnia reduces cell death by inhibiting apoptosis signal-regulating kinase 1 *(ASK-1)* and intracellular caspase-3 activity. *EGFR,* Epidermal growth factor receptor.

Nuclear factor kappa-B (NF-κB) is a key transcriptional protein in injury, inflammation, and repair, and several effects of HC may be mediated via this pathway. HCA inhibits NF-κB at key steps of the cell signaling pathway, including inhibition of degradation of IκBα, which binds NF-κB and prevents translocation to the nucleus,[68] and also by inhibition of the activation of an upstream protein IKK-β and downstream DNA binding in the nucleus.[69,70] This mechanism prevents the release of inflammatory cytokines in response to injury and may play a key role in the mechanisms underlying protection in models of VILI, and potentially other "sterile" injury models.[25,69,71] However, HC-mediated inhibition of NF-κB retards pulmonary epithelial wound healing,[70] and mediates the reduced production of innate immune cytokines from endotoxin-stimulated macrophages,[72] potentially

via a mechanism involving via heat shock factor 1 (HSF1) protein. In summary, the effects of HC-mediated inhibition of NF-κB in the setting of sepsis are complex, and may represent a double-edged sword.[6]

Mechanical stretch has been shown to activate "shedding" of endogenous ligands, such as tumor necrosis factor receptor (TNFR), by the metalloprotease ADAM-17.[73] Mitogen-activated protein kinase (MAPK), which plays a key role in the pathogenesis of stretch-induced lung injury, is activated via the epidermal growth factor receptor (EGFR) pathway, which in turn is activated via ADAM-17 cleavage products. HCA inhibits stretch-induced activation of ADAM-17, reducing EGFR and p44/42 MAPK activation, and decreasing VILI in vivo. These studies reveal an important novel therapeutic target.[73] In addition, sustained HC can induce micro RNAs such as MiR-183 that lead to mitochondrial dysfunction.[74]

When examining the molecular mechanisms of action of HC, it is important to consider its effects in the setting of hypoxia, a common feature of respiratory diseases. In this regard, in a series of elegant studies, Selfridge and colleagues[75] examined the effect of HC on hypoxia inducible factor (HIF), the main regulator of the hypoxia response. HC was demonstrated to reduce HIF activation, by decreasing HIF-1α protein stability, in an at least partially pH-dependent manner, suggesting that HC can modulate the response to hypoxia, thereby affecting the pathophysiology of diseases where HIF is implicated.

ROLE IN CLINICAL ARDS

Prevalence of Hypercapnia

Notwithstanding the widespread use of protective ventilatory strategies, the prevalence of HC in patients with ARDS has remained unclear. The Large observational study to UNderstand the Global impact of Severe Acute respiratory FailurE (LUNG SAFE) study was undertaken in 459 intensive care units (ICUs) in 50 countries in five continents[76] in the winter of 2014 in both hemispheres. The results showed that ARDS continues to represent a global public health problem, occurring in 10% of patients admitted to ICUs. ARDS was underrecognized by clinicians, while the use of contemporary evidence-based ventilatory strategies and adjuncts was lower than expected. Of most concern, ARDS continues to confer a high mortality, with 40% of patients with ARDS dying in hospital. The LUNG SAFE study also provided interesting insights regarding the prevalence of HC (Fig. 17.2). Of particular interest, approximately 20% of patients had significant HC (PaCO$_2$ $\geq$50 mm Hg) on day 1 of ARDS, and the proportion of patients with permissive HC increased with increasing ARDS severity. Nevertheless, median arterial CO$_2$ tension was in the normal range at all three levels of ARDS severity (see Fig. 17.2). In addition, approximately one-third of patients received a tidal volume of $\geq$8 mL/kg. These data suggest that there appear to be limits to the degree of HC that clinicians are prepared to tolerate to facilitate lower tidal volumes in patients with ARDS. Indeed, ongoing concerns regarding HC may constitute a barrier to the institution of protective lung ventilation strategies by clinicians.

Benefit vs. Harm in ARDS

Protective ventilation using lower tidal volumes is a proven intervention that reduces mortality in ARDS.[3,77] A key 'enabler' of lung protective ventilation has been the reduction of tidal and minute ventilation, and the 'tolerance' of the resultant HC—this 'permissive HC' was advocated in seminal studies from the early 1990s.[4,5] Of the subsequent five major prospective randomized controlled trials (RCTs) of protective ventilatory strategies, two RCTs demonstrated an impact of ventilator strategy on mortality,[3,77] although three RCTs did not.[78–80] While to some extent, HC developed in all of the trials, there was much variability (Table 17.1).

In the absence of clinical trials examining the impact of HC independent of changes in tidal volume, the potential for HC to impact on outcome remains unclear. Of interest, a subsequent analysis of the ARMA trial[3] suggested that there might be an independent effect of hypercapnic acidosis.[81] Mortality was examined as a function of HCA severity on the day of enrollment using multivariate analysis and controlling for other comorbidities and severity of lung injury. It was found that HCA reduced 28-day mortality in patients randomized to the higher V$_t$ but not in those receiving lower V$_t$.[81]

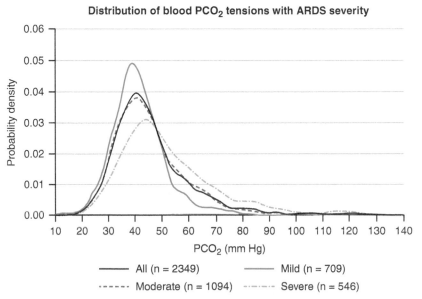

Fig. 17.2 The frequency distribution of arterial carbon dioxide tension in patients with acute respiratory distress syndrome *(ARDS)* in the LUNG SAFE study. The profiles of PaCO$_2$ varied, depending on ARDS severity. (Modified from Bellani G, Laffey JG, Pham T, et al. Epidemiology, patterns of care, and mortality for patients with acute respiratory distress syndrome in intensive care units in 50 countries. *JAMA.* 2016;315[8]:788-800.)

TABLE 17.1 Ventilatory Strategies and Management of CO_2 in Clinical Trials.

Trial	Mortality Benefit	Control Group, $PaCO_2$ (mm Hg, Mean ± SD)	Protective Ventilation Group, $PaCO_2$ (mm Hg, Mean ± SD)	Buffering Permitted
'ARMA' ARDSnet Trial, 2000[3]	Yes	35.8 ± 8.0	40.0 ± 10.0	Yes
Amato et al., 1998[77]	Yes	36.0 ± 1.5	58.0 ± 3.0	No
Stewart et al., 1998[80]	No	46.0 ± 10.0	54.5 ± 15.0	No
Brochard et al., 1998[78]	No	41.0 ± 7.5	59.5 ± 19.0	No
Brower et al., 1999[79]	No	40.1 ± 1.6	50.3 ± 3.5	Yes

In contrast, Nin et al. found that a $PaCO_2$ of over 50 mm Hg in ARDS patients during the first 48 hours was associated with a higher ICU mortality in a secondary analysis of three noninterventional cohort studies, and suggested that "severe" HC ($PaCO_2 \geq 50$ mm Hg) can no longer be considered "safe."[82] Criticisms of these conclusions include the fact that the investigators did not adjust for severity of ARDS, lung compliance, or baseline $PaCO_2$ values, and they did not include pH in the model collinearity issues.[83] Other analyses of prospective cohort studies show no effect of HC in patients with ARDS.[83] A further study in a large cohort of critically ill patients found that increasing levels of $PaCO_2$ (up to 65 mm Hg) were associated with increasing levels of ICU mortality during the first 24 hours of admission.[84]

A number of clinical studies of HC in other settings suggest that it is safe and may have some beneficial effects. Sixty patients undergoing pancreaticoduodenal surgery were randomized to receive standard ventilation, protective ventilation, and protective ventilation with HC. Patients undergoing protective ventilation demonstrated decreased postoperative lactate profiles and improved postoperative oxygenation, reduced hospital stay, and developed less atelectasis.[85] The subgroup undergoing protective ventilation with HC also had a reduced lactate, but no additional beneficial effects. In a study of 50 patients undergoing lung lobectomy, patients were randomized to a $PaCO_2$ range of 35–45 mm Hg or of 60–70 mm Hg.[86] Patients randomized to the higher CO_2 levels were shown to have lower TNF-α in bronchoalveolar lavage (BAL); lower IL-1, IL-6, and IL-8 in both serum and BAL; a higher serum IL-10; decreased protein and white cell count; increased postoperative oxygenation index values (PaO_2/FiO_2); and decreased airway pressures.[86]

In summary, the evidence linking HC to harm or benefit in patients with ARDS remains inconclusive. The finding of an "association" between HC and outcome does not imply "cause-and-effect," and potential confounders exist in even the most careful analyses. Nevertheless, concerns regarding more severe levels of HC are supported by experimental studies demonstrating dose–response effects, and reinforce the need for careful titration of low tidal volume strategies and the degree of HC that is required to facilitate the strategy.

Extracorporeal CO_2 Removal

Studies such as the LUNG SAFE study[76] raise the possibility that concerns regarding HC may constitute a barrier to the institution of protective lung ventilation strategies.

Advances in extracorporeal device technologies have made selective extracorporeal CO_2 removal ($ECCO_2$-R) devices a less-invasive, and potentially more feasible option. The rationale to integrate $ECCO_2$-R to the management of severe ARDS is to allow more 'protective' ventilation (low V_t) while avoiding extreme levels of respiratory acidosis. Arterial CO_2 tensions are generally maintained in the range 45–55 mm Hg rather than targeting normocapnia with this approach.

Initial clinical studies suggest promise. Terragni et al.[9] demonstrated, in a small cohort of ARDS patients ($n = 10$), that application of $ECCO_2$-R can further reduce lung injury by allowing very low V_t (3.7–4.6 mL/kg). Subsequently, Bein et al.[8] showed that combining $ECCO_2$-R with a very low V_t ventilation strategy (3 mL/kg ideal body weight [IBW]) in patients with established severe ARDS was safe. Importantly, a subset of patients with more severe hypoxemia ($PaO_2/FiO_2 \leq 150$ mm Hg) had significantly higher ventilator-free days when a combination of $ECCO_2$-R and very low V_t was used (41 vs. 28 days). Furthermore, Fanelli and colleagues[87] have demonstrated the safety and the feasibility of $ECCO_2$-R in patients with moderate ARDS using low blood flow to allow ultraprotective mechanical ventilation (4 mL/kg predicted body weight [PBW]). The recently reported SUPERNOVA study, a prospective observational study of 3 $ECCO_2$-R devices, provided further evidence for the safety and feasibility of $ECCO_2$-R. SUPERNOVA highlighted the potential for $ECCO_2$-R to permit further reduction of tidal volumes in patients with ARDS.[88]

A key unknown at present is whether any potential benefit of utilizing $ECCO_2$-R to permit further reductions in tidal volume will produce a benefit that is outweighed by any complications (e.g., thrombosis, bleeding)[89] related to the extracorporeal circuit. The potential to integrate $ECCO_2$-R into continuous renal replacement circuits may improve the risk–benefit ratio for hypercapnic patients with acute kidney injury.[90]

Large-scale clinical trials of $ECCO_2$-R are currently in progress, such as the REST Trial (NCT02654327) that will hopefully clarify these issues.

CONTROVERSIES AND AREAS OF UNCERTAINTY

Permissive Hypercapnia and Intracranial Pressure Regulation

Intracranial pressure increases due to augmentation of cerebral blood volume can be induced by HC.[91] For patients with head trauma, it is recommended that $PaCO_2$ be maintained at normal levels and HC avoided due to the increased vasodilation and CBF. "Brain-directed" ventilatory strategies differ from that of lung protective ventilation with higher tidal volumes, FiO_2 and low or no positive end-expiratory pressure (PEEP) in an effort to avoid HC.[92] However, intracranial hypertension constitutes a relative rather than an absolute contraindication to HC. Therefore, a balance should be sought between lung-protective and brain-protective ventilation strategies in terms of permissive HC. The use of an intracranial pressure monitor or an oximetry catheter placed in the jugular vein may facilitate the gradual titration HC in patients with brain trauma, and identify those in which HC should be avoided.

Permissive Hypercapnia and Pulmonary Vascular Tone

HC and the associated acidosis increases vasoconstriction in pulmonary vessels.[93–95] However, clinical conditions predisposing to pulmonary hypertension constitute a relative rather than absolute contraindication to permissive HC. Where concerns exist regarding pulmonary hypertension, a useful approach is to measure pulmonary pressures and titrate the degree of HC accordingly. In this context, monitoring with transthoracic echocardiography or placement of a pulmonary artery catheter may be indicated.

Permissive Hypercapnia—The Role of Buffering

Buffering of the acidosis induced by HC remains a common, albeit controversial, clinical practice. The evidence that hypercapnic acidosis is directly deleterious, especially where pH is >7.2, is weak. Specific concerns exist regarding sodium bicarbonate, the "buffer" used most frequently in the clinical setting. Although the physiochemical effect of $NaHCO_3$ is to increase the strong ion difference by increasing extracellular Na^+,[96] the net effect is the generation of CO_2.[97] Hence, $NaHCO_3$ is an inappropriate therapy in patients with hypercapnic acidosis. Tromethamine (THAM) has been suggested as an alternative buffer,[98] as its use reverses severe acidosis and also reduces $PaCO_2$; however, pulmonary CO_2 emission is also reduced, indicating a risk for increased $PaCO_2$ if THAM administration is ceased.[99] THAM is currently unavailable in the United States.

PERMISSIVE HYPERCAPNIA AT THE BEDSIDE—PRACTICAL ISSUES

The utilization and management of HC in the critically ill patient with ARDS requires a number of practical considerations.

First, there is considerable evidence that patients generally tolerate hypercapnic acidosis to pH values of 7.2 and even lower very well. The reported levels of $PaCO_2$ and pH in the study of Hickling et al.[100] reflect reasonable initial goals ($PaCO_2$ 67 mm Hg, mean pH 7.2). However, a more useful approach is to individualize $PaCO_2$ and pH goals in each patient, with great care required in settings where HC may have deleterious effects, such as the setting of combined lung and head injury.

Secondly, rapid induction of hypercapnic acidosis in ARDS patients should be avoided, as it can have profound adverse hemodynamic effects. Therefore, care should be taken to ensure the degree of HC should be gradually titrated upwards over a period of at least several hours, until the ventilatory goals to minimize the potential for VILI have been achieved.

Thirdly, in regard to altering the ventilatory strategy to protect the lung, the first priority in ARDS patients is to reduce V_t in order to reduce plateau pressures below 30 cm H_2O where possible. Tidal volumes should be reduced to 6 mL/kg IBW and may need to be decreased further if plateau pressures remain unacceptably high.[3] It is important to remember, that 30% of patients ventilated with the ARDSnet strategy still have significant hyperinflation and may benefit from very low V_t ventilation (3 mL/kg IBW).[101] To prevent excessive HC and acidosis in these situations, or where there are specific concerns regarding HC, application of selective CO_2 removal by $ECCO_2$-R is an increasingly feasible option.[8]

Fourthly, the effect of the disease process on the optimal ventilatory strategy must be considered. ARDS is characterized by a predominance of alveoli with short time constants due to low compliance with normal airways resistance. Therefore it is possible to ventilate at relatively high ventilatory rates and therefore minimize the degree of HC in these patients, with relatively low risk of auto-PEEP.

AUTHORS' RECOMMENDATIONS

- Permissive HC is a common consequence of lung protective ventilation that has been associated with improved outcome in ARDS patients.
- Evidence also supports the use of permissive HC strategies in other forms of respiratory failure, including acute severe asthma and COPD, and in pediatric intensive care.
- HC is a potent biologic agent and there is substantial evidence from laboratory studies that HC attenuates lung and systemic organ injury. However, recent experimental data suggest that HC may be harmful by delaying wound repair and suppressing innate immune responses to bacterial infection.
- The potential for HC to exert deleterious physiologic effects in cases of raised intracranial pressure or pulmonary hypertension should be considered.
- There is no clinical evidence to support the clinical practice of buffering hypercapnic acidosis with bicarbonate.
- A clearer understanding of the effects and mechanisms of action of HC is central to determining its safety and therapeutic utility.
- The potential for extracorporeal CO_2 removal technologies to facilitate even greater reductions in tidal and minute ventilation is clear, but awaits definitive studies.

REFERENCES

1. Dreyfuss D, Saumon G. Ventilator-induced lung injury: lessons from experimental studies. *Am J Respir Crit Care Med.* 1998;157(1):294-323.
2. Pinhu L, Whitehead T, Evans T, Griffiths M. Ventilator-associated lung injury. *Lancet.* 2003;361(9354):332-340.

3. Acute Respiratory Distress Syndrome Network; Brower RG, Matthay MA, et al. Ventilation with lower tidal volumes as compared with traditional tidal volumes for acute lung injury and the acute respiratory distress syndrome. *N Engl J Med*. 2000;342(18):1301-1308.

4. Hickling KG, Henderson SJ, Jackson R. Low mortality associated with low volume pressure limited ventilation with permissive hypercapnia in severe adult respiratory distress syndrome. *Intensive Care Med*. 1990;16(6):372-377.

5. Hickling KG, Walsh J, Henderson S, Jackson R. Low mortality rate in adult respiratory distress syndrome using low-volume, pressure-limited ventilation with permissive hypercapnia: a prospective study. *Crit Care Med*. 1994;22(10):1568-1578.

6. Curley G, Contreras MM, Nichol AD, et al. Hypercapnia and acidosis in sepsis: a double-edged sword? *Anesthesiology*. 2010; 112(2):462-472.

7. Laffey JG, Kavanagh BP. Biological effects of hypercapnia (review). *Intensive Care Med*. 2000;26(1):133-138.

8. Bein T, Weber-Carstens S, Goldmann A, et al. Lower tidal volume strategy (approximately 3 ml/kg) combined with extracorporeal CO_2 removal versus 'conventional' protective ventilation (6 ml/kg) in severe ARDS: the prospective randomized Xtravent-study. *Intensive Care Med*. 2013;39(5):847-856.

9. Terragni PP, Del Sorbo L, Mascia L, et al. Tidal volume lower than 6 ml/kg enhances lung protection: role of extracorporeal carbon dioxide removal. *Anesthesiology*. 2009;111(4):826-835.

10. Daristotle L, Berssenbrugge AD, Engwall MJ, Bisgard GE. The effects of carotid body hypocapnia on ventilation in goats. *Respir Physiol*. 1990;79(2):123-135.

11. Putnam RW, Filosa JA, Ritucci NA. Cellular mechanisms involved in CO(2) and acid signaling in chemosensitive neurons. *Am J Physiol Cell Physiol*. 2004;287(6):C1493-C1526.

12. Forster HV, Martino P, Hodges M, et al. The carotid chemoreceptors are a major determinant of ventilatory CO_2 sensitivity and of $PaCO_2$ during eupneic breathing. *Adv Exp Med Biol*. 2008;605:322-326.

13. Borison HL, Hurst JH, McCarthy LE, Rosenstein R. Arterial hydrogen ion versus CO_2 on depth and rate of breathing in decerebrate cats. *Respir Physiol*. 1977;30(3):311-325.

14. Fukuda Y. Difference between actions of high PCO_2 and low $[HCO^{-3}]$ on neurons in the rat medullary chemosensitive areas in vitro. *Pflugers Arch*. 1983;398(4):324-330.

15. Detweiler ND, Vigil KG, Resta TC, et al. Role of acid-sensing ion channels in hypoxia- and hypercapnia-induced ventilatory responses. *PLoS One*. 2018;13(2):e0192724.

16. Beltrán-Castillo S, Olivares MJ, Contreras RA, et al. D-serine released by astrocytes in brainstem regulates breathing response to CO_2 levels. *Nat Commun*. 2017;8(1):838.

17. Kregenow DA, Swenson ER. The lung and carbon dioxide: implications for permissive and therapeutic hypercapnia. *Eur Respir J*. 2002;20(1):6-11.

18. Linde LM, Simmons DH, Lewis N. Pulmonary hemodynamics in respiratory acidosis in dogs. *Am J Physiol*. 1963;205(5):1008-1012.

19. Bommakanti N, Isbatan A, Bavishi A, et al. Hypercapnic acidosis attenuates pressure-dependent increase in whole-lung filtration coefficient (Kf). *Pulm Circ*. 2017;7(3):719-726.

20. Laffey JG, Engelberts D, Kavanagh BP. Buffering hypercapnic acidosis worsens acute lung injury. *Am J Respir Crit Care Med*. 2000;161(1):141-146.

21. Shibata K, Cregg N, Engelberts D, et al. Hypercapnic acidosis may attenuate acute lung injury by inhibition of endogenous xanthine oxidase. *Am J Resp Crit Care Med*. 1998;158:1578-1584.

22. van den Elshout FJ, van Herwaarden CL, Folgering HT. Effects of hypercapnia and hypocapnia on respiratory resistance in normal and asthmatic subjects. *Thorax*. 1991;46(1):28-32.

23. Rodarte JR, Hyatt RE. Effect of acute exposure to CO_2 on lung mechanics in normal man. *Respir Physiol*. 1973;17(2):135-145.

24. Laffey JG, Engelberts D, Duggan M, et al. Carbon dioxide attenuates pulmonary impairment resulting from hyperventilation. *Crit Care Med*. 2003;31(11):2634-2640.

25. Contreras M, Ansari B, Curley G, et al. Hypercapnic acidosis attenuates ventilation-induced lung injury by a nuclear factor-kappaB-dependent mechanism. *Crit Care Med*. 2012;40(9): 2622-2630.

26. Laffey JG, Honan D, Hopkins N, Hyvelin JM, Boylan JF, McLoughlin P. Hypercapnic acidosis attenuates endotoxin-induced acute lung injury. *Am J Respir Crit Care Med* 2004;169:46-56.

27. Chonghaile MN, Higgins BD, Costello J, Laffey JG. Hypercapnic acidosis attenuates lung injury induced by established bacterial pneumonia. *Anesthesiology*. 2008;109(5):837-848.

28. Costello J, Higgins B, Contreras M, et al. Hypercapnic acidosis attenuates shock and lung injury in early and prolonged systemic sepsis. *Crit Care Med*. 2009;37(8):2412-2420.

29. Yang W, Yue Z, Cui X, et al. Comparison of the effects of moderate and severe hypercapnic acidosis on ventilation-induced lung injury. *BMC Anesthesiol*. 2015;15:67.

30. Laffey JG, Jankov RP, Engelberts D, et al. Effects of therapeutic hypercapnia on mesenteric ischemia-reperfusion injury. *Am J Respir Crit Care Med*. 2003;168(11):1383-1390.

31. Tan J, Liu Y, Jiang T, et al. Effects of hypercapnia on acute cellular rejection after lung transplantation in rats. *Anesthesiology*. 2018; 128(1):130-139.

32. Hummler HD, Banke K, Wolfson MR, et al. The effects of lung protective ventilation or hypercapnic acidosis on gas exchange and lung injury in surfactant deficient rabbits. *PLoS One*. 2016; 11(2):e0147807.

33. Turner MJ, Saint-Criq V, Patel W, et al. Hypercapnia modulates cAMP signalling and cystic fibrosis transmembrane conductance regulator-dependent anion and fluid secretion in airway epithelia. *J Physiol*. 2016;594(6):1643-1661.

34. Briva A, Vadász I, Lecuona E, et al. High CO_2 levels impair alveolar epithelial function independently of pH. *PLoS One*. 2007;2(11):e1238.

35. Chen J, Lecuona E, Briva A, et al. Carbonic anhydrase II and alveolar fluid reabsorption during hypercapnia. *Am J Respir Cell Mol Biol*. 2008;38(1):32-37.

36. Puthucheary ZA, Rawal J, McPhail M, et al. Acute skeletal muscle wasting in critical illness. *JAMA*. 2013;310(15):1591-1600.

37. Herridge MS, Cheung AM, Tansey CM, et al. One-year outcomes in survivors of the acute respiratory distress syndrome. *N Engl J Med*. 2003;348(8):683-693.

38. Jonville S, Delpech N, Denjean A. Contribution of respiratory acidosis to diaphragmatic fatigue at exercise. *Eur Respir J*. 2002; 19(6):1079-1086.

39. Juan G, Calverley P, Talamo C, et al. Effect of carbon dioxide on diaphragmatic function in human beings. *N Engl J Med*. 1984;310(14):874-879.

40. Jung B, Sebbane M, Le Goff C, et al. Moderate and prolonged hypercapnic acidosis may protect against ventilator-induced diaphragmatic dysfunction in healthy piglet: an in vivo study. *Crit Care*. 2013;17(1):R15.

41. Schellekens WJ, van Hees HW, Kox M, et al. Hypercapnia attenuates ventilator-induced diaphragm atrophy and modulates dysfunction. *Crit Care*. 2014;18(1):R28.

42. Twose P, Jones U, Wise MP. Effect of hypercapnia on respiratory and peripheral skeletal muscle loss during critical illness—a pilot study. *J Crit Care.* 2018;45:105-109.

43. Cullen DJ, Eger EI 2nd. Cardiovascular effects of carbon dioxide in man. *Anesthesiology.* 1974;41(4):345-349.

44. Tang WC, Weil MH, Gazmuri RJ, et al. Reversible impairment of myocardial contractility due to hypercarbic acidosis in the isolated perfused rat heart. *Crit Care Med.* 1991;19(2):218-224.

45. Akça O, Doufas AG, Morioka N, et al. Hypercapnia improves tissue oxygenation. *Anesthesiology.* 2002;97(4):801-806.

46. Mas A, Saura P, Joseph D, et al. Effect of acute moderate changes in $PaCO_2$ on global hemodynamics and gastric perfusion. *Crit Care Med.* 2000;28(2):360-365.

47. Hering R, Kreyer S, Putensen C. Effects of lung protective mechanical ventilation associated with permissive respiratory acidosis on regional extra-pulmonary blood flow in experimental ARDS. *BMC Anesthesiol.* 2017;17(1):149.

48. Wang Z, Su F, Bruhn A, et al. Acute hypercapnia improves indices of tissue oxygenation more than dobutamine in septic shock. *Am J Respir Crit Care Med.* 2008;177(2):178-183.

49. Kitakaze M, Takashima S, Funaya H, et al. Temporary acidosis during reperfusion limits myocardial infarct size in dogs. *Am J Physiol.* 1997;272(5 Pt 2):H2071-H2078.

50. Yang HJ, Dey D, Sykes J, et al. Arterial CO_2 as a potent coronary vasodilator: a preclinical PET/MR validation study with implications for cardiac stress testing. *J Nucl Med.* 2017;58(6):953-960.

51. Torbati D, Mangino MJ, Garcia E, et al. Acute hypercapnia increases the oxygen-carrying capacity of the blood in ventilated dogs. *Crit Care Med.* 1998;26(11):1863-1867.

52. Hood VL, Tannen RL. Protection of acid-base balance by pH regulation of acid production. *N Engl J Med.* 1998;339(12):819-826.

53. Greif R, Akça O, Horn EP, et al. Supplemental perioperative oxygen to reduce the incidence of surgical-wound infection. *N Engl J Med.* 2000;342(3):161-167.

54. Akça O, Liem E, Suleman MI, et al. Effect of intra-operative end-tidal carbon dioxide partial pressure on tissue oxygenation. *Anaesthesia.* 2003;58(6):536-542.

55. Hager H, Reddy D, Mandadi G, et al. Hypercapnia improves tissue oxygenation in morbidly obese surgical patients. *Anesth Analg.* 2006;103(3):677-681.

56. Akça O, Kurz A, Fleischmann E, et al. Hypercapnia and surgical site infection: a randomized trial. *Br J Anaesth.* 2013;111(5):759-767.

57. Hare GM, Kavanagh BP, Mazer CD, et al. Hypercapnia increases cerebral tissue oxygen tension in anesthetized rats. *Can J Anaesth.* 2003;50(10):1061-1068.

58. Nakahata K, Kinoshita H, Hirano Y, et al. Mild hypercapnia induces vasodilation via adenosine triphosphate-sensitive K^+ channels in parenchymal microvessels of the rat cerebral cortex. *Anesthesiology.* 2003;99(6):1333-1339.

59. Vannucci RC, Brucklacher RM, Vannucci SJ. Effect of carbon dioxide on cerebral metabolism during hypoxia-ischemia in the immature rat. *Pediatr Res.* 1997;42(1):24-29.

60. Tregub PP, Kulikov VP, Rucheikin NY, et al. Proliferative and synthetic activity of nerve cells after combined or individual exposure to hypoxia and hypercapnia. *Bull Exp Biol Med.* 2015;159(3):334-336.

61. Ding HG, Deng YY, Yang RQ, et al. Hypercapnia induces IL-1beta overproduction via activation of NLRP3 inflammasome: implication in cognitive impairment in hypoxemic adult rats. *J Neuroinflammation.* 2018;15(1):4.

62. Corfield DR, McKay LC. Regional cerebrovascular responses to hypercapnia and hypoxia. *Adv Exp Med Biol.* 2016;903:157-167.

63. Reinhard M, Schwarzer G, Briel M, et al. Cerebrovascular reactivity predicts stroke in high-grade carotid artery disease. *Neurology.* 2014;83(16):1424-1431.

64. Raichle ME, Posner JB, Plum F. Cerebral blood flow during and after hyperventilation. *Arch Neurol.* 1970;23(5):394-403.

65. Wang N, Gates KL, Trejo H, et al. Elevated CO_2 selectively inhibits interleukin-6 and tumor necrosis factor expression and decreases phagocytosis in the macrophage. *FASEB J.* 2010;24(7):2178-2190.

66. Casalino-Matsuda SM, Nair A, Beitel GJ, et al. Hypercapnia inhibits autophagy and bacterial killing in human macrophages by increasing expression of Bcl-2 and Bcl-xL. *J Immunol.* 2015; 194(11):5388-5396.

67. O'Croinin DF, Nichol AD, Hopkins N, et al. Sustained hypercapnic acidosis during pulmonary infection increases bacterial load and worsens lung injury. *Crit Care Med.* 2008;36(7):2128-2135.

68. Takeshita K, Suzuki Y, Nishio K, et al. Hypercapnic acidosis attenuates endotoxin-induced nuclear factor-κB activation. *Am J Respir Cell Mol Biol.* 2003;29(1):124-132.

69. Masterson C, O'Toole D, Leo A, et al. Effects and mechanisms by which hypercapnic acidosis inhibits sepsis-induced canonical nuclear factor-κB signaling in the lung. *Crit Care Med.* 2016; 44(4):e207-e217.

70. O'Toole D, Hassett P, Contreras M, et al. Hypercapnic acidosis attenuates pulmonary epithelial wound repair by an NF-kappaB dependent mechanism. *Thorax.* 2009;64(11):976-982.

71. Wu SY, Li MH, Ko FC, et al. Protective effect of hypercapnic acidosis in ischemia-reperfusion lung injury is attributable to upregulation of heme oxygenase-1. *PLoS One.* 2013;8(9):e74742.

72. Lu Z, Casalino-Matsuda SM, Nair A, et al. A role for heat shock factor 1 in hypercapnia-induced inhibition of inflammatory cytokine expression. *FASEB J.* 2018;32(7):3614-3622.

73. Otulakowski G, Engelberts D, Gusarova GA, et al. Hypercapnia attenuates ventilator-induced lung injury via a disintegrin and metalloprotease-17. *J Physiol.* 2014;592(20):4507-4521.

74. Vohwinkel CU, Lecuona E, Sun H, et al. Elevated CO(2) levels cause mitochondrial dysfunction and impair cell proliferation. *J Biol Chem.* 2011;286(43):37067-37076.

75. Selfridge AC, Cavadas MA, Scholz CC, et al. Hypercapnia suppresses the HIF-dependent adaptive response to hypoxia. *J Biol Chem.* 2016;291(22):11800-11808.

76. Bellani G, Laffey JG, Pham T, et al. Epidemiology, patterns of care, and mortality for patients with acute respiratory distress syndrome in intensive care units in 50 countries. *JAMA.* 2016; 315(8):788-800.

77. Amato MB, Barbas CS, Medeiros DM, et al. Effect of protective-ventilation strategy on mortality in the acute respiratory distress syndrome. *N Engl J Med.* 1998;338(6):347-354.

78. Brochard L, Roudot-Thoraval F, Roupie E, et al. Tidal volume reduction for prevention of ventilator-induced lung injury in acute respiratory distress syndrome. *Am J Respir Crit Care Med.* 1998;158(6):1831-1838.

79. Brower RG, Shanholtz CB, Fessler HE, et al. Prospective, randomized, controlled clinical trial comparing traditional versus reduced tidal volume ventilation in acute respiratory distress syndrome patients. *Crit Care Med.* 1999;27(8):1492-1498.

80. Stewart TE, Meade MO, Cook DJ, et al. Evaluation of a ventilation strategy to prevent barotrauma in patients at high risk for acute respiratory distress syndrome. *N Engl J Med.* 1998;338(6):355-361.

81. Kregenow DA, Rubenfeld G, Hudson L, et al. Permissive hypercapnia reduces mortality with 12 ml/kg tidal volumes in acute lung injury. *Am J Resp Crit Care Med.* 2003;167:A616.

82. Nin N, Muriel A, Peñuelas O, et al. Severe hypercapnia and outcome of mechanically ventilated patients with moderate or severe acute respiratory distress syndrome. *Intensive Care Med.* 2017;43(2):200-208.

83. Muthu V, Agarwal R, Sehgal IS, et al. 'Permissive' hypercapnia in ARDS: is it passé? *Intensive Care Med.* 2017;43(6):952-953.

84. Tiruvoipati R, Pilcher D, Buscher H, et al. Effects of hypercapnia and hypercapnic acidosis on hospital mortality in mechanically ventilated patients. *Crit Care Med.* 2017;45(7):e649-e656.

85. Kuzkov VV, Rodionova LN, Ilyina YY, et al. Protective ventilation improves gas exchange, reduces incidence of atelectases, and affects metabolic response in major pancreatoduodenal surgery. *Front Med (Lausanne).* 2016;3:66.

86. Gao W, Liu DD, Li D, Cui GX. Effect of therapeutic hypercapnia on inflammatory responses to one-lung ventilation in lobectomy patients. *Anesthesiology.* 2015;122(6):1235-1252.

87. Fanelli V, Ranieri MV, Mancebo J, et al. Feasibility and safety of low-flow extracorporeal carbon dioxide removal to facilitate ultra-protective ventilation in patients with moderate acute respiratory distress syndrome. *Crit Care.* 2016;20:36.

88. Combes A, Fanelli V, Pham T, Ranieri VM; European Society of Intensive Care Medicine Trials Group and the "Strategy of Ultra-Protective lung ventilation with Extracorporeal CO_2 Removal for New-Onset moderate to severe ARDS" (SUPERNOVA) investigators. Feasibility and safety of extracorporeal CO_2 removal to enhance protective ventilation in acute respiratory distress syndrome: the SUPERNOVA study. *Intensive Care Med.* 2019;45(5):592–600. doi:10.1007/s00134-019-05567-4.

89. Peperstraete H, Eloot S, Depuydt P, et al. Low flow extracorporeal CO_2 removal in ARDS patients: a prospective short-term cross-over pilot study. *BMC Anesthesiol.* 2017;17(1):155.

90. Fanelli V, Cantaluppi V, Alessandri F, et al. Extracorporeal CO_2 removal may improve renal function of patients with ARDS and acute kidney injury: an open-label, interventional clinical trial. *Am J Respir Crit Care Med.* 2018;198(5):687-690.

91. Marx P, Weinert G, Pfiester P, Kuhn H. The influence of hypercapnia and hypoxia on intracranial pressure and on CSF electrolyte concentrations. In: Schürmann K, Kasner M, Reulen HJ, Voth D, eds. *Brain Edema/Cerebello Pontine Angle Tumors. Advances in Neurosurgery.* Berlin: Springer; 1973.

92. Lapinsky SE, Posadas-Calleja JG, McCullagh I. Clinical review: ventilatory strategies for obstetric, brain-injured and obese patients. *Crit Care.* 2009;13(2):206.

93. Green M, Widdicombe JG. The effects of ventilation of dogs with different gas mixtures on airway calibre and lung mechanics. *J Physiol.* 1966;186(2):363-381.

94. Brimioulle S, Lejeune P, Vachiery JL, et al. Effects of acidosis and alkalosis on hypoxic pulmonary vasoconstriction in dogs. *Am J Physiol.* 1990;258(2 Pt 2):H347-H353.

95. Cutaia M, Rounds S. Hypoxic pulmonary vasoconstriction. Physiologic significance, mechanism, and clinical relevance. *Chest.* 1990;97(3):706-718.

96. Stewart PA. Modern quantitative acid-base chemistry. *Can J Physiol Pharmacol.* 1983;61(12):1444-1461.

97. Goldsmith DJ, Forni LG, Hilton PJ. Bicarbonate therapy and intracellular acidosis. *Clin Sci (Lond).* 1997;93(6):593-598.

98. Weber T, Tschernich H, Sitzwohl C, et al. Tromethamine buffer modifies the depressant effect of permissive hypercapnia on myocardial contractility in patients with acute respiratory distress syndrome. *Am J Respir Crit Care Med.* 2000;162(4 Pt 1):1361-1365.

99. Höstman S, Kawati R, Perchiazzi G, Larsson A. THAM administration reduces pulmonary carbon dioxide elimination in hypercapnia—an experimental porcine study. *Acta Anaesthesiol Scand.* 2018;62(6):820-828.

100. Hickling KG, Walsh J, Henderson S, Jackson R. Low mortality rate in adult respiratory distress syndrome using low-volume, pressure-limited ventilation with permissive hypercapnia: a prospective study. *Crit Care Med.* 1994;22:1568-1578.

101. Terragni PP, Rosboch G, Tealdi A, et al. Tidal hyperinflation during low tidal volume ventilation in acute respiratory distress syndrome. *Am J Respir Crit Care Med.* 2007;175(2):160-166.

18

Does Patient Positioning Make a Difference in ARDS?

Amy L. Bellinghausen, Robert L. Owens, and Atul Malhotra

INTRODUCTION

Despite clinicians' best efforts, many of the proposed therapies for acute respiratory distress syndrome (ARDS) have shown either no benefit or have caused harm. These interventions include medications aimed at altering lung physiology, such as surfactant administration, and specialized ventilatory modes attempting to minimize lung injury while maintaining adequate gas exchange.[1,2] Low tidal volume (V_t) ventilation and high positive end-expiratory pressure (PEEP) have shown benefit, but the dosing of these interventions is uncertain. Muscle relaxants may also be effective, but more research is needed.[3] One of the handful of interventions that appears to improve mortality is prone positioning, an intervention that is underutilized in the intensive care unit (ICU) population.[4] This chapter discusses the physiologic justification for such an approach, as well as the supporting literature. Other positioning strategies in patients with ARDS are also discussed.

PRONE POSITIONING IN ARDS

Mechanisms of Possible Benefit

In the supine position, mediastinal structures preferentially exert pressure on the lungs, particularly the well-perfused lower lobes.[5] This situation can theoretically result in increased dependent atelectasis, with subsequent ventilation/perfusion mismatching (Fig. 18.1). In contrast, by turning the patient prone, the weight of the heart is removed from the lungs, and instead rests primarily on the sternum. Additionally, in the prone position, the abdominal viscera are pulled anteriorly, rather than compressing the lower pulmonary lobes.[6,7] Gravity appears to be a less important determinant of regional perfusion than ventilation; it has been shown that in both the prone and supine states, blood flows preferentially to the dorsal portions of the lung.[8] The improvement in V/Q (ventilation/perfusion) matching with better ventilation of these dorsal segments appears to be the major mechanism by which prone positioning improves oxygenation.

Offloading of weight from extrapulmonary structures is not the only mechanism by which prone positioning increases resting lung volumes.[9] Although it is convenient and safe to nurse critically ill patients supine, few individuals actually sleep in this position. It has been observed that the human thoracic cage and lungs have evolved to function best in the prone position, which is the typical orientation for the majority of mammals. While prone, there is improved shape matching of the lung and chest wall (due to the asymmetric shape of the lung), resulting in more homogeneous aeration, and increased functional residual capacity (FRC) compared with supine positioning.[10,11]

Both decreased compression of the lung by the heart and abdomen, as well as better conformational matching of the lung and chest wall contribute to increased lung volume, more homogeneous aeration, and better V/Q matching in the prone vs. supine position. These mechanisms appear to be the primary reasons by which prone positioning ("proning") improves oxygenation. However, improving oxygenation in ARDS does not guarantee better patient outcomes.[12] Therefore, investigators have sought to determine whether prone ventilation might mitigate development of ventilator-induced lung injury (VILI).

Proposed mechanisms of decreasing VILI include decreased shear stress and reduced alveolar hyperinflation, resulting in less overdistension on controlled mechanical ventilation. Animal studies also show attenuation of VILI by prone positioning.[13] Although direct evidence of reduced VILI in humans is lacking, bronchoalveolar lavage fluid from proned ARDS patients shows reduced inflammatory markers compared with patients in the supine position.[14] Reduced VILI may explain why patients with improved gas exchange during proning do not consistently show improved survival.[15]

Hemodynamic effects of prone positioning are variable. Proning may exert beneficial effects on the right ventricle, by decreasing pulmonary vascular tone and lowering pulmonary vascular resistance (PVR), independent of its beneficial effect on oxygenation.[16] A potential mechanism of reduced PVR would be via lung recruitment in ARDS if prone positioning helps to restore FRC. Another case series demonstrated that, in patients with preload reserve, prone positioning significantly increased cardiac output (presumably by improving right ventricular [RV] function).[17]

Finally, prone positioning results in a relatively more anterior position of the trachea and oropharynx compared with the lung, which may assist in secretion clearance and the possible prevention of ventilator-associated pneumonia (VAP).

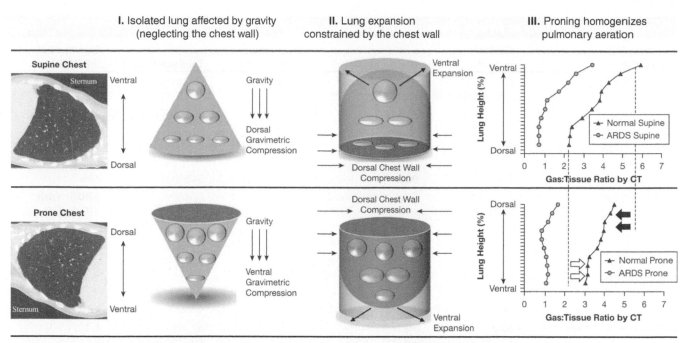

I. Isolated lung affected by gravity (neglecting the chest wall)

II. Lung expansion constrained by the chest wall

III. Proning homogenizes pulmonary aeration

Fig. 18.1 Lung and Chest Wall Interaction with Gravity in Prone and Supine Positions. Column I shows an isolated lung (cone) and alveolar units (circles) removed from the chest wall, and illustrates the differential effects of gravity in the prone vs. the supine position. Column II shows the effect of compression of the lung by the rigid chest wall, again in both prone and supine orientations. Column III displays the experimental data supporting the model. *ARDS*, acute respiratory distress syndrome; *CT*, computed tomography. (Modified from Gattinoni L, Taccone P, Carlesso E, Marini JJ. Prone position in acute respiratory distress syndrome: rational, indications, and limits. *Am J Respir Crit Care Med.* 2013;188[11]:1286-1293. From Scholten et al.[48])

Decreased risk of VAP with prone positioning has been demonstrated in a porcine model.[18] However, to date, studies in humans have shown inconsistent differences in rates of VAP in prone vs. other positions.[19–21]

Evidence/Clinical Trials

Some of the first experimental data in proning were gathered by Christie and Beams in 1922, who reported a decrease in vital capacity for supine compared with prone ventilation in normal individuals.[22] In the 1970s prone positioning emerged as a potential therapy for the management of the patient with ARDS.[23] Table 18.1 outlines five major randomized trials of prone ventilation in adults with ARDS and acute lung injury. Other randomized controlled trials (RCTs) have also been conducted, but generally were limited to specific population subsets or had small numbers of participants, and are therefore not discussed in depth.[14,24–30]

Gattinoni and colleagues studied 304 patients with ARDS, randomized to conventional ventilation vs. prone positioning for 7 hours per day.[31] The study was published in 2001: hence the mean tidal volumes were 10 mL/kg predicted body weight in both groups, with mean peak airway pressures of > 32 cm H_2O. The mean ratio of partial pressure of arterial oxygen to the fraction of inspired oxygen (PaO_2/FiO_2 or PF ratio) was < 130 in both groups. Although there was a significant improvement in oxygenation in the prone group, this did not translate into a mortality benefit (60-day mortality was 62% vs. 58% in the prone vs. conventional groups,

nonsignificant). Subsequent investigations by Mancebo et al.[32] and Taccone et al.[33] also failed to show a benefit of proning, although the average hours spent in the prone position were increased to 17 and 18 hours, respectively. The "duration of pronation" has been controversial for decades; on the one hand, clinicians argue that if prone positioning is lung protective, then the bulk of the time should be spent with the patient prone rather than supine. On the other hand, some have argued that the benefits of prone positioning may be predicated on the use of open lung protective ventilation (i.e., low V_t and high PEEP; Fig. 18.2), in which case the risk of supine ventilation may be less critical.[36]

Guérin and colleagues randomized 791 patients with acute respiratory failure to prone vs. supine positioning between 1998 and 2002 at 21 general ICUs in France. Although the study called for recruitment of patients with clinical and radiologic evidence of ARDS and with PF ratios < 300, the mean PF ratio in the study was 150.[21] Static compliance of the respiratory system averaged approximately 40 mL/cm H_2O in both groups—indicating relatively compliant lungs. Pre-ARDSNET tidal volumes were 10–11 mL/kg, with driving pressures that averaged 20 cm H_2O and PEEP < 8 cm H_2O. Patients were proned for a median of 4 days for a median of 8 hours. One-quarter of patients in the intervention group were proned, on average, for less than the 8-hour target. Patients in the control group were allowed to cross over and undergo prone ventilation, at physician discretion. There was no difference in mortality at 28 or 60 days, more pressure

TABLE 18.1 Trials of Prone Ventilation in ARDS.

Variable	Gattinoni et al.[31]	Guérin et al.[21]	Mancebo et al.[32]	Taccone et al.[33]	Guérin et al. (PROSEVA)[34]
Prone group mortality, %	50.7 (ICU mortality)	32.4 (28 days)	43 (ICU mortality)	31 (28 days)	**16 (28 days)**
Control group mortality, %	48 (ICU mortality)	31.5 (28 days)	58 (ICU mortality)	32.8 (28 days)	**32.8 (28 days)**
RR of mortality (prone/control)	1.05 ($P = .65$)	1.02 ($P = .77$)	0.74 ($P = .12$)	0.97 ($P = .72$)	**0.48 ($P < .001$)**
Patients, No.	304	**802**	142	342	466
Targeted disease	ALI[a] and ARDS[a]	Respiratory failure with PaO_2/FiO_2 < 300 mm Hg	ARDS[a]	ARDS[a]	**ARDS[a] with PaO_2/FiO_2 < 150 mm Hg**
PaO_2/FiO_2 at enrollment, mm Hg	128	153	139	113	**100**
Enrollment early in disease course?	No	No	Yes, < 2 days of intubation	Yes, < 3 days	**Yes, < 1.5 days**
SAPS II	40	**46**	43	41	**46**
V_t delivered, mL/kg	10.3	7.9	8.5	8	**6.1**
Patients paralyzed, %	Not reported	21	45	Not reported	**87**
Mean increase in PaO_2/FiO_2 on prone positioning, mm Hg	19	18	32[b]	44	**59**
Average time prone, hours/day	7	8	17	**18**	17
Average days prone	**10**	4	**10**	8.4	4
Significant reduction in ventilator days?[c]	No	No	No	No	**Yes**
Difficulty enrolling?	**Yes**	No	**Yes**	No	No
Crossover (supine to prone), %	8	**21**	8	12	7

[a]ALI and ARDS were defined according to the American-European Consensus Conference Definition of ARDS.[35]
[b]This value was estimated based on graphic data presented in the text.
[c]Not all trials reported ventilator days or ICU length of stay; absence of reporting was taken to imply no significant difference.
Bold text indicates the most extreme value across all five trials.
ALI, acute lung injury; *ICU,* intensive care unit; *PROSEVA,* Proning Severe ARDS Patients; *RR,* relative risk; *SAPS II,* Simplified Acute Physiology Score II; V_t, tidal volume.
From Scholten et al.[48]

Group by High vs. Low V_t	Study name	Risk ratio	Lower limit	Upper limit	P-Value		Relative weight
High	Gattinoni, 2001	1.106	0.900	1.360	0.337		32.46
High	Guerin, 2004	1.020	0.862	1.207	0.819		45.08
High	Mancebo, 2006	0.786	0.551	1.120	0.183		12.30
High	Taccone, 2009 (mod)	0.852	0.575	1.262	0.424		10.15
High		0.996	0.876	1.132	0.949		
Low	Voggenreiter, 2005	0.304	0.035	2.659	0.282		1.56
Low	Fernandez, 2008	0.724	0.362	1.446	0.360		13.40
Low	Taccone, 2009 (sev)	0.814	0.588	1.128	0.216		40.82
Low	Guerin, 2013	0.534	0.394	0.724	0.000		44.23
Low		0.655	0.499	0.860	0.002		
Overall		0.834	0.683	1.017	0.073		

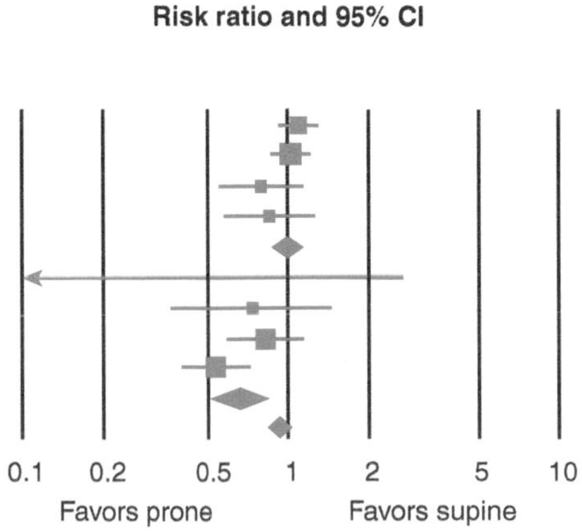

Risk ratio and 95% CI

0.1   0.2   0.5   1   2   5   10
Favors prone   Favors supine

Fig. 18.2 Effect of Prone Positioning on Mortality, Overall and Stratified by Mean Baseline Tidal Volume. High tidal volume (V_t) was defined as > 8 mL/kg predicted body weight (*PBW*) and low V_t as ≤ 8 mL/kg PBW. *CI,* confidence interval. (From Beitler et al.[36])

sores and episodes of endotracheal tube obstruction occurred, but there were fewer VAPs in the prone group.

A 2008 meta-analysis of the five major trials of prone positioning in ARDS[37] raised the tantalizing question that, buried in the cohort of patients that were labeled "ARDS," there was a group that had elevated rates of mortality, secondary to hypoxemia and VILI that may well benefit from prone positioning. No study, to date, had rigorously applied limited "stretch"/open lung strategies in both the control and intervention arm.

The PROSEVA trial, another French multicenter RCT led by Guérin and colleagues,[34] was published in 2013. A total of 466 patients were recruited into the trial and randomized to conventional low-stretch mechanical ventilation (pressure controlled) vs. the same ventilator strategy plus prone positioning for 16 hours per day. The key difference in this trial vs. previous studies was that randomization occurred >12 hours after presentation (to eliminate non-ARDS causes of hypoxemia), PF ratios were below 150 in all patients, patients were turned prone for 16 hours per day, and this continued until hypoxemia began to resolve (PF ratio > 150 on < 10 cm H_2O PEEP). Rigorous attention was paid to ensuring that plateau pressures and tidal volumes were restricted. There were some baseline differences between the groups. Patients in the control group were slightly older, had higher SAP II and SOFA scores, received more vasopressors and renal replacement therapy, and were more likely to receive corticosteroids. No data were presented regarding sedative dose, vasopressor dose, or fluid balance in either group. Compared with the previous French study, patients were recruited earlier, had worse oxygenation, lower compliance (mean 35–36 mL/cm H_2O), lower V_ts (mean 6.1 mL/kg predicted body weight), and higher PEEP (mean 10 cm H_2O). There was a dramatic difference in outcomes: the 28-day mortality was 16.0% in the prone group and 32.8% in the supine group (absolute risk reduction [ARR] 16.8%, number needed to treat [NNT] 6; $P < .001$). Unadjusted 90-day mortality was 23.6% in the prone group vs. 41.0% in the supine group (ARR 17.4%, NNT 6; $P < .001$). It is highly unlikely that this beneficial treatment signal could be accounted for by baseline variations, and, since the study was published, prone positioning has become the de facto standard of care in this setting.

Practical Considerations

One of the factors that may dissuade clinicians from proning is the fear of complications. Loss of airway, dislodgement of central lines, and pressure ulcers are all potential consequences of a turn.[38] Another concern is that prone positioning may limit the ability to perform necessary therapeutic procedures. Aside from the possibility of repositioning the patient supine at any time, these fears may be more theoretical than actual, with studies and case reports demonstrating the feasibility of many interventions while prone, including bronchoscopy, interfacility transport, and extracorporeal membrane oxygenation (ECMO).[39–41] Furthermore, proning is an intervention that can be used even in resource-limited

settings.[42] Traditionally, recent sternotomy has been viewed as an absolute contraindication to prone positioning; however, a small case series of 10 patients demonstrated the feasibility of proning for acute respiratory failure after coronary artery bypass graft surgery.[43]

A concern during prone positioning is the potential for increasing intra-abdominal pressure (IAP). In a series of 16 patients, proning was shown to increase IAP from a mean of 12 ± 4 to 14 ± 5 mm Hg ($P < .05$). More reassuring was that effective renal blood flow index and glomerular filtration rate (determined by para-aminohippurate and inulin clearance) did not change with prone positioning.[44] However, in a retrospective analysis of 82 patients undergoing prone positioning for ARDS, the 41 patients with abdominal obesity had significantly higher rates of renal failure and hypoxic hepatitis.[45] A potential strategy to mitigate the IAP rise associated with proning is use of an air-cushioned mattress.[46]

Another question that may arise when initiating proning is whether to use a specially designed bed or to roll patients manually with blankets or patient slings. One complication that seems to be more frequent in those using automatic rotating beds is conjunctival edema, which, in one case series, occurred in every patient undergoing that therapy.[47] Other considerations include cost, accessibility, and staff experience with prone positioning. To our knowledge, there are no major outcome data for these expensive technologies to facilitate proning.

During proning, there is little consensus about the optimal strategy for ventilation. As discussed above, low V_t appears to be important for the benefits of proning to be realized.[36] Beyond that finding, an approach to ventilation of the prone patient has not been agreed upon. Interactions with neuromuscular blockade and PEEP management while prone are areas where more study is needed.[48] However, animal data suggest that the beneficial effects of prone positioning and PEEP on lung compliance may be independent and complimentary.[49] Low PEEP is often provided in prone positioning trials and there may be incremental benefit to higher PEEP strategies in this context.

Of note, most of the research on prone positioning has been done as an empiric strategy rather than as a rescue therapy. Clinical experience, as well as evidence, suggests that the lung is maximally recruitable in early ARDS and less so as the disease progresses. As such, we generally advocate for early prone positioning rather than as a rescue or salvage therapy. Similarly, the application of high PEEP strategies are likely to be more helpful in early vs. late ARDS. However, the optimal setting of PEEP in the context of a prone ARDS patient requires further study.

When should prone positional therapy be discontinued? In PROSEVA, prone positioning was continued until there was a sustained improvement in oxygenation ($PaO_2/FiO_2 \geq 150$ mm Hg with PEEP ≤ 10 cm H_2O and $FiO_2 \leq 60\%$ for at least 4 hours after supine positioning).[21] A suggested course of action is to terminate prone positioning once there is clear evidence of clinical improvement and a trend toward reversal of the underlying process. Clearly, bedside judgment is helpful in this context. It is also unclear when neuromuscular blockade and deep sedation should be discontinued and whether or not to allow the patient to breathe spontaneously in the prone position.

OTHER POSITIONING STRATEGIES

Head of Bed Elevation

Head of bed (HOB) elevation has increasingly become the standard of care for mechanically ventilated patients. This assertion was primarily driven by trials demonstrating increased risk of VAP in patients with HOB flat during the first 24 hours after intubation.[19,50,51] However, subsequent studies have demonstrated increases in oxygenation and end-expiratory lung volume in some patients with ARDS after HOB elevation, particularly in the "seated" position (HOB 45–60 degrees, legs down at 45 degrees).[52,53] The underlying mechanism is thought to be either caudal displacement of the abdominal viscera and diaphragm, improving lung recruitment, or an increase in lung/chest wall compliance.[54] Unfortunately, the optimal degree and duration of HOB elevation have not been well established.

Frequent Turns

Physiologically, the human organism was not meant to lie still. This situation results in many well-established complications, including muscle atrophy, deep venous thrombosis, and pressure sores. Researchers for decades have sought to determine if frequent repositioning has cardiopulmonary benefit.[55,56] Small trials have demonstrated a decrease in V/Q mismatch in early ARDS.[57] There are some data that oscillating beds or continuous lateral rotational therapy may decrease risk of lower respiratory tract infection in mechanically ventilated or trauma patients, but no mortality benefit has been demonstrated.[58–60] A recent Cochrane review determined that the current evidence was insufficient to recommend for or against frequent turns to improve pulmonary function or mortality in ARDS.[61] Given the cost and time-consuming nature of oscillating beds or frequent turns, more evidence is needed before recommending this practice.

Lateral Position

Although ARDS is defined as a bilateral process, some patients (especially those with underlying lung disease) have markedly more pathology on one side compared with the other. In such cases, positioning the patient with the good lung down (GLD) has been advised as a potential strategy for maximizing perfusion to the less-diseased lung. Although physiologically this approach seems sound (gravitational forces acting on blood flow promote increased circulation in dependent regions), confirmatory empirical evidence is limited. Of note, the GLD approach may be problematic in unilateral lung disease, in cases of bleeding, or profuse edema where the diseased lung may compromise the healthier side. Furthermore, anecdotal and case series evidence has shown that lateral turns in critically ill patients may precipitate adverse hemodynamic changes.[62,63] Although generally

transient, such changes have the potential to result in a cascade of adverse outcomes.

AUTHORS' RECOMMENDATIONS

- Evidence currently supports early prone positioning in patients with severe ARDS.
- There are no available data to support prone positioning as a rescue strategy in later-stage ARDS.
- Prone positioning should be coupled with a lung protective ("low-stretch") ventilation strategy and should be continued for at least 16 hours each day.
- Complications of proning are generally minimal and can be mitigated by advanced planning and experienced staff.
- Cessation of proning should be considered once there is a clear improvement in clinical course, gas exchange, and respiratory mechanics.
- Other positioning strategies in ARDS are not well supported, although head of bed elevation in intubated patients has been shown to decrease risk of VAP and improve lung mechanics.

REFERENCES

1. Spragg RG, Lewis JF, Wurst W, et al. Treatment of acute respiratory distress syndrome with recombinant surfactant protein C surfactant. *Am J Respir Crit Care Med.* 2003; 167(11):1562-1566.
2. Lall R, Hamilton P, Young D, et al. A randomised controlled trial and cost-effectiveness analysis of high-frequency oscillatory ventilation against conventional artificial ventilation for adults with acute respiratory distress syndrome. The OSCAR (OSCillation in ARDS) study. *Health Technol Assess.* 2015;19(23):1-177.
3. Papazian L, Forel JM, Gacouin A, et al. Neuromuscular blockers in early acute respiratory distress syndrome. *N Engl J Med.* 2010;363(12):1107-1116.
4. Guérin C, Beuret P, Constantin JM, et al. A prospective international observational prevalence study on prone positioning of ARDS patients: the APRONET (ARDS Prone Position Network) study. *Intensive Care Med.* 2018;44(1): 22-37.
5. Albert RK, Hubmayr RD. The prone position eliminates compression of the lungs by the heart. *Am J Respir Crit Care Med.* 2000;161(5):1660-1665.
6. Gattinoni L, Pelosi P, Vitale G, Pesenti A, D'Andrea L, Mascheroni D. Body position changes redistribute lung computed-tomographic density in patients with acute respiratory failure. *Anesthesiology.* 1991;74(1):15-23.
7. Mutoh T, Guest RJ, Lamm WJ, Albert RK. Prone position alters the effect of volume overload on regional pleural pressures and improves hypoxemia in pigs in vivo. *Am Rev Respir Dis.* 1992;146:300-306.
8. Glenny RW, Lamm WJ, Albert RK, Robertson HT. Gravity is a minor determinant of pulmonary blood flow distribution. *J Appl Physiol.* 1991;71(2):620-629.
9. Aguirre-Bermeo H, Turella M, Bitondo M, et al. Lung volumes and lung volume recruitment in ARDS: a comparison between supine and prone position. *Ann Intensive Care.* 2018;8(1):25.

10. Mure M, Domino KB, Lindahl SG, Hlastala MP, Altemeier WA, Glenny RW. Regional ventilation-perfusion distribution is more uniform in the prone position. *J Appl Physiol*. 2000;88(3):1076-1083.

11. Lumb AB, Nunn JF. Respiratory function and ribcage contribution to ventilation in body positions commonly used during anesthesia. *Anesth Analg*. 1991;73(4):422-426.

12. Acute Respiratory Distress Syndrome Network. Ventilation with lower tidal volumes as compared with traditional tidal volumes for acute lung injury and the acute respiratory distress syndrome. *N Engl J Med*. 2000;342(18):1301-1308.

13. Broccard A, Shapiro RS, Schmitz LL, Adams AB, Nahum A, Marini JJ. Prone positioning attenuates and redistributes ventilator-induced lung injury in dogs. *Crit Care Med*. 2000;28(2):295-303.

14. Chan MC, Hsu JY, Liu HH, et al. Effects of prone position on inflammatory markers in patients with ARDS due to community-acquired pneumonia. *J Formos Med Assoc*. 2007; 106(9):708-716.

15. Albert RK, Keniston A, Baboi L, Ayzac L, Guérin C. Prone position-induced improvement in gas exchange does not predict improved survival in the acute respiratory distress syndrome. *Am J Respir Crit Care Med*. 2014;189(4):494-496.

16. Zochios V, Parhar K, Vieillard-Baron A. Protecting the right ventricle in ARDS: the role of prone ventilation. *J Cardiothorac Vasc Anesth*. 2018;32(5):2248-2251.

17. Jozwiak M, Teboul JL, Anguel N, et al. Beneficial hemodynamic effects of prone positioning in patients with acute respiratory distress syndrome. *Am J Respir Crit Care Med*. 2013;188(12):1428-1433.

18. Zanella A, Cressoni M, Epp M, Hoffmann V, Stylianou M, Kolobow T. Effects of tracheal orientation on development of ventilator-associated pneumonia: an experimental study. *Intensive Care Med*. 2012;38(4):677-685.

19. Alexiou VG, Ierodiakonou V, Dimopoulos G, Falagas ME. Impact of patient position on the incidence of ventilator-associated pneumonia: a meta-analysis of randomized controlled trials. *J Crit Care*. 2009;24(4):515-522.

20. Ayzac L, Girard R, Baboi L, et al. Ventilator-associated pneumonia in ARDS patients: the impact of prone positioning. A secondary analysis of the PROSEVA trial. *Intensive Care Med*. 2016;42(5):871-878.

21. Guérin C, Gaillard S, Lemasson S, et al. Effects of systematic prone positioning in hypoxemic acute respiratory failure: a randomized controlled trial. *JAMA*. 2004;292(19):2379-2387.

22. Christie CD, Beams AJ. The estimation of normal vital capacity: with especial reference to the effect of posture. *Arch Intern Med*. 1922;30(1):34-39.

23. Douglas WW, Rehder K, Beynen FM, Sessler AD, Marsh HM. Improved oxygenation in patients with acute respiratory failure: the prone position. *Am Rev Respir Dis*. 1977;115(4): 559-566.

24. Papazian L, Gainnier M, Marin V, et al. Comparison of prone positioning and high-frequency oscillatory ventilation in patients with acute respiratory distress syndrome. *Crit Care Med*. 2005;33(10):2162-2171.

25. Fridrich P, Krafft P, Hochleuthner H, Mauritz W. The effects of long-term prone positioning in patients with trauma-induced adult respiratory distress syndrome. *Anesth Analg*. 1996;83(6):1206-1211.

26. Beuret P, Carton MJ, Nourdine K, Kaaki M, Tramoni G, Ducreux JC. Prone position as prevention of lung injury in comatose patients: a prospective, randomized, controlled study. *Intensive Care Med*. 2002;28(5):564-569.

27. Curley MA, Hibberd PL, Fineman LD, et al. Effect of prone positioning on clinical outcomes in children with acute lung injury: a randomized controlled trial. *JAMA*. 2005;294(2): 229-237.

28. Voggenreiter G, Aufmkolk M, Stiletto RJ, et al. Prone positioning improves oxygenation in post-traumatic lung injury— a prospective randomized trial. *J Trauma*. 2005;59(2): 333-343.

29. Demory D, Michelet P, Arnal JM, et al. High-frequency oscillatory ventilation following prone positioning prevents a further impairment in oxygenation. *Crit Care Med*. 2007;35(1): 106-111.

30. Fernandez R, Trenchs X, Klamburg J, et al. Prone positioning in acute respiratory distress syndrome: a multicenter randomized clinical trial. *Intensive Care Med*. 2008;34(8): 1487-1491.

31. Gattinoni L, Tognoni G, Pesenti A, et al. Effect of prone positioning on the survival of patients with acute respiratory failure. *N Engl J Med*. 2001;345(8):568-573.

32. Mancebo J, Fernández R, Blanch L, et al. A multicenter trial of prolonged prone ventilation in severe acute respiratory distress syndrome. *Am J Respir Crit Care Med*. 2006;173(11): 1233-1239.

33. Taccone P, Pesenti A, Latini R, et al. Prone positioning in patients with moderate and severe acute respiratory distress syndrome: a randomized controlled trial. *JAMA*. 2009; 302(18):1977-1984.

34. Guérin C, Reignier J, Richard JC, et al. Prone positioning in severe acute respiratory distress syndrome. *N Engl J Med*. 2013;368(23):2159-2168.

35. Bernard GR, Artigas A, Brigham KL, et al. The American-European Consensus Conference on ARDS. Definitions, mechanisms, relevant outcomes, and clinical trial coordination. *Am J Respir Crit Care Med*. 1994;149(3 Pt 1):818-824.

36. Beitler JR, Shaefi S, Montesi SB, et al. Prone positioning reduces mortality from acute respiratory distress syndrome in the low tidal volume era: a meta-analysis. *Intensive Care Med*. 2014;40(3):332-341.

37. Alsaghir AH, Martin CM. Effect of prone positioning in patients with acute respiratory distress syndrome: a meta-analysis. *Crit Care Med*. 2008;36(2):603-609.

38. Lee JM, Bae W, Lee YJ, Cho YJ. The efficacy and safety of prone positional ventilation in acute respiratory distress syndrome: updated study-level meta-analysis of 11 randomized controlled trials. *Crit Care Med*. 2014;42(5):1252-1262.

39. Lucchini A, De Felippis C, Pelucchi G, et al. Application of prone position in hypoxaemic patients supported by venovenous ECMO. *Intensive Crit Care Nurs*. 2018;48:61-68.

40. Kalchiem-Dekel O, Shanholtz CB, Jeudy J, Sachdeva A, Pickering EM. Feasibility, safety, and utility of bronchoscopy in patients with ARDS while in the prone position. *Crit Care*. 2018;22(1):54.

41. Hersey D, Witter T, Kovacs G. Transport of a prone position acute respiratory distress syndrome patient. *Air Med J*. 2018;37(3):206-210.

42. Laux T, Ghali B, Seth B, Jajoo S. Feasibility of prone ventilation in resource-limited setting in rural-based hospital in India: a pilot study. Presented at C45 Critical Care: Against the Wind-ARDS from Identification to Management to Outcomes. *Am J Respir Crit Care Med*. 2018;197:A5069.

43. Brüssel T, Hachenberg T, Roos N, Lemzem H, Konertz W, Lawin P. Mechanical ventilation in the prone position for acute respiratory failure after cardiac surgery. *J Cardiothorac Vasc Anesth*. 1993;7(5):541-546.

44. Hering R, Wrigge H, Vorwerk R, et al. The effects of prone positioning on intraabdominal pressure and cardiovascular and renal function in patients with acute lung injury. *Anesth Analg*. 2001;92(5):1226-1231.

45. Weig T, Janitza S, Zoller M, et al. Influence of abdominal obesity on multiorgan dysfunction and mortality in acute respiratory distress syndrome patients treated with prone positioning. *J Crit Care*. 2014;29(4):557-561.

46. Michelet P, Roch A, Gainnier M, Sainty JM, Auffray JP, Papazian L. Influence of support on intra-abdominal pressure, hepatic kinetics of indocyanine green and extravascular lung water during prone positioning in patients with ARDS: a randomized crossover study. *Crit Care*. 2005;9(3):R251-R257.

47. Bajwa AA, Arasi L, Canabal JM, Kramer DJ. Automated prone positioning and axial rotation in critically ill, nontrauma patients with acute respiratory distress syndrome (ARDS). *J Intensive Care Med*. 2010;25(2):121-125.

48. Scholten EL, Beitler JR, Prisk GK, Malhotra A. Treatment of ARDS with prone positioning. *Chest*. 2017;151(1):215-224.

49. Keenan JC, Cortes-Puentes GA, Zhang L, Adams AB, Dries DJ, Marini JJ. PEEP titration: the effect of prone position and abdominal pressure in an ARDS model. *Intensive Care Med Exp*. 2018;6(1):3.

50. Kollef MH. Ventilator-associated pneumonia. A multivariate analysis. *JAMA*. 1993;270(16):1965-1970.

51. Drakulovic MB, Torres A, Bauer TT, Nicolas JM, Nogué S, Ferrer M. Supine body position as a risk factor for nosocomial pneumonia in mechanically ventilated patients: a randomised trial. *Lancet*. 1999;354(9193):1851-1858.

52. Dellamonica J, Lerolle N, Sargentini C, et al. Effect of different seated positions on lung volume and oxygenation in acute respiratory distress syndrome. *Intensive Care Med*. 2013;39(6):1121-1127.

53. Richard JC, Maggiore SM, Mancebo J, Lemaire F, Jonson B, Brochard L. Effects of vertical positioning on gas exchange and lung volumes in acute respiratory distress syndrome. *Intensive Care Med*. 2006;32(10):1623-1626.

54. Klingstedt C, Hedenstierna G, Lundquist H, Strandberg A, Tokics L, Brismar B. The influence of body position and differential ventilation on lung dimensions and atelectasis formation in anaesthetized man. *Acta Anaesthesiol Scand*. 1990;34(4):315-322.

55. Toscani V, Davis VB, Stevens E, Whedon GD, Deitrick JE, Shorr E. Modification of the effects of immobilization upon metabolic and physiologic functions of normal men by the use of an oscillating bed. *Am J Med*. 1949;6(6):684-711.

56. Sanders CE. Cardiovascular and peripheral vascular diseases: treatment by a motorized oscillating bed. *JAMA*. 1936;106(11):916-918.

57. Bein T, Reber A, Metz C, Jauch KW, Hedenstierna G. Acute effects of continuous rotational therapy on ventilation-perfusion inequality in lung injury. *Intensive Care Med*. 1998;24(2):132-137.

58. Fink MP, Helsmoortel CM, Stein KL, Lee PC, Cohn SM. The efficacy of an oscillating bed in the prevention of lower respiratory tract infection in critically ill victims of blunt trauma. A prospective study. *Chest*. 1990;97(1):132-137.

59. Schieren M, Piekarski F, Dusse F, et al. Continuous lateral rotational therapy in trauma—a systematic review and meta-analysis. *J Trauma Acute Care Surg*. 2017;83(5):926-933.

60. Delaney A, Gray H, Laupland KB, Zuege DJ. Kinetic bed therapy to prevent nosocomial pneumonia in mechanically ventilated patients: a systematic review and meta-analysis. *Crit Care*. 2006;10(3):R70.

61. Hewitt N, Bucknall T, Faraone NM. Lateral positioning for critically ill adult patients. *Cochrane Database Syst Rev*. 2016;(5):CD007205.

62. Winslow EH, Clark AP, White KM, Tyler DO. Effects of a lateral turn on mixed venous oxygen saturation and heart rate in critically ill adults. *Heart Lung*. 1990;19(5 Pt 2):557-561.

63. Thomas PJ, Paratz JD, Lipman J, Stanton WR. Lateral positioning of ventilated intensive care patients: a study of oxygenation, respiratory mechanics, hemodynamics, and adverse events. *Heart Lung*. 2007;36(4):277-286.

19

Do Inhaled Vasodilators in ARDS Make a Difference?

Francois Lamontagne, Paige Guyatt, and Maureen O. Meade

INTRODUCTION

Inhaled vasodilators have a compelling physiologic rationale in the management of critically ill patients with acute respiratory distress syndrome (ARDS). A 25-year accumulation of rigorous research has helped to clarify their role in this setting, which is significantly more limited than original reports suggested.

PHYSIOLOGIC RATIONALE

Lung imaging studies in patients with ARDS show alveoli that are poorly aerated due to exudative edema, hyaline membranes, and microatelectasis that are not homogeneously distributed throughout the lung parenchyma. Instead, patchy areas of lung tissue are relatively preserved and remain compliant, allowing them to receive disproportionately large fractions of the minute ventilation.[1,2] The more diseased lung regions, located predominantly in the dependent areas of the lungs, may be poorly ventilated and yet receive much of the right ventricular cardiac output, resulting in a significant mismatch.

Heart–lung interactions can occasionally contribute to the pathology of ARDS. Laboratory research shows that hypoxia-induced vasoconstriction can result in pulmonary hypertension.[3,4] This is compounded by the dysregulation of constricting and dilating mediators, which can further increase pulmonary vascular resistance.[5] In severe ARDS, these effects may lead to right ventricular failure, a plausible independent predictor for death.[6]

Vasodilators delivered through the ventilator will preferentially reach the relatively more compliant lung regions, which are also most amenable to participate in gas exchange. Theoretically, the selective vasodilatation of vessels perfusing aerated lung tissue would redistribute blood flow from poorly ventilated regions, reducing the shunt fraction and at the same time correcting pulmonary hypertension. Improved oxygenation would reduce the mortality risk that is directly attributable to respiratory and right ventricular failure, while quicker resolution of ARDS would reduce the complications and morbidities associated with prolonged mechanical ventilation.[7] Unfortunately these are not the effects observed in randomized clinical trials.

The following discussion will focus mainly on inhaled nitric oxide (NO), which is by far the most extensively studied inhaled vasodilator in the context of ARDS. Additional data are available for nebulized prostaglandins, specifically epoprostenol, alprostadil, and dinoprostone.

NITRIC OXIDE

In 1993, Rossaint et al. completed a prospective cohort study of 10 adults with ARDS and observed that inhaled NO, in comparison to intravenous prostacyclin, improved oxygenation.[8] This report supported the potential benefit of selective pulmonary vasodilatation. Other preclinical and clinical observational studies supported this effect of inhaled NO on arterial oxygenation.[9–11] Added to further laboratory investigations finding additional benefits of NO on platelet and leukocyte function,[12] these results inspired the conduct of several randomized clinical trials and systematic reviews.

Systematic reviews have consistently challenged the potential for inhaled NO to improve survival in adult ARDS.[13–16] Among the included randomized trials, study populations varied. Most included adults with moderate to severe ARDS; however, some included children,[17–19] less severe ARDS,[20,21] or patients with a demonstrated favorable physiologic response to inhaled NO.[22] Protocols for the dose and duration of therapy also varied from 1 to 80 ppm and from less than 1 day to 28 days, respectively. One trial was a dose-finding study.[22] Lastly, efforts to minimize bias ranged across the studies: ten had concealed allocation,[17,18,20–28] five studies blinded caregivers,[18,21,23,26,28] and six reported on the use of alternative experimental therapies for ARDS.[20,21,23–25,29]

Despite the nuances of study populations, therapeutic protocols, and methodologic rigor, the results related to mortality were strikingly consistent. The relative similarity of patients, methods, and the results supports the decision to statistically aggregate results for this outcome. With or without statistical pooling, a visual review of the meta-analytical results provides a strong impression (Fig. 19.1). The aggregate results further suggest that inhaled NO does not improve survival despite a demonstration of improved oxygenation. The trends are more in keeping with increased mortality (relative risk 1.06; 95% CI 0.93 to 1.22).[14] Furthermore, the pooled results consistently suggest that inhaled NO is not beneficial in terms of ventilator-free days (mean difference −0.57; 95% CI −1.82 to 0.69).[14]

Analysis I.I
Comparison I Mortality: iNO versus control group, outcome I Longest follow-up mortality
(complete case analysis): iNO versus control

Review: Inhaled nitric oxide for acute respiratory distress syndrome (ARDS) and acute lung injury in children and adults

Comparison: I Mortality: iNO versus control group

Outcome: I Longest follow up mortality (complete case analysis): iNO versus control

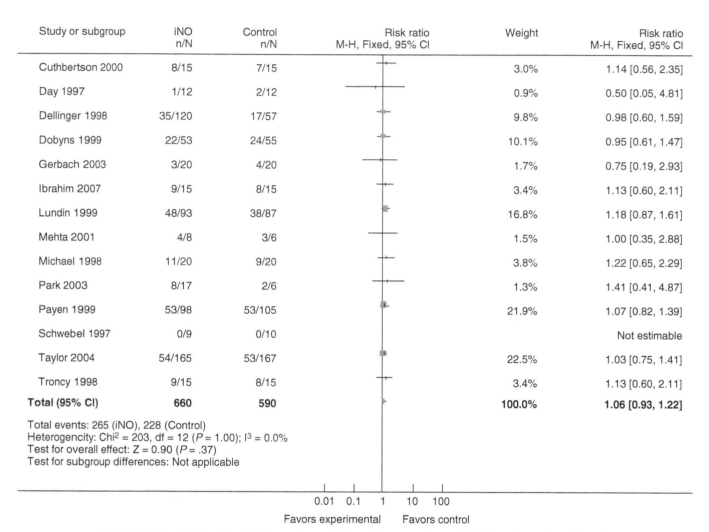

Study or subgroup	iNO n/N	Control n/N	Risk ratio M-H, Fixed, 95% CI	Weight	Risk ratio M-H, Fixed, 95% CI
Cuthbertson 2000	8/15	7/15		3.0%	1.14 [0.56, 2.35]
Day 1997	1/12	2/12		0.9%	0.50 [0.05, 4.81]
Dellinger 1998	35/120	17/57		9.8%	0.98 [0.60, 1.59]
Dobyns 1999	22/53	24/55		10.1%	0.95 [0.61, 1.47]
Gerbach 2003	3/20	4/20		1.7%	0.75 [0.19, 2.93]
Ibrahim 2007	9/15	8/15		3.4%	1.13 [0.60, 2.11]
Lundin 1999	48/93	38/87		16.8%	1.18 [0.87, 1.61]
Mehta 2001	4/8	3/6		1.5%	1.00 [0.35, 2.88]
Michael 1998	11/20	9/20		3.8%	1.22 [0.65, 2.29]
Park 2003	8/17	2/6		1.3%	1.41 [0.41, 4.87]
Payen 1999	53/98	53/105		21.9%	1.07 [0.82, 1.39]
Schwebel 1997	0/9	0/10			Not estimable
Taylor 2004	54/165	53/167		22.5%	1.03 [0.75, 1.41]
Troncy 1998	9/15	8/15		3.4%	1.13 [0.60, 2.11]
Total (95% CI)	**660**	**590**		**100.0%**	**1.06 [0.93, 1.22]**

Total events: 265 (iNO), 228 (Control)
Heterogencity: Chi^2 = 203, df = 12 (P = 1.00); I^3 = 0.0%
Test for overall effect: Z = 0.90 (P = .37)
Test for subgroup differences: Not applicable

0.01   0.1   1   10   100
Favors experimental   Favors control

Fig. 19.1 Inhaled nitric oxide (*iNO*) for acute respiratory distress syndrome (*ARDS*) and acute lung injury in children and adults (Review). (Copyright 2013 The Cochrane Collaboration. Published by John Wiley & Sons, Ltd.)

The systematic reviews also consistently suggest a statistically significant increase in the risk of renal dysfunction with inhaled NO therapy in the four studies that evaluated this outcome (relative risk 1.59; 95% CI 1.17 to 2.16).[14–16] One unblinded and three blinded trials observed this effect.[21–23,26] A subsequent propensity-matched cohort study of 547 patients confirmed this finding, reporting that inhaled NO was associated with a 59% increase in the use of renal replacement therapy in ARDS.[27]

The generalizability of these results to clinical practice is high. The studies included patients across the spectrum of

ARDS that clinicians commonly considered (prior to the publication of these studies) for inhaled NO therapy. Moreover, the treatment effects were strikingly similar across studies, notwithstanding the variations in populations, drug administration protocols, and methodologic quality.

In parallel to these systematic reviews, data on the long-term quality of life outcomes and costs of inhaled NO have emerged. Using the dataset of a previously published trial of inhaled NO in ARDS,[21] Angus et al.[30] reported a cost-effectiveness analysis suggesting that inhaled NO did not modify long-term outcomes nor post-hospital discharge costs. In contrast, a separate retrospective analysis of the same dataset observed positive effects of inhaled NO on the long-term pulmonary function of ARDS survivors who had participated in the trial.[31] At 6 months, the 51 survivors treated with inhaled NO (vs. 41 who were not treated with inhaled NO) had a greater mean (standard deviation [SD]) (1) total lung capacity (TLC: 5.54 [1.42] vs. 4.81 [1.0], $P = .026$); (2) percentage of predicted forced expiratory volume in 1 second (FEV$_1$: 80.2 [21.2] vs. 69.5 [29.0], $P = .042$); (3) percentage of predicted forced vital capacity (FVC: 83.8 [19.4] vs. 69.8 [27.4], $P = .02$); (4) percentage of predicted FEV$_1$/FVC (96.1 [13.8] vs. 87.9 [19.8], $P = .03$); and (5) percentage of predicted total lung capacity (93.3 [18.2] vs. 76.1 [21.8], $P < .001$). Medjo et al.[32] reported on a prospective observational study of inhaled NO in 16 children with ARDS who were compared to historical controls. Although oxygenation improved for up to 4 hours with inhaled NO, values had returned to baseline 24 hours after the onset of therapy and survival was not improved.

In summary, current clinical trials do not support a role for inhaled NO in the routine management of patients with acute lung injury and ARDS. In fact, meta-analyses suggest this approach to patient care is more likely to cause harm.[13–16]

PROSTAGLANDINS

Bearing the same physiologic rationale as inhaled NO in ARDS, three vasodilating prostaglandin molecules are a focus of interest in ARDS research: epoprostenol (also known as prostacyclin, or PGI$_2$), alprostadil (PGE$_1$), and dinoprostone (PGE$_2$). Additionally, epoprostenol blocks platelet aggregation and neutrophil migration and dinoprostone has anti-inflammatory properties. For these reasons, many investigators have hypothesized that nebulized prostaglandins would serve as selective vasodilators and, therefore, useful adjuncts in the context of ARDS.

The body of literature evaluating a role for inhaled prostaglandins in the management of patients with ARDS is limited. Dahlem et al.[33] reported that among 14 children with ARDS randomized to nebulized prostacyclin or placebo, oxygenation did improve with prostacyclin (median change in oxygen index –2.5, interquartile range –5.8 to –0.2) but mortality was unchanged. Other uncontrolled trials led to similar results. In a dose-finding study, Van Heerden et al.[34] treated 9 adult patients suffering from ARDS with inhaled prostacyclin. PaO$_2$/FiO$_2$ increased, but prostacyclin had no effect on hemodynamic variables or on platelet function. Sawheny et al.[35] treated 20 patients with ARDS and elevated pulmonary arterial pressures with prostacyclin. The mean PaO$_2$/FiO$_2$ ratio increased from 177 (SD 60) to 213 (SD 67) but PaCO$_2$, peak and plateau airway pressures, systemic blood pressure, and heart rate did not change significantly. More recently, Kallett and colleagues[36] determined that 60% of patients experience improved oxygenation with inhaled prostacyclin. Using a different prostaglandin, Meyer et al.[37] treated 15 adult patients with acute lung injury with inhaled dinoprostone. The mean PaO$_2$/FiO$_2$ ratio increased from 105 (standard error [SE] 9) to 160 (SE 17) ($P < .05$) after 4 hours and to 189 (SE 25) ($P < .05$) after 24 hours.

In contrast, Camamo et al.[38] reviewed the charts of 27 patients treated with epoprostenol or alprostadil for a primary or secondary diagnosis of ARDS and found no statistically significant improvement in oxygenation. Similarly, Domenighetti et al.,[39] in a prospective uncontrolled trial of nebulized prostacyclin to 15 consecutive patients with ARDS and severe hypoxemia, found no improvement in oxygenation.

COMPARISONS OF INHALED NITRIC OXIDE AND PROSTAGLANDIN

In contrast to the original 10-patient study reported by Rossaint and colleagues,[40,41] direct comparisons of nebulized epoprostenol and inhaled NO have consistently observed similar clinical effects between the two agents. Various groups titrated doses of both agents sequentially and observed nearly identical effects on pulmonary arterial pressure and distribution of blood flow. Torbic and colleagues[42] retrospectively compared vasodilator effects in 105 patients, and found no difference in the change in PaO$_2$/FiO$_2$, duration of mechanical ventilation, or intensive care unit or hospital lengths of stay. They did observe that inhaled NO was 4.5 to 17 times more expensive than nebulized epoprostenol. More recently, Ammar and colleagues[43] compared inhaled nitric oxide and epoprostenol in a retrospective, propensity-matched cohort study of 102 patients with ARDS and found no difference in oxygenation effects, ventilator free days, or survival.

RECONCILING THE RATIONALE WITH CLINICAL RESEARCH FINDINGS

This discordance between physiologic outcomes and survival is not without precedent in critical care. In a landmark study of low tidal volume ventilation conducted by the ARDS Network, patients ventilated with low tidal volumes had lower oxygen levels but an increased survival rate when compared with those patients receiving traditionally larger tidal volumes.[44] A disconnect between effects of inhaled NO on physiologic outcomes and survival fits with the understanding that ARDS patients seldom die of respiratory failure.[45] Yet for the minority of patients with profound and refractory hypoxemia threatening immediate survival the question remains unanswered. There are insufficient research data in this specific at-risk subgroup to conclude that inhaled NO is, on balance, more likely to benefit or to harm.

There are a number of plausible explanations for the lack of benefit of inhaled NO and, probably, prostaglandins in most patients with ARDS. It is conceivable that the purported physiologic benefits are offset by relatively hidden deleterious effects on other organ systems. Contrary to common belief, recent experiments have shown that inhaled NO does not act strictly within the pulmonary vasculature: rather, it reacts with various molecules to produce nitrosothiol compounds that share many properties of NO donors but have longer half-lives.[46–49] This evidence, in keeping with the unexpected association between inhaled NO administration and renal dysfunction, suggests that the pharmacodynamic effects of inhaled NO are probably more complex than originally understood. The data on inhaled prostaglandins are less clear, but the same principles may apply.

SUMMARY

The use of inhaled vasodilators appeals to our current understanding of ARDS physiopathology. Caregivers expect that by limiting ventilation–perfusion mismatch, these medications will improve survival. Also there are hypotheses related to pleiotropic effects on leukocyte migration, platelet adhesion, and overall inflammation. Inhaled vasodilator therapies, therefore, have been subjected to wide and rapid dissemination.[50] A careful examination of randomized trials, however, reveals disappointing results. In the case of NO, where the overall trend is indicative of harm, there are now sufficient data—in quantity and quality—to suggest that inhaled NO should not be used in the routine management of patients with ARDS, as noted in current clinical practice guidelines.[51] Whether or not this therapy can make a difference in the setting of severe, life-threatening refractory hypoxemia is uncertain but any potential benefit should be weighed against the risk for extrapulmonary side effects such as renal failure, and its high cost. Less data are available to address the potential role for nebulized prostaglandin therapy, but the learnings from NO research warrant caution.

AUTHORS' RECOMMENDATIONS

- There is a compelling physiologic rationale behind the use of inhaled pulmonary vasodilators in the treatment of hypoxemia and right heart failure, secondary to hypoxic pulmonary vasoconstriction.
- Studies of inhaled nitric oxide (NO) and inhaled prostaglandins demonstrate improved oxygenation.
- There is no evidence that inhaled vasodilators reduce mortality.
- In the case of inhaled NO, the trend is towards worse, rather than improved outcomes. This includes an increase in the incidence of acute kidney injury.
- Inhaled NO is not cost-effective. Inhaled prostaglandins are significantly less expensive, but clinical efficacy has not been demonstrated.
- Inhaled vasodilators may have some value as "rescue therapy" in extreme situations, but this is not currently supported by data.

REFERENCES

1. Gattinoni L, Pesenti A, Bombino M, et al. Relationships between lung computed tomographic density, gas exchange, and PEEP in acute respiratory failure. *Anesthesiology.* 1988;69:824-832.
2. Maunder RJ, Shuman WP, McHugh JW, et al. Preservation of normal lung regions in the adult respiratory distress syndrome: analysis by computed tomography. *JAMA.* 1986;255:2463-2465.
3. Tomashefski JF Jr, Davies P, Boggis C, Greene R, Zapol WM, Reid LM. The pulmonary vascular lesions of the adult respiratory distress syndrome. *Am J Pathol.* 1983;112:112-126.
4. Zapol WM, Snider MT. Pulmonary hypertension in severe acute respiratory failure. *N Engl J Med.* 1977;296:476-480.
5. Moloney ED, Evans TW. Pathophysiology and pharmacological treatment of pulmonary hypertension in acute respiratory distress syndrome. *Eur Respir J.* 2003;21:720-727.
6. Boissier F, Katsahian S, Razazi K, et al. Prevalence and prognosis of cor pulmonale during protective ventilation for acute respiratory distress syndrome. *Intensive Care Med.* 2013;39:1725-1733.
7. Siobal MS, Hess DR. Are inhaled vasodilators useful in acute lung injury and acute respiratory distress syndrome? *Respir Care.* 2010;55:144-157.
8. Rossaint R, Falke KJ, López F, Slama K, Pison U, Zapol WM. Inhaled nitric oxide for the adult respiratory distress syndrome. *N Engl J Med.* 1993;328:399-405.
9. Bigatello LM, Hurford WE, Kacmarek RM, Roberts JD, Zapol WM. Prolonged inhalation of low concentrations of nitric oxide in patients with severe adult respiratory distress syndrome: effects on pulmonary hemodynamics and oxygenation. *Anesthesiology.* 1994;80:761-770.
10. Rossaint R, Gerlach H, Schmidt-Ruhnke H, et al. Efficacy of inhaled nitric oxide in patients with severe ARDS. *Chest.* 1995;107:1107-1115.
11. Puybasset L, Stewart T, Rouby JJ, et al. Inhaled nitric oxide reverses the increase in pulmonary vascular resistance induced by permissive hypercapnia in patients with acute respiratory distress syndrome. *Anesthesiology.* 1994;80:1254-1267.
12. Bigatello LM, Hurford WE, Hess D. Use of inhaled nitric oxide for ARDS. *Respir Care Clin N Am.* 1997;3:437-458.
13. Adhikari NK, Burns KE, Friedrich JO, Granton JT, Cook DJ, Meade MO. Effect of nitric oxide on oxygenation and mortality in acute lung injury: systematic review and meta-analysis. *BMJ.* 2007;334:779-787.
14. Afshari A, Brok J, Møller AM, Wetterslev J. Inhaled nitric oxide for acute respiratory distress syndrome (ARDS) and acute lung injury in children and adults. *Cochrane Database Syst Rev.* 2010; CD002787.
15. Ruan SY, Huang TM, Wu HY, Wu HD, Yu CJ, Lai MS. Inhaled nitric oxide therapy and risk for renal dysfunction: a systematic review and meta-analysis of randomized trials. *Crit Care.* 2015; 19:137.
16. Gebistorf F, Karam O, Wetterslev J, Afshari A. Inhaled nitric oxide for acute respiratory distress syndrome (ARDS) in children and adults. *Cochrane Database Syst Rev.* 2016;(6):CD002787.
17. Day RW, Allen EM, Witte MK. A randomized, controlled study of the 1-hour and 24-hour effects of inhaled nitric oxide therapy in children with acute hypoxemic respiratory failure. *Chest.* 1997;112:1324-1331.
18. Dobyns EL, Cornfield DN, Anas NG, et al. Multicenter randomized controlled trial of the effects of inhaled nitric oxide therapy on gas exchange in children with acute hypoxemic respiratory failure. *J Pediatr.* 1999;134:406-412.
19. Ibrahim T, El-Mohamady H. Inhaled nitric oxide and prone position: How far they can improve oxygenation in pediatric patients with acute respiratory distress syndrome? *J Med Sci.* 2007;7:390-395.
20. Troncy E, Collet JP, Shapiro S, et al. Inhaled nitric oxide in acute respiratory distress syndrome: a pilot randomized controlled study. *Am J Respir Crit Care Med.* 1998;157:1483-1488.

21. Taylor RW, Zimmerman JL, Dellinger RP, et al. Low-dose inhaled nitric oxide in patients with acute lung injury: a randomized controlled trial. *JAMA*. 2004;291:1603-1609.

22. Lundin S, Mang H, Smithies M, Stenqvist O, Frostell C. Inhalation of nitric oxide in acute lung injury: results of a European multi-centre study. The European Study Group of Inhaled Nitric Oxide. *Intensive Care Med*. 1999;25:911-919.

23. Dellinger RP, Zimmerman JL, Taylor RW, et al. Effects of inhaled nitric oxide in patients with acute respiratory distress syndrome: results of a randomized phase II trial. Inhaled Nitric Oxide in ARDS Study Group. *Crit Care Med*. 1998; 26:15-23.

24. Gerlach H, Keh D, Semmerow A, et al. Dose-response characteristics during long-term inhalation of nitric oxide in patients with severe acute respiratory distress syndrome: a prospective, randomized, controlled study. *Am J Respir Crit Care Med*. 2003;167:1008-1015.

25. Park KJ, Lee YJ, Oh YJ, et al. Combined effects of inhaled nitric oxide and a recruitment maneuver in patients with acute respiratory distress syndrome. *Yonsei Med J*. 2003;44:219-226.

26. Payen D, Vallet B; Groupe d'étude du NO dans l'ARDS. Results of the French prospective multicentric randomized double-blind placebo-controlled trial on inhaled nitric oxide (NO) in ARDS [abstract]. *Intensive Care Med*. 1999;25:S166.

27. Ruan SY, Wu HY, Lin HH, Wu HD, Yu CJ, Lai MS. Inhaled nitric oxide and the risk of renal dysfunction in patients with acute respiratory distress syndrome: a propensity-matched cohort study. *Crit Care*. 2016;20:389.

28. Schwebel C, Beuret P, Perdrix JP, et al. Early inhaled nitric oxide inhalation in acute lung injury: results of a double-blind randomized study [abstract]. *Intensive Care Med*. 1997;23:S2.

29. Mehta S, Simms HH, Levy MM, et al. Inhaled nitric oxide improves oxygenation acutely but not chronically in acute respiratory syndromes: a randomized controlled trial. *J Appl Res*. 2001;1:73-84.

30. Angus DC, Clermont G, Linde-Zwirble WT, et al. Healthcare costs and long-term outcomes after acute respiratory distress syndrome: a phase III trial of inhaled nitric oxide. *Crit Care Med*. 2006;34:2883-2890.

31. Dellinger RP, Trzeciak SW, Criner GJ, et al. Association between inhaled nitric oxide treatment and long-term pulmonary function in survivors of acute respiratory distress syndrome. *Crit Care*. 2012;16:R36.

32. Medjo B, Atanaskovic-Markovic M, Nikolic D, Cuturilo G, Djukic S. Inhaled nitric oxide therapy for acute respiratory distress syndrome in children. *Indian Pediatr*. 2012;49(7):573-576.

33. Dahlem P, van Aalderen WM, de Neef M, Dijkgraaf MG, Bos AP. Randomized controlled trial of aerosolized prostacyclin therapy in children with acute lung injury. *Crit Care Med*. 2004;32:1055-1060.

34. van Heerden PV, Barden A, Michalopoulos N, Bulsara MK, Roberts BL. Dose-response to inhaled aerosolized prostacyclin for hypoxemia due to ARDS. *Chest*. 2000;117:819-827.

35. Sawheny E, Ellis AL, Kinasewitz GT. Iloprost improves gas exchange in patients with pulmonary hypertension and ARDS. *Chest*. 2013;144:55-62.

36. Kallett RH, Burns G, Zhuo H, et al. Severity of hypoxemia and other factors that influence the response to aerosolized prostacyclin in ARDS. *Respir Care*. 2017;62:1014-1022.

37. Meyer J, Theilmeier G, Van Aken H, et al. Inhaled prostaglandin E_1 for treatment of acute lung injury in severe multiple organ failure. *Anesth Analg*. 1998;86:753-758.

38. Camamo JM, McCoy RH, Erstad BL. Retrospective evaluation of inhaled prostaglandins in patients with acute respiratory distress syndrome. *Pharmacotherapy*. 2005;25:184-190.

39. Domenighetti G, Stricker H, Waldispuehl B. Nebulized prostacyclin (PGI_2) in acute respiratory distress syndrome: impact of primary (pulmonary injury) and secondary (extrapulmonary injury) disease on gas exchange response. *Crit Care Med*. 2001;29:57-62.

40. Eichelbrönner O, Reinelt H, Wiedeck H, et al. Aerosolized prostacyclin and inhaled nitric oxide in septic shock—different effects on splanchnic oxygenation? *Intensive Care Med*. 1996; 22:880-887.

41. Walmrath D, Schneider T, Schermuly R, Olschewski H, Grimminger F, Seeger W. Direct comparison of inhaled nitric oxide and aerosolized prostacyclin in acute respiratory distress syndrome. *Am J Respir Crit Care Med*. 1996;153:991-996.

42. Torbic H, Szumita PM, Anger KE, Nuccio P, LaGambina S, Weinhouse G. Inhaled epoprostenol vs inhaled nitric oxide for refractory hypoxemia in critically ill patients. *J Crit Care*. 2013;28:844-848.

43. Ammar MA, Bauer SR, Bass SN, Sasidhar M, Mullin R, Lam SW. Noninferiority of inhaled epoprostenol to inhaled nitric oxide for the treatment of ARDS. *Ann Pharmacother*. 2015;49:1105-1112.

44. The Acute Respiratory Distress Syndrome Network; Brower RG, Matthay MA, et al.. Ventilation with lower tidal volumes as compared with traditional tidal volumes for acute lung injury and the acute respiratory distress syndrome. *N Engl J Med*. 2000;342:1301-1308.

45. Montgomery AB, Stager MA, Carrico CJ, Hudson LD. Causes of mortality in patients with the adult respiratory distress syndrome. *Am Rev Respir Dis*. 1985;132:485-489.

46. Fox-Robichaud A, Payne D, Hasan SU, et al. Inhaled NO as a viable antiadehesive therapy for ischemia/reperfusion injury of distal microvascular beds. *J Clin Invest*. 1998;101:2497-2505.

47. Keaney Jr JF, Simon DI, Stamler JS, et al. NO forms an adduct with serum albumin that has endothelium-derived relaxing factor-like properties. *J Clin Invest*. 1993;91:1582-1589.

48. Kubes P, Payne D, Grisham MB, Jourd-Heuil D, Fox-Robichaud A. Inhaled NO impacts vascular but not extravascular compartments in postischemic peripheral organs. *Am J Physiol*. 1999; 277:H676-H682.

49. Jia L, Bonaventura C, Bonaventura J, Stamler JS. S-nitrosohaemoglobin: a dynamic activity of blood involved in vascular control. *Nature*. 1996;380:221-226.

50. Beloucif S, Payen D. A European survey of the use of inhaled nitric oxide in the ICU. Working Group on Inhaled NO in the ICU of the European Society of Intensive Care Medicine. *Intensive Care Med*. 1998;24:864-877.

51. Claesson J, Freundlich M, Gunnarsson I, et al. Scandinavian clinical practice guideline on fluid and drug therapy in adults with acute respiratory distress syndrome. *Acta Anaesthesiol Scand*. 2016;60:697-709.

20

Does ECMO Work?

Jesse M. Raiten, William J. Vernick, and Jacob T. Gutsche

INTRODUCTION

Interest in extracorporeal membrane oxygenation (ECMO) for respiratory support has dramatically increased in the past decade, aided by advancements in extracorporeal technology, publication of a small number of randomized trials, and continued high mortality of patients suffering from severe acute respiratory distress syndrome (ARDS) and shock. In the United States, utilization has increased dramatically and the number of centers performing ECMO has risen sharply; some clinicians are calling for more widespread and earlier application of ECMO, which has previously been considered a therapy of last resort.[1,2]

The development of modern ECMO, also called extracorporeal life support, for cardiopulmonary support can be traced to the original heart/lung machine designed by Dr Gibbon.[3] The original cardiopulmonary bypass (CPB) machine was insufficient for prolonged extracorporeal support due to damage and activation of blood components during direct exposure to gas during exchange. Significant advancements in technology, materials, and design of the oxygenator, pump, and circuit technology have facilitated the increased durability of ECMO circuits and reduced the damage to blood components. In this chapter, we briefly review ECMO techniques for support of the patient with ARDS and provide a detailed review of the ECMO evidence.

BASICS OF ECMO

A basic ECMO circuit consists of inflow and outflow cannula, tubing, a pump, and a membrane oxygenator/heat exchanger. The oxygen and carbon dioxide levels in the blood pumped through the ECMO circuit are controlled by altering the oxygen content and flow rate (sweep) of gas infused through the membrane oxygenator.

There are two basic types of ECMO: venoarterial (VA), which supports the heart and/or lungs, and venovenous (VV), which supports the lungs only. For patients with pulmonary failure, ECMO has the capability to temporarily support cardiopulmonary function as the patient recovers or is bridged to transplantation.[4] ECMO cannulae may be inserted directly into the central vessels, usually in patients failing to wean from cardiopulmonary bypass, or into peripheral vessels. A third type of peripheral ECMO, adds a venous outflow cannula to oxygenate blood returning to the right atrium which would provide oxygenated blood to the myocardial and carotid circulation.[5]

In general, VV ECMO is used in patients with ARDS patients who do not have severe cardiac dysfunction. Even patients receiving significant doses of vasopressors can be supported with VV ECMO and, after ECMO implementation, the pressor requirement usually decreases after correction of metabolic abnormalities.[6] Although ECMO remains challenging to manage and is still associated with relatively high morbidity and mortality, increased experience and durability of ECMO circuits have allowed care teams to support patients for several weeks to months.

In patients with severe ARDS and severe cardiac dysfunction, peripheral VA ECMO may be considered. In peripheral VA ECMO, blood is usually drained from a femoral vein and returned to the femoral artery. Most ECMO circuits are designed to flow to a maximum of 7 L/min, which may not be sufficient to fully empty the heart, particularly in large patients. Blood that returns to the heart, bypassing the ECMO circuit, may be ejected in a patient with residual cardiac function. With a peripheral cannulation strategy, blood has three ways to bypass the ECMO circuit and contribute to hypoxia:

- Bronchial blood flow, which usually accounts for about 2% of the cardiac output, returns to the left atrium via the pulmonary veins.
- Venous blood flow that has perfused the pericardium may also return directly to the cardiac chambers via the thebesian veins.
- Finally, blood that returns to the heart, having bypassed the venous drainage cannula, may be ejected through the aortic valve in the case of residual cardiac function.

If this blood is poorly oxygenated due to inadequate pulmonary function, it may compete with the blood flowing into the aorta from the peripheral arterial cannula. This can be a serious complication, known as differential hypoxia (alternate terminology includes north-south syndrome, proximal-distal syndrome, and harlequin syndrome). For this reason, peripheral VA ECMO should not be considered for patients with ARDS, with the exception of patients with severe cardiac dysfunction. There are no modern studies analyzing the utility of VA ECMO in patients with severe ARDS with severe cardiac dysfunction, and the mortality in this group is 50% according to data voluntarily reported to the Extracorporeal Life Support Organization (ELSO).[7]

HISTORY, EVOLUTION, AND CURRENT STATUS OF ECMO

Extracorporeal circulatory support in the adult population has become commonplace in the setting of refractory cardiogenic shock where VA ECMO is recommended by the American Heart Association to bridge patients either to recovery or ventricular assist device.[8] ECMO for respiratory support though, particularly in the setting of the 2009 H1NI pandemic (where it was widely used), has been controversial, despite being recommended in Europe.[9] Since 2013 there has been a dramatic increase in ECMO usage worldwide, attributable to two important events. The first was the publication of the CESAR trial in 2009, which randomized patients with severe respiratory failure to either conventional medical therapy in general hospitals vs. ECMO support in specialized medical centers (70 centers in the UK, 180 patients, 6-month monitoring period).[10] The second event was the 2009 influenza A (H1N1) worldwide pandemic that prompted dramatically increased VV ECMO usage worldwide as emergent salvage therapy for patients with severe viral pneumonia/ARDS unresponsive to mechanical ventilation. The first reported publication attesting to the success of ECMO in this group came from Australia/New Zealand,[11] quickly followed by data reporting usage of ECMO from Europe,[12,13] South America,[14] Canada,[15] Taiwan,[16] and Hong Kong.[17] Gattinoni et al.[18] published a report that emphasized the explosion in use of ECMO, and found that from early 2009 through May 2011, there were more than 1000 papers on ECMO reported on Medline, with the majority of ECMO usage not being H1N1 related, but from other causes of respiratory failure and cardiac failure. The trend of increased ECMO implementation has continued, as demonstrated in a 2014 study. which reported a significant (433%) increase in ECMO utilization in adults within the United States alone from 2006 to 2011.[19] Using data from the Nationwide Inpatient Sample (NIS), part of the Healthcare Cost and Utilization Project (HCUP), sponsored by the Agency for Healthcare Research and Quality (AHRQ), in addition to summary datasets from the ECMO registry of the ELSO (Ann Arbor, MI), Sauer et al.[19] calculated ECMO utilization rates, survival rates, and overall costs in patients ≥ 18 years old. In terms of ECMO utilization, there was no significant difference from 1999 to 2007. Survival rates from 2006 to 2011 showed a trend towards improvement, but this was not statistically significant. Patients in 2011 were twice as likely to be categorized as critically ill as those in 2006. Analysis of the ELSO registry showed survival rates of 41%, with no significant change from 2006. There were also no significant changes in costs incurred due to ECMO between 2006 and 2011.[19]

ECMO PHYSIOLOGY/GAS EXCHANGE

As per the extracorporeal life support (ECLS) Registry, the most rapidly growing aspect of ECMO remains VV ECMO, spurred on by the results of the CESAR trial and the H1N1 pandemic in 2009–2010.[10,11] In the key data published, average ECMO use ranged from 9 to 10 days in duration and was initiated in the first 7 days of mechanical ventilation, with mortality rates ranging from 21 to 37%.[10,11] In general, VV ECMO is considered in patients with life-threatening but potentially reversible respiratory failure who otherwise do not have contraindications to extracorporeal life support.[20] The Murray Score played a key role in determining the need for ECMO support in the CESAR trial and is based on the severity assessment of respiratory failure. It uses four criteria: ratio of partial pressure of arterial oxygen to the fraction of inspired oxygen (PaO_2/FiO_2); positive end-expiratory pressure (PEEP); dynamic lung compliance; and the number of quadrants infiltrated on a chest radiograph.[21,22] In this trial, a Murray Score > 3.0 was the key criterion for patient enrollment, in addition to uncompensated hypercapnia with pH < 7.20.[23]

As per the 2013 ELSO guidelines, VV ECMO indication recommendations vary based on the impending mortality risk. In patients with a 50% risk of mortality (PaO_2/FiO_2 < 150 or FiO_2 > 90% and/or Murray Score 2–3), ECMO should be considered. When anticipated mortality approaches ≥80% (PaO_2/FiO_2 < 100 on FiO_2 > 90% and/or Murray Score 3–4 despite optimal care for 6 hours or more), VV ECMO is indicated. In addition to ARDS, the ELSO Guidelines for VV ECMO in acute respiratory failure also recommend ECMO for severe air leak syndromes, CO_2 retention in mechanically ventilated patients despite high plateau pressure (P_{plat} > 30 cm H_2O) and miscellaneous conditions, such as patients listed for lung transplantation who need airway support as well patients with acute respiratory failure unresponsive to optimal care.[24,25]

CONTRAINDICATIONS

Aside from the inability to anticoagulate for ECMO, there are no specific, absolute contraindications. Well-established conditions that are recognized to have poor outcomes on ECMO, as per ELSO, are considered to be relative contraindications and include high pressure ventilation (end-expiratory P_{plat} > 30 cm H_2O) for >7 days, high FiO_2 requirements (>0.8) for >7 days, nonrecoverable conditions such as major CNS bleeding or trauma, malignancy, immunosuppression, and limited vascular access.[24]

Age and body mass index (BMI), as contraindications, vary by center and country. Age > 65 years old is considered a contraindication in some countries.[26] BMI does present practical limitations related to cannulation and maximum pump flows. Tulman et al.[27] suggest that patients with BMI > 35 might develop early hemolysis due to flow-related issues resulting from elevated driveline pressures.

VV ECMO CANNULATION STRATEGIES

Ideally, the VV ECMO cannula configuration should maximize flow and minimize recirculation and, as Sidebotham et al.[28] emphasize, the former can be maximized by IVC placement of a long, multiport (> 50 cm) 23F to 29F drainage cannula in the IVC and the latter minimized by returning oxygenated blood directly to the right atrium and directed flow through the tricuspid valve.

Ventilator settings on VV ECMO can vary based on clinical pathophysiology. Current ELSO guidelines recommend, in general, "rest settings", with FiO_2 as low as possible ($< 40\%$) and the avoidance of $P_{plat} > 25$ mm Hg.[29] Typical rest settings consist of pressure-controlled ventilation, with low respiratory rates, very low tidal volumes, low FiO_2, peak inspiratory pressure < 25 cm H_2O and PEEP of 10–15 cm H_2O. There are no published data in non-ECMO patients or ECMO patients to suggest that these so-called rest settings provide any improvement in long-term lung function or survival advantage.

ECMO: THE EVIDENCE FOR ITS USE IN ARDS

There is a surprising paucity of high-quality evidence supporting the use of ECMO in patients with ARDS (Table 20.1). Of the five randomized controlled trials (RCTs) that have been published,[10,30–33] two RCTs were performed before 1994.[30,33] Technological advances in ECMO equipment, therapeutic improvements, and a substantial increase in practitioner experience since then justifiably question the applicability of these trials to modern practice. Furthermore, the management of ARDS has evolved since these trials to include low stretch ventilation, use of muscle relaxants, and prone positioning.[34–36] Even without the numerous RCTs that

have been conducted for therapies for other common ICU conditions—such as shock and ventilator management—there is a rapidly growing interest in studying and developing ECMO programs dedicated to the treatment of acute respiratory failure. Inevitably, as the use of ECMO grows in this patient population, so will a body of evidence to ultimately support or refute its use.

The CESAR trial[10] randomized 180 adult patients with severe but potentially reversible respiratory failure to either conventional management or referral to a center for consideration of ECMO. When patients were randomized into the ECMO group, they were transferred to an ECMO-capable hospital. If their hemodynamics were stable, they were managed for up to 12 hours with a standard ARDS treatment protocol (pressure-restricted mechanical ventilation, PEEP, prone positioning, etc.). If they did not improve with this strategy, then VV ECMO was initiated. The primary outcome was death or severe disability at 6 months following randomization. Based on statistically significant results, the authors concluded that patient transfer to an ECMO-capable center led to improved survival without severe disability.[10] Furthermore, a financial analysis demonstrated that the costs of referral to an ECMO center, given the improved outcomes, made this approach financially justifiable and appropriately considered as cost-effective.

There are several important considerations with this study. First, of the 90 patients assigned for consideration of ECMO, 22 ultimately did not receive ECMO. Secondly, although a lung protective ventilation strategy was recommended, it was not mandated, and therefore ventilation strategies could differ between patients. This study must therefore not be considered as a pure trial comparing ECMO with traditional mechanical ventilation, but more in the context of conventional management vs. management at an ECMO-designated center. Furthermore, the primary endpoint was death or

---

TABLE 20.1   **Clinical Trials of ECMO for the Treatment of ARDS.**

Study	Study Design	Control	Intervention	Conclusions
ECMO in severe ARDS[30]	Prospective RCT, nonblinded	Mechanical ventilation	Mechanical ventilation plus partial VA ECMO	Mortality unchanged
CESAR trial[10]	Prospective RCT, nonblinded	Mechanical ventilation (non-standardized protocol)	Transfer to ECMO capable hospital, option for ECMO initiation	Improved survival without disability if transferred to ECMO capable facility
ELOIA[31]	Prospective RCT, nonblinded	Mechanical ventilation (standardized protocol)	Mechanical ventilation plus VV ECMO	Mortality not statistically changed
XTRAVENT[32]	Prospective RCT, nonblinded	Mechanical ventilation (6 mL/kg)	Mechanical ventilation (3 mL/kg) plus $ECCO_2$ removal	Mortality not statistically changed
PCIRV/ECCO$_2$ REMOVAL[33]	Prospective RCT, nonblinded	Mechanical ventilation	Mechanical ventilation plus $ECCO_2$ removal	Mortality not statistically changed

$ECCO_2$, extracorporeal CO_2 removal; *ECMO*, extracorporeal membrane oxygenation; *PCIRV*, pressure control inverse ratio ventilation; *RCT*, randomized controlled trial; *VA ECMO*, venoarterial extracorporeal membrane oxygenation; *VV ECMO*, venovenous extracorporeal membrane oxygenation

severe disability at 6 months. ECMO may be associated with considerable morbidity; therefore, including severe disability in the primary endpoint was an important factor from a quality-of-life perspective. Additionally, the risks associated with transport of a critically ill patient to a specialized ECMO center were built into the study.[37] Although transport was provided by a specialized ECMO team, patients were not transported while on ECMO.

Combes and colleagues[31] published a multicenter controlled trial of ECMO vs. conventional therapy + ECMO in severe ARDS in 2018 (known as the ELOIA trial). This multicenter RCT enrolled 249 patients with severe ARDS, which was defined as a PaO_2/FiO_2 ratio of <50 mm Hg for more than 3 hours, a PaO_2/FiO_2 ratio of <80 mm Hg for more than 6 hours, or an arterial pH of <7.25 with PCO_2 >60 mm Hg for more than 6 hours. Patients were randomized to either continuous VV ECMO or conventional treatment, and the primary endpoint was mortality at 60 days. Crossover was allowed from the control group to the ECMO group, and 28% of patients initially assigned to the control group did cross over due to refractory hypoxemia. At 60 days, mortality in the ECMO group was 35% and in the control group, was 46%; this did not meet statistical significance, and the authors concluded that the use of ECMO was not associated with significantly lower mortality in patients with very severe early ARDS. The frequency of complications was similar between the groups, with the exception of a greater rate of transfusion from bleeding events in the ECMO group.

The ELOIA trial[31] had important differences from the CESAR trial.[10] The ELOIA trial ensured standardized ECMO management and mechanical ventilation strategies were maintained throughout, while the CESAR trial did not. Furthermore, ventilation strategies in the ELOIA trial ensured what was considered "best practice," including lung protective ventilation with low tidal volumes, recruitment maneuvers, prone positioning, and use of neuromuscular blocking agents.

The ELOIA trial's primary endpoint of mortality at 60 days failed to reach statistical significance; however, this was complicated by the large crossover rate from the control to the ECMO group for refractory hypoxemia.[38] These patients had an increased mortality rate compared with patients in the control group who did not cross over to receive ECMO. The high crossover rate also contributed to early termination of the trial, for futility, based on interval analysis by the data safety monitoring board.[39] Enrollment in the trial had also been slow, although 64 units were involved in the study: fewer than 1 patient per unit per year was enrolled. The decision to terminate patient enrollment early was controversial, and the editors of the *New England Journal of Medicine*, where the trial was published, concluded that ECMO probably has some benefit for patients with severe ARDS.[40] Without crossover, it is likely that the absolute risk reduction between the intervention and control groups would have achieved statistical significance.[41] ARDS may manifest as impaired oxygenation, impaired ventilation, or difficulty with both oxygenation

and ventilation. Traditional VV ECMO facilitates oxygen delivery and CO_2 removal. A simpler version of AV ECMO allows for CO_2 removal by using a pumpless machine (iLA AV, Novalung, Heilbronn, Germany) and lower blood flow rates. Bein and colleagues[32] compared traditional mechanical ventilation strategies (6 mL/kg) with a lower tidal volume strategy (3 mL/kg) combined with CO_2 removal via pumpless ECMO. Their primary outcome measure was ventilator-free days at the 28-day and 60-day marks. Overall, there was no significant difference between the study and control groups for all patients, but a post hoc analysis did show that ARDS patients with increased hypoxia (PaO_2/FiO_2 < 150 at baseline) who were randomized to the study group did have a statistically shorter ventilator requirement. Among patients treated with low tidal volumes and ECMO for CO_2 removal, there was a reduction in analgesic and sedative use, they spent more time in spontaneous ventilation, and the proinflammatory cytokine interleukin-6 (IL-6) was reduced.[32] It should be noted that this study was limited to hemodynamically stable patients in order to allow proper function of the pumpless ECMO circuit, and many patients with severe ARDS being considered for ECMO are unstable hemodynamically.

Although it may be valuable at this point only for historical perspective, one of the first trials of ECMO for respiratory failure was published in 1979 by Zapol and colleagues.[30] Ninety patients with severe arterial hypoxemia were randomized to receive either conventional mechanical ventilation or VA ECMO. Most patients suffered from bacterial or viral pneumonia, but others had pulmonary emboli or posttraumatic acute respiratory failure. Survival was not statistically different between the two groups. Similarly, Morris and colleagues'[33] 1994 study of pressure-controlled inverse ratio ventilation and extracorporeal CO_2 removal for ARDS did not find any survival difference between the control and ECMO study groups.

Since studies before the year 2000, ECMO strategies and equipment have undergone considerable improvement and many centers have gained experience with its use in patients with respiratory failure. It has been argued that it would be unethical to conduct another trial evaluating ECMO for ARDS in which ECMO is not considered conventional care.[39] With the increasing use of ECMO for ARDS, and improving technology, there are numerous opportunities for future studies. Notably, questions remain about the timing of ECMO initiation in ARDS, as well as sedation requirements, patients' ability to ambulate, the use of spontaneous ventilation while on ECMO to reduce diaphragmatic dysfunction, and how long patients can be managed on ECMO and still have a chance for lung recovery.

FACTORS COMPLICATING THE STUDY OF ECMO

Timing of Initiation

The lack of-high powered clinical trials supporting the use of ECMO has made it difficult for intensivists to understand the appropriate timing or indications for ECMO support. It appears clear that some patients with severe ARDS and refractory hypoxemia may be salvaged with ECMO.[31] What is unclear is the timing of initiation.

There are no data to support the use of ECMO for patients with mild or moderate ARDS. In patients with severe ARDS, it is reasonable to assume that they should have reasonable attempts at utilizing low stretch ventilation, muscle relaxants, and prone positioning prior to considering ECMO. In our experience, some patients experience severe hemodynamic instability due to severe hypoxemia and severe acidosis due to impaired gas exchange, which may allow a narrow window of time to consider the implementation of ECMO. This is particularly important for hospitals caring for patients with no ECMO support or a regional hospital able to deploy a mobile team who can implement ECMO.[42] Once the patient becomes hemodynamically unstable, transport may become life threatening, and the physician and family are faced with the decision of keeping the patient and hoping for a recovery or a high-risk transport to an ECMO-capable hospital.

ECMO Centers

ECMO is a resource-intensive therapy that can require complex management strategies, complicated screening practices, and highly trained personnel available to manage patients. In addition, higher-volume centers are more likely to have consultants with greater exposure to patients on ECMO who may understand the implications on pharmacokinetics, organ function, and the complicated profile associated with these patients. In the United States, there has been a rapid rise in the number of centers performing ECMO; some of these have low volumes of patients requiring ECMO, with virtually no oversight on competence or outcomes. This is in sharp contrast to organ transplant, ventricular assist device, and cardiac surgery outcomes, which enforce or encourage participation in outcomes tracking and public reporting.[43–45] For highly complex procedures and management of severely ill patients, the evidence seems clear that greater individual and institutional experience is associated with improved outcomes.[46–50] Although public reporting of ECMO outcomes is not likely in the near future, the ELSO does have a voluntary database for reporting ECMO site outcomes. To assess the impact of hospital volume on ECMO outcomes, Barbaro and colleagues[51] used the ELSO database to stratify hospitals by volume of patients placed on ECMO annually and compared the survival to discharge of ECMO patients within hospitals with <6, 6–14, 15–30, and >30 cases per year. The authors found that mortality rates varied widely among centers (33–92%) and that ECMO mortality rates were lower in higher-volume centers. Based on this study and pediatric literature,[52–54] concluding that higher-volume ECMO centers have lower mortality, it is reasonable to conclude that patients requiring ECMO should be managed at high-volume centers.

AUTHORS' RECOMMENDATIONS

- The incorporation of low stretch ventilation, early muscle relaxants, and prone positioning should all be considered first-line therapies for ARDS (conventional care).
- Venovenous extracorporeal membrane oxygenation (VV ECMO) was developed in the 1970s, but its use in ARDS has rapidly expanded in the 2010s, particularly after publication of the CESAR trial.
- It is widely believed that a cohort of patients with severe ARDS would probably die without ECMO—this was demonstrated during the H1N1 influenza epidemic of 2009-10.
- To date, a mortality benefit of utilizing ECMO has not been demonstrated in ARDS. The major RCT (ELOIA) was terminated early, with a 28% crossover (to ECMO) rate probably confounding the data.
- ECMO should be considered salvage therapy in patients with refractory hypoxemia or a severe respiratory acidosis that is affecting hemodynamic instability or end-organ function.
- Any mortality benefit for ECMO is likely to be achieved in high-volume centers that have expertise in both conventional strategies and the use of ECMO.

REFERENCES

1. McCarthy FH, McDermott KM, Kini V, et al. Trends in U.S. extracorporeal membrane oxygenation use and outcomes: 2002-2012. *Semin Thorac Cardiovasc Surg.* 2015;27(2):81-88.
2. Schmidt M, Pham T, Arcadipane A, et al. International ECMO Network (ECMONet), and the LIFEGARDS Study Group. Mechanical Ventilation Management during ECMO for ARDS: An International Multicenter Prospective Cohort. *Am J Respir Crit Care Med.* 2019;30. doi:10.1164/rccm.201806-1094OC. [Epub ahead of print.]
3. Castillo JG, Silvay G. John H. Gibbon Jr. and the 60th anniversary of the first successful heart-lung machine. *J Cardiothorac Vasc Anesth.* 2013;27(2):203-207.
4. Maslach-Hubbard A, Bratton SL. Extracorporeal membrane oxygenation for pediatric respiratory failure: history, development and current status. *World J Crit Care Med.* 2013; 2(4):29-39.
5. Zhao J, Wang D, Ballard-Croft C, et al. Hybrid extracorporeal membrane oxygenation using Avalon Elite double lumen cannula ensures adequate heart/brain oxygen supply. *Ann Thorac Surg.* 2017;104(3):847-853.
6. Gutsche JT, Mikkelsen ME, McCarthy FH, et al. Veno-venous extracorporeal life support in hemodynamically unstable patients with ARDS. *Anesth Analg.* 2017;124(3):846-848.
7. Extracorporeal Life Support Organization. *Extracorporeal Life Support Organization ECLS Registry Report International Summary.* July 2018. Available at https://www.elso.org/Registry/RegistryPublications.aspx
8. Peura JL, Colvin-Adams M, Francis GS, et al. Recommendations for the use of mechanical circulatory support: device strategies and patient selection: a scientific statement from the American Heart Association. *Circulation.* 2012;126(22):2648-2667.
9. Patroniti N, Zangrillo A, Pappalardo F, et al. The Italian ECMO network experience during the 2009 influenza A(H1N1) pandemic: preparation for severe respiratory emergency outbreaks. *Intensive Care Med.* 2011;37(9):1447-1457.

10. Peek GJ, Mugford M, Tiruvoipati R, et al. Efficacy and economic assessment of conventional ventilatory support versus extracorporeal membrane oxygenation for severe adult respiratory failure (CESAR): a multicentre randomised controlled trial. *Lancet*. 2009;374(9698):1351-1363.

11. Australia and New Zealand Extracorporeal Membrane Oxygenation (ANZ ECMO) Influenza Investigators; Davies A, Jones D, et al. Extracorporeal membrane oxygenation for 2009 influenza A(H1N1) acute respiratory distress syndrome. *JAMA*. 2009; 302(17):1888-1895.

12. Roch A, Lepaul-Ercole R, Grisoli D, et al. Extracorporeal membrane oxygenation for severe influenza A (H1N1) acute respiratory distress syndrome: a prospective observational comparative study. *Intensive Care Med*. 2010;36(11):1899-1905.

13. Norfolk SG, Hollingsworth CL, Wolfe CR, et al. Rescue therapy in adult and pediatric patients with pH1N1 influenza infection: a tertiary center intensive care unit experience from April to October 2009. *Crit Care Med*. 2010;38(11):2103-2107.

14. Ugarte S, Arancibia F, Soto R. Influenza A pandemics: clinical and organizational aspects: the experience in Chile. *Crit Care Med*. 2010;38(4 suppl):e133-e137.

15. Freed DH, Henzler D, White CW, et al. Extracorporeal lung support for patients who had severe respiratory failure secondary to influenza A (H1N1) 2009 infection in Canada. *Can J Anaesth*. 2010;57(3):240-247.

16. Kao TM, Wu UI, Chen YC. Rapid diagnostic tests and severity of illness in pandemic (H1N1) 2009, Taiwan. *Emerg Infect Dis*. 2010;16(7):1181-1183.

17. Liong T, Lee KL, Poon YS, et al. The first novel influenza A (H1N1) fatality despite antiviral treatment and extracorporeal membrane oxygenation in Hong Kong. *Hong Kong Med J*. 2009;15(5):381-384.

18. Gattinoni L, Carlesso E, Langer T. Clinical review: extracorporeal membrane oxygenation. *Crit Care*. 2011;15(6):243.

19. Sauer CM, Yuh DD, Bonde P. Extracorporeal membrane oxygenation use has increased by 433% in adults in the United States from 2006 to 2011. *ASAIO J*. 2015;61(1):31-36.

20. Blum JM, Lynch WR, Coopersmith CM. Clinical and billing review of extracorporeal membrane oxygenation. *Chest*. 2015;147(6):1697-1703.

21. Sidebotham D, McGeorge A, McGuinness S, Edwards M, Willcox T, Beca J. Extracorporeal membrane oxygenation for treating severe cardiac and respiratory disease in adults. Part 1—overview of extracorporeal membrane oxygenation. *J Cardiothorac Vasc Anesth*. 2009;23(6):886-892.

22. Peek GJ, Clemens F, Elbourne D, et al. CESAR: conventional ventilatory support vs extracorporeal membrane oxygenation for severe adult respiratory failure. *BMC Health Serv Res*. 2006;6:163.

23. Murray JF, Matthay MA, Luce JM, Flick MR. An expanded definition of the adult respiratory distress syndrome. *Am Rev Respir Dis*. 1988;138(3):720-723.

24. Extracorporeal Life Support Organization. *Adult Respiratory Failure Supplement to the ELSO General Guidelines*. Version 1.3. Available at: www.elso.org. Accessed December 8, 2014.

25. Kornfield ZN, Horak J, Gibbs RM, et al. CASE 2—2015: extracorporeal membrane oxygenation as a bridge to clinical recovery in life-threatening autoimmune acute respiratory distress syndrome. *J Cardiothorac Vasc Anesth*. 2015;29(1): 221-228.

26. Oliver WC. Anticoagulation and coagulation management for ECMO. *Semin Cardiothorac Vasc Anesth*. 2009;13(3):154-175.

27. Tulman DB, Stawicki SP, Whitson BA, et al. Veno-venous ECMO: a synopsis of nine key potential challenges, considerations, and controversies. *BMC Anesthesiol*. 2014;14:65.

28. Sidebotham D, Allen SJ, McGeorge A, Ibbott N, Willcox T. Venovenous extracorporeal membrane oxygenation in adults: practical aspects of circuits, cannulae, and procedures. *J Cardiothorac Vasc Anesth*. 2012;26(5):893-909.

29. Extracorporeal Life Support Organization. *General Guidelines for all ECLS Cases*. Version 1.3. Available at https://www.elso.org/Resources/Guidelines.aspx. Accessed March 1, 2018.

30. Zapol WM, Snider MT, Hill JD, et al. Extracorporeal membrane oxygenation in severe acute respiratory failure. A randomized prospective study. *JAMA*. 1979;242(20):2193-2196.

31. Combes A, Hajage D, Capellier G, et al. Extracorporeal membrane oxygenation for severe acute respiratory distress syndrome. *N Engl J Med*. 2018;378(21):1965-1975.

32. Bein T, Weber-Carstens S, Goldmann A, et al. Lower tidal volume strategy ($\approx$3 ml/kg) combined with extracorporeal CO_2 removal versus 'conventional' protective ventilation (6 ml/kg) in severe ARDS: the prospective randomized Xtravent-study. *Intensive Care Med*. 2013;39(5):847-856.

33. Morris AH, Wallace CJ, Menlove RL, et al. Randomized clinical trial of pressure-controlled inverse ratio ventilation and extracorporeal CO_2 removal for adult respiratory distress syndrome. *Am J Respir Crit Care Med*. 1994;149(2 Pt 1):295-305.

34. Acute Respiratory Distress Syndrome Network; Brower RG, Matthay MA, et al. Ventilation with lower tidal volumes as compared with traditional tidal volumes for acute lung injury and the acute respiratory distress syndrome. *N Engl J Med*. 2000;342(18):1301-1308.

35. Papazian L, Forel JM, Gacouin A, et al. Neuromuscular blockers in early acute respiratory distress syndrome. *N Engl J Med*. 2010;363(12):1107-1116.

36. Guérin C, Reignier J, Richard JC, et al. Prone positioning in severe acute respiratory distress syndrome. *N Engl J Med*. 2013;368(23):2159-2168.

37. Zwischenberger JB, Lynch JE. Will CESAR answer the adult ECMO debate? *Lancet*. 2009;374(9698):1307-1308.

38. Hardin CC, Hibbert K. ECMO for severe ARDS. *N Engl J Med*. 2018;378(21):2032-2034.

39. Bartlett RH. Extracorporeal membrane oxygenation for acute respiratory distress syndrome: EOLIA and beyond. *Crit Care Med*. 2019;47(1):114-117.

40. Harrington D, Drazen JM. Learning from a trial stopped by a data and safety monitoring board. *N Engl J Med*. 2018;378(21): 2031-2032.

41. Gattinoni L, Vasques F, Quintel M. Use of ECMO in ARDS: does the EOLIA trial really help? *Crit Care*. 2018;22(1):171.

42. Gutsche J, Vernick W, Miano TA; Penn Lung Rescue. One-year experience with a mobile extracorporeal life support service. *Ann Thorac Surg*. 2017;104(5):1509-1515.

43. Shahian DM, Grover FL, Prager RL, et al. The Society of Thoracic Surgeons voluntary public reporting initiative: the first 4 years. *Ann Surg*. 2015;262(3):526-535, discussion 533-535.

44. Kirklin JK, Naftel DC, Pagani FD, et al. Sixth INTERMACS annual report: a 10,000-patient database. *J Heart Lung Transplant*. 2014;33(6):555-564.

45. Salkowski N, Snyder JJ, Zaun DA, et al. A scientific registry of transplant recipients bayesian method for identifying underperforming transplant programs. *Am J Transplant*. 2014;14(6):1310-1317.

46. Birkmeyer JD, Siewers AE, Finlayson EV, et al. Hospital volume and surgical mortality in the United States. *N Engl J Med*. 2002; 346(15):1128-1137.

47. Cowan Jr JA, Dimick JB, Thompson BG, Stanley JC, Upchurch Jr GR. Surgeon volume as an indicator of outcomes after carotid endarterectomy: an effect independent of specialty practice and hospital volume. *J Am Coll Surg*. 2002;195(6):814-821.

48. Billingsley KG, Morris AM, Dominitz JA, et al. Surgeon and hospital characteristics as predictors of major adverse outcomes following colon cancer surgery: understanding the volume-outcome relationship. *Arch Surg*. 2007;142(1):23-31, discussion 32.

49. Kahn JM, Goss CH, Heagerty PJ, Kramer AA, O'Brien CR, Rubenfeld GD. Hospital volume and the outcomes of mechanical ventilation. *N Engl J Med*. 2006;355(1):41-50.

50. Walkey AJ, Wiener RS. Hospital case volume and outcomes among patients hospitalized with severe sepsis. *Am J Respir Crit Care Med*. 2014;189(5):548-555.

51. Barbaro RP, Odetola FO, Kidwell KM, et al. Association of hospital-level volume of extracorporeal membrane oxygenation cases and mortality. Analysis of the extracorporeal life support organization registry. *Am J Respir Crit Care Med*. 2015;191(8):894-901.

52. Freeman CL, Bennett TD, Casper TC, et al. Pediatric and neonatal extracorporeal membrane oxygenation: does center volume impact mortality? *Crit Care Med*. 2014;42(3):512-519.

53. Karamlou T, Vafaeezadeh M, Parrish AM, et al. Increased extracorporeal membrane oxygenation center case volume is associated with improved extracorporeal membrane oxygenation survival among pediatric patients. *J Thorac Cardiovasc Surg*. 2013;145(2): 470-475.

54. Jen HC, Shew SB. Hospital readmissions and survival after nonneonatal pediatric ECMO. *Pediatrics*. 2010;125(6): 1217-1223.

What Lessons Have We Learned From Epidemiologic Studies of ARDS?

Jordan Anthony Kempker and Greg S. Martin

What lessons have we learned from epidemiologic studies of ARDS? To answer this titular question, we first must set a common foundation for readers. ARDS is defined elsewhere in this book, and epidemiology can be defined as "the study of the occurrence and distribution of health-related events, states, and processes in specified populations, including the study of the determinants influencing such processes, and the application of this knowledge to control relevant health problems."[1] With this in mind, we will approach this chapter by distilling several salient lessons from current observational and population-based studies that can be applied to the practice and interpretation of evidence-based critical care medicine. The first lesson takes a brief detour from this objective to provide a context for the heterogeneity of the data apparent in the subsequent sections and can be skipped by readers who do not wish to delve into the weeds of epidemiology. The subsequent lessons address what we know about (1) the burden of ARDS, (2) how physicians perform in the recognition and treatment of ARDS, (3) the discernible trends in burden and outcomes, (4) whether there are true biologic phenotypes of the syndrome, and (5) the possibility of ARDS prevention. Certain lessons generally found under the rubric of epidemiology—such as risk factors, natural history, analysis of case definitions, and long-term outcomes—have been intentionally given minimal or no treatment in this chapter given their coverage elsewhere in this book.

LESSON 1: CRITICAL CARE EPIDEMIOLOGY IS CHALLENGING

There are several factors that contribute to the variability found in epidemiologic studies of ARDS and their clarification can help replace confusion with nuanced understanding.

First, there is unavoidable heterogeneity in the epidemiology of ARDS due to the lack of specificity of the clinical definition. Precise and reliable epidemiology requires a precise and reliable case definition of disease and this is not currently possible for ARDS, as it lacks a practical gold standard definition.[2] Unfortunately, although these inadequacies of the Berlin criteria have limited impact on clinical practice because we lack ARDS-specific therapies, they introduce complex heterogeneity into epidemiologic disease estimates. Specifically, the clinical criteria for ARDS inevitably captures ARDS mimickers such as cardiogenic pulmonary edema, pulmonary contusion, and alveolar

hemorrhage, among others.[2] Descriptive epidemiology of ARDS will therefore inevitably differ to the degrees that these ARDS mimickers have different natural histories, respond differently to therapies, and are distributed in a particular population.

Secondly, the epidemiology of ARDS depends on the availability and utilization of critical care resources. Specifically, most studies capture patients who are admitted to the ICU and/or are mechanically ventilated. Therefore, the number and types of cases captured will depend on the availability of these resources and the manner in which they are allocated. For example, a study population drawn from an environment with a large number of available critical care beds and ventilators that are liberally allocated will capture a higher burden of ARDS than a population with a similar underlying ARDS burden that is restricted either by available resources or their allocation.

Thirdly, the epidemiology of ARDS depends on a causal chain that begins with the prevalence of predisposing chronic conditions and includes the incidences of and survival from the requisite inciting, inflammatory injuries for ARDS. Specifically, populations with a higher prevalence of chronic conditions that are risk factors for the acute, inflammatory conditions that cause ARDS may have higher incidences of ARDS. Examples include populations with a higher prevalence of conditions such as immunosuppression or indwelling medical devices that predispose to an underlying cause of ARDS (e.g., sepsis) or conditions such as chronic alcoholism that predispose more specifically to the development of ARDS. Independent of these chronic predisposing conditions, the incidence of ARDS is also directly proportional to the incidences of the acute conditions of sepsis, trauma, and aspiration, among others, in a population. These can depend on such factors as the local patterns of infection, immunization, and risk for major trauma.

Finally, given that ARDS generally almost invariably occurs 1–7 days after the inciting, inflammatory event, populations with higher short-term survival from these acute conditions may demonstrate a higher burden of ARDS.

All of these factors, along with the seasonal variations in ARDS incidence, contribute to the heterogeneity of results from epidemiologic studies of ARDS and urge us to interpret all results within the context of the population in which they were studied. A final point from this section is that the above concepts apply to much of critical care epidemiology. One could easily substitute such words as *sepsis, shock,* or *delirium* for ARDS in the above paragraphs. This lesson from the epidemiology of ARDS is that the study of many of the defining syndromes in critical care is difficult, fraught with an imprecision that leads to difficulty in understanding the burdens of disease and in developing and testing new therapies.

LESSON 2: ARDS IS RARE IN THE POPULATION BUT COMMON IN THE ADULT ICU

Knowing the burden of ARDS helps critical care physicians contextualize their individual experiences of ARDS in the larger scope of the population and participate in the development of appropriate institutional and public health plans for the allocation of resources to this problem. At a general population level, the majority of epidemiologic results describe ARDS as a rare disease (Table 21.1). With the exception of the 1999–2000 King

TABLE 21.1 Summary of Published Incidence Estimates of Acute Respiratory Distress Syndrome (ARDS).

Year (Timespan of Study Sample)	Location of Study Sample	Severity of ARDS	Estimate
Incidence per 100,000 Person-Years			
2007[28]	Finland	Moderate, severe	5.0
2008–2009[29]	Spain	Moderate, severe	7.2
2010[22]	Iceland	Moderate, severe	9.6
2005[30]	Netherlands	Moderate, severe	24.0
2008[17]	Olmsted Co., Minnesota, USA	Moderate, severe	38.0
1999–2000[31]	King Co., Washington, USA	Moderate, severe	58.7
1999[32]	Southern, Western, and Tasmania, Australia	Moderate, severe	28.0
2007[33]	Vitória, Brazil	Moderate, severe	6.3
Incidence Among Admissions to Intensive Care Unit			
2008–2009 (1 year)[29]	Spain	All	2%
2005 (3 days)[30]	Netherlands	All	12%
2006 (10 summer/ fall weeks)[34]	Ireland	All	19%
1999 (2 winter months)[35]	10 European countries	All	7%
2014 (4 winter weeks)[5]	50 countries worldwide	All	10%

County, Washington, USA estimate, all of the incidence estimates for moderate–severe ARDS fit within the definitions of a rare disease from the US Food and Drug Administration (FDA) (i.e., affecting <200,000 persons per year, extrapolated using above estimates with 2018 US population estimates) and the European Union (<1 case per 2000 persons per year).[3,4]

In contrast, within the critical care unit ARDS is a common problem. The two epidemiologic metrics relevant to understanding the burden of ARDS within the ICU are (1) the ICU incidence of ARDS, derived as the number of ARDS cases per ICU admission per unit of time and (2) the ICU prevalence of ARDS, derived as the number of ARDS cases per ICU bed averaged over a period of time. In the current literature, the incidence of cases of ARDS is most commonly reported and estimates have varied (see Table 22.1). The largest and most recent study, gathered over 4 winter weeks from ICUs reporting any cases of ARDS across 50 countries worldwide, reported an average ICU incidence of ARDS of 10%.[5] This most recent study (Large observational study to UNderstand the Global impact of Severe Acute respiratory FailurE [LUNG SAFE]) also reported the ICU prevalence of ARDS at 0.42 case per ICU bed over 4 weeks, with substantial regional variation (lowest regional average of 0.27 case/ICU bed in Asia to highest regional average of 0.57 case per ICU bed in Oceania).[5] Prevalence estimates exceed those of incidence due to duration of mechanical ventilation, ICU length of stay, and ICU mortality in ARDS relative to other common ICU problems. Point estimates from two large, recent studies demonstrate a substantially longer duration of mechanical ventilation in ARDS patients than in mechanically ventilated patients at high risk of developing ARDS: median (interquartile range) days of invasive mechanical ventilation among survivors 8 (4–15) vs. 2 (1–4), respectively.[5,6] Thus, in our opinion, the ICU prevalence represents a critical metric of the burden of ARDS in the ICU because it captures the high amount of ICU resources used and occupied by these very ill patients, further translating into a large economic burden for a hospital system and for society.

As a point of comparison with pediatric ARDS, a recent meta-analysis has summarized the main findings regarding the population and ICU incidence of ARDS among children (between <36 weeks and <18 years of age).[7] This study demonstrated a marked heterogeneity of the estimated incidence of ARDS, making it difficult to draw generalizable comments about this population. The pooled estimates of incidences were 3.5 cases per 100,000 children per year and 2.3% of admissions to pediatric ICU.

LESSON 3: THERE ARE DIFFERENT ARDS PHENOTYPES

With a variety of acute conditions that can precede ARDS, it is not surprising that there are several characteristics upon which ARDs can be differentially categorized and described. These include late vs. early onset, direct vs. indirect mechanisms of lung injury, and trauma vs. nontrauma, with considerable overlap between different categorization schemes.

First, we summarize three studies that approach the categorization of ARDS along different axes yet appear to demonstrate that there may be inflammatory and noninflammatory phenotypes of ARDS. One analysis of patients from two ARDSnet trials demonstrated that patients with nontrauma-related ARDS had a higher prevalence of chronic illness and higher severity of acute illness, notably characterized by more circulatory shock and higher odds of mortality. Interestingly, while the higher odds of mortality remained significant when adjusting for APACHE III score, they became insignificant when adjusting baseline biomarkers of capillary barrier dysfunction.[8] Another analysis approached the same dataset without the preconceived categorizations of trauma and nontrauma, utilizing the statistical technique of *latent class analysis* to identify unobserved (latent) distinct categorizations of disease from baseline clinical and physiologic characteristics. This analysis revealed two distinguishable ARDS phenotypes. One phenotype was comparatively defined by increased inflammatory markers, acidosis, and circulatory shock, with up to a three times higher prevalence of vasopressor use. Sepsis was the most frequent inciting event in this inflammatory phenotype, while trauma was more common in the noninflammatory phenotype. Furthermore, the inflammatory phenotype was associated with higher mortality, fewer ventilator-free days, and fewer organ failure-free days.[9] Finally, a third study comparing sepsis and nonsepsis (including trauma, aspiration, and transfusion-related) ARDS, demonstrated that sepsis-related ARDS patients had higher APACHE III scores, a higher proportion of pre-ICU hospital stay >48 hours, a higher proportion of circulatory shock at ARDS diagnosis, and a higher mortality that was not significant when adjusting for acute and chronic illness severity.[10] While this last study did not examine inflammatory markers, the characteristics of the sepsis ARDS appear consistent with the other categorizations of inflammatory ARDS. This inflammatory vs. noninflammatory dichotomy may also be present specifically within trauma-related ARDS. One study using latent class analysis on a prospective cohort of trauma patients identified two classes of ARDS phenotypes within this trauma population seemingly defined by early vs. late onset (dichotomized by onset within 48 hours of trauma). Early onset was associated with higher severity of thoracic trauma, lower systolic blood pressure, with higher concentrations of biomarkers of proinflammatory endothelial injury and permeability, but no differences in mortality.[11]

While these data are still speculative, they may have important clinical implications. The latent class analysis of two ARDSnet trials demonstrated that the effect of a higher positive end-expiratory pressure (PEEP) strategy was different between patients recategorized as inflammatory and noninflammatory ARDS. Specifically, when compared with the lower PEEP strategy, the higher PEEP strategy was associated with a higher mortality in the inflammatory ARDS phenotype but a lower mortality among the noninflammatory phenotype.[9] While these data are not yet definitive and must be considered hypothesis-generating at this point, prior physiologic studies and broader meta-analyses in ARDS have demonstrated potentially differential effects of PEEP by ARDS characteristics.[12,13] A final word on these inflammatory and noninflammatory phenotypes within the data is that it is possible that the noninflammatory phenotype actually represents a group of ARDS mimickers with better outcomes than true pathophysiologic ARDS. Until the development of a reliable biomarker for ARDS, this heterogeneity among ARDS study groups will continue to be a challenge in epidemiology and clinical trials.

LESSON 4: ARDS IS UNDERRECOGNIZED AND TREATMENT STRATEGIES UNDERUTILIZED

This section relies on the findings of the largest and most comprehensive recent study on ARDS epidemiology in 50 countries over 4 winter weeks: LUNG SAFE.[5] In this study 34% of ARDS was recognized by clinicians at the time of fulfillment of Berlin criteria, with 60% recognized later in their clinical course. Although this is evidence for inappropriately delayed diagnosis, it is tempered by the fact that 17% of patients no longer met Berlin criteria 24 hours after initial fulfillment. Some of the factors associated with increased recognition were systems level (higher nurse–patient ratios, higher physician–patient ratios) and others were more relevant to individual patient factors (ratio of partial pressure of arterial oxygen to the fraction of inspired oxygen [PaO_2/FiO_2], presence of pneumonia, or pancreatitis as inciting factors). Factors associated with lower recognition included cardiac failure as the inciting cause of ARDS. Importantly, there were treatment differences associated with physician recognition. Patients with ARDS recognized by physicians had lower average tidal volumes, higher average PEEP, and substantially more use of adjunctive treatments (44% vs. 22%). When looking at just the severe ARDS patients in this study in whom most trials of adjunctive therapy more accurately apply, physician recognition was still associated with more frequent use of adjunctive therapies (60% vs. 43%).[5]

Other epidemiologic data lend support to the finding that provider and hospital experience with ARDS may be associated with better outcomes, such as studies that examine the associations between hospital case volume and outcomes. One US study using national-level administrative data and one French study demonstrated that higher average annual hospital case volume of ARDS were associated with lower hospital case-fatality rates.[14,15] These limited data may lead one to speculate that increased exposure to ARDS increases recognition and therapeutic attention, and thus better outcomes. Practical and proactive responses to these speculations may include increased education of providers through campaigns similar to the Surviving Sepsis campaign, simplifying ARDS through checklists, or the regionalization of ARDS care to more experienced treatment centers.

LESSON 5: ARDS MAY BE PREVENTABLE

Concepts regarding the prevention of ARDS have been tested since the 1980s with early steroid therapy; however, they seem to have gained wider interest in the past decade. In 2007, one single-center observational study demonstrated that quality improvement initiatives to reduce tidal volumes in all mechanically ventilated patients and adopt restrictive transfusion practices in three ICUs paralleled significant reductions in the ICU incidence of ARDS over 4 years.[16] Then, in 2011, another group published the 8-year decline in population incidence of ARDS in Olmsted County, Minnesota, that paralleled hospital-wide initiatives precisely aimed at reducing hospital-acquired ARDS and included decreased blood product transfusions, increased procurement of male predominant plasma for transfusion products, low tidal volume ventilation in all ventilated patients, and improved treatment in sepsis and pneumonia.[17] This provocative epidemiologic study further demonstrated that the declines in ARDS incidence were primarily from declines in hospital-acquired ARDS.

These and other findings perhaps helped spur the development of the Prevention and Early Treatment of Acute Lung Injury (PETAL) trial network and the consensus development of tools such as the Checklist for Lung Injury Prevention (CLIP) that was used as the baseline cointervention for the clinical trial of aspirin to prevent ARDS.[18,19] While the epidemiologic studies support the implementation of *system-wide*, nonharmful strategies for ARDS prevention, they have set a bar that may be elusive for the testing and application of *individual-level* strategies for prevention. The differences between systems- and individual-level approaches lie in the difficulty in predicting ARDS for individuals and the low ICU incidence of ARDS: these factors, respectively, translate into generally low overall ARDS event rates for preventive trials and unpredictable heterogeneity of ARDS rates among trial arms, making differences difficult to detect. In response, the Lung Injury Prediction Score (LIPS) was developed to improve prediction in clinical trials.[6,20,21] However, in validation studies, a LIPS ≥ 4 had variable discriminatory power for predicting ARDS in at-risk patients (areas under the curve of 0.84 and 0.62).[6,20,21] Furthermore, in patients already with risk for ARDS who additionally had a LIPS ≥ 4, the overall incidence of ARDS was low (7.0–9.5%).[18] These low event rates and the unavoidable heterogeneity in the population require large sample sizes for adequate trial power and therefore will continue to make the study of individual-level prediction difficult.

LESSON 6: THE TRENDS IN ARDS INCIDENCE AND MORTALITY ARE UNKNOWN

One of the fundamental questions of descriptive epidemiology is: are we doing better? Not surprisingly, the above-mentioned challenges in examining the burden of ARDS within a fixed time period are compounded when studying trends in ARDS over time. Among studies examining both incidence and outcomes there are inconsistent findings. One aforementioned study from 2001 to 2008 in Olmsted County, Minnesota, demonstrated decreases in incidence but not in case fatality.[17] In contrast, a study of nationwide incidence in Iceland from 1988 to 2010 documented increases in population incidence of ARDS with decreases in case fatality.[22] Similar to these

findings, a study of nationwide incidence in Taiwan from 1997 to 2011 observed increases in incidence and decreases in case fatality.[23] Yet another study demonstrated decreases in ICU incidence of ARDS with stable case fatality.[24]

Among studies only examining outcomes, there have been three meta-analyses with net trials that demonstrated declines in mortality.[25] Another meta-analysis inclusive of observational and experimental studies from 1994 to 2006 without individual-level data for confounding adjustment demonstrated higher variability in ARDS mortality rates but still an overall pooled significant decline of about 1% per year.[26] Another meta-analysis including studies over the same time period but with different exclusion criteria (did not include retrospective studies and combined outcomes of intervention and control arms of trials rather than only using control arm mortality rates) did not demonstrate decreases in ARDS case fatality rates over time. Furthermore, this study demonstrated higher mortality from observational than experimental studies, calling into question the generalizability of the ARDSnet meta-analyses to the general population.[27]

CONCLUSION

In summary, there are several lessons to be distilled from epidemiologic studies of ARDS. While the precise epidemiologic study of ARDS is challenging due to the lack of a gold standard diagnostic test, we observe that ARDS is rare in the population but a prevalent and persistent problem in ICUs. Under the current clinical definition of ARDS, there are probably different phenotypes of ARDS, perhaps characterized by the level of underlying inflammation, which may have therapeutic implications. ARDS appears to be underrecognized, with proven treatment strategies underutilized, and there is provocative early evidence that ARDS can be prevented using systems-level strategies. Finally, the question of whether or not ARDS mortality is improving remains difficult to answer given conflicting results in the current literature.

AUTHORS' RECOMMENDATIONS
- There is much heterogeneity in the epidemiologic estimates of acute respiratory distress syndrome (ARDS) due to the lack of a highly specific gold standard case definition, differences in the prevalence of underlying risk factors and inciting inflammatory events, and dependence on the availability and allocation of critical care resources.
- ARDS is a rare disease in the general population but a very common one in the intensive care unit (ICU), afflicting between 2% and 19% of ICU admissions and consuming a large amount of ICU resources due to long durations of mechanical ventilation.
- There are probably inflammatory and noninflammatory phenotypes of ARDS and it is yet to be determined whether these may respond differently to ventilator strategies.
- ARDS is underrecognized by physicians, resulting in the underutilization of beneficial treatment strategies and suggesting the development of strategies to improve early recognition.

- ARDS may be preventable through systems-based strategies of reducing transfusions, high quality of care for underlying causes of ARDS, and more ubiquitous use of lung protective ventilation.
- Temporal trends in ARDS mortality are unknown and likely to be modest, suggesting that we may improve through larger campaigns for early recognition, treatment, and prevention.

REFERENCES

1. Porta M. *A Dictionary of Epidemiology*. 6th ed. New York: Oxford University Press; 2014.
2. Ranieri VM, Rubenfeld GD, Thompson BT, et al. Acute respiratory distress syndrome: the Berlin definition. *JAMA*. 2012;307(23): 2526-2533.
3. US Food and Drug Administration. Developing products for rare diseases & conditions. 2018. Available at: https://www.fda.gov/ForIndustry/DevelopingProductsforRareDiseasesConditions/default.htm. Accessed May 23, 2018.
4. European Commission. Rare diseases. Available at: https://ec.europa.eu/health/rare_diseases/overview_en.
5. Bellani G, Laffey JG, Pham T, et al. Epidemiology, patterns of care, and mortality for patients with acute respiratory distress syndrome in intensive care units in 50 countries. *JAMA*. 2016;315(8):788-800.
6. Neto AS, Barbas CSV, Simonis FD, et al. Epidemiological characteristics, practice of ventilation, and clinical outcome in patients at risk of acute respiratory distress syndrome in intensive care units from 16 countries (PRoVENT): an international, multicentre, prospective study. *Lancet Respir Med*. 2016; 4(11):882-893.
7. Schouten LR, Veltkamp F, Bos AP, et al. Incidence and mortality of acute respiratory distress syndrome in children: a systematic review and meta-analysis. *Crit Care Med*. 2016;44(4):819-829.
8. Calfee CS, Eisner MD, Ware LB, et al. Trauma-associated lung injury differs clinically and biologically from acute lung injury due to other clinical disorders. *Crit Care Med*. 2007;35(10): 2243-2250.
9. Calfee CS, Delucchi K, Parsons PE, et al. Subphenotypes in acute respiratory distress syndrome: latent class analysis of data from two randomised controlled trials. *Lancet Respir Med*. 2014;2(8):611-620.
10. Sheu CC, Gong MN, Zhai R, et al. Clinical characteristics and outcomes of sepsis-related vs non-sepsis-related ARDS. *Chest*. 2010;138(3):559-567.
11. Reilly JP, Bellamy S, Shashaty MG, et al. Heterogeneous phenotypes of acute respiratory distress syndrome after major trauma. *Ann Am Thorac Soc*. 2014;11(5):728-736.
12. Briel M, Meade M, Mercat A, et al. Higher vs lower positive end-expiratory pressure in patients with acute lung injury and acute respiratory distress syndrome: systematic review and meta-analysis. *JAMA*. 2010;303(9):865-873.
13. Gattinoni L, Pelosi P, Suter PM, et al. Acute respiratory distress syndrome caused by pulmonary and extrapulmonary disease. Different syndromes? *Am J Respir Crit Care Med*. 1998; 158(1):3-11.
14. Ike JD, Kempker JA, Kramer MR, Martin GS. The association between acute respiratory distress syndrome hospital case volume and mortality in a U.S. cohort, 2002-2011. *Crit Care Med*. 2018;46(5):764-773.
15. Dres M, Austin PC, Pham T, et al. Acute respiratory distress syndrome cases volume and ICU mortality in medical patients. *Crit Care Med*. 2018;46(1):e33-e40.
16. Yilmaz M, Keegan MT, Iscimen R, et al. Toward the prevention of acute lung injury: protocol-guided limitation of large tidal volume ventilation and inappropriate transfusion. *Crit Care Med*. 2007;35(7):1660-1666; quiz 1667.
17. Li G, Malinchoc M, Cartin-Ceba R, et al. Eight-year trend of acute respiratory distress syndrome: a population-based study in Olmsted County, Minnesota. *Am J Respir Crit Care Med*. 2011;183(1):59-66.
18. Kor DJ, Carter RE, Park PK, et al. Effect of aspirin on development of ARDS in at-risk patients presenting to the emergency department: the LIPS—a randomized clinical trial. *JAMA*. 2016;315(22):2406-2414.
19. Litell JM, Gajic O, Sevransky J, et al. Multicenter consensus development of a checklist for lung injury prevention. *Crit Care*. 2012;16(Suppl 1):P504.
20. Gajic O, Dabbagh O, Park PK, et al. Early identification of patients at risk of acute lung injury: evaluation of lung injury prediction score in a multicenter cohort study. *Am J Respir Crit Care Med*. 2011;183(4):462-470.
21. Trillo-Alvarez C, Cartin-Ceba R, Kor DJ, et al. Acute lung injury prediction score: derivation and validation in a population-based sample. *Eur Respir J*. 2011;37(3):604-609.
22. Sigurdsson MI, Sigvaldason K, Gunnarsson TS, et al. Acute respiratory distress syndrome: nationwide changes in incidence, treatment and mortality over 23 years. *Acta Anaesthesiol Scand*. 2013;57(1):37-45.
23. Chen W, Chen YY, Tsai CF, et al. Incidence and outcomes of acute respiratory distress syndrome: a nationwide registry-based study in Taiwan, 1997 to 2011. *Medicine*. 2015;94(43):e1849.
24. Pierrakos C, Vincent JL. The changing pattern of acute respiratory distress syndrome over time: a comparison of two periods. *Eur Respir J*. 2012;40(3):589-595.
25. Cooke CR, Erickson SE, Watkins TR, et al. Age-, sex-, and race-based differences among patients enrolled versus not enrolled in acute lung injury clinical trials. *Crit Care Med*. 2010;38(6): 1450-1457.
26. Zambon M, Vincent JL. Mortality rates for patients with acute lung injury/ARDS have decreased over time. *Chest*. 2008;133(5): 1120-1127.
27. Phua J, Badia JR, Adhikari NK, et al. Has mortality from acute respiratory distress syndrome decreased over time? A systematic review. *Am J Respir Crit Care Med*. 2009;179(3):220-227.
28. Linko R, Okkonen M, Pettilä V, et al. Acute respiratory failure in intensive care units. FINNALI: a prospective cohort study. *Intensive Care Med*. 2009;35(8):1352-1361.
29. Villar J, Blanco J, Añón JM, et al. The ALIEN study: incidence and outcome of acute respiratory distress syndrome in the era of lung protective ventilation. *Intensive Care Med*. 2011; 37(12):1932-1941.
30. Wind J, Versteegt J, Twisk J, et al. Epidemiology of acute lung injury and acute respiratory distress syndrome in The Netherlands: a survey. *Respir Med*. 2007;101(10):2091-2098.
31. Rubenfeld GD, Caldwell E, Peabody E, et al. Incidence and outcomes of acute lung injury. *N Engl J Med*. 2005;353(16):1685-1693.
32. Bersten AD, Edibam C, Hunt T, Moran J. Incidence and mortality of acute lung injury and the acute respiratory

distress syndrome in three Australian States. *Am J Respir Crit Care Med*. 2002;165(4):443-448.

33. Caser EB, Zandonade E, Pereira E, et al. Impact of distinct definitions of acute lung injury on its incidence and outcomes in Brazilian ICUs: prospective evaluation of 7,133 patients. *Crit Care Med*. 2014;42(3):574-582.

34. Irish Critical Care Trials Group. Acute lung injury and the acute respiratory distress syndrome in Ireland: a prospective

audit of epidemiology and management. *Crit Care*. 2008; 12(1):R30.

35. Brun-Buisson C, Minelli C, Bertolini G, et al. Epidemiology and outcome of acute lung injury in European intensive care units. Results from the ALIVE study. *Intensive Care Med*. 2004;30(1):51-61.

22

What Are the Long-Term Outcomes after ARDS?

Catherine L. Hough

INTRODUCTION

It has been five decades since the original description of the acute respiratory distress syndrome (ARDS). Early reports had a narrow focus, primarily describing pulmonary pathophysiology, mechanical ventilation and intensive care unit (ICU) treatments, and short-term outcomes, such as in-hospital mortality.[1] Currently, research and clinical care encompass a broader and longer view of ARDS patients and their recovery, recognizing the far-reaching impacts of survival from and recovery after ARDS.

It is now clear that physical, mental health, and cognitive impairments—the recognized domains of the Post Intensive Care Syndrome (PICS)—have a lasting impact on most survivors of ARDS as they struggle to return home, return to work, cope with disability and financial strain, and avoid rehospitalization and death. Most aspects of ARDS long-term outcomes appear to be common across survivors of acute and critical illness.

This chapter will focus on aspects of survivorship that are important after ARDS, including (1) survival after hospital discharge, (2) respiratory outcomes, (3) health-related quality of life, and (4) PICS.

SURVIVAL AFTER HOSPITAL DISCHARGE

ARDS is associated with high initial mortality, with 20%–45% of patients dying before hospital discharge.[2-4] The risk of death after discharge is also high. A single-center study of 493 hospital survivors of ARDS reported 1-year mortality of 22%.[5] ARDS hospital survivors were more likely to die in the first year if they were older, had higher severity of illness (measured by organ failures and APACHE II score) and/or key comorbidities (HIV, cancer, and chronic kidney disease). Patients were more likely to survive to 1 year if they lived at home at the time of admission, and if ARDS was trauma-related. Discharge destination was also associated with 1-year mortality, with home or inpatient rehabilitation associated with lower risk than discharge to a nursing home or hospice.

The attributable risk of ARDS on longer term mortality among hospital survivors remains unclear. A single-center study of 127 patients with ARDS associated with sepsis or trauma and 127 critically ill controls (without ARDS but matched for ARDS risk factor and other key covariates) found no association between ARDS and 5-year survival (Cox hazard ratio of 1.0, 95% confidence interval [CI] 0.47–2.09).[6] More recently, a single center study of 252 patients with ARDS and 252 matched hospitalized controls found an association between ARDS and increased late mortality. This study demonstrated a significantly increased risk of death among ARDS patients who survived initial hospitalization, and showed that increased risk persisted 90 days and 6 months later.[7] Unadjusted 5-year mortality was approximately 40% for hospital survivors with ARDS compared to 20% among those without (adjusted Cox hazard ratio 1.70, 95% CI 1.29–2.25).

Why might the conclusions of these two studies differ? It is possible that the Davidson study, with only 31 deaths observed, was underpowered to detect a true association between ARDS and late mortality. It is also possible that the different conclusions were based on key differences in control patients. Controls were all critically ill in the Davidson study, while only 28 of the 252 controls in the Biehl study required mechanical ventilation. Wunsch et al. have demonstrated previously that mechanical ventilation is an independent risk factor for mortality after hospital discharge among Medicare beneficiaries.[8] This finding suggests that mechanical ventilation could be in the causal pathway between ARDS and late mortality, and identifies an important topic for additional study.

RESPIRATORY OUTCOMES AFTER ARDS

Early follow-up studies of survivors of ARDS focused on lung recovery, including assessment of respiratory symptoms, chest imaging, and pulmonary function.

Symptoms

Dyspnea on exertion may be the most common respiratory symptom after ARDS. In a study where patients were surveyed a median of 15 months after ARDS, 36% reported shortness of breath.[9] Other symptoms included cough, wheezing, and chest tightness. The severity of symptoms generally improved over time. A study of 30 ARDS survivors found that the three patients with progressive dyspnea all had upper airway obstruction explaining worsening symptoms.[10] These reports suggest that symptomatic improvement is to be expected after ARDS, and that progressive respiratory symptoms during recovery indicate clinical evaluation for alternative etiologies.

Imaging

While all patients with ARDS have bilateral lung infiltrates on chest radiograph or computed tomography (CT) at the time of diagnosis, marked improvement in imaging occurs along with resolution of respiratory failure. Of 85 patients across multiple reports with chest imaging performed around 3 months after ARDS onset, only 16 (19%) chest radiographs were found to have persistent abnormalities. Reticular patterns and bilateral basilar interstitial infiltrates were most commonly reported.[11] Herridge reported similar results, with 20% of patients' chest radiographs demonstrating persistent abnormalities at 1 year.[12]

Persistent abnormalities are recognized more commonly on CT, however. For example, a study of 27 survivors imaged between 3 and 9 months after ARDS found persistent ground glass opacities in 17 (63%) patients occupying less than 1% of the lung parenchyma.[13] Reticular changes with parenchymal distortion were detected in 23 (85%) patients in the same study, primarily in small anterior lung regions.

It appears that these minor radiographic abnormalities do not change significantly after the first year. In a more recent study, high resolution CT imaging of 24 5-year survivors in the Herridge Toronto cohort described persistent abnormalities in 18 patients (75%), which were minor and predominantly located in anterior lung regions.[14] Fibrotic changes, consisting of intralobular septal thickening in 9 patients and honeycombing in 5 were the most common; ground glass opacities and decreased attenuation consistent with emphysema or mosaicism were also noted. This investigation found no association between lung imaging and pulmonary symptoms, pulmonary function testing, or health-related quality of life.

Pulmonary Function Testing

There have been a number of prospective studies that performed repeated pulmonary function testing of ARDS survivors during the early months and years of recovery. The longest study of pulmonary function after ARDS was performed by Herridge et al. in Toronto.[12] At 3 months after ARDS, most of the 71 patients who completed testing demonstrated mild or moderate reductions in forced vital capacity (FVC) (median 72% predicted, interquartile range 57%–96%), forced expiratory volume in 1 second (FEV1) (median 75% predicted, interquartile range 58%–92%), and diffusing capacity (median 63% predicted, interquartile range 54%–77%).

Across the cohort, all test results improved between 3 and 12 months post-ARDS, with most patients ultimately reaching the normal range of at least 80% predicted on spirometric measures (FVC and FEV1). Diffusing capacity improved at 12 months but continued to be at least mildly impaired for most patients. Among the 64 patients who survived to 5-year assessment, measures of pulmonary function were in the normal range for most, and abnormalities in the 25 percentile were mild (70%–78% predicted).[15] While the overall tendency is one of marked improvement in pulmonary function to normal or near normal, there was a small minority of ARDS survivors with severe pulmonary impairment that did not improve over time, particularly as reported in older series.[16]

It is plausible that ventilator-induced lung injury contributes to respiratory impairment after ARDS. The persistent fibrotic changes in the nondependent lung regions—regions most at risk of overdistension—are consistent with this hypothesis. Therefore, it may follow that respiratory outcomes are improved in the era of lung protective treatments, including low tidal volume ventilation and extracorporeal membrane oxygenation (ECMO). However, given the mortality benefit associated with lung protection, it is difficult to compare outcomes before and after implementation of low tidal volume ventilation. Needham studied long-term outcomes of >200 patients enrolled in an ARDS Network trial (in which low tidal volume was protocolized and achieved with high adherence),[2] and found impairments in FVC and FEV1 at 6 months; as noted in other reports, these abnormalities resolved in most patients by 12 months.[17] Additionally, a recent study of 21 survivors of severe ARDS treated with ECMO reported similar follow-up abnormalities on imaging in addition to potentially improved pulmonary function and reduced symptom burden.[18] The patients included in this ECMO cohort were generally young and without comorbidities, potentially quite different than those included in prior cohorts. For these reasons, the impact of ventilation strategies on respiratory outcomes of ARDS survivors remains unclear.

The studies cited cannot inform the independent contribution of ARDS on respiratory symptoms, imaging, and pulmonary function testing among survivors is unknown because only ARDS patients were included. While ARDS may be causally associated with many of the respiratory abnormalities detected among survivors, there are also many non-ARDS factors that could contribute. For example, premorbid pulmonary exposures and conditions (e.g., tobacco, air pollution, and underlying pulmonary disease) may be risk factors for ARDS while known ARDS risk factors (e.g., pneumonia or chest trauma) may affect respiratory outcomes even without ARDS; and ICU treatments and complications (e.g., method of mechanical ventilation, pulmonary emboli, and neuromuscular weakness) may also impact outcomes. Therefore, the direct relationship between ARDS and long-term respiratory outcomes remains unknown.

In conclusion, most survivors have rapid improvement in respiratory function with the resolution of symptoms, the clearance of infiltrates on chest radiograph and of mild fibrotic changes on chest CT, and the normalization of spirometric measures of lung function and diffusing capacity within the first year post-ARDS. However, a sizeable minority of patients have continued respiratory symptoms and abnormalities on pulmonary function testing.

HEALTH-RELATED QUALITY OF LIFE AFTER ARDS

The first prospective study of health-related quality of life followed 52 survivors in Seattle over the first 12 months after ARDS. This investigation, conducted in the early 1990s, had patients complete questionnaires at hospital discharge, and 3, 6, and 12 months later.[19] This Seattle cohort was characterized by significant impairments in health-related quality of life (measured by the Sickness Impact Profile) that were not explained by the resolution of respiratory symptoms or abnormalities on pulmonary function testing. Larger cohorts—including the Toronto cohort and the Needham ALTOS cohort—confirmed these findings and identified profound reductions in both physical and mental health-related quality of life at 3 months after ARDS, with marked improvement but not full recovery at 12 months.[12,15,17] Physical health domains consistently revealed greater impairment than measures of mental health, with scores a full standard deviation below age- and sex-adjusted norms at 12 months after ARDS. There may be additional improvement in physical health-related quality of life after the first year, but loss to follow-up over time makes interpretation challenging.[15]

Several studies have attempted to investigate the independent association between ARDS and impaired health-related quality of life. Davidson et al. compared standard form (SF-36) scores between survivors of ARDS and matched survivors of critical illness without ARDS. ARDS survivors had significantly lower SF-36 scores in 7 of 8 domains, with the largest decrement in the domain of physical function.[20] While this study suggests that ARDS is associated with worse outcomes, it could not determine if health-related quality of life was worse *before* the onset of critical illness among the patients with ARDS compared to those without.

In an attempt to account for pre-ARDS health-related quality of life, Biehl used SF-12 surveys for 41 patients with ARDS (54% completed by patient) and for 57 with risk factors but without ARDS (75% completed by patient) during the index hospitalization.[21] There were no significant differences in either baseline physical or mental component scores between those with or without ARDS, suggesting that premorbid health-related quality of life may be less likely to drive the observed differences. In contrast, Brown et al. did not detect a difference in SF-12 scores at 6 months between ARDS and non-ARDS groups. However, only 26 patients with ARDS completed the 6 months follow-up, limiting the power of the study. Interestingly, initial severity of illness was not associated with health utility among survivors of ARDS.[22]

In summary, studies suggest that most survivors experience marked impairment in health-related quality of life in the first year after ARDS, particularly in domains reflecting physical health. These impairments may be worse in ARDS survivors than in those with critical illness without ARDS, and this relationship between ARDS and impaired health-related quality of life appears unlikely to be fully explained by premorbid differences. Most patients experience significant improvement over the first year, and others may continue to improve in the years that follow. However, even among 5-year survivors, most continue to experience impaired health-related quality of life.

POST INTENSIVE CARE SYNDROME AFTER ARDS

Studies of ARDS survivors led the way to the recognition of the multiple post-ICU morbidities experienced by patients after critical illness. To promote recognition of this constellation of new or worsening impairments, the term "Post Intensive Care Syndrome (PICS)" was coined at a 2010 stakeholder conference convened by the Society of Critical Care Medicine.[23] PICS in survivors encompasses three domains: physical impairments, cognitive impairments, and mental health. Family members are also at risk for difficulties; PICS-F is recognized in family members of patients experiencing critical illness who are at risk for problems with mental health. A wealth of data from dozens of observational studies of ARDS survivors and their family members has provided the background and the motivation for recognizing PICS, which was recently reviewed by Herridge and colleagues.[24]

Physical Impairments After ARDS

Physical impairment is ubiquitous among survivors of ARDS. During critical illness and early recovery, patients may be too weak to sit upright or to lift limbs up from the bed. Over one-third of patients may demonstrate objective weakness on manual muscle testing at hospital discharge; this number is reduced to 14% at 1 year.[25] One year later, nearly all ARDS patients still describe loss of muscle mass, weakness, and fatigue.[12] Six minute walk testing—an integrative test of cardiopulmonary function, ability to walk, and endurance—reveals profound impairment in the first months after ARDS with improvement over the first year for most patients. However, most patients have marked impairments in walking speed and endurance that persist beyond 1 year, with most walking less than 70% of predicted distance.[15] Impairment in activities of daily living is seen after ARDS as well, particularly in the first months of recovery.[26] Risk factors for physical impairment after ARDS include age, comorbidity, duration of mechanical ventilation, and duration of bedrest.[27,28] It remains unclear if ARDS is an independent risk factor for physical impairment, although certainly patients with ARDS are likely to endure more time on mechanical ventilation and in bed. One study suggested that premorbid disability is more common among patients who develop ARDS than those who do not, likely increasing the prevalence of disability in the post-ARDS population as well.[21]

There are multiple potential mechanisms that might contribute to physical impairment. These include muscle atrophy, which is common among critically ill patients with multiple organ failure,[29] critical illness neuropathy and myopathy,[30] and other conditions (e.g., heterotopic ossification of joints, entrapment neuropathies, and pain) that affect strength and function.[24] It is to be hoped that an increased focus on mobility and rehabilitation during and after critical illness will lead to long-term physical recovery of ARDS survivors. However, to date, few effective strategies have been identified,[31–33] with the strongest signal for benefit seen in the use of a rehabilitation package that included a manual, regular phone follow-up, and two visits to a follow-up clinic.[34] Significant work remains to identify opportunities to prevent and treat physical impairment during and after ARDS.

Mental Health and Cognitive Impairment After ARDS

Mental health impairment is also common among survivors of ARDS.[35] Symptoms of anxiety are perhaps most prevalent, seen in 38%–62% of survivors 1 year or more after critical illness.[28,36] Depression is common as well, with moderate-to-severe symptoms in 26%–41%.[15,25] Symptoms of posttraumatic stress are similarly common.[28,36] Mental health impairment is most common among patients with a history of psychiatric morbidity before critical illness. The magnitude of physical functional impairment during recovery may also be an important risk factor.[37] While severity of critical illness is not consistently associated with mental health impairment after ARDS, demographic factors, such as female sex, younger age, unemployment, and substance use may be.[25] Patients with signs of acute stress disorder during their hospitalization may be at highest risk for symptoms of posttraumatic stress.[38]

Preliminary evidence suggests that mental health outcomes—especially posttraumatic stress—may be improved by strategies that minimize sedation during mechanical ventilation.[39,40] The use of ICU diaries may also be valuable.[41] Considerable ongoing research is exploring other interventions (e.g., psychological interventions during critical illness and coping and mindfulness skills training afterwards) in the hope of improving mental health after the ICU stay.[42,43] While there is no standard of care regarding screening and treatment of mental health impairment after ARDS, care providers should be able to recognize, treat, and make referrals for patients struggling with anxiety, depression, and posttraumatic stress symptoms after hospital discharge.

The vast majority of ARDS survivors experience impairment in cognitive function. At the time of initial hospital discharge, studies have uncovered cognitive impairment in 70%–100% of patients. There is dramatic improvement over time, but persistent impairment is found in 46%-80% of patients at 1 year, 20%–47% at 2 years, and 20% 5 years after ARDS.[44] Memory and executive function are frequently affected. Research is actively investigating potential mechanisms, risk factors, and strategies for improving outcomes.

However, at this time, there are no evidence-based approaches that have been demonstrated to reduce cognitive impairment after ARDS.

CONCLUSION

Like other survivors of critical illness, patients are at risk for ongoing morbidity and mortality in the months and years after ARDS. It remains unclear if ARDS itself is independently associated with poorer long-term outcomes when adjusting for patient demographics, baseline health, and risk factors for the development of ARDS. Most patients have full pulmonary recovery, with mild or no symptoms and minimal radiographic and pulmonary function testing abnormalities detectable after the first year. Physical and cognitive impairments are generally most severe early in recovery and improve over 2–5 years. Mental health impairments are less common, and follow a less predictable pattern of recovery. Little is known about how to prevent, rehabilitate, and cope with new impairments after ARDS. Additional research is ongoing and much needed.

AUTHOR'S RECOMMENDATIONS

- ARDS patients and families should be provided with information and support for the broad range of impairments commonly seen in the months and years after critical illness.
- Pulmonary symptoms should improve over time; worsening of symptoms is not explained by ARDS recovery alone and should be evaluated by a clinician.
- ARDS survivors should be evaluated for physical, cognitive, and mental health impairments during recovery and connected with clinical and supportive resources.
- Additional research is needed to understand the role of ARDS in the long-term outcomes of its survivors, and to investigate effective approaches for the prevention of, rehabilitation from, and adaptation to post-ARDS impairments.

REFERENCES

1. Ashbaugh DG, Bigelow DB, Petty TL, Levine BE. Acute respiratory distress in adults. *Lancet.* 1967;2(7511):319-323.
2. National Heart, Lung, and Blood Institute Acute Respiratory Distress Syndrome (ARDS) Clinical Trials Network, Rice TW, Wheeler AP, et al. Initial trophic vs full enteral feeding in patients with acute lung injury: the EDEN randomized trial. *JAMA.* 2012;307(8):795-803.
3. Bellani G, Laffey JG, Pham T, et al. Epidemiology, patterns of care, and mortality for patients with acute respiratory distress syndrome in intensive care units in 50 countries. *JAMA.* 2016;315(8):788-800.
4. Ranieri VM, Rubenfeld GD, Thompson BT, et al. Acute respiratory distress syndrome: the Berlin Definition. *JAMA.* 2012;307(23):2526-2533.
5. Wang CY, Calfee CS, Paul DW, et al. One-year mortality and predictors of death among hospital survivors of acute respiratory distress syndrome. *Intensive Care Med.* 2014;40(3):388-396.

6. Davidson TA, Rubenfeld GD, Caldwell ES, Hudson LD, Steinberg KP. The effect of acute respiratory distress syndrome on long-term survival. *Am J Respir Crit Care Med.* 1999;160(6):1838-1842.

7. Biehl M, Ahmed A, Kashyap R, Barwise A, Gajic O. The Incremental burden of acute respiratory distress syndrome: long-term follow-up of a population-based nested case-control study. *Mayo Clin Proc.* 2018;93(4):445-452.

8. Wunsch H, Guerra C, Barnato AE, Angus DC, Li G, Linde-Zwirble WT. Three-year outcomes for Medicare beneficiaries who survive intensive care. *JAMA.* 2010;303(9):849-856.

9. Weinert CR, Gross CR, Kangas JR, Bury CL, Marinelli WA. Health-related quality of life after acute lung injury. *Am J Respir Crit Care Med.* 1997;156(4 Pt 1):1120-1128.

10. Elliott CG, Rasmusson BY, Crapo RO. Upper airway obstruction following adult respiratory distress syndrome. An analysis of 30 survivors. *Chest.* 1988;94(3):526-530.

11. Lee CM, Hudson LD. Long-term outcomes after ARDS. *Semin Respir Crit Care Med.* 2001;22(3):327-336.

12. Herridge MS, Cheung AM, Tansey CM, et al. One-year outcomes in survivors of the acute respiratory distress syndrome. *N Engl J Med.* 2003;348(8):683-693.

13. Desai SR, Wells AU, Rubens MB, Evans TW, Hansell DM. Acute respiratory distress syndrome: CT abnormalities at long-term follow-up. *Radiology.* 1999;210(1):29-35.

14. Wilcox ME, Patsios D, Murphy G, et al. Radiologic outcomes at 5 years after severe ARDS. *Chest.* 2013;143(4):920-926.

15. Herridge MS, Tansey CM, Matte A, et al. Functional disability 5 years after acute respiratory distress syndrome. *N Engl J Med.* 2011;364(14):1293-1304.

16. Peters JI, Bell RC, Prihoda TJ, Harris G, Andrews C, Johanson WG. Clinical determinants of abnormalities in pulmonary functions in survivors of the adult respiratory distress syndrome. *Am Rev Respir Dis.* 1989;139(5):1163-1168.

17. Needham DM, Dinglas VD, Bienvenu OJ, et al. One year outcomes in patients with acute lung injury randomised to initial trophic or full enteral feeding: prospective follow-up of EDEN randomised trial. *BMJ.* 2013;346:f1532.

18. Linden VB, Lidegran MK, Frisen G, Dahlgren P, Frenckner BP, Larsen F. ECMO in ARDS: a long-term follow-up study regarding pulmonary morphology and function and health-related quality of life. *Acta Anaesthesiol Scand.* 2009;53(4):489-495.

19. McHugh LG, Milberg JA, Whitcomb ME, Schoene RB, Maunder RJ, Hudson LD. Recovery of function in survivors of the acute respiratory distress syndrome. *Am J Respir Crit Care Med.* 1994;150(1):90-94.

20. Davidson TA, Caldwell ES, Curtis JR, Hudson LD, Steinberg KP. Reduced quality of life in survivors of acute respiratory distress syndrome compared with critically ill control patients. *JAMA.* 1999;281(4):354-360.

21. Biehl M, Kashyap R, Ahmed AH, et al. Six-month quality-of-life and functional status of acute respiratory distress syndrome survivors compared to patients at risk: a population-based study. *Crit Care.* 2015;19:356.

22. Brown SM, Wilson E, Presson AP, et al. Predictors of 6-month health utility outcomes in survivors of acute respiratory distress syndrome. *Thorax.* 2017;72(4):311-317.

23. Needham DM, Davidson J, Cohen H, et al. Improving long-term outcomes after discharge from intensive care unit: report from a stakeholders' conference. *Crit Care Med.* 2012;40(2):502-509.

24. Herridge MS, Moss M, Hough CL, et al. Recovery and outcomes after the acute respiratory distress syndrome (ARDS) in patients and their family caregivers. *Intensive Care Med.* 2016;42(5):725-738.

25. Needham DM, Dinglas VD, Morris PE, et al. Physical and cognitive performance of patients with acute lung injury 1 year after initial trophic versus full enteral feeding. EDEN trial follow-up. *Am J Respir Crit Care Med.* 2013;188(5):567-576.

26. Hopkins RO, Weaver LK, Pope D, Orme JF, Bigler ED, Larson LV. Neuropsychological sequelae and impaired health status in survivors of severe acute respiratory distress syndrome. *Am J Respir Crit Care Med.* 1999;160(1):50-56.

27. Herridge MS, Chu LM, Matte A, et al. The RECOVER Program: disability risk groups and 1-year outcome after 7 or more days of mechanical ventilation. *Am J Respir Crit Care Med.* 2016;194(7):831-844.

28. Fan E, Dowdy DW, Colantuoni E, et al. Physical complications in acute lung injury survivors: a two-year longitudinal prospective study. *Crit Care Med.* 2014;42(4):849-859.

29. Puthucheary ZA, Rawal J, McPhail M, et al. Acute skeletal muscle wasting in critical illness. *JAMA.* 2013;310(15):1591-1600.

30. Hough CL. Neuromuscular sequelae in survivors of acute lung injury. *Clin Chest Med.* 2006;27(4):691-703.

31. Elliott D, McKinley S, Alison J, et al. Health-related quality of life and physical recovery after a critical illness: a multi-centre randomised controlled trial of a home-based physical rehabilitation program. *Crit Care.* 2011;15(3):R142.

32. Denehy L, Skinner EH, Edbrooke L, et al. Exercise rehabilitation for patients with critical illness: a randomized controlled trial with 12 months of follow-up. *Crit Care.* 2013;17(4):R156.

33. Morris PE, Berry MJ, Files DC, et al. Standardized rehabilitation and hospital length of stay among patients with acute respiratory failure: a randomized clinical trial. *JAMA.* 2016;315(24):2694-2702.

34. Jones C, Skirrow P, Griffiths RD, et al. Rehabilitation after critical illness: a randomized, controlled trial. *Crit Care Med.* 2003;31(10):2456-2461.

35. Davydow DS, Desai SV, Needham DM, Bienvenu OJ. Psychiatric morbidity in survivors of the acute respiratory distress syndrome: a systematic review. *Psychosom Med.* 2008;70(4):512-519.

36. Mikkelsen ME, Christie JD, Lanken PN, et al. The adult respiratory distress syndrome cognitive outcomes study: long-term neuropsychological function in survivors of acute lung injury. *Am J Respir Crit Care Med.* 2012;185(12):1307-1315.

37. Brown SM, Wilson EL, Presson AP, et al. Understanding patient outcomes after acute respiratory distress syndrome: identifying subtypes of physical, cognitive and mental health outcomes. *Thorax.* 2017;72(12):1094-1103.

38. Davydow DS, Zatzick D, Hough CL, Katon WJ. A longitudinal investigation of posttraumatic stress and depressive symptoms over the course of the year following medical-surgical intensive care unit admission. *Gen Hosp Psychiatry.* 2013;35(3):226-232.

39. Kress JP, Gehlbach B, Lacy M, Pliskin N, Pohlman AS, Hall JB. The long-term psychological effects of daily sedative interruption on critically ill patients. *Am J Respir Crit Care Med.* 2003;168(12):1457-1461.

40. Treggiari MM, Romand JA, Yanez ND, et al. Randomized trial of light versus deep sedation on mental health after critical illness. *Crit Care Med.* 2009;37(9):2527-2534.

41. Jones C, Backman C, Capuzzo M, et al. Intensive care diaries reduce new onset post traumatic stress disorder following critical illness: a randomised, controlled trial. *Crit Care*. 2010; 14(5):R168.

42. Cox CE, Hough CL, Jones DM, et al. Effects of mindfulness training programmes delivered by a self-directed mobile app and by telephone compared with an education programme for survivors of critical illness: a pilot randomised clinical trial. *Thorax*. 2019;74(1):33-42.

43. Cox CE, Hough CL, Carson SS, et al. Effects of a telephone- and web-based coping skills training program compared with an education program for survivors of critical illness and their family members. A randomized clinical trial. *Am J Respir Crit Care Med*. 2018;197(1):66-78.

44. Wilcox ME, Brummel NE, Archer K, Ely EW, Jackson JC, Hopkins RO. Cognitive dysfunction in ICU patients: risk factors, predictors, and rehabilitation interventions. *Crit Care Med*. 2013;41(9 Suppl. 1):S81-S98.

23

How Do I Approach Fever in the Intensive Care Unit and Should Fever Be Treated?

Anne M. Drewry

Fever, generally described as a pyrogen-mediated elevation of core body temperature,[1] is common in critically ill patients and accompanies both infectious and noninfectious processes.[2–6] Although fever is inconsistently defined, a core body temperature of $\geq 38.3°C$ is most frequently used in the literature and in the American College of Critical Care Medicine and Infectious Diseases Society of America guidelines.[7] However, this threshold is somewhat arbitrary and may not be applicable to all patients, especially those who are elderly or immunocompromised. Furthermore, accurate detection of fever depends on where it is measured and the type of thermometer used. Core thermometers (pulmonary artery catheter, esophageal, bladder, and rectal) are more reliable than peripheral thermometers (oral, axillary, temporal artery, and tympanic membrane) and are preferred in critically ill patients unless contraindicated.[7,8]

The mechanisms by which fevers are generated are not entirely understood. The classic model of fever generation proposes that exogenous pyrogens (known as pathogen-associated molecular patterns) bind to pattern recognition receptors and activate host macrophages to release circulating substances that alter activity in the thermoregulatory regions of the preoptic area (POA) of the rostral hypothalamus (Fig. 23.1).[9–13] Endogenous pyrogens, such as inflammatory cytokines released from immune cells also induce the expression of prostaglandin E_2 (PGE_2) in endothelial cells around the POA and further modulate the hypothalamic temperature control center.[14,15] PGE_2 reduces cyclic adenosine monophosphate (cAMP) levels in the POA, and reduced activity of cAMP triggers efferent neural signals that generate fever.[12,13] Thus temperature regulation and generation of fever are controlled predominantly via a PGE_2-dependent pathway. However, it is possible that other mechanisms, such as stimulation of the hepatic branch of the vagus nerve, contribute to fever; however, such suggestions are controversial.[12,13,16]

In infection, fever may modulate the host defense response,[4,16] affecting cellular innate immunity, CD4 T cells, or B cells.[17] Fever also decreases inflammatory cytokine levels, such as tumor necrosis factor-α,[17,18] delays expression of interferon-γ,[18] rapidly increases expression of cytoprotective heat shock proteins,[4,16,19–21] and inhibits nuclear factor-κB.[22] These changes can limit the deleterious effects of infection, thereby reducing organ dysfunction and improving survival.[20,22,23] Fever may also affect pathogens by inhibiting their growth[24] or increasing antibiotic susceptibility.[25] These effects suggest that fever is an adaptive response to infection.

Conversely, an elevated body temperature also has several detrimental effects. Fever increases energy expenditure and oxygen demand and decreases vascular tone, resulting in an imbalance between oxygen demand and supply.[26,27] Thus controlling fever may decrease (1) global oxygen demand when oxygen supply is limited; (2) the risk of oxygen supply/demand mismatch; (3) the metabolic rate, and with it catabolism; and (4) the risk of septic encephalopathy, thereby decreasing the need for sedatives and antipsychotic drugs. These possibilities provide a rationale for treating fever.[4,16]

The overall balance of fever's potential beneficial and adverse effects likely depends on the underlying etiology of the fever as well as on patient comorbidities and concurrent diagnoses. For example, in patients with neurological injury, fever may be particularly harmful.[28–32] A metaanalysis of 39 studies assessing the impact of fever on clinical outcome in patients with neurological injury and stroke found that fever was consistently associated with higher mortality, worse disability, and longer hospital stays.[31] Likewise, a more recent multicenter retrospective cohort study demonstrated that peak temperatures above 39°C were associated with an increased risk of death compared with normothermia in patients with stroke or traumatic brain injury.[32] Alternatively, in critically ill patients with sepsis, observational studies demonstrate that fever is less predictive of poor outcomes and may even be associated with improved survival.[33–36] A metaanalysis of 42 studies in 2017 found a significant negative linear correlation between temperature and mortality in septic patients and demonstrated that mean temperature was highest in the lowest mortality quartile.[36] This trend,

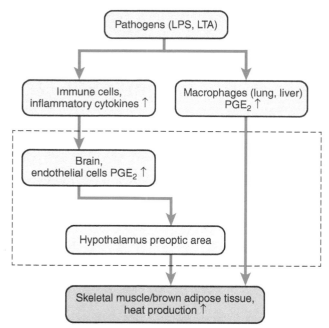

Pathogens (LPS, LTA)

Immune cells, inflammatory cytokines ↑

Macrophages (lung, liver) PGE₂ ↑

Brain, endothelial cells PGE₂ ↑

Hypothalamus preoptic area

Skeletal muscle/brown adipose tissue, heat production ↑

Fig. 23.1 Lipopolysaccharide, a main component of the outer membrane of gram-negative bacteria, is a pathogen-associated molecular pattern recognized by pattern recognition receptors such as toll-like receptor 4 on immune cells. In the lung and liver, prostaglandin E_2 (PGE_2), synthesized by activated macrophages, is released into the circulation and circulates to the preoptic area (POA) in the rostral pole of the hypothalamus, the brain's thermoregulatory center. In addition to PGE_2 from the lung and liver, PGE_2 is also expressed by local brain endothelial cells. Inflammatory cytokines released from immune cells induce PGE_2 expression in such endothelial cells around POA. PGE_2 diffuses into the parenchyma and signals the hypothalamic temperature control center. It also reduces cyclic adenosine monophosphate (cAMP) levels in the POA, and reduced activity of cAMP causes fever. Thus temperature and generation of fever are controlled predominantly via a PGE_2-dependent pathway. *LPS*, Lipopolysaccharide; *LTA*, lipoteichoic acid.

however, may not be applicable in noninfectious critically ill patients. A large retrospective study using two independent cohorts (Australia and New Zealand, N = 269,078; United Kingdom, N = 366,973) examined the relationship between peak temperature in the first 24 hours after intensive care unit (ICU) admission and hospital mortality in patients with and without infection. In infected critically ill patients, elevated temperatures were associated with decreased hospital mortality compared with normal body temperature (36.5°C–36.9°C).[33] Conversely, in patients without infection, elevated temperatures were less protective, and fevers above 40.0°C were associated with increased mortality. A prospective observational cohort study of critically ill patients in Korea and Japan (N = 1425) demonstrated similar results in that a maximum body temperature greater than 39.5°C was independently predictive of 28-day mortality in patients without sepsis but not in those with sepsis.[37]

This evidence alone is not sufficient to determine if fever directly impacts mortality in these patient populations or if it is simply a marker for other factors (e.g., disease severity, inflammatory state, and immune function) that ultimately drive outcome. To determine whether actively treating or preventing fever is beneficial requires review evidence from randomized controlled trials (RCTs).

CRITICALLY ILL PATIENTS WITH NEUROLOGICAL DISEASE

Elevated brain temperatures exacerbate neuroinflammation, cerebral hypermetabolism, permeability of the blood-brain barrier, and neuronal injury.[28,38] Not surprisingly, fever has been linked with poor outcomes in various types of neurological injury, including ischemic stroke,[32,39,40] intracranial hemorrhage,[32,41–44] traumatic brain injury,[32,45–47] and cardiac arrest.[48] Based primarily on these observational data, the 2018 American Heart Association/American Stroke Association guidelines for management of patients with ischemic stroke recommend pharmacological treatment of fevers greater than 38°C.[49] Similar recommendations exist for subarachnoid hemorrhage.[50] Although fever control is not explicitly addressed in the most recent Brain Trauma Foundation guidelines for management of traumatic brain injury,[51] it is generally considered to be the standard of care in this population as well. In a 2018 survey of 68 neurotrauma centers in Europe and Israel, 98% of centers reported that they routinely treat fever in patients with brain injury.[52] Because the benefits of fever control are well accepted in patients with acute neurological disease, the vast majority of randomized trials of temperature management in these patients have focused on comparing induced hypothermia with maintenance of normothermia or standard care; this topic will be reviewed elsewhere. Specific to fever treatment, pertinent ongoing debate involves whether afebrile patients with brain injury should receive prophylactic antipyretic therapy (Table 23.1).[53–60]

The largest RCT of prophylactic antipyretic therapy in patients with neurological injury is the Paracetamol (Acetaminophen) in Stroke (PAIS) trial.[58] This study enrolled 1400 patients with a diagnosis of ischemic stroke or intracerebral hemorrhage and a body temperature between 36°C and 39°C within 12 hours of symptom onset. Although febrile patients could be enrolled, the majority of included patients were afebrile, with a mean (standard deviation) baseline temperature of 36.9°C (0.6°C). Patients were randomized to receive acetaminophen (6 g daily) or placebo for 3 days. Overall, there were no differences between the two groups with respect to the primary outcome variable, improvement beyond expectation on the modified Rankin scale at 3 months, nor in any of the secondary outcomes, including 3-month mortality. However, a post hoc analysis, performed in the 661 patients with a baseline body temperature of 37°C–39°C, showed that a significantly greater percentage of patients treated with acetaminophen improved beyond expectation compared with those treated with placebo; adjusted odds ratio (OR) = 1.43 (95% confidence interval [CI] = 1.02, 1.97). Initial planned enrollment was 2500 patients, but the study was stopped early due to lack of funding, thereby reducing statistical power. Moreover, few patients with severe stroke were included in the study, limiting the generalizability of the results.

TABLE 23.1   Randomized Controlled Trials of Prophylactic Fever Control in Patients With Neurological Disease.

Study, Year	Setting	Main Inclusion Criteria	Sample Size (*N*)	Intervention	Duration	Main Clinical Findings
Dippel, 2001[53]	Acute stroke care unit	Acute ischemic stroke within 24 hours; baseline body temperature 36.0°C–39.0°C	75	Acetaminophen 500 mg or 1 g rectally every 4 hours	5 days	Lower temperature in the treatment group; no difference in mortality or mRS score at 1 month
Koennecke, 2001[54]	Not specified	Acute ischemic stroke; baseline temperature <37.5°C	42	Acetaminophen 1 g enterally or rectally every 6 hours	5 days	Less frequent fever in the treatment group; no difference in change in mRS score from admission to discharge
Kasner, 2002[55]	Not specified	Acute ischemic or hemorrhagic stroke within 24 hours; baseline temperature <38.5°C	39	Acetaminophen 650 mg enterally or rectally every 4 hours	24 hours	No differences in temperature, mortality, or change in NIHSS from baseline to 24 hours
Dippel, 2003[56]	Acute stroke care unit	Acute ischemic stroke within 24 hours; baseline temperature 36.0°C–39.0°C	75	Acetaminophen 1 g or ibuprofen 400 mg enterally every 4 hours	5 days	Lower temperature in the acetaminophen group; no difference in mortality or mRS score at 1 month
Broessner, 2009[57]	Neuro ICU	Subarachnoid hemorrhage, intracerebral hemorrhage, or cerebral infarction; baseline temperature ≥35.5°C	102	Endovascular maintenance of normothermia with a target temperature of 36.5°C	7 days (intracerebral hemorrhage, cerebral infarction) or 14 days (subarachnoid hemorrhage)	Less fever burden and more infections complications in the treatment group; no difference in neurological outcomes or mortality at 30 days or 6 months
PAIS, 2009[58]	Not specified	Acute ischemic stroke or intracerebral hemorrhage within 12 hours, baseline temperature 36.0°C–39.0°C	1400	Acetaminophen 1 g rectally every 4 hours	3 days	No difference in percentage of patients with mRS score improvement beyond expectation; no difference in 3-month mortality
Saxena, 2015[59]	Trauma ICU	Traumatic brain injury within 72 hours; baseline temperature 36.0°C–38.9°C	41	Acetaminophen 1 g IV every 4 hours	72 hours	No difference in temperature, intracranial pressure, or 28-day mortality
PAIS 2, 2017[60]	Not specified	Acute ischemic stroke or intracerebral hemorrhage within 12 hours; temperature ≥36.5°C	256	Acetaminophen 1 g enterally or rectally every 4 hours	72 hours	Lower temperature in the treatment group; no difference in improvement in mRS score or mortality at 90 days

ICU, intensive care unit; *IV*, intravenous; *mRS*, modified Rankin Scale; *NIHSS*, National Institutes of Health Stroke Scale.

The PAIS 2 study was subsequently performed to confirm the subgroup finding in the original PAIS trial that acetaminophen improved outcomes in stroke patients with body temperatures 37°C–39°C.[60] The enrollment criteria were similar to PAIS, except that the criterion for baseline body temperature was changed to ≥36.5°C instead of 36°C–39°C. Planned enrollment was 1500 patients, but enrollment was stopped at 256 patients due to slow recruitment and lack of funding. Results demonstrated no differences in mortality or functional outcomes between the two groups. Subsequently, a metaanalysis of seven studies of prophylactic pharmacological antipyresis in acute stroke patients also found no differences in outcomes between those prophylactically treated with and without acetaminophen.[60,61]

In patients with traumatic brain injury, a comparative cohort study with historical controls found that maintenance of normothermia via intravascular cooling lowered fever burden and reduced intracranial pressure,[62] suggesting that prevention of fever may yield better outcomes. To our knowledge, however, there has been only one small randomized trial assessing prophylactic administration of antipyretic therapy in this population to date.[59] A total of 41 mechanically ventilated patients with traumatic brain injury were randomized to treatment with acetaminophen (1 g intravenous [IV]) or placebo every 4 hours for 3 days. Results demonstrated no significant differences in adverse effects (e.g., cerebral hypoperfusion or hepatic abnormalities), mean body temperature, or clinical outcomes.

In summary, in patients with neurological disease, we concur with international guidelines and recommend that fever be treated.[49–51] Although there is little randomized evidence supporting this recommendation, preclinical data and observational studies showing worse outcomes in febrile patients are compelling. Additional research is needed to validate this practice and to provide insight into the optimal method of antipyresis and the appropriate temperature threshold at which to initiate treatment. Currently available evidence, however, does not support a benefit of prophylactic fever treatment. Therefore we do not recommend treatment with scheduled antipyretic medication or physical cooling to prevent fever in afebrile patients.

CRITICALLY ILL PATIENTS WITH SEPSIS

Septic patients are theoretically the most likely to benefit from the immune-modulating effects of fever; despite this, fever is frequently treated in septic patients in ICU. In an international survey of ICU practitioners in 23 countries, 70% of respondents reported controlling fever in patients with septic shock most or all of the time.[63] Several randomized trials have explored the impact of antipyretic therapy on outcomes in critically ill patients with sepsis (Table 23.2).[64–70]

Bernard et al.[66] performed a large ($N = 455$) RCT comparing ibuprofen with placebo in patients with severe sepsis. Ibuprofen significantly decreased core temperature, heart rate, oxygen consumption, and lactate level. In addition, potential drug-induced adverse events, including renal dysfunction and gastrointestinal bleeding, did not differ between the two groups. There was, however, no significant difference in organ failure or 30-day mortality between study groups (ibuprofen vs. placebo, 37% vs. 40%, respectively). Notably, the main premise of the study was that septic patients might benefit from administration of ibuprofen through its amelioration of the cardiovascular and pulmonary effects of prostaglandin and thromboxane. Fever control was not the primary goal, and patients were not required to be febrile to be enrolled in the study. Furthermore, administration of acetaminophen was not controlled by the study protocol; up to 33% of study patients and 44% of controls received acetaminophen at some point during the study.

Schortgen et al.[68] conducted an RCT to evaluate the safety and efficacy of fever control by external cooling in febrile patients with septic shock. This RCT enrolled 200 critically ill patients who had infection with a core body temperature greater than 38.3°C and required vasopressor infusion, ventilator support, and sedation. The intervention group ($n = 101$) had external cooling to normothermia for 48 hours, whereas controls ($n = 99$) had usual care without cooling. This study successfully attained rapid, significant fever control by external cooling. Because there was no difference in adverse events between the two groups, fever control by external cooling was demonstrated to be safe. However, the primary outcome variable, the number of patients reaching a 50% decrease in the dose of vasopressors within 48 hours, was not significantly different between the two groups. The patients who had external cooling had significantly decreased 14-day mortality compared with patients without external cooling (19% vs. 34%; $P = .013$), but ICU and hospital mortality were similar among the two groups. External cooling can cause shivering and thus increase the need for sedation and even neuromuscular paralysis. Although the use of sedation and neuromuscular paralysis was similar between groups, it is unclear if sedation or neuromuscular blockade was managed by a protocol. Importantly, the groups differed at baseline; initial vasopressor doses in patients without external cooling were higher than those in patients with external cooling. The adjusted analyses confirmed the efficacy of cooling; nonetheless, post hoc statistical adjustment of baseline differences in the primary outcome variable (vasopressor dose) between study groups is always a concern in the interpretation of RCTs.

Most recently, Young et al.[70] evaluated treatment with acetaminophen in 700 critically ill patients with a diagnosis of sepsis and a fever ≥38.0°C. Patients were randomized to receive acetaminophen 1 g IV or placebo every 6 hours for 28 days or until ICU discharge, fever resolution, cessation of antimicrobial therapy, or death. Patients in both groups received physical cooling as needed for temperatures ≥39.5°C. There were no significant differences in the primary outcome variable, the number of ICU-free days to day 28, in secondary outcomes including 28- and 90-day mortality, ICU- and hospital length of stay, and days free from mechanical ventilation, vasopressor, or renal replacement therapy. Acetaminophen effectively lowered body temperature, and there were no differences in liver dysfunction or other adverse events between the two groups. Interestingly, acetaminophen was associated with a shorter median ICU length of stay among survivors and a longer ICU stay among nonsurvivors. This longer time to death in patients treated with acetaminophen was consistent with the study by Schortgen et al.,[68] which also demonstrated a delay in death of patients who underwent cooling, suggesting that any mortality benefit associated with antipyresis occurs early and may be offset by later adverse effects of fever control.

A metaanalysis published in 2017 identified eight randomized studies and six observational studies that examined the impact of antipyretic therapy on 28-day or hospital mortality in critically ill septic patients.[71] Pooled results demonstrated that antipyretic therapy neither reduced mortality in randomized

TABLE 23.2 Randomized Controlled Trials of Fever Control in Critically Ill Septic Patients.

Study, Year	Setting	Main Inclusion Criteria	Sample Size (N)	Intervention	Duration	Main Clinical Findings
Bernard, 1991[64]	ICU	Severe sepsis	30	Ibuprofen 800 mg rectally every 4 hours	12 hours	Lower temperature, heart rate, and peak airway pressures in the treatment group; no difference in 30-day mortality
Haupt, 1991[65]	Medical ICU	Severe sepsis	29	Ibuprofen 600 mg or 800 mg IV once, then ibuprofen 800 mg rectally every 6 hours	24 hours	Lower temperature in the treatment group; no difference in hospital mortality
Bernard, 1997[66]	Medical/ Surgical ICU	Severe sepsis	455	Ibuprofen 10 mg/kg (maximum dose 800 mg) IV every 6 hours	48 hours	Lower temperature and heart rate in the treatment group; no difference in 30-day mortality
Memis, 2004[67]	ICU	Severe sepsis; positive culture data	40	Lornoxicam 8 mg IV every 12 hours	72 hours	No differences in temperature, hemodynamic parameters, or hospital mortality
Schortgen, 2012[68]	Medical/ Surgical ICU	Septic shock; fever (two consecutive values ≥38.3°C or a single value ≥39.5°C)	200	External cooling to achieve normothermia (36.5°C–37.0°C)	48 hours	Lower temperature, vasopressor requirements, and 14-day mortality in the treatment group; no difference in hospital mortality
Janz, 2015[69]	Medical ICU	Severe sepsis	51	Acetaminophen 1000 mg enterally every 6 hours	3 days	Lower temperature in the treatment group; no difference in hospital mortality
Young, 2015[70]	Medical/ Surgical ICU	Sepsis; fever (≥38.3°C)	700	Acetaminophen 1000 mg IV every 6 hours	28 days or until fever resolution or cessation of antimicrobial therapy	No difference in ICU-free days or mortality at 28 or 90 days

ICU, intensive care unit; *IV*, intravenous.

studies (relative risk [RR] = 0.93 [95% CI = 0.77, 1.13], I^2 = 0.0%) nor in observational studies (OR = 0.90 [95% CI = 0.54, 1.51], I^2 = 76.1%). Subgroup analyses of patients with shock (two studies) and of febrile patients (five studies) also showed no difference in mortality between those treated with or without antipyretics.

Overall, the totality of the evidence suggests that while antipyretic therapy is generally safe in critically ill septic patients, it does not significantly improve long-term mortality. Early mortality may be decreased by antipyretic therapy (both pharmacological and physical cooling), but the patient-centeredness of this outcome is questionable and should not drive clinical decisions. Thus, given the lack of proven benefit, we recommend that fever should not be routinely treated in critically ill septic patients. That said, the decision to control fever should be individualized to patient circumstances and other potential benefits should be considered, such as pain control and relief of discomfort, which were not analyzed in these studies.

CRITICALLY ILL PATIENTS WITHOUT SEPSIS OR NEUROLOGICAL DISEASE

Among fevers in critically ill patients, approximately 50% are noninfectious.[2,6,72] Common causes of noninfectious fevers, apart from neurological injury, include surgery, trauma, atelectasis, ischemia, inflammatory disorders, drug reaction, and transfusion.[72,73] Despite the differential prognostic significance of fever in patients with and without infection,[33,37] most randomized studies of fever control in critically ill patients have been limited to septic patients[64–70] or have included mixed populations of infected and noninfected patients.[74–76]

As with RCTs in septic patients, RCTs in mixed populations of ICU patients have consistently demonstrated no long-term clinical benefit for antipyretic therapy.[74–76] Further randomized trials are needed to determine whether fever control in noninfected patients is of value and to identify the patients who are most likely to benefit. In the absence of additional evidence, we recommend that fever should not be routinely treated in non-infected patients without neurological injury, similar to the recommendation for septic patients. The exception to this, however, is in the case of exceptionally high fever. Sustained fevers greater than 40°C may lead to multiorgan failure, with the brain, liver, and kidneys being most susceptible to hyperthermia-related abnormalities.[77] We recommend treating all fevers greater than 40°C, regardless of underlying etiology and infection status.

AUTHORS' RECOMMENDATIONS
- There is substantial evidence that fever is harmful in critically ill patients with neurological injury; therefore, fever control is recommended despite the lack of evidence supporting this practice.
- Evidence does not support prophylactic treatment with antipyretic therapy to prevent fever in afebrile patients with neurological injury.
- In septic patients, several large-scale trials and a meta-analysis have shown no improvement in 28-day and/or hospital mortality with antipyretic therapy; thus routine antipyretic therapy in not recommended.
- Decisions to control fever in critically ill patients should be individualized and based on patient comorbidities, cardiovascular reserve, degree of discomfort due to fever, and potential adverse effects of antipyretic therapy.
- Fever >40°C should be treated, regardless of underlying etiology, to avoid hyperpyrexia-induced organ dysfunction.

REFERENCES

1. Mackowiak PA. Concepts of fever. *Arch Intern Med.* 1998;158(17):1870-1881.
2. Niven DJ, Léger C, Stelfox HT, Laupland KB. Fever in the critically ill: a review of epidemiology, immunology, and management. *J Intensive Care Med.* 2012;27(5):290-297.
3. Niven DJ, Stelfox HT, Shahpori R, Laupland KB. Fever in adult ICUs: an interrupted time series analysis*. *Crit Care Med.* 2013;41(8):1863-1869.
4. Schortgen F. Fever in sepsis. *Minerva Anestesiol.* 2012;78(11):1254-1264.
5. Laupland KB. Fever in the critically ill medical patient. *Crit Care Med.* 2009;37(7 Suppl):S273-278.
6. Circiumaru B, Baldock G, Cohen J. A prospective study of fever in the intensive care unit. *Intensive Care Med.* 1999;25(7):668-673.
7. O'Grady NP, Barie PS, Bartlett JG, et al. Guidelines for evaluation of new fever in critically ill adult patients: 2008 update from the American College of Critical Care Medicine and the Infectious Diseases Society of America. *Crit Care Med.* 2008;36(4):1330-1349.
8. Niven DJ, Gaudet JE, Laupland KB, et al. Accuracy of peripheral thermometers for estimating temperature: a systematic review and meta-analysis. *Ann Intern Med.* 2015;163(10):768-777.
9. Kawai T, Akira S. The role of pattern-recognition receptors in innate immunity: update on Toll-like receptors. *Nat Immunol.* 2010;11(5):373-384.
10. Ivanov AI, Pero RS, Scheck AC, Romanovsky AA. Prostaglandin E(2)-synthesizing enzymes in fever: differential transcriptional regulation. *Am J Physiol Regul Integr Comp Physiol.* 2002;283(5):R1104-1117.
11. Steiner AA, Ivanov AI, Serrats J, et al. Cellular and molecular bases of the initiation of fever. *PLoS Biol.* 2006;4(9):e284.
12. Nakamura K. Central circuitries for body temperature regulation and fever. *Am J Physiol Regul Integr Comp Physiol.* 2011;301(5):R1207-1228.
13. Hasday JD, Thompson C, Singh IS. Fever, immunity, and molecular adaptations. *Compr Physiol.* 2014;4(1):109-148.
14. Matsumura K, Cao C, Ozaki M, et al. Brain endothelial cells express cyclooxygenase-2 during lipopolysaccharide-induced fever: light and electron microscopic immunocytochemical studies. *J Neurosci.* 1998;18(16):6279-6289.
15. Yamagata K, Matsumura K, Inoue W, et al. Coexpression of microsomal-type prostaglandin E synthase with cyclooxygenase-2 in brain endothelial cells of rats during endotoxin-induced fever. *J Neurosci.* 2001;21(8):2669-2677.
16. Launey Y, Nesseler N, Mallédant Y, Seguin P. Clinical review: fever in septic ICU patients–friend or foe? *Crit Care.* 2011;15(3):222.
17. Ozveri ES, Bekraki A, Cingi A, et al. The effect of hyperthermic preconditioning on the immune system in rat peritonitis. *Intensive Care Med.* 1999;25(10):1155-1159.
18. Jiang Q, Cross AS, Singh IS, et al. Febrile core temperature is essential for optimal host defense in bacterial peritonitis. *Infect Immun.* 2000;68(3):1265-1270.
19. Murapa P, Ward MR, Gandhapudi SK, et al. Heat shock factor 1 protects mice from rapid death during Listeria monocytogenes infection by regulating expression of tumor necrosis factor alpha during fever. *Infect Immun.* 2011;79(1):177-184.
20. Hasday JD, Singh IS. Fever and the heat shock response: distinct, partially overlapping processes. *Cell Stress Chaperones.* 2000;5(5):471-480.
21. Sucker C, Zacharowski K, Thielmann M, Hartmann M. Heat shock inhibits lipopolysaccharide-induced tissue factor activity in human whole blood. *Thromb J.* 2007;5:13.
22. Sun Z, Andersson R. NF-kappaB activation and inhibition: a review. *Shock.* 2002;18(2):99-106.
23. Villar J, Ribeiro SP, Mullen JB, et al. Induction of the heat shock response reduces mortality rate and organ damage in a sepsis-induced acute lung injury model. *Crit Care Med.* 1994;22(6):914-921.
24. Small PM, Täuber MG, Hackbarth CJ, Sande MA. Influence of body temperature on bacterial growth rates in experimental pneumococcal meningitis in rabbits. *Infect Immun.* 1986;52(2):484-487.
25. Mackowiak PA, Marling-Cason M, Cohen RL. Effects of temperature on antimicrobial susceptibility of bacteria. *J Infect Dis.* 1982;145(4):550-553.
26. Manthous CA, Hall JB, Olson D, et al. Effect of cooling on oxygen consumption in febrile critically ill patients. *Am J Respir Crit Care Med.* 1995;151(1):10-14.
27. Haupt MT, Rackow EC. Adverse effects of febrile state on cardiac performance. *Am Heart J.* 1983;105(5):763-768.

28. Polderman KH. Induced hypothermia and fever control for prevention and treatment of neurological injuries. *Lancet.* 2008;371(9628):1955-1969.

29. Saini M, Saqqur M, Kamruzzaman A, et al. Effect of hyperthermia on prognosis after acute ischemic stroke. *Stroke.* 2009;40(9):3051-3059.

30. Hajat C, Hajat S, Sharma P. Effects of poststroke pyrexia on stroke outcome : a meta-analysis of studies in patients. *Stroke.* 2000;31(2):410-414.

31. Greer DM, Funk SE, Reaven NL, et al. Impact of fever on outcome in patients with stroke and neurologic injury: a comprehensive meta-analysis. *Stroke.* 2008;39(11):3029-3035.

32. Saxena M, Young P, Pilcher D, et al. Early temperature and mortality in critically ill patients with acute neurological diseases: trauma and stroke differ from infection. *Intensive Care Med.* 2015;41(5):823-832.

33. Young PJ, Saxena M, Beasley R, et al. Early peak temperature and mortality in critically ill patients with or without infection. *Intensive Care Med.* 2012;38:437-444.

34. Sundén-Cullberg J, Rylance R, Svefors J, et al. Fever in the emergency department predicts survival of patients with severe sepsis and septic shock admitted to the ICU. *Crit Care Med.* 2017;45(4):591-599.

35. Drewry AM, Ablordeppey EA, Murray ET, et al. Monocyte function and clinical outcomes in febrile and afebrile patients with severe sepsis. *Shock.* 2018;50(4):381-387.

36. Rumbus Z, Matics R, Hegyi P, et al. Fever is associated with reduced, hypothermia with increased mortality in septic patients: a meta-analysis of clinical trials. *PLoS One.* 2017;12(1):e0170152.

37. Lee BH, Inui D, Suh GY, et al. Association of body temperature and antipyretic treatments with mortality of critically ill patients with and without sepsis: multi-centered prospective observational study. *Crit Care.* 2012;16(1):R33.

38. Mrozek S, Vardon F, Geeraerts T. Brain temperature: physiology and pathophysiology after brain injury. *Anesthesiol Res Pract.* 2012;2012:989487.

39. Castillo J, Dávalos A, Marrugat J, Noya M. Timing for fever-related brain damage in acute ischemic stroke. *Stroke.* 1998;29(12):2455-2460.

40. Azzimondi G, Bassein L, Nonino F, et al. Fever in acute stroke worsens prognosis. A prospective study. *Stroke.* 1995;26(11):2040-2043.

41. Fernandez A, Schmidt JM, Claassen J, et al. Fever after subarachnoid hemorrhage: risk factors and impact on outcome. *Neurology.* 2007;68(13):1013-1019.

42. Oddo M, Frangos S, Milby A, et al. Induced normothermia attenuates cerebral metabolic distress in patients with aneurysmal subarachnoid hemorrhage and refractory Fever. *Stroke.* 2009;40(5):1913-1916.

43. Naidech AM, Bendok BR, Bernstein RA, et al. Fever burden and functional recovery after subarachnoid hemorrhage. *Neurosurgery.* 2008;63(2):212-217; discussion 217-218.

44. Schwarz S, Häfner K, Aschoff A, Schwab S. Incidence and prognostic significance of fever following intracerebral hemorrhage. *Neurology.* 2000;54(2):354-361.

45. Jiang JY, Gao GY, Li WP, et al. Early indicators of prognosis in 846 cases of severe traumatic brain injury. *J Neurotrauma.* 2002;19(7):869-874.

46. Stocchetti N, Rossi S, Zanier ER, et al. Pyrexia in head-injured patients admitted to intensive care. *Intensive Care Med.* 2002;28(11):1555-1562.

47. Jones PA, Andrews PJ, Midgley S, et al. Measuring the burden of secondary insults in head-injured patients during intensive care. *J Neurosurg Anesthesiol.* 1994;6(1):4-14.

48. Zeiner A, Holzer M, Sterz F, et al. Hyperthermia after cardiac arrest is associated with an unfavorable neurologic outcome. *Arch Intern Med.* 2001;161(16):2007-2012.

49. Powers WJ, Rabinstein AA, Ackerson T, et al. 2018 guidelines for the early management of patients with acute ischemic stroke: a guideline for healthcare professionals from the American Heart Association/American Stroke Association. *Stroke.* 2018;49(3):e46-e110.

50. Steiner T, Juvela S, Unterberg A, et al. European Stroke Organization guidelines for the management of intracranial aneurysms and subarachnoid haemorrhage. *Cerebrovasc Dis.* 2013;35(2):93-112.

51. Carney N, Totten AM, O'Reilly C, et al. Guidelines for the Management of Severe Traumatic Brain Injury, Fourth Edition. Neurosurgery 2017;80(10):6-15.

52. Huijben JA, Volovici V, Cnossen MC, et al. Variation in general supportive and preventive intensive care management of traumatic brain injury: a survey in 66 neurotrauma centers participating in the Collaborative European NeuroTrauma Effectiveness Research in Traumatic Brain Injury (CENTER-TBI) study. *Crit Care.* 2018;22(1):90.

53. Dippel DW, van Breda EJ, van Gemert HM, et al. Effect of paracetamol (acetaminophen) on body temperature in acute ischemic stroke: a double-blind, randomized phase II clinical trial. *Stroke.* 2001;32(7):1607-1612.

54. Koennecke HC, Leistner S. Prophylactic antipyretic treatment with acetaminophen in acute ischemic stroke: a pilot study. *Neurology.* 2001;57(12):2301-2303.

55. Kasner SE, Wein T, Piriyawat P, et al. Acetaminophen for altering body temperature in acute stroke: a randomized clinical trial. *Stroke.* 2002;33(1):130-134.

56. Dippel DW, van Breda EJ, van der Worp HB, et al. Effect of paracetamol (acetaminophen) and ibuprofen on body temperature in acute ischemic stroke PISA, a phase II double-blind, randomized, placebo-controlled trial [ISRCTN98608690]. *BMC Cardiovasc Disord.* 2003;3:2.

57. Broessner G, Beer R, Lackner P, et al. Prophylactic, endovascularly based, long-term normothermia in ICU patients with severe cerebrovascular disease: bicenter prospective, randomized trial. *Stroke.* 2009;40(12):e657-665.

58. den Hertog HM, van der Worp HB, van Gemert HM, et al. The Paracetamol (Acetaminophen) In Stroke (PAIS) trial: a multicentre, randomised, placebo-controlled, phase III trial. *Lancet Neurol.* 2009;8(5):434-440.

59. Saxena MK, Taylor C, Billot L, et al. The effect of paracetamol on core body temperature in acute traumatic brain injury: a randomised, controlled clinical trial. *PLoS One.* 2015;10(12):e0144740.

60. de Ridder IR, den Hertog HM, van Gemert HM, et al. PAIS 2 (Paracetamol [Acetaminophen] in Stroke 2): Results of a randomized, double-blind placebo-controlled clinical trial. *Stroke.* 2017;48(4):977-982.

61. Den Hertog HM, van der Worp HB, Tseng MC, Dippel DW. Cooling therapy for acute stroke. *Cochrane Database Syst Rev.* 2009(1):CD001247.

62. Puccio AM, Fischer MR, Jankowitz BT, et al. Induced normo-thermia attenuates intracranial hypertension and reduces fever burden after severe traumatic brain injury. *Neurocrit Care.* 2009;11(1):82-87.

63. Niven DJ, Laupland KB, Tabah A, et al. Diagnosis and management of temperature abnormality in ICUs: a EUROBACT investigators' survey. *Crit Care*. 2013;17(6): R289.

64. Bernard GR, Reines HD, Halushka PV, et al. Prostacyclin and thromboxane A2 formation is increased in human sepsis syndrome. Effects of cyclooxygenase inhibition. *Am Rev Respir Dis*. 1991;144(5):1095-1101.

65. Haupt MT, Jastremski MS, Clemmer TP, et al. Effect of ibuprofen in patients with severe sepsis: a randomized, double-blind, multicenter study. The Ibuprofen Study Group. *Crit Care Med*. 1991;19(11):1339-1347.

66. Bernard GR, Wheeler AP, Russell JA, et al. The effects of ibuprofen on the physiology and survival of patients with sepsis. The Ibuprofen in Sepsis Study Group. *N Engl J Med*. 1997;336(13):912-918.

67. Memiş D, Karamanlioğlu B, Turan A, et al. Effects of lornoxicam on the physiology of severe sepsis. *Crit Care*. 2004;8(6): R474-482.

68. Schortgen F, Clabault K, Katsahian S, et al. Fever control using external cooling in septic shock: a randomized controlled trial. *Am J Respir Crit Care Med*. 2012;185(10):1088-1095.

69. Janz DR, Bastarache JA, Rice TW, et al. Randomized, placebo-controlled trial of acetaminophen for the reduction of oxidative injury in severe sepsis: the Acetaminophen for the Reduction of Oxidative Injury in Severe Sepsis trial. *Crit Care Med*. 2015;43(3):534-541.

70. Young P, Saxena M, Bellomo R, et al. Acetaminophen for fever in critically ill patients with suspected infection. *N Engl J Med*. 2015;373(23):2215-2224.

71. Drewry AM, Ablordeppey EA, Murray ET, et al. Antipyretic therapy in critically ill septic patients: a systematic review and meta-analysis. *Crit Care Med*. 2017;45(5):806-813.

72. Peres Bota D, Lopes Ferreira F, Mélot C, Vincent JL. Body temperature alterations in the critically ill. *Intensive Care Med*. 2004;30(5):811-816.

73. Barie PS, Hydo LJ, Eachempati SR. Causes and consequences of fever complicating critical surgical illness. *Surg Infect (Larchmt)*. 2004;5(2):145-159.

74. Gozzoli V, Schöttker P, Suter PM, Ricou B. Is it worth treating fever in intensive care unit patients? Preliminary results from a randomized trial of the effect of external cooling. *Arch Intern Med*. 2001;161(1):121-123.

75. Schulman CI, Namias N, Doherty J, et al. The effect of antipyretic therapy upon outcomes in critically ill patients: a randomized, prospective study. *Surg Infect (Larchmt)*. 2005;6(4):369-375.

76. Morris PE, Promes JT, Guntupalli KK, et al. A multi-center, randomized, double-blind, parallel, placebo-controlled trial to evaluate the efficacy, safety, and pharmacokinetics of intravenous ibuprofen for the treatment of fever in critically ill and non-critically ill adults. *Crit Care*. 2010;14(3):R125.

77. Mackowiak PA, Boulant JA. Fever's glass ceiling. *Clin Infect Dis*. 1996;22(3):525-536.

24

What Fluids Should Be Given to the Critically Ill Patient? What Fluids Should Be Avoided?

Anders Perner

Many critically ill patients are hypovolemic, which may result in impaired cardiac output and organ perfusion, leading to poor outcome. Fluid therapy is a mainstay in their management. Indeed, a third of patients in intensive care units (ICUs) worldwide receive fluid for resuscitation each day.[1] Therefore differences in patient outcomes among different types of fluids will affect global health, and differences in direct and related costs will affect health-care expenditure.

When deciding what fluid to give to a critically ill patient, clinicians may choose between colloid and crystalloid solutions, and if the latter is chosen between saline and buffered salt solutions. Blood products may be considered for resuscitation of hemorrhagic shock for their oxygen carrying and hemostatic properties and for their colloidal effects.

CRYSTALLOIDS

Crystalloids are salt solutions used for intravenous infusion. Presently, none of the commercially available solutions contain electrolyte and buffer concentrations comparable with those of plasma; bicarbonate is very rarely found in these solutions.

Isotonic saline (0.9% sodium chloride) is still frequently used despite concentrations of sodium and chloride (154 mmol/L) well above those found in plasma. Alternatives are so-called buffered (or 'balanced') salt solutions including lactate-buffered (Ringer's lactate or Hartmann's), acetate-buffered (Ringer's acetate), and acetate-gluconate-buffered (Plasmalyte) solutions. The concentrations of electrolytes in these buffered solutions more closely resemble those of plasma, and most preparations include sodium, chloride, potassium, and calcium. However, bicarbonate is normally not included because bicarbonate-containing fluids, particularly those in plastic containers, have a shorter shelf-life. Instead, solutions are buffered with lactate or different combinations of acetate, gluconate, and malate. The concentrations of these buffers exceed those in plasma by many fold; it appears, therefore, less appropriate to label these fluids 'balanced'— 'buffered' is a more neutral term.

COLLOIDS

Colloid solutions contain large molecules that prolong the time the fluid remains in circulation. The molecules used to provide the colloidal and, therefore, the volume-expanding properties of these solutions are human albumin or synthetically modified sugars or collagens. The most frequently used synthetic colloid solutions are hydroxyethyl starch (HES), gelatin, and dextrans.

Colloid solutions have been extensively administered for volume expansion in critically ill patients, but clinical practice has varied, mainly because of regional differences in the types of colloid solutions available.[1] Moreover, in recent years, results of large trials have examined the efficacy of and adverse events associated with colloids in critically ill patients.[2-4] These trials raise questions regarding the clinical value of colloids and have clearly raised some serious concerns regarding the use of some colloids in groups of critically ill patients.

In the following section, what fluids to give to critically ill patients and what fluids to avoid is described. Recommendations are based on data from recently updated high-quality systematic reviews and recently conducted high-quality randomized trials. These findings allow evidence-based choices to be made and are likely to improve care and outcome and reduce costs.

IN GENERAL ICU PATIENTS, WHAT FLUIDS SHOULD I GIVE AND WHAT SHOULD I AVOID?

The short answer is to give crystalloids and avoid the synthetic colloids (HES, gelatins, and dextrans).

The systematic review by the Cochrane Collaboration comparing crystalloid with colloid solutions showed that crystalloids were associated with lower mortality rates relative to HES solutions. No differences in mortality were noted when crystalloids were compared with the other colloid solutions analyzed (albumin, gelatins, and dextrans).[5] The increased mortality with the use of HES most likely reflects adverse effects on renal function and hemostasis, resulting in an increased use of renal replacement therapy and increased bleeding (Table 24.1). A recently published large randomized trial, the Colloids vs. Crystalloids for the Resuscitation of the Critically Ill (CRISTAL) trial,[6] was not included in the Cochrane analysis. The CRISTAL trial compared any crystalloid to any colloid solution in ICU patients with shock. The results suggested that, relative to crystalloids (mainly

TABLE 24.1 Characteristics and Results of the Trials With Low Risk of Bias Randomizing Critically Ill Patients to Colloids Versus Crystalloids.*

Trial	The SAFE Trial	The 6S Trial	The CHEST
Colloid solution	4% Albumin	6% Tetrastarch in Ringer's acetate	6% Tetrastarch in saline
Crystalloid comparator	Saline	Ringer's acetate	Saline
Patients	Adult ICU patients	Adult ICU patients with severe sepsis	Adult ICU patients
Number of patients randomized	7000	805	7000
Outcomes	**Relative Risks (95% Confidence Intervals)**		
Mortality	0.99 (0.91–1.09)	1.17 (1.01–1.36)	1.06 (0.96–1.18)
Renal replacement therapy	Similar duration of therapy in the two groups	1.35 (1.01–1.80)	1.21 (1.00–1.45)
Bleeding	—	1.55 (1.16–2.08)	—
Use of blood transfusion	Higher volume of red blood cells given in the albumin vs. the saline group	1.28 (1.12–1.47)	Higher volume of red blood cells given in the HES vs. the saline group
Adverse reactions	Not reported	1.56 (0.97–2.53)	1.86 (1.46–2.38)

*The definitions of adverse reactions differed between trials.
CHEST, Crystalloid vs. Hydroxyethyl Starch Trial; *HES*, hydroxyethyl starch; *ICU*, intensive care unit; *SAFE*, Saline vs. Albumin Fluid Evaluation; *6S*, Scandinavian Starch for Severe Sepsis/Septic Shock.

saline), colloids (mainly HES) improved 90-day mortality, a secondary outcome measure. The primary outcome measure, 28-day mortality, did not differ between the groups, and the trial had high risk of bias in several domains (unblinded, uncertain allocation concealment, and baseline imbalance).[7] Moreover, the results differed from those of high-quality trials,[2–4] and the editor argued in an accompanying editorial for cautious interpretation of these findings, advocating for crystalloids as the first-line fluid in patients with shock.[8]

The interpretation of the Cochrane meta-analyses on crystalloid vs. gelatin and dextran solutions was hampered by low-quality trial data and a limited number of patients and events, and thus wide confidence intervals on the point estimates.[5] Because gelatins and dextrans have been associated with adverse events that are similar to those observed with HES, these synthetic colloids should probably be avoided in critically ill patients. This recommendation is substantiated by the fact that no patient group in any low-risk-of-bias trial has been shown to benefit from any colloid solution, including the trial using human albumin (see Table 24.1), although the latter showed that albumin is safe to administer to critically ill patients, excluding those with trauma.[2] As a blood product fractionated from human plasma, albumin is an expensive and limited resource; thus, it is of limited value in many health-care systems. The same may be said of red blood cells, plasma, and platelets, but these products have a larger potential for harm than albumin, and their safety has not been fully ensured in large trials in the critically ill. Liberal transfusion of red blood cells may even increase the mortality of general ICU patients, as observed in the Transfusion Requirement in Critical Care (TRICC) trial.[9] Thus blood products should only be used for patients with severe anemia

or bleeding or as a prophylactic in high-risk patients with severely impaired hemostasis.

Overall, the recommendations of the European Society of Intensive Care Medicine Task Force on colloids support the notion that crystalloid solutions should be preferred over colloids in most critically ill patients.[10]

The choice between the different crystalloid solutions is more difficult because the two large trials done in this area are difficult to interpret and they show somewhat differing results (Table 24.2). The recent Isotonic Solutions and Major Adverse Renal Events Trial (SMART) cluster randomized five ICUs in a single US hospital to unmasked use of either 0.9% saline or buffered solutions for all patients except those with contraindications against the allocated solution; for these patients the alternative was available.[11] The ICUs crossed over every month so that all five ICUs had months with saline use and months with buffered solution use. In all units, patients admitted around the time of the cross-overs received both solutions. The primary result of the SMART trial indicated fewer major adverse kidney events at day 30—a composite of mortality, new use of renal replacement therapy, and an elevation of the creatinine level to more than 200% of baseline—in the buffered vs. the saline group. The other large trial, the Saline vs. Plasma-Lyte 148 (PL-148) for ICU fluid Therapy (SPLIT) trial, cluster randomized four ICUs in four hospitals in New Zealand to masked use of either 0.9% saline or buffered solutions for all patients except those with established renal replacement therapy.[12] The staff and patients were blinded to the intervention and cross-over was done every 7 weeks, but the patients in the ICUs at cross-over continued their allocated fluid. The primary result of the SPLIT trial indicated no differences in rates of acute kidney injury

TABLE 24.2 Characteristics and Results of the Trials Randomizing Critically Ill Patients to Saline Versus Buffered Salt Solutions.

Trial	The SMART Trial	The SPLIT Trial
Buffered solution	Lactate- or acetate/gluconate-buffered solutions	Acetate/gluconate-buffered solution
Saline solution	0.9% Saline	0.9% Saline
Blinding	No	Clinical and trial staff and patients
Patients	Adult ICU patients	Adult ICU patients
Number of clusters randomized (ICUs/ hospitals)	5/1	4/4
Number of patients randomized	15,802	2278
Outcomes	**Adjusted Odd Ratios (95% CIs)**	**Relative Risks (95% CIs)**
Mortality	0.90 (0.80–1.01)	0.88 (0.67–1.17)
New renal replacement therapy	0.84 (0.68–1.02)	0.96 (0.62–1.50)
Acute kidney injury	0.91 (0.82–1.01)	1.04 (0.80–1.36)

CI, Confidence interval; *ICU*, intensive care unit; *SMART*, Isotonic Solutions and Major Adverse Renal Events Trial; *SPLIT*, Saline vs. Plasma-Lyte 148 (PL-148) for ICU fluid Therapy.

between the two groups; neither were there any differences in the use of renal replacement therapy or in mortality.[12] Presently, at least two large randomized trials with individual patient allocation are ongoing, the Plasma-Lyte 148 vs. Saline (PLUS) trial and the Balanced Solution vs. Saline in Intensive Care Study (BASICS). Given the uncertainty, it appears appropriate to await the results of these trials, which include more patient-important outcome measures, before making strong recommendations of one crystalloid solution over the other.

With the lack of high-quality evidence, the choice of crystalloid solution may be guided by specific patient characteristics. 0.9% saline may be preferred in patients at risk of brain edema because the higher plasma concentrations of sodium may reduce brain swelling and intracranial pressure in these patients. Conversely, severe acidosis may be worsened by saline-induced hyperchloremia. A buffered crystalloid solution may be the better choice in these patients.

IN PATIENTS WITH SEPSIS, WHAT FLUIDS SHOULD I GIVE AND WHAT SHOULD I AVOID?

Again, the short answer is give crystalloids and avoid the synthetic colloids (HES, gelatins, and dextrans).

There are high-quality data to guide clinicians on choice of fluids in patients with sepsis. An updated systematic review showed that crystalloids are superior to HES with respect to mortality, use of renal replacement therapy and blood products, and adverse reactions.[13] There are no high-quality data on the other synthetic colloids, but they have the same registered adverse events as HES; they should, therefore, be avoided in sepsis.

Regarding albumin, there are now two large trials comparing albumin with crystalloids in patients with sepsis: the subgroup analysis of the Saline vs. Albumin Fluid Evaluation (SAFE) trial and the recent Albumin Italian Outcome Sepsis (ALBIOS) trial.[2,14] Neither showed significantly improved

mortality, use of life support, or length of ICU or hospital stay with albumin as compared with saline. The lack of benefit is supported by a recently updated systematic review that included trials of patients with sepsis regardless of severity.[15] Extensive subgroup and sensitivity analysis was applied to challenge the overall result; the conclusions remained unchanged. Because albumin is an expensive and limited resource, it may be reasonable to avoid its use in patients with sepsis before we have identified subgroups of patients (e.g., early shock) who will benefit from albumin.

IN TRAUMA PATIENTS, WHAT FLUIDS SHOULD I GIVE AND WHAT SHOULD I AVOID?

Saline or isotonic buffered salt solutions should be used in patients with trauma, in particular in those with obvious traumatic brain injury, whereas colloids should be avoided. The latter is particularly true for albumin. All the buffered crystalloids have concentrations of sodium below that of saline, and Ringer's lactate and Hartmann solutions are hypotonic, which may worsen brain edema.

The best evidence on the choice of fluid in trauma comes from the predefined subgroup analysis of the 1186 patients with trauma in the SAFE study.[2] Albumin increased 28-day mortality in these patients, an effect that may have been mediated by increased intracranial pressure in those with traumatic brain injury.[16,17] If this is an effect caused by albumin crossing a leaky blood-brain barrier, then the same may apply for the synthetic colloid solutions. In addition, the synthetic colloids directly impair coagulation, and HES as compared with saline was shown to increase the use of blood products in patients with blunt trauma.[18] In the latter trial, there were no data on bleeding, but a nonsignificant 86% relative risk increase in mortality with HES was observed.[19] In addition, HES has been shown to increase bleeding in patients with severe sepsis and those undergoing surgery.[20,21] There are presently not enough high-quality data to support that any of the synthetic colloids can be used safely in trauma; therefore all synthetic colloids (HES, gelatins, and dextrans) should be avoided in these patients.

IN PATIENTS WITH HEMORRHAGIC SHOCK, WHAT FLUIDS SHOULD I GIVE AND WHAT SHOULD I AVOID?

A crystalloid solution should be used in patients with life-threatening bleeding, and blood products, including red blood cells, plasma, and platelets, should be considered early. Synthetic colloids (HES, gelatins, and dextrans) should be avoided because they impair hemostasis and increase the rate of bleeding. The synthetic colloids induce coagulopathy, and HES and gelatin have been shown to increase bleeding compared with crystalloids in patients undergoing surgery.[21,22] Furthermore, HES has been shown to increase bleeding in severe sepsis.[20] Balanced blood component therapy mimicking full blood should be considered early in patients with hemorrhagic shock, including those with trauma,[23] but there are still no high-quality data supporting this approach.

IN PATIENTS WITH BURN INJURY, WHAT FLUIDS SHOULD I GIVE AND WHAT SHOULD I AVOID?

There are no data from high-quality trials that can inform us on the choice of fluids in patients with burn injury. Patients with burn injury likely represent a specific entity because of the large leak of fluids in the burned areas. These patients receive high volumes of fluid, and lactate-buffered solution has traditionally been used. There are no updated systematic reviews comparing crystalloid and colloid therapy for these patients, but there are at least three smaller randomized trials, two comparing lactate-buffered solution with albumin[24,25] and one comparing lactate-buffered solution with HES.[26] Taken together, the trial results do not support the use of colloids for patients with burn injury, but the quality of the evidence is very low. Therefore, it is difficult to give strong recommendations, but high fluid volumes are often needed, and these patients are at increased risk of dysnatremias and acidosis. Thus, high volume saline resuscitation should probably be avoided.

CONCLUSIONS

In recent years, an increasing number of critically ill patients have been randomized into fluid trials. Taken together the trials with low risk of bias indicate that crystalloid solutions should be used for most critically ill patients; the choice between the crystalloid solutions remains less clear. No critically ill patients should be given HES, and gelatins and dextrans should be avoided because of lack of safety data and concerns about serious adverse events. Patients with traumatic brain injury should not be given albumin. Moreover, there are no high-quality data showing an overall benefit of albumin, which is an expensive and limited resource.

> **AUTHORS' RECOMMENDATIONS**
> - Crystalloid solutions should be used for critically ill patients.
> - Either 0.9% saline or buffered salt solutions may be used, but their differing effects on brain edema, acidosis, and dysnatremias should be considered.
> - HES should not be given because of its life-threatening adverse events.
> - Gelatins and dextrans should not be used because their safety has not been adequately assessed.
> - The use of albumin should be limited because it is an expensive and limited resource without apparent benefit for patients.

REFERENCES

1. Finfer S, Liu B, Taylor C, et al. Resuscitation fluid use in critically ill adults: an international cross-sectional study in 391 intensive care units. *Crit Care*. 2010;14:R185.
2. Finfer S, Bellomo R, Boyce N, et al. A comparison of albumin and saline for fluid resuscitation in the intensive care unit. *N Engl J Med*. 2004;350:2247-2256.
3. Perner A, Haase N, Guttormsen AB, et al. Hydroxyethyl starch 130/0.42 versus Ringer's acetate in severe sepsis. *N Engl J Med*. 2012;367:124-134.
4. Myburgh JA, Finfer S, Bellomo R, et al. Hydroxyethyl starch or saline for fluid resuscitation in intensive care. *N Engl J Med*. 2012;367:1901-1911.
5. Perel P, Roberts I, Ker K. Colloids versus crystalloids for fluid resuscitation in critically ill patients. *Cochrane Database Syst Rev*. 2013;(2):CD000567.
6. Annane D, Siami S, Jaber S, et al. Effects of fluid resuscitation with colloids vs crystalloids on mortality in critically ill patients presenting with hypovolemic shock: the CRISTAL randomized trial. *JAMA*. 2013;310:1809-1817.
7. Perner A, Haase N, Wetterslev J. Mortality in patients with hypovolemic shock treated with colloids or crystalloids. *JAMA*. 2014;311:1067.
8. Seymour CW, Angus DC. Making a pragmatic choice for fluid resuscitation in critically ill patients. *JAMA*. 2013;310:1803-1804.
9. Hébert PC, Wells G, Blajchman MA, et al. A multicenter, randomized, controlled clinical trial of transfusion requirements in critical care. *N Engl J Med*. 1999;340:409-417.
10. Reinhart K, Perner A, Sprung CL, et al. Consensus statement of the ESICM task force on colloid volume therapy in critically ill patients. *Intensive Care Med*. 2012;38:368-383.
11. Semler MW, Self WH, Wanderer JP, et al. Balanced crystalloids versus saline in critically ill adults. *N Engl J Med*. 2018;378:829-839.
12. Young P, Bailey M, Beasley R, et al. Effect of a buffered crystalloid solution vs saline on acute kidney injury among patients in the intensive care unit: the SPLIT randomized clinical trial. *JAMA*. 2015;314:1701-1710.
13. Haase N, Perner A, Hennings LI, et al. Hydroxyethyl starch 130/0.38–0.45 versus crystalloid or albumin in patients with sepsis: systematic review with meta-analysis and trial sequential analysis. *BMJ*. 2013;346:f839.
14. Caironi P, Tognoni G, Masson S, et al. Albumin replacement in patients with severe sepsis or septic shock. *N Engl J Med*. 2014;370:1412-1421.

15. Patel A, Laffan MA, Waheed U, Brett SJ. Randomised trials of human albumin for adults with sepsis: systematic review and meta-analysis with trial sequential analysis of all-cause mortality. *BMJ*. 2014;349:g4561.

16. Myburgh J, Cooper DJ, Finfer S, et al. Saline or albumin for fluid resuscitation in patients with traumatic brain injury. *N Engl J Med*. 2007;357:874-884.

17. Cooper DJ, Myburgh J, Heritier S, et al. Albumin resuscitation for traumatic brain injury: is intracranial hypertension the cause of increased mortality? *J Neurotrauma*. 2013;30:512-518.

18. James MF, Michell WL, Joubert IA, et al. Resuscitation with hydroxyethyl starch improves renal function and lactate clearance in penetrating trauma in a randomized controlled study: the FIRST trial (Fluids in Resuscitation of Severe Trauma). *Br J Anaesth*. 2011;107:693-702.

19. James MFM, Michell WL, Joubert IA, et al. Reply from the authors. *Br J Anaesth*. 2012;108:160-161.

20. Haase N, Wetterslev J, Winkel P, Perner A. Bleeding and risk of death with hydroxyethyl starch in severe sepsis: post hoc analyses of a randomized clinical trial. *Intensive Care Med*. 2013;39:2126-2134.

21. Rasmussen KC, Johansson PI, Højskov M, et al. Hydroxyethyl starch reduces coagulation competence and increases blood loss during major surgery: results from a randomized controlled trial. *Ann Surg*. 2014;259:249-254.

22. Mittermayr M, Streif W, Haas T, et al. Hemostatic changes after crystalloid or colloid fluid administration during major orthopedic surgery: the role of fibrinogen administration. *Anesth Analg*. 2007;105:905-917.

23. Johansson PI, Sørensen AM, Larsen CF, et al. Low hemorrhage-related mortality in trauma patients in a Level I trauma center employing transfusion packages and early thromboelastography-directed hemostatic resuscitation with plasma and platelets. *Transfusion*. 2013;53:3088-3099.

24. Goodwin CW, Dorethy J, Lam V, Pruitt BA Jr. Randomized trial of efficacy of crystalloid and colloid resuscitation on hemodynamic response and lung water following thermal injury. *Ann Surg*. 1983;197:520-531.

25. Cooper AB, Cohn SM, Zhang HS, et al. Five percent albumin for adult burn shock resuscitation: lack of effect on daily multiple organ dysfunction score. *Transfusion*. 2006;46:80-89.

26. Béchir M, Puhan MA, Fasshauer M, et al. Early fluid resuscitation with hydroxyethyl starch 130/0.4 (6%) in severe burn injury: a randomized, controlled, double-blind clinical trial. *Crit Care*. 2013;17:R299.

25

Should Blood Glucose Be Tightly Controlled in the Intensive Care Unit?

Olivier Lheureux and Jean-Charles Preiser

Before 2001, the hyperglycemia found in most critically ill patients was considered as a component of the stress response. Current understanding was completely changed by the publication of the first Leuven study article in 2001.[1] This investigation compared an intensive insulin regimen targeting a blood glucose (BG) level within the range of 80–110 mg/dL with a "conventional" management cohort in whom BG was treated only when above 200 mg/dL. Van den Berghe and colleagues, the authors of the study, demonstrated a 4% decrease in the absolute mortality of critically ill patients randomized to intensive insulin therapy (IIT). These unexpectedly impressive results triggered a huge wave of enthusiasm. Recommendations to implement tight glucose control (TGC) in intensive care units (ICUs) were rapidly issued by several health-care agencies (Joint Commission on Accreditation of Healthcare Organization, the Institute for Healthcare Improvement, and the Volunteer Hospital Organization). Simultaneously, several different teams tried to reproduce the results and to examine the underlying mechanisms of the findings of the Leuven team. Overall, the results of the Leuven study have not been reproduced. Nonetheless, these follow-up studies have led to several controversies and raised important but yet unanswered questions for the physicians taking care of critically ill patients, including "What is the optimal value of BG?", "What are the risks associated with hypoglycemia?", and "What categories of patient might benefit from TGC by IIT?"

PATHOPHYSIOLOGY AND MECHANISM OF ACTION

It has long been recognized that critically ill patients tend to be hyperglycemic.[2] For many years, this abnormality was believed to be a part of the host response to critical illness. Thus hyperglycemia was viewed as a biomarker of the severity of illness. The Leuven studies started with the hypothesis that hyperglycemia was not just a biomarker. Rather, these investigators postulated that elevations in serum glucose contributed to the pathophysiology of critical illness. This proposal spawned the current field of investigation. The initial question might be reframed as, "What is the optimal BG concentration in a critically ill patient?" Further exploration and investigation of this question are warranted.

The physiology behind "stress hyperglycemia" is complex. The elaboration of glucose, primarily by the liver, is known to be an essential component of the host's response. This reflects the energy demand that results from injury, ischemia, or other deleterious processes. White blood cells, the main effectors of the inflammatory response, are more or less obligate glucose users. Because the blood supply to injured tissue often has been interrupted or diminished, delivery is primarily through mass action across the intracellular matrix. Increases in concentration facilitate this movement. Gluconeogenesis, the process whereby the liver synthesizes glucose, is driven primarily by the direct action of glucagon and epinephrine on hepatocytes. This is enhanced by cortisol and perhaps by inflammatory cytokines. In addition, these hormones and cytokines limit the peripheral response to insulin to some extent. This latter effect has been termed "insulin resistance," although there are no data in nonseptic patients or animals to indicate that the direct responses of the insulin signaling pathway are impaired. At some point, the process becomes maladaptive in the critically ill patients. This is especially true in sepsis and multiorgan dysfunction. Thus, the question asked earlier must be expanded to examine the time course of stress hyperglycemia as well as the actual glucose concentration.

In experimental conditions, concentrations of glucose higher than 300 mg/dL clearly are deleterious.[3] However, new insights into the cellular mechanisms of glucose toxicity suggest a link between glucose, cytopathic hypoxia, and the production of reactive oxygen and nitrogen species.[4,5] These concentrations, unfortunately, are clinically irrelevant, and only clinical data can be used to define the optimal value for TGC. Indeed, the ultimate proof that hyperglycemia is an independent risk factor for poor outcome in critically ill patients is lacking.[6] Importantly, insulin exerts effects other than the promotion of glucose metabolism and utilization. These include vasodilatory, anti-inflammatory, and antiapoptotic activities that can be viewed as a homeostatic control mechanism limiting some of the processes that occur in inflammation and other potentially injurious responses. Such a role for insulin might explain some of the beneficial but unexpected effects of IIT.

PRESENTATION OF AVAILABLE DATA BASED ON SYSTEMATIC REVIEW

It has been difficult to replicate the results of the Leuven study.[1] This leaves several practical questions unanswered. First, it is unclear just what constitutes "normoglycemia" in critical illness.[7] Retrospective data and the two Leuven studies clearly indicate that a BG higher than 180 mg/dL cannot be considered acceptable.[1,8] However, the optimal target for BG concentration is still unknown. Interestingly, several retrospective trials found that patients with BG levels lower than 150 mg/dL had a better outcome than those with higher levels.[9,10]

To solve the issues of the external validity of the Leuven study and the optimal BG target, large single-center and multicenter prospective trials of TGC by IIT comparing two ranges of BG were launched. The designs of these trials (Table 25.1) were similar. All aimed to compare the effects of insulin therapy titrated to restore and maintain BG between 80 and 110 mg/dL for adult studies. In two mixed pediatric ICUs, the BG target in the IIT group was the same as in the adult studies in the HALF-PINT study[11] and was between 72 and 126 mg/dL in the CHiP trial.[12] However, they differed in the target range of BG for the control (nonintensive insulin therapy) group. The Normoglycemia in Intensive

Care Evaluation-Survival Using Glucose Algorithm Regulation (NICE-SUGAR)[13] and GluControl trials[14] used a target value of 140–180 mg/dL; both the Leuven studies,[1,8] the VISEP study,[15] and two other single-center large-scale trials[16,17] used a target value of 180–200 mg/dL, the CGAO-REA study[18] used a target value of less than 180 mg/dL, and a target of BG level less than 150 mg/dL was encouraged in the COIITSS trial.[19] Finally, the two pediatric studies used different target values of 180–215 mg/dL and 150–180 mg/dL.

The results of these trials are summarized in Table 25.1. Basically, there was no significant difference in the vital outcomes between the two groups, with the notable exceptions of the Leuven I study[1] and the NICE-SUGAR study,[13] in opposite directions. Not surprisingly, TGC by IIT is associated with a four- to six-fold increase in the incidence of hypoglycemia. This represents the major concern when starting IIT and is the major cause of an increased workload.[20] In a post hoc analysis of the NICE-SUGAR study, investigators demonstrated a strong, dose-dependent association between the risk of death and moderate (41–70 mg/dL) and severe (<40 mg/dL) hypoglycemia.[21] Similarly, Kalfon et al.[22] showed that severe hypoglycemia (<40 mg/dL) and multiple hypoglycemic episodes (≥3) were associated with increased 90-day mortality. Macrae et al.[12] were unable to demonstrate an improvement of the primary outcome (number of days alive

TABLE 25.1 Summary of the Prospective Large-Scale Randomized Controlled Trials of Tight Glucose Control by Intensive Insulin Therapy.

	Study	Number of Subjects (Intervention/No Intervention)	Study Design	Intervention (Blood Glucose Target)	Control (Blood Glucose Target)	Primary Outcome Variable
Single center	van der Bergeh et al. (Leuven I), 2001	765/783	Single-blind	80–110 mg/dL	180–200 mg/dL	ICU mortality
	van der Bergeh et al. (Leuven II), 2006	595/605	Single-blind	80–110 mg/dL	180–200 mg/dL	ICU mortality
	Arabi, 2008	266/257	Single-blind	80–110 mg/dL	180–200 mg/dL	ICU mortality
	De La Rosa, 2008	254/250	Single-blind	80–110 mg/dL	180–200 mg/dL	28-day mortality
Multicenter	Brunkhorst et al., 2008 (VISEP)	247/289	Single-blind	80–110 mg/dL	180–200 mg/dL	28-day mortality and SOFA
	Finfer et al., 2009 (NICE-SUGAR)	3054/3050	Single-blind	80–110 mg/dL	140–180 mg/dL	90-day mortality
	Preiser et al., 2009 (GluControl)	542/536	Single-blind	80–110 mg/dL	140–180 mg/dL	ICU mortality
	Annane et al., 2010 (COIITSS)	255/254	Open label multifactorial	80–110 mg/dL	<150 mg/dL	In-hospital mortality
	Kalfon et al., 2014	1336/1312	Single-blind	80–110 mg/dL	<180 mg/dL	90-day mortality
	Macrae et al., 2014	694/675	Single-blind	72–126 mg/dL	180–215 mg/dL	Number of days alive and free from MV at 30 days
	Agus et al., 2017	360/353	Single-blind	80–110 mg/dL	150–180 mg/dL	Number of ICU-free days today 28

ICU, intensive care unit; *NICE-SUGAR,* Normoglycemia in Intensive Care Evaluation—Survival Using Glucose Algorithm Regulation; *SOFA,* Sequential Organ Failure Assessment.

and free from mechanical ventilation at 30 days) but uncovered a decrease in the length of stay and health-care costs. In the GluControl[14] and VISEP[15] studies, the rate of hypoglycemia and mortality in patients who experienced at least one such episode (defined as BG < 40 mg/dL) were higher than in patients who did not experience hypoglycemia. In contrast, in both Leuven studies, hypoglycemic patients had no detectable differences in outcomes compared with patients without hypoglycemic episodes.[1,8] This does not exclude the possibility that long-lasting hypoglycemia, with consequent decreases in glucose availability for tissues that are glucose dependent, may be deleterious or even life threatening. The most typical example is the injured brain; using cerebral microdialysis, Oddo et al.[23] demonstrated that TGC was associated with a greater risk of brain energy crisis and death. These data suggest that TGC may result in hypoglycemia and neuroglycopenia at a time of increased cerebral metabolic demand. More recently, the concept of relative hypoglycemia has emerged to illustrate the relationship between the control of premorbid glycemia and dysglycemia in ICU.[24] In diabetic patients, the authors used HbA$_{1C}$ at admission to estimate premorbid baseline BG concentration and defined relative hypoglycemia when glycemic distance (the difference between BG concentrations in ICU and baseline BG concentration) was greater than 30%.

Systematic reviews and meta-analyses including data on glucose control recorded in the ICU and in other patients are also available. The design and main results of the nine meta-analyses[25-33] are summarized in Table 25.2. These analyses yielded different results, including the overall effects on mortality. The meta-analyses by Pittas et al.[25] and Gandhi et al.[26] revealed decreased short-term mortality (respective relative risks [95% confidence interval] of 0.85 [0.75–0.97] and 0.69 [0.51–0.94]). In contrast, the seven other studies[27-33] showed no significant effect on mortality and an increased risk of hypoglycemia.

INTERPRETATION OF DATA

The results of the different large-scale individual trials can be summarized as follows: in critically ill patients staying in an ICU, TGC by IIT improved survival in one proof-of-concept study only (Leuven I[1]). There are multiple potential explanations for the discrepant results between this and other studies. These include differences in the study population and treatment protocol, especially with regard to the amount of intravenous glucose, which was higher in Leuven I than in the other settings. Another possible factor that could explain differences in the outcome data is the quality of glucose control. Unfortunately, currently, there is no agreement on the best index to assess and compare the quality of glucose control.[34] Finally, the statistical power of each of these individual studies is probably too low. The rate of hypoglycemia in virtually all studies is increased five-fold.[27] Most hypoglycemic episodes are classified as a nonserious adverse event. However, this interpretation may be questioned following the publication of data from a retrospective cohort of 102 patients with at least one episode of severe hypoglycemia (<40 mg/dL) matched with 306 control patients from a

TABLE 25.2 Summary of Meta-analyses on Insulin Therapy.

Study	Number of Trials Included/ Retrieved	Number of Subjects (Intervention/No Intervention)	Intervention	Control	Outcomes
Pittas et al., 2004	35/941	Not indicated: total of 8432	Insulin therapy	No insulin	Short-term or hospital mortality
Gandhi et al., 2008	34/445	2192/2163	Intravenous perioperative insulin	Higher blood glucose target	Mortality and 11 outcome variables
Wiener et al., 2008	29/1358	4127/4188	Tight glucose control	Usual care	Short-term mortality, septicemia, new need for dialysis, hypoglycemia
Griesdale et al., 2009	26/54	Not indicated: total of 13,567	Intensive insulin therapy	Conventional glycemic control	Mortality risk and hypoglycemia risk
Marik et al., 2010	7/59	Not indicated: total of 11,412	Intensive insulin therapy	Less strict glucose control	28-day mortality
Song et al., 2014	12/26	2094/2006	Tight glucose control	Higher blood glucose target	28 days, 90 days, ICU, hospital mortality
Srinivasan et al., 2014	4/33	Not indicated: total of 3288	Intensive insulin therapy	Conventional glycemic control	30-day mortality
Zhao et al., 2018	5/58	1931/2002	Intensive insulin therapy	Conventional glycemic control	30-day mortality rates and acquired infections
Chen et al., 2018	6/170	1980/2050	Intensive insulin therapy	Usual care	Hospital mortality

cohort of 5365 patients.[35] In this study, hypoglycemia was found to be an independent risk predictor of mortality, possibly related to neuroglycopenia.

In contrast to studies that included patients who were not critically ill,[25,26] the meta-analysis that focused on critically ill patients[27] did not demonstrate an advantage of TGC. The meta-analysis by Pittas et al.[25] included patients with stroke, acute myocardial infarction, and diabetes. The results of the large trials of the effects of glucose-insulin-potassium (GIK) after acute myocardial infarction in patients with diabetes, a different intervention than TGC, were included and substantially influenced the overall results. Incidentally, most large trials of GIK during myocardial ischemia were conducted before the 1990s and involved populations with diabetes and acute myocardial infarction. The positive results of some of these studies in all probability reflect the metabolic effects of insulin. This includes the ability to promote the use of glucose as a primary myocardial energy substrate. In myocytes, the delivery of insulin increases glycolytic substrate and ultimately adenosine triphosphate (ATP) synthesis. This attenuated ischemia-induced decreases in ATP. However, these effects are unrelated to glucose control because BG in the GIK studies actually was not corrected.

The meta-analysis by Gandhi et al.[26] focused on perioperative glucose control. Most of the included studies involved coronary artery bypass surgery and patients who were not critically ill. The authors of this meta-analysis acknowledged that the available mortality data represent only 40% of the optimal information size required to reliably detect a treatment effect. Further, methodologic and reporting biases may weaken inferences.[26]

In the meta-analysis of Wiener et al.,[27] only studies performed in ICUs and aiming to reach a predefined BG level were included. This analysis, however, included studies of various sizes that targeted different BG levels. When evaluating the data from the largest individual prospective studies that used a target of 80–110 mg/dL BG in the intensive treatment arm,[1,8,13,16,17] the Leuven I study still appears as the outlier (Table 25.1). The aggregation of individual data from participants in each of these prospective studies could solve the remaining questions.[36] Griesdale et al.[28] analyzed this point in their meta-analysis. When they looked at the effect of IIT according to the type of ICU, they demonstrated a possible benefit among the surgical ICU patients although they did not find any effect on the overall risk of death. The lower mortality rate of surgical patients than that of other patients demonstrates that this is a distinct group and makes it difficult for an extrapolation to whole ICU patients.

Marik and Preiser[29] raised the question of any variables that would differ between Leuven I and the other studies. They identified the route of administration of calories—a positive effect of IIT was noted when a large amount of calories was administrated intravenously. The explanation could be the reduction of the toxicity due to an important hyperglycemia with excessive cellular glucose uptake.

Song et al.[30] performed a subgroup meta-analysis of studies in septic patients. This was pertinent because septic patients

are "insulin-resistant" with an important modification of their metabolism and because hyperglycemia in sepsis correlated with an unfavorable prognosis.[37] However, they failed to demonstrate a positive effect of insulin for these patients. Currently, the recommendations of the Surviving Sepsis Campaign is to treat the hyperglycemia with a target less than 180 mg/dL without minimum value and avoiding hypoglycemia, in agreement with other protocol recommendations.[38–40]

In pediatric population, the meta-analyses showed the same conclusions in terms of mortality and hypoglycemia rate.[31–33]

CONCLUSION

- IIT titrated to restore and maintain BG between 80 and 110 mg/dL was found to improve survival of critically ill patients in one pioneering proof-of-concept study performed in a surgical ICU.[1] This result was not confirmed in any of the subsequent trials.[8,13–17] The underlying reasons for this discrepancy are under investigation and could be linked to the fact that this study analyzed a particular subgroup of patients.
- Studies using IIT reveal a high rate of hypoglycemia that may alter outcome.[41]
- The effects of severe hyperglycemia (>180 mg/dL) are well documented.
- The choice of intermediate target appears logical to minimize the risks for hypoglycemia.
- A BG target below 180 mg/dL is presently recommended by the Surviving Sepsis Campaign.[42]

AUTHORS' RECOMMENDATIONS
- Severe hyperglycemia is harmful.
- IIT titrated to achieve a BG level between 80 and 110 mg/dL was found to improve survival in one study.
- IIT is labor intensive and increases the risk for hypoglycemia.
- Particularities of the case mix, usual care, and quality of glucose control in the unit where IIT was found beneficial compared with other ICUs might explain the differences in the effects of IIT.

REFERENCES

1. Van den Berghe G, Wouters P, Weekers F, et al. Intensive insulin therapy in the critically ill patients. *N Engl J Med*. 2001;345(19):1359-1367.
2. Dungan KM, Braithwaite SS, Preiser JC. Stress hyperglycemia. *Lancet*. 2009;373(9677):1798-1807.
3. Brownlee M. Biochemistry and molecular cell biology of diabetic complications. *Nature* 2001;414(6865):813-820.
4. Szabó C, Biser A, Benko R, et al. Poly(ADP-Ribose) polymerase inhibitors ameliorate nephropathy of type 2 diabetic Leprdb/db mice. *Diabetes*. 2006;55(11):3004-3012.
5. Ceriello A. Oxidative stress and diabetes-associated complications. *Endocr Pract*. 2006;12(suppl 1):S60-S62.
6. Corstjens AM, van der Horst IC, Zijlstra JG, et al. Hyperglycaemia in critically ill patients: marker or mediator of mortality? *Crit Care*. 2006;10(3):216.

7. Preiser JC. Restoring normoglycemia: not so harmless. *Crit Care.* 2008;12(1):116.

8. Van den Berghe G, Wilmer A, Hermans G, et al. Intensive insulin therapy in the medical ICU. *N Engl J Med.* 2006;354(5):449-461.

9. Krinsley JS. Effect of an intensive glucose management protocol on the mortality of critically ill adult patients. *Mayo Clin Proc.* 2004;79(8):992-1000.

10. Finney SJ, Zekveld C, Elia A, Evans TW. Glucose control and mortality in critically ill patients. *JAMA.* 2003;290(15): 2041-2047.

11. Agus MS, Wypij D, Hirschberg EL, et al. Tight glycemic control in critically ill children. *N Engl J Med.* 2017;376(8):729-741.

12. Macrae D, Grieve R, Allen E, et al. A randomized trial of hyperglycemic control in pediatric intensive care. *N Engl J Med.* 2014;370(2):107-118.

13. NICE-SUGAR Study Investigators, Finfer S, Chittock DR, et al. Intensive versus conventional glucose control in critically ill patients. *N Engl J Med.* 2009;360(13):1283-1297.

14. Preiser JC, Devos P, Ruiz-Santana S, et al. A prospective randomised multi-centre controlled trial on tight glucose control by intensive insulin therapy in adult intensive care units: the Glucontrol study. *Intensive Care Med.* 2009;35(10):1738-1748.

15. Brunkhorst FM, Engel C, Bloos F, et al. Intensive insulin therapy and pentastarch resuscitation in severe sepsis. *N Engl J Med.* 2008;358(2):125-139.

16. De La Rosa Gdel C, Donado JH, Restrepo AH, et al. Strict glycaemic control in patients hospitalised in a mixed medical and surgical intensive care unit: a randomised clinical trial. *Crit Care.* 2008;12(5):R120.

17. Arabi YM, Dabbagh OC, Tamim HM, et al. Intensive versus conventional insulin therapy: a randomized controlled trial in medical and surgical critically ill patients. *Crit Care Med.* 2008;36(12):3190-3197.

18. Kalfon P, Giraudeau B, Ichai C, et al. Tight computerized versus conventional glucose control in the ICU: a randomized controlled trial. *Intensive Care Med.* 2014;40(2):171-181.

19. COIITSS Study Investigators, Annane D, Cariou A, et al. Corticosteroid treatment and intensive insulin therapy for septic shock in adults: a randomized controlled trial. *JAMA.* 2010;303(4):341-348.

20. Aragon D. Evaluation of nursing work effort and perceptions about blood glucose testing in tight glycemic control. *Am J Crit Care.* 2006;15(4):370-377.

21. NICE-SUGAR Study Investigators, Finfer S, Liu B, et al. Hypoglycemia and risk of death in critically ill patients. *N Engl J Med.* 2012;367(12):1108-1118.

22. Kalfon P, Le Manach Y, Ichai C, et al. Severe and multiple hypoglycemic episodes are associated with increased risk of death in ICU patients. *Crit Care.* 2015;19:153.

23. Oddo M, Schmidt JM, Carrera E, et al. Impact of tight glycemic control on cerebral glucose metabolism after severe brain injury: a microdialysis study. *Crit Care Med.* 2008;36(12):3233-3238.

24. Di Muzio F, Presello B, Glassford NJ, et al. Liberal versus conventional glucose targets in critically ill diabetic patients: an exploratory safety cohort assessment. *Crit Care Med.* 2016;44(9):1683-1691.

25. Pittas AG, Siegel RD, Lau J. Insulin therapy for critically ill hospitalized patients: a meta-analysis of randomized controlled trials. *Arch Intern Med.* 2004;164(18):2005-2011.

26. Gandhi GY, Murad MH, Flynn DN, et al. Effect of perioperative insulin infusion on surgical morbidity and mortality: systematic review and meta-analysis of randomized trials. *Mayo Clin Proc.* 2008;83(4):418-430.

27. Wiener RS, Wiener DC, Larson RJ. Benefits and risks of tight glucose control in critically ill adults: a meta-analysis. *JAMA.* 2008;300(8):933-944.

28. Griesdale DE, de Souza RJ, van Dam RM, et al. Intensive insulin therapy and mortality among critically ill patients: a meta-analysis including NICE-SUGAR study data. *CMAJ.* 2009;180(8):821-827.

29. Marik PE, Preiser JC. Toward understanding tight glycemic control in the ICU: a systematic review and metaanalysis. *Chest.* 2010;137(3):544-551.

30. Song F, Zhong LJ, Han L, et al. Intensive insulin therapy for septic patients: a meta-analysis of randomized controlled trials. *Biomed Res Int.* 2014;2014:698265.

31. Srinivasan V, Agus MS. Tight glucose control in critically ill children—a systematic review and meta-analysis. *Pediatr Diabetes.* 2014;15(2):75-83.

32. Zhao Y, Wu Y, Xiang B. Tight glycemic control in critically ill patients: a meta-analysis and systematic review of randomized controlled trials. *Pediatr Res.* 2018;84(1):22-27.

33. Chen L, Li T, Fang F, et al. Tight glycemic control in critically ill patients: a systematic review and meta-analysis. *Crit Care.* 2018;22(1):57.

34. Eslami S, de Keizer NF, de Jonge E, et al. A systematic review on quality indicators for tight glycaemic control in critically ill patients: need for an unambiguous indicator reference subset. *Crit Care.* 2008;12(6):R139.

35. Krinsley JS, Grover A. Severe hypoglycemia in critically ill patients: risk factors and outcomes. *Crit Care Med.* 2007;35(10):2262-2267.

36. Stewart LA, Tierney JF. To IPD or not to IPD? Advantages and disadvantages of systematic reviews using individual patient data. *Eval Health Prof.* 2002;25(1):76-97.

37. Leonidou L, Michalaki M, Leonardou A, et al. Stress-induced hyperglycemia in patients with severe sepsis: a compromising factor for survival. *Am J Med Sci.* 2008;336(6):467-471.

38. Ichai C, Preiser JC, Société Française d'Anesthésie-Réanimation, et al. International recommendations for glucose control in adult non diabetic critically ill patients. *Crit Care.* 2010;14(5):R166.

39. Qaseem A, Humphrey LL, Chou R, et al. Use of intensive insulin therapy for the management of glycemic control in hospitalized patients: a clinical practice guideline from the American College of Physicians. *Ann Intern Med.* 2011;154(4):260-267.

40. Jacobi J, Bircher N, Krinsley J, et al. Guidelines for the use of an insulin infusion for the management of hyperglycemia in critically ill patients. *Crit Care Med.* 2012;40(12):3251-3276.

41. Krinsley JS, Preiser JC. Moving beyond tight glucose control to safe effective glucose control. *Crit Care.* 2008;12(3):149.

42. Dellinger RP, Levy MM, Rhodes A, et al. Surviving Sepsis Campaign: international guidelines for management of severe sepsis and septic shock: 2012. *Crit Care Med.* 2013;41(2):580-637.

26

Is There a Role for Therapeutic Hypothermia in Critical Care?

Tomas Drabek and Patrick M. Kochanek

Despite its long history,[1] the widespread clinical application of hypothermia is a relatively new phenomenon. Two seminal clinical trials published in 2002 demonstrated the benefits of therapeutic hypothermia (TH) after cardiac arrest (CA).[2,3] Recent findings suggest that even ultra-mild hypothermia (36°C) may have favorable physiologic effects and that avoidance of hyperthermia may be a desirable clinical goal. In this chapter, we focus on mild to moderate hypothermia that does not require the use of cardiopulmonary bypass and can be accomplished in an intensive care unit (ICU).

TEMPERATURE MONITORING

The normal body temperature in healthy individuals (measured in the oral cavity) is 36.8 ± 0.4°C with normal diurnal variations of 0.5°C. Rectal temperatures are usually 0.4°C higher than oral readings.[4] Lower-esophageal temperature closely reflects the core temperature, as well as rectal and bladder temperatures. The temperature measured via pulmonary artery catheters most closely correlates with brain temperature during rapid cooling.[5] Clinically, measuring heat radiating from the tympanic membrane (tympanic temperature) is often used as a surrogate for deep brain temperature. In clinical practice, temperatures of 33°C–36°C are usually referred to as mild hypothermia, 28°C–32°C as moderate hypothermia, and below 28°C as deep hypothermia.[6]

COOLING METHODS

Traditionally, external cooling with ice packs applied over great vessels or ice-water soaked cloth blankets has been used to treat hyperthermia and, eventually, induce hypothermia. Gastric, peritoneal, or pulmonary lavage was used to rewarm drowning victims and, in reverse, for cooling. Recently, cooling of CA victims with a rapid large volume (30 mL/kg) intravenous (IV) infusion of ice-cold (4°C) solutions has been shown to decrease the core temperature from 35.5°C to 33.8°C within 30 minutes without any observed changes in vital signs, electrolytes, arterial blood gases, or coagulation parameters.[2,7] However, this method is not effective for maintaining hypothermia.[8] Methods used to achieve hypothermia are listed in Box 26.1.

COMPLICATIONS ASSOCIATED WITH THERAPEUTIC HYPOTHERMIA

Hypothermia initiates temperature-dependent physiologic changes in the circulatory, respiratory, neurologic, immunologic, and coagulation systems. It also has profound metabolic effects. TH may induce sinus tachycardia, decrease cardiac output, and increase systemic vascular resistance, central venous pressure, and myocardial perfusion.[9] As currently used mild hypothermia is well tolerated. Hypothermia also induces the release of endogenous catecholamines; a minimal temperature change (0.7°C–1.2°C) is associated with a four- to seven-fold increase in norepinephrine levels.[10] Ventricular ectopy was more frequent at 33°C than at 36°C.[11] Bradycardia during TH is associated with good neurologic outcome at hospital discharge and should not be aggressively treated if other hemodynamic parameters are favorable.[12]

The impact of hypothermia on coagulation is a result of platelet or clotting factor depletion or dysfunction. The magnitude of changes is often difficult to assess because clinical laboratories adjust the temperatures of all samples to a standard of 37°C.[13] Reed et al. cooled plasma containing clotting factors equivalent to 100% of normal to 35°C, 33°C, and 31°C.[14] Partial thromboplastin time in these samples was prolonged as if Factor IX had been depleted to 39%, 16%, and 2.5% of normal, respectively. Thromboelastography (TEG) may be a useful tool in the setting of post-CA TH.[15,16]

TEG measurements performed on hypothermic (32°C) swine demonstrated a deficit in thrombin availability and/or a delay in thrombin generation or activation. This change, however, was not associated with a decrease in clot strength or an increase in clot lysis.[17] Bleeding time, one indicator of platelet function, was prolonged two and a half-fold in a sample from a cold (32°C) versus warm extremity (37°C) in baboons.[18] In a similar experiment in human volunteers, clotting times were longer at 22°C than at 37°C.[19] Concurrent acidosis further impaired coagulation.[20] Trials indicate that neither mild nor moderate TH is associated with bleeding complications in patients with severe traumatic brain injury (TBI).[21,22] A tendency toward higher bleeding was observed in CA patients treated with TH.[23]

Hypothermia may lead to leukopenia and an increased risk of infection. Studies in patients after CA, TBI, or acute

BOX 26.1   **Some Methods for Inducing Hypothermia.**

Surface cooling devices
Intravascular cooling catheters
Cooling helmets
Nasopharyngeal cooling
Neck cooling
Esophageal cooling
Direct cooling of blood in the carotid arteries
Extracorporeal circulation

BOX 26.2   **Possible Mechanisms Underlying Central Nervous System Protection by Hypothermia.**

Maintenance of physiologic ATP concentrations
Suppression of glutamate release
Reduction of seizures
Attenuation of oxidative or nitrative stress
Prevention of energy failure
Limitation of cytoskeletal damage
Increased levels of neurotrophins
Prevention of anoxic depolarization
Regulation of gene expression
Attenuation of apoptosis
Limitation of blood-brain barrier injury
Reduction in vasogenic edema
Intracranial pressure[36,37]

stroke showed an increased risk of pneumonia, especially when the duration of TH was prolonged.[2,3,22,24,25] A 2014 metaanalysis confirmed that TH was associated with an increased risk for pneumonia and sepsis (RR, 1.44 [95% CI, 1.10–1.90]; 1.80 [95% CI, 1.04–3.10], respectively) but overall the prevalence of infections was not increased (RR, 1.21 [95% CI, 0.95–1.54]).[26]

Electrolyte disorders, although common in TH, are usually minor.[27,28] Magnesium supplementation may be especially important given its known protective role in neuronal and myocardial injury.[27,29,30]

Hypothermia-induced decreases in insulin sensitivity may lead to hyperglycemia. This abnormality could enhance susceptibility to infection and might also exacerbate secondary brain injury.[31] Tight glycemic control may be warranted with glucose target level of >150 mg/dL.[32]

Drug metabolism is profoundly altered by hypothermia.[33] Mild to moderate hypothermia decreases systemic clearance of cytochrome P450-metabolized drugs by approximately 7%–22% per degree below 37°C.[34] Hypothermia decreases the potency and efficacy of certain drugs.[34] Hypothermia-mediated effects are an important factor when dosing and monitoring patients undergoing TH.

MECHANISM OF ACTION OF HYPOTHERMIA

Hypothermia was originally believed to provide protection because the cerebral metabolic rate is decreased by 5%–7% for each degree that body temperature is decreased.[35] However, this observation does not explain the effects of even small temperature changes on physiology and neuroprotection. Protection by hypothermia in experimental central nervous system (CNS) injury might involve a myriad of mechanisms listed in Box 26.2. One or any combination of these could underlie the different outcomes in the wide variety of CNS injuries.

HYPOTHERMIA IN CARDIAC ARREST

Several randomized human trials assessed the efficacy of TH after CA. Following a small study,[38] two studies published in 2002 clearly established the value of TH in CA. Bernard et al.[2] studied 77 patients after CA due to ventricular fibrillation (VF); 49% of the hypothermic patients survived with good

neurologic outcome, a finding significantly different from those who were not treated (26%, P = .046, odds ratio for good outcome = −5.25; 95% CI, 1.47–18.76; P = .011). In the European multicenter Hypothermia After Cardiac Arrest trial, 55% of patients randomized to the hypothermia group (32°C–34°C for 24 hours) after resuscitation from VF-induced CA showed favorable neurologic outcome compared with 39% in controls (RR, 1.68; 95% CI, 1.29–2.07; number needed to treat = 6).[3] The similar results in these two trials led to International Liaison Committee on Resuscitation recommending the use of cooling (32°C–34°C for 12–24 hours) in unconscious adult patients with spontaneous circulation after out-of-hospital VF-associated CA. Further, the committee recommended this cooling regimen be considered for unconscious adult patients with spontaneous circulation after out-of-hospital CA from any other rhythm or CA in hospital.[39,40] Improvements in cognitive and neurophysiological outcomes have not been detected.[25,41–44]

Current recommendations have been adjusted to reflect conflicting results.[45–51] It remains for future trials to determine if the benefits originally reported can be extended to other settings. Data from in-hospital CA are emerging,[52] but the initial results are not compelling.[53] TH for CA induced by hanging and in children following drowning also is not promising.[54,55] Other data on the pediatric population similarly failed to demonstrate a benefit from TH.[56–59] However, success in infants undergoing TH for 72 hours after CA have suggested the need to evaluate this treatment time in children after CA.[60]

THERAPEUTIC HYPOTHERMIA IN ISCHEMIC STROKE

Preclinical studies addressing focal brain ischemia have shown up to 90% lesion reduction with hypothermia.[61,62] Importantly, it was found that brain temperatures in stroke patients seem to exceed core temperature by at least 1°C (1.0°C–2.1°C).[63] Unfortunately, studies aimed at reducing body temperature in stroke victims have proven to be challenging. A study involving 3790 patients demonstrated that preventing hyperthermia in stroke patients improved outcome[64] but a pharmacologic approach to hypothermia did not adequately decrease body temperature.[65] Studies document that use of TH following acute ischemic stroke decreases intracranial pressure (ICP) but increases occur during rewarming. Additional studies have revealed that TH did not affect clinical outcomes or lesion size at 1 month.

Thus, there currently are no robust data to support the use of TH in patients with ischemic stroke and the European Stroke Organisation does not recommend routine use of hypothermia in stroke patients, or use of antipyretics to prevent hyperthermia.[66]

HYPOTHERMIA FOR SPINAL CORD INJURY

There are a limited number of studies addressing the use of TH following traumatic spinal cord injury (SCI). Animal studies are mixed but overall suggest beneficial effects.[67] Several case series using whole-body hypothermia for SCI have been published documenting feasibility.[68,69] Currently, there is emerging evidence suggesting that TH might be beneficial after traumatic SCI, but definitive studies are still lacking.

HYPOTHERMIA FOR TRAUMATIC BRAIN INJURY

In contrast to CA, the onset of neuronal death in TBI occurs early in the course of the syndrome,[70] and there are distinct pathophysiologic differences between children and adults. Several published meta-analyses yielded conflicting results: some indicated improved neurologic outcome and mortality,[71] whereas some did not.[72–74] Metaanalyses in pediatric TBI are conflicting.[75–77] Hypothermia does appear to be effective in reducing increased ICP; however, favorable neurologic outcome could not be achieved in all patients.[78] Hypothermia did not seem to negatively affect the outcomes in patients with coagulopathy following severe TBI and seems safe in this population.[79]

In a 2008 international multicenter trial, TH did not improve the neurologic outcome and indeed even seemed to increase mortality. Technical issues complicated interpretation.[80] Other studies reported similar results.[81,82] Hypothermia also reduced phenytoin metabolism in TBI patients; caution is advised, especially during rewarming.[83] It is also associated with an increased incidence of pulmonary infections.[24] Fever control may be considered instead of TH in TBI patients with noncritical severity.[84]

In conclusion, TH has not, to date, been convincingly shown to improve outcomes in TBI.

HYPOTHERMIA FOR ACUTE MYOCARDIAL INFARCTION

In a small multicenter study of patients with AMI undergoing primary percutaneous coronary intervention, endovascular cooling (33°C for 3 hours) did not affect median infarct size.[85] Extending the duration of TH (33°C) from 24 hours to 48 hours in CA survivors showed no difference in myocardial injury[86] and failed to improve key echocardiographic signs of myocardial recovery.[87]

These studies are in contrast with the combined results of COOL-MI and ICE-IT trials and of the RAPID MI-ICE[88] and CHILL-MI[89] trials suggesting that TH reduced infarct size following AMI.[90,91] In contrast, the SHOCK-COOL trial did not show a benefit in AMI patients with cardiogenic shock.[92]

HYPOTHERMIA FOR HYPOXIC-ISCHEMIC ENCEPHALOPATHY

The data from 11 randomized controlled trials comprising 1505 near-term infants were summarized in a 2016 Cochrane review that was consistent with earlier results.[93] TH resulted in a statistically significant and clinically important reduction in the combined outcome of mortality or major neurodevelopmental disability to 18 months of age. Some adverse effects of TH included an increased sinus bradycardia and significant thrombocytopenia.[93] Initiation of TH past 6 hours may still confer benefits.[94] Cooling for longer than 72 hours, cooling to lower than 33.5°C, or both did not reduce early ICU mortality,[95] or death or moderate or severe disability at 18 months of age.[96] Unfortunately, these benefits were not seen in a metaanalysis of seven trials from low- and middle-income countries.[97] The current regimen of cooling for 72 hours at 33.5°C should be followed.

HYPOTHERMIA IN OTHER CLINICAL SCENARIOS

Moderate hypothermia did not improve outcomes in comatose patients with severe bacterial meningitis and may even be harmful.[98]

In patients with sepsis, spontaneous[99,100] or induced[101] hypothermia was associated with worse outcomes. However, cooling to normothermia lowered vasopressor requirement and 14-day mortality in septic shock.[102] Antipyretic therapy decreased body temperature (by 0.4°C) but did not significantly improve hospital mortality.[103]

In a large multicenter trial (IHAST), intraoperative TH did not improve the neurologic outcome after craniotomy among patients with aneurysmal subarachnoid hemorrhage and good preoperative neurologic status.[104]

In a small pilot trial, TH prevented the development of perihemorrhagic edema after large intracranial hemorrhage and its complications.[105] In a metaanalysis of patients with hemorrhagic stroke, TH did not significantly reduce mortality or poor outcomes but led to a decreased incidence of delayed cerebral ischemia.[106]

A large randomized study of TH added to standard care was not associated with significantly better 90-day outcomes than standard care alone in patients with convulsive status epilepticus.[107]

CONCLUSION

TH in ICU represents a promising multifaceted therapy for several medical conditions. While extremely powerful, it requires careful titration of its depth, duration, and rewarming. To date, TH (33°C or 36°C) is a generally accepted treatment for out-of-hospital CA in adults. Hospitals adopting a target temperature of 36°C need to be aware that this target may not be easy to achieve and requires adequate sedation and muscle-relaxant to avoid fever. Indeed, anecdotally, it can be easier to maintain mild hypothermia (33°C–34°C) than to clamp temperature at 36°C. There is strong efficacy for treatment of hypoxic ischemic encephalopathy in term newborns. The current technology to induce and maintain TH allows for precise temperature control. Future studies should focus on optimizing hypothermic treatment to the full benefit of patients.

AUTHORS' RECOMMENDATIONS

- Targeted temperature management at 32°C–36°C is neuroprotective in comatose patients who survive out-of-hospital CA and suggested in patients after in-hospital CA irrespective of the presenting rhythm. A strict control of the temperature must be maintained to avoid hyperthermia (>37.5°C) and severe hypothermia (<32°C) in children. Prehospital cooling is not recommended. In adults and children, it is unclear whether TH at 33°C–34°C is more efficacious than rigorous prevention of fever by clamping temperature at 36°C.
- Mild TH (33.5°C–34.5°C for 72 hours) is an accepted treatment of term newborns (≥35 weeks of gestation) suffering hypoxic-ischemic insults in the perinatal period.
- Based on studies in experimental models and clinical studies, mild TH may have other potential uses as a neuroprotectant in neurointensive care such as in stroke, TBI, SCI, and other conditions. However, further studies are needed to determine potential benefits in these scenarios.
- The mechanisms underlying the beneficial effects of TH appear to be multifactorial and are only beginning to be understood in the clinical setting.
- Optimization of cooling methods, duration and depth of TH, approach to rewarming, and minimization and management of side effects are needed to maximize the therapeutic potential of hypothermia.

REFERENCES

1. Bohl MA, Martirosyan NL, Killeen ZW, et al. The history of therapeutic hypothermia and its use in neurosurgery. *J Neurosurg.* 2018;1-15.
2. Bernard SA, Gray TW, Buist MD, et al. Treatment of comatose survivors of out-of-hospital cardiac arrest with induced hypothermia. *N Engl J Med.* 2002;346:557-563.
3. Hypothermia after Cardiac Arrest Study Group. Mild therapeutic hypothermia to improve the neurologic outcome after cardiac arrest. *N Engl J Med.* 2002;346:549-556.
4. Fauci AS, Braunwald E, Kasper DL, et al. Alterations in body temperature. *Harrison's Principles of Internal Medicine.* 17th ed. New York: McGraw-Hill; 2008:117-121.
5. Janata A, Weihs W, Bayegan K, et al. Therapeutic hypothermia with a novel surface cooling device improves neurologic outcome after prolonged cardiac arrest in swine. *Crit Care Med.* 2008;36:895-902.
6. Safar PJ, Kochanek PM. Therapeutic hypothermia after cardiac arrest. *N Engl J Med.* 2002;346:612-613.
7. Kim F, Olsufka M, Carlbom D, et al. Pilot study of rapid infusion of 2 L of 4 degrees C normal saline for induction of mild hypothermia in hospitalized, comatose survivors of out-of-hospital cardiac arrest. *Circulation.* 2005;112:715-719.
8. Kliegel A, Janata A, Wandaller C, et al. Cold infusions alone are effective for induction of therapeutic hypothermia but do not keep patients cool after cardiac arrest. *Resuscitation.* 2007; 73:46-53.
9. Frank SM, Satitpunwaycha P, Bruce SR, et al. Increased myocardial perfusion and sympathoadrenal activation during mild core hypothermia in awake humans. *Clin Sci (Lond).* 2003;104:503-508.
10. Frank SM, Higgins MS, Fleisher LA, et al. Adrenergic, respiratory, and cardiovascular effects of core cooling in humans. *Am J Physiol.* 1997;272:R557-R562.
11. Thomsen JH, Kjaergaard J, Graff C, et al. Ventricular ectopic burden in comatose survivors of out-of-hospital cardiac arrest treated with targeted temperature management at 33 degrees C and 36 degrees C. *Resuscitation.* 2016;102:98-104.
12. Staer-Jensen H, Sunde K, Olasveengen TM, et al. Bradycardia during therapeutic hypothermia is associated with good neurologic outcome in comatose survivors of out-of-hospital cardiac arrest. *Crit Care Med.* 2014;42:2401-2408.
13. Brinkman AC, Ten Tusscher BL, de Waard MC, et al. Minimal effects on ex vivo coagulation during mild therapeutic hypothermia in post cardiac arrest patients. *Resuscitation.* 2014;85(10):1359-1363.
14. Johnston T.D.; Chen Y.; Reed R.L. 2nd. Functional equivalence of hypothermia to specific clotting factor deficiencies. *J Trauma* (1994) 37 413–417
15. Trąbka-Zawicki A, Tomala M, Zeliaś A, et al. Adaptation of global hemostasis to therapeutic hypothermia in patients with out-of-hospital cardiac arrest: thromboelastography study. *Cardiol J.* 2017 [Epub ahead of print].
16. Jacob M, Hassager C, Bro-Jeppesen J, et al. The effect of targeted temperature management on coagulation parameters and bleeding events after out-of-hospital cardiac arrest of presumed cardiac cause. *Resuscitation.* 2015;96:260-267.
17. Martini WZ. The effects of hypothermia on fibrinogen metabolism and coagulation function in swine. *Metabolism.* 2007;56:214-221.
18. Watts DD, Trask A, Soeken K, et al. Hypothermic coagulopathy in trauma: effect of varying levels of hypothermia on enzyme speed, platelet function, and fibrinolytic activity. *J Trauma.* 1998;44:846-854.
19. Valeri CR, MacGregor H, Cassidy G, et al. Effects of temperature on bleeding time and clotting time in normal male and female volunteers. *Crit Care Med.* 1995;23:698-704.
20. Dirkmann D, Hanke AA, Gorlinger K, Peters J. Hypothermia and acidosis synergistically impair coagulation in human whole blood. *Anesth Analg.* 2008;106:1627-1632.
21. Clifton GL, Miller ER, Choi SC, et al. Lack of effect of induction of hypothermia after acute brain injury. *N Engl J Med.* 2001; 344:556-563.
22. Marion DW, Penrod LE, Kelsey SF, et al. Treatment of traumatic brain injury with moderate hypothermia. *N Engl J Med.* 1997; 336:540-546.
23. Stockmann H, Krannich A, Schroeder T, Storm C. Therapeutic temperature management after cardiac arrest and the risk of

bleeding: systematic review and meta-analysis. *Resuscitation*. 2014;85(11):1494-1503.

24. O'Phelan KH, Merenda A, Denny KG, et al. Therapeutic temperature modulation is associated with pulmonary complications in patients with severe traumatic brain injury. *World J Crit Care Med*. 2015;4:296-301.

25. Dankiewicz J, Nielsen N, Linder A, et al. Infectious complications after out-of-hospital cardiac arrest–a comparison between two target temperatures. *Resuscitation*. 2017;113:70-76.

26. Geurts M, Macleod MR, Kollmar R, et al. Therapeutic hypothermia and the risk of infection: a systematic review and meta-analysis. *Crit Care Med*. 2014;42:231-242.

27. Polderman KH, Peerdeman SM, Girbes AR. Hypophosphatemia and hypomagnesemia induced by cooling in patients with severe head injury. *J Neurosurg*. 2001;94:697-705.

28. Aibiki M, Kawaguchi S, Maekawa N. Reversible hypophosphatemia during moderate hypothermia therapy for brain-injured patients. *Crit Care Med*. 2001;29:1726-1730.

29. Shechter M, Hod H, Rabinowitz B, et al. Long-term outcome of intravenous magnesium therapy in thrombolysis-ineligible acute myocardial infarction patients. *Cardiology*. 2003;99:205-210.

30. McIntosh TK, Vink R, Yamakami I, Faden AI. Magnesium protects against neurological deficit after brain injury. *Brain Res*. 1989;482:252-260.

31. Rovlias A, Kotsou S. The influence of hyperglycemia on neurological outcome in patients with severe head injury. *Neurosurgery*. 2000;46:335-342; discussion 342-343.

32. Vespa P, Boonyaputthikul R, McArthur DL, et al. Intensive insulin therapy reduces microdialysis glucose values without altering glucose utilization or improving the lactate/pyruvate ratio after traumatic brain injury. *Crit Care Med*. 2006;34:850-856.

33. Anderson KB, Poloyac SM, Kochanek PM, Empey PE. Effect of hypothermia and targeted temperature management on drug disposition and response following cardiac arrest: a comprehensive review of preclinical and clinical investigations. *Ther Hypothermia Temp Manag*. 2016;6:169-179.

34. Tortorici MA, Kochanek PM, Poloyac SM. Effects of hypothermia on drug disposition, metabolism, and response: a focus of hypothermia-mediated alterations on the cytochrome P450 enzyme system. *Crit Care Med*. 2007;35:2196-2204.

35. Rosomoff HL, Holaday DA. Cerebral blood flow and cerebral oxygen consumption during hypothermia. *Am J Physiol*. 1954;179:85-88.

36. Polderman KH. Induced hypothermia and fever control for prevention and treatment of neurological injuries. *Lancet*. 2008;371:1955-1969.

37. Schwab S, Schwarz S, Spranger M, et al. Moderate hypothermia in the treatment of patients with severe middle cerebral artery infarction. *Stroke*. 1998;29:2461-2466.

38. Hachimi-Idrissi S, Corne L, Ebinger G, et al. Mild hypothermia induced by a helmet device: a clinical feasibility study. *Resuscitation*. 2001;51:275-281.

39. ECC Committee of the AHA. 2005 American Heart Association Guidelines for Cardiopulmonary Resuscitation and Emergency Cardiovascular Care. Part 4: advanced life support. *Circulation*. 2005;112:III-25-54.

40. Deakin CD, Morrison LJ, Morley PT, et al. Part 8: advanced life support: 2010 International Consensus on Cardiopulmonary Resuscitation and Emergency Cardiovascular Care Science with Treatment Recommendations. *Resuscitation*. 2010;81 Suppl 1:e93-e174.

41. Nielsen N, Wetterslev J, Cronberg T, et al. Targeted temperature management at 33 degrees C versus 36 degrees C after cardiac arrest. *N Engl J Med*. 2013;369:2197-2206.

42. Cronberg T, Lilja G, Horn J, et al. Neurologic function and health-related quality of life in patients following targeted temperature management at 33 degrees C vs 36 degrees C after out-of-hospital cardiac arrest: a randomized clinical trial. *JAMA Neurol*. 2015;72:634-641.

43. Arvidsson L, Lindgren S, Martinell L, et al. Target temperature 34 vs. 36 degrees C after out-of-hospital cardiac arrest - a retrospective observational study. *Acta Anaesthesiol Scand*. 2017;61:1176-1183.

44. Bray JE, Stub D, Bloom JE, et al. Changing target temperature from 33 degrees C to 36 degrees C in the ICU management of out-of-hospital cardiac arrest: a before and after study. *Resuscitation*. 2017;113:39-43.

45. Nolan JP, Soar J, Cariou A, et al. European Resuscitation Council and European Society of Intensive Care Medicine guidelines for post-resuscitation care 2015: section 5 of the European Resuscitation Council guidelines for resuscitation 2015. *Resuscitation*. 2015;95:202-222.

46. Donnino MW, Andersen LW, Berg KM, et al. Temperature management after cardiac arrest: an advisory statement by the Advanced Life Support Task Force of the International Liaison Committee on Resuscitation and the American Heart Association Emergency Cardiovascular Care Committee and the Council on Cardiopulmonary, Critical Care, Perioperative and Resuscitation. *Circulation*. 2015;132:2448-2456.

47. Geocadin RG, Wijdicks E, Armstrong MJ, et al. Practice guideline summary: reducing brain injury following cardiopulmonary resuscitation: report of the Guideline Development, Dissemination, and Implementation Subcommittee of the American Academy of Neurology. *Neurology*. 2017;88:2141-2149.

48. Cariou A, Payen JF, Asehnoune K, et al. Targeted temperature management in the ICU: guidelines from a French expert panel. *Ann Intensive Care*. 2017;7:70.

49. Vargas M, Servillo G, Sutherasan Y, et al. Effects of in-hospital low targeted temperature after out of hospital cardiac arrest: a systematic review with meta-analysis of randomized clinical trials. *Resuscitation*. 2015;91:8-18.

50. Arrich J, Holzer M, Havel C, et al. Hypothermia for neuroprotection in adults after cardiopulmonary resuscitation. *Cochrane Database Syst Rev*. 2016;2:CD004128.

51. Kirkegaard H, Soreide E, de Haas I, et al. Targeted temperature management for 48 vs 24 hours and neurologic outcome after out-of-hospital cardiac arrest: a randomized clinical trial. *JAMA*. 2017;318:341-350.

52. Dankiewicz J, Schmidbauer S, Nielsen N, et al. Safety, feasibility, and outcomes of induced hypothermia therapy following in-hospital cardiac arrest-evaluation of a large prospective registry. *Crit Care Med*. 2014;42(12):2537-2545.

53. Chan PS, Berg RA, Tang Y, et al. Association between therapeutic hypothermia and survival after in-hospital cardiac arrest. *JAMA*. 2016;316:1375-1382.

54. Hsu CH, Haac BE, Drake M, et al. EAST multicenter trial on targeted temperature management for hanging-induced cardiac arrest. *J Trauma Acute Care Surg*. 2018;85:37-47.

55. Moler FW, Hutchison JS, Nadkarni VM, et al. Targeted temperature management after pediatric cardiac arrest due to drowning: outcomes and complications. *Pediatr Crit Care Med*. 2016;17:712-720.

56. Scholefield B, Duncan H, Davies P, et al. Hypothermia for neuroprotection in children after cardiopulmonary arrest. *Cochrane Database Syst Rev*. 2013;2:CD009442.

57. Moler FW, Silverstein FS, Holubkov R, et al. Therapeutic hypothermia after out-of-hospital cardiac arrest in children. *N Engl J Med*. 2015;372:1898-1908.

58. Meert K, Telford R, Holubkov R, et al. Exploring the safety and efficacy of targeted temperature management amongst infants with out-of-hospital cardiac arrest due to apparent life threatening events. *Resuscitation*. 2016;109:40-48.

59. Moler FW, Silverstein FS, Holubkov R, et al. Therapeutic hypothermia after in-hospital cardiac arrest in children. *N Engl J Med*. 2017;376:318-329.

60. Fink EL, Clark RSB, Berger RP, et al. 24 vs. 72 hours of hypothermia for pediatric cardiac arrest: a pilot, randomized controlled trial. *Resuscitation*. 2018;126:14-20.

61. Xue D, Huang ZG, Smith KE, Buchan AM. Immediate or delayed mild hypothermia prevents focal cerebral infarction. *Brain Res*. 1992;587:66-72.

62. Maier CM, Ahern K, Cheng ML, et al. Optimal depth and duration of mild hypothermia in a focal model of transient cerebral ischemia: effects on neurologic outcome, infarct size, apoptosis, and inflammation. *Stroke*. 1998;29:2171-2180.

63. Schwab S, Schwarz S, Aschoff A, et al. Moderate hypothermia and brain temperature in patients with severe middle cerebral artery infarction. *Acta Neurochir Suppl*. 1998;71:131-134.

64. Hajat C, Hajat S, Sharma P. Effects of poststroke pyrexia on stroke outcome: a meta-analysis of studies in patients. *Stroke*. 2000;31:410-414.

65. Kasner SE, Wein T, Piriyawat P, et al. Acetaminophen for altering body temperature in acute stroke: a randomized clinical trial. *Stroke*. 2002;33:130-134.

66. Ntaios G, Dziedzic T, Michel P, et al. European Stroke Organisation (ESO) guidelines for the management of temperature in patients with acute ischemic stroke. *Int J Stroke*. 2015;10:941-949.

67. Batchelor PE, Skeers P, Antonic A, et al. Systematic review and meta-analysis of therapeutic hypothermia in animal models of spinal cord injury. *PLoS One*. 2013;8:e71317.

68. Levi AD, Casella G, Green BA, et al. Clinical outcomes using modest intravascular hypothermia after acute cervical spinal cord injury. *Neurosurgery*. 2010;66:670-677.

69. Dididze M, Green BA, Dietrich WD, et al. Systemic hypothermia in acute cervical spinal cord injury: a case-controlled study. *Spinal Cord*. 2013;51:395-400.

70. Berger RP, Adelson PD, Richichi R, Kochanek PM. Serum biomarkers after traumatic and hypoxemic brain injuries: insight into the biochemical response of the pediatric brain to inflicted brain injury. *Dev Neurosci*. 2006;28:327-335.

71. Crossley S, Reid J, McLatchie R, et al. A systematic review of therapeutic hypothermia for adult patients following traumatic brain injury. *Crit Care*. 2014;18:R75.

72. Watson HI, Shepherd AA, Rhodes JKJ, Andrews PJD. Revisited: a systematic review of therapeutic hypothermia for adult patients following traumatic brain injury. *Crit Care Med*. 2018;46:972-979.

73. Lewis SR, Evans DJ, Butler AR, et al. Hypothermia for traumatic brain injury. *Cochrane Database Syst Rev*. 2017;9:CD001048.

74. Zhu Y, Yin H, Zhang R, et al. Therapeutic hypothermia versus normothermia in adult patients with traumatic brain injury: a meta-analysis. *SpringerPlus*. 2016;5:801.

75. Zhang BF, Wang J, Liu ZW, et al. Meta-analysis of the efficacy and safety of therapeutic hypothermia in children with acute traumatic brain injury. *World Neurosurg*. 2015;83:567-573.

76. Tasker RC, Vonberg FW, Ulano ED, Akhondi-Asl A. Updating evidence for using hypothermia in pediatric severe traumatic brain injury: conventional and Bayesian meta-analytic perspectives. *Pediatr Crit Care Med*. 2017;18:355-362.

77. Li P, Yang C. Moderate hypothermia treatment in adult patients with severe traumatic brain injury: a meta-analysis. *Brain Injury*. 2014;28:1036-1041.

78. Adelson PD, Ragheb J, Kanev P, et al. Phase II clinical trial of moderate hypothermia after severe traumatic brain injury in children. *Neurosurgery*. 2005;56:740-754; discussion 740-754.

79. Hifumi T, Kuroda Y, Kawakita K, et al. Therapeutic hypothermia in patients with coagulopathy following severe traumatic brain injury. *Scand J Trauma, Resusc Emerg Med*. 2017;25:120.

80. Hutchison JS, Ward RE, Lacroix J, et al. Hypothermia therapy after traumatic brain injury in children. *N Engl J Med*. 2008;358:2447-2456.

81. Maekawa T, Yamashita S, Nagao S, et al. Prolonged mild therapeutic hypothermia versus fever control with tight hemodynamic monitoring and slow rewarming in patients with severe traumatic brain injury: a randomized controlled trial. *J Neurotrauma*. 2015;32(7):422-429.

82. Andrews PJ, Sinclair HL, Rodriguez A, et al. Hypothermia for intracranial hypertension after traumatic brain injury. *N Engl J Med*. 2015;373:2403-2412.

83. Empey PE, Velez de Mendizabal N, et al. Therapeutic hypothermia decreases phenytoin elimination in children with traumatic brain injury. *Crit Care Med*. 2013;41:2379-2387.

84. Hifumi T, Kuroda Y, Kawakita K, et al. Fever control management is preferable to mild therapeutic hypothermia in traumatic brain injury patients with abbreviated injury scale 3-4: a multi-center, randomized controlled trial. *J Neurotrauma*. 2016;33:1047-1053.

85. Dixon SR, Whitbourn RJ, Dae MW, et al. Induction of mild systemic hypothermia with endovascular cooling during primary percutaneous coronary intervention for acute myocardial infarction. *J Am Coll Cardiol*. 2002;40:1928-1934.

86. Grejs AM, Gjedsted J, Thygesen K, et al. The extent of myocardial injury during prolonged targeted temperature management after out-of-hospital cardiac arrest. *Am J Med*. 2017;130:37-46.

87. Grejs AM, Nielsen BRR, Juhl-Olsen P, et al. Effect of prolonged targeted temperature management on left ventricular myocardial function after out-of-hospital cardiac arrest - a randomised, controlled trial. *Resuscitation*. 2017;115:23-31.

88. Gotberg M, Olivecrona GK, Koul S, et al. A pilot study of rapid cooling by cold saline and endovascular cooling before reperfusion in patients with ST-elevation myocardial infarction. *Circ Cardiovasc Interv*. 2010;3:400-407.

89. Erlinge D, Gotberg M, Lang I, et al. Rapid endovascular catheter core cooling combined with cold saline as an adjunct to percutaneous coronary intervention for the treatment of acute myocardial infarction. The CHILL-MI trial: a randomized controlled study of the use of central venous catheter core cooling combined with cold saline as an adjunct to percutaneous coronary intervention for the treatment of acute myocardial infarction. *J Am Coll Cardiol*. 2014;63:1857-1865.

90. Erlinge D, Gotberg M, Grines C, et al. A pooled analysis of the effect of endovascular cooling on infarct size in patients with ST-elevation myocardial infarction. *EuroIntervention*. 2013;8:1435-1440.

91. Erlinge D, Gotberg M, Noc M, et al. Therapeutic hypothermia for the treatment of acute myocardial infarction-combined analysis of the RAPID MI-ICE and the CHILL-MI trials. *Ther Hypothermia Temp Manag.* 2015;5:77-84.

92. Fuernau G, Beck J, Desch S, et al. Mild hypothermia in cardiogenic shock complicating myocardial infarction—the randomized SHOCK-COOL trial. *Circulation.* 2018 [Epub ahead of print].

93. Jacobs SE, Berg M, Hunt R, et al. Cooling for newborns with hypoxic ischaemic encephalopathy. *Cochrane Database Syst Rev.* 2013;1:CD003311.

94. Laptook AR, Shankaran S, Tyson JE, et al. Effect of therapeutic hypothermia initiated after 6 hours of age on death or disability among newborns with hypoxic-ischemic encephalopathy: a randomized clinical trial. *JAMA.* 2017;318:1550-1560.

95. Shankaran S, Laptook AR, Pappas A, et al. Effect of depth and duration of cooling on deaths in the NICU among neonates with hypoxic ischemic encephalopathy: a randomized clinical trial. *JAMA.* 2014;312:2629-2639.

96. Shankaran S, Laptook AR, Pappas A, et al. Effect of depth and duration of cooling on death or disability at age 18 months among neonates with hypoxic-ischemic encephalopathy: a randomized clinical trial. *JAMA.* 2017;318:57-67.

97. Pauliah SS, Shankaran S, Wade A, et al. Therapeutic hypothermia for neonatal encephalopathy in low- and middle-income countries: a systematic review and meta-analysis. *PLoS One.* 2013;8:e58834.

98. Mourvillier B, Tubach F, van de Beek D, et al. Induced hypothermia in severe bacterial meningitis: a randomized clinical trial. *JAMA.* 2013;310:2174-2183.

99. Kushimoto S, Gando S, Saitoh D, et al. The impact of body temperature abnormalities on the disease severity and outcome in patients with severe sepsis: an analysis from a multicenter, prospective survey of severe sepsis. *Crit Care.* 2013;17:R271.

100. Rumbus Z, Matics R, Hegyi P, et al. Fever is associated with reduced, hypothermia with increased mortality in septic patients: a meta-analysis of clinical trials. *PLoS One.* 2017;12:e0170152.

101. Gao Y, Zhu J, Yin C, et al. Effects of target temperature management on the outcome of septic patients with fever. *Biomed Res Int.* 2017;2017:3906032.

102. Schortgen F, Clabault K, Katsahian S, et al. Fever control using external cooling in septic shock: a randomized controlled trial. *Am J Respir Crit Care Med.* 2012;185:1088-1095.

103. Drewry AM, Ablordeppey EA, Murray ET, et al. Antipyretic therapy in critically ill septic patients: a systematic review and meta-analysis. *Crit Care Med.* 2017;45:806-813.

104. Todd MM, Hindman BJ, Clarke WR, et al. Mild intraoperative hypothermia during surgery for intracranial aneurysm. *N Engl J Med.* 2005;352:135-145.

105. Staykov D, Wagner I, Volbers B, et al. Mild prolonged hypothermia for large intracerebral hemorrhage. *Neurocrit Care.* 2013;18:178-183.

106. Yao Z, You C, He M. Effect and feasibility of therapeutic hypothermia in patients with hemorrhagic stroke: a systematic review and meta-analysis. *World Neurosurg.* 2018;111:404-412.e2.

107. Legriel S, Lemiale V, Schenck M, et al. Hypothermia for neuroprotection in convulsive status epilepticus. *N Engl J Med.* 2016;375:2457-2467.

27

How Do I Manage the Morbidly Obese Critically Ill Patient?

Ali A. El Solh

INTRODUCTION

Obesity is a chronic metabolic condition with important public health implications. It has been linked to increased morbidity and mortality from acute and chronic medical problems, including hypertension, cardiovascular diseases, dyslipidemia, diabetes mellitus, arthritis, sleep apnea, and certain forms of cancer.

Although far from being ideal, the most convenient method of quantifying and defining the degree of obesity is via the body mass index (BMI), which is the ratio of a person's weight (in kilograms) to height (in meters) squared.[1] In 1998, the World Health Organization committee and the National Institutes of Health put forward a classification that became the worldwide standard for comparison of obesity rates both within and across populations. The consensus defined "morbid obesity"—also termed "clinically severe obesity"—as a BMI of ≥ 40 kg/m^2 or a BMI of >35 kg/m^2 and significant comorbidities.[2]

While the US prevalence of obesity has leveled in the last decade, compared with some European countries, the prevalence of obesity in the United States is three times higher than in France, and one and a half times higher than in the United Kingdom. According to the latest National Health and Nutrition Examination Survey (NHANES), the age-adjusted obesity prevalence was 35.7% in the United States in 2010 with no sex differences. Extreme obesity has more than doubled since the 1988–1994 NHANES, shifting from 2.9% to 6.3% in 2010 for grade 3 (severe) obesity and reaching 15.2% for grade 2 obesity.[3] The age-adjusted prevalence of overweight and obesity combined (BMI ≥ 25 kg/m^2) was 68.8% in 2010 with a mean BMI of 28.7 kg/m^2 in the US population.[3] With such a global epidemic, it is not surprising that an increasing number of morbidly obese patients are admitted to an intensive care unit (ICU). Hence, what are the special considerations in the management of the morbidly obese patients in the ICU?

Critically ill obese patients present the intensive care physicians with unique challenges that only a thorough knowledge of the peculiar pathophysiologic changes that occur in this population will allow for anticipation of complications and effective delivery of care.

AIRWAY MANAGEMENT

Morbid obesity has been considered one of the risk factors for difficult intubation.[4] In two series of morbidly obese patients undergoing upper abdominal surgery, the incidence of difficult intubation was estimated at 13% and 24%, respectively.[5,6] More recently, the magnitude of this risk was challenged. A study of over 90,000 Danish patients undergoing intubation for surgery put the frequency of difficult intubation closer to 6.4% in those with BMI ≥ 35 kg/m^2 vs. 5.2% in the overall population.[7] In the Australian Incident Monitoring Study, limited neck mobility and mouth opening accounted for most cases of difficult intubation in obese subjects.[8] Other studies added to the preceding list a short sternomental distance, a receding mandible, a large neck circumference, and a Mallampati score of ≥ 3 as predictors of difficult intubation.[9,10] Although these multivariate predictive models have yet to be tested in an ICU setting, neither obesity nor BMI predicted problems with tracheal intubation.[10,11] One of the reasons for the observed differences among these studies is the lack of consensus on the definition of the term "difficult intubation."[12] Nonetheless, the increased bulk of soft tissues in the upper airway make the morbidly obese, particularly those with obstructive sleep apnea, prone to partial obstruction. Hiremath et al.[13] found that 8 of 15 individuals with Cormack and Lehane grade 4 laryngoscopic views had apnea-hypopnea indices consistent with previously undiagnosed sleep apnea syndrome, whereas only 2 matched controls without a difficult laryngoscopic view had similar scores. Within this context, the American Society of Anesthesiology advocates awake intubation in morbidly obese patient if both difficult mask ventilation and difficult intubation are anticipated.[14]

Emergent airway management of the critically ill morbidly obese is frequently complicated by the patient's limited physiologic reserve. Morbidly obese patients are more prone to hypoxemia due to reductions in expiratory reserve volume, functional residual capacity, and maximum voluntary ventilation.[15] Severely obese patients undergoing surgery have significantly lower nadir SpO$_2$ (oxygen saturation by pulse oximetry) during intubation compared with normal and overweight patients despite similar preoxygenation duration and baseline SpO$_2$ readings.[16] Moreover, the increased intra-abdominal pressure is thought to place the obese patient at a higher risk of aspiration of gastric content.[17] These levels are considered traditionally to place the adult obese patient at risk for aspiration pneumonitis. Given these physiologic changes, a rapid sequence induction (RSI) has been advocated.[18] However, the use of RSI in fasted patients with no risk factors for aspiration other than obesity is debatable. Obese patients without symptoms of gastroesophageal reflux have a resistance gradient between the stomach and the gastroesophageal junction similar to that in nonobese subjects.[19] In addition, there are several drawbacks for RSI that could prove deleterious in these patients. First, there is a distinct risk of the scenario "cannot intubate and cannot ventilate" situation because the ability to mask ventilate is not tested before the administration of the muscle relaxant. Secondly, while cricoid pressure may or may not decrease the risk of aspiration,[20] there is evidence that it may worsen the quality of laryngeal exposure.[21] Finally, the application of cricoid pressure can lead to a complete airway occlusion occurring between 6% and 11% of the time.[22]

In short, the degree of obesity or neck size that justifies advanced interventions for intubation remains unknown. The experience and ability of the laryngoscopist are probably the most important determinants for establishing an airway in the morbidly obese patient.

In patients who require tracheostomy, morbidly obese patients present a unique surgical challenge because of increased submental and anterior cervical adipose tissue. The initial goal of securing a stable airway can be compromised by the size discrepancy and curvature mismatch between a standard-size tracheostomy tube and the increased distance between skin and trachea. Standard tracheotomy tubes are typically too short and too curved. One study of 427 critically ill morbidly obese patients undergoing surgical tracheostomy reported a complication rate of 25%, the majority of which were minor.[23] Life-threatening complications occurred in 10% and were related to tube obstruction and extratracheal tube placement. Some surgeons advocate performing a Bjork flap at the time of surgery to prevent tube misplacement in the pretracheal fascia. Others favor a cervical lipectomy in combination with tracheostomy.[24] As to whether morbidly obese patients will benefit from the application of these techniques in reducing the rate of extratracheal placement, there are no studies, to our knowledge, that provide a conclusive answer.

Percutaneous dilational tracheostomy (PDT) remains controversial for these patients. Obese patients with large and thick necks were traditionally considered poor candidates for PDT[25]; however, PDT has been performed in these patients with low rates of complications.[26] A large retrospective study of more than 3000 cases of PDT that included 16% with BMI ≥ 35 kg/m² reaffirmed the safety of this procedure in this high-risk group. The authors postulated that the introduction of extra-long tracheostomy tubes in obese patients may have contributed to the low complication rate in this high-risk group.[27] In the absence of large randomized trials, no recommendation could be made regarding PDT in this population; however, it should be noted that the outcome of PDT depends largely on the skills and the experience of the operator.

Despite substantial investigation, the optimal timing of tracheotomy for critically ill obese patients requiring mechanical ventilation continues to be debated between those who support early intervention, citing the benefits of early liberation from mechanical ventilation, and those who argue against this approach for lack of supportive evidence. To date, no randomized trial of tracheotomy time has been completed in the morbidly obese patients. One retrospective study of 102 morbidly obese patients requiring artificial ventilation did suggest a reduced duration of mechanical ventilation and ICU length of stay and a lower incidence of nosocomial pneumonia in those who underwent early tracheostomy (≤9 days) compared with late tracheostomy.[28] However, no difference in hospital mortality was observed. Because of the possibility of selection bias in retrospective designs, a consensus on when a tracheostomy should be performed in these patients awaits a randomized clinical trial.

RESPIRATORY

The most prominent pulmonary function test abnormalities associated with obesity consist of decreased expiratory reserve volume (ERV) and functional residual capacity (FRC), whereas the vital capacity and total lung capacity (TLC) are essentially unchanged[15,29] (Fig. 27.1). Relative to nonobese subjects, the total respiratory system compliance is decreased because of the greater degree of chest wall compression and cephalad displacement of the diaphragm. In the supine and Trendelenburg positions, FRC may fall below the closing capacity, leading to small airway collapse, atelectasis, ventilation perfusion mismatch and hypoxemia.[30] These alterations in

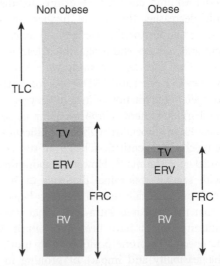

Fig. 27.1 Lung volumes in obese and nonobese patients. Obese patients tend to have higher respiratory rates and lower tidal volumes (*TV*). Expiratory reserve volume (*ERV*) is decreased in obesity. Functional residual capacity (*FRC*) (the sum of *ERV* and residual volume [*RV*]) is usually decreased as well, but to a lesser extent, since RV is usually relatively well preserved. *TLC*, Total lung capacity.

pulmonary function carry important implications in the treatment of obese patients requiring mechanical ventilation. As lung volumes are reduced and airway resistance is increased, a tidal volume based on a patient's actual body weight is likely to result in high airway pressures, alveolar overdistention, and barotrauma. The current consensus would favor that the initial tidal volume be calculated according to ideal body weight and then adjusted according to the desired plateau pressure and systemic arterial blood gases.[31]

The role of positive end-expiratory pressure (PEEP) on respiratory mechanics and blood gases in postoperative mechanically ventilated morbidly obese subjects has been tested by a number of studies. Pelosi et al.[32] applied PEEP of 10 cm H_2O to 9 anesthetized-paralyzed morbidly obese subjects after abdominal surgery and found a significant reduction in respiratory system elastance and resistance. This reduction was attributed to alveolar recruitment and/or to the reopening of closed airways. The authors also found a small but significant improvement in arterial oxygenation, which was correlated with the amount of recruited volume. In a similar group of subjects, Koutsoukou and colleagues[33] found that the PEEP used (4–16 cm H_2O) caused a significant reduction in elastance and resistance of the respiratory system. However, PEEP had no significant effect on gas exchange. In both studies, oxygenation remained markedly abnormal even after the application of PEEP, probably reflecting residual atelectasis. In fact, the extent of atelectasis, which was correlated with the amount of venous admixture, was not reduced by inflation of the lungs with conventional tidal volume, or even with a doubled tidal volume.[34]

In patients with acute respiratory distress syndrome (ARDS), prone positioning has been suggested as an important recruitment strategy to improve gas exchange. By allowing the weight of the mediastinal structure to be supported by the sternum, less pulmonary tissue is subjected to collapsing forces. The delivered tidal volume and peak pressure are dispersed to more alveoli, decreasing the risk of further alveolar injury from stretch and strain forces. Proning also ameliorates $\dot{V}/Q$ mismatching and reduces shunting, which lead to improved oxygenation.[35] One case control study with morbidly obese patients (BMI $\geq$ 35 kg/m²) and ARDS (ratio of partial pressure of arterial oxygen to the fraction of inspired oxygen [Pao_2/Fio_2] $\leq$ 200 mm Hg) documented improvement in oxygenation and decreased 90-day mortality without significant increase in duration of mechanical ventilation, length of stay, or incidence of nosocomial pneumonia.[36] However, abdominally obese patients (with sagittal abdominal diameter $\geq$ 26 cm) were at higher risk of renal failure and hypoxic hepatitis.[37] It is speculated that the increased intra-abdominal pressure from prone positioning might have been the culprit. Given the limited data specific to prone positioning in morbidly obese patients, the feasibility and impact of proning in morbidly patients with ARDS will probably be impacted by the degree of familiarity of nursing and physicians with proning and the availability of appropriate resources.

The rate of reintubation postextubation in the severely obese patients has been reported at 8% to 14% among patients undergoing mechanical ventilation for more than 48 hours.[38,39] Earlier investigations suggested that the prophylactic use of noninvasive ventilation (NIV) in morbidly obese patients during the first 24 hours postoperatively reduced pulmonary dysfunction after gastroplasty and accelerated reestablishment of preoperative pulmonary function. Joris and colleagues[40] demonstrated that the application of bilevel positive airway pressure set at 12 and 4 cm H_2O significantly improved the peak expiratory flow rate, the forced vital capacity, and the oxygen saturation on the first postoperative day. This improvement was attributed to a combined effect of improved lung inflation, prevention of alveolar collapse, and reduced inspiratory threshold load. In a parallel study of 50 morbidly obese patients admitted to a medical ICU with acute respiratory failure, patients who were successfully treated with NIV had a shorter hospital stay and a lower mortality.[41] The reduction in the rate of respiratory failure was more pronounced when NIV was instituted immediately postextubation.[42] Subgroup analysis of hypercapnic patients showed reduced hospital mortality in the NIV group compared with controls. In contrast, patients who failed a trial of NIV and those who required invasive mechanical ventilation demonstrated a longer ICU and hospital length of stay and higher mortality (31%).[41]

DEEP VENOUS THROMBOSIS PROPHYLAXIS

Morbid obesity carries a moderate-to-high risk category for venous thromboembolic disease (VTE).[43,44] Increased venous stasis, decreased mobility, and possible hypercoagulable state are among the factors that predispose morbidly obese patients in the ICU to increased risk for VTE.[45] Unfortunately, limited data exist on the effective prophylactic regimens of anticoagulation in the critically ill morbidly obese patients. These patients are typically excluded from trials because of the equivocal results of the diagnostic tests used to confirm or exclude thromboembolic disease.

Studies evaluating the effectiveness of VTE prophylaxis in obese hospitalized patients are listed in Table 27.1.[46–60] Despite the absence of well-designed randomized controlled trials in critically ill morbidly obese patients, the use of prophylaxis is indicated. Pharmacokinetic and epidemiologic studies suggest that the standard fixed doses of thromboprophylaxis are suboptimal in obese patients. A high-dose thromboprophylaxis (heparin 7500 U three times a day instead of standard dosing of 5000 U two to three times a day or enoxaparin 40 mg twice a day instead of 40 mg once a day) approximately halves the odds of symptomatic VTE in patients with weight >100 kg or BMI > 40 kg/m², with no increased risk of bleeding.[49] Alternatively, a weight-based regimen dosing (0.5 mg/kg twice daily) proved to be sufficient in achieving antifactor Xa levels within the appropriate prophylactic range (0.2–0.59 IU/mL) without additional adverse effects.[61] However, there is no universal consensus on the optimal regimens (mechanical or pharmacologic) and duration of VTE prophylaxis in these patients.

TABLE 27.1 Evidence of Efficacy of VTE Prophylaxis in Hospitalized Obese Patients.

Author Year	Study Design	Intervention	Outcome
Samama 1999[50]	Randomized, controlled trial	738 hospitalized medical patients >40 years old, including 20% of obese patients randomized to enoxaparin 40 mg/day or placebo	RR 0.37 (97.6% CI 0.22–0.63) with enoxaparin 40 mg/day. Major hemorrhage in 1.7% vs. 1.1% in the placebo group
Kalfarentzos 2001[51]	Randomized, controlled trial	60 patients undergoing bariatric surgery, randomized to 5700 IU or 9500 IU of nadroparin	No incidence of DVT in both groups receiving nadroparin. Major hemorrhage reported in 6.7% in the group receiving higher dose of nadroparin
Scholten 2002[52]	Prospective noncontrolled study	481 patients undergoing bariatric surgery receiving prophylaxis with 30 mg SC q12h or 40 mg q12h of enoxaparin	Incidence of symptomatic VTE of 5.4% with enoxaparin 30 mg q12h, and of 0.6% with 40 mg q12h. Major hemorrhage in 1.0% and 0.25% in the two groups of enoxaparin, respectively
Gonzalez 2004[53]	Prospective noncontrolled study	380 patients undergoing bariatric surgery with SCD	Incidence of symptomatic DVT of 0.26%. No PE reported
Alikhan 2003[54]	Randomized, controlled trial	866 hospitalized obese medical patients 40 years old randomized to enoxaparin 40 mg/day or placebo	RR 0.49 (95% CI 0.18–1.36) with enoxaparin 40 mg/day
Shepherd 2003[55]	Prospective noncontrolled study	700 patients undergoing bariatric surgery receiving prophylaxis with continuous intravenous UH during the perioperative period	Incidence of DVT and symptomatic PE of 0% and 0.4%, respectively. Postoperative hemorrhage in 2.3%
Miller 2004[56]	Retrospective cohort	255 patients undergoing bariatric surgery receiving prophylaxis with LDUH 5000 IU or 7500 IU q8h	Overall incidence of VTE of 1.2%. Prospective hemorrhage in 2.4%
Shepherd 2004[57]	Prospective noncontrolled study	19 patients undergoing bariatric surgery receiving prophylaxis with continuous intravenous UH during the perioperative period	No symptomatic VTE confirmed. Major hemorrhage in 10.5%
Leizorovicz 2004	Randomized, controlled trial	3706 hospitalized medical patients >40 years old, including 30% of obese patients randomized to dalteparin 5000 IU/day or placebo	RR 0.55 (95% CI 0.38–0.80) with dalteparin 5000 IU/day. Major hemorrhage in 0.49% vs. 0.16% in the placebo group
Kucher 2005[58]	Subgroup analysis of randomized, controlled trial	1118 hospitalized obese medical patients >40 years old, randomized to dalteparin 5000 IU/day or placebo	VTE occurred in 2.8% of the dalteparin and 4.3% of the placebo group. RR 0.64 (95% CI 0.32–1.28) with dalteparin 5000 IU/day
Hamad 2005[59]	Multicentric retrospective cohort	668 patients undergoing bariatric surgery receiving prophylaxis with enoxaparin 30 mg (daily or q12h) or 40 mg (daily or q12h) or no prophylaxis	Overall incidence of objectively confirmed symptomatic PE of 0.9%, and DVT of 0.1%; highest incidence without prophylaxis. Major hemorrhage in 0.9%
Quebbemann 2005[60]	Prospective noncontrolled study	822 patients undergoing bariatric surgery receiving prophylaxis with continuous intravenous UH at 400U/h from the preoperative period until discharge	Overall incidence of objectively confirmed symptomatic VTE of 0.1%. Major hemorrhage in 1.3%
Cossu 2007[46]	Retrospective cohort	151 patients underwent surgery for morbid obesity. In the first 65 cases, prophylaxis consisted of a single intravenous injection of heparin sodium (2500–5000 IU) at the time of induction of anesthesia. Later cases (86 cases) adjusted according to PT, TT, and aPTT	Two cases of VTE in the first group and one in the second group. Major bleeding occurred in 2.33%

Continued

TABLE 27.1		Evidence of Efficacy of VTE Prophylaxis in Hospitalized Obese Patients.—cont'd		
Author Year	**Study Design**	**Intervention**	**Outcome**
Raftopoulos 2008[48]	Retrospective cohort	(Group A) Enoxaparin 1 hour prior to surgery followed by enoxaparin 30 mg SC twice a day until discharge from hospital. (Group B) No preoperative heparin, then enoxaparin 30 mg SC twice a day followed by a 10-day course of enoxaparin 40 mg SC once a day at home after hospital discharge	VTE event occurred in Group A (1.14%) vs. Group B (0%). The incidence of significant bleeding was lower in Group B (Group A [5.3%] vs. Group B [0.56%], $P = .02$)
Borkgren-Okonek 2008[47]	Prospective open trial	223 undergoing Roux-en-Y gastric bypass assigned to receive enoxaparin 40 mg (BMI < 50 kg/m²) or 60 mg (BMI > 50 kg/m²) q12h during hospitalization and once daily for 10 days after discharge	One patient developed nonfatal VTE (0.45%). Four patients required transfusion (1.79%)
Wang 2014[49]	Retrospective cohort	9241 inpatients with weight > 100 kg comparing high-dose thromboprophylaxis (heparin 7500 U three times daily or enoxaparin 40 mg twice daily) to standard doses (heparin 5000 U two or three times daily or enoxaparin 40 mg once daily)	The rate of VTE was 1.48% for those who received standard doses compared with 0.77% for those who received high doses. High-dose thromboprophylaxis did not increase bleeding (OR 0.84, 95% CI 0.66–1.07, $P = .15$)

aPTT, activated partial thromboplastin time; *BMI*, body mass index; *CI*, confidence interval; *DVT*, deep vein thrombosis; *LDUH*, low-dose unfractionated heparin; *OR*, odds ratio; *PE*, pulmonary embolism; *PT*, prothrombin time; *RR*, relative risk; *SC*, subcutaneous; *SCD*, sequential compression device; *TT*, thrombin time; *UH*, unfractionated heparin; *VTE*, venous thromboembolic disease.

PHARMACOTHERAPY

A number of factors underlie the rate and extent of drug distribution in the morbidly obese, including degree of tissue perfusion, binding of drugs to plasma proteins, and permeability of tissue membranes. In general, the extent to which obesity influences the volume of distribution of a drug depends on its lipid solubility.[62] Early work with barbiturates clearly demonstrated the close correlation between lipid solubility and drug distribution. In this instance, loading is based on total body weight (TBW). However, lipophilic compounds do not always have larger volumes of distribution. Conversely, the volume of distribution (V_d) for some hydrophilic drugs in adipose tissue may be only a fraction of the V_d in other tissues. This is because the water content in adipose tissue is 20–50% of that in other tissues.[63] Hence, distribution of these drugs may warrant adjusting the dose in proportion to the excess in body weight with the use of a dosing weight correction factor (DWCF).

Adjusted body weight (ABW) = DWCF (TBW − IBW) + IBW

In the case of the least liposoluble drugs (atracurium, H_2 blockers) and specific lipophilic drugs (methylprednisolone), distribution is restricted to lean mass, and loading is usually based on ideal body weight (IBW).

The influence of pathophysiologic and histologic changes associated with obesity on hepatic and renal metabolism has yet to be fully elucidated. Previous evidence has suggested that hepatic oxidative metabolism is not different from that in lean individuals but more recent investigations have pointed to an increased activity of cytochrome P450 enzymes. Kotlyar and Carson[64] have provided strong evidence that the condition of obesity significantly increases hepatic CYP2E1 activity while decreasing hepatic CYP3A4 activities. On the same note, the use of the creatinine clearance equations to assess renal function in the morbidly obese can be misleading. In a study involving 12 men and 31 women who weighed > 195% of their IBW, creatinine clearance was overestimated by 51–61 mL/min/1.73 m² when using TBW and underestimated by 36–40 mL/min/1.73 m² when using IBW.[65] Salazar and Corcoran[66] proposed alternative formulas based on animal models for creatinine clearance in obese subjects. However, these equations have not been validated in critically ill morbidly obese patients. A formula derived from the Modification of Diet in Renal Disease (MDRD) Study group[67] [GFR = 170 × (serum creatinine [SCr])$^{-0.999}$ × (age, years)$^{-0.176}$ × 0.762 (if female) × 1.18 (if black) × (blood urea nitrogen [BUN])$^{-0.17}$ × (albumin)$^{+0.318}$] has the advantage of predicting glomerular filtration rate (GFR) rather than creatinine clearance. Data obtained in an intensive care unit from a morbidly obese patient using ^{51}Cr-ethylenediaminetetraacetic acid clearance as the gold standard suggest close estimation of the MDRD formula to the actual GFR.[68] Comprehensive reviews of this topic have been published elsewhere[63,69] but some of the commonly used drugs are detailed below.

Sedatives and Analgesics

There are no established guidelines for the optimal drug of choice for sedation in the critically ill morbidly obese patients. Midazolam, lorazepam, and propofol are currently the three sedatives most commonly administered in the ICU. Propofol is a hypnotic agent with a rapid onset and offset. Both V_d and clearance are increased in obese patients and correlate with ABW.[70] Because propofol is emulsified in a soybean base, it may increase CO_2 production.

The lipophilic benzodiazepines demonstrate increased V_d and increased elimination half-life in obese patients.[68] Midazolam has the shortest half-life among benzodiazepines but its sedative effect might be prolonged in morbidly obese individuals because of its accumulation in the adipose tissue. When combined with propofol or fentanyl, its clearance might decrease due to competitive inhibition of CYP3A4.[71] Dose calculations for continuous benzodiazepines infusion in obese patients should follow IBW because clearance is not significantly different from nonobese patients. Nonetheless, daily discontinuation with retitration to a target sedation endpoint is advocated in order to reduce the duration of mechanical ventilation and ICU length of stay. Dexmedetomidine is considered a viable alternative because it is not associated with respiratory depression. In morbidly obese patients undergoing bariatric surgery, both intraoperative and postoperative infusions of dexmedetomidine lead to significant opioid sparing in early and extended postoperative recovery phases, better pain control, and a lower incidence of postoperative nausea-vomiting.[72]

The synthetic opioids (remifentanil, fentanyl, and alfentanil) are lipophilic compounds with a rapid onset of action and minimal histamine-related vasodilation. Their cardiovascular responses to endotracheal intubation in morbidly obese patients are comparable.[73] Fentanyl is often administered to patients who are hemodynamically unstable or morphine allergic, in ICU, on pharmacoeconomic grounds. Similar pharmacokinetics of fentanyl in obese and nonobese patients was documented, suggesting dosing based on IBW. A more recent investigation observed that the relationship between TBW and the fentanyl doses required to achieve and to maintain postoperative analgesic endpoints had a nonlinear profile[74] (Table 27.2). In contrast, pharmacokinetic data suggest that remifentanil should be based on IBW.[75] All short-acting opioids are associated with rapid-onset tachyphylaxis (acute opioid tolerance). As for morphine dosing, a 10-fold variation in dosing requirement was reported that was unrelated to age, gender, or body surface area.[76,77]

Neuromuscular Blockade

Atracurium and vecuronium both have a limited V_d, but while vecuronium, rocuronium, and cisatracurium dosing is based on IBW, the hyposensitivity to atracurium observed in obese individuals necessitates calculation of the dose based on TBW.[63] There are no studies demonstrating a reduction in neuromuscular complications when intermittent dosing techniques are used instead of continuous infusions. Periodic monitoring with the train of four should be conducted routinely to adjust the

TABLE 27.2 Proposed Dosing of Commonly Used Drugs in Obese Patients.

Drug	Initial	Maintenance
Lidocaine	TBW	IBW
Digoxin	IBW	IBW
Beta-blockers	IBW	IBW
Aminoglycosides	ABW	ABW
Vancomycin	ABW	ABW
Atracurium	TBW	TBW
Vencuronium	IBW	IBW
Fentanyl	$52/(1+[196.4 \times e^{-0.025TBW}-53.66]/100)$	
Phenytoin	TBW	IBW
Corticosteroids	IBW	IBW
Cyclosporine	IBW	IBW
Aminophylline	IBW	IBW
Heparin[a]	ABW	
Argatroban		ABW
Enoxaparin[a]	TBW	TBW

[a]Dosing for treatment of venous thromboembolism.
IBW, ideal body weight; *TBW*, total body weight; *ABW*, adjusted body weight.
Male: IBW= 50 kg + 2.3 kg per inch of height > 5 ft
Female: IBW= 45.5 kg + 2.3 kg per inch of height > 5 ft
ABW = IBW + 0.4 (TBW – IBW)

rate of infusion. However, increased adiposity around the wrist may require more milliamperes to produce the desired result. Reversal of nondepolarizing neuromuscular blockade produced by rocuronium, vecuronium, and pipecuronium can be safely accomplished by sugammadex at a dose of 1.5 mg/kg of IBW.[78]

Antimicrobial Agents

Physiologic alterations seen in obesity commonly impact the pharmacokinetics (PK) and pharmacodynamics (PD) of antibiotics and may result in suboptimal dosing. An indirect but important way of evaluating the effects of obesity on antimicrobial PK is to estimate pharmacodynamics target attainment (PTA) after administration in the clinical setting. Given that the V_d of piperacillin and clearance of piperacillin is increased in obese patients,[79] intermittent infusion of piperacillin/tazobactam may result in suboptimal PTA.[80] Prolonged infusion dosing strategies may help decrease variability in PD achievement, especially in the critically ill with fluctuating renal function and unpredictable plasma levels. A similar argument can be made for both meropenem and doripenem when treating less-susceptible pathogens; however, dose escalation for carbapenems is not warranted based on BMI alone.[81,82] As for cephalosporins, several studies have signaled concerns when used for surgical prophylaxis because of inadequate tissue penetration and subtherapeutic levels in obese patients.[83] Higher doses may be needed, yet there are limited studies assessing the efficacy of such a strategy. For cases requiring vancomycin infusion, increasing BMI was associated with a significantly higher proportion of obese patients reaching troughs less than 20 mg/L, even after controlling for dose, serum creatinine, and age.[84] Weight-normalized V_d does not scale proportionally in a comparison of morbidly obese patients with obese patients, implying that lower loading doses would be an appropriate adjustment for patient groups with increasing BMIs. A recommended approach would be to reduce the loading dose (if indicated) to 20–25 mg/kg TBW (instead of 25–30 mg/kg load) and to reduce the starting maintenance dose using the ABW formula [ABW = IBW + 0.4(TBW–IBW)], and then to adjust according to therapeutic drug monitoring (TDM). Similarly, initial dosing of aminoglycosides should be based on ABW, with subsequent dosing adjusted based on TDM. Given the relatively wide therapeutic index of daptomycin and clinical experience of tolerability as well as data supporting the use of higher daptomycin doses (up to 10–12 mg/kg) for adequate PK/PD target attainment, dosing obese patients with ABW0.4 is reasonable to ensure treatment efficacy while balancing the risk of muscle toxicity.[85] For multidrug resistant bacteria, colistin (polymyxin E) should be dosed using IBW with a limit of 360 mg/day to reduce the risks of nephrotoxicity while it may be appropriate to dose polymyxin B using ABW0.4, limiting the daily dose to 2 million units (200 mg).[86] Oxazolidinones do not appear to require dose adjustment. Dose adjustments do not appear also to be necessary for dalbavancin and oritavancin.

Anticoagulants

Morbid obesity had little to no effect on the weight-based heparin dosing protocols that use the total body weight in systemic anticoagulation.[87] Large studies evaluating the safety and efficacy of using weight-based dosing of low molecular weight heparins (LMWHs) for the treatment of venous thromboembolism in these critically ill morbid obese patients are limited. Pharmacokinetic studies suggest that body mass does not appear to have a significant effect on the response to LMWHs in obese patients with normal renal function.[88] Nonetheless, monitoring of anti-Xa activity should be considered. Although the timing of the blood sampling in relation to the dose and the optimal range of values has yet to be clearly defined, a peak anti-Xa level, drawn 4 hours after a dose is given, is considered the most useful.[89] For twice-daily administration, a target of anti-Xa level of 0.6–1.0 IU/mL has been recommended. The range at 4 hours for those treated with a once-daily dose is less certain, but a level of 1.0–2.0 IU/mL is suggested.

Our treatment options have been expanded recently by the addition of an oral direct thrombin inhibitor and two Xa inhibitors. Unfortunately, studies focusing on dosing in obesity are lacking. Dabigatran is approved in the United States for prevention of stroke and systemic embolism in nonvalvular atrial fibrillation (AF).[90] The RE-LY trial noted a 20% decrease in trough concentrations in patients weighing >100 kg; however, dose adjustments have not been recommended.[91] Rivaroxaban is approved for prevention of stroke and systemic embolism in nonvalvular AF, DVT, and pulmonary embolism (PE) treatment and reduction of recurrence, and DVT prophylaxis after knee and hip surgery.[92–94] A phase

2 study demonstrated that a TBW > 120 kg was not associated with clinically significant changes in PK or PD parameters; thus, dose adjustments are not warranted.[95] Studies with rivaroxaban have a small proportion of patients with a BMI of >28 kg/m^2 or weights exceeding >100 kg; however, subgroup analyses have shown dose modifications are not needed.[92,96] Two other agents, apixaban and edoxaban, have received FDA approval for the prevention of stroke and systemic embolism in nonvalvular AF.[97,98] Cumulative analysis of available trials involving these two compounds found that high BMI was not associated with inferior effectiveness or safety and a dose adjustment is not required.[99]

NUTRITIONAL CARE

There are few data for any specific feeding strategy of critically ill morbidly obese patients. Generally, the energy expenditure of morbidly obese patients is increased due to an increase in lean body mass.[100] Inadequate nutritional intake combined with elevated basal insulin concentrations suppresses lipid mobilization from body stores, causing accelerated proteolysis, which in turn forces rapid loss of muscle mass and early deconditioning. Conversely, aggressively high caloric formulas have been associated with increased carbon dioxide production,[101] which increases the work of breathing and may prolong the need for mechanical ventilation. Hence, the need to accurately determine energy requirements in this patient population cannot be overemphasized. The current guidelines favor enteral nutritional support within 48 hours after admission to an ICU.[102]

The most challenging question is how to assess energy requirements of obese patients. Several predictive equations have been developed to estimate energy requirements, but adapting these formulas for obese patients is problematic. Estimates of energy expenditure in the critically ill have been traditionally derived from the Harris-Benedict equation, but several studies have shown its inaccuracies when it comes to whether ideal or actual body weight should be used.[103] In morbidly obese individuals, indirect calorimetry is considered the method of choice to determine energy expenditure if the inspired oxygen is less than 60%.[102] Whether any of these measures translate into improved outcome cannot be determined in the absence of randomized clinical trials.[104]

Hypocaloric high-protein enteral or parenteral nutrition has allowed the achievement of a net protein anabolism and avoidance of overfeeding complications such as hyperglycemia, while burning excess fat.[8] Widely accepted recommendations consist of no more than 60–70% of requirements or administration of 11–14 kcal/kg current body weight/day or 22–25 kcal/kg ideal weight/day, with 2–2.5 g/kg ideal weight/day of proteins.[105] Several studies evaluated the use of hypocaloric high-protein nutritional support in critically ill obese patients.[106] Overall, these studies showed a preserved nitrogen balance and decreased morbidity, but they were limited by the small number of patients and lack of mortality benefit. Furthermore, the hypocaloric high-protein diet has not been evaluated in patients with renal or liver disease, so the use of

TABLE 27.3 Weight and Aperture Diameter Limitations per Imaging Modality.

Imaging Modality	Maximum Aperture Diameter (cm)	Weight Limit (lb)
Fluoroscopy	63	700
Vertical field MRI	55	550
Cylindrical bore MRI	70	550

MRI, magnetic resonance imaging.

hypocaloric nutritional support in obese patients with these conditions is not advocated at present.

DIAGNOSTIC IMAGING

Selection of the appropriate imaging modality is paramount to obtain a precise diagnosis in critically ill obese patients. Radiography can be limited by X-ray beam attenuation that results in decreased image contrast and amplification of noise and increased exposure time, resulting in motion artifacts. Raising kilovoltage (kVp) and milliamps (mAs) helps in improving the image quality.[107] Use of multiple cassettes may be needed to cover the entire chest or abdomen.

Ultrasound image quality is affected by fat to a greater degree than any other imaging modality.[107] The ultrasound beam is attenuated by fat at a rate of 0.63 dB/cm. Use of the lowest frequency transducer (1.5–2.0 MHz) may partially overcome the increased image attenuation. For fluoroscopy, computed tomography (CT), and magnetic resonance imaging (MRI), the weight and aperture diameter limitations of the imaging modality should be obtained prior to transporting these patients out of the ICU (Table 27.3). MRI scanners with a high signal-to-noise ratio and strong gradients ($\geq$1.5 T) cannot accommodate patients weighing 350 lb (159 kg). Vertical field open MRI systems are needed for patients up to 550 lb (250 kg) and can offer a range of vertical apertures from 40 to 55 cm.

INTRAVENOUS ACCESS

Morbid obesity poses a particular challenge for intravenous access. Possible explanations for complications related to central venous catheter placement in obese patients include loss of anatomic landmarks, increased depth of insertion, need for multiple needle passes, increased duration of cannulation, and difficulty in maintaining proper angle during insertion. As a result, the femoral route has been used more frequently than subclavian or internal jugular access. Despite the fact that an increased risk of blood stream infection has been suggested when femoral placement was attempted in these patients,[108] two studies have shown that the risk of infection and mechanical complications were similar between internal jugular and femoral routes.[109] The use of two-dimensional ultrasound guidance for cannulation of the internal jugular veins unequivocally decreases the risk of failed catheter placement, improves first-pass success, and facilitates faster placement compared with the landmark method.[110] Chlorhexidine dressings[111] and antiseptic-impregnated catheters[112] are recommended, especially if a femoral route is the only accessible insertion site.

OUTCOMES OF CRITICALLY ILL OBESE PATIENTS

Since 2001, there have been numerous reports trying to elucidate the relationship between BMI and critical care outcome. Earlier studies of morbidly obese patients in critical care setting (BMI > 40 kg/m²) reported higher mean length of stay in ICU and longer duration of mechanical ventilation compared with nonobese patients (BMI < 30 kg/m²).[113–115] There was also a higher in-hospital mortality of the obese vs. the nonobese patients.

These dire prognostications for critically obese patients have been subsequently challenged by parallel investigations.[116] More contemporary studies have demonstrated that underweight was independently associated with a higher hazard of 60-day in-hospital death, while overweight and morbidly obese with a lower hazard.[116] A further understanding of the role of morbid obesity on critical outcomes was derived from the National Heart, Lung, and Blood Institute's multicenter, randomized trials of the Acute Respiratory Distress Syndrome Network (ARD-net), which attempted to address the effect of obesity on the course of ventilated patients with acute lung injury (ALI). A secondary analysis of pooled data from three studies revealed that the unadjusted outcomes across BMI groups did not differ significantly for any of the dependent variables (28-day mortality, achievement of unassisted ventilation, 180-day mortality rate, or ventilator-free days).[117] The authors acknowledged that improved outcomes in the study population could have been the result of increased intensity of care of the study population and standardized weaning procedures that were used. In line with these findings, three systematic reviews concluded that obesity was associated with comparable or lower risk of death compared with normal weight.[118–120] It is not clear what the exact nature of such pathophysiologic mechanisms beyond the obesity paradox is or which body composition component in obesity is more or less protective in disease states. However, several potential hypotheses have been advanced to explain this obesity paradox. A time discrepancy between the long-term harmful effects vs. short-time survival advantages imparted by obesity has been suggested in that it takes years to decades of exposure to such risk factors to develop a debilitating illness, whereas under the unique circumstances of a disease state, obesity can confer a short-term advantage against the ravages of an acute critical care illness. Alternatively, specific hormonal mechanisms could play a role in the relation between obesity and mortality. Bornstein and colleagues[121] reported a positive association between leptin concentrations and survival of septic patients, suggesting that leptin could play a role in the adaptive response to critical illness.

Morbidly obese patients requiring admission to surgical or trauma units have more adverse events than their nonobese counterparts. Morbid obesity was reported as an independent risk factor for death in surgical patients who required 4 days or more in ICU stay, indicating that complications of health-care processes may be the key to improved outcomes in this cohort.[122] The increased mortality was attributed to more organ failures, the need for more vasopressors, and failed extubation. However, these complications were not higher in obese cardiac patients who required bypass graft surgery than in nonobese patients,[123] although the risks of sternal wound infection were substantially increased in the obese and severely obese individual.[124,125] The introduction of extracorporeal devices (ECD) has added a new dimension to the intensive care management of acute cardiac and/or respiratory failure in adult patients who fail conventional treatment. Despite the fact that ECD support presents unique challenges, including percutaneous cannulation, no association was established between BMI and mortality.[126]

In trauma patients, obesity seems to be associated with poorer outcomes.[127–129] In blunt trauma, obese patients sustain different type of injuries than lean patients, with a higher frequency of thoracoabdominal wounds and fewer traumatic brain injuries. Moreover, obese trauma patients had more than twofold increase in risk of acquiring a bloodstream, urinary tract, or respiratory tract infection after hospital admission[130] including sepsis, ventilator-associated pneumonia, and catheter-associated bacteremia.[131] Further studies are needed to clarify whether obesity is deleterious in this population or not and to assess the possible differences in outcome between various surgical interventions.

CONCLUSION

The treatment of the critically ill morbidly obese patient remains a daunting task for critical care practitioners. Despite the growing global obesity epidemic, the management approach to the morbidly obese in intensive care settings is based mainly on expert opinion. Future randomized controlled trials are needed to guide clinicians in providing care to this unique population.

AUTHORS' RECOMMENDATIONS
- The critical care aspects of the morbidly obese are multi-faceted and require a true multidisciplinary approach for optimal outcomes. Unfortunately, there are no randomized controlled studies addressing the management of critically ill morbidly obese patients in the ICU setting. The following recommendations are based on best-available evidence extrapolated from other critical settings and practice management of morbidly obese patients.
- There are several physical signs that can alert one to the possibility of a patient having a difficult airway in the morbidly obese, but none of these are highly predictive. Life-threatening cases in morbidly obese airway management result not from failure of intubation but from failure of ventilation.
- The respiratory system is by far the most affected by the excess weight. Reduction in FRC and ERV predispose these patients to ventilation–perfusion mismatching, leading to arterial hypoxemia, most notably in the supine position.

- Because the lung volumes may be reduced and airway resistance increased, mechanical ventilation should be initiated with a tidal volume calculated according to the IBW to avoid alveolar overdistention and barotrauma. The addition of PEEP is highly recommended to facilitate alveolar recruitment and prevent atelectasis.
- Application of NIV immediately postextubation might reduce the rate of respiratory failure and decrease mortality in hypercarbic patients.
- When using unfractionated heparin to treat DVT or PE in the obese, ABW is safe and appropriate.
- Consensus guidelines recommend enteral feeding with 11–14 kcal/kg ABW per day and protein intake of 2.0–2.5 g/kg IBW per day.
- It is recommended that a discussion with the radiology department regarding patient's weight and body diameter is performed before the patient is transferred out of ICU.
- Overall, the impact of morbid obesity on critical care outcome remains controversial, with the worst outcome reported in obese trauma patients.

REFERENCES

1. Kral JG, Heymsfield S. Morbid obesity: definitions, epidemiology, and methodological problems. *Gastroenterol Clin North Am.* 1987;16(2):197-205.
2. Gastrointestinal surgery for severe obesity: National Institutes of Health Consensus Development Conference Statement. *Am J Clin Nutr.* 1992;55(2 suppl):615S-619S.
3. Flegal KM, Carroll MD, Kit BK, Ogden CL. Prevalence of obesity and trends in the distribution of body mass index among US adults, 1999-2010. *JAMA.* 2012;307(5):491-497.
4. Joshi R, Hypes CD, Greenberg J, et al. Difficult airway characteristics associated with first-attempt failure at intubation using video laryngoscopy in the intensive care unit. *Ann Am Thorac Soc.* 2017;14(3):368-375.
5. Buckley FP, Robinson NB, Simonowitz DA, Dellinger EP. Anaesthesia in the morbidly obese. A comparison of anaesthetic and analgesic regimens for upper abdominal surgery. *Anaesthesia.* 1983;38(9):840-851.
6. Dominguez-Cherit G, Gonzalez R, Borunda D, et al. Anesthesia for morbidly obese patients. *World J Surg.* 1998;22(9):969-973.
7. Lundstrøm LH, Moller AM, Rosenstock C, et al. High body mass index is a weak predictor for difficult and failed tracheal intubation: a cohort study of 91,332 consecutive patients scheduled for direct laryngoscopy registered in the Danish Anesthesia Database. *Anesthesiology.* 2009;110(2):266-274.
8. Williamson JA, Webb RK, Van der Walt JH, Runciman WB. The Australian Incident Monitoring Study. Pneumothorax: an analysis of 2000 incident reports. *Anaesth Intensive Care.* 1993;21(5):642-645.
9. Naguib M, Malabarey T, AlSatli RA, et al. Predictive models for difficult laryngoscopy and intubation. A clinical, radiologic and three-dimensional computer imaging study. *Can J Anaesth.* 1999;46(8):748-759.
10. Brodsky JB, Lemmens HJ, Brock-Utne JG, et al. Morbid obesity and tracheal intubation. *Anesth Analg.* 2002;94(3):732-736.
11. Gaszynski T. Standard clinical tests for predicting difficult intubation are not useful among morbidly obese patients. *Anesth Analg.* 2004;99(3):956.

12. Collins JS, Lemmens HJ, Brodsky JB. Obesity and difficult intubation: where is the evidence? *Anesthesiology.* 2006;104(3):617; author reply 618-619.

13. Hiremath AS, Hillman DR, James AL, et al. Relationship between difficult tracheal intubation and obstructive sleep apnoea. *Br J Anaesth.* 1998;80(5):606-611.

14. Apfelbaum JL, Hagberg CA, Caplan RA, et al. Practice guidelines for management of the difficult airway: an updated report by the American Society of Anesthesiologists Task Force on Management of the Difficult Airway. *Anesthesiology.* 2013;118(2):251-270.

15. Salome CM, King GG, Berend N. Physiology of obesity and effects on lung function. *J Appl Physiol.* 2010;108(1):206-211.

16. Juvin P, Lavaut E, Dupont H, et al. Difficult tracheal intubation is more common in obese than in lean patients. *Anesth Analg.* 2003;97(2):595-600.

17. Dority J, Hassan ZU, Chau D. Anesthetic implications of obesity in the surgical patient. *Clin Colon Rectal Surg.* 2011; 24(4):222-228.

18. Freid EB. The rapid sequence induction revisited: obesity and sleep apnea syndrome. *Anesthesiol Clin North America.* 2005; 23(3):551-564, viii.

19. Zacchi P, Mearin F, Humbert P, et al. Effect of obesity on gastroesophageal resistance to flow in man. *Dig Dis Sci.* 1991; 36(10):1473-1480.

20. Butler J, Sen A. Best evidence topic report. Cricoid pressure in emergency rapid sequence induction. *Emerg Med J.* 2005; 22(11):815-816.

21. Haslam N, Parker L, Duggan JE. Effect of cricoid pressure on the view at laryngoscopy. *Anaesthesia.* 2005;60(1):41-47.

22. Allman KG. The effect of cricoid pressure application on airway patency. *J Clin Anesth.* 1995;7(3):197-199.

23. El Solh AA, Jaafar W. A comparative study of the complications of surgical tracheostomy in morbidly obese critically ill patients. *Crit Care.* 2007;11(1):R3.

24. Gross ND, Cohen JI, Andersen PE, Wax MK. 'Defatting' tracheotomy in morbidly obese patients. *Laryngoscope.* 2002; 112(11):1940-1944.

25. Byhahn C, Lischke V, Meininger D, et al. Peri-operative complications during percutaneous tracheostomy in obese patients. *Anaesthesia.* 2005;60(1):12-15.

26. Mansharamani NG, Koziel H, Garland R, et al. Safety of bedside percutaneous dilatational tracheostomy in obese patients in the ICU. *Chest.* 2000;117(5):1426-1429.

27. Dennis BM, Eckert MJ, Gunter OL, et al. Safety of bedside percutaneous tracheostomy in the critically ill: evaluation of more than 3,000 procedures. *J Am Coll Surg.* 2013;216(4):858-865; discussion 865-857.

28. Alhajhusain A, Ali AW, Najmuddin A, et al. Timing of tracheotomy in mechanically ventilated critically ill morbidly obese patients. *Crit Care Res Pract.* 2014;2014:840638.

29. Jones RL, Nzekwu MM. The effects of body mass index on lung volumes. *Chest.* 2006;130(3):827-833.

30. Holley HS, Milic-Emili J, Becklake MR, Bates DV. Regional distribution of pulmonary ventilation and perfusion in obesity. *J Clin Invest.* 1967;46(4):475-481.

31. El-Solh AA. Clinical approach to the critically ill, morbidly obese patient. *Am J Respir Crit Care Med.* 2004;169(5): 557-561.

32. Pelosi P, Ravagnan I, Giurati G, et al. Positive end-expiratory pressure improves respiratory function in obese but not in normal subjects during anesthesia and paralysis. *Anesthesiology.* 1999;91(5):1221-1231.

33. Koutsoukou A, Koulouris N, Bekos B, et al. Expiratory flow limitation in morbidly obese postoperative mechanically ventilated patients. *Acta Anaesthesiol Scand.* 2004;48(9): 1080-1088.

34. Rothen HU, Sporre B, Engberg G, et al. Re-expansion of atelectasis during general anaesthesia: a computed tomography study. *Br J Anaesth.* 1993;71(6):788-795.

35. Fernandez R, Trenchs X, Klamburg J, et al. Prone positioning in acute respiratory distress syndrome: a multicenter randomized clinical trial. *Intensive Care Med.* 2008;34(8):1487-1491.

36. De Jong A, Molinari N, Sebbane M, et al. Feasibility and effectiveness of prone position in morbidly obese patients with ARDS: a case-control clinical study. *Chest.* 2013; 143(6):1554-1561.

37. Weig T, Janitza S, Zoller M, et al. Influence of abdominal obesity on multiorgan dysfunction and mortality in acute respiratory distress syndrome patients treated with prone positioning. *J Crit Care.* 2014;29(4):557-561.

38. Blouw EL, Rudolph AD, Narr BJ, Sarr MG. The frequency of respiratory failure in patients with morbid obesity undergoing gastric bypass. *AANA J.* 2003;71(1):45-50.

39. Gaszyńsnki T, Gaszyński W, Strzelczyk J. Critical respiratory events in morbidly obese. *Twój Magazyn Medyczny Chirurgia.* 2003;3:55-58.

40. Joris JL, Sottiaux TM, Chiche JD, et al. Effect of bi-level positive airway pressure (BiPAP) nasal ventilation on the postoperative pulmonary restrictive syndrome in obese patients undergoing gastroplasty. *Chest.* 1997;111(3):665-670.

41. Duarte AG, Justino E, Bigler T, Grady J. Outcomes of morbidly obese patients requiring mechanical ventilation for acute respiratory failure. *Crit Care Med.* 2007;35(3):732-737.

42. El-Solh AA, Aquilina A, Pineda L, et al. Noninvasive ventilation for prevention of post-extubation respiratory failure in obese patients. *Eur Respir J.* 2006;28(3):588-595.

43. Rocha AT, de Vasconcellos AG, da Luz Neto ER, et al. Risk of venous thromboembolism and efficacy of thromboprophylaxis in hospitalized obese medical patients and in obese patients undergoing bariatric surgery. *Obes Surg.* 2006;16(12):1645-1655.

44. Eichinger S, Hron G, Bialonczyk C, et al. Overweight, obesity, and the risk of recurrent venous thromboembolism. *Arch Intern Med.* 2008;168(15):1678-1683.

45. Overby DW, Kohn GP, Cahan MA, et al. Prevalence of thrombophilias in patients presenting for bariatric surgery. *Obes Surg.* 2009;19(9):1278-1285.

46. Cossu ML, Pilo L, Piseddu G, et al. Prophylaxis of venous thromboembolism in bariatric surgery. *Chir Ital.* 2007;59(3): 331-335.

47. Borkgren-Okonek MJ, Hart RW, Pantano JE, et al. Enoxaparin thromboprophylaxis in gastric bypass patients: extended duration, dose stratification, and antifactor Xa activity. *Surg Obes Relat Dis.* 2008;4(5):625-631.

48. Raftopoulos I, Martindale C, Cronin A, Steinberg J. The effect of extended post-discharge chemical thromboprophylaxis on venous thromboembolism rates after bariatric surgery: a prospective comparison trial. *Surg Endosc.* 2008;22(11): 2384-2391.

49. Wang TF, Milligan PE, Wong CA, et al. Efficacy and safety of high-dose thromboprophylaxis in morbidly obese inpatients. *Thromb Haemost.* 2014;111(1):88-93.

50. Samama MM, Cohen AT, Darmon JY, et al. A comparison of enoxaparin with placebo for the prevention of venous thromboembolism in acutely ill medical patients. Prophylaxis in

Medical Patients with Enoxaparin Study Group. *N Engl J Med.* 1999;341(11):793-800.

51. Kalfarentzos F, Stavropoulou F, Yarmenitis S, et al. Prophylaxis of venous thromboembolism using two different doses of low-molecular-weight heparin (nadroparin) in bariatric surgery: a prospective randomized trial. *Obes Surg.* 2001;11(6):670-676.

52. Scholten DJ, Hoedema RM, Scholten SE. A comparison of two different prophylactic dose regimens of low molecular weight heparin in bariatric surgery. *Obes Surg.* 2002;12(1):19-24.

53. Gonzalez QH, Tishler DS, Plata-Munoz JJ, et al. Incidence of clinically evident deep venous thrombosis after laparoscopic Roux-en-Y gastric bypass. *Surg Endosc.* 2004;18(7):1082-1084.

54. Alikhan R, Cohen AT, Combe S, et al. Prevention of venous thromboembolism in medical patients with enoxaparin: a subgroup analysis of the MEDENOX study. *Blood Coagul Fibrinolysis.* 2003;14(4):341-346.

55. Shepherd MF, Rosborough TK, Schwartz ML. Heparin thromboprophylaxis in gastric bypass surgery. *Obes Surg.* 2003;13(2):249-253.

56. Miller MT, Rovito PF. An approach to venous thromboembolism prophylaxis in laparoscopic Roux-en-Y gastric bypass surgery. *Obes Surg.* 2004;14(6):731-737.

57. F Shepherd M, Rosborough TK, Schwartz ML. Unfractionated heparin infusion for thromboprophylaxis in highest risk gastric bypass surgery. *Obes Surg.* 2004;14(5):601-605.

58. Kucher N, Leizorovicz A, Vaitkus PT, et al. Efficacy and safety of fixed low-dose dalteparin in preventing venous thromboembolism among obese or elderly hospitalized patients: a subgroup analysis of the PREVENT trial. *Arch Intern Med.* 2005;165(3):341-345.

59. Hamad GG, Choban PS. Enoxaparin for thromboprophylaxis in morbidly obese patients undergoing bariatric surgery: findings of the prophylaxis against VTE outcomes in bariatric surgery patients receiving enoxaparin (PROBE) study. *Obes Surg.* 2005;15(10):1368-1374.

60. Quebbemann B, Akhondzadeh M, Dallal R. Continuous intravenous heparin infusion prevents peri-operative thromboembolic events in bariatric surgery patients. *Obes Surg.* 2005;15(9):1221-1224.

61. Ludwig KP, Simons HJ, Mone M, et al. Implementation of an enoxaparin protocol for venous thromboembolism prophylaxis in obese surgical intensive care unit patients. *Ann Pharmacother.* 2011;45(11):1356-1362.

62. Ritschel WA, Kaul S. Prediction of apparent volume of distribution in obesity. *Methods Find Exp Clin Pharmacol.* 1986;8(4):239-247.

63. Erstad B. Drug dosing in the critically ill obese patient. In: El Solh AA, ed. *Critical Care Management of the Obese Management.* West Sussex, UK: Wiley-Blackwell; 2012:197-207.

64. Kotlyar M, Carson SW. Effects of obesity on the cytochrome P450 enzyme system. *Int J Clin Pharmacol Ther.* 1999;37(1):8-19.

65. Dionne RE, Bauer LA, Gibson GA, et al. Estimating creatinine clearance in morbidity obese patients. *Am J Hosp Pharm.* 1981;38(6):841-844.

66. Salazar DE, Corcoran GB. Predicting creatinine clearance and renal drug clearance in obese patients from estimated fat-free body mass. *Am J Med.* 1988;84(6):1053-1060.

67. Levey AS, Bosch JP, Lewis JB, et al. A more accurate method to estimate glomerular filtration rate from serum creatinine: a new prediction equation. Modification of Diet in Renal Disease Study Group. *Ann Intern Med.* 1999;130(6):461-470.

68. Greenblatt DJ, Abernethy DR, Locniskar A, et al. Effect of age, gender, and obesity on midazolam kinetics. *Anesthesiology.* 1984;61(1):27-35.

69. Medico CJ, Walsh P. Pharmacotherapy in the critically ill obese patient. *Crit Care Clin.* 2010;26(4):679-688.

70. Servin F, Farinotti R, Haberer JP, Desmonts JM. Propofol infusion for maintenance of anesthesia in morbidly obese patients receiving nitrous oxide. A clinical and pharmacokinetic study. *Anesthesiology.* 1993;78(4):657-665.

71. Oda Y, Mizutani K, Hase I, et al. Fentanyl inhibits metabolism of midazolam: competitive inhibition of CYP3A4 in vitro. *Br J Anaesth.* 1999;82(6):900-903.

72. Singh PM, Panwar R, Borle A, et al. Perioperative analgesic profile of dexmedetomidine infusions in morbidly obese undergoing bariatric surgery: a meta-analysis and trial sequential analysis. *Surg Obes Relat Dis.* 2017;13(8):1434-1446.

73. Salihoglu Z, Demiroluk S, Demirkiran, Kose Y. Comparison of effects of remifentanil, alfentanil and fentanyl on cardiovascular responses to tracheal intubation in morbidly obese patients. *Eur J Anaesthesiol.* 2002;19(2):125-128.

74. Shibutani K, Inchiosa Jr MA, Sawada K, Bairamian M. Pharmacokinetic mass of fentanyl for postoperative analgesia in lean and obese patients. *Br J Anaesth.* 2005;95(3):377-383.

75. Egan TD, Huizinga B, Gupta SK, et al. Remifentanil pharmacokinetics in obese versus lean patients. *Anesthesiology.* 1998;89(3):562-573.

76. Bennett R, Batenhorst R, Graves DA, et al. Variation in postoperative analgesic requirements in the morbidly obese following gastric bypass surgery. *Pharmacotherapy.* 1982;2(1):50-53.

77. Rand CS, Kuldau JM, Yost RL. Obesity and post-operative pain. *J Psychosom Res.* 1985;29(1):43-48.

78. Abd El-Rahman AM, Othman AH, El Sherif FA, et al. Comparison of three different doses sugammadex based on ideal body weight for reversal of moderate rocuronium-induced neuromuscular blockade in laparoscopic bariatric surgery. *Minerva Anestesiol.* 2017;83(2):138-144.

79. Chung EK, Cheatham SC, Fleming MR, et al. Population pharmacokinetics and pharmacodynamics of piperacillin and tazobactam administered by prolonged infusion in obese and nonobese patients. *J Clin Pharmacol.* 2015;55(8):899-908.

80. Alobaid AS, Brinkmann A, Frey OR, et al. What is the effect of obesity on piperacillin and meropenem trough concentrations in critically ill patients? *J Antimicrob Chemother.* 2016;71(3):696-702.

81. Cheatham SC, Fleming MR, Healy DP, et al. Steady-state pharmacokinetics and pharmacodynamics of meropenem in morbidly obese patients hospitalized in an intensive care unit. *J Clin Pharmacol.* 2014;54(3):324-330.

82. Chung EK, Fleming MR, Cheatham SC, Kays MB. Population pharmacokinetics and pharmacodynamics of doripenem in obese, hospitalized patients. *Ann Pharmacother.* 2017;51(3):209-218.

83. Toma O, Suntrup P, Stefanescu A, et al. Pharmacokinetics and tissue penetration of cefoxitin in obesity: implications for risk of surgical site infection. *Anesth Analg.* 2011;113(4):730-737.

84. Richardson J, Scheetz M, O'Donnell EP. The association of elevated trough serum vancomycin concentrations with obesity. *J Infect Chemother.* 2015;21(7):507-511.

85. Bookstaver PB, Bland CM, Qureshi ZP, et al. Safety and effectiveness of daptomycin across a hospitalized obese population: results of a multicenter investigation in the southeastern United States. *Pharmacotherapy.* 2013;33(12):1322-1330.

86. Kassamali Z, Jain R, Danziger LH. An update on the arsenal for multidrug-resistant Acinetobacter infections: polymyxin antibiotics. *Int J Infect Dis.* 2015;30:125-132.

87. Spruill WJ, Wade WE, Huckaby WG, Leslie RB. Achievement of anticoagulation by using a weight-based heparin dosing protocol for obese and nonobese patients. *Am J Health Syst Pharm.* 2001;58(22):2143-2146.

88. Nutescu EA, Spinler SA, Wittkowsky A, Dager WE. Low-molecular-weight heparins in renal impairment and obesity: available evidence and clinical practice recommendations across medical and surgical settings. *Ann Pharmacother.* 2009;43(6):1064-1083.

89. Duplaga BA, Rivers CW, Nutescu E. Dosing and monitoring of low-molecular-weight heparins in special populations. *Pharmacotherapy.* 2001;21(2):218-234.

90. Faria R, Spackman E, Burch J, et al. Dabigatran for the prevention of stroke and systemic embolism in atrial fibrillation: a NICE single technology appraisal. *Pharmacoeconomics.* 2013;31(7):551-562.

91. Connolly SJ, Ezekowitz MD, Yusuf S, et al. Dabigatran versus warfarin in patients with atrial fibrillation. *N Engl J Med.* 2009;361(12):1139-1151.

92. Patel MR, Mahaffey KW, Garg J, et al. Rivaroxaban versus warfarin in nonvalvular atrial fibrillation. *N Engl J Med.* 2011; 365(10):883-891.

93. Lassen MR, Ageno W, Borris LC, et al. Rivaroxaban versus enoxaparin for thromboprophylaxis after total knee arthroplasty. *N Engl J Med.* 2008;358(26):2776-2786.

94. Eriksson BI, Borris LC, Friedman RJ, et al. Rivaroxaban versus enoxaparin for thromboprophylaxis after hip arthroplasty. *N Engl J Med.* 2008;358(26):2765-2775.

95. Kubitza D, Becka M, Zuehlsdorf M, Mueck W. Body weight has limited influence on the safety, tolerability, pharmacokinetics, or pharmacodynamics of rivaroxaban (BAY 59-7939) in healthy subjects. *J Clin Pharmacol.* 2007;47(2):218-226.

96. Turpie AG, Lassen MR, Eriksson BI, et al. Rivaroxaban for the prevention of venous thromboembolism after hip or knee arthroplasty. Pooled analysis of four studies. *Thromb Haemost.* 2011;105(3):444-453.

97. Lopes RD, Alexander JH, Al-Khatib SM, et al. Apixaban for Reduction In Stroke and Other ThromboemboLic Events in atrial fibrillation (ARISTOTLE) trial: design and rationale. *Am Heart J.* 2010;159(3):331-339.

98. Hurst KV, O'Callaghan JM, Handa A. Risk impact of edoxaban in the management of stroke and venous thromboembolism. *Vasc Health Risk Manag.* 2016;12: 329-335.

99. Tittl L, Endig S, Marten S, et al. Impact of BMI on clinical outcomes of NOAC therapy in daily care—results of the prospective Dresden NOAC Registry (NCT01588119). *Int J Cardiol.* 2018;262:85-91.

100. Breen HB, Ireton-Jones CS. Predicting energy needs in obese patients. *Nutr Clin Pract.* 2004;19(3):284-289.

101. Dickerson RN. Specialized nutrition support in the hospitalized obese patient. *Nutr Clin Pract.* 2004;19(3):245-254.

102. Choban P, Dickerson R, Malone A, et al. A.S.P.E.N. Clinical guidelines: nutrition support of hospitalized adult patients with obesity. *JPEN J Parenter Enteral Nutr.* 2013;37(6): 714-744.

103. Ireton-Jones CS, Turner Jr WW. Actual or ideal body weight: which should be used to predict energy expenditure? *J Am Diet Assoc.* 1991;91(2):193-195.

104. Frankenfield DC, Coleman A, Alam S, Cooney RN. Analysis of estimation methods for resting metabolic rate in critically ill adults. *JPEN J Parenter Enteral Nutr.* 2009;33(1):27-36.

105. Mesejo A, Vaquerizo Alonso C, Acosta Escribano J, et al. [Guidelines for specialized nutritional and metabolic support in the critically-ill patient. Update. Consensus of the Spanish Society of Intensive Care Medicine and Coronary Units–Spanish Society of Parenteral and Enteral Nutrition (SEMICYUC-SENPE): introduction and methodology]. *Med Intensiva.* 2011;35(suppl 1):1-6.

106. Dickerson RN, Medling TL, Smith AC, et al. Hypocaloric, high-protein nutrition therapy in older vs. younger critically ill patients with obesity. *JPEN J Parenter Enteral Nutr.* 2013; 37(3):342-351.

107. Uppot RN. Impact of obesity on radiology. *Radiol Clin North Am.* 2007;45(2):231-246.

108. Parienti JJ, Thirion M, Mégarbane B, et al. Femoral vs. jugular venous catheterization and risk of nosocomial events in adults requiring acute renal replacement therapy: a randomized controlled trial. *JAMA.* 2008;299(20):2413-2422.

109. Timsit JF, Bouadma L, Mimoz O, et al. Jugular versus femoral short-term catheterization and risk of infection in intensive care unit patients. Causal analysis of two randomized trials. *Am J Respir Crit Care Med.* 2013;188(10):1232-1239.

110. Hind D, Calvert N, McWilliams R, et al. Ultrasonic locating devices for central venous cannulation: meta-analysis. *BMJ.* 2003;327(7411):361.

111. Thokala P, Arrowsmith M, Poku E, et al. Economic impact of Tegaderm chlorhexidine gluconate (CHG) dressing in critically ill patients. *J Infect Prev.* 2016;17(5):216-223.

112. Lai NM, Chaiyakunapruk N, Lai NA, et al. Catheter impregnation, coating or bonding for reducing central venous catheter-related infections in adults. *Cochrane Database Syst Rev.* 2016;3:CD007878.

113. El-Solh A, Sikka P, Bozkanat E, et al. Morbid obesity in the medical ICU. *Chest.* 2001;120(6):1989-1997.

114. Bercault N, Boulain T, Kuteifan K, et al. Obesity-related excess mortality rate in an adult intensive care unit: a risk-adjusted matched cohort study. *Crit Care Med.* 2004;32(4): 998-1003.

115. Goulenok C, Monchi M, Chiche JD, et al. Influence of overweight on ICU mortality: a prospective study. *Chest.* 2004;125(4):1441-1445.

116. Sasabuchi Y, Yasunaga H, Matsui H, et al. The dose-response relationship between body mass index and mortality in subjects admitted to the ICU with and without mechanical ventilation. *Respir Care.* 2015;60(7):983-991.

117. O'Brien Jr JM, Welsh CH, Fish RH, et al. Excess body weight is not independently associated with outcome in mechanically ventilated patients with acute lung injury. *Ann Intern Med.* 2004;140(5):338-345.

118. Akinnusi ME, Pineda LA, El Solh AA. Effect of obesity on intensive care morbidity and mortality: a meta-analysis. *Crit Care Med.* 2008;36(1):151-158.

119. Hogue Jr CW, Stearns JD, Colantuoni E, et al. The impact of obesity on outcomes after critical illness: a meta-analysis. *Intensive Care Med.* 2009;35(7):1152-1170.

120. Oliveros H, Villamor E. Obesity and mortality in critically ill adults: a systematic review and meta-analysis. *Obesity.* 2008;16(3):515-521.

121. Bornstein SR, Licinio J, Tauchnitz R, et al. Plasma leptin levels are increased in survivors of acute sepsis: associated loss of

diurnal rhythm, in cortisol and leptin secretion. *J Clin Endocrinol Metab.* 1998;83(1):280-283.

122. Nasraway Jr SA, Albert M, Donnelly AM, et al. Morbid obesity is an independent determinant of death among surgical critically ill patients. *Crit Care Med.* 2006;34(4):964-970; quiz 971.

123. Devarajan J, Vydyanathan A, You J, et al. The association between body mass index and outcome after coronary artery bypass grafting operations. *Eur J Cardiothorac Surg.* 2016;50(2):344-349.

124. Birkmeyer NJ, Charlesworth DC, Hernandez F, et al. Obesity and risk of adverse outcomes associated with coronary artery bypass surgery. Northern New England Cardiovascular Disease Study Group. *Circulation.* 1998;97(17):1689-1694.

125. Moulton MJ, Creswell LL, Mackey ME, et al. Obesity is not a risk factor for significant adverse outcomes after cardiac surgery. *Circulation.* 1996;94(9 suppl):II87-92.

126. Swol J, Buchwald D, Strauch JT, et al. Effect of body mass index on the outcome of surgical patients receiving extracorporeal devices (VV ECMO, pECLA) for respiratory failure. *Int J Artif Organs.* 2017;40:102-108.

127. Brown CV, Neville AL, Rhee P, et al. The impact of obesity on the outcomes of 1,153 critically injured blunt trauma patients. *J Trauma.* 2005;59(5):1048-1051; discussion 1051.

128. Neville AL, Brown CV, Weng J, et al. Obesity is an independent risk factor of mortality in severely injured blunt trauma patients. *Arch Surg.* 2004;139(9):983-987.

129. Byrnes MC, McDaniel MD, Moore MB, et al. The effect of obesity on outcomes among injured patients. *J Trauma.* 2005; 58(2):232-237.

130. Bochicchio GV, Joshi M, Bochicchio K, et al. Impact of obesity in the critically ill trauma patient: a prospective study. *J Am Coll Surg.* 2006;203(4):533-538.

131. Yaegashi M, Jean R, Zuriqat M, et al. Outcome of morbid obesity in the intensive care unit. *J Intensive Care Med.* 2005; 20(3):147-154.

28

How Do I Safely Transport the Critically Ill Patient?

Bairbre Aine McNicholas and John James Bates

INTRODUCTION

The provision of intensive care during transport to and from the intensive care unit (ICU) presents a major challenge. Available data[1,2] suggest that critical care transport is becoming increasingly common, driven by the centralization of specialties and an expanding number of diagnostic and therapeutic options outside of the ICU. The bulk of critical care transports happen within the hospital itself. Observational data[1,3,4] suggest that critical care transport is a high-risk but worthwhile activity and that this risk can be minimized by adequate planning, proper equipment, and appropriate staffing. Prehospital transport of the critically ill patient presents more problems because prior planning is more difficult.

Clinical data on the transport of the critically ill patient are derived mainly from cohort trials and can provide guidelines in terms of personnel (physicians, nurses, and paramedics), mode of transport (air or road), and specific treatments (prehospital tracheal intubation and advanced life support).

INTRAHOSPITAL TRANSPORT OF THE CRITICALLY ILL

Adverse Effects

Several observational studies suggest that significant physiologic disturbances (large variations in heart rate, blood pressure [BP], or oxygen saturation) occur during 53–68% of intrahospital transports.[5–7] Physiologic variability is also common in stationary critically ill patients, occurring in 60% of such patients in a study by Hurst and colleagues compared with 66% in transported patients.[6] Many of these physiologic changes can be safely managed by an appropriately trained transport team, but serious adverse events do occur. Prospective observational studies have found an adverse event rate of 36–45.8%.[8,9] A large multicenter cohort study showed an odds ratio (OR) for the occurrence of adverse events on intrahospital transports of 1.9. These events included pneumothorax, ventilator-associated pneumonia, and atelectasis. Increased length of stay was noted in the same study but not a difference in mortality.[10]

Damm and colleagues[11] found a cardiac arrest rate of 1.6% in a prospective observational study of 123 intrahospital transports.

Waydhas and colleagues[12] found that a reduction in the ratio of partial pressure of arterial oxygen to the fraction of inspired oxygen (PaO_2/FiO_2) occurred in 83.7% of patients when transported using a transport ventilator and that this was severe (>20% reduction from baseline) in 42.8%. Furthermore, these changes persisted for >24 hours in 20.4% of transports. Two large cohort studies using logistic regression analysis[13,14] found out-of-unit transport to be an independent risk factor for ventilator-associated pneumonia (OR 3.1[13] and 3.8[14]) in ICU patients. Intrahospital transport is also one of the factors associated with unplanned extubation.[15]

When compared with APACHE (Acute Physiology and Chronic Health Evaluation) II and III matched controls, patients requiring intrahospital transport were found to have a higher mortality rate (28.6% vs. 11.4%) and a longer ICU length of stay.[16] None of the excess mortality was directly attributable to complications of the transport, and the authors concluded that the findings reflected a higher severity of illness in patients who required transportation. However, serious adverse events did occur in 5.9% of transports.

Predicting Adverse Events During Intrahospital Transport

Factors associated with an increased risk for adverse events during transport include pretransport secondary insults in head-injured patients, high injury severity score,[17] and high Therapeutic Interventions Severity Score (TISS) but not APACHE II score.[18] Age over 43 years old and an $FiO_2 > 0.5$ are predictive of respiratory deterioration on transport.[19]

The number of intravenous pumps and infusions, as well as the time spent outside the unit, has been shown to correlate with the number of technical mishaps.[20] The Australian ICU Incident Monitoring Study,[21] found that 39% of transport problems were equipment related, with 61% relating to patient or staff management issues. Factors limiting harm were rechecking of the patient and equipment, skilled assistance, and prior experience.

Hemodynamic variability is more frequent in patients being transferred to the ICU from the operating room than those transported for diagnostic procedures outside the ICU. This is probably related to emergence from anesthesia.[22]

Risk-to-Benefit Ratio of Intrahospital Transport

Observational studies suggest that the therapeutic yield for intrahospital transport is high. Hurst and colleagues found that the results of diagnostic testing facilitated by the transport resulted in a change in treatment in 39% of patients.[6] Out-of-unit radiologic studies in ICU patients tend to be high yield. For instance, computed tomography (CT) scanning of the thorax has been shown in observational studies to change the clinical course in 26–57% of cases.[23,24]

Management of the Transport

A cohort study has found that transport ventilators reduce variability in blood gas parameters when compared with manual bagging.[25] While several older studies found manual ventilation to be as good or better than use of a transport ventilator,[26–28] the performance characteristics of transport ventilators has improved significantly over time[29–31] and the performance of many modern transport ventilators is comparable to that of ICU ventilators.[32] Changes in blood gas parameters have been shown to correlate with hemodynamic disturbances (arrhythmias, hypotension).[25]

Capnometry (end-tidal carbon dioxide [$EtCO_2$]) monitoring reduces partial pressure of arterial carbon dioxide ($PaCO_2$) variability in adults.[33] In children, manual ventilation without $EtCO_2$ monitoring resulted in only 31% of readings falling within the intended range.[34]

A single randomized controlled trial (RCT) found that hypothermia was common in trauma patients undergoing intrahospital transport (average temperature on return to the unit was 34.7°C) and that this was prevented by active warming during transport.[35]

Who should accompany the critically ill patient during transport? Specialized transport teams have been found to have a lower rate of complications than historical controls.[36,37] Interestingly, physician attendance was not clearly correlated with a reduced risk for mishap in an observational study of 125 transports.[18]

The implementation of a pretransport checklist has been found to reduce the rate of serious adverse events from 9.1–5.2%.[38]

INTERHOSPITAL TRANSFER

The interhospital transfer is a secondary transport from one institution of initial or standard care for further therapy to an institution of advanced and/or maximum care, while maintaining the intensive medical therapy already in progress[39]; 1.5% of emergency department (ED) admissions, 5% of hospital admissions, and approximately 4.5% of critical care stays are associated with an interhospital transfer.[40–42] The number of interhospital transfers of critically ill patients is increasing[2] because of a reduction in the number of hospitals, centralization of specialist services, and reconfiguration of health-care services between acute and elective medicine.

Adverse Effects

The benefits of transport to the patient need to be weighed against the considerable risks of the transport process from a human and organizational aspect. These include clinical deterioration, lack of adequate medical resources during transfer, delays in time-sensitive care, transportation risk, poor handoff communication, and neglected patient preference with patient's care being conducted in a hospital remote from home and social support.[40] There are few RCTs on this subject, and conclusions have to be drawn from nonrandomized, cohort, or uncontrolled studies. This results in difficulty determining accurate rates of adverse events, thus preventing firm conclusions regarding the attributable mortality, morbidity, or risk factors associated with the interhospital transport of critically ill patients.[43,44]

Time delays can occur from triaging, accepting, and organizing the transport logistics. These can be deleterious for conditions such as ST-segment elevation myocardial infarction (STEMI), where institution of nonpercutaneous coronary intervention (non-PCI)-based therapy in a remote hospital may be in the patient's interest, or sepsis, where a time-sensitive treatment can be initiated in any hospital and bypassing rural hospitals is associated with increased mortality.[45,46] Risks associated with the transfer include motor vehicle accidents[47] diversion for other emergencies encountered en route,[48] and helicopter emergency medical service (HEMS) accidents. HEMS have a crash rate per 10,000 missions ranging between 0.4 and 3.05 and fatal crash rates between 0.04 and 2.12.[49]

Various published audits and descriptive studies have shown that the interhospital transport of critically ill patients is associated with an increased morbidity and mortality during and after the journey.[50–54] Critical events can include changes in heart rate, hypotension, hypertension, increased intracranial pressure, arrhythmias, cardiac arrest, hypoxemia, hypocapnia, and hypercapnia.[55] Events leading to mortality can include airway-related events, cardiopulmonary arrest, sustained hypotension, and loss of crucial intravenous access.[56] These risks need to be balanced against the survival advantage in transfer to regional centers of expertise.[57–59] Critical events occur in 4–17.1% of interhospital transfers, with 24–70% of incidents avoidable.[50,55,60–62] Patients undergoing interhospital transport after cardiac arrest have a rearrest rate of 6% during the transfer.[63] Rates of critical events range from 5.1% to 6.5% for air and ground ambulance, respectively,[61] with time being a critical factor, increasing the risk of a critical event by 2–10% for every 15 minutes duration of transfer.[60,61] Reductions in rates of adverse events have resulted from better trained and equipped personnel, which has made interhospital transfer safer.[39,57,62,64] The use of mobile ICUs or specialist retrieval teams has been shown to reduce risk related to transfer.[57,65]

Prediction of Adverse Events

Independent predictors of critical events during transport include female sex, older age, higher FiO_2, multiple injury, assisted ventilation, hemodynamic instability, inadequate stabilization before transport, transport in a fixed-wing aircraft, and increased duration of transport.[19,61,66] The APACHE II, TISS, and Rapid Acute Physiology scoring systems and the Pediatric Risk of Mortality (PRISM) score do not correlate with the likelihood of critical events during transport.[19,55,67–69]

Planning of the Transport

Adequate training of the transport team and improving provider communication during the transfer is important to reduce the complications associated with interhospital transfer. Guidelines have been developed to address this issue,[39,70,71] but inadequate assessment and resuscitation remain a problem. The use of a centralized and specialized patient retrieval service for severely injured patients requiring interhospital transfer results in improved outcomes, probably by improving team expertise, logistical coordination, and facilitating optimal destination choice.[59] Improving provider communication both for referring and receiving physicians is also important to reduce complications during transfer as well as reducing repeated testing and diagnostic uncertainty at the time of transfer.[50,72–74] Retrievalists may have greater exposure to critically ill patients than the providers in some referring hospitals and can potentially extend the abilities of inexperienced doctors in those hospitals as well as optimizing patients prior to transfer.[39,75,76] Expansion of telemedicine, such as video conferencing and computer-based data transmission between referral and retrieving hospitals, is likely to improve communication for patients who are being selected for interhospital transfer to both optimize patients for transfer as well as preventing over-triage of patients.[77,78]

Selection of Personnel

It is recommended that a minimum of two people, in addition to the vehicle operators, accompany a critically ill patient during transport. The team leader can be a nurse or physician, depending on clinical and local circumstances. It is imperative that the team leader has adequate training in transport medicine and advanced life support. Adequately trained nurses have been shown to be as safe at transporting critically ill children as doctors.[64,79]

Appropriately staffed and equipped specialist retrieval teams have been shown to be superior to occasional teams at transferring critically ill adults[57,65,80] and children.[81] Vos and colleagues demonstrated a 60% reduction in critical incidents during interhospital transport undertaken by a specialist retrieval team. In another cohort study, mortality was increased (23% vs. 9%) in children transported by a nonspecialized team, a difference that remained after adjustment for severity of illness.[56] Fatigue amongst personnel involved in transport is understudied, but given the challenging environment, length of missions, and frequent night work, unsurprisingly, high levels of fatigue are experienced by providers.[82]

Mode of Transport

The choice between the three options of road, helicopter, and fixed-wing transport are affected by three main factors: distance, patient status, and weather conditions. A prospective cohort study has demonstrated that air transport is faster than ground transport, and for transfers of less than 225 km, helicopter transport is faster than fixed-wing transport.[83] The majority of transports are conducted by ground transportation,[84] but helicopter transfers frequently carry sicker patients and have a faster transfer time. However, the speed of the overall transfer is dependent on the logistics required to facilitate this transfer. A prospective observational study examining transfer of stroke patients found that time to transfer from referral to neurologist to arrival at stroke center was faster by ground transportation, although distance to stroke center was shorter for ground transportation than helicopter.[85] There have been no RCTs to allow comparison between helicopter and ground transportation. Some, but not all, observational series have reported improved mortality for helicopter transfers compared with ground transportation.[84,86,87] HEMS have the advantage of highly skilled crews and may offer no mortality benefit when crew expertise is controlled for.[88] Difficulties encountered with air transport include narrow cabin, airsickness, lack of medical equipment, poor coordination, noise, aircraft turbulence, and low air pressure. In one series of HEMS patients in a combat environment, 30% of those being transported within 8 hours of surgery experienced in-flight deterioration and 9% required urgent intervention on arrival.[52] Finally, speed at which transfers occur using ground transport can influence the vibration injury that patients are exposed to, which may be particularly important in neonates and brain injury.[53]

Equipment and Monitoring

Comprehensive lists of equipment and medications needed for transport of critically ill patients are available elsewhere; they are beyond the scope of this chapter and should reflect the scope of practice of the retrievalist.[57,89,90] Greater numbers of extremely ill patients are being transferred, leading to the expansion of mobile ICUs that can deliver nitric oxide,[91] extracorporeal membrane oxygenation (ECMO), and mechanical circulatory assist devices.[58,92–99] Introduction of mobile ICUs with specialized retrieval teams has led to a reduction in the rates of adverse events compared with standard ambulance transport.[62]

It is generally accepted that the standard of organ support and monitoring available in the ICU should be continued during the transport to the greatest extent possible. An RCT of near-continuous noninvasive BP monitoring compared with intermittent BP monitoring during interhospital transport of critically ill children found less organ dysfunction and a shorter ICU stay in the intervention group.[100] A bispectral index (BIS) monitor can be used for the assessment of sedation levels during critical care transfer and is highly sensitive in the detection of unwanted awakening of patients during transfers.[101]

Improvement in technology for capillary blood testing producing reproducible and comparable test results to reference methods will allow for laboratory tests during critical care transport.[102] Uncontrolled observational studies have shown that point-of-care blood gas analysis during interhospital transfer allows early identification and treatment of changes in gas exchange and metabolic parameters.[103]

Retrospective studies of transports of infants being transferred for therapeutic hypothermia have found that the use of a purpose-built cooling device was associated with better temperature control and faster time to achieving target temperature than passive cooling and these are increasingly used.[103,104] Additional equipment that may be potentially used in the future during interhospital transfer includes point-of-care ultrasound as intensivists' experience with the use of this modality increases.[105]

PREHOSPITAL TRANSPORT

Most research in the area of prehospital transport has focused on patients with trauma or out-of-hospital cardiac arrest (OOHCA), due to the potential for early appropriate intervention to improve outcome.

Retrieval Systems

Four main infrastructural factors have been addressed in clinical studies:

1. Mode of transport
2. Prehospital personnel
3. Prehospital time
4. Receiving care facility

Mode of Transport

The comparison between road and helicopter transport has been the focus of several large cohort studies in the past decade.[106–113] Five of six studies demonstrated a survival advantage for severely injured patients with physiologic instability transported by helicopter[106,108–113] with an OR of death of 0.41–0.68,[106,108,110] although a Cochrane review in 2015 could not determine an accurate composite estimate of improved survival.[114] The reason for the survival advantage is less clear. A survival advantage is seen in the absence of reduced prehospital time.[108,112,115] It has been suggested that the benefit might be due to HEMS crews transporting a greater proportion of patients to level I or II trauma centers[107] or the greater expertise and experience of HEMS crews compared with ground emergency medical services.[112]

Prehospital Personnel

One RCT[116] and a systematic review of controlled nonrandomized studies[117] have addressed the issue of physician- vs. paramedic-delivered prehospital care. The RCT found a 35% reduction in mortality in the physician-treated group. In the systematic review, 9 of 19 studies involving trauma patients and 4 of 5 studies involving OOHCA patients also demonstrated a reduction in mortality in the physician-treated group.[117] The largest of these controlled studies involved 14,702 trauma patients and showed an OR for death of 0.7 in the physician-treated group.[118] The evidence indicates that physicians tend to treat patients more aggressively and can improve physiologic stability in 33% at the scene (with 66% remaining unchanged and only 1% deteriorating).[119] Physicians also have fewer prehospital tracheal intubation failures than nonphysicians.[120]

Prehospital Time

Severely injured patients have been shown in cohort trials to suffer an increased mortality,[121] length of stay, and complications[122] with prehospital times of more than 60 minutes. Time from injury to arrival at definitive care may not be as important

in highly developed trauma systems with the capability to provide aggressive care in the prehospital phase.[108,112,123] Prolonged scene time is particularly associated with mortality in patients with hypotension, penetrating injury, or flail chest.[124]

Receiving Care Facility

Several large cohort studies have found a reduction in mortality for severely injured trauma patients when they are transferred directly to a level 1 trauma center.[125–127] The largest of these centers treated more than 6000 patients from 15 regions in the United States. Patients treated primarily in level 1 trauma centers had a lower in-hospital (OR 0.8, confidence interval [CI] 0.66–0.98) and 1-year mortality (OR 0.75, CI 0.60–0.95). Subgroup analysis suggested that the mortality benefit was primarily confined to more severely injured patients.[127]

Specific Interventions in the Prehospital Setting

Whether advanced life support (ALS) measures (endotracheal intubation, intravenous cannulation, and fluid and drug administration) delivered at the scene and in transit are of benefit to patients when compared with basic life support (BLS) is unclear,[128] but it is likely that benefit depends on the expertise of the provider and the patient population.[124,129]

Three before and after studies of ALS vs. BLS (the Ontario Prehospital Advanced Life Support [OPALS] studies) looked at the effect of the institution of ALS in prehospital care in patients with OOHCA,[130] respiratory distress,[131] and major trauma.[132] No improvement in mortality was observed amongst patients with cardiac arrest or trauma. For trauma patients with a Glasgow Coma Scale (GCS) < 9, mortality was increased in the ALS phase. There was a small mortality benefit in patients with respiratory distress.

Similarly, a meta-analysis[128] of 15 observational and cohort studies comparing ALS with BLS for trauma patients demonstrated an increased mortality in ALS patients (OR 2.59). The same authors subsequently published a large observational study comparing different prehospital systems in Canada. After correction for confounders using logistic regression analysis, they found a 21% increase in mortality for patients treated with on-site ALS ($P = .01$).[133]

One RCT and many observational studies have looked specifically at the effect of prehospital tracheal intubation on outcome. The RCT compared prehospital rapid sequence induction (RSI) by intensive care paramedics vs. intubation in hospital for patients ($n = 312$) with traumatic brain injury (TBI) (GCS <9).[134] The authors found an improvement in neurologic outcome at 6 months (risk ratio for good outcome of 1.28 in the intervention group). Two other cohort studies found an improvement in outcome in severe TBI where intubation prehospital was performed by expert providers.[124,129] Other observational studies have found an increase in mortality with prehospital intubation,[135–137] particularly in hypotensive patients where an adjusted OR of death of 2.89–9.99 has been observed.[138,139]

A prospective observational study of 1320 trauma patients who underwent airway interventions by an anesthesiologist on arrival in a level I trauma center found that 31% of those who had undergone tracheal intubation met the criteria for failed intubation, with 12% having unrecognized esophageal intubation on arrival.[140] A prospective observational study found a decrease in the rate of unrecognized misplaced intubations from 9% to 0% after the introduction of continuous $EtCO_2$ monitoring in the prehospital setting.[141] A meta-analysis of the success rate of prehospital tracheal intubation has found that physicians have a better success rate than nonphysicians (0.988 vs. 0.917) and that the use of muscle relaxants improves the success rate (0.96 vs. 0.88).[120] Prehospital tracheal intubation is a complex intervention and its value is probably related to many factors, including the skill of the provider, patient population, access to drugs to facilitate the intervention, and other aspects of the prehospital trauma system.

A single retrospective cohort study found an association between prehospital red cell transfusion and 24-hour survival (adjusted OR 4.92) in trauma patients.[142]

An RCT of the use of a mechanical compression device in OOHCA found no survival advantage associated with use of the device.[143]

AUTHORS' RECOMMENDATIONS
- Transport of the critically ill patient is a necessary and important part of clinical practice. It is often overlooked.
- The risk to the patient of the transport itself can be reduced by appropriate planning and training of personnel and attention to pretransport stabilization of the patient.
- Transport of critically ill patients is best undertaken by experienced specialist transport teams wherever possible. This is especially true for pediatric critical care transports.
- The prehospital interventions that are associated with improved outcome are as follows:
  - helicopter transport of severely injured trauma patients
  - presence of a physician on the prehospital transport team
  - transfer directly to a level 1 trauma center
  - the use of continuous $EtCO_2$ monitoring for prehospital endotracheal intubation
  - the use of prehospital RSI by trained prehospital crews for TBI with GCS < 9

REFERENCES

1. Mackenzie PA, Smith EA, Wallace PG. Transfer of adults between intensive care units in the United Kingdom: postal survey. *BMJ*. 1997;314(7092):1455-1456.
2. Fried MJ, Bruce J, Colquhoun R, Smith G. Inter-hospital transfers of acutely ill adults in Scotland. *Anaesthesia*. 2010; 65(2):136-144.
3. Gentleman D, Jennett B. Audit of transfer of unconscious head-injured patients to a neurosurgical unit. *Lancet*. 1990;335(8685): 330-334.
4. Koppenberg J, Taeger K. Interhospital transport: transport of critically ill patients. *Curr Opin Anaesthesiol*. 2002;15(2):211-215.
5. Evans A, Winslow EH. Oxygen saturation and hemodynamic response in critically ill, mechanically ventilated adults during intrahospital transport. *Am J Crit Care*. 1995;4(2):106-111.
6. Hurst JM, Davis Jr K, Johnson DJ, Branson RD, Campbell RS, Branson PS. Cost and complications during in-hospital transport of critically ill patients: a prospective cohort study. *J Trauma*. 1992;33(4):582-585.
7. Indeck M, Peterson S, Smith J, Brotman S. Risk, cost, and benefit of transporting ICU patients for special studies. *J Trauma*. 1988;28(7):1020-1025.
8. Picetti E, Antonini MV, Lucchetti MC, et al. Intra-hospital transport of brain-injured patients: a prospective, observational study. *Neurocrit Care*. 2013;18(3):298-304.
9. Parmentier-Decrucq E, Poissy J, Favory R, et al. Adverse events during intrahospital transport of critically ill patients: incidence and risk factors. *Ann Intensive Care*. 2013;3(1):10.
10. Schwebel C, Clec'h C, Magne S, et al. Safety of intrahospital transport in ventilated critically ill patients: a multicenter cohort study. *Crit Care Med*. 2013;41(8):1919-1928.
11. Damm C, Vandelet P, Petit J, et al. [Complications during the intrahospital transport in critically ill patients]. *Ann Fr Anesth Reanim*. 2005;24(1):24-30.
12. Waydhas C, Schneck G, Duswald KH. Deterioration of respiratory function after intra-hospital transport of critically ill surgical patients. *Intensive Care Med*. 1995;21(10): 784-789.
13. Bercault N, Wolf M, Runge I, Fleury JC, Boulain T. Intrahospital transport of critically ill ventilated patients: a risk factor for ventilator-associated pneumonia—a matched cohort study. *Crit Care Med*. 2005;33(11):2471-2478.
14. Kollef MH, Von Harz B, Prentice D, et al. Patient transport from intensive care increases the risk of developing ventilator-associated pneumonia. *Chest*. 1997;112(3):765-773.
15. Christie JM, Dethlefsen M, Cane RD. Unplanned endotracheal extubation in the intensive care unit. *J Clin Anesth*. 1996;8(4): 289-293.
16. Szem JW, Hydo LJ, Fischer E, Kapur S, Klemperer J, Barie PS. High-risk intrahospital transport of critically ill patients: safety and outcome of the necessary "road trip." *Crit Care Med*. 1995; 23(10):1660-1666.
17. Andrews PJ, Piper IR, Dearden NM, Miller JD. Secondary insults during intrahospital transport of head-injured patients. *Lancet*. 1990;335(8685):327-330.
18. Smith I, Fleming S, Cernaianu A. Mishaps during transport from the intensive care unit. *Crit Care Med*. 1990;18(3):278-281.
19. Marx G, Vangerow B, Hecker H, et al. Predictors of respiratory function deterioration after transfer of critically ill patients. *Intensive Care Med*. 1998;24(11):1157-1162.
20. Doring BL, Kerr ME, Lovasik DA, Thayer T. Factors that contribute to complications during intrahospital transport of the critically ill. *J Neurosci Nurs*. 1999;31(2):80-86.
21. Beckmann U, Gillies DM, Berenholtz SM, Wu AW, Pronovost P. Incidents relating to the intra-hospital transfer of critically ill patients. An analysis of the reports submitted to the Australian Incident Monitoring Study in Intensive Care. *Intensive Care Med*. 2004;30(8):1579-1585.
22. Insel J, Weissman C, Kemper M, Askanazi J, Hyman AI. Cardiovascular changes during transport of critically ill and postoperative patients. *Crit Care Med*. 1986;14(6): 539-542.
23. Roddy LH, Unger KM, Miller WC. Thoracic computed tomography in the critically ill patient. *Crit Care Med*. 1981;9(7):515-518.
24. Voggenreiter G, Aufmkolk M, Majetschak M, et al. Efficiency of chest computed tomography in critically ill patients with multiple traumas. *Crit Care Med*. 2000;28(4):1033-1039.

25. Braman SS, Dunn SM, Amico CA, Millman RP. Complications of intrahospital transport in critically ill patients. *Ann Intern Med*. 1987;107(4):469-473.

26. Gervais HW, Eberle B, Konietzke D, Hennes HJ, Dick W. Comparison of blood gases of ventilated patients during transport. *Crit Care Med*. 1987;15(8):761-763.

27. Weg JG, Haas CF. Safe intrahospital transport of critically ill ventilator-dependent patients. *Chest*. 1989;96(3):631-635.

28. Dockery WK, Futterman C, Keller SR, Sheridan MJ, Akl BF. A comparison of manual and mechanical ventilation during pediatric transport. *Crit Care Med*. 1999;27(4):802-806.

29. Zanetta G, Robert D, Guérin C. Evaluation of ventilators used during transport of ICU patients—a bench study. *Intensive Care Med*. 2002;28(4):443-451.

30. Chipman DW, Caramez MP, Miyoshi E, Kratohvil JP, Kacmarek RM. Performance comparison of 15 transport ventilators. *Respir Care*. 2007;52(6):740-751.

31. Blakeman TC, Branson RD. Inter- and intra-hospital transport of the critically ill. *Respir Care*. 2013;58(6):1008-1023.

32. Boussen S, Gainnier M, Michelet P. Evaluation of ventilators used during transport of critically ill patients: a bench study. *Respir Care*. 2013;58(11):1911-1922.

33. Palmon SC, Liu M, Moore LE, Kirsch JR. Capnography facilitates tight control of ventilation during transport. *Crit Care Med*. 1996;24(4):608-611.

34. Tobias JD, Lynch A, Garrett J. Alterations of end-tidal carbon dioxide during the intrahospital transport of children. *Pediatr Emerg Care*. 1996;12(4):249-251.

35. Scheck T, Kober A, Bertalanffy P, et al. Active warming of critically ill trauma patients during intrahospital transfer: a prospective, randomized trial. *Wien Klin Wochenschr*. 2004;116(3):94-97.

36. Stearley HE. Patients' outcomes: intrahospital transportation and monitoring of critically ill patients by a specially trained ICU nursing staff. *Am J Crit Care*. 1998;7(4):282-287.

37. Kue R, Brown P, Ness C, Scheulen J. Adverse clinical events during intrahospital transport by a specialized team: a preliminary report. *Am J Crit Care*. 2011;20(2):153-161; quiz 162.

38. Choi HK, Shin SD, Ro YS, Kim DK, Shin SH, Kwak YH. Before- and after-intervention trial for reducing unexpected events during the intrahospital transport of emergency patients. *Am J Emerg Med*. 2012;30(8):1433-1440.

39. Blecha S, Dodoo-Schittko F, Brandstetter S, et al. Quality of inter-hospital transportation in 431 transport survivor patients suffering from acute respiratory distress syndrome referred to specialist centers. *Ann Intensive Care*. 2018;8(1):5.

40. Feazel L, Schlichting AB, Bell GR, et al. Achieving regionalization through rural interhospital transfer. *Am J Emerg Med*. 2015; 33(9):1288-1296.

41. Iwashyna TJ, Christie JD, Moody J, Kahn JM, Asch DA. The structure of critical care transfer networks. *Med Care*. 2009;47(7):787-793.

42. Reimer AP, Schiltz N, Koroukian SM, Madigan EA. National incidence of medical transfer: patient characteristics and regional variation. *J Health Hum Serv Adm*. 2016;38(4): 509-528.

43. Fan E, MacDonald RD, Adhikari NK, et al. Outcomes of inter-facility critical care adult patient transport: a systematic review. *Crit Care*. 2006;10(1):R6.

44. Strauch U, Bergmans DC, Habers J, et al. QUIT EMR trial: a prospective, observational, multicentre study to evaluate quality and 24 hours post-transport morbidity of interhospital transportation of critically ill patients: study protocol. *BMJ Open*. 2017;7(3):e012861.

45. Mohr NM, Harland KK, Shane DM, et al. Rural patients with severe sepsis or septic shock who bypass rural hospitals have increased mortality: an instrumental variables approach. *Crit Care Med*. 2017;45(1):85-93.

46. Park JH, Ahn KO, Shin SD, et al. The first-door-to-balloon time delay in STEMI patients undergoing interhospital transfer. *Am J Emerg Med*. 2016;34(5):767-771.

47. Maguire BJ, Hunting KL, Smith GS, Levick NR. Occupational fatalities in emergency medical services: a hidden crisis. *Ann Emerg Med*. 2002;40(6):625-632.

48. Raman S, Ramnarayan P. Impact of stops for road traffic accidents on the inter-hospital transport of critically ill children. *Emerg Med J*. 2014;31(7):589-590.

49. Hinkelbein J, Schwalbe M, Genzwuerker HV. Helicopter emergency medical services accident rates in different international air rescue systems. *Open Access Emerg Med*. 2010;2:45-49.

50. Ligtenberg JJ, Arnold LG, Stienstra Y, et al. Quality of interhospital transport of critically ill patients: a prospective audit. *Crit Care*. 2005;9(4):R446-R451.

51. Nicholson BD, Dhindsa HS, Roe MT, Chen AY, Jollis JG, Kontos MC. Relationship of the distance between non-PCI hospitals and primary PCI centers, mode of transport, and reperfusion time among ground and air interhospital transfers using NCDR's ACTION Registry-GWTG: a report from the American Heart Association Mission: Lifeline Program. *Circ Cardiovasc Interv*. 2014;7(6):797-805.

52. Lehmann R, Oh J, Killius S, Cornell M, Furay E, Martin M. Interhospital patient transport by rotary wing aircraft in a combat environment: risks, adverse events, and process improvement. *J Trauma*. 2009;66(suppl 4):S31-S34; discussion S34-S36.

53. Blaxter L, Yeo M, McNally D, et al. Neonatal head and torso vibration exposure during inter-hospital transfer. *Proc Inst Mech Eng H*. 2017;231(2):99-113.

54. Henning R, McNamara V. Difficulties encountered in transport of the critically ill child. *Pediatr Emerg Care*. 1991;7(3):133-137.

55. Waydhas C. Intrahospital transport of critically ill patients. *Crit Care*. 1999;3(5):R83-R89.

56. Orr RA, Felmet KA, Han Y, et al. Pediatric specialized transport teams are associated with improved outcomes. *Pediatrics*. 2009; 124(1):40-48.

57. Gebremichael M, Borg U, Habashi NM, et al. Interhospital transport of the extremely ill patient: the mobile intensive care unit. *Crit Care Med*. 2000;28(1):79-85.

58. Peek GJ, Mugford M, Tiruvoipati R, et al. Efficacy and economic assessment of conventional ventilatory support versus extracorporeal membrane oxygenation for severe adult respiratory failure (CESAR): a multicentre randomised controlled trial. *Lancet*. 2009;374(9698):1351-1363.

59. Kennedy MP, Gabbe BJ, McKenzie BA. Impact of the introduction of an integrated adult retrieval service on major trauma outcomes. *Emerg Med J*. 2015;32(11):833-839.

60. Singh JM, MacDonald RD, Ahghari M. Critical events during land-based interfacility transport. *Ann Emerg Med*. 2014; 64(1):9-15.e2.

61. Singh JM, MacDonald RD, Bronskill SE, Schull MJ. Incidence and predictors of critical events during urgent air-medical transport. *CMAJ*. 2009;181(9):579-584.

62. Wiegersma JS, Droogh JM, Zijlstra JG, Fokkema J, Ligtenberg JJ. Quality of interhospital transport of the critically ill: impact of a Mobile Intensive Care Unit with a specialized retrieval team. *Crit Care*. 2011;15(1):R75.

63. Hartke A, Mumma BE, Rittenberger JC, Callaway CW, Guyette FX. Incidence of re-arrest and critical events during prolonged transport of post-cardiac arrest patients. *Resuscitation*. 2010; 81(8):938-942.

64. van Lieshout EJ, Binnekade J, Reussien E, et al. Nurses versus physician-led interhospital critical care transport: a randomized non-inferiority trial. *Intensive Care Med*. 2016;42(7):1146-1154.

65. Lucchini A, De Felippis C, Elli S, et al. Mobile ECMO team for inter-hospital transportation of patients with ARDS: a retrospective case series. *Heart Lung Vessel*. 2014;6(4):262-273.

66. Holena DN, Wiebe DJ, Carr BG, et al. Lead-time bias and interhospital transfer after injury: trauma center admission vital signs underpredict mortality in transferred trauma patients. *J Am Coll Surg*. 2017;224(3):255-263.

67. Rhee KJ, Mackenzie JR, Burney RE, et al. Rapid acute physiology scoring in transport systems. *Crit Care Med*. 1990;18(10):1119-1123.

68. Reimer AP, Dalton JE. Predictive accuracy of medical transport information for in-hospital mortality. *J Crit Care*. 2018;44:238-242.

69. Orr RA, Venkataraman ST, Cinoman MI, Hogue BL, Singleton CA, McCloskey KA. Pretransport Pediatric Risk of Mortality (PRISM) score underestimates the requirement for intensive care or major interventions during interhospital transport. *Crit Care Med*. 1994;22(1):101-107.

70. Newton SM, Fralic M. Interhospital transfer center model: components, themes, and design elements. *Air Med J*. 2015;34(4):207-212.

71. Warren J, Fromm Jr RE, Orr RA, Rotello LC, Horst HM; American College of Critical Care Medicine. Guidelines for the inter- and intrahospital transport of critically ill patients. *Crit Care Med*. 2004;32(1):256-262.

72. Reimer AP, Madigan E. Developing a fully integrated medical transport record to support comparative effectiveness research for patients undergoing medical transport. *EGEMS (Wash DC)*. 2013;1(3):1024.

73. Lyphout C, Bergs J, Stockman W, et al. Patient safety incidents during interhospital transport of patients: a prospective analysis. *Int Emerg Nurs*. 2018;36:22-26.

74. Usher MG, Fanning C, Wu D, et al. Information handoff and outcomes of critically ill patients transferred between hospitals. *J Crit Care*. 2016;36:240-245.

75. Baker T, Kumar K, Kennedy M. Learning on the fly: how rural junior doctors learn during consultations with retrieval physicians. *Emerg Med Australas*. 2017;29(3):342-347.

76. Wilcox SR, Ries M, Bouthiller TA, Berry ED, Dowdy TL, DeGrace S. The importance of ground critical care transport. *J Intensive Care Med*. 2017;32(2):163-169.

77. Rosenfeld BA, Dorman T, Breslow MJ, et al. Intensive care unit telemedicine: alternate paradigm for providing continuous intensivist care. *Crit Care Med*. 2000;28(12):3925-3931.

78. Tang A, Hashmi A, Pandit V, et al. A critical analysis of secondary overtriage to a Level I trauma center. *J Trauma Acute Care Surg*. 2014;77(6):969-973.

79. King BR, King TM, Foster RL, McCans KM. Pediatric and neonatal transport teams with and without a physician: a comparison of outcomes and interventions. *Pediatr Emerg Care*. 2007;23(2):77-82.

80. Bellingan G, Olivier T, Batson S, Webb A. Comparison of a specialist retrieval team with current United Kingdom practice for the transport of critically ill patients. *Intensive Care Med*. 2000;26(6):740-744.

81. Vos GD, Nissen AC, H M Nieman F, et al. Comparison of interhospital pediatric intensive care transport accompanied by a referring specialist or a specialist retrieval team. *Intensive Care Med*. 2004;30(2):302-308.

82. Myers JA, Haney MF, Griffiths RF, Pierse NF, Powell DM. Fatigue in air medical clinicians undertaking high-acuity patient transports. *Prehosp Emerg Care*. 2015;19(1):36-43.

83. Goldstein L, Doig CJ, Bates S, Rink S, Kortbeek JB. Adopting the pre-hospital index for interfacility helicopter transport: a proposal. *Injury*. 2003;34(1):3-11.

84. Brown JB, Stassen NA, Bankey PE, Sangosanya AT, Cheng JD, Gestring ML. Helicopters improve survival in seriously injured patients requiring interfacility transfer for definitive care. *J Trauma*. 2011;70(2):310-314.

85. Hesselfeldt R, Gyllenborg J, Steinmetz J, Do HQ, Hejselbæk J, Rasmussen LS. Is air transport of stroke patients faster than ground transport? A prospective controlled observational study. *Emerg Med J*. 2014;31(4):268-272.

86. Arfken CL, Shapiro MJ, Bessey PQ, Littenberg B. Effectiveness of helicopter versus ground ambulance services for interfacility transport. *J Trauma*. 1998;45(4):785-790.

87. Kim OH, Roh YI, Kim HI, et al. Reduced mortality in severely injured patients using hospital-based helicopter emergency medical services in interhospital transport. *J Korean Med Sci*. 2017;32(7):1187-1194.

88. Borst GM, Davies SW, Waibel BH, et al. When birds can't fly: an analysis of interfacility ground transport using advanced life support when helicopter emergency medical service is unavailable. *J Trauma Acute Care Surg*. 2014;77(2):331-336; discussion 336-337.

89. Boyd LR, Borawski J, Lairet J, Limkakeng Jr AT. Critical Care Air Transport Team severe traumatic brain injury short-term outcomes during flight for Operation Iraqi Freedom/Operation Enduring Freedom. *J R Army Med Corps*. 2017; 163(5):342-346.

90. Barillo DJ, Renz E, Broger K, Moak B, Wright G, Holcomb JB. An emergency medical bag set for long-range aeromedical transportation. *Am J Disaster Med*. 2008;3(2):79-86.

91. Buskop C, Bredmose PP, Sandberg M. A 10-year retrospective study of interhospital patient transport using inhaled nitric oxide in Norway. *Acta Anaesthesiol Scand*. 2015;59(5):648-653.

92. Yeo HJ, Cho WH, Park JM, Kim D. Interhospital transport system for critically ill patients: mobile extracorporeal membrane oxygenation without a ventilator. *Korean J Thorac Cardiovasc Surg*. 2017;50(1):8-13.

93. Burrell AJC, Pilcher DV, Pellegrino VA, Bernard SA. Retrieval of adult patients on extracorporeal membrane oxygenation by an intensive care physician model. *Artif Organs*. 2018;42(3): 254-262.

94. Broman LM, Holzgraefe B, Palmér K, Frenckner B. The Stockholm experience: interhospital transports on extracorporeal membrane oxygenation. *Crit Care*. 2015;19:278.

95. Bryner B, Cooley E, Copenhaver W, et al. Two decades' experience with interfacility transport on extracorporeal membrane oxygenation. *Ann Thorac Surg*. 2014;98(4): 1363-1370.

96. Lee SG, Son BS, Kang PJ, et al. The feasibility of extracorporeal membrane oxygenation support for inter-hospital transport and as a bridge to lung transplantation. *Ann Thorac Cardiovasc Surg*. 2014;20(1):26-31.

97. Lunz D, Philipp A, Judemann K, et al. First experience with the deltastream(R) DP3 in venovenous extracorporeal membrane oxygenation and air-supported inter-hospital transport. *Interact Cardiovasc Thorac Surg*. 2013;17(5):773-777.

98. Isgrò S, Patroniti N, Bombino M, et al. Extracorporeal membrane oxygenation for interhospital transfer of severe acute respiratory distress syndrome patients: 5-year experience. *Int J Artif Organs.* 2011;34(11):1052-1060.

99. Australia and New Zealand Extracorporeal Membrane Oxygenation (ANZ ECMO) Influenza Investigators; Davies A, Jones D, et al. Extracorporeal membrane oxygenation for 2009 influenza A(H1N1) acute respiratory distress syndrome. *JAMA.* 2009;302(17):1888-1895.

100. Stroud MH, Prodhan P, Moss M, Fiser R, Schexnayder S, Anand K. Enhanced monitoring improves pediatric transport outcomes: a randomized controlled trial. *Pediatrics.* 2011;127(1):42-48.

101. Prottengeier J, Moritz A, Heinrich S, Gall C, Schmidt J. Sedation assessment in a mobile intensive care unit: a prospective pilot-study on the relation of clinical sedation scales and the bispectral index. *Crit Care.* 2014;18(6):615.

102. Cao J, Edwards R, Chairez J, Devaraj S. Validation of capillary blood analysis and capillary testing mode on the epoc Point of Care system. *Pract Lab Med.* 2017;9:24-27.

103. Vos G, Engel M, Ramsay G, et al. Point-of-care blood analyzer during the interhospital transport of critically ill children. *Eur J Emerg Med,* 2006;13(5):304-307.

104. Sharma A. Provision of therapeutic hypothermia in neonatal transport: a longitudinal study and review of literature. *Cureus.* 2015;7(5):e270.

105. Blanco P, Miralles Aguiar F, Vallejo A. Point-of-care ultrasonography in critical care medicine: a one way directional road. *J Ultrasound.* 2016;19(2):157-158.

106. Hannay RS, Wyrzykowski AD, Ball CG, Laupland K, Feliciano DV. Retrospective review of injury severity, interventions and outcomes among helicopter and nonhelicopter transport patients at a Level 1 urban trauma centre. *Can J Surg.* 2014;57(1):49-54.

107. Rose MK, Cummings GR, Rodning CB, Brevard SB, Gonzalez RP. Is helicopter evacuation effective in rural trauma transport? *Am Surg.* 2012;78(7):794-797.

108. Desmettre T, Yeguiayan JM, Coadou H, et al. Impact of emergency medical helicopter transport directly to a university hospital trauma center on mortality of severe blunt trauma patients until discharge. *Crit Care.* 2012;16(5):R170.

109. Galvagno Jr SM, Haut ER, Zafar SN, et al. Association between helicopter vs ground emergency medical services and survival for adults with major trauma. *JAMA.* 2012;307(15):1602-1610.

110. Sullivent EE, Faul M, Wald MM. Reduced mortality in injured adults transported by helicopter emergency medical services. *Prehosp Emerg Care.* 2011;15(3):295-302.

111. Brown JB, Stassen NA, Bankey PE, Sangosanya AT, Cheng JD, Gestring ML. Helicopters and the civilian trauma system: national utilization patterns demonstrate improved outcomes after traumatic injury. *J Trauma.* 2010;69(5):1030-1034; discussion 1034-1036.

112. Brown JB, Gestring ML, Guyette FX, et al. Helicopter transport improves survival following injury in the absence of a time-saving advantage. *Surgery.* 2016;159(3):947-959.

113. Bekelis K, Missios S, Mackenzie TA. Prehospital helicopter transport and survival of patients with traumatic brain injury. *Ann Surg.* 2015;261(3):579-585.

114. Galvagno Jr SM, Sikorski R, Hirshon JM, et al. Helicopter emergency medical services for adults with major trauma. *Cochrane Database Syst Rev.* 2015;(12):CD009228.

115. Ryb GE, Dischinger P, Cooper C, Kufera JA. Does helicopter transport improve outcomes independently of emergency medical system time? *J Trauma Acute Care Surg.* 2013;74(1):149-154; discussion 154-156.

116. Baxt WG, Moody P. The impact of a physician as part of the aeromedical prehospital team in patients with blunt trauma. *JAMA.* 1987;257(23):3246-3250.

117. Bøtker MT, Bakke SA, Christensen EF. A systematic review of controlled studies: do physicians increase survival with prehospital treatment? *Scand J Trauma Resusc Emerg Med.* 2009;17:12.

118. Roudsari BS, Nathens AB, Cameron P, et al. International comparison of prehospital trauma care systems. *Injury.* 2007;38(9):993-1000.

119. Reid BO, Rehn M, Uleberg O, Krüger AJ. Physician-provided prehospital critical care, effect on patient physiology dynamics and on-scene time. *Eur J Emerg Med.* 2018;25(2):114-119.

120. Crewdson K, Lockey DJ, Røislien J, Lossius HM, Rehn M. The success of pre-hospital tracheal intubation by different pre-hospital providers: a systematic literature review and meta-analysis. *Crit Care.* 2017;21(1):31.

121. Sampalis JS, Lavoie A, Williams JI, Mulder DS, Kalina M. Impact of on-site care, prehospital time, and level of in-hospital care on survival in severely injured patients. *J Trauma.* 1993;34(2):252-261.

122. Báez AA, Lane PL, Sorondo B, Giráldez EM. Predictive effect of out-of-hospital time in outcomes of severely injured young adult and elderly patients. *Prehosp Disaster Med.* 2006;21(6):427-430.

123. Ingalls N, Zonies D, Bailey JA, et al. A review of the first 10 years of critical care aeromedical transport during Operation Iraqi Freedom and Operation Enduring Freedom: the importance of evacuation timing. *JAMA Surg.* 2014;149(8):807-813.

124. Brown JB, Rosengart MR, Forsythe RM, et al. Not all prehospital time is equal: influence of scene time on mortality. *J Trauma Acute Care Surg.* 2016;81(1):93-100.

125. Härtl R, Gerber LM, Iacono L, Ni Q, Lyons K, Ghajar J. Direct transport within an organized state trauma system reduces mortality in patients with severe traumatic brain injury. *J Trauma.* 2006;60(6):1250-1256; discussion 1256.

126. Sampalis JS, Denis R, Fréchette P, Brown R, Fleiszer D, Mulder D. Direct transport to tertiary trauma centers versus transfer from lower level facilities: impact on mortality and morbidity among patients with major trauma. *J Trauma.* 1997;43(2):288-295; discussion 295-296.

127. MacKenzie EJ, Rivara FP, Jurkovich GJ, et al. A national evaluation of the effect of trauma-center care on mortality. *N Engl J Med.* 2006;354(4):366-378.

128. Liberman M, Mulder D, Sampalis J. Advanced or basic life support for trauma: meta-analysis and critical review of the literature. *J Trauma.* 2000;49(4):584-599.

129. Meizoso JP, Valle EJ, Allen CJ, et al. Decreased mortality after prehospital interventions in severely injured trauma patients. *J Trauma Acute Care Surg.* 2015;79(2):227-231.

130. Stiell IG, Wells GA, Field B, et al. Advanced cardiac life support in out-of-hospital cardiac arrest. *N Engl J Med.* 2004;351(7):647-656.

131. Stiell IG, Spaite DW, Field B, et al. Advanced life support for out-of-hospital respiratory distress. *N Engl J Med.* 2007;356(21):2156-2164.

132. Stiell IG, Nesbitt LP, Pickett W, et al. The OPALS Major Trauma Study: impact of advanced life-support on survival and morbidity. *CMAJ.* 2008;178(9):1141-1152.

133. Liberman M, Mulder D, Lavoie A, Denis R, Sampalis JS. Multicenter Canadian study of prehospital trauma care. *Ann Surg.* 2003;237(2):153-160.

134. Bernard SA, Nguyen V, Cameron P, et al. Prehospital rapid sequence intubation improves functional outcome for patients with severe traumatic brain injury: a randomized controlled trial. *Ann Surg.* 2010;252(6):959-965.

135. Eckstein M, Chan L, Schneir A, Palmer R. Effect of prehospital advanced life support on outcomes of major trauma patients. *J Trauma.* 2000;48(4):643-648.

136. Stockinger ZT, McSwain Jr NE. Prehospital endotracheal intubation for trauma does not improve survival over bag-valve-mask ventilation. *J Trauma.* 2004;56(3):531-536.

137. Wang HE, Peitzman AB, Cassidy LD, Adelson PD, Yealy DM. Out-of-hospital endotracheal intubation and outcome after traumatic brain injury. *Ann Emerg Med.* 2004;44(5):439-450.

138. Chou D, Harada MY, Barmparas G, et al. Field intubation in civilian patients with hemorrhagic shock is associated with higher mortality. *J Trauma Acute Care Surg.* 2016;80(2):278-282.

139. Crewdson K, Rehn M, Brohi K, Lockey DJ. Pre-hospital emergency anaesthesia in awake hypotensive trauma patients: beneficial or detrimental? *Acta Anaesthesiol Scand.* 2018;62(4):504-514.

140. Cobas MA, De la Peña MA, Manning R, Candiotti K, Varon AJ. Prehospital intubations and mortality: a level 1 trauma center perspective. *Anesth Analg.* 2009;109(2):489-493.

141. Silvestri S, Ralls GA, Krauss B, et al. The effectiveness of out-of-hospital use of continuous end-tidal carbon dioxide monitoring on the rate of unrecognized misplaced intubation within a regional emergency medical services system. *Ann Emerg Med.* 2005;45(5):497-503.

142. Brown JB, Sperry JL, Fombona A, Billiar TR, Peitzman AB, Guyette FX. Pre-trauma center red blood cell transfusion is associated with improved early outcomes in air medical trauma patients. *J Am Coll Surg.* 2015;220(5):797-808.

143. Gates S, Lall R, Quinn T, et al. Prehospital randomised assessment of a mechanical compression device in out-of-hospital cardiac arrest (PARAMEDIC): a pragmatic, cluster randomised trial and economic evaluation. *Health Technol Assess.* 2017;21(11):1-176.

29

What Are the Causes of and How Do I Treat Critical Illness Neuropathy/Myopathy?

Frank Brunkhorst and Hubertus Axer

NEUROMUSCULAR WEAKNESS

Neuromuscular weakness is a significant complication of critical illness, sepsis, and multiorgan dysfunction.[1,2] The major clinical hallmark is muscular weakness; therefore, the entity is referred to as intensive care unit-acquired weakness (ICUAW). Underlying abnormalities include an axonal defect in peripheral nerves (i.e., critical illness polyneuropathy [CIP]),[3] a loss of thick myosin filaments in the muscles (i.e., critical illness myopathy [CIM]),[4] or global mechanisms of muscle wasting and cachexia.[5,6] In most cases a combination of these three conditions contributes to this complication.

CIP and CIM are significant complications of ICU stay as they are associated with a prolonged requirement for mechanical ventilation, increased hospital length of stay, longer rehabilitation, and increased mortality in excess of that imposed by the specific form of critical illness.[7,8] Therefore, CIP and CIM impose a significant economic burden and impact post-ICU quality of life.[9]

CIP and CIM share the major clinical symptoms of muscle weakness and early muscle atrophy.[10] In addition, CIP is characterized by a loss of deep tendon reflexes and a distal loss of sensitivity to light touch, pain, temperature, and vibration due to the impairment of sensory nerve fibers.[11] As many critical ill patients are mechanically ventilated, careful clinical neurologic evaluation may be difficult and failure to wean may be a first sign in the ICU.[12] In addition, there are other differential causes of neuromuscular weakness in the ICU (Table 29.1) that should be investigated.

Incidence rates of CIP depend on the specific patient population studied, diagnostic criteria used, timing of diagnosis, and severity of critical illness.[11] Between 50%[13] and 100%[14] of patients with severe sepsis, septic shock, and prolonged mechanical ventilation develop CIP/CIM. About 70% of patients with severe sepsis and multiorgan dysfunction develop electrophysiologic criteria consistent with CIP and about 30% manifest clinical signs.[15] About 25% of patients who undergo 7 or more days of mechanical ventilation have clinical signs of CIP.[16] Furthermore, axonal polyneuropathy is related to the severity of multiorgan dysfunction in these patients.[17]

Data differentiating CIP from CIM indicate that CIM may occur more frequently than CIP.[18] Other studies have found similar proportions of patients diagnosed with CIP, CIM, and a combination of both.[13] It appears that CIM carries a better prognosis than CIP[19] because muscles regenerate faster than nerves.[20]

WHAT ARE THE CAUSES OF CIP AND CIM?

The pathophysiology of CIP is complex, multifactorial, and poorly understood.[11] The strong association between sepsis and CIP suggests that both share common pathophysiologic principles.[21] In general, inflammatory cascades have neurotoxic effects, impaired microcirculation causes ischemic defects of muscle and nerve, metabolic effects (especially hyperglycemia) cause nerve impairment, and hypercatabolic conditions lead to depletion of muscle proteins. Table 29.2 summarizes the major pathophysiologic factors that are believed to underlie CIP and CIM.

Several clinical risk factors associated with the proposed pathophysiologic mechanisms have also been associated with CIP and CIM. First, sepsis and inflammation are major risk factors. In addition, conditions associated with the severity of the disease such as mechanical ventilation, multiorgan failure, or APACHE (Acute Physiology and Chronic Health Evaluation) score contribute. Catabolic states, administration of parenteral nutrition, and muscular inactivity are involved. Hyperglycemia is a risk factor for the development of neuromuscular weakness.[25] The use of nondepolarizing neuromuscular blocking agents[34] and the use of corticosteroids have been implicated in the development of CIM,[16,35–37] although some studies have been unable to confirm these findings.[38,39] A study[40] on patients with severe acute respiratory distress syndrome (ARDS) found that early administration of neuromuscular blocking agents improved 90-day survival and increased the time off the ventilator without increasing muscle weakness. Box 29.1 shows a summary of the clinical risk factors associated with the development of CIP and CIM.

HOW CIP AND CIM CAN BE DETECTED

Most studies quantify weakness using the Medical Research Council (MRC) muscle strength score.[51] The MRC score is a semiquantitative estimation of muscle strength between 0 and 5 (where 0 = no visible/palpable contraction; 1 = visible/palpable contraction without movement; 2 = movement of the limb but not against gravity; 3 = movement against

TABLE 29.1   Differential Diagnoses of CIP and CIM.

Neuromuscular Weakness	Impairment
Central paresis	Encephalitis
	Cerebral ischemia (e.g., due to endocarditis, vasculitis, and others)
	Cervical or thoracic paraplegia (ischemic, inflammatory)
Impairment of neuromuscular transmission	Myasthenia gravis
	Drug induced (e.g., aminoglycosides and other antibiotics, anesthetics)
Peripheral nerve lesions	GBS
	Toxic polyneuropathy (drugs: e.g., chemotherapeutics)
	Paraneoplastic polyneuropathy (malignoma)
	CMV
	Porphyria
Myopathy	Rhabdomyolysis (inflammatory, drug induced)
	Steroid myopathy
	Hypokalemic paresis

CIM, critical illness myopathy; CIP, critical illness polyneuropathy; CMV, cytomegalovirus; GBS, Guillain-Barré syndrome.

TABLE 29.2   Potential Pathophysiologic Mechanisms Underlying CIP and CIM.

	Mechanism
Inflammatory activity	Direct and indirect neurotoxic effects caused by inflammatory cascades[22–24] (e.g., TNF and IL-6)
Metabolic disturbance	Hyperglycemia and relative insulin deficiency cause nerve lesions[25,26]
	Mitochondrial dysfunction[25,27]
	Oxidative stress[28]
Disturbance of microcirculation	Increased microvascular permeability, endoneural edema, and extravasation of inflammatory cells cause hypoxic nerve lesions[29,30]
Reduction of electrical excitability of nerve and muscle membrane	Sodium channelopathy[31]
Hypercatabolism	Cytosines and hormones (also steroids) activate muscle proteolysis[32]
	Muscle protein fractional synthetic rate is depressed[6]
	TNF-induced muscle degradation[33]

CIM, critical illness myopathy; CIP, critical illness polyneuropathy; IL-6, interleukin-6; TNF, tumor necrosis factor.

BOX 29.1   Risk Factors Associated with the Development of CIP and CIM.

Sepsis and systemic inflammation[7,35,41]
Severity of disease (APACHE)[7,35]
Mechanical ventilation[16,42,43]
Multiorgan failure[16,44]
Parenteral nutrition[7,45]
Catabolic state[7,46]
High blood glucose[25,26,42,47]
Drug induced, e.g., aminoglycosides,[17,42] nondepolarizing neuromuscular blocking agents,[34,48] glucocorticoids[16,36,37]
Female sex,[16] hypogonadism in men[49]
Muscular inactivity[43,50]

APACHE, Acute Physiology and Chronic Health Evaluation; CIM, critical illness myopathy; CIP, critical illness polyneuropathy.

gravity but not against resistance; 4 = movement against gravity and resistance; 5 = normal).[52] To obtain the MRC score, strength from six muscle groups (abduction of the arm, flexion of the forearm, extension of the wrist, flexion of the hip, extension of the knee, and dorsal flexion of the foot) are quantified bilaterally and the individual scores are summed. Thus, patients with significant weakness have MRC sum scores ≤ 48 and patients with severe weakness have scores ≤ 36.[52] However, patients have to be cooperative and alert for a complete and reliable neurologic status and, in many critically ill patients, clinical evaluation may be limited by sedation or confusion.[53]

Electrophysiologic measurements of CIP consist of a nerve conduction study (NCS) characterized by a reduction in the amplitude of compound muscle action potential (CMAP) and sensory nerve action potential (SNAP) with a less pronounced reduction in conduction velocity (Figs. 29.1 and 29.2).[38,54] Reduced CMAP and SNAP amplitudes are consistent with axonal damage to peripheral nerves in CIP,[29] although reduced CMAP amplitudes also develop in myopathies such as CIM.[46] NCS can detect CIP early in the course of the disease: that is, in the first week after the onset of sepsis.[55]

Electromyography (EMG) signs of axonal denervation include spontaneous activity in the relaxed muscle. The earliest these changes appear is about 14 days after axonal damage. The media time to develop denervation on EMG was found to be 21 days after ICU admission.[10] Spontaneous activity can also be found in CIM at earlier time points.[56]

However, if a differentiation between CIP and CIM is needed for prognostic reasons, other assessments are required.[18] One such test is direct muscle stimulation (DMS). An advantage of DMS is that it does not require patient cooperation.[57] Muscle action potentials are recorded after direct electrical stimulation of the muscle and following electrical stimulation of the nerve.[58] The ratio of the amplitudes of these two may indicate the relative contributions of neuropathy and myopathy. DMS may be valuable in the first week of muscular weakness development[59] and may identify type II muscle fiber atrophy.[60]

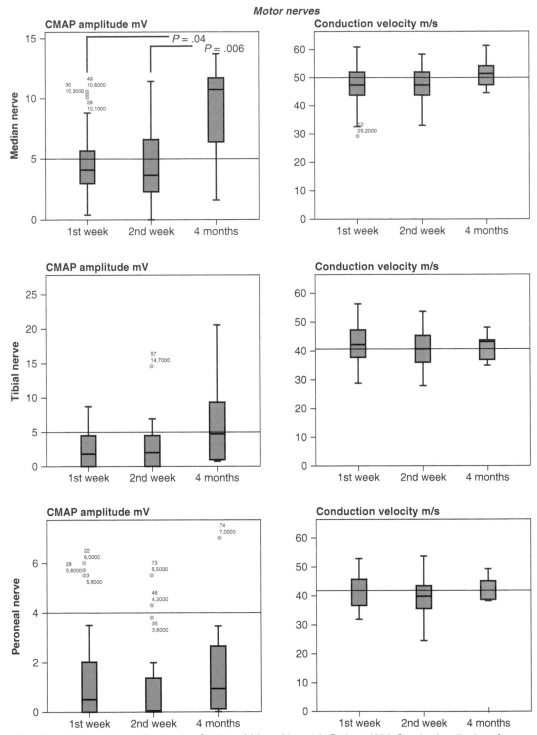

Fig. 29.1 Follow-up Nerve Conduction Studies of Motor Nerves in Patients With Sepsis. Amplitudes of compound potentials are considerably decreased, while conduction velocity is marginally impaired. *Horizontal lines* show the normative values of the measurements. *CMAP,* compound muscle action potential.

Other tests that may differentiate nerve impairment from muscle impairment include muscle biopsy,[36,61] muscle ultrasound,[12] and skin biopsies.[62,63] Nevertheless, NCS represents the method of choice for early and simple detection of CIP. Use of peroneal nerve NCS has been suggested as a highly sensitive and specific screening method for CIP.[64,65]

HOW TO TREAT CIP AND CIM

Currently, no specific therapy related to CIP and CIM has been established.[66] Given that sepsis is a major risk factor for the development of CIP and CIM, early sepsis management per established guidelines[67] is the major strategy to prevent

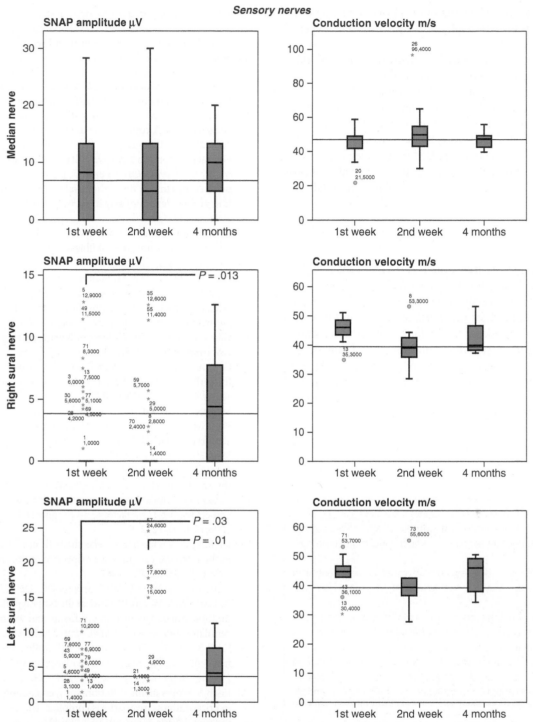

Fig. 29.2 Follow-up Nerve Conduction Studies of Sensory Nerves in Patients With Sepsis. *SNAP,* sensory nerve action potential.

CIP and CIM. Further preventive strategies include the reduction or avoidance of other known risk factors.[68]

Several studies have indicated that intensive insulin therapy may lead to a substantial reduction of CIP.[25,26,68,69] However, intensive insulin therapy also increases the risk of hypoglycemia-associated complications,[70] which means that this strategy cannot, per se, be recommended.

Intravenous immunoglobulin (IVIG) therapy has been shown to reduce mortality in patients with sepsis and septic shock in small trials.[51] Small, retrospective analyses of patients with severe sepsis and multiorgan dysfunction suggested that IVIG treatment prevented the development of CIP[71] and led to a reduction of mortality.[72] However, a 2013 prospective study was unable to demonstrate that IVIG altered the development of CIP/CIM in patients with severe sepsis and multiorgan dysfunction.[73]

Therefore, the therapeutic management of patients with CIP and CIM is supportive, relying on early physiotherapy, daily trials of decreased ventilatory support, reduction of sedation, and optimization of nutrition to prevent hypercatabolism.

In addition, nondepolarizing neuromuscular blocking agents and glucocorticoids should only be used in critically ill patients and only when absolutely necessary.[34]

A new approach to limit immobilization involves a reduction in deep sedation in mechanically ventilated patients. This strategy is designed to facilitate rehabilitation therapy and early mobilization in the ICU.[74–76] However, there are no randomized controlled trials that examine the value of early physical therapy with respect to the development of CIP and CIM.[77]

CONCLUSIONS

ICUAW, CIP, and CIM are frequent and significant complications in critically ill patients. These conditions lead to prolonged duration of mechanical ventilation, increased hospital length of stay, a need for more rehabilitation, and increased mortality. Clinical risk factors include sepsis and inflammation, mechanical ventilation, multiorgan dysfunction, a catabolic state, parenteral nutrition, and hyperglycemia. Diagnostic procedures focus on the clinical detection of muscle weakness and electrophysiologic measurements. Therapy is supportive, paralleling early sepsis management, and includes early physiotherapy, daily trials of decreased ventilatory support with reduction of sedation, and optimized nutrition.

AUTHORS' RECOMMENDATIONS
- CIP and CIM are important complications of critically ill patients, especially those with sepsis and multiorgan dysfunction.
- The clinical hallmark is symmetric muscle weakness. The first symptom may be the failure of weaning from the ventilator.
- Diagnostic principles are based upon clinical evaluation of muscle strength and electrophysiologic measurements (nerve conduction studies, direct muscle stimulation).
- Supportive but unproven therapeutic strategies include early physiotherapy, daily trials of decreased ventilatory support with reduction of sedation, and optimized nutrition.

REFERENCES

1. Kress JP, Hall JB. ICU-acquired weakness and recovery from critical illness. *N Engl J Med*. 2014;370:1626-1635.
2. Zink W, Kollmar R, Schwab S. Critical illness polyneuropathy and myopathy in the intensive care unit. *Nat Rev Neurol*. 2009;5:372-379.
3. Latronico N, Bolton CF. Critical illness polyneuropathy and myopathy: a major cause of muscle weakness and paralysis. *Lancet Neurol*. 2011;10:931-941.
4. Lacomis D. Neuromuscular disorders in critically ill patients: review and update. *J Clin Neuromuscul Dis*. 2011;12:197-218.
5. Schefold JC, Bierbrauer J, Weber-Carstens S. Intensive care unit-acquired weakness (ICUAW) and muscle wasting in critically ill patients with severe sepsis and septic shock. *J Cachexia Sarcopenia Muscle*. 2010;1:147-157.
6. Puthucheary ZA, Rawal J, McPhail M, et al. Acute skeletal muscle wasting in critical illness. *JAMA*. 2013;310:1591-1600.
7. Garnacho-Montero J, Madrazo-Osuna J, García-Garmendia JL, et al. Critical illness polyneuropathy: risk factors and clinical consequences. A cohort study in septic patients. *Intensive Care Med*. 2001;27:1288-1296.
8. Garnacho-Montero J, Amaya-Villar R, García-Garmendía JL, Madrazo-Osuna J, Ortiz-Leyba C. Effect of critical illness polyneuropathy on the withdrawal from mechanical ventilation and the length of stay in septic patients. *Crit Care Med*. 2005;33:349-354.
9. Grimm A, Günther A, Witte OW, Axer H. [Critical illness polyneuropathy and critical illness myopathy]. *Med Klin Intensivmed Notfmed*. 2012;107:649-659.
10. Hund E, Genzwürker H, Böhrer H, Jakob H, Thiele R, Hacke W. Predominant involvement of motor fibres in patients with critical illness polyneuropathy. *Br J Anaesth*. 1997;78:274-278.
11. Hermans G, De Jonghe B, Bruyninckx F, Van den Berghe G. Clinical review: critical illness polyneuropathy and myopathy. *Crit Care*. 2008;12:238.
12. Grimm A, Teschner U, Porzelius C, et al. Muscle ultrasound for early assessment of critical illness neuromyopathy in severe sepsis. *Crit Care*. 2013;17:R227.
13. Stevens RD, Dowdy DW, Michaels RK, Mendez-Tellez PA, Pronovost PJ, Needham DM. Neuromuscular dysfunction acquired in critical illness: a systematic review. *Intensive Care Med*. 2007;33:1876-1891.
14. Latronico N, Fenzi F, Recupero D, et al. Critical illness myopathy and neuropathy. *Lancet*. 1996;347:1579-1582.
15. Visser LH. Critical illness polyneuropathy and myopathy: clinical features, risk factors and prognosis. *Eur J Neurol*. 2006;13:1203-1212.
16. De Jonghe B, Sharshar T, Lefaucheur JP, et al. Paresis acquired in the intensive care unit: a prospective multicenter study. *JAMA*. 2002;288:2859-2867.
17. Leijten FS, De Weerd AW, Poortvliet DC, De Ridder VA, Ulrich C, Harink-De Weerd JE. Critical illness polyneuropathy in multiple organ dysfunction syndrome and weaning from the ventilator. *Intensive Care Med*. 1996;22:856-861.
18. Koch S, Spuler S, Deja M, et al. Critical illness myopathy is frequent: accompanying neuropathy protracts ICU discharge. *J Neurol Neurosurg Psychiatry*. 2011;82:287-293.
19. Koch S, Wollersheim T, Bierbrauer J, et al. Long-term recovery in critical illness myopathy is complete, contrary to polyneuropathy. *Muscle Nerve*. 2014;50:431-436.
20. Khan J, Harrison TB, Rich MM. Mechanisms of neuromuscular dysfunction in critical illness. *Crit Care Clin*. 2008;24:165-177.
21. Witt NJ, Zochodne DW, Bolton CF, et al. Peripheral nerve function in sepsis and multiple organ failure. *Chest*. 1991;99:176-184.
22. Mohammadi B, Schedel I, Graf K, et al. Role of endotoxin in the pathogenesis of critical illness polyneuropathy. *J Neurol*. 2008;255:265-272.
23. Verheul GA, de Jongh-Leuvenink J, Op de Coul AA, van Landeghem AA, van Puyenbroek MJ. Tumor necrosis factor and interleukin-6 in critical illness polyneuromyopathy. *Clin Neurol Neurosurg*. 1994;96:300-304.

24. Druschky A, Herkert M, Radespiel-Tröger M, et al. Critical illness polyneuropathy: clinical findings and cell culture assay of neurotoxicity assessed by a prospective study. *Intensive Care Med.* 2001;27:686-693.

25. Van den Berghe G, Schoonheydt K, Becx P, Bruyninckx F, Wouters PJ. Insulin therapy protects the central and peripheral nervous system of intensive care patients. *Neurology.* 2005;64:1348-1353.

26. van den Berghe G, Wouters P, Weekers F, et al. Intensive insulin therapy in the critically ill patients. *N Engl J Med.* 2001;345:1359-1367.

27. Carré JE, Orban JC, Re L, et al. Survival in critical illness is associated with early activation of mitochondrial biogenesis. *Am J Respir Crit Care Med.* 2010;182:745-751.

28. Reid MB, Moylan JS. Beyond atrophy: redox mechanisms of muscle dysfunction in chronic inflammatory disease. *J Physiol.* 2011;589:2171-2179.

29. Bolton CF. Neuromuscular manifestations of critical illness. *Muscle Nerve.* 2005;32:140-163.

30. Fenzi F, Latronico N, Refatti N, Rizzuto N. Enhanced expression of E-selectin on the vascular endothelium of peripheral nerve in critically ill patients with neuromuscular disorders. *Acta Neuropathol.* 2003;106:75-82.

31. Rich MM, Pinter MJ. Crucial role of sodium channel fast inactivation in muscle fibre inexcitability in a rat model of critical illness myopathy. *J Physiol.* 2003;547:555-566.

32. Mitch WE, Goldberg AL. Mechanisms of muscle wasting. The role of the ubiquitin-proteasome pathway. *N Engl J Med.* 1996;335:1897-1905.

33. Li YP, Reid MB. NF-kappaB mediates the protein loss induced by TNF-alpha in differentiated skeletal muscle myotubes. *Am J Physiol Regul Integr Comp Physiol.* 2000;279:R1165-R1170.

34. Murray MJ, Brull SJ, Bolton CF. Brief review: nondepolarizing neuromuscular blocking drugs and critical illness myopathy. *Can J Anaesth.* 2006;53:1148-1156.

35. de Letter MA, Schmitz PI, Visser LH, et al. Risk factors for the development of polyneuropathy and myopathy in critically ill patients. *Crit Care Med.* 2001;29:2281-2286.

36. Kerbaul F, Brousse M, Collart F, et al. Combination of histopathological and electromyographic patterns can help to evaluate functional outcome of critical ill patients with neuromuscular weakness syndromes. *Crit Care.* 2004;8:R358-R366.

37. Ruff RL. Acute illness myopathy. *Neurology.* 1996;46:600-601.

38. Bednarik J, Lukas Z, Vondracek P. Critical illness polyneuromyopathy: the electrophysiological components of a complex entity. *Intensive Care Med.* 2003;29:1505-1514.

39. Hough CL, Steinberg KP, Taylor Thompson B, Rubenfeld GD, Hudson LD. Intensive care unit-acquired neuromyopathy and corticosteroids in survivors of persistent ARDS. *Intensive Care Med.* 2009;35:63-68.

40. Papazian L, Forel JM, Gacouin A, et al. Neuromuscular blockers in early acute respiratory distress syndrome. *N Engl J Med.* 2010;363:1107-1116.

41. Thiele RI, Jakob H, Hund E, et al. Sepsis and catecholamine support are the major risk factors for critical illness polyneuropathy after open heart surgery. *Thorac Cardiovasc Surg.* 2000;48:145-150.

42. Nanas S, Kritikos K, Angelopoulos E, et al. Predisposing factors for critical illness polyneuromyopathy in a multidisciplinary intensive care unit. *Acta Neurol Scand.* 2008;118:175-181.

43. Levine S, Nguyen T, Taylor N, et al. Rapid disuse atrophy of diaphragm fibers in mechanically ventilated humans. *N Engl J Med.* 2008;358:1327-1335.

44. Bednarík J, Vondracek P, Dusek L, Moravcova E, Cundrle I. Risk factors for critical illness polyneuromyopathy. *J Neurol.* 2005;252:343-351.

45. Waldhausen E, Mingers B, Lippers P, Keser G. Critical illness polyneuropathy due to parenteral nutrition. *Intensive Care Med.* 1997;23:922-923.

46. Trojaborg W, Weimer LH, Hays AP. Electrophysiologic studies in critical illness associated weakness: myopathy or neuropathy—a reappraisal. *Clin Neurophysiol.* 2001;112:1586-1593.

47. Bercker S, Weber-Carstens S, Deja M, et al. Critical illness polyneuropathy and myopathy in patients with acute respiratory distress syndrome. *Crit Care Med.* 2005;33:711-715.

48. Leatherman JW, Fluegel WL, David WS, Davies SF, Iber C. Muscle weakness in mechanically ventilated patients with severe asthma. *Am J Respir Crit Care Med.* 1996;153:1686-1690.

49. Sharshar T, Bastuji-Garin S, De Jonghe B, et al. Hormonal status and ICU-acquired paresis in critically ill patients. *Intensive Care Med.* 2010;36:1318-1326.

50. Ochala J, Gustafson AM, Diez ML, et al. Preferential skeletal muscle myosin loss in response to mechanical silencing in a novel rat intensive care unit model: underlying mechanisms. *J Physiol.* 2011;589:2007-2026.

51. Fan E, Cheek F, Chlan L, et al. An official American Thoracic Society Clinical Practice guideline: the diagnosis of intensive care unit-acquired weakness in adults. *Am J Respir Crit Care Med.* 2014;190:1437-1446.

52. Hermans G, Clerckx B, Vanhullebusch T, et al. Interobserver agreement of Medical Research Council sum-score and handgrip strength in the intensive care unit. *Muscle Nerve.* 2012;45:18-25.

53. Axer H, Romeike B, Brunkhorst F, et al. Neurological sequelae of sepsis. II. Neuromuscular weakness. *Open Crit Care Med J.* 2011;4:8-14.

54. Lacomis D. Electrophysiology of neuromuscular disorders in critical illness. *Muscle Nerve.* 2013;47:452-463.

55. Khan J, Harrison TB, Rich MM, Moss M. Early development of critical illness myopathy and neuropathy in patients with severe sepsis. *Neurology.* 2006;67:1421-1425.

56. Young GB, Hammond RR. A stronger approach to weakness in the intensive care unit. *Crit Care.* 2004;8:416-418.

57. Rich MM, Bird SJ, Raps EC, McCluskey LF, Teener JW. Direct muscle stimulation in acute quadriplegic myopathy. *Muscle Nerve.* 1997;20:665-673.

58. Lefaucheur JP, Nordine T, Rodriguez P, Brochard L. Origin of ICU acquired paresis determined by direct muscle stimulation. *J Neurol Neurosurg Psychiatry.* 2006;77:500-506.

59. Weber-Carstens S, Koch S, Spuler S, et al. Nonexcitable muscle membrane predicts intensive care unit-acquired paresis in mechanically ventilated, sedated patients. *Crit Care Med.* 2009;37:2632-2637.

60. Bierbrauer J, Koch S, Olbricht C, et al. Early type II fiber atrophy in intensive care unit patients with nonexcitable muscle membrane. *Crit Care Med.* 2012;40:647-650.

61. Howard RS, Tan SV, Z'Graggen WJ. Weakness on the intensive care unit. *Pract Neurol.* 2008;8:280-295.

62. Axer H, Grimm A, Pausch C, et al. The impairment of small nerve fibers in severe sepsis and septic shock. *Crit Care.* 2016;20:64.

63. Skorna M, Kopacik R, Vlckova E, Adamova B, Kostalova M, Bednarik J. Small nerve fiber pathology in critical illness documented by serial skin biopsies. *Muscle Nerve.* 2015;52(1):28-33.

64. Moss M, Yang M, Macht M, et al. Screening for critical illness polyneuromyopathy with single nerve conduction studies. *Intensive Care Med.* 2014;40:683-690.

65. Latronico N, Nattino G, Guarneri B, et al. Validation of the peroneal nerve test to diagnose critical illness polyneuropathy and myopathy in the intensive care unit: the multicentre Italian CRIMYNE-2 diagnostic accuracy study. *F1000Res.* 2014;3:127.

66. Hermans G, Van den Berghe G. Clinical review: intensive care unit acquired weakness. *Crit Care.* 2015;19:274.

67. Rhodes A, Evans LE, Alhazzani W, et al. Surviving Sepsis Campaign: International Guidelines for Management of Sepsis and Septic Shock: 2016. *Intensive Care Med.* 2017;43:304-377.

68. Hermans G, De Jonghe B, Bruyninckx F, Van den Berghe G. Interventions for preventing critical illness polyneuropathy and critical illness myopathy. *Cochrane Database Syst Rev.* 2014;1:CD006832.

69. Hermans G, Schrooten M, Van Damme P, et al. Benefits of intensive insulin therapy on neuromuscular complications in routine daily critical care practice: a retrospective study. *Crit Care.* 2009;13:R5.

70. Brunkhorst FM, Engel C, Bloos F, et al. Intensive insulin therapy and pentastarch resuscitation in severe sepsis. *N Engl J Med.* 2008;358:125-139.

71. Mohr M, Englisch L, Roth A, Burchardi H, Zielmann S. Effects of early treatment with immunoglobulin on critical illness polyneuropathy following multiple organ failure and gram-negative sepsis. *Intensive Care Med.* 1997;23:1144-1149.

72. Alejandria MM, Lansang MA, Dans LF, Mantaring JB. Intravenous immunoglobulin for treating sepsis and septic shock. *Cochrane Database Syst Rev.* 2002;(1):CD001090.

73. Brunner R, Rinner W, Haberler C, et al. Early treatment with IgM-enriched intravenous immunoglobulin does not mitigate critical illness polyneuropathy and/or myopathy in patients with multiple organ failure and SIRS/sepsis: a prospective, randomized, placebo-controlled, double-blinded trial. *Crit Care.* 2013;17:R213.

74. Needham DM. Mobilizing patients in the intensive care unit: improving neuromuscular weakness and physical function. *JAMA.* 2008;300:1685-1690.

75. Jolley SE, Bunnell AE, Hough CL. ICU-acquired weakness. *Chest.* 2016;150:1129-1140.

76. Zorowitz RD. ICU-acquired weakness: a rehabilitation perspective of diagnosis, treatment, and functional management. *Chest.* 2016;150:966-971.

77. Mehrholz J, Pohl M, Kugler J, Burridge J, Mückel S, Elsner B. Physical rehabilitation for critical illness myopathy and neuropathy. *Cochrane Database Syst Rev.* 2015;(3):CD010942.

What is Sepsis? What is Septic Shock? What are MODS and Persistent Critical Illness?

Daniel E. Leisman and Clifford S. Deutschman

INTRODUCTION

Sepsis is a syndrome of enormous global consequence.[1] The incidence in the United States is estimated to be 1.5 million/year, resulting in 250,000 to 300,000 in-hospital deaths every year.[2,3] Fewer than half of sepsis survivors remain alive for 2 years following hospital discharge.[4] Those who do often endure functional and cognitive limitations.[5] Sepsis incidence continues to rise[6] and the burden may be greatest in lower- and middle-income nations.[7,8] Nonetheless, a comprehensive understanding of sepsis pathobiology has proven elusive. This problem reflects, in part, the difficulty in identifying patients with sepsis. Responsibility for dealing with this problem has been assumed, at different times, by three different panels of experts. In this chapter, we review the work of these task forces with emphasis on the most recent one.[9]

HISTORICAL PERSPECTIVE

The word "sepsis" has been in use for several millennia.[10] Across the centuries it has been associated with a number of different pathologic processes. However, its importance as a distinct entity correlates directly with the development of critical care medicine as a unique medical specialty—only the ability to resuscitate and support the sickest patients led to the identification of an infection-induced syndrome of profound organ dysfunction.[11] Importantly, similar abnormalities were also observed in response to severe noninfectious illnesses such as trauma or rupture of an abdominal aortic aneurysm.[12,13] Initially, the myriad definitions for many of the terms used in describing these new syndromes made it difficult to identify patients with extreme responses to infection and virtually impossible to compare therapeutic approaches to the disorder. Therefore, in 1991, Roger Bone, then at Rush Medical College in Chicago, convened a group of experts and charged them with developing standardized terminology in order to "eliminate confusion in communication … for both clinicians and researchers" so that "the ability to compare protocols and evaluate therapeutic interventions would be improved."[14] The results of this conference were published in 1992 and have been referred to as "Sepsis-1."[14]

Sepsis-1

The first formalized "definition" of sepsis detailed in the recommendations published in 1993 reflected the then prevailing view that sepsis was the manifestation of a systemic inflammatory response to infection.[14] Thus, *sepsis* could be identified by the presence or suspicion of infection and a "systemic inflammatory response syndrome" (SIRS). SIRS, in turn, was said to be present if patients displayed two or more of four abnormalities in heart rate, respiratory rate, body temperature, and white blood cell count—the so-called "SIRS criteria." Sepsis that was associated with cardiovascular, pulmonary, hepatic, renal, hematocoagulative, or neurologic dysfunction was called "severe sepsis." Finally, the specific case of sepsis-induced hypotension unresponsive to fluid resuscitation was termed "septic shock." The report also addressed the terms "bacteremia"—bacteria in the blood, a possible cause of, but distinct from, sepsis—and recommended that the term "septicemia" be abandoned because it was used in a number of different ways and because it inadequately described the spectrum of organisms that infect the blood. The latter two recommendations remain valid today.

Sepsis-2

Following publication, concerns regarding the limitations of Sepsis-1 arose almost immediately.[15] Three specific criticisms were most often invoked. First, it was felt that the term "sepsis" actually described infection, and therefore lacked specificity. For example, nearly every febrile child with pharyngitis or otitis meets two SIRS criteria, but this presentation clearly does not reflect the deadly clinical entity that we call sepsis. This concern gave rise to a second criticism: the invention of a new disorder, "severe sepsis," to describe "sepsis + organ dysfunction." Many felt that the disorder most practitioners referred to as "sepsis" was now called "severe sepsis," introduced an unnecessary and confusing new term. Finally, while severe sepsis was defined as "sepsis + organ dysfunction," criteria as to what actually constituted organ dysfunction were not included.[15] As a result of these concerns, a second consensus conference, charged with updating Sepsis-1, was convened in 2001.[16] Sepsis-2 broadened the list of diagnostic criteria for sepsis and clarified operational criteria for organ dysfunction based on measures used to construct two scoring systems: the "MODS" (multiple organ dysfunction syndrome) and "SOFA" (sequential organ failure assessment) scores.[17,18] Sepsis-2 acknowledged concerns with the prior definition, including with the SIRS criteria but, in the absence of evidence, did not offer an alternative. Thus, while Sepsis-2 provided criteria for organ dysfunction, the conceptual framework for sepsis—i.e., systemic inflammation in reponse to infection—remained essentially unchanged from the concept in 1991.

Sepsis-3

Definitions

The decade following the publication of Sepsis-2 in 2003 was characterized by a number of important findings that dramatically impacted sepsis recognition and care. They included:

- *A better understanding of the pathobiology of sepsis*[19]
- *Failure of a number of highly touted clinical trials of drugs believed to specifically target sepsis*[20]
- *Recognition that sepsis-associated mortality could be reduced via implementation of a bundle of relatively simple supportive measures—the Surviving Sepsis Campaign (SSC)*[21]
- *Identification, in sepsis survivors, of a number of life-altering conditions: muscle weakness, respiratory insufficiency, and, most importantly, neuropsychologic abnormalities such as cognitive dysfunction and post-traumatic stress disorder.*[5]

A new consensus conference, Sepsis-3, was convened in 2014 and the results of those deliberations were published in 2016.[9] From the onset, Sepsis-3 differed dramatically from the first two conferences. Perhaps the most dramatic difference was semantic. The Sepsis-3 participants recognized that what were referred to in Sepsis-1/2 as "definitions" were, in fact, not definitions at all. From the *Merriam-Webster English Dictionary*, a definition is "the essential nature of a thing" or, more succinctly, "what something *is*." Clearly, the essential nature of sepsis is unknown: this recognition was both liberating and confining. It freed the task force members to devise a "definition" of sepsis that included the most up-to-date investigative evidence. Thus, a new definition emerged:

> *Sepsis is defined as a life-threatening organ dysfunction caused by a dysregulated host response to infection.*[9]

The new definition eliminated the term "severe sepsis," because its key characteristic, organ dysfunction, was now included in the definition of sepsis. However, while "severe sepsis" was jettisoned, it was felt that the term "septic shock" could not be so easily eliminated. The discussion centered on the actual nature of septic shock. On the one hand, septic shock could easily be viewed as sepsis with dysfunction

primarily manifested in the cardiovascular system. Thus, one could argue that "septic shock" was already included in the new definition of sepsis. However, some felt that, in contrast to "severe sepsis," the term "septic shock" was well-accepted and entrenched in the vocabulary of critical care. At the very least, the term connoted a syndrome more likely to result in death than sepsis. In addition, several task force members expressed the view that septic shock encompassed more than just cardiovascular dysfunction.[9] Several individuals voiced the opinion that septic shock was characterized by a wide range of metabolic abnormalities, while others strongly believed that shock was a dysfunction on a cellular level and therefore could be present in any organ or tissue. The ultimate definition encompassed all three concepts:

> *Septic shock is defined as a subset of sepsis in which underlying circulatory and cellular metabolism abnormalities are profound enough to substantially increase mortality.*[9]

PATHOBIOLOGY

A Response to Infection

The syndrome that we identify as "sepsis" can occur in response to insults other than infection, including trauma, burns, major surgery, and cardiac arrest.[22] Seminal work by Tracey et al. showed that lipopolysaccharide (LPS) strongly stimulated tumor necrosis factor alpha (TNF-α), which is sufficient to induce acute circulatory collapse, even in the absence of LPS.[19] This excess of inflammation in response to both pathogen-associated molecular patterns (PAMPs) such as LPS, and damage-associated molecular patterns (DAMPs) like TNF-α, occurs in response to infectious and noninfectious insults and may represent a final common pathway for severe insults that produce organ dysfunction. Thus, the Sepsis-3 task force chose to limit their consideration to the specific response to infection, reflecting a decision to retain focus and to provide a reasonable starting point for epidemiologic characterization.

The Dysregulated Host Response

One of the fundamental problems with the SIRS criteria was that many of the findings they encompassed—fever, tachycardia, and leukocytosis—are normal adaptive responses to infection. In fact, failure to mount this response (e.g., absence of fever) is a poor prognostic sign.[23] Thus, differentiating a "regulated" (i.e., adaptive) response from a "dysregulated" (i.e., maladaptive) host response represents a defining characteristic of sepsis.

In a landmark 1996 paper, Godin and Buchman postulated that sepsis pathobiology represented "an uncoupling of biological oscillators."[22] In this paradigm, "normal" physiology does not represent a homeostatic "steady state" but rather the tight coupling of biologic oscillators that generate inherently self-organizing systems that exhibit natural variation over time.[22] These oscillations reflect the input of small perturbations in the immediate environment and of more remote changes that are somewhat larger: e.g., heart rate oscillates by several beats/second in response to local pH or ion concentrations and more substantially in response to a change of blood flow to the kidneys or to skeletal muscle. This second source of variability requires the transfer of information, and pathology occurs if communication is disrupted. Phrased another way, system elements (like tissues and organs) that lose the ability to "talk to each other," can generate a potentially irreversible, self-amplifying disruption that can have a greater impact on overall function than alterations in any discrete element in the system. This paradigm is evident in sepsis, which is characterized by *loss* of variability in heart rate, neutrophil function, and diurnal hormone secretion.[24] These examples are not randomly chosen: they reflect changes in the three systems responsible for communication between anatomically remote systems that must coordinate their function—the immune, endocrine, and neural systems. Evidence suggests sepsis produces profound dysfunction in each.

Immune Dysfunction

Knowledge acquired after the publication of the Sepsis-1 consensus conference increasingly suggested that viewing sepsis as a disorder of excessive systemic inflammation was problematic. Additional data demonstrated that, in addition to a hyperinflammatory state, the sepsis phenotype contained an anti-inflammatory component. However, while patients with sepsis can exhibit both pro- and anti-inflammatory characteristics, and in fact may even concurrently display both, it would appear that even that description is incomplete.[25] Thus, while the elaboration and secretion of inflammatory mediators by a host of immune and nonimmune cells is often elevated,[25] the effector arms of both the innate and adaptive immune systems may become profoundly dysfunctional.[26] There are also aspects of immune function that are unique to sepsis. These findings suggest that the immune phenotype of sepsis is neither hyperinflammatory nor immunosuppressed—or even an amalgam of the two. Rather, the authors hypothesize that sepsis reflects a unique phenotype with some well-described elements and others that remain undiscovered or unexplored. Further supporting this hypothesis is the fact that, between the publication of Sepsis-1 in 1993 and the convening of the Sepsis-3 in 2014, over 100 randomized clinical trials (RCTs) of novel therapeutics intended to modulate inflammation or immunity were conducted in sepsis patients; all ultimately failed to demonstrate a consistent benefit.[20] Clearly, the "dysregulated host response" that characterizes sepsis involves more than simply described inflammatory states.

Endocrinopathy

The endocrinopathy of sepsis has been well-described.[27] In general, infection causes physiologic perturbations that induce the neuroendocrine stress response. Sepsis, and all critical illness, alters this response in a biphasic manner, with distinct acute and chronic phases.[27] The acute response is marked by inactivation of peripheral anabolic pathways and hyperstimulation of hypothalamic–pituitary function. Manifestations include decreased tissue activity. For example, glucocorticoid (GC) activity is depressed by a decrease in tissue levels of the active GC receptor (GR) alpha isoform and an increase in the inactive GR beta isoform,[28–30] as well as decreased peripheral conversion of thyroxine (T_4) to triiodothyronine (T_3).[27] In response, levels of pituitary hormones such as thyroid-stimulating hormone (TSH) or adrenocorticotropic hormone (ACTH) increase.[27] The chronic phase of sepsis-induced endocrinopathy is characterized by marked central suppression.[27] Release of ACTH, growth hormone (GH), and TSH ceases to be pulsatile, further compromising peripheral effects.[27] These abnormalities are linked to manifestations such as the "euthyroid sick syndrome" and wasting syndrome, and whether this endocrine profile persists or resolves is prognostic.[27,31,32]

Neural Pathways

Sepsis also impairs both afferent and efferent neural signaling, evidenced by bidirectional disruption of the inflammatory reflex.[19] Described by Tracey in 2002, the inflammatory reflex represents a prototypical model of neuroimmune crosstalk, whereby hardwired neural circuits directly regulate peripheral inflammation.[33] In brief, DAMP (damage-associated molecular pattern) stimulation activates afferent vagus impulses to nucleus tractus solitarius in the brainstem. These signals contribute to characteristic responses such as fever and sickness behavior. This signaling also reflexively triggers anti-inflammatory efferent vagus signaling. Sepsis impairs efferent vagus signaling.[24] Central cholinergic deficiency has been implicated. Sepsis-induced neural disruptions are not limited to inflammatory pathways. The orexinergic nervous system, a central neural circuit essential to regulating arousal and many basic physiologic functions, becomes hypoactive in experimental sepsis.[34] Instilling orexin into cerebral ventricles of mice not only corrects these abnormalities but also normalizes centrally depressed pituitary hormone levels in the chronic phase of sepsis-induced endocrinopathy, suggesting that dysfunctional orexinergic activation contributes to many physiologic aberrancies in sepsis.[34]

Taken together, sepsis disrupts all three of the major physiologic communication systems. An important clinical implication of this framework is that restoration of a specific organ function—whether in response to treatment (e.g., antibiotics) or exogenously (e.g., dialysis)—does not guarantee restoration of normal intercellular or interorgan relationships, which may prevent recovery even in the absence of the instigating stimulus. Indeed, persistent critical illness is a common phenomenon in sepsis patients.[35]

Organ Dysfunction

Organ dysfunction should not be confused with the mere absence of a function observed in normal physiology. For example, one in four patients presenting with sepsis-induced hypotension are oliguric and have decreased glomerular filtration rates (GFRs). However, in the setting of a distributive shock process, these changes could be adaptive: limiting further relative intravascular volume depletion may take precedence over the creation of electrolyte or acid-base disturbances. Indeed, this early form of renal "dysfunction" is not predictive of an inability to resolve hypotension with intravenous fluid resuscitation.[36] In contrast, oliguria and loss of GFR in patients with sepsis who have been sufficiently resuscitated, perhaps several days into an intensive care unit (ICU) stay, carry a poor prognosis.[37] At some point, an organ that inadequately performs an essential physiologic task—e.g., respiratory gas-exchange, urine production, bilirubin metabolism, blood circulation, etc.—becomes maladaptive. The clinical criteria for identifying sepsis that were derived and validated by the Sepsis-3 task force rely on the SOFA score to operationalize organ dysfunction at the bedside. This approach is more fully examined in Chapter 31 of this volume.

Septic Shock: Truly Distinct from Sepsis?

A substantive distinction between sepsis and septic shock is in some ways historical. Indeed, "septic shock" may actually have preceded "sepsis" as a distinct entity. Blalock's 1934 antecedent of the most commonly used system to classify shock today delineated four etiologic causes of shock: hematogenic (hypovolemic), cardiogenic, neurogenic, and vasogenic (most often septic). Vasogenic shock has been renamed "distributive shock," referring to a volume inadequate to fill a low-resistance, high-capacitance vascular system. In both Sepsis-1 and Sepsis-2, septic shock was "defined" as infection-induced cardiovascular dysfunction (or more specifically, sepsis-induced hypotension) that did not resolve with intravenous fluid resuscitation. The Sepsis-3 task force spent a significant amount of time discussing septic shock. One group advocated retention of the previous description, in which septic shock was a distinct entity characterized by cardiovascular dysfunction. Some clinicians pointed out that, using this approach, septic shock was simply sepsis, where the dysfunctional organ is the cardiovascular system. This postulate is consistent with some, but not all, pathobiologic aspects of sepsis-induced organ dysfunction and specifically, with PAMP—mediated acute circulatory insufficiency.[19] Other clinicians, however, took the view that shock is a metabolic and/or cellular phenomenon. Ultimately, the task force recognized that the understanding was insufficient to truly determine whether sepsis and septic shock are distinct pathobiologic entities: indeed, the main feature distinguishing the two was the markedly greater mortality associated with septic shock. Ultimately, all these views were incorporated into the Sepsis-3 definition of septic shock as "a subset of sepsis in which underlying circulatory and cellular metabolism abnormalities are profound enough to substantially increase mortality."

A Unifying Hypothesis—Mitochondrial Dysfunction and Bioenergetic Reprioritization

Sepsis alters mitochondrial function in virtually all cells and tissues investigated. There are four key changes. First, sepsis impairs the function of the electron transport chain. Abnormalities in all four complexes have been reported in both animal models and in clinical sepsis.[38] These impairments decrease net adenosine triphosphate (ATP) production and cellular oxygen utilization (Vo_2).[39] Indeed, resuscitated sepsis is associated with normal or elevated O_2 tension and decreased Vo_2.[39] Second, there is a reprogramming of metabolism to favor aerobic glycolysis (i.e., glycolysis-predominant metabolism despite available oxygen), resulting in hyperlactemia.[40] Sepsis-induced aerobic glycolysis has been compared to the Warburg effect, where cancer cells convert their metabolism to aerobic glycolysis.[41] The third key change is the powerful induction of mitochondrially generated reactive oxygen species (ROS) and reactive nitrogen species (RNS).[42] These free radicals further impair oxidative phosphorylation by depleting mitochondrial reducing agents, hindering electron transfer. In addition to producing a self-potentiating feedback loop by augmenting ROS production, free radicals also damage mitochondrial DNA and membranes.[42] Membrane damage is particularly important because mitochondrial contents that leak into cytosol can activate caspases, which in turn may induce programmed cell death.[42] Caspase activation is also involved in activation of the inflammasome, a signaling platform that triggers maturation of proinflammatory cytokines (e.g., interleukin 1 beta [IL-1β]) and, via caspase-1, may activate pyroptosis, a form of "incendiary" cell death that results in the release of DAMPS.[43] Pyroptosis does not arise from normal "wear-and-tear" because of autophagy, a process whereby damaged mitochondria are degraded and recycled.[43] However, the fourth key mitochondrial change is a disruption of autophagy and biogenesis, the processes by which mitochondria repair and replicate themselves.[42] The level of impairment of autophagy and biogenesis reliably correlates with organ injury and mortality in preclinical and clinical sepsis.[42] Importantly, all four of these mitochondrial changes potentiate each other, leading to profound mitochondrial and thus cellular metabolic dysfunction.

The ultimate effect is an energy crisis; mitochondria cannot produce sufficient ATP to meet full cellular demand. This *bioenergetic disturbance* elicits three particularly important manifestations:

- Insufficient ATP generation to meet demand for tissue- or organ-specific functions of cells leads to reprioritized energy allocation; essentially, cells "decide" to pursue self-survival over tasks that contribute to the health of the organism. Thus, while actual cell death is unusual in sepsis (save in high-turnover cell types such as those of hematopoietic origin or the intestinal epithelia),[44,45] the contribution of some cells to organ-specific action is reduced: that is, there is reduced contraction in cardiomyocytes and vascular smooth muscle, protein synthesis in hepatocytes, filtration and resorption in nephrons, synaptic transmission between neurons, absorption across the intestinal epithelium, etc.
- Because many key signal transduction mechanisms involve energy-dependent phosphorylation, bioenergetic

failure also impedes cells from appropriately propagating afferent and efferent responses to internal and external stimuli, representing a collapse of cell communication. For example, while IL-6 levels are elevated in sepsis, signal transduction within the cytosol from IL-6 receptor stimulation is impaired.[46]

- Maintaining barriers and (specific concentrations across them) is an energy-intensive process required for intracellular and systemic homeostasis.

Sepsis-3 Clinical Criteria

The new definition of sepsis contained the concepts that were believed to best describe the nature of sepsis—initiated by infection, mediated by a dysregulated host response, characterized by organ dysfunction, often culminating in death. Similarly, the definition of septic shock included cardiovascular abnormalities, metabolic dysregulation, and cellular dysfunction, and emphasized that the entity was even more deadly than sepsis. However, neither definition could be used by the clinician at the bedside to identify the patient with sepsis. Indeed, it was recognized that, while Sepsis-1/2 did not provide definitions, they did represent attempts to provide *clinical criteria* that could be directly applied to diagnosis and care. Unfortunately, these initial clinical criteria were not data-driven; rather, they represented consensus expert opinion as to what clinical characteristics were present in the patient with sepsis. Therefore, the Sepsis-3 task force also set out to use large databases to derive and validate clinical criteria for sepsis and septic shock. The results of these data-driven exercises were published at the same time as the paper summarizing the findings of the task force as a whole.[9,47,48] (They are described in detail in Chapter 31 of this text.)

AUTHORS' RECOMMENDATIONS

- Sepsis is defined as a life-threatening organ dysfunction caused by a dysregulated host response to infection.
- Septic shock is defined as sepsis in which cellular and metabolic abnormalities are profound enough to substantially increase mortality, although the extent to which septic shock truly represents a disorder distinct from sepsis is unclear.
- The pathobiology of sepsis is complex and reflects the uncoupling of physiologic networks that maintain homeostasis. This phenomenon appears driven by profound dysfunction in all three of the body's major communication systems: the immune, endocrine, and nervous systems.
- Organ dysfunction is the hallmark of sepsis, but adaptively decreased function should not be confused with true dysfunction.
- Sepsis induces profound mitochondrial dysfunction, producing a cellular energy crisis. This widespread cellular dysfunction may prove to be a unifying pathology in the sepsis syndrome.
- Sepsis and septic shock can be identified clinically using criteria described in Chapter 31.

REFERENCES

1. Fleischmann C, Scherag A, Adhikari NK, et al. Assessment of global incidence and mortality of hospital-treated sepsis. Current estimates and limitations. *Am J Respir Crit Care Med.* 2016;193(3):259-272.
2. Liu V, Escobar GJ, Greene JD, et al. Hospital deaths in patients with sepsis from 2 independent cohorts. *JAMA.* 2014;312(1):90-92.
3. Torio CMA, Andrews RMA. National inpatient hospital costs: the most expensive conditions by payer, 2011. *Statistical Brief No. 160.* Rockville, MD: Agency for Healthcare Research and Quality; 2013.
4. Prescott HC, Osterholzer JJ, Langa KM, Angus DC, Iwashyna TJ. Late mortality after sepsis: propensity matched cohort study. *BMJ.* 2016;353:i2375.
5. Odden AJ, Rohde JM, Bonham C, et al. Functional outcomes of general medical patients with severe sepsis. *BMC Infect Dis.* 2013;13:588.
6. Meyer N, Harhay MO, Small DS, et al. Temporal trends in incidence, sepsis-related mortality, and hospital-based acute care after sepsis. *Crit Care Med.* 2018;46(3):354-360.
7. Machado FR, Azevedo LCP. Sepsis: a threat that needs a global solution. *Crit Care Med.* 2018;46(3):454-459.
8. Rudd KE, Seymour CW, Aluisio AR, et al. Association of the quick Sequential (Sepsis-Related) Organ Failure Assessment (qSOFA) score with excess hospital mortality in adults with suspected infection in low- and middle-income countries. *JAMA.* 2018;319(21):2202-2211.
9. Singer M, Deutschman CS, Seymour CW, et al. The Third International Consensus Definitions for Sepsis and Septic Shock (Sepsis-3). *JAMA.* 2016;315(8):801-810.
10. Funk DJ, Parrillo JE, Kumar A. Sepsis and septic shock: a history. *Crit Care Clin.* 2009;25(1):83-101, viii.
11. Siegel JH, Cerra FB, Peters D, et al. The physiologic recovery trajectory as the organizing principle for the quantification of hormonometabolic adaptation to surgical stress and severe sepsis. *Adv Shock Res.* 1979;2:177-203.
12. Eiseman B, Beart R, Norton L. Multiple organ failure. *Surg Gynecol Obstet.* 1977;144(3):323-326.
13. Tilney NL, Bailey GL, Morgan AP. Sequential system failure after rupture of abdominal aortic aneurysms: an unsolved problem in postoperative care. *Ann Surg.* 1973;178(2):117-122.
14. Bone RC, Balk RA, Cerra FB, et al. Definitions for sepsis and organ failure and guidelines for the use of innovative therapies in sepsis. The ACCP/SCCM Consensus Conference Committee. American College of Chest Physicians/Society of Critical Care Medicine. *Chest.* 1992;101(6):1644-1655.
15. Vincent JL. Dear SIRS, I'm sorry to say that I don't like you. *Crit Care Med.* 1997;25(2):372-374.
16. Levy MM, Fink MP, Marshall JC, et al. 2001 SCCM/ESICM/ACCP/ATS/SIS International Sepsis Definitions Conference. *Crit Care Med.* 2003;31(4):1250-1256.
17. Marshall JC, Cook DJ, Christou NV, Bernard GR, Sprung CL, Sibbald WJ. Multiple organ dysfunction score: a reliable descriptor of a complex clinical outcome. *Crit Care Med.* 1995;23(10):1638-1652.
18. Ferreira FL, Bota DP, Bross A, Mélot C, Vincent JL. Serial evaluation of the SOFA score to predict outcome in critically ill patients. *JAMA.* 2001;286(14):1754-1758.

19. Deutschman CS, Tracey KJ. Sepsis: current dogma and new perspectives. *Immunity.* 2014;40(4):463-475.

20. Marshall JC. Sepsis: rethinking the approach to clinical research. *J Leukoc Biol.* 2008;83(3):471-482.

21. Dellinger RP, Levy MM, Rhodes A, et al. Surviving Sepsis Campaign: International Guidelines for Management of Severe Sepsis and Septic Shock: 2012. *Crit Care Med.* 2013;41(2):580-637.

22. Godin PJ, Buchman TG. Uncoupling of biological oscillators: a complementary hypothesis concerning the pathogenesis of multiple organ dysfunction syndrome. *Crit Care Med.* 1996;24(7):1107-1116.

23. Sundén-Cullberg J, Rylance R, Svefors J, Norrby-Teglund A, Björk J, Inghammar M. Fever in the emergency department predicts survival of patients with severe sepsis and septic shock admitted to the ICU. *Crit Care Med.* 2017;45(4):591-599.

24. Rassias AJ, Holzberger PT, Givan AL, Fahrner SL, Yeager MP. Decreased physiologic variability as a generalized response to human endotoxemia. *Crit Care Med.* 2005;33(3):512-519.

25. Angus DC, van der Poll T. Severe sepsis and septic shock. *N Engl J Med.* 2013;369(9):840-851.

26. Hotchkiss RS, Monneret G, Payen D. Sepsis-induced immuno-suppression: from cellular dysfunctions to immunotherapy. *Nat Rev Immunol.* 2013;13(12):862-874.

27. Ingels C, Gunst J, Van den Berghe G. Endocrine and metabolic alterations in sepsis and implications for treatment. *Crit Care Clin.* 2018;34(1):81-96.

28. Abraham MN, Jimenez DM, Fernandes TD, Deutschman CS. Cecal ligation and puncture alters glucocorticoid receptor expression. *Crit Care Med.* 2018;46(8):e797-e804.

29. Peeters RP, Hagendorf A, Vanhorebeek I, et al. Tissue mRNA expression of the glucocorticoid receptor and its splice variants in fatal critical illness. *Clin Endocrinol (Oxf).* 2009;71(1):145-153.

30. Molijn GJ, Spek JJ, van Uffelen JC, et al. Differential adaptation of glucocorticoid sensitivity of peripheral blood mononuclear leukocytes in patients with sepsis or septic shock. *J Clin Endocrinol Metab.* 1995;80(6):1799-1803.

31. Van den Berghe G. Non-thyroidal illness in the ICU: a syndrome with different faces. *Thyroid.* 2014;24(10):1456-1465.

32. Marquardt DJ, Knatz NL, Wetterau LA, Wewers MD, Hall MW. Failure to recover somatotropic axis function is associated with mortality from pediatric sepsis-induced multiple organ dysfunction syndrome. *Pediatr Crit Care Med.* 2010;11(1):18-25.

33. Tracey KJ. The inflammatory reflex. *Nature.* 2002;420(6917):853-859.

34. Deutschman CS, Raj NR, McGuire EO, Kelz MB. Orexinergic activity modulates altered vital signs and pituitary hormone secretion in experimental sepsis. *Crit Care Med.* 2013;41(11):e368-e375.

35. Iwashyna TJ, Hodgson CL, Pilcher D, et al. Timing of onset and burden of persistent critical illness in Australia and New Zealand: a retrospective, population-based, observational study. *Lancet Respir Med.* 2016;4(7):566-573.

36. Leisman DE, Doerfler ME, Schneider SM, Masick KD, D'Amore JA, D'Angelo JK. Predictors, prevalence, and outcomes of early crystalloid responsiveness among initially hypotensive patients with sepsis and septic shock. *Crit Care Med.* 2018;46(2):189-198.

37. Plataki M, Kashani K, Cabello-Garza J, et al. Predictors of acute kidney injury in septic shock patients: an observational cohort study. *Clin J Am Soc Nephrol.* 2011;6(7):1744-1751.

38. Ruggieri AJ, Levy RJ, Deutschman CS. Mitochondrial dysfunction and resuscitation in sepsis. *Crit Care Clin.* 2010;26(3):567-575, x-xi.

39. Singer M. The role of mitochondrial dysfunction in sepsis-induced multi-organ failure. *Virulence.* 2014;5(1):66-72.

40. Kraut JA, Madias NE. Lactic acidosis. *N Engl J Med.* 2014;371(24):2309-2319.

41. Vander Heiden MG, Cantley LC, Thompson CB. Understanding the Warburg effect: the metabolic requirements of cell proliferation. *Science.* 2009;324(5930):1029-1033.

42. Arulkumaran N, Deutschman CS, Pinsky MR, et al. Mitochondrial function in sepsis. *Shock.* 2016;45(3):271-281.

43. Schroder K, Tschopp J. The inflammasomes. *Cell.* 2010;140(6):821-832.

44. Hotchkiss RS, Swanson PE, Freeman BD, et al. Apoptotic cell death in patients with sepsis, shock, and multiple organ dysfunction. *Crit Care Med.* 1999;27(7):1230-1251.

45. Takasu O, Gaut JP, Watanabe E, et al. Mechanisms of cardiac and renal dysfunction in patients dying of sepsis. *Am J Respir Crit Care Med.* 2013;187(5):509-517.

46. Abcejo AS, Andrejko KM, Raj NR, Deutschman CS. Failed interleukin-6 signal transduction in murine sepsis: attenuation of hepatic glycoprotein 130 phosphorylation. *Crit Care Med.* 2009;37(5):1729-1734.

47. Shankar-Hari M, Phillips GS, Levy ML, et al. Developing a new definition and assessing new clinical criteria for septic shock: for the Third International Consensus Definitions for Sepsis and Septic Shock (Sepsis-3). *JAMA.* 2016;315(8):775-787.

48. Seymour CW, Liu VX, Iwashyna TJ, et al. Assessment of clinical criteria for sepsis: for the Third International Consensus Definitions for Sepsis and Septic Shock (Sepsis-3). *JAMA.* 2016;315(8):762-774.

How Do I Identify the Patient With "Sepsis"?

Craig M. Coopersmith and Katherine Lyn Nugent

SEPSIS-1 AND SEPSIS-2

The ability to identify a patient with sepsis is directly related to the ability to define sepsis. It has been acknowledged that, as recently as the 1980s, the lack of a consensus definition of sepsis limited the ability of medical providers to identify and treat septic patients. In 1992, an American College of Chest Physicians (ACCP)/Society of Critical Care Medicine (SCCM) consensus conference provided the first comprehensive approach to defining sepsis.[1] A critical portion of the definition was the use of the systemic inflammatory response syndrome (SIRS) criteria. SIRS was a response to a variety of severe clinical insults (infectious and not-infectious) and contained four elements:

- heart rate >90 beats per minute
- respiratory rate >20 breaths per minute or a pCO_2 <34 mm Hg
- white blood cell count >12,000/mm^3 or <4,000 mm^3, and
- temperature >38°C or <34°C.

Sepsis was defined as at least two of four SIRS criteria in the setting of suspected infection. Severe sepsis was defined as sepsis plus organ dysfunction, hypoperfusion or hypotension. Septic shock was defined as sepsis plus hypotension resistant to fluid resuscitation in the presence of perfusion abnormalities including, but not limited to, lactic acidosis, oliguria or an acute alteration in mental status.

Eleven years later, a second attempt was made to define sepsis via a consensus conference involving the SCCM, ACCP, the European Society of Intensive Care Medicine (ESCIM), the American Thoracic Society (ATS), and the Surgical Infection Society (SIS).[2] Despite the passage of time and new insights into the pathophysiology of sepsis, little changed in the definition of sepsis as the authors concluded that apart from expanding the lists of signs and symptoms of sepsis to better reflect bedside experience, a lack of new evidence precluded updating the definition. Of note, the authors did propose use of the predisposition, insult/infection, response, organ dysfunction (PIRO) staging system as an intellectual construct for future sepsis research. Although the elements within this hypothesis-generating model would be incorporated into future thought on sepsis, PIRO did not gain widespread usage.

The definitions from these two consensus conferences (now termed Sepsis-1 and Sepsis-2) served the medical community well for nearly a quarter century. Indeed, an explosion of sepsis studies used this common framework for the disease. Unfortunately, numerous limitations to the definitions were identified over time. First, the "definition" of sepsis was not actually a definition. The term "definition" is described in the dictionary as "the essential nature of a thing" or, more succinctly, "what something is." Sepsis-1 and Sepsis-2 did not meet this criterion—in reality, they were bedside tools for identifying patients with the syndrome. By analogy, an elevated troponin is a biomarker for a myocardial infarction, but it does not define the disorder.

Other problems also existed with Sepsis-1 and Sepsis-2. First, the term "severe sepsis" was controversial because it implied that there was also a nonsevere form of the disease. Considering the high mortality associated with sepsis, the possibility that a clinician might conclude that there is a nonsevere form of sepsis has potential direct effects on patient outcome. Medical providers might not see this as an acute, time-sensitive condition, leading to delays in treatment and increased mortality.

Finally, the concept of SIRS came under significant criticism for a variety of reasons.[3] Studies indicated that at least 50% of patients developed SIRS at some point during their hospitalization, limiting its utility for specifically identifying patients with sepsis.[4] Perhaps more concerning was the finding that in a retrospective analysis of over 100,00 patients admitted to the intensive care unit (ICU), 1 out of 8 did not have two SIRS criteria despite confirmed infection and similar organ dysfunction as patients with two or more SIRS criteria.[5] Intellectually, there was also a concern that SIRS generally represented an adaptive response to any inflammatory insult, whereas sepsis represents a maladaptive response to infection. It seems questionable to define a disease in large part by a body's appropriate response to an insult.

SEPSIS-3: AN INTELLECTUAL ADVANCE

Based upon these concerns, as well as those that Sepsis-1 and Sepsis-2 focused disproportionately on systemic inflammation in the pathophysiology of the disease process, SCCM and ESICM assembled the Third International Consensus Definitions Task Force for Sepsis and Septic shock (Sepsis-3).[6] This task force redefined sepsis as "life-threatening organ dysfunction caused by a dysregulated host response to infection." A number of changes to the concept of sepsis were made explicit (and implicit) in this new definition. First, after being part of how sepsis was defined for a quarter century, the SIRS criteria were eliminated from the new definition of sepsis. SIRS, as a concept, has face validity for the diagnosis of infection, but this is distinct from diagnosing sepsis. Next, the new definition recharacterized the disorder. The physiologic state formerly termed "sepsis" (with SIRS but without organ dysfunction) now represents "systemic infection" alone and not "sepsis" given the concept of organ dysfunction was absent from the previous definition. This change not only eliminated a significant population of patients from being classified as septic when they lacked organ dysfunction but also highlighted the characterization of sepsis as preventable; infected patients treated rapidly with antibiotics might never develop organ dysfunction.

The next change in Sepsis-3 was the elimination of the term, "severe sepsis." Sepsis is now life threatening by definition, acknowledging its severity at all times. Notably, no change was made to the definition of infection, which the task force felt was beyond its scope, and continues to refer to "a pathologic process caused by the invasion of normally sterile tissue or fluid or body cavity by pathogenic or potentially pathogenic microorganisms."

Sepsis-3 also redefined septic shock as a subset of sepsis in which underlying circulatory and cellular/metabolic abnormalities are profound enough to substantially increase mortality. Similar to sepsis, the "definition" of septic shock in Sepsis-1 and Sepsis-2 was actually a bedside tool to recognize the disease, and the redefinition of septic shock more accurately reflects the essential nature of the disorder. In addition, Sepsis-3 extends the definition of septic shock by emphasizing the pathobiological role of cellular and metabolic abnormalities in circulatory dysfunction.

SEPSIS-3 AT THE BEDSIDE

While the definitions of sepsis and septic shock represent an intellectual advance, they are unhelpful at the bedside. As such, in order to rapidly identify patients with sepsis, clinical criteria were required. To be useful to the bedside clinician, these criteria must reflect the components of the definition—a threat to life, organ dysfunction, and abnormal host response to infection—while simultaneously differentiating patients with sepsis from those without with acceptable sensitivity and specificity. Additionally, high criterion validity (as achieved by more complex scoring systems involving a larger number of clinical or laboratory variables) needed to be balanced with the value placed on low encumbrance for the bedside clinician. Furthermore, a high value was placed on the timeliness of identification. This last was critical given the link between syndrome identification and management. Considering this direct link between sepsis and septic shock management and outcomes,[7–10] the clinical criteria for sepsis and septic shock had to be simple enough that bedside clinicians could rapidly identify at-risk patients.

The clinical criteria used for the recognition of sepsis are the presence of suspected or confirmed infection and a Sequential Organ Failure Assessment (SOFA, also known as the Sepsis-related Organ Failure Assessment) score of ≥ 2. The baseline SOFA score is assumed to be zero in patients not known to have preexisting organ dysfunction, even if no history is available. The SOFA score wasn't created for use in Sepsis-3. Rather, it was unveiled in 1994[11] as a simple, easily determined index composed of objective, routinely measured variables. The SOFA score could be followed over time to map the natural course of a disease or to assess the influence of therapeutic interventions. The score is comprised of a combination of laboratory values, physical exam characteristics, and clinical interventions aimed at grading the level of dysfunction of six different organ systems (Table 31.1).

While the SOFA score was not designed to predict outcomes, a rise in the SOFA score 24 hours after the initial score is calculated has been associated with an increased probability of mortality.[12] SOFA is more complicated than SIRS, but is relatively easy to calculate and represents a reasonable approach to the quantification of organ dysfunction, allowing for rapid clinical operationalization of the new sepsis definition. The Sepsis-3 criteria were explicitly compared to SIRS and, in the data sets examined, had both superior sensitivity and specificity.

The clinical criteria for septic shock allow for identification of this state by utilizing a construct in which patients have
(1) hypotension requiring vasopressors to maintain a mean arterial pressure >65 mm Hg and
(2) a serum lactate >2 mmol/L despite adequate fluid resuscitation.

It is important to note that, in contrast to previous approaches to septic shock, the Sepsis-3 clinical criteria were derived and validated via analysis of over 3 million hospital charts.[13] In this analysis, mortality was 42% in patients meeting all criteria. In those who were hypotensive/vasopressor dependent but had a lactate < 2 mmol/L, mortality was 30%, while patients not requiring vasopressors who had an elevated lactate had a mortality rate of 26%. It is important to note which criteria are used when reading the literature because the change from Sepsis-1 to Sepsis-3 alters which patients are identified as septic. This difference has the potential to change clinical trial results when different criteria are applied to an identical patient cohort.[14]

qSOFA: A NEW SCREENING TOOL FOR SEPSIS

Perhaps the most misunderstood aspect of Sepsis-3 was the introduction of the quick Sequential (Sepsis-related) Organ Failure Assessment (qSOFA) score.[7] This new screening tool has three components:
- systolic hypotension (<100 mm Hg),
- tachypnea (respiratory rate ≥ 22 breaths per minute), and
- altered mentation (as assessed by a Glasgow Coma Scale of 13 or less).

TABLE 31.1 The SOFA Score.

SOFA Score	1	2	3	4
Respiration PaO$_2$/FiO$_2$[a] mmHg	<400	<300	<200 ——with respiratory support——	<100
Coagulation Platelets ×10^3/mm^3	<150	<100	<50	<20
Liver Bilirubin, mg/dl (μmol/l)	1.2–1.9 (20–32)	2.0–5.9 (33–101)	6.0–11.9 (102–204)	>12.0 (<204)
Cardiovascular Hypotension	MAP <70 mmHg	Dopamine ≤ 5 or dobutamine (any dose)[a]	Dopamine >5 or epinephrine ≤0.1 or norepinephrine ≤0.1	Dopamine >15 or epinephrine >0.1 or norepinephrine >0.1
Central Nervous System Glasgow Coma Score	13–14	10–12	6–9	<6
Renal Creatinine, mg/dl (μmol/l) or urine output	1.2–1.9 (110–170)	2.0–3.4 (171–299)	3.5–4.9 (300–440) or <500 ml/day	>5.0 (>440) or <200 ml/day

[a]Adrenergic agents administered for at least 1 h (doses given are in μg/kg • min)

qSOFA was derived from a large electronic health record and validated in several additional databases. Overall, more than 7 million patient charts were examined. From the initial dataset, patients with suspected, presumed or documented infection were identified. Because there is no "gold standard" for diagnosing sepsis, the combination of death and/or ICU stay ≥3 days served as a proxy. Each of the variables compiled in Sepsis-2 for their value in identifying patients with sepsis was examined, alone or in combination, for the ability to predict the proxy. Patients in whom 2 of the 3 components of qSOFA were present had a 3- to 14-fold increase in in-hospital mortality across baseline risk deciles relative to patients whose qSOFA score was <2. Adding a serum lactate level ≥2.0 mmol/L to the three qSOFA variables did not increase predictive validity. Of note, the qSOFA score was derived and validated in over 7 million patient charts.

Importantly, qSOFA is a screening tool to be used to identify septic patients in whom further work up may be warranted. It is not intended to be an alternative to the SOFA score as an approach to clinical criteria for sepsis. Indeed, the utility of qSOFA varied by location within the hospital. In patients outside of the ICU, the qSOFA score was found to have similar areas under the curve for in-hospital mortality as SOFA. In contrast, for patients inside the ICU, SOFA had a predictive validity that was superior to qSOFA. Of note, in the datasets examined, the SIRS score had a lower predictive validity for in-hospitality mortality than qSOFA and SOFA regardless of whether the patient was in the ICU or not.

A key attribute of qSOFA is its simplicity. In contrast to SOFA or other more complex scoring systems, qSOFA consists of only three elements, each of which is easily measured at the bedside. No laboratory tests are needed. However, while the simplicity of qSOFA is attractive, it has generated significant criticism.[15,16] Much of it surrounded a concern that patients are quite ill by the time they have a qSOFA score of 2, which could delay intervention. Further, the primary outcome driving the development and validation of qSOFA was in-hospital mortality, one of only multiple outcomes of interest in sepsis screening, especially in the emergency department. Finally, while emergency medicine providers use screening tools to not only identify patients with possible sepsis but also to assist with triaging the sickest patients from a large census, to initiate time-sensitive interventions, and to help with disposition planning, sSOFA was derived and validated in patients with suspected, presumed or documented infection. The validity of qSOFA in evaluation of patients with other underlying disorders has not been tested. In addition, the clinical criteria derived in Sepsis-3 do not include any treatment recommendations for the management of sepsis or septic shock.

WHAT HAS HAPPENED SINCE SEPSIS-3?

The Sepsis-3 manuscript has been viewed over 2.5 million times on the JAMA website and has been cited over 2000 times.[6] Because the original clinical criteria were based on analysis of a large database in a manner that had not previously been performed, the authors explicitly stated that clinical criteria and qSOFA required additional validation. There were over 150 publications on qSOFA in the first 2 years following the publication of Sepsis-3. Most are directed at comparing the Sepsis-3 criteria, either SOFA or qSOFA, with other approaches, most often Sepsis-1 (i.e., SIRS). Some[17,18] have supported the results of aspects of Sepsis-3,[7] others[12,17,19] have not. A number of studies have compared Sepsis-3 criteria to approaches other than Sepsis-1.[15,20,21] Many have focused on outcomes other than those used in Sepsis-3. Perhaps the most salient with respect to Sepsis-3 criteria in the ICU examined patients in the Case Mix Programme Database, a national clinical audit for adult admissions to general ICUs in England.[22] Among patients admitted to the ICU for infection, 197,724 met Sepsis-2 criteria for severe sepsis while 197,142 met Sepsis-3 criteria and 189,243 met both definitions, a 92% overlap. Differences in mortality and ICU length of stay were not statistically significant. What this study illustrates is an issue that arises with virtually all such reports—difficulty in comparing false positives (patients who met either set of criteria but did not meet outcome criteria) and false negatives (patients who did not meet either set of criteria but did meet outcome criteria).

The need to validate Sepsis-3 criteria in middle- and low-income countries was specifically cited as a deficit by the Sepsis-3 Task Force. A 2018 metaanalysis of nine studies of qSOFA in low- and middle-income countries demonstrated that qSOFA identified patients at risk of death beyond that explained by baseline factors and was superior to SIRS.[23] In a single institution study, Matics and Sanchez-Pinto validated an age-adjusted qSOFA score.[24]

CONCLUSION

Identifying patients with sepsis is problematic, especially given the lack of a gold-standard for comparison. Thus, inter-observer variability becomes important. The difficulty is exemplified by the results of a survey distributed to 94 physicians (the majority of whom were critical care medicine specialists). When asked to evaluate five clinical vignettes of patients with suspected or confirmed infection and organ dysfunction, the variable results demonstrated the subjective nature of diagnosing sepsis regardless of participants' perceived confidence in sepsis-related definitions or clinical experience.[25] Further complicating matters is the fact that there is more than one set of clinical criteria currently in use. It has been proposed that different definitions may be useful for different purposes including clinical care, clinical trials, basic research, surveillance, and quality improvement/audit.[26] The usefulness of these definitions can be measured by six criteria that vary widely depending upon the context of the definition (1) reliability, (2) content validity, (3) construct validity, (4) criterion validity, (5) measurement burden and (6) timeliness.[27] Ultimately, different classification criteria may identify different incidences of sepsis with different mortalities.[28] Each definition has inherent strengths and weaknesses, and an approach using more than one set of clinical criteria may balance the sensitivity and specificity needed in identifying septic patients.[29]

> **AUTHORS' RECOMMENDATIONS**
> * The Sepsis-3 formulation provided new, clinically validated criteria for identifying patients likely to have sepsis or septic shock. These criteria have been designed to supersede SIRS-based criteria. The new clinical criteria are based on use of the SOFA score.
> * A prompt designed to alert clinicians of a need for additional evaluation, qSOFA, was also derived and validated *de novo*.
> * Studies conducted since the publication of Sepsis-3 have examined the value of SOFA and qSOFA relative to Sepsis-1 criteria and a number of additional assessment methods.
> * Current data suggest that Sepsis-3 criteria are effective in low- and middle-income countries. A single study suggests the value of an age-adjusted qSOFA score in children.

REFERENCES

1. Bone RC, Balk RA, Cerra FB, et al. Definitions for sepsis and organ failure and guidelines for the use of innovative therapies in sepsis. The ACCP/SCCM Consensus Conference Committee. American College of Chest Physicians/Society of Critical Care Medicine. *Chest.* 1992;101(6):1644-1655.
2. Levy MM, Fink MP, Marshall JC, et al. 2001 SCCM/ESICM/ACCP/ATS/SIS International Sepsis Definitions Conference. *Crit Care Med.* 2003;31(4):1250-1256.
3. Vincent JL. Dear SIRS, I'm sorry to say that I don't like you... *Crit Care Med.* 1997;25(2):372-374.
4. Churpek MM, Zadravecz FJ, Winslow C, Howell MD, Edelson DP. Incidence and prognostic value of the systemic inflammatory response syndrome and organ dysfunctions in ward patients. *Am J Respir Crit Care Med.* 2015;192(8):958-964.
5. Kaukonen KM, Bailey M, Pilcher D, Cooper DJ, Bellomo R. Systemic inflammatory response syndrome criteria in defining severe sepsis. *N Engl J Med.* 2015;372(17):1629-1638.
6. Singer M, Deutschman CS, Seymour CW, et al. The third international consensus definitions for sepsis and septic shock (Sepsis-3). *JAMA.* 2016;315(8):801-810.
7. Seymour CW, Liu VX, Iwashyna TJ, et al. Assessment of clinical criteria for sepsis: for the Third International Consensus Definitions for Sepsis and Septic Shock (Sepsis-3). *JAMA.* 2016;315(8):762-774.
8. Levy MM, Gesten FC, Phillips GS, et al. Mortality changes associated with mandated public reporting for sepsis. The results of the New York State Initiative. *Am J Respir Crit Care Med.* 2018;198(11):1406-1412.
9. Ferrer R, Martin-Loeches I, Phillips G, et al. Empiric antibiotic treatment reduces mortality in severe sepsis and septic shock from the first hour: results from a guideline-based performance improvement program. *Crit Care Med.* 2014;42(8):1749-1755.
10. Kumar A, Roberts D, Wood KE, et al. Duration of hypotension before initiation of effective antimicrobial therapy is the critical determinant of survival in human septic shock. *Crit Care Med.* 2006;34(6):1589-1596.
11. Vincent JL, Moreno R, Takala J, et al. The SOFA (Sepsis-related Organ Failure Assessment) score to describe organ dysfunction/failure. On behalf of the Working Group on Sepsis-Related Problems of the European Society of Intensive Care Medicine. *Intensive Care Med.* 1996;22(7):707-710.

12. Raith EP, Udy AA, Bailey M, et al. Prognostic accuracy of the SOFA score, SIRS criteria, and qSOFA score for in-hospital mortality among adults with suspected infection admitted to the intensive care unit. *JAMA*. 2017;317(3):290-300.

13. Shankar-Hari M, Phillips GS, Levy ML, et al. Developing a new definition and assessing new clinical criteria for septic shock: for the Third International Consensus Definitions for Sepsis and Septic Shock (Sepsis-3). *JAMA*. 2016;315(8):775-787.

14. Russell JA, Lee T, Singer J, Boyd JH, Walley KR. The Septic Shock 3.0 definition and trials: a vasopressin and septic shock trial experience. *Crit Care Med*. 2017;45(6):940-948.

15. Churpek MM, Snyder A, Han X, et al. Quick sepsis-related organ failure assessment, systemic inflammatory response syndrome, and early warning scores for detecting clinical deterioration in infected patients outside the intensive care unit. *Am J Respir Crit Care Med*. 2017;195(7):906-911.

16. Hwang SY, Jo IJ, Lee SU, et al. Low accuracy of positive qSOFA criteria for predicting 28-day mortality in critically ill septic patients during the early period after emergency department presentation. *Ann Emerg Med*. 2018;71(1):1-9.e2.

17. Fang X, Wang Z, Yang J, et al. Clinical evaluation of Sepsis-1 and Sepsis-3 in the ICU. *Chest*. 2018;153(5):1169-1176.

18. Freund Y, Lemachatti N, Krastinova E, et al. Prognostic accuracy of Sepsis-3 criteria for in-hospital mortality among patients with suspected infection presenting to the emergency department. *JAMA*. 2017;317(3):301-308.

19. Song JU, Sin CK, Park HK, Shim SR, Lee J. Performance of the quick Sequential (sepsis-related) Organ Failure Assessment score as a prognostic tool in infected patients outside the intensive care unit: a systematic review and meta-analysis. *Crit Care*. 2018;22:28.

20. Wang JY, Chen YX, Guo SB, Mei X, Yang P. Predictive performance of quick Sepsis-related Organ Failure Assessment for mortality and ICU admission in patients with infection at the ED. *Am J Emerg Med*. 2016;34:1788-1793.

21. Chen YX, Wang JY, Guo SB. Use of CRB-65 and quick Sepsis-related Organ Failure Assessment to predict site of care and mortality in pneumonia patients in the emergency department: a retrospective study. *Crit Care*. 2016;20(1):167.

22. Shankar-Hari M, Harrison DA, Rubenfeld GD, Rowan K. Epidemiology of sepsis and septic shock in critical care units: comparison between sepsis-2 and sepsis-3 populations using a national critical care database. *Br J Anaesth*. 2017;119:626-636.

23. Rudd KE, Seymour CW, Aluisio AR, et al. Association of the quick Sequential (Sepsis-Related) Organ Failure Assessment (qSOFA) score with excess hospital mortality in adults with suspected infection in low- and middle-income countries. *JAMA*. 2018;319(21):2202-2211.

24. Matics TJ, Sanchez-Pinto LN. Adaptation and validation of a pediatric sequential organ failure assessment score and evaluation of the sepsis-3 definitions in critically ill children. *JAMA Pediatr*. 2017;171(10):e172352.

25. Rhee C, Kadri SS, Danner RL, et al. Diagnosing sepsis is subjective and highly variable: a survey of intensivists using case vignettes. *Crit Care*. 2016;20:89.

26. Seymour CW, Coopersmith CM, Deutschman CS, et al. Application of a framework to assess the usefulness of alternative sepsis criteria. *Crit Care Med*. 2016;44:e122-e130.

27. Angus DC, Seymour CW, Coopersmith CM, et al. A framework for the development and interpretation of different sepsis definitions and clinical criteria. *Crit Care Med*. 2016;44(3):e113-e121.

28. Donnelly JP, Safford MM, Shapiro NI, Baddley JW, Wang HE. Application of the Third International Consensus Definitions for Sepsis (Sepsis-3) Classification: a retrospective population-based cohort study. *Lancet Infect Dis*. 2017;17(6):661-670.

29. Serafim R, Gomes JA, Salluh J, Póvoa P. A comparison of the quick-SOFA and systemic inflammatory response syndrome criteria for the diagnosis of sepsis and prediction of mortality: a systematic review and meta-analysis. *Chest*. 2018;153(3):646-655.

Is There Immune Suppression in the Critically Ill Patient - Pro?

Kenneth E. Remy and Isaiah R. Turnbull

In his seminal 1876 work defining germ theory, Dr. Robert Koch described experiments in which he established the causative role of infecting microorganisms in septic shock.[1] Infection was accepted as the cause of sepsis until 1957, when bacterial endotoxin was discovered and demonstrated to recapitulate the pathophysiology of septic shock in the absence of a live replicating bacterial infection.[2] The link between septic shock and the immune system was established 30 years later when Cerami and colleagues demonstrated that endotoxin activated macrophages to release the inflammatory cytokine tumor necrosis factor (TNF-alpha), which was found to be a primary endogenous mediator of endotoxic shock.[3] Subsequent studies established elevated levels of inflammatory cytokines in the blood of patients with sepsis. The prevailing theory for the pathogenesis of sepsis at that time was that bacterial infection induced an inflammatory cytokine storm that caused septic shock.[4] Subsequently, sepsis researchers sought to treat sepsis by attenuating the inflammatory response. Unfortunately, in more than 50 clinical trials, antiinflammatory strategies have failed to improve sepsis survival.[5–11]

The failure of antiinflammatory strategies alone to improve sepsis outcomes led to a reevaluation of the role of the immune system in the pathogenesis of sepsis.[12] Mounting evidence suggests that immunosuppression is the primary immune derangement in the septic patient and that the pathophysiology of sepsis results as much or more from an immunocompromised state than from a systemic inflammatory response.[13,14]

In this chapter, we will review clinical data demonstrating that sepsis results in functional immunosuppression, decreasing the ability of patients to clear their primary infections and increasing susceptibility to secondary infection. We will describe the immunologic mechanism underlying this immunosuppression and the related metrics for assessing the immunologic state. Lastly, we will present emerging data for next-generation immune adjuvant therapies to reverse sepsis-induced immunosuppression.

SEPSIS INDUCES CLINICAL IMMUNOSUPPRESSION

At the cellular level, the host response to infection is complex and varies depending on type of infection, bacterial load, and host genetic factors.[12] Cells of the innate immune system, including granulocytes, macrophages, dendritic cells and innate lymphoid cells such as natural killer cells, express germ-line encoded receptors that recognize both pathogen-associated molecular patterns (PAMPS) and host-derived molecules associated with tissue damage (damage-associated molecular patterns or DAMPS).[15] The proximal signaling mechanisms of the innate immune system form a positive feedback loop that serves to amplify the response to minor injuries and infections in order to facilitate early clearance of infecting organisms and damaged tissue. This innate inflammatory response activates the adaptive immune system, inducing the proliferation of antigen specific T-cells and B-cells that acutely combat infection and provide long-term memory cells, improving future immunity.[16] Under normal physiologic conditions, progression of the immune response leads to activation of negative feedback pathways that downregulate inflammation. It was hypothesized that in response to severe infections such as sepsis, the positive feedback loops of the innate immune response drove an exaggerated activation of the inflammatory response that extended beyond the local environment, leading to a systemic inflammatory response syndrome (SIRS).[17] The exaggerated inflammation of the SIRS response was hypothesized to induce an exaggerated negative feedback response, termed the "compensatory antiinflammatory response syndrome" (CARS), reflecting pathologic downregulation of immune function.[18] The SIRS-CARS model seeks to describe the cellular and molecular function of the immune system during sepsis as a concurrent dysregulation of pro- and anti-inflammatory pathways. Regardless of the balance of SIRS and CARS, clinical data suggests septic patients are functionally immunosuppressed, defined as the inability to clear primary infections and increased susceptibility to secondary infection.

Clinical evidence demonstrates that sepsis causes a functionally immunocompromised state. Daviaud et al. reported that, in single cohort study of 543 patients, up to 80% of the deaths from sepsis that occurred within 3 days of ICU admission were attributable to infection-related multiple organ dysfunction, despite the fact that 93% of patients received adequate antimicrobial therapy.[19] Autopsy studies of patients confirm the immunosuppressed state of the septic patient, with persistent foci of infection and microabscesses identified in 80% of patients.[20] With ongoing sepsis, infectious burden increased, with increased frequency of positive blood cultures and increased infections with opportunistic organisms.[21] The Surviving Sepsis Campaign (SSC) guidelines recognize that sepsis may be associated with defects in the host antimicrobial response, affirming that prolonged courses of antibiotics may be required in septic patients whose clinical response may be slow despite appropriate antimicrobial therapy.[22]

The suppression of antiinfective immunity is reflected in the incidence and impact of secondary infections in septic patients. Between 13%–39% of critically ill septic patients will develop a secondary infection while in the ICU.[23,24] These secondary infections have a significant clinical impact, accounting for 10% of the attributable mortality from sepsis.[25] Overall, 10% of patients discharged from the ICU after sepsis will have an unplanned hospital admission within 30 days; 69% of these admissions will be for infection.[26] Sepsis-induced defects in immune function are persistent: as compared to patients with noninfectious critical illness, septic patients are 3.8-fold more likely to be readmitted to the hospital for infection within 1 year.[27]

Sepsis also results in increased susceptibility to nonvirulent and latent pathogens. This fact was first recognized as a response to the widespread use of penicillin-based antibiotics. These agents were effective at treating gram-positive microbes but left septic patients susceptible to gram-negative organisms that previously had rarely caused infection. This change was first recognized in a landmark paper by Altemeirer et al,[28] who identified a relationship between immunosuppression and the development of gram-negative sepsis. The immunosuppressive effects of sepsis on the immune system also leave patients susceptible to infection with opportunistic organisms. Common ICU pathogens such as *Pseudomonas aeruginosa, Acinetobacter baumannii, Stenotrophomonas maltophillia,* and *candida species* rarely cause clinically significant infections in immunocompetent hosts. In the setting of sepsis, these organisms can become pathogenic, rapidly upregulating virulence factors and antibiotic resistance genes.

Sepsis is also associated with the reactivation of latent viruses. The immune system most often eradicates viral infections, but some viruses are suppressed and lie dormant within the host. During times of impaired host immunity, such as during the treatment of hematologic malignancies or after transplantation, latent viruses escape immune surveillance mechanisms and begin replicating, leading to higher mortality and morbidity.[29,30] Several studies have demonstrated that a significant percentage of adult patients with sepsis and clinical evidence of immune suppression develop viral reactivation.[30] Limaye and colleagues examined the incidence of reactivation of cytomegalovirus (CMV) in 120 previously immunocompetent critically ill patients, many of whom had sepsis.[31–33] CMV viremia occurred in 33% of patients and was associated with prolonged hospitalization and death. More recently, viral DNAemia was detected in 28/73 (38%) of children admitted with sepsis-induced organ failure.[29] These findings directly correlated with immune suppression and with a high risk for the subsequent development of secondary infection. Consistent with this, a study reported herpes reactivation viremia in 68% of a cohort of critically ill patients, and found that viremia was associated with a significant increased risk of mortality in critically ill patients.[34]

MECHANISMS OF IMMUNOSUPPRESSION IN SEPSIS

Mechanistic studies demonstrate that sepsis induces pleiotropic defects in both innate and adaptive immune function, extending across both myeloid and lymphoid cell populations (Box 32.1).[35] As early as 1972, Alexander and Meakins[36] reported that sepsis caused abnormalities in the ability of neutrophils to kill bacteria. Subsequent studies have found that sepsis is associated with changes in neutrophil production of reactive oxygen species and phagocytosis.[37–39] Defects in myeloid cell function during sepsis also extend to monocytes. In patients with postoperative sepsis, there is an immediate suppression of both proinflammatory and antiinflammatory cytokines by monocytes in response to lipopolysaccharide stimulation.[40] Survival among these patients correlated with a recovery of the proinflammatory, but not the antiinflammatory, response. Monocytes from septic patients have decreased levels of cell surface markers associated with activation, notably monocyte human leukocyte antigen type DR (mHLA-DR).[41] These monocytes produce only small amounts of tumor necrosis factor-α (TNF-α) and interleukin-1 (IL-1) in response to bacterial challenges.[42]

Sepsis also alters the differentiation of myeloid cells. Recent studies have demonstrated that sepsis is associated with expansion and peripheral mobilization of incompletely differentiated myeloid suppressor cells (MDSC) from the bone marrow. MDSC are incompletely differentiated myeloid cells that are mobilized out of the bone marrow as part of the hematopoietic response to sepsis. Ex-vivo studies have demonstrated that MDSC suppress the activation of T-cells and release immunosuppressive IL-10, decreasing the function of both macrophages and dendritic cells.[43,44] Studies of lung tissue from septic patients demonstrated increased numbers of MDSCs in the lung as compared to healthy controls.[45] Clinical studies suggest a functional role for MDSC in sepsis, finding that the magnitude of MDSC expansion in sepsis

---

BOX 32.1   Mechanisms of Immunosuppression in Sepsis.

Lymphocyte (CD4 T-cells, B-cells) and dendritic cell apoptosis
Switch to T_H2, or immunosuppressive, cytokine profile and release of anti-inflammatory mediators
Lymphocyte anergy increased proportion of regulatory T cells
Monocyte deactivation evidenced by decreased expression of mHLA-DR
Impairment of neutrophil functions
Expansion of immature myeloid suppressor cell populations

mHLA-DR, monocyte human leukocyte antigen type DR.

correlated with adverse outcomes, including mortality and increased rates of secondary infections.[46]

Foundational work by Hotchkiss et al. established sepsis-induced apoptosis as a key underlying immunosuppressive mechanism.[47] In both animal and human studies, sepsis induced apoptosis in both lymphocytes and gastrointestinal epithelial cells (Fig. 32.1).[47–49] Examination of the spleens of patients who died from sepsis revealed a profound depletion of B cells, CD4 T-cells, and follicular dendritic cells from both the innate and adaptive immune systems that was not observed in the spleens of patients who died following trauma.[47] Studies in a clinically relevant mouse model of sepsis (cecal ligation and puncture, CLP) confirm the contribution of lymphocyte apoptosis to the observed pathophysiology.[50] Mice were injected with either apoptotic or necrotic cells before CLP and survival was recorded. Mice receiving adoptively transferred apoptotic cells had greater mortality compared with mice that received necrotic cells. Significantly, mice that received apoptotic as opposed to necrotic cells also exhibited T_H2 cytokine profiles and decreased IFN-γ production by spleen cells, suggesting that apoptosis caused immunosuppression. Interventions that block sepsis-induced lymphocyte apoptosis were associated with improved outcomes in animal models of sepsis including CLP and pneumonia.[51–54]

Although controversial, some investigators have reported that T-regulatory (CD4$^+$ and CD25$^+$) cells play an important role in sepsis-induced immunosuppression. T-regulatory cells modulate the immune response to pathogens by acting on other T-cells and antigen-presenting cells.[55] T-regulatory cells release cytokines like IL-10, TGF-β, and IL-4 and thereby mediate responses in CD4 and CD8 T cells. One study revealed that the proportion of circulating T-regulatory cells was increased in septic patients immediately after diagnosis and persisted only in non-survivors.[56] This increase in T-regulatory cells was also observed in clinically relevant animal models of sepsis.[57–60] T-regulatory cells may be important in the switch from a hyperinflammatory state to immune dysfunction. One study demonstrated improved survival in mice subjected to CLP who were treated with an antibody to the glucocorticoid-induced TNF receptor that is highly expressed on T-regulatory cells.[59] This antibody restored CD4+ T-cell proliferation and increased T_H1 and T_H2 cytokines and reversed the adaptive immune dysfunction seen in sepsis. T-regulatory cells thus may prove to play a crucial role in the development and treatment of immune dysfunction in severe sepsis.

DIAGNOSING IMMUNOSUPPRESSION IN THE SEPTIC PATIENT

The host immune response to sepsis is complex and involves many circulating mediators and cells. Various cytokines and their correlation with mortality have been studied. Baseline circulating IL-6 and soluble-TNF receptor have been shown to correlate with disease severity and 28-day all-cause mortality[61] and may help in determining when an antiinflammatory therapy may benefit. Levels of antiinflammatory cytokines such as IL-10 may be more helpful in determining whether a patient is immunosuppressed (Box 32.2). Both elevated and sustained levels of IL-10[62,63] and high IL-10/TNF-α ratios are

---

BOX 32.2 Possible Diagnostic Markers of Sepsis Induced Immunosuppression.

Increased initial and sustained IL-10 levels
High IL-10/TNF-α ratios
Decreased mHLA-DR expression

IL-10, interleukin-10; *mHLA-DR*, monocyte human leukocyte antigen type DR; *TNF-α*; tumor necrosis factor-α.

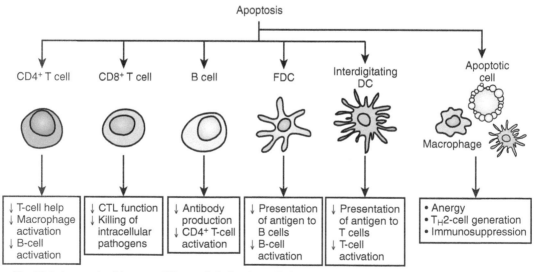

Fig. 32.1 Apoptosis of Immune Effector Cells Lead to a Defective Immune Response to Infection. *CTL*, cytotoxic T lymphocyte; *DC*, dendritic cell; *FDC*, follicular dendritic cell. (From Hotchkiss RS, Nicholson DW. Apoptosis and caspases regulate death and inflammation in sepsis. *Nat Rev Immunol.* 2006;6:813-822.)

predictive of poor outcomes.[64] IL-10 correlates with the decreased expression of mHLA-DR in septic patients (another marker of sepsis induced immunosuppression, see following section) and may mediate this finding.[65] IL-10 may prove to be a useful marker of immune dysfunction but needs to be evaluated in larger clinical trials. For both pro- and anti-inflammatory cytokines, changes in circulating mediator levels may not correlate with biological activity. Sepsis is associated with changes in cytokine receptor levels[66] and alterations in intracellular signaling pathways[67] that make the biological consequence of circulating cytokine levels difficult to interpret.

Another possibility for evaluating the robustness of the immune response is quantitation of the mHLA-DR cell surface expression in the septic patient. mHLA-DR expression was reduced in patients who develop nosocomial infections after trauma, surgery, and pancreatitis.[68] Patients who recovered from these complications also recovered mHLA-DR expression.[68] This finding became apparent only 48 hours after the onset of sepsis.[69] Therefore, measuring mHLA-DR expression in critically ill patients with concern for sepsis sequentially over time may help to identify patients in the early phases of sepsis. However, monitoring mHLA-DR is difficult because there is no reliable, standardized testing system at this time.

Procalcitonin has been widely investigated as a serum marker to differentiate SIRS from sepsis. Several small trials indicate that procalcitonin predicts mortality in critically ill patients.[70–72] A 2007 metaanalysis reviewed the available clinical data and concluded that procalcitonin cannot be used to distinguish sepsis from SIRS and that more studies are needed.[70]

POTENTIAL THERAPIES AIMED AT SEPSIS-INDUCED IMMUNOSUPPRESSION

Antiinflammatory therapies, including TNF-α antagonists, IL-1 receptor antagonists, antiendotoxin antibodies, and corticosteroids, have not been shown to decrease overall mortality in patients with sepsis. Data suggest that new approaches aimed at stimulating the immune system will succeed where interventions based on inhibiting the immune response have failed.[11] In septic patients with decreased expression of HLA-DR, treatment with GM-CSF was associated with a decrease in the number of ICU days and decreased Acute Physiology and Chronic Health Evaluation (APACHE –II) score.[73] Based upon these encouraging results, a large multicenter trial of GM-CSF was completed in 2015, assessing both restoration of immune function and improvement in clinical outcomes from sepsis; results of this trial are pending.[74] Treatment with IFN-γ improved mHLA-DR expression and mortality in a small group of septic patients but has not been studied in a large clinical trial[75] and case report suggests that IFN-gamma can be effective in treating staphylococcal sepsis.[76] The potential for IFN-gamma treatment to improve outcomes from sepsis is currently being evaluated in a large randomized controlled trial.[77]

Blockade of the interaction between the inhibitory receptor PD-1 and its cognate receptor PD-L1 is also being evaluated as a potential therapeutic avenue in sepsis.[14] PD-1 is an inhibitory costimulatory molecule expressed by T-cells. It is expressed after persistent antigenic stimulation of a T-cell; ligation of PD-1 by its cognate ligand results in T-cell anergy with abrogation of proliferation and cytokine secretion.[14] An increased proportion of splenocytes from septic patients expressed PD-1, and its ligand PD-L1 was upregulated on antigen presenting cells and macrophage isolated from septic patients.[66] In animal models, several groups have demonstrated blockade of PD-1/PD-L1 interactions improved survival.[78–80] Antibodies blocking the PD-1/PD-L1 interaction have been used successfully as an immunostimulant in cancer patients.[81] Clinical studies to evaluate the efficacy of PD-1 modulation in sepsis are under development.

Researchers are also initiating clinical trials of the cytokine IL-7 as an immunomodulator. IL-7 acts broadly on cells of the adaptive immune system, driving the proliferation and survival of T-cells, B-cells and innate lymphoid cells including natural killer cells. IL-7 increased lymphocyte counts in cancer patient and in HIV+ patients with persistently low CD4+ T-cell counts. Therapeutic exogenous IL-7 lead to a predominate increase in CD4+ and CD8+ T-cells with no significant increase in B-cell numbers.[82] In ex-vivo studies, IL-7 reversed sepsis-induced lymphocyte hyporesponsiveness. Ex-vivo treatment of lymphocytes isolated from septic patients with IL-7 increased levels of the antiapoptotic molecule BCL-2 relative to that seen in healthy controls.[83] Ex-vivo IL-7 treatment improved sepsis-induced deficits in lymphocyte IFN-gamma production.[83] IL-7 treatment improved sepsis survival and lymphocyte function in a clinically relevant animal model of sepsis.[84] In a recent phase-IIb clinical trial, IL-7 treatment was well tolerated in septic patients and reversed sepsis-induced lymphopenia.[85] These results make a compelling case for a larger trial of IL-7 as an immune adjuvant in sepsis.

CONCLUSION

Previous theories regarding the pathophysiology of sepsis failed to appropriately characterize sepsis-associated immune dysfunction. Most deaths in sepsis occur after the initial hyperdynamic, proinflammatory phase when patients are unable to clear either primary infection or develop secondary, nosocomial infections. This period of hypoinflammation or immunosuppression is an important cause of mortality, and patients who recover immune function tend to resolve their infections and ultimately survive. Lymphocyte apoptosis, T-cell anergy, increased proportion of T-regulatory cells, monocyte deactivation, decreased HLA-DR expression, a T_H2 cytokine profile, and neutrophil impairment are all hallmarks of immunosuppression in sepsis. Diagnostic modalities that will enable the physician to track a patient's immune status and tailor treatment accordingly need to be developed. The goal is to be able to administer immune-stimulating therapies during periods of immune suppression and several promising candidates are under development.

AUTHORS' RECOMMENDATIONS

- Septic patients develop an immunosuppressed state characterized by loss of delayed hypersensitivity, inability to clear primary infections, and susceptibility to secondary infections.
- Most deaths in sepsis occur late in the course of the syndrome, and survivors show evidence of immune recovery.
- Mechanisms of immunosuppression in sepsis include lymphocyte, dendritic cell, and gut apoptosis, a switch from a T_H1 to a T_H2 cytokine profile, release of anti-inflammatory mediators, lymphocyte anergy, and monocyte deactivation.
- Diagnostic modalities aimed at monitoring the immune response in sepsis may help tailor future therapies intended to modulate the immune system.

REFERENCES

1. Koch R, Cheyne WW. *Investigations into the Etiology of Traumatic Infective Diseases*. London, UK: The New Sydenham Society; 1880.
2. Schweinburg FB, Fine J. Evidence for a lethal endotoxemia as the fundamental feature of irreversibility in three types of traumatic shock. *J Exp Med*. 1960;112:793-800.
3. Cerami A, Ikeda Y, Le Trang N, Hotez PJ, Beutler B. Weight loss associated with an endotoxin-induced mediator from peritoneal macrophages: the role of cachectin (tumor necrosis factor). *Immunol Lett*. 1985;11(3-4):173-177.
4. Baue AE. The horror autotoxicus and multiple-organ failure. *Arch Surg*. 1992;127(12):1451-1462.
5. Zeni F, Freeman B, Natanson C. Anti-inflammatory therapies to treat sepsis and septic shock: a reassessment. *Crit Care Med*. 1997;25(7):1095-1100.
6. Fisher Jr CJ, Slotman GJ, Opal SM, et al. Initial evaluation of human recombinant interleukin-1 receptor antagonist in the treatment of sepsis syndrome: a randomized, open-label, placebo-controlled multicenter trial. *Crit Care Med*. 1994;22(1):12-21.
7. Abraham E, Wunderink R, Silverman H, et al. Efficacy and safety of monoclonal antibody to human tumor necrosis factor alpha in patients with sepsis syndrome. a randomized, controlled, double-blind, multicenter clinical trial. Tnf-Alpha Mab Sepsis Study Group. *JAMA*. 1995;273(12):934-941.
8. Ziegler EJ, Fisher Jr CJ, Sprung CL, et al. Treatment of gram-negative bacteremia and septic shock with Ha-1a human monoclonal antibody against endotoxin. A randomized, double-blind, placebo-controlled trial. The Ha-1a Sepsis Study Group. *N Engl J Med*. 1991;324(7):429-436.
9. Bone RC, Fisher Jr CJ, Clemmer TP, Slotman GJ, Metz CA, Balk RA. A controlled clinical trial of high-dose methylprednisolone in the treatment of severe sepsis and septic shock. *N Engl J Med*. 1987;317(11):653-658.
10. Fisher Jr CJ, Agosti JM, Opal SM, et al. Treatment of septic shock with the tumor necrosis factor receptor:Fc fusion protein. The Soluble TNF Receptor Sepsis Study Group. *N Engl J Med*. 1996;334(26):1697-1702.
11. Delano MJ, Ward PA. Sepsis-induced immune dysfunction: can immune therapies reduce mortality? *J Clin Invest*. 2016;126(1):23-31.
12. Hotchkiss RS, Karl IE. The pathophysiology and treatment of sepsis. *N Engl J Med*. 2003;348(2):138-150.
13. Hotchkiss RS, Monneret G, Payen D. Sepsis-induced immunosuppression: from cellular dysfunctions to immunotherapy. *Nat Rev Immunol*. 2013;13(12):862-874.
14. Hotchkiss RS, Monneret G, Payen D. Immunosuppression in sepsis: a novel understanding of the disorder and a new therapeutic approach. *Lancet Infect Dis*. 2013;13(3):260-268.
15. Matzinger P. The danger model: a renewed sense of self. *Science*. 2002;296(5566):301-305.
16. Oberholzer A, Oberholzer C, Moldawer LL. Sepsis syndromes: understanding the role of innate and acquired immunity. *Shock*. 2001;16(2):83-96.
17. Bone RC, Balk RA, Cerra FB, et al. Definitions for sepsis and organ failure and guidelines for the use of innovative therapies in sepsis. The ACCP/SCCM Consensus Conference Committee. American College of Chest Physicians/Society of Critical Care Medicine. *Chest*. 1992;101(6):1644-1655.
18. Bone RC. Sir Isaac Newton, sepsis, SIRS, and CARS. *Crit Care Med*. 1996;24(7):1125-1128.
19. Daviaud F, Grimaldi D, Dechartres A, et al. Timing and causes of death in septic shock. *Ann Intensive Care*. 2015;5(1):16.
20. Torgersen C, Moser P, Luckner G, et al. Macroscopic postmortem findings in 235 surgical intensive care patients with sepsis. *Anesth Analg*. 2009;108(6):1841-1847.
21. Otto GP, Sossdorf M, Claus RA, et al. The late phase of sepsis is characterized by an increased microbiological burden and death rate. *Crit Care*. 2011;15(4):R183.
22. Rhodes A, Evans LE, Alhazzani W, et al. Surviving Sepsis Campaign: international guidelines for management of sepsis and septic shock: 2016. *Crit Care Med*. 2017;45(3):486-552.
23. Zhao GJ, Li D, Zhao Q, et al. Incidence, risk factors and impact on outcomes of secondary infection in patients with septic shock: an 8-year retrospective study. *Sci Rep*. 2016;6:38361.
24. van Vught LA, Klein Klouwenberg PM, Spitoni C, et al. Incidence, risk factors, and attributable mortality of secondary infections in the intensive care unit after admission for sepsis. *JAMA*. 2016;315(14):1469-1479.
25. van der Poll T, van de Veerdonk FL, Scicluna BP, Netea MG. The immunopathology of sepsis and potential therapeutic targets. *Nat Rev Immunol*. 2017;17(7):407-420.
26. Sun A, Netzer G, Small DS, et al. Association between index hospitalization and hospital readmission in sepsis survivors. *Crit Care Med*. 2016;44(3):478-487.
27. Wang T, Derhovanessian A, De Cruz S, Belperio JA, Deng JC, Hoo GS. Subsequent infections in survivors of sepsis: epidemiology and outcomes. *J Intensive Care Med*. 2014;29(2):87-95.
28. Altemeier WA, Todd JC, Inge WW. Gram-negative septicemia: a growing threat. *Ann Surg*. 1967;166(4):530-542.
29. Davila S, Halstead ES, Hall MW, et al. Viral DNAemia and immune suppression in pediatric sepsis. *Pediatr Crit Care Med*. 2018;19(1):e14-e22.
30. Walton AH, Muenzer JT, Rasche D, et al. Reactivation of multiple viruses in patients with sepsis. *PLoS One*. 2014;9(2):e98819.
31. La Rosa C, Limaye AP, Krishnan A, Longmate J, Diamond DJ. Longitudinal assessment of cytomegalovirus (CMV)-specific immune responses in liver transplant recipients at high risk for late CMV disease. *J Infect Dis*. 2007;195(5):633-644.
32. Limaye AP, Boeckh M. CMV in critically ill patients: pathogen or bystander? *Rev Med Virol*. 2010;20(6):372-379.
33. Limaye AP, Huang ML, Leisenring W, Stensland L, Corey L, Boeckh M. Cytomegalovirus (CMV) DNA load in plasma for

the diagnosis of CMV disease before engraftment in hematopoietic stem-cell transplant recipients. *J Infect Dis.* 2001; 183(3):377-382.

34. Ong DSY, Bonten MJM, Spitoni C, et al. Epidemiology of multiple herpes viremia in previously immunocompetent patients with septic shock. *Clin Infect Dis.* 2017;64(9): 1204-1210.

35. Hotchkiss RS., Moldawer LL, Opal SM, Reinhart K, Turnbull IR, Vincent JL. Sepsis and septic shock. *Nat Rev Dis Primers.* 2016;2:16045.

36. Alexander JW, Meakins JL. A physiological basis for the development of opportunistic infections in man. *Ann Surg.* 1972; 176(3):273-287.

37. Kaufmann I, Hoelzl A, Schliephake F, et al. Polymorphonuclear leukocyte dysfunction syndrome in patients with increasing sepsis severity. *Shock.* 2006;26(3):254-261.

38. Demaret J, Venet F, Friggeri A, et al. Marked alterations of neutrophil functions during sepsis-induced immunosuppression. *J Leukoc Biol.* 2015;98(6):1081-1090.

39. Vespasiano MC, Lewandoski JR, Zimmerman JJ. Longitudinal analysis of neutrophil superoxide anion generation in patients with septic shock. *Crit Care Med.* 1993;21(5):666-672.

40. Weighardt H, Heidecke CD, Emmanuilidis K, et al. Sepsis after major visceral surgery is associated with sustained and interferon-gamma-resistant defects of monocyte cytokine production. *Surgery.* 2000;127(3):309-315.

41. Astiz M, Saha D, Lustbader D, Lin R, Rackow E. Monocyte response to bacterial toxins, expression of cell surface receptors, and release of anti-inflammatory cytokines during sepsis. *J Lab Clin Med.* 1996;128(6):594-600.

42. Manjuck J, Saha DC, Astiz M, Eales LJ, Rackow EC. Decreased response to recall antigens is associated with depressed costimulatory receptor expression in septic critically ill patients. *J Lab Clin Med.* 2000;135(2):153-160.

43. Ost M, Singh A, Peschel A, Mehling R, Rieber N, Hartl D. Myeloid-derived suppressor cells in bacterial infections. *Front Cell Infect Microbiol.* 2016;6:37.

44. Cuenca AG, Delano MJ, Kelly-Scumpia KM, et al. A paradoxical role for myeloid-derived suppressor cells in sepsis and trauma. *Mol Med.* 2011;17(3-4):281-292.

45. Delano MJ, Scumpia PO, Weinstein JS, et al. Myd88-dependent expansion of an immature Gr-1(+)Cd11b(+) population induces T cell suppression and Th2 polarization in sepsis. *J Exp Med.* 2007;204(6):1463-1474.

46. Mathias B, Delmas AL, Ozrazgat-Baslanti T, et al. Human myeloid-derived suppressor cells are associated with chronic immune suppression after severe sepsis/septic shock. *Ann Surg.* 2017;265(4):827-834.

47. Hotchkiss RS, Swanson PE, Freeman BD, et al. Apoptotic cell death in patients with sepsis, shock, and multiple organ dysfunction. *Crit Care Med.* 1999;27(7):1230-1251.

48. Hotchkiss RS, Tinsley KW, Swanson PE, et al. Depletion of dendritic cells, but not macrophages, in patients with sepsis. *J Immunol.* 2002;168(5):2493-2500.

49. Hotchkiss RS, Tinsley KW, Swanson PE, et al. Sepsis-induced apoptosis causes progressive profound depletion of B and CD4+ T lymphocytes in humans. *J Immunol.* 2001;166(11): 6952-6963.

50. Hotchkiss RS, Chang KC, Grayson MH, et al. Adoptive transfer of apoptotic splenocytes worsens survival, whereas adoptive transfer of necrotic splenocytes improves survival in sepsis. *Proc Natl Acad Sci U S A.* 2003;100(11):6724-6729.

51. Hotchkiss RS, Chang KC, Swanson PE, et al. Caspase inhibitors improve survival in sepsis: a critical role of the lymphocyte. *Nat Immunol.* 2000;1(6):496-501.

52. Coopersmith CM, Stromberg PE, Dunne WM, et al. Inhibition of intestinal epithelial apoptosis and survival in a murine model of pneumonia-induced sepsis. *JAMA.* 2002;287(13): 1716-1721.

53. Hotchkiss RS, Swanson PE, Knudson CM, et al. Overexpression of Bcl-2 in transgenic mice decreases apoptosis and improves survival in sepsis. *J Immunol.* 1999;162(7):4148-4156.

54. Hotchkiss RS, Dunne WM, Swanson PE, et al. Role of apoptosis in pseudomonas aeruginosa pneumonia. *Science.* 2001; 294(5548):1783.

55. Venet F, Chung CS, Monneret G, et al. Regulatory T cell populations in sepsis and trauma. *J Leukoc Biol.* 2008;83(3):523-535.

56. Venet F, Pachot A, Debard AL, et al. Increased percentage of CD4+CD25+ regulatory T cells during septic shock is due to the decrease of CD4+CD25- lymphocytes. *Crit Care Med.* 2004;32(11):2329-2331.

57. MacConmara MP, Maung AA, Fujimi S, et al. Increased CD4+ CD25+ T regulatory cell activity in trauma patients depresses protective Th1 immunity. *Ann Surg.* 2006;244(4):514-523.

58. Wisnoski N, Chung CS, Chen Y, Huang X, Ayala A. The contribution of CD4+ CD25+ T-regulatory-cells to immune suppression in sepsis. *Shock.* 2007;27(3):251-257.

59. Scumpia PO, Delano MJ, Kelly-Scumpia KM, et al. Treatment with GITR agonistic antibody corrects adaptive immune dysfunction in sepsis. *Blood.* 2007;110(10):3673-3681.

60. Scumpia PO, Delano MJ, Kelly KM, et al. Increased natural CD4+CD25+ regulatory T cells and their suppressor activity do not contribute to mortality in murine polymicrobial sepsis. *J Immunol.* 2006;177(11):7943-7949.

61. Oberholzer A, Souza SM, Tschoeke SK, et al. Plasma cytokine measurements augment prognostic scores as indicators of outcome in patients with severe sepsis. *Shock.* 2005;23(6):488-493.

62. Monneret G, Finck ME, Venet F, et al. The anti-inflammatory response dominates after septic shock: association of low monocyte HLA-DR expression and high interleukin-10 concentration. *Immunol Lett.* 2004;95(2):193-198.

63. Gogos CA, Drosou E, Bassaris HP, Skoutelis A. Pro- versus anti-inflammatory cytokine profile in patients with severe sepsis: a marker for prognosis and future therapeutic options. *J Infect Dis.* 2000;181(1):176-180.

64. van Dissel JT, van Langevelde P, Westendorp RG, Kwappenberg K, Frölich M. Anti-inflammatory cytokine profile and mortality in febrile patients. *Lancet.* 1998;351(9107):950-953.

65. Lekkou A, Karakantza M, Mouzaki A, Kalfarentzos F, Gogos CA. Cytokine production and monocyte HLA-DR expression as predictors of outcome for patients with community-acquired severe infections. *Clin Diagn Lab Immunol.* 2004;11(1):161-167.

66. Boomer JS, To K, Chang KC, et al. Immunosuppression in patients who die of sepsis and multiple organ failure. *JAMA.* 2011;306(23):2594-2605.

67. Abcejo AS, Andrejko KM, Raj NR, Deutschman CS. Failed interleukin-6 signal transduction in murine sepsis: attenuation of hepatic glycoprotein 130 phosphorylation. *Crit Care Med.* 2009;37(5):1729-1734.

68. Muehlstedt SG, Lyte M, Rodriguez JL. Increased IL-10 production and HLA-DR suppression in the lungs of injured patients precede the development of nosocomial pneumonia. *Shock.* 2002;17(6):443-450.

69. Monneret G, Elmenkouri N, Bohe J, et al. Analytical requirements for measuring monocytic human lymphocyte antigen DR by flow cytometry: application to the monitoring of patients with septic shock. *Clin Chem.* 2002;48(9):1589-1592.

70. Tang BM, Eslick GD, Craig JC, McLean AS. Accuracy of procalcitonin for sepsis diagnosis in critically ill patients: systematic review and meta-analysis. *Lancet Infect Dis.* 2007;7(3):210-217.

71. Novotny A, Emmanuel K, Matevossian E, et al. Use of procalcitonin for early prediction of lethal outcome of postoperative sepsis. *Am J Surg.* 2007;194(1):35-39.

72. Jensen JU, Heslet L, Jensen TH, Espersen K, Steffensen P, Tvede M. Procalcitonin increase in early identification of critically ill patients at high risk of mortality. *Crit Care Med.* 2006;34(10):2596-2602.

73. Meisel C, Schefold JC, Pschowski R, et al. Granulocyte-macrophage colony-stimulating factor to reverse sepsis-associated immunosuppression: a double-blind, randomized, placebo-controlled multicenter trial. *Am J Respir Crit Care Med.* 2009;180(7):640-648.

74. U.S. National Library of Medicine. Does GM-CSF restore neutrophil phagocytosis in critical illness? *ClinicalTrials.gov (website).* 2018. Available at: http://clinicaltrials.gov/show/NCT01653665. Accessed November 14, 2018.

75. Döcke WD, Randow F, Syrbe U, et al. Monocyte deactivation in septic patients: restoration by ifn-gamma treatment. *Nat Med.* 1997;3(6):678-681.

76. Nalos M, Santner-Nanan B, Parnell G, Tang B, McLean AS, Nanan R. Immune effects of interferon gamma in persistent staphylococcal sepsis. *Am J Respir Crit Care Med.* 2012;185(1):110-112.

77. U.S. National Library of Medicine. The effects of interferon-gamma on sepsis-induced immunoparalysis. *ClinicalTrials.gov (website).* 2017. Available at https://clinicaltrials.gov/ct2/show/NCT01649921. Accessed November 14, 2018.

78. Huang X, Venet F, Wang YL, et al. PD-1 expression by macrophages plays a pathologic role in altering microbial clearance and the innate inflammatory response to sepsis. *Proc Natl Acad Sci U S A.* 2009;106(15):6303-6308.

79. Brahmamdam P, Inoue S, Unsinger J, Chang KC, McDunn JE, Hotchkiss RS. Delayed administration of anti-PD-1 antibody reverses immune dysfunction and improves survival during sepsis. *J Leukoc Biol.* 2010;88(2):233-240.

80. Zhang Y, Zhou Y, Lou J, et al. PD-L1 blockade improves survival in experimental sepsis by inhibiting lymphocyte apoptosis and reversing monocyte dysfunction. *Crit Care.* 2010;14(6):R220.

81. Topalian SL, Hodi FS, Brahmer JR, et al. Safety, activity, and immune correlates of anti-PD-1 antibody in cancer. *N Engl J Med.* 2012;366(26):2443-2454.

82. Lundström W, Fewkes NM, Mackall CL. IL-7 in human health and disease. *Semin Immunol.* 2012;24(3):218-224.

83. Venet F, Foray AP, Villars-Méchin A, et al. IL-7 restores lymphocyte functions in septic patients. *J Immunol.* 2012;189(10):5073-5081.

84. Unsinger J, McGlynn M, Kasten KR, et al. IL-7 promotes T cell viability, trafficking, and functionality and improves survival in sepsis. *J Immunol.* 2010;184(7):3768-3779.

85. Francois, B., et al. "Interleukin-7 Restores Lymphocytes in Septic Shock: The Iris-7 Randomized Clinical Trial." *JCI Insight.* 2018;3(5):e98960.

33

Is There Immune Suppression in the Critically Ill Patient—Con?

Jean-Marc Cavaillon and Evangelos J. Giamarellos-Bourboulis

INTRODUCTION

The systemic inflammatory response syndrome (SIRS) is regularly observed in critically ill patients. Naturally occurring mechanisms aimed to dampen overzealous inflammation lead to an opposing phenomenon known as the compensatory anti-inflammatory response syndrome (CARS).[1] CARS is associated with an alteration in blood leukocyte immune status in critically ill patients. The phenomenon has been regularly described using words such as immunoparalysis,[2] immunodepression,[3] anergy,[4] or immunosuppression.[5–9] This characterization is misleading. The authors suggest that immune failure influences patient outcome in a manner similar to that observed in organ failure. For example, posttraumatic immunosuppression has been suggested to be one of the leading causes of postsurgical mortality,[10] and reversing immunosuppression has been proposed as a potentially major advance in the treatment of sepsis.[11] However, to the best of our knowledge, immunosuppression is not an appropriate term to qualify the immune status of critically ill patients because (1) immune cells within tissues of critically ill or sepsis patients are rarely hyporeactive or desensitized, (2) reprogramming of blood leukocytes (or from lymphoid organs) does not correspond to a global functional extinction, and (3) the nature of the agonist used to activate the immune cells influences the observation. Indeed, CARS corresponds to a reprogramming of circulating immune cells,[12] reminiscent of the phenomenon of endotoxin tolerance, itself associated to trained innate immunity.[13]

REPROGRAMMING OF CIRCULATING BLOOD LEUKOCYTES

An altered immune status is regularly associated with an increased frequency of nosocomial infections among intensive care unit (ICU) patients. In particular, viral reactivation (cytomegalovirus, herpes simplex virus, Epstein–Barr virus, etc.) has been reported to influence the length of hospital stay, disease severity, and, eventually, outcome.[14–20] However, evidence supporting nosocomial infection as the major cause of death in sepsis remains weak.[21] Indeed, in a Dutch investigation, the overall contribution of secondary infections to short-term mortality was shown to be quite modest.[22] As stated by Derek Angus and Steven Opal:

> Early hopes that immune suppression would be a unifying and common feature of all patients with sepsis who have poor outcomes are not supported by this study. However, immune dysfunction does appear to have an important role in a subset of patients.[23]

Most interestingly, in a study of solid organ transplant patients, recipients with sepsis had a significantly lower risk of death at 28 days than nontransplanted patients[24]; rather, this study suggested that the immunosuppression associated with transplantation may provide a survival advantage to the transplant recipients with sepsis through the modulation of the inflammatory response.

Although CARS has been regularly claimed to take place after the occurrence of SIRS, we postulated in 2001 that the two responses occurred almost concomitantly,[25] a distinction that is illustrated by the significant positive correlations observed between proinflammatory and anti-inflammatory cytokines measured in the bloodstream. The altered immune status is illustrated by a major lymphopenia[26,27] associated with a significant apoptosis of lymphocytes and dendritic cells.[28] In contrast, spontaneous and induced apoptosis of neutrophils is reduced.[29–31]

The immune alteration can be demonstrated in vivo by reduced delayed-type hypersensitivity assessed by skin test reactivity.[32] Analyses performed ex vivo have demonstrated a lower capacity of monocytes and lymphocytes to produce cytokines in response to certain agonists.[33] In addition, the lymphocyte proliferative response to mitogens is decreased,[34–36] illustrating a generalized metabolic defect at the level of both glycolysis and oxidative metabolism in leukocytes from patients. Another hallmark of this alteration is the lower expression of human leukocyte antigen DR isotype (HLA-DR).[37–41] Of note, the expression of many other cell surface markers is either decreased (e.g., tumor necrosis factor receptor [TNFR] p75, CD14, Toll-like receptor 4 [TLR4], transferrin receptor [CD71], coactivation marker CD86, and fractalkine receptor [CX3CR1]), or increased (TNFR p50, CD40, CD48, CD64, CD69, triggering receptor expressed on myeloid cells-1 [TREM-1], tissue factor, programmed death-1 [PD1], and PD-ligand-1 [PDL1]).

NATURE OF THE ACTIVATING SIGNAL

Most interestingly, whenever ex vivo cytokine production by monocytes is assessed by using endotoxin as a triggering agent, the production of most proinflammatory cytokines (e.g., tumor necrosis factor [TNF] and interleukin-1 [IL-1] and IL-6) is shown to be decreased while that of anti-inflammatory cytokines (e.g., IL-10, IL-1Ra) is shown to be enhanced. However, when whole heat-killed bacteria (e.g., *Staphylococcus aureus*) were used instead of endotoxin, a normal production of inflammatory cytokines was observed in patients with trauma,[42] patients with sepsis,[43] patients successfully resuscitated after cardiac arrest,[44] or in patients with stroke-related brain death.[45] When neutrophil IL-1β production from sepsis patients was assessed, lipopolysaccharide (LPS)-induced secretion was significantly reduced but that induced by *S. aureus* was unchanged as compared with healthy controls.[46] Similarly, when IκBα expression was analyzed in the cytoplasm of peripheral blood mononuclear cells (PBMCs) from trauma patients, an altered expression was found in response to LPS, as compared with healthy controls, while similar no differences were observed for heat-killed *S. aureus*.[47] In patients with orthopedic trauma, TNF-α production of whole blood upon stimulation with LPS or peptidoglycan induced different profiles, with a reduced production on day 1 postsurgery in response to LPS and an unaltered production in response to peptidoglycan.[48] While studying ex vivo IL-12 production by blood dendritic cells in patients with aneurysmal subarachnoid hemorrhage, Asehnoune et al.[49] reported that the responses to TLR3 and TLR4 agonists were significantly decreased as compared with healthy controls, but the response to a TLR7/8 agonist was unchanged. Most interestingly, in a murine model of hemorrhagic shock, Asehnoune et al.[50] showed that the ex vivo production of TNF in response to LPS was altered, whereas that was not the case in response to heat-killed *S. aureus*. In patients with sepsis, it was reported that monocyte-dependent indoleamine 2,3-dioxygenase activity was reduced in response to LPS, but was unchanged in response to interferon gamma (IFN-γ).[51] A similar discrepancy was observed for lymphocyte-derived cytokines (i.e., IL-2, IL-5, and IL-10), the production of which was decreased in sepsis patients when concanavalin A was used as a T-cell activator but not when phytohemagglutinin was used.[52] These results further illustrate that the nature of the activator used to stimulate the cells greatly influences the read out. One may speculate that the different signaling pathways are not modified/reprogrammed similarly after a first activation.

UNALTERED FUNCTIONS OF CIRCULATING LEUKOCYTES

Monocytes from SIRS and sepsis patients display an altered capacity to produce TNF and other inflammatory cytokines in response to LPS, but other functions such as phagocytosis are not altered. Monocytes of sepsis patients do not display a major alteration of their phagocytosis of fluorescein isothiocyanate (FITC)—of green fluorescent protein (GFP)-labeled *Escherichia coli*.[53,54] Furthermore, Biswas and colleagues showed that, during sepsis, monocytes display enhanced antimicrobial activity, enhanced metalloproteinase-9 and -19 mRNA production, and enhanced vascular endothelial growth factor alpha (VEGF-α) release when compared with monocytes of patients who had recovered from sepsis.[54] We also found that the ex vivo production of macrophage migration inhibitory factor (MIF) was enhanced when analyzing PBMCs from sepsis patients as compared with healthy controls.[55] Of interest is the work of Chaudry's group, demonstrating that altered ex vivo splenocyte proliferation, as well as IL-2 and IL-3 release in response to concanavalin A observed in male mice undergoing trauma hemorrhage, was not observed in female animals. The phenomenon was shown to be regulated by both male and female hormones.[56,57]

TISSUE IMMUNE CELLS AS THE MAIN SOURCE OF INFLAMMATORY CYTOKINES

As illustrated in Table 33.1, during sterile or infectious inflammation, tissues are a major source of inflammatory cytokines,

TABLE 33.1 Some Examples of Tissues as the Main Source of Inflammatory Cytokines Following Different Types of Aggression in Animal Models.

Organ	Nature of Insult	Increased Cytokines	References
Liver	*S. hemolyticus*	↑ IFNγ, IL-2, IL-10, IL-12 mRNAs	*Vallespi et al., Int Immunopharmacol, 2004;4:343*
	LPS injection	↑ TNF-α (mRNA + protein)	*Qin et al., Glia, 2007;55:453*
	CLP	↑ TNF-α, IL-1β, CXCL1 gene expression	*Hviid et al., Innate Immun, 2012;18:717*
	P. aeruginosa	↑ Lipid peroxidation	*Toufekoula et al., Crit Care, 2013;17:R6*
	Gut IR	↑ TNF-α, IL-1β, IL-6 gene expression	*Collange et al., Eur J Vasc Endovasc Surg, 2015;49:60*
Spleen	LPS	↑ TNF-α production	*Fitting et al., J Infect Dis, 2004;189:1295*
	E. coli	↑ IL-1α, IL-1β	*Ge et al., J Infect Dis, 1997;176:1313*
	N. meningitidis	↑ IL-1β, TNF-α production	*Hellerud et al., Shock, 2015;44:458*

TABLE 33.1   Some Examples of Tissues as the Main Source of Inflammatory Cytokines Following Different Types of Aggression in Animal Models.—cont'd

Organ	Nature of Insult	Increased Cytokines	References
Lungs	Hemorrhage	↑ IL-1β, IL-6, IL-10, IFN-γ gene expression	Shenkar et al., Am J Respir Cell Mol Biol, 1994;10:290
	S. haemolyticus	↑ IFNγ, IL-2, IL-10, IL-12 mRNAs	Vallespi et al., Int Immunopharmacol, 2004;10-11:1343
	Hemorrhage	↑ NF-κB activation (Alv. MØ)	Papia et al., Shock, 2011;35:171
	CLP	↑ TNF-α, IL-6, CXCL1 gene expression	Hviid et al., Innate Immun, 2012;18:717
	Gut IR	↑ IL-1β, IL-6 gene expression	Collange et al., Eur J Vasc Endovasc Surg, 2015;49:60
Heart	LPS	↑ TNF-α, IL-1β, IL-6, MCP-1 production	Kadokami et al., Am J Physiol Heart Circ, 2001;280:H2281
	CLP	↑ TNF-α mRNA expression	Zhou et al., Oncotarget, 2017;8:47317
	Heart IR	Mast cell derived TNF	Frangogiannis et al., Circulation, 1998;98:699
Brain	LPS	↑ TNF-α (mRNA + protein)	Qin et al., Glia, 2007;55:453
	LPS, IL-1β, TNFα,	↑ hypothalamic and hippocampal TNF mRNA	Skelly et al., Plos One, 2013;8:e69123
	Laparotomy	↑ hippocampus IL-1β and IL-8 mRNA	Huang et al., J Neuroinflammation, 2018;15:147
Gut	Abdominal aortic surgery	High levels of TNF-α in portal vein	Cabié et al., Cytokine, 1993;5:448
	Brain injury	TNF in intestine	Jin et al., Cytokine, 2008;44:135
	Kidney IR	↑ inflammatory cytokine genes	Park et al., Lab Invest, 2011;91:63
	Liver IR	Production of IL-17 by Paneth cells causes MOF	Park et al., Hepatology 2011;53:1662
	Gut IR	↑ TNF-α, IL-1β, IL-6 gene expression	Collange et al., Eur J Vasc Endovasc Surg, 2015;49:60
Kidney	LPS	↑ TNF-α (endothelial cells)	Kita et al., Int J Exp Pathol, 1993;74:471
	LPS	↑ IL-1α (endothelial cells)	Laszik et al., Circ Shock, 1994;43:115
	LPS	↑ TNF-α, iNOS gene expression	Zager et al., Kidney Int, 2007;71:496
	E. coli	↑ TNF-α, IL-6 gene expression	Muller et al., J Clin Endocrinol Metab, 2001;86:396
	Intestinal IR	↑ inflammatory cytokine genes	Lee et al., Am J Physiol, 2013;304:G12
Muscle	E. coli	↑ TNF-α, IL-6 gene expression	Muller et al., J Clin Endocrinol Metab, 2001;86:396
Adipose tissue	Sepsis	↑ TNF-α & iNOS activity	Annane et al., Lancet, 2000;355:1143
	LPS	↑ IL-1α, IL-1β, TNF-α, IL-6 gene expression	Starr et al., Aging Cell, 2013;12:194
	anti-CD40+IL-2	Cytokine storm	Mirsoian et al., J Exp Med, 2014;211:2373
Bone marrow	LPS	in situ detection of TNF	Schmauder-Chock et al., Histochem J, 1994;26:142
	LPS	↑ G-CSF, KC, MIP-2	Zhang et al., Shock, 2005;23:344
	Sepsis	Hemophagocytosis	François et al., Am J Med, 1997;103:114
			Stéphan et al., Clin Infect Dis, 1997;25:1159
			Strauss et al., Crit Care Med, 2004;32:1316
			Schaer et al., Eur J Haematol, 2006;77:462
			Raschke et al., Chest, 2011;140:933

CLP, cecal ligature and puncture; IR, ischemia–reperfusion.

and numerous instances illustrate that remote tissues that are not initially concerned by the insult are producing inflammatory mediators. This is particularly the case in models of ischemia–reperfusion. This process is also illustrated after LPS injection, infections or organ injury, when all tissues are involved. In addition, a crosstalk between organs contributes to perpetuate the ongoing inflammatory process.[58] Each organ has its own specificity in terms of cytokine production as a reflection of its constitutive cells and concentration of different natural mediators in the local environment.

ENHANCED ACTIVATION WITHIN TISSUES

In contrast to the observations with circulating or lymphoid tissues (particularly the spleen) cells, leukocytes derived from organs may not display any alteration in immune status (Table 33.2). Murine in vivo models of endotoxin tolerance demonstrated a decrease in detectable TNF in the bloodstream, but an associated increase in TNF production within the renal cortex.[59] In ex vivo murine models of endotoxin tolerance, we reported that alveolar macrophages do not undergo tolerization because of their specific microenvironment and the local influence of B lymphocytes, natural killer (NK) cells, granulocyte–macrophage colony-stimulating factor GM-CSF, IFN-γ, and IL-18.[60] Most importantly, this observation was confirmed in human volunteers injected with endotoxin.[61,62] In accordance with these experimental models, in patients with acute respiratory distress syndrome, spontaneous and LPS-induced IL-1 production by alveolar macrophages was enhanced when compared with healthy subjects.[63] When signaling molecules were studied in neutrophils from a hemorrhage murine model or after LPS administration, activation was observed in the cells derived from the lungs but not in the cells derived from the

TABLE 33.2 Some Examples of ex Vivo Proofs of Activated Tissue-Derived Leukocytes.

Organ	Cells	Nature of In Vivo Insult	Increased Ex Vivo Observation	References
Lungs	Alv. MØ	ARDS	↑ IL-1 production	Jacobs et al., Am Rev Respir Dis, 1989; 140:1686
	Alv. MØ	ARDS	TNF mRNA expression	Tran Van Nhieu et al., Am Rev Respir Dis, 1993; 147:1585
	Alv. MØ	ARDS	NF-κB activation	Schwartz et al., Crit Care Med, 1996;24:1285
	Alv. MØ	ARDS	NF-κB activation	Moine et al., Shock, 2000; 13:85
	Alv. MØ	Irradiation	↑ TNF-α and IL-8 production	Cavaillon et al., J Endotoxin Res, 2001;7:85
	Alv. MØ	CLP	↑ MIP-2 production	Guo et al., J Immunol, 2006;177:1306
	Alv. MØ	Trauma/CLP	↑ TNF-α and IL-6 production	Suzuki et al., Cytokine, 2006;34:76
	Alv. MØ	LPS	↑ TNF-α production	Smith et al., J Clin Immunol, 1994;14:141
	Alv. MØ	LPS	↑ TNF-α & IL-6 production	Hoogerwerf et al., Am J Respir Cell Mol Biol, 2010;42:349
	Neutrophils	Chronic bronchial sepsis	High spontaneous IL-8 production	Pang et al., Am J Respir Crit Care Med, 1997; 155:726
	Neutrophils	Hemorrhage	NF-κB and CREB activation	Shenkar et al., J Immunol, 1999;163:954
	Sputum PMN	Cystic fibrosis	High spontaneous IL-8 production	Petit-Bertron et al., Cytokine, 2008;41:54
Peritoneum	Per. MØ	Peritonitis	↑ IL-1 production	Fieren et al., Eur J Clin Invest, 1990;20:453
	Per. MØ	CLP	↑ TNF-α production	Ellaban et al., Cell Immunol, 2004;231:103
	Per. Dendritic ¢	CLP	↑ IL-12 production	Ding et al., Shock, 2004; 22:137
	Peyer's patch ¢	Fracture	↑ Proliferation	Buzdon et al., J Surg Res, 1999;82:201

TABLE 33.2 Some Examples of ex Vivo Proofs of Activated Tissue-Derived Leukocytes.—cont'd

Organ	Cells	Nature of In Vivo Insult	Increased Ex Vivo Observation	References
Gut	Lymphocytes	Trauma/hemorrhage	↑ IL-6 production	Wang et al., J Surg Res, 1998;79:39
	Lymphocytes	LPS	↑ IFN-γ production; proliferation	Nüssler et al., Shock, 2001;16:454
	Peyer's patch ¢	fracture	↑ proliferation	Buzdon et al., J Surg Res, 1999;82:201
Liver	Kupffer cells	Trauma/CLP	↑ TNF-α and IL-6 production	Suzuki et al., Cytokine, 2006;34:76
	Kupffer cells	Fracture	↑ TNF-α and MCP-1 production	Neunaber et al., Immunol Lett, 2013;152:159
Brain	Microglial cells	CLP	↑ TNF-α production	Singer et al., Am J Respir Crit Care Med, 2018; 197:747

ARDS, acute respiratory distress syndrome; *CREB,* cAMP response element binding protein; *MOF,* multiorgan failure.

blood.[64,65] One of the most convincing demonstrations was reported by Chaudry's group when analyzing the murine model of peritonitis alone or associated with trauma hemorrhage.[66] They showed that the ex vivo production of TNF in response to LPS was reduced among peripheral blood mononuclear cells and spleen cells, whereas the production by alveolar macrophages and liver Kupffer cells was enhanced. In a murine model of sepsis, it was reported that spontaneous IL-12 production was reduced when analyzing splenic dendritic cells, whereas in peritoneal dendritic cells, it was enhanced.[67] Similarly, in human peritonitis, LPS + IFN-γ induced more IL-1 production in peritoneal macrophages when compared with infection-free donors.[68] In the skin, it was demonstrated that resident memory CD8+ T lymphocytes maintain Ag-dependent "sensing and alarming" functions (assessed in terms of IFN-γ production) after sepsis, which is in contrast to the reduced activity seen in splenic CD8+ T lymphocytes.[69] An important question was recently addressed concerning microglial cells. In a murine model of sepsis, it was reported that ex vivo activation of isolated microglial cells was associated with an increase in TNF release in response to LPS when compared with control animals.[70] This later result is reminiscent of the long-lasting detection of TNF after LPS injection[71] and the nuclear factor kappa B (NF-κB) upregulation in the hypothalamus of rats injected with repeated doses of LPS.[72] While adipose tissues contribute to inflammatory cytokine production upon LPS injection or after sepsis,[73,74] their involvement appears to increase with age.[75] However, to our knowledge, the nature of the reprogramming within these tissues has, thus far, been poorly studied. Another compartment in which an ongoing activation process has been regularly reported in sepsis is in bone marrow. Indeed, hemophagocytosis has been regularly found in 60–65% of septic and SIRS patients.[76–78] High levels of ferritin have been proposed as a marker of poor outcome and for macrophage activation-like syndrome, although its frequency remains below the one reported following direct bone marrow cell analysis.[79]

AUTHORS' RECOMMENDATIONS
- Despite the worldwide use of the word immunosuppression to qualify the immune status of SIRS and septic patients and proposals to boost the immune system, we consider that this represents an oversimplification of the process and a risky therapeutic approach.[45]
- While many parameters are indeed associated with altered immunity, a more careful analysis reveals that:
  - the observation is mainly achieved with cells from the bloodstream and lymphoid tissues
  - the nature of the agonists used to investigate reactivity of these cells influences the results
  - different cellular functions may be reduced, unchanged, or even enhanced
  - the location of the immune cells greatly influences their functional status.
- Therefore, the immune status of leukocytes reflects an adapted compartmentalized appropriate response aimed to prevent an overzealous inflammatory reaction and to maintain an anti-infectious process, as observed in the different models of endotoxin tolerance.[80]
- Instead of immunosuppression, the word "reprogramming" or "trained innate immunity"[13] better reflects the immune status of circulating leukocytes in SIRS and septic patients, although the word "reprogramming" may better reflect the intrinsic events occurring within the leukocytes to prevent them from an overzealous response while favoring their anti-inflammatory properties and maintaining their anti-infectious functions.[81]

REFERENCES

1. Adib-Conquy M, Cavaillon JM. Compensatory anti-inflammatory response syndrome. *Thromb Haemost.* 2009;101:36-47.
2. Volk HD, Reinke P, Döcke WD. Clinical aspects: from systemic inflammation to "immunoparalysis". *Chem Immunol.* 2000;74: 162-177.
3. Angele MK, Faist E. Clinical review: immunodepression in the surgical patient and increased susceptibility to infection. *Crit Care.* 2002;6:298-305.

4. Dawson CW, Ledgerwood AM, Rosenberg JC, Lucas CE. Anergy and altered lymphocyte function in the injured patient. *Am Surg.* 1982;48:397-401.

5. Gaze WH, Krone SM, Larsson DG, et al. Influence of humans on evolution and mobilization of environmental antibiotic resistome. *Emerg Infect Dis.* 2013;19:e120871.

6. Chopra SS, Haacke N, Meisel C, et al. Postoperative immunosuppression after open and laparoscopic liver resection: assessment of cellular immune function and monocytic HLA-DR expression. *J Soc Laparoendoscopic Surg.* 2013;17:615-621.

7. Roquilly A, Gautreau L, Segain JP, et al. CpG-ODN and MPLA prevent mortality in a murine model of post-hemorrhage-*Staphyloccocus aureus* pneumonia. *PLoS One.* 2010;5:e13228.

8. Kokhaei P, Barough MS, Hassan ZM. Cimetidine effects on the immunosuppression induced by burn injury. *Int Immunopharmacol.* 2014;22:273-276.

9. Fattahi F, Ward PA. Understanding immunosuppression after sepsis. *Immunity.* 2017;47:3-5.

10. Islam MN, Bradley BA, Ceredig R. Sterile post-traumatic immunosuppression. *Clin Transl Immunology.* 2016;5:e77.

11. Hotchkiss RS, Monneret G, Payen D. Immunosuppression in sepsis: a novel understanding of the disorder and a new therapeutic approach. *Lancet Infect Dis.* 2013;13:260-268.

12. Cavaillon JM, Adrie C, Fitting C, Adib-Conquy M. Reprogramming of circulatory cells in sepsis and SIRS. *J Endotoxin Res.* 2005;11:311-320.

13. Netea MG, Quintin J, van der Meer JW. Trained immunity: a memory for innate host defense. *Cell Host Microbe.* 2011;9:355-361.

14. Luyt CE, Combes A, Deback C, et al. Herpes simplex virus lung infection in patients undergoing prolonged mechanical ventilation. *Am J Respir Crit Care Med.* 2007;175:935-942.

15. Kutza AS, Muhl E, Hackstein H, Kirchner H, Bein G. High incidence of active cytomegalovirus infection among septic patients. *Clin Infect Dis.* 1998;26:1076-1082.

16. Linssen CF, Jacobs JA, Stelma FF, et al. Herpes simplex virus load in bronchoalveolar lavage fluid is related to poor outcome in critically ill patients. *Intensive Care Med.* 2008;34 2202-2209.

17. Limaye AP, Kirby KA, Rubenfeld GD, et al. Cytomegalovirus reactivation in critically ill immunocompetent patients. *JAMA.* 2008;300:413-422.

18. Heininger A, Haeberle H, Fischer I, et al. Cytomegalovirus reactivation and associated outcome of critically ill patients with severe sepsis. *Crit Care.* 2011;15:R77.

19. Brenner T, Rosenhagen C, Hornig I, et al. Viral infections in septic shock (VISS-trial)—crosslinks between inflammation and immunosuppression. *J Surg Res.* 2012;176:571-582.

20. Walton AH, Muenzer JT, Rasche D, et al. Reactivation of multiple viruses in patients with sepsis. *PLoS One.* 2014;9:e98819.

21. Goldenberg NM, Leligdowicz A, Slutsky AS, Friedrich JO, Lee WL. Is nosocomial infection really the major cause of death in sepsis? *Crit Care.* 2014;18:540.

22. van Vught LA, Klein Klouwenberg PM, Spitoni C, et al. Incidence, risk factors, and attributable mortality of secondary infections in the intensive care unit after admission for sepsis. *JAMA.* 2016;315:1469-1479.

23. Angus DC, Opal S. Immunosuppression and secondary infection in sepsis: part, not all, of the story. *JAMA.* 2016;315:1457-1459.

24. Kalil AC, Syed A, Rupp ME, et al. Is bacteremic sepsis associated with higher mortality in transplant recipients than in nontransplant patients? A matched case-control propensity-adjusted study. *Clin Infect Dis.* 2015;60:216-222.

25. Cavaillon JM, Adib-Conquy M, Clo®z-Tayarani I, Fitting C. Immunodepression in sepsis and SIRS assessed by ex vivo cytokine production is not a generalized phenomenon: a review. *J Endotoxin Res.* 2001;7:85-93.

26. Roth G, Moser B, Krenn C, et al. Susceptibility to programmed cell death in T-lymphocytes from septic patients: a mechanism for lymphopenia and Th2 predominance. *Biochem Biophys Res Commun.* 2003;308:840-846.

27. Venet F, Davin F, Guignant C, et al. Early assessment of leukocyte alterations at diagnosis of septic shock. *Shock.* 2010; 34:358-363.

28. Le Tulzo Y, Pangault C, Gacouin A, et al. Early circulating lymphocyte apoptosis in human septic shock is associated with poor outcome. *Shock.* 2002;18:487-494.

29. Jia SH, Li Y, Parodo J, et al. Pre-B cell colony-enhancing factor inhibits neutrophil apoptosis in experimental inflammation and clinical sepsis. *J Clin Invest.* 2004;113:1318-1327.

30. Keel M, Ungethüm U, Steckholzer U, et al. Interleukin-10 counterregulates proinflammatory cytokine-induced inhibition of neutrophil apoptosis during severe sepsis. *Blood.* 1997;90:3356-3363.

31. Parlato M, Souza-Fonseca-Guimaraes F, Philippart F, et al. CD24-triggered caspase-dependent apoptosis via mitochondrial membrane depolarization and reactive oxygen species production of human neutrophils is impaired in sepsis. *J Immunol.* 2014;192:2449-2459.

32. MacLean LD, Meakins JL, Taguchi K, Duignan JP, Dhillon KS, Gordon J. Host resistance in sepsis and trauma. *Ann Surg.* 1975;182:207-217.

33. Muñoz C, Carlet J, Fitting C, et al. Dysregulation of in vitro cytokine production by monocytes during sepsis. *J Clin Invest.* 1991;88:1747-1754.

34. Zellweger R, Ayala A, DeMaso CM, Chaudry IH. Trauma-hemorrhage causes prolonged depression in cellular immunity. *Shock.* 1995;4:149-153.

35. Napolitano LM, Koruda MJ, Meyer AA, Baker CC. The impact of femur fracture with associated soft tissue injury on immune function and intestinal permeability. *Shock.* 1996;5: 202-207.

36. Venet F, Chung CS, Kherouf H, et al. Increased circulating regulatory T cells (CD4(+)CD25 (+)CD127 (−)) contribute to lymphocyte anergy in septic shock patients. *Intensive Care Med.* 2009;35:678-686.

37. Hershman MJ, Cheadle WG, Wellhausen SR, Davidson PF, Polk Jr HC. Monocyte HLA-DR antigen expression characterizes clinical outcome in the trauma patients. *Br J Surg.* 1990;77:204-207.

38. Monneret G, Lepape A, Voirin N, et al. Persisting low monocyte human leukocyte antigen-DR expression predicts mortality in septic shock. *Intensive Care Med.* 2006;32:1175-1183.

39. Haveman JW, van den Berg AP, Verhoeven EL, et al. HLA-DR expression on monocytes and systemic inflammation in patients with ruptured abdominal aortic aneurysms. *Crit Care.* 2006;10:R119.

40. Lukaszewicz AC, Grienay M, Resche-Rigon M, et al. Monocytic HLA-DR expression in intensive care patients: interest for prognosis and secondary infection prediction. *Crit Care Med.* 2009;37:2746-2752.

41. Venet F, Tissot S, Debard AL, et al. Decreased monocyte human leukocyte antigen-DR expression after severe burn injury: correlation with severity and secondary septic shock. *Crit Care Med.* 2007;35:1910-1917.

42. Cavaillon JM, Adib-Conquy M. Bench-to-bedside review: endotoxin tolerance as a model of leukocyte reprogramming in sepsis. *Crit Care*. 2006;10:233.

43. Adib-Conquy M, Adrie C, Fitting C, Gattolliat O, Beyaert R, Cavaillon JM. Up-regulation of MyD88s and SIGIRR, molecules inhibiting Toll-like receptor signaling, in monocytes from septic patients. *Crit Care Med*. 2006;34:2377-2385.

44. Adrie C, Adib-Conquy M, Laurent I, et al. Successful cardiopulmonary resuscitation after cardiac arrest as a "sepsis like" syndrome. *Circulation*. 2002;106:562-568.

45. Cavaillon JM, Eisen D, Annane D. Is boosting the immune system in sepsis appropriate? *Crit Care*. 2014;18:216.

46. Antonakos N, Tsaganos T, Oberle V, et al. Decreased cytokine production by mononuclear cells after severe gram-negative infections: early clinical signs and association with final outcome. *Crit Care*. 2017;21:48.

47. Adib-Conquy M, Asehnoune K, Moine P, Cavaillon JM. Long-term impaired expression of nuclear factor-kB and IkBa in peripheral blood mononuclear cells of trauma patients. *J Leukoc Biol*. 2001;70:30-38.

48. Reikerås O, Sun J, Wang JE, Foster SJ, Aasen AO. Differences in LPS and PepG induced release of inflammatory cytokines in orthopedic trauma. *J Invest Surg*. 2008;21(5):255-260.

49. Roquilly A, Braudeau C, Cinotti R, et al. Impaired blood dendritic cell numbers and functions after aneurysmal subarachnoid hemorrhage. *PLoS One*. 2013;8:e71639.

50. Asehnoune K, Fitting C, Edouard AR, et al. beta2-Adrenoceptor blockade partially restores ex vivo TNF production following hemorrhagic shock. *Cytokine*. 2006;34:212-218.

51. Tattevin P, Monnier D, Tribut O, et al. Enhanced indoleamine 2,3-dioxygenase activity in patients with severe sepsis and septic shock. *J Infect Dis*. 2010;201:956-966.

52. Souza-Fonseca-Guimaraes F, Parlato M, Philippart F, et al. Toll-like receptors expression and interferon-gamma production by NK cells in human sepsis. *Crit Care*. 2012;16:R206.

53. Danikas DD, Karakantza M, Theodorou GL, Sakellaropoulos GC, Gogos CA. Prognostic value of phagocytic activity of neutrophils and monocytes in sepsis. Correlation to CD64 and CD14 antigen expression. *Clin Exp Immunol*. 2008;154:87-97.

54. Shalova IN, Lim JY, Chittezhath M, et al. Human monocytes undergo functional re-programming during sepsis mediated by hypoxia-inducible factor-1alpha. *Immunity*. 2015;42:484-498.

55. Maxime V, Fitting C, Annane D, Cavaillon JM. Corticoids normalize leukocyte production of macrophage migration inhibitory factor in septic shock. *J Infect Dis*. 2005;191:138-144.

56. Angele MK, Ayala A, Cioffi WG, Bland KI, Chaudry IH. Testosterone: the culprit for producing splenocyte immune depression after trauma hemorrhage. *Am J Physiol*. 1998;274(6 Pt 1):C1530-C1536.

57. Knöferl MW, Jarrar D, Angele MK, et al. 17 beta-Estradiol normalizes immune responses in ovariectomized females after trauma-hemorrhage. *Am J Physiol Cell Physiol*. 2001;281:C1131-C1138.

58. Cavaillon JM, Annane D. Compartmentalization of the inflammatory response in sepsis and SIRS. *J Endotoxin Res*. 2006;12:151-170.

59. Zager RA, Johnson AC, Lund S. 'Endotoxin tolerance': TNF-alpha hyper-reactivity and tubular cytoresistance in a renal cholesterol loading state. *Kidney Int*. 2007;71:496-503.

60. Philippart F, Fitting C, Cavaillon JM. Lung microenvironment contributes to the resistance of alveolar macrophages to develop tolerance to endotoxin. *Crit Care Med*. 2012;40:2987-2996.

61. Smith PD, Suffredini AF, Allen JB, Wahl LM, Parrillo JE, Wahl SM. Endotoxin administration to humans primes alveolar macrophages for increased production of inflammatory mediators. *J Clin Immunol*. 1994;14:141-148.

62. Hoogerwerf JJ, de Vos AF, van't Veer C, et al. Priming of alveolar macrophages upon instillation of lipopolysaccharide in the human lung. *Am J Respir Cell Mol Biol*. 2010;42:349-356.

63. Jacobs RF, Tabor DR, Burks AW, Campbell GD. Elevated interleukin-1 release by human alveolar macrophages during adult respiratory distress syndrome. *Am Rev Respir Dis*. 1989;140:1686-1692.

64. Shenkar R, Abraham E. Mechanisms of lung neutrophil activation after hemorrhage or endotoxemia: roles of reactive oxygen intermediates, NF-κB and cyclic AMP response element binding protein. *J Immunol*. 1999;163:954-962.

65. Abraham E, Arcaroli J, Shenkar R. Activation of extracellular signal-regulated kinases, NF-κB, and cyclic adenosine 5′-monophosphate response element-binding protein in lung neutrophils occurs by differing mechanisms after hemorrhage or endotoxemia. *J Immunol*. 2001;166:522-530.

66. Suzuki T, Shimizu T, Szalay L, et al. Androstenediol ameliorates alterations in immune cells cytokine production capacity in a two-hit model of trauma-hemorrhage and sepsis. *Cytokine*. 2006;34:76-84.

67. Ding Y, Chung CS, Newton S, et al. Polymicrobial sepsis induces divergent effects on splenic and peritoneal dendritic cell function in mice. *Shock*. 2004;22:137-144.

68. Fieren MW, Van den Bemd GJ, Bonta IL. Endotoxin-stimulated peritoneal macrophages obtained from continuous ambulatory peritoneal dialysis patients show an increased capacity to release interleukin-1 beta in vitro during infectious peritonitis. *Eur J Clin Invest*. 1990;20:453-457.

69. Danahy DB, Anthony SM, Jensen IJ, et al. Polymicrobial sepsis impairs bystander recruitment of effector cells to infected skin despite optimal sensing and alarming function of skin resident memory CD8 T cells. *PLoS Pathog*. 2017;13:e1006569.

70. Singer BH, Dickson RP, Denstaedt SJ, et al. Bacterial dissemination to the brain in sepsis. *Am J Respir Crit Care Med*. 2018;197:747-756.

71. Qin L, Wu X, Block ML, et al. Systemic LPS causes chronic neuroinflammation and progressive neurodegeneration. *Glia*. 2007;55:453-462.

72. Adzic M, Djordjevic J, Mitic M, Brkic Z, Lukic I, Radojcic M. The contribution of hypothalamic neuroendocrine, neuroplastic and neuroinflammatory processes to lipopolysaccharide-induced depressive-like behaviour in female and male rats: involvement of glucocorticoid receptor and C/EBP-β. *Behav Brain Res*. 2015;291:130-139.

73. Starr ME, Saito M, Evers BM, Saito H. Age-associated increase in cytokine production during systemic inflammation—II: the role of IL-1β in age-dependent IL-6 upregulation in adipose tissue. *J Gerontol A Biol Sci Med Sci*. 2015;70:1508-1515.

74. Annane D, Sanquer S, Sébille V, et al. Compartmentalised inducible nitric-oxide synthase activity in septic shock. *Lancet*. 2000;355:1143-1148.

75. Mirsoian A, Bouchlaka MN, Sckisel GD, et al. Adiposity induces lethal cytokine storm after systemic administration of stimulatory immunotherapy regimens in aged mice. *J Exp Med*. 2014;211:2373-2383.

76. Raschke RA, Garcia-Orr R. Hemophagocytic lymphohistiocytosis: a potentially underrecognized association with systemic inflammatory response syndrome, severe sepsis, and septic shock in adults. *Chest*. 2011;140:933-938.

77. François B, Trimoreau F, Vignon P, Fixe P, Praloran V, Gastinne H. Thrombocytopenia in the sepsis syndrome: role of hemophagocytosis and macrophage colony-stimulating factor. *Am J Med*. 1997;103:114-120.

78. Strauss R, Neureiter D, Westenburger B, Wehler M, Kirchner T, Hahn EG. Multifactorial risk analysis of bone marrow histiocytic hyperplasia with hemophagocytosis in critically ill medical patients—a postmortem clinicopathologic analysis. *Crit Care Med*. 2004;32:1316-1321.

79. Kyriazopoulou E, Leventogiannis K, Norrby-Teglund A, et al. Macrophage activation-like syndrome: an immunological entity associated with rapid progression to death in sepsis. *BMC Med*. 2017:15:172.

80. Foster SL, Hargreaves DC, Medzhitov R. Gene-specific control of inflammation by TLR-induced chromatin modifications. *Nature*. 2007;447:972-978.

81. Boraschi D, Italiani P. Innate immune memory: time for adopting a correct terminology. *Front Immunol*. 2018;9:799.

34

Does the Timing of Antibiotic Administration Matter in Sepsis?

Ithan D. Peltan and Vincent X. Liu

INTRODUCTION

Well-designed observational studies link lower sepsis mortality with earlier antibiotic initiation, leading advocacy and regulatory bodies to embrace antibiotic initiation time as a measure of sepsis care quality.[1-4] However, citing limitations in the observational data supporting early antibiotics and the fact that sepsis—in contrast to simple infection—is a syndrome that can persist or progress despite eradication of the inciting organism, others argue that an emphasis on very early antibiotics is premature and potentially harmful.[4-6] In this chapter, we critically review the evidence underlying the premise that sepsis mortality increases with each hour of antibiotic delay. Overall, we find that although more research is needed to fully inform treatment and policy decisions, prompt, appropriate antibiotic initiation is the single most important action clinicians can take today to improve sepsis outcomes.

HOW DO WE MEASURE THE TIMING OF ANTIBIOTICS IN SEPSIS?

Quantifying "time to antibiotics" (TTA) requires choosing a reliable onset time (often called "time zero") and end time. While supported by some data,[7] defining an onset time for sepsis based on physiologic criteria (shock onset) or diagnosis recognition (sepsis onset) is problematic. These criteria are (1) difficult to capture accurately; (2) unlikely to represent the true physiologic onset time of sepsis or shock; and (3) reliant on arbitrary thresholds. In the emergency department (ED), where the vast majority of sepsis patients are identified,[8] the Surviving Sepsis Campaign therefore endorses using ED arrival for "time zero" because it is: (1) clinically meaningful[2,8]; (2) easily and reproducibly measurable; (3) recognizes opportunities to accelerate both sepsis evaluation and treatment; and (4) represents a patient-centered care interval.[3,9] However, ED arrival time cannot be used in non-ED settings and further may encourage indiscriminate antibiotic initiation when there is initial diagnostic uncertainty of sepsis.

Defining a reliable TTA endpoint is simpler, but still not easy. The clinically meaningful event is, of course, effective antibiotic initiation. Adjudication of this event, however, is difficult and resource intensive. Worse, not all sepsis patients ultimately have a microbiologically-confirmed pathogen, so assessing antibiotic appropriateness in these patients requires time-consuming and partially subjective adjudication to establish presumed effectiveness based on the clinical syndrome and risk factors. By comparison, the administration time of the first antibiotic is objective and much easier to measure, but may underestimate the benefit from fast initiation of effective antibiotics. Importantly, if applied for incentives or penalties (including public reporting), ending the TTA interval based on the administration time of the first antibiotic could incentivize rapid, indiscriminate antibiotic initiation. On the other hand, using effective antibiotic initiation to end the TTA window could encourage unnecessarily broad-spectrum regimens.

WHAT IS THE EVIDENCE THAT ANTIBIOTIC TIMING MATTERS IN SEPSIS?

It seems obvious that earlier causative pathogen eradication should improve sepsis outcomes. However, whereas early theories blamed sepsis pathogenesis on exuberant inflammation and uncontrolled infection, current evidence suggests that poor sepsis outcomes often result from progressive multiorgan failure despite infection control, secondary infections resulting from acquired immunoparalysis, or chronic critical illness.[10-12] It is becoming clear that sepsis behaves as a nonlinear system where the modification of a single contributing pathway may exert unpredictable effects on the trajectory of organ failure due to the complexity of interacting disease pathways.[13] Theoretical considerations aside, however, both preclinical and observational clinical data indicate early antibiotics are a critical determinant of sepsis outcomes.

Preclinical Data

Preclinical data on antibiotic timing in sepsis are surprisingly limited. In one study of mice given lethal intraperitoneal doses of Enterobacteriaceae, survival was 100% with immediate antibiotics but decreased to 90% when treatment occurred at 60 minutes, 55% at 90 minutes, 30% at 120 minutes, and <10% at 3 hours.[14] Mortality rose rapidly in another trial when antibiotics were started in mice more than 12 hours after intraperitoneal infection.[15] Interestingly, the mice developed shock over approximately the same time frame. More recently, survival decreased in a stepwise fashion for mice with abdominal sepsis given antibiotics as soon as early physiologic deterioration was detected rather than after a 2- or 4-hour delay.[16]

Clinical Data

Numerous observational studies have examined the association of antibiotic timing and sepsis mortality. Due to the serious challenges that indication bias poses for such analyses, we focus here on studies employing methods to mitigate this problem (Table 34.1).

Kumar et al.[7] reported the findings of the first large study on this subject in 2006.[7] Among 2154 patients, hospital mortality increased by 7.6% with each elapsed hour between hypotension onset and appropriate antibiotic initiation. After adjustment, the odds of mortality increased 12% per hour (95% confidence interval [CI] 10–14%). However, the elapsed intervals between hypotension and antibiotic administration were long by contemporary standards (mean 13.5 hours), raising concern that these findings may no longer be generalizable to modern sepsis care.

Whereas some subsequent studies failed to identify a statistically significant benefit,[17–20] larger studies consistently show improved adjusted mortality with earlier antibiotics, albeit with less impressive effects on absolute mortality. In a propensity score-based analysis of 2796 sepsis patients treated in 77 Spanish intensive care units (ICUs), the odds of mortality were 49% higher (95% CI 11–100%) among patients whose antibiotics were started > 6 hours vs. < 1 hour after presentation.[21] TTAs between 1 and 6 hours also showed a trend toward improved outcomes, but did not reach statistical significance. In a study of 17,990 patients from 177 Surviving Sepsis Campaign ICUs, most (72%) sepsis patients presented to the ED and had antibiotic timing measured from ED triage.[8] Beyond 2 hours, each elapsed hour was associated with increasing hospital mortality, although the hour-upon-hour increase was not linear.

Liu et al.[2] reported a 9% (95% CI 5–13%) increase in the odds of hospital mortality with each hour that door-to-antibiotic time increased for 35,000 ED patients with sepsis who received antibiotics within 6 hours of triage. Their findings suggested that the mortality risk plateaued between 2 and 5 hours, with an abrupt rise for the minority of patients receiving antibiotics more than 5 hours after triage (Fig. 34.1). The effect was stronger for patients with septic shock than for sepsis or systemic inflammatory response syndrome (SIRS) plus infection. Another study of 2683 patients meeting Sepsis-3 criteria, arriving at the ED entrance via ambulance, found that both the time from ambulance arrival to first antibiotics (odds ratio [OR] 1.03 per hour, 95% CI 1.01–1.05) and door-to-antibiotic time (OR 1.03, 95% CI 1.00–1.05) were significantly associated with hospital mortality.[22]

The largest analysis to date evaluated 49,331 ED sepsis cases enrolled in the New York State sepsis registry.[1] The adjusted odds of death increased 4% for each hour antibiotics were started after sepsis bundle initiation (95% CI 3–6%) or ED arrival (95% CI 2–5%). By contrast, time to fluid initiation,

another hallmark of contemporary early sepsis care, was not associated with mortality. In an analysis evaluating the robustness of their results to unmeasured confounding, the authors determined that a hypothetical confounder would need to exhibit a twofold difference in frequency between early vs. late antibiotic patients and exert an effect on mortality at least sevenfold stronger than that observed for antibiotics to abrogate these findings.

Although careful risk adjustment reduces the likelihood that analyses based on observational data will yield false-positive results or even invert the true relationship, residual confounding and bias remain a persistent concern. In this context, alternative analytic approaches bolster our confidence in the suggested benefit of early antibiotics. For instance, the benefits of earlier antibiotics persist using an alternate unit of measure: hospital-level sepsis mortality and 8-hour antibiotic initiation rates correlate inversely.[23] Kalil et al.[24] compared discordant early goal directed therapy (EGDT) studies and noted that positive EGDT studies included a cointervention that accelerated antibiotic initiation, while negative EGDT trials showed no difference in standardized antibiotic timing among treatment groups. Meta-regression across these studies suggested a 10% increase in the relative mortality risk per hour of elapsed antibiotic time. Finally, the finding that mortality is increased when septic patients' second dose of antibiotics is delayed provides indirect evidence of benefit, since adverse consequences from early interruption of coverage makes sense only if early antibiotic initiation is important.[25]

So far, only one published randomized trial is available to inform the antibiotic timing debate. A 2018 study assigned ambulance-transported patients with infection plus SIRS, sepsis, or septic shock to prehospital ceftriaxone or standard care, producing a 96-minute difference in median antibiotic initiation time between the 1535 intervention and 1137 control patients.[26] Mortality at 28 days did not differ significantly between treatment arms (7.8% vs. 8.2%, respectively). However, the study was critically underpowered for the primary outcome; the study would have needed to enroll over 10,000 subjects per group to detect the predicted 15% relative risk reduction given the relatively low observed mortality rate. Other factors that probably impact outcome validity in this innovative study include nonrandomized selection of treatment assignment for at least 10–15% of subjects, ceftriaxone's relatively narrow spectrum, and the fact that over 20% of patients were already on antibiotics prior to randomization.

WHAT ARE THE LIMITATIONS OF EXISTING EVIDENCE ON EARLY ANTIBIOTICS' BENEFITS?

Biologic plausibility and robust, consistent findings from multiple large observational studies employing high-quality methods support causal inference.[27] However, observational studies cannot ultimately establish causality,[27] so the possibility that a randomized trial of antibiotic timing might not

TABLE 34.1 Studies Reporting Adjusted Estimates of the Association between time to Antibiotics (TTA) and Mortality in Adult Sepsis.

First Author (Year)	SYNDROME[a]				N	ANTIBIOTIC TIMING WINDOW AND DELAY UNITS				Outcome	Adjusted Risk per Unit of Antibiotic Delay (95% CI)[b]
	SIRS	Sepsis	Septic Shock	Other		Time Zero	Endpoint	Maximum	Units		
Garnacho-Montero (2003)[77]	X	X	X		406	ICU arrival	Effective	None	>24 h[c]	Hospital morality —Non-surgical sepsis —Surgical sepsis	8.14 (1.98–33.5) 2.70 (1.30–5.56)
Larché (2003)[78]			X	Cancer	88	ICU arrival	First	None	>2 h[c]	30-day mortality	7.05 (1.17–42.21)
Kumar (2006)[7]			X		2154	Shock onset	Effective	None	Hours	Hospital mortality	1.12 (1.10–1.14)
Garnacho-Montero (2006)[79]	X	X	X		224	ED arrival	Effective	None	Hours	Hospital morality	1.09 (1.04–1.19)
Gaieski (2010)[80]		X	X		261	ED triage EGDT ED triage EGDT	First First Effective Effective	None	>1 h[c]	Hospital mortality	1.96 (0.82–4.76) 1.72 (0.93–3.23) 3.33 (1.20–9.09) 2.00 (1.09–3.70)
Ferrer (2009)[21]		X	X		2796	Sepsis presentation	First	24 h	>6 h vs. <1 h[c]	Hospital mortality	1.49 (1.11–2.00)
Puskarich (2011)[17]			X		291	ED triage ED triage	First First	6 h	>3 h[c] Shock recognition[c]	Hospital mortality	0.66 (0.27–1.63) 2.59 (1.17–5.74)
Ferrer (2014)[8]		X	X		17,990	Presentation	First	6 h	1–2 h vs. <.1 h[c] 2–3 h vs. <.1 h[c] 3–4 h vs. <.1 h[c] 4–5 h vs. <1 h[c] 5–6 h vs. <1 h[c] >6 h vs. <1 h[c]	In-hospital mortality	1.07 (0.87–1.18) 1.14 (1.02–1.26) 1.19 (1.04–1.35) 1.24 (1.06–1.45) 1.47 (1.22–1.76) 1.52 (1.36–1.70)
Joo (2014)[81]		X	X		591	ED arrival	First	None	>3 h[c]	Hospital mortality	1.85 (1.15–2.94)
Yokota (2014)[82]		X	X		1281	Sepsis diagnosis	First	None	>1 h[c]	Hospital mortality	1.30 (0.99–1.70)

Continued

TABLE 34.1   Studies Reporting Adjusted Estimates of the Association between Time to Antibiotics (TTA) and Mortality in Adult Sepsis.—cont'd

First Author (Year)	SYNDROME[a]				ANTIBIOTIC TIMING WINDOW AND DELAY UNITS						Adjusted Risk per Unit of Antibiotic Delay (95% CI)[b]
	SIRS	Sepsis	Septic Shock	Other	N	Time Zero	Endpoint	Maximum	Units	Outcome	
de Groot (2015)[19]				Suspected infection, ED triage score ≥ 3/5	1,168	ED arrival	First	ED DC	>3 h vs. <1 h[c]	28-day mortality	5.31 (0.43–68.2)
										—PIRO score 1–7	0.86 (0.28–2.63)
										—PIRO score 8–14	1.11 (0.40–3.08)
										—PIRO score >14	
Garnacho-Montero (2015)[83]		X	X		638	ED arrival	First	None	>ICU admit[c]	Hospital mortality	3.45 (1.59–769)
										—Sepsis	2.50 (1.54–4.17)
										—Septic shock	
Ryoo (2015)[84]			X		426	Shock onset	First	None	Hours	28-day mortality	1.15 (0.87–1.52)
Karvellas (2016)[84a]			X	Cholangitis	133	Shock onset	First	None	Hours	Hospital mortality	1.15 (1.07-1.25)
Seymour (2017)[22]		X	X		2,683	ED arrival	First	24 h	Hours	In-hospital mortality	1.03 (1.00-1.05)
Seymour (2017)[1]		X	X		49,331	ED arrival Sepsis bundle initiation	First	12 h	Hours	Hospital mortality	1.04 (1.02-1.05) 1.04 (1.03-1.06)
Morneau (2017)[85]	X	X		Cancer	100	ED arrival	Effective	6 h	Hours	Hospital mortality	1.16 (1.04-1.34)
Peltan (2017)[86]		X	X		421	ED arrival	First	ED DC	Hours	Hospital mortality	1.20 (1.00-1.44)
Liu (2017)[2]		X	X		35,000	ED arrival	First	6 h	Hours	Hospital mortality	1.09 (1.05-1.13)
Rhee (2018)[87]		X	X		851	Sepsis onset	First	None	>3 h	In-hospital mortality	1.94 (1.04-3.62)

[a]For studies that employed the 2001 International Sepsis Definitions Conference,[88] simple sepsis is classified here as "SIRS" and severe sepsis as "sepsis."
[b]Published odds ratio (OR) and confidence interval (CI) values were inverted as needed to consistently reflect comparison of longer vs. shorter time to antibiotics.
[c]Binary exposure.
DC, discharge; ED, emergency department; EGDT, early goal directed therapy; OR, odds ratio; SIRS, systemic inflammatory response syndrome.

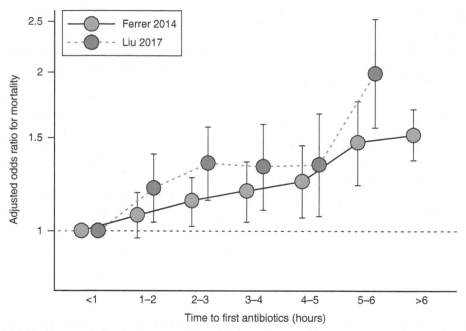

Fig. 34.1 Hourly association between sepsis antibiotic timing and mortality. Association between risk-adjusted hospital mortality and time to first antibiotics from case recognition for 17,990 ICU sepsis patients[8] or emergency department (ED) arrival for 35,000 sepsis patients.[2] The reference group is patients who received antibiotics <1 hour from ED arrival. (From Liu VX, Fielding-Singh V, Greene JD, et al. The timing of early antibiotics and hospital mortality in sepsis. *Am J Respir Crit Care Med.* 2017;196:856–863. With permission of the American Thoracic Society.)

confirm the observational data is an ever-present concern. Since most physicians lack equipoise to delay antibiotics after diagnosing sepsis, randomized trials to measure the "true" effect of antibiotic timing on sepsis outcomes would require designs that alter the location of randomization (e.g., prehospital rather than ED),[26] unit of randomization (e.g. hospital rather than patient), and/or intervention (e.g., randomizing process interventions to speed antibiotics rather than randomizing individual patient's antibiotic timing).[28]

In the meantime, it is useful to understand the limitations inherent to observational data on antibiotic timing. Most importantly, because patients with more acute sepsis receive antibiotics faster,[2,29] observational studies on this subject suffer from "indication bias."[30] While statistical methods to reduce such bias may be technically complex,[6] failure to address the problem can weaken or even reverse a beneficial association of antibiotic timing and mortality.[2] Given this issue, it is unsurprising that a 2015 meta-analysis that pooled crude mortality data did not show any association with early antibiotics.[20] However, even after risk adjustment, observational data remain imperfect. First, and most fundamentally, rapid antibiotics may simply be a marker for unmeasured cointerventions that actually benefit patients. Secondly, many published studies are severely underpowered and prone to false-negative results. Finally, it is possible that the antibiotic/outcome association is nonlinear or that antibiotic delay only exerts meaningful harm beyond a certain threshold. In fact, two studies with large multicenter cohorts suggest the hour-by-hour increase was nonlinear (see Fig. 34.1).

Perhaps the greatest limitation to understanding how antibiotic timing influences sepsis outcomes is fundamental to the sepsis concept itself: it is a syndrome, not a single disease.[5] Having lumped together diverse infections and organ failure patterns,[31] research into the syndrome's treatment implicitly assumes all patients will exhibit the same response to therapy.[32] This assumption is increasingly belied by the identification of sepsis endotypes predictive of distinct clinical trajectories[33] and is the likely reason that scores of antisepsis therapies tested in clinical trials have failed to benefit patients.[34] We suspect that antibiotic timing is an important outcome determinant for all sepsis patients, but that the time course over which the benefit is maximized varies between patients and is dependent on the characteristics of the infection, the host, and on the host–pathogen interaction.

WHAT ARE THE POTENTIAL ADVERSE EFFECTS OF EARLY ANTIBIOTICS?

While few would consider withholding antibiotics among patients with severe infection within an individual clinical encounter and the overwhelming weight of existing data favor early antibiotics, it is important to consider whether potential harms resulting from widespread early antibiotics alter the risk–benefit profile across larger populations. When evaluating these potential harms, we are primarily concerned with the *excess* harms that result from delivering (or trying to deliver) antibiotics earlier, rather than all the adverse effects due to appropriate antibiotics.

Too Early Antibiotics

Clinicians and researchers have long worried that antibiotic-induced bacterial lysis could release harmful amounts of pathogen-associated molecular patterns (PAMPs).[35] For instance, early reports described clinical deterioration after chloramphenicol for typhoid,[36] and antibiotic treatment of disseminated spirochetal infections frequently triggers a Jarisch-Herxheimer reaction.[37] On this basis, as recently as 1978, a review in *The Lancet* of gram-negative infection treatment argued "antibiotics should be withheld from patients already in shock until the peripheral circulation and renal function have been reestablished."[38] However, in comparison to animal studies showing antibiotic-induced release of pro-inflammatory PAMPs modulates outcomes, human data remain limited and inconclusive.[39,40] Antiendotoxin therapy's inability to improve sepsis outcomes provides indirect evidence that, even if early antibiotics do increase PAMP release,[41] the effect is not clinically important for sepsis *in general.*

Bacterial meningitis may represent one exception. Endotoxin levels in cerebrospinal fluid increase after antibiotics,[42] and steroids improve outcomes if given prior to antibiotics, presumably due to reduced central nervous system inflammation.[43] Nevertheless, most but not all observational studies report worse outcomes with delayed antibiotics for meningitis.[44,45] Thus, current evidence supports giving antibiotics early and steroids even earlier for meningitis. The overall role of steroids in sepsis remains unresolved and is further addressed in Chapter 73.

Drivers of Mistargeted Treatment

Most of the theoretical harms postulated to result from earlier antibiotics assume a concomitant increase in antibiotic mistargeting. Mistargeting includes undertreatment and two forms of overtreatment: unnecessarily broad-spectrum treatment and entirely unnecessary treatment. Cognitive biases can contribute to this problem, including altered pretest probability (availability heuristic), difficulty making alternative diagnoses (anchoring, diagnostic momentum, and premature closure), and overweighting early antibiotics' benefits and neglecting potential harms (commission bias).[46] Notably, incorporating antibiotic initiation thresholds into sepsis-related public reporting and government mandates is likely to exacerbate the severity of commission bias.[4,47] For example, when a 4-hour standard for door-to-antibiotic time in community-acquired pneumonia was incorporated into pay-for-performance programs, unnecessary antibiotic administration for ED patients with poorly defined respiratory symptoms increased as hospitals and physicians sought to avoid censure and reimbursement penalties.[48,49]

Consequences of Mistargeted Treatment

The consequences of undertreatment are straightforward: clinicians rushing to start antibiotics may target the wrong infection or miss drug-resistant pathogen (DRP) risk factors and, to the patient's detriment, choose an ineffective empiric regimen.[50–52] While few data exist to quantify either the marginal overtreatment or harm with faster antibiotic initiation, increased overtreatment has diverse putative consequences and victims, including sepsis patients themselves, uninfected "bystanders," and the population as a whole. Key potential consequences include:

- Delayed treatment of the true disease: for uninfected patients, anchoring and premature closure may delay diagnosis and treatment of the real problem, including sepsis mimics such as heart failure and pulmonary embolism that require specific, preferably early, treatment.[53,54]
- Acquisition of DRPs: selective pressure from antibiotics increases subsequent DRP infections.[55] DRP infections, in turn, exhibit poorer prognosis because early empiric regimens are more often ineffective.[56]
- *Clostridium difficile* colitis: antibiotic administration disrupts the barrier function of normal gut flora and selects for pathogenic *C. difficile* strains.[57] The number of different antibiotics, their cumulative dose, and the treatment duration are all associated with *C. difficile* risk.[58]
- Other adverse drug events (ADEs): in one study, about 20% of hospitalized patients who received antibiotics for 24 hours or more experienced at least one antibiotic-associated ADE or infection, with similar rates among patients receiving unnecessary antibiotics (Table 34.2).[59] While most of these ADEs were clinically meaningful, however, the most common ADE was gastrointestinal upset. Most of the

TABLE 34.2 Classification and Examples of Antibiotic-Associated Adverse Drug Events.

Classification	Examples
Antibiotic-associated infections	*C. difficile* colitis, methicillin-resistant *Staphylococcus aureus* pneumonia in patient without history of colonization
Systemic	Anaphylaxis, drug fever, serotonin syndrome
Neurologic	Seizure, peripheral neuropathy
Dermatologic	Rash, Stevens-Johnson syndrome, DRESS
Cardiac	Q_t interval prolongation
Gastrointestinal	Antibiotic-associated diarrhea, nausea/vomiting
Hematologic	Thrombocytopenia, agranulocytosis, eosinophilia
Pulmonary	Pulmonary fibrosis
Renal	Acute kidney failure, acute interstitial nephritis
Hepatobiliary	Acute liver failure or injury, cholestasis
Musculoskeletal	Tendinitis, tendon rupture
Drug interactions	Serotonin syndrome, altered levels or effects of other drugs

DRESS, Drug Reaction with Eosinophilia and Systemic Symptoms.

feared antibiotic complications were rare: for example, only one of 1488 patients developed anaphylaxis. Renal failure is a larger problem, especially when nephrotoxic antibiotics are given together.[60]

- Dysbiosis: increasing evidence points to disruption of the normal microbiome as a driver of critical illness and multiorgan failure.[61,62] Antibiotics interrupt beneficial functions and increase pathogenicity; conversely, aiding microbiome recovery and suppressing overgrowth of pathogens seems to improve critical illness outcomes.[63–65] Unnecessary antibiotics, therefore, prolong illness and increase subsequent severe infection.[66]

Antibiotic overtreatment also exerts effects beyond the antibiotic recipient, including both "innocent bystanders" and the overall population. Redesigning care to accelerate antibiotic delivery for sepsis may drain resources from other patients.[67] Patients cared for on hospital wards where antibiotic utilization is high suffer higher *C. difficile* incidence.[68] Most importantly, and beyond the treated patient's risk of DRPs, population-level increases in antibacterial resistance are a concern for any intervention prone to increasing overtreatment. One must, however, consider this problem in context: 30–50% of ward patients[69,70] and over 70% of ICU patients[71] already receive antibiotics on any given day. Moreover, 85% of antibiotics are prescribed in the outpatient setting, including 30% that are inappropriate.[72,73] Any effect on antibiotic utilization from interventions to speed antibiotics for sepsis is therefore likely to be small relative to current utilization and exert a proportionately modest effect on population-level DRP infection incidence.

CONCLUSIONS AND FUTURE DIRECTIONS

Patients, clinicians, and policymakers deserve high-quality data about both the benefits and harms of early antibiotics in sepsis to guide clinical care and policy creation.[74] Evidence from large, high-quality, contemporary observational studies indicate that each elapsed hour until antibiotic administration is associated with a relative 3–10% increase in mortality. However, studies using innovative designs to examine the unconfounded association between antibiotic timing and sepsis outcomes are still needed. Approaches to this evidence gap might include advanced epidemiologic methods to mitigate the problem of confounding by indication[75,76] and appropriately powered randomized trials targeting care processes or treatment sites. Given the heterogeneity inherent to the sepsis syndrome, understanding how the impact of early antibiotics varies across clinical phenotypes and molecular endotypes is necessary to identify patient subgroups in whom diagnosis clarification, pathogen confirmation, and/or adjunctive preantibiotic therapies are warranted. Finally, both the frequency of antibiotic mistargeting caused by efforts to initiate sepsis antibiotics rapidly and the magnitude of harms per mistargeting event are largely hypothetical. Research to quantify these harms is urgently needed.

AUTHORS' RECOMMENDATIONS
- Sepsis patients should receive appropriate antibiotics as soon as possible to reduce mortality and morbidity.
- ED arrival offers a replicable, efficient, and meaningful start point to measure antibiotic timing in community-acquired sepsis. First antibiotic initiation time is a clinically validated surrogate endpoint for effective antibiotic initiation.
- Caution should be employed when incorporating rapid antibiotic initiation into sepsis regulatory mandates to avoid incentivizing mistargeted treatment.
- Future research should employ innovative methods to measure the unconfounded association between antibiotic timing and sepsis outcomes and quantify the harms associated with an emphasis on early antibiotics.

REFERENCES

1. Seymour CW, Gesten F, Prescott HC, et al. Time to treatment and mortality during mandated emergency care for sepsis. *N Engl J Med.* 2017;376:2235-2244.
2. Liu VX, Fielding-Singh V, Greene JD, et al. The timing of early antibiotics and hospital mortality in sepsis. *Am J Respir Crit Care Med.* 2017;196:856-863.
3. Levy MM, Evans LE, Rhodes A. The Surviving Sepsis Campaign bundle: 2018 update. *Intensive Care Med.* 2018;44(6):925-928.
4. Rhee C, Gohil S, Klompas M. Regulatory mandates for sepsis care—reasons for caution. *N Engl J Med.* 2014;370:1673-1676.
5. Singer M, Deutschman CS, Seymour CW, et al. The Third International Consensus Definitions for Sepsis and Septic Shock (Sepsis-3). *JAMA.* 2016;315:801-810.
6. Singer M. Antibiotics for sepsis: does each hour really count, or is it incestuous amplification? *Am J Respir Crit Care Med.* 2017;196:800-802.
7. Kumar A, Roberts D, Wood KE, et al. Duration of hypotension before initiation of effective antimicrobial therapy is the critical determinant of survival in human septic shock. *Crit Care Med.* 2006;34:1589-1596.
8. Ferrer R, Martín-Loeches I, Phillips G, et al. Empiric antibiotic treatment reduces mortality in severe sepsis and septic shock from the first hour: results from a guideline-based performance improvement program. *Crit Care Med.* 2014;42:1749-1755.
9. Statement from SSC Leadership on Time Zero in the Emergency Department. *Surviving Sepsis Campaign.* 2013. Available at: http://www.survivingsepsis.org/SiteCollectionDocuments/Time-Zero.pdf. Accessed April 19, 2016.
10. Angus DC, van der Poll T. Severe sepsis and septic shock. *N Engl J Med.* 2013;369:840-851.
11. Boomer JS, To K, Chang KC, et al. Immunosuppression in patients who die of sepsis and multiple organ failure. *JAMA.* 2011;306:2594-2605.
12. Prescott HC, Angus DC. Enhancing recovery from sepsis: a review. *JAMA.* 2018;319:62-75.
13. Seely AJ, Christou NV. Multiple organ dysfunction syndrome: exploring the paradigm of complex nonlinear systems. *Crit Care Med.* 2000;28:2193-2200.
14. Greisman SE, DuBuy JB, Woodward CL. Experimental gram-negative bacterial sepsis: prevention of mortality not preventable by antibiotics alone. *Infect Immun.* 1979;25:538-557.

15. Kumar A, Haery C, Paladugu B, et al. The duration of hypotension before the initiation of antibiotic treatment is a critical determinant of survival in a murine model of *Escherichia coli* septic shock: association with serum lactate and inflammatory cytokine levels. *J Infect Dis*. 2006;193:251-258.
16. Lewis AJ, Griepentrog JE, Zhang X, et al. Prompt administration of antibiotics and fluids in the treatment of sepsis: a murine trial. *Crit Care Med*. 2018;46:e426-e434.
17. Puskarich MA, Trzeciak S, Shapiro NI, et al. Association between timing of antibiotic administration and mortality from septic shock in patients treated with a quantitative resuscitation protocol. *Crit Care Med*. 2011;39:2066-2071.
18. Bloos F, Thomas-Rüddel D, Rüddel H, et al. Impact of compliance with infection management guidelines on outcome in patients with severe sepsis: a prospective observational multicenter study. *Crit Care*. 2014;18:R42.
19. de Groot B, Ansems A, Gerling DH, et al. The association between time to antibiotics and relevant clinical outcomes in emergency department patients with various stages of sepsis: a prospective multi-center study. *Crit Care*. 2015;19:194.
20. Sterling SA, Miller WR, Pryor J, et al. The impact of timing of antibiotics on outcomes in severe sepsis and septic shock: a systematic review and meta-analysis. *Crit Care Med*. 2015;43:1907-1915.
21. Ferrer R, Artigas A, Suarez D, et al. Effectiveness of treatments for severe sepsis: a prospective, multicenter, observational study. *Am J Respir Crit Care Med*. 2009;180:861-866.
22. Seymour CW, Kahn JM, Martin-Gill C, et al. Delays from first medical contact to antibiotic administration for sepsis. *Crit Care Med*. 2017;45:759-765.
23. Yu DT, Black E, Sands KE, et al. Severe sepsis: variation in resource and therapeutic modality use among academic centers. *Crit Care*. 2003;7:R24-34.
24. Kalil AC, Johnson DW, Lisco SJ, Sun J. Early goal-directed therapy for sepsis: a novel solution for discordant survival outcomes in clinical trials. *Crit Care Med*. 2017;45:607-614.
25. Leisman D, Wie B, Doerfler M, et al. Association of fluid resuscitation initiation within 30 minutes of severe sepsis and septic shock recognition with reduced mortality and length of stay. *Ann Emerg Med*. 2016;68:298-311.
26. Alam N, Oskam E, Stassen PM, et al. Prehospital antibiotics in the ambulance for sepsis: a multicentre, open label, randomised trial. *Lancet Respir Med*. 2018;6:40-50.
27. Weiss NS, Koepsell TR. *Epidemiologic Methods: Studying the Occurrence of Illness*. New York: Oxford University Press; 2003.
28. Ferrer R, Martínez ML, Gomà G, et al. Improved empirical antibiotic treatment of sepsis after an educational intervention: the ABISS-Edusepsis study. *Crit Care*. 2018;22:167.
29. Amaral AC, Fowler RA, Pinto R, et al. Patient and organizational factors associated with delays in antimicrobial therapy for septic shock. *Crit Care Med*. 2016;44:2145-2153.
30. Kyriacou DN, Lewis RJ. Confounding by indication in clinical research. *JAMA*. 2016;316:1818-1819.
31. Knox DB, Lanspa MJ, Kuttler KG, et al. Phenotypic clusters within sepsis-associated multiple organ dysfunction syndrome. *Intensive Care Med*. 2015;41:814-822.
32. Prescott HC, Calfee CS, Thompson BT, et al. Toward smarter lumping and smarter splitting: rethinking strategies for sepsis and acute respiratory distress syndrome clinical trial design. *Am J Respir Crit Care Med*. 2016;194:147-155.
33. Burnham KL, Davenport EE, Radhakrishnan J, et al. Shared and distinct aspects of the sepsis transcriptomic response to fecal peritonitis and pneumonia. *Am J Respir Crit Care Med*. 2017;196:328-339.
34. Vincent JL. Individual gene expression and personalised medicine in sepsis. *Lancet Respir Med*. 2016;4:242-243.
35. Periti P, Mazzei T. Antibiotic-induced release of bacterial cell wall components in the pathogenesis of sepsis and septic shock: a review. *J Chemother*. 1998;10:427-448.
36. Reilly J, Compagnon A, Tuornier P, et al. Les accidents du traitement des fievres typhoides par la chloromycetine. *Ann Med (Paris)*. 1950;51:597-629.
37. Butler T. The Jarisch-Herxheimer reaction after antibiotic treatment of spirochetal infections: a review of recent cases and our understanding of pathogenesis. *Am J Trop Med Hyg*. 2017;96:46-52.
38. Hopkin DA. Frapper fort ou frapper doucement: a gram-negative dilemma. *Lancet*. 1978;2:1193-1194.
39. Holzheimer RG. Antibiotic induced endotoxin release and clinical sepsis: a review. *J Chemother*. 2001;13 Spec No 1:159-172.
40. Nau R, Eiffert H. Modulation of release of proinflammatory bacterial compounds by antibacterials: potential impact on course of inflammation and outcome in sepsis and meningitis. *Clin Microbiol Rev*. 2002;15:95-110.
41. Angus DC, Birmingham MC, Balk RA, et al. E5 murine monoclonal antiendotoxin antibody in gram-negative sepsis: a randomized controlled trial. E5 Study Investigators. *JAMA*. 2000;283:1723-1730.
42. Arditi M, Ables L, Yogev R. Cerebrospinal fluid endotoxin levels in children with *H. influenzae* meningitis before and after administration of intravenous ceftriaxone. *J Infect Dis*. 1989;160:1005-1011.
43. de Gans J, van de Beek D, European Dexamethasone in Adulthood Bacterial Meningitis Study Investigators. Dexamethasone in adults with bacterial meningitis. *N Engl J Med*. 2002;347:1549-1556.
44. Glimåker M, Johansson B, Grindborg Ö, et al. Adult bacterial meningitis: earlier treatment and improved outcome following guideline revision promoting prompt lumbar puncture. *Clin Infect Dis*. 2015;60:1162-1169.
45. Buckingham SC, McCullers JA, Luján-Zilbermann J, et al. Early vancomycin therapy and adverse outcomes in children with pneumococcal meningitis. *Pediatrics*. 2006;117:1688-1694.
46. Croskerry P. The importance of cognitive errors in diagnosis and strategies to minimize them. *Acad Med*. 2003;78:775-780.
47. Lanspa MJ, Yarbrough PM. Unintended consequences of quality-of-care measures. *Ann Am Thorac Soc*. 2018;15:552-553.
48. Kanwar M, Brar N, Khatib R, Fakih MG. Misdiagnosis of community-acquired pneumonia and inappropriate utilization of antibiotics: side effects of the 4-h antibiotic administration rule. *Chest*. 2007;131:1865-1869.
49. Wachter RM, Flanders SA, Fee C, Pronovost PJ. Public reporting of antibiotic timing in patients with pneumonia: lessons from a flawed performance measure. *Ann Intern Med*. 2008;149:29-32.
50. Capp R, Chang Y, Brown DFM. Effective antibiotic treatment prescribed by emergency physicians in patients admitted to the intensive care unit with severe sepsis or septic shock: where is the gap? *J Emerg Med*. 2011;41:573-580.
51. Vazquez-Guillamet C, Scolari M, Zilberberg MD, et al. Using the number needed to treat to assess appropriate antimicrobial therapy as a determinant of outcome in severe sepsis and septic shock. *Crit Care Med*. 2014;42:2342-2349.
52. Kumar A, Ellis P, Arabi Y, et al. Initiation of inappropriate antimicrobial therapy results in a fivefold reduction of survival in human septic shock. *Chest*. 2009;136:1237-1248.

53. Matsue Y, Damman K, Voors AA, et al. Time-to-furosemide treatment and mortality in patients hospitalized with acute heart failure. *J Am Coll Cardiol.* 2017;69:3042-3051.

54. Smith SB, Geske JB, Maguire JM, et al. Early anticoagulation is associated with reduced mortality for acute pulmonary embolism. *Chest.* 2010;137:1382-1390.

55. Webb BJ, Jones B, Dean NC. Empiric antibiotic selection and risk prediction of drug-resistant pathogens in community-onset pneumonia. *Curr Opin Infect Dis.* 2016;29:167-177.

56. Zilberberg MD, Shorr AF, Micek ST, et al. Multi-drug resistance, inappropriate initial antibiotic therapy and mortality in Gram-negative severe sepsis and septic shock: a retrospective cohort study. *Crit Care.* 2014;18:596.

57. Leffler DA, LaMont JT. *Clostridium difficile* infection. *N Engl J Med.* 2015;372:1539-1548.

58. Stevens V, Dumyati G, Fine LS, et al. Cumulative antibiotic exposures over time and the risk of *Clostridium difficile* infection. *Clin Infect Dis.* 2011;53:42-48.

59. Tamma PD, Avdic E, Li DX, et al. Association of adverse events with antibiotic use in hospitalized patients. *JAMA Intern Med.* 2017;177:1308-1315.

60. Filippone EJ, Kraft WK, Farber JL. The nephrotoxicity of vancomycin. *Clin Pharmacol Ther.* 2017;102:459-469.

61. Cho I, Blaser MJ. The human microbiome: at the interface of health and disease. *Nat Rev Genet.* 2012;13:260-270.

62. Klingensmith NJ, Coopersmith CM. The gut as the motor of multiple organ dysfunction in critical illness. *Crit Care Clin.* 2016;32:203-212.

63. Modi SR, Collins JJ, Relman DA. Antibiotics and the gut microbiota. *J Clin Invest.* 2014;124:4212-4218.

64. Price R, MacLennan G, Glen J; SuDDICU Collaboration. Selective digestive or oropharyngeal decontamination and topical oropharyngeal chlorhexidine for prevention of death in general intensive care: systematic review and network meta-analysis. *BMJ.* 2014;348:g2197.

65. Manzanares W, Lemieux M, Langlois PL, Wischmeyer PE. Probiotic and synbiotic therapy in critical illness: a systematic review and meta-analysis. *Crit Care.* 2016;20:1-19.

66. Prescott HC, Dickson RP, Rogers MAM, et al. Hospitalization type and subsequent severe sepsis. *Am J Respir Crit Care Med.* 2015;192:581-588.

67. Volchenboum SL, Mayampurath A, Göksu-Gürsoy G, et al. Association between in-hospital critical illness events and outcomes in patients on the same ward. *JAMA.* 2016;316:2674-2675.

68. Brown K, Valenta K, Fisman D, et al. Hospital ward antibiotic prescribing and the risks of *Clostridium difficile* infection. *JAMA Intern Med.* 2015;175:626-633.

69. Ansari F, Erntell M, Goossens H, Davey P. The European surveillance of antimicrobial consumption (ESAC) point-prevalence survey of antibacterial use in 20 European hospitals in 2006. *Clin Infect Dis.* 2009;49:1496-1504.

70. Magill SS, Edwards JR, Beldavs ZG, et al. Prevalence of antimicrobial use in US acute care hospitals, May-September 2011. *JAMA.* 2014;312:1438-1446.

71. Vincent J-L, Rello J, Marshall J, et al. International study of the prevalence and outcomes of infection in intensive care units. *JAMA.* 2009;302:2323-2329.

72. Ashiru-Oredope D, Bhattacharya A, Budd E, et al. English Surveillance Programme for Antimicrobial Utilisation and Resistance (ESPAUR): Report 2014. *govuk.* 2014. Available at: https://assets.publishing.service.gov.uk/government/uploads/system/uploads/attachment_data/file/362374/ESPAUR_Report_2014__3_.pdf. Accessed Jun 27, 2018.

73. Fleming-Dutra KE, Hersh AL, Shapiro DJ, et al. Prevalence of inappropriate antibiotic prescriptions among US ambulatory care visits, 2010-2011. *JAMA.* 2016;315:1864-1873.

74. X Liu V, Fielding-Singh V, Iwashyna TJ, et al. Reply: the timing of early antibiotics and hospital mortality in sepsis. *Am J Respir Crit Care Med.* 2017;196:935-936.

75. Walkey AJ, Drainoni ML, Cordella N, Bor J. Advancing quality improvement with regression discontinuity designs. *Ann Am Thorac Soc.* 2018;15:523-529.

76. Iwashyna TJ, Kennedy EH. Instrumental variable analyses: exploiting natural randomness to understand causal mechanisms. *Ann Am Thorac Soc.* 2013;10:255-260.

77. Garnacho-Montero J, Garcia-Garmendia JL, Barrero-Almodovar A, et al. Impact of adequate empirical antibiotic therapy on the outcome of patients admitted to the intensive care unit with sepsis. *Crit Care Med.* 2003;31:2742-2751.

78. Larché J, Azoulay E, Fieux F, et al. Improved survival of critically ill cancer patients with septic shock. *Intensive Care Med.* 2003;29:1688-1695.

79. Garnacho-Montero J, Aldabo-Pallas T, Garnacho-Montero C, et al. Timing of adequate antibiotic therapy is a greater determinant of outcome than are TNF and IL-10 polymorphisms in patients with sepsis. *Crit Care.* 2006;10:R111.

80. Gaieski DF, Mikkelsen ME, Band RA, et al. Impact of time to antibiotics on survival in patients with severe sepsis or septic shock in whom early goal-directed therapy was initiated in the emergency department. *Crit Care Med.* 2010;38:1045-1053.

81. Joo YM, Chae MK, Hwang SY, et al. Impact of timely antibiotic administration on outcomes in patients with severe sepsis and septic shock in the emergency department. *Clin Exp Emerg Med.* 2014;1:35-40.

82. Yokota PKO, Marra AR, Martino MDV, et al. Impact of appropriate antimicrobial therapy for patients with severe sepsis and septic shock—a quality improvement study. *PLoS One.* 2014;9:e104475.

83. Garnacho-Montero J, Gutiérrez-Pizarraya A, Escoresca-Ortega A, et al. Adequate antibiotic therapy prior to ICU admission in patients with severe sepsis and septic shock reduces hospital mortality. *Crit Care.* 2015;19:302.

84. Ryoo SM, Kim WY, Sohn CH, et al. Prognostic value of timing of antibiotic administration in patients with septic shock treated with early quantitative resuscitation. *Am J Med Sci.* 2015;349:328-333.

84a. Karvellas CJ, Abraldes JG, Zepeda-Gomez S, et al. The impact of delayed biliary decompression and anti-microbial therapy in 260 patients with cholangitis-associated septic shock. *Aliment Pharmacol Ther.* 2016;44(7):755-766. doi: 10.1111/apt.13764.

85. Morneau K, Chisholm GB, Tverdek F, et al. Timing to antibiotic therapy in septic oncologic patients presenting without hypotension. *Support Care Cancer.* 2017;25:3357-3363.

86. Peltan ID, Mitchell KH, Rudd KE, et al. Physician variation in time to antimicrobial treatment for septic patients presenting to the emergency department. *Crit Care Med.* 2017;45:1011-1018.

87. Rhee C, Filbin MR, Massaro AF, et al. Compliance with the national SEP-1 quality measure and association with sepsis outcomes: a multicenter retrospective cohort study. *Crit Care Med.* 2018;46(10):1585-1591.

88. Levy MM, Fink MP, Marshall JC, et al. 2001 SCCM/ESICM/ACCP/ATS/SIS International Sepsis Definitions Conference. *Crit Care Med.* 2003;31:1250-1256.

35

What is the Role of Vasopressors and Inotropes in Septic Shock?

David Devlin, Clifford S. Deutschman, and Patrick J. Neligan

This chapter briefly summarizes the hemodynamic derangement associated with sepsis and sequentially evaluates the various vasopressor agents and inotropes that have been investigated and are in current use for the treatment of septic shock.

HEMODYNAMIC DERANGEMENT IN SEPSIS

Early sepsis is characterized by hypoperfusion, manifesting as cold (hypodynamic shock) or warm (hyperdynamic shock) extremities, oliguria, confusion, lactic acidosis, and increased oxygen extraction (reduced mixed venous oxygen saturation [SvO_2]). Current conventional therapy involves early administration of broad-spectrum antibiotics and an initial empirical fluid load of 30 mL/kg.[1] While the actual endpoint remains controversial, the goal of ongoing fluid therapy is to increase mean arterial pressure (MAP) to >65 mm Hg. Most patients respond to antibiotics and fluids, and vasopressor therapy is usually relatively short.[2,3] Failure to respond to initial fluid therapy is an indication for vasopressor therapy.[4]

Established (late-stage) septic shock is a complex disorder characterized by various cardiovascular and neurohormonal anomalies. Although the hemodynamic consequences are easily described, the underlying mechanisms are incompletely understood. The major features of established septic shock are:
1. Vasoplegia from multiple complex mechanisms:
   a. endothelial-related, such as the increased production of inducible nitric oxide synthase (iNOS), the elaboration of free oxygen species, hydrogen sulfide, and production of prostanoids, such as PGI2, IL-1b, and TNF-a
   b. Loss of sympathetic vascular tone, caused by hyperpolarization of vascular smooth muscle cells, through dysregulation of ATP-sensitive potassium channels is also a contributing factor.
2. Endocrine dysfunction
   a. a reduction in the expression of adrenergic and angiotensin receptors on vascular smooth muscle leading to a relative resistance to catecholamines and angiotensin.
   b. An increase in the intracellular abundance of an inactive form of the glucocorticoid receptor (GRβ) and a decrease in the active GRα.[5–7]
   c. Endocrine dysfunction, including but not limited to subacute depletion of circulating vasopressin and reduced expression of VP1 receptors.

3. Biventricular systolic and/or diastolic cardiac dysfunction. This abnormality reflects mitochondrial dysfunction and perhaps microcirculatory changes. Ejection fraction is reduced but cardiac output may be maintained via an increase in left ventricular end diastolic volume (ventricular dilatation), reduced afterload secondary to vasoplegia and a compensatory increase in heart rate.
4. Microcirculatory failure with dysregulation and maldistribution of blood flow, arteriovenous shunting, oxygen utilization defects, and widespread capillary leak.

Initial therapy for both sepsis and septic shock follow the recommendations put forth by the Surviving Sepsis Campaign (SSC).[1] This approach has been remarkably effective,[2,3] despite ongoing controversies regarding the components and timing of the bundles.

VASOPRESSOR THERAPY

Hypotension and tissue hypoperfusion, unresponsive to intravenous fluid in sepsis, are indications for vasopressor therapy.[4] However, the trigger for initiating these agents is controversial. Vasopressors/inotropes have been used to target MAP, peripheral perfusion, microcirculation, cardiac output, stroke volume, and SvO_2. Currently, norepinephrine (noradrenaline/NE) is recommended as the initial vasoactive agent. NE to achieve a MAP of 65 mm Hg is strongly recommended by the SSC but this goal is a general one and should be adjusted for individual patients—for example, a patient with pre-existing hypertension may require a higher MAP.

Norepinephrine

NE has pharmacologic effects on α_1-, β_1-, and $\beta2$ adrenergic receptors. Its affinity for β_1 and α receptors exceeds that for β_2 receptors. These β_1 and α effects are reflected in a mild increase in cardiac output and a more substantial increase in blood pressure. The increase in peripheral resistance prevents any β1-mediated increase in heart rate. The main beneficial effect of NE is to increase organ perfusion by increasing vascular tone,[8,9] although NE increases renal perfusion and splanchnic blood flow in sepsis.[10,11] A study directly comparing NE to dopamine (DA), targeting a blood pressure at a MAP >65 mm Hg in patients with shock (septic, cardiogenic and other), demonstrated that NE was associated with substantial improvements in oxygen delivery, organ perfusion, and oxygen consumption.[12] What the study did not show was a difference in 28-day mortality in the NE group in septic shock. The DA group had more complications, principally atrial fibrillation in sepsis and DA-treated patients had higher mortality in cardiogenic and hypovolemic shock.

Martin and colleagues[13] used stepwise logistic regression analysis in a prospective, observational cohort study of 97 patients with septic shock. Hospital mortality rates were significantly lower in the 57 patients treated with NE (62% vs. 82%; $P < .001$; relative risk, 0.68; 95% confidence interval [CI], 0.54–0.87) as opposed to high-dose DA, epinephrine (EPI), or both. Limitations that cast significant doubt on these results include its observational nonblinded design, probable selection bias, and a weak endpoint (hospital mortality). These data confirmed the work by Goncalves and colleagues.[14]

The timing of NE administration was examined in a retrospective analysis in 213 patients with septic shock in two intensive care units (ICUs).[15] Patients whose NE was started within 2 hours of onset of septic shock (Early-NE) were compared to patients in who NE was initiated after 2 hours (Late-NE). Twenty-eight-day mortality was significantly higher in the Late-NE group (odds ratio [OR] for death = 1.86; 95% CI, 1.04–3.34; $P = .035$). Each 1-hour delay in NE initiation during the first 6 hours was associated with a 5.3% increase in mortality. Both the duration of hypotension and of NE administration were significantly shorter in the Early-NE group.

In conclusion, use of NE is associated with rapid achievement of SSC hemodynamic goals, particularly when administered early. Thus, it is the agent of choice in septic shock.

Dopamine

DA stimulates dopaminergic, β-adrenergic and α-adrenergic receptors. The affinity of DA for these receptors is in that order. Thus, preferential binding is reflected in an apparent predominance of DA-mediated effects at low doses, β-mediated effects at moderate doses and α-mediated effects at high doses. The latter effects may also reflect conversion of DA to NE in the myocardium. Thus, the agent is a mixed inotrope and vasoconstrictor. At all dose ranges, DA is a potent chronotrope. DA may be a useful agent in patients with compromised systolic function, but it causes more tachycardia and is more arrhythmogenic and has been, in metaanalysis, associated with higher mortality than NE.[12,16]

DA is a potent diuretic but does not directly affect renal filtration or resorption.[17] Thus, a high-quality prospective trial[17] and a metaanalysis demonstrated that the use of "renal-dose" dopamine does not change mortality, risk for developing renal failure, or the need for renal replacement therapy.[18]

DA has complex neuroendocrine effects; it may interfere with thyroid and pituitary[19] function and may also be immunosuppressive.[20] The effects of these DA-mediated responses on outcomes is unknown.

In the Sepsis Occurrence in Acutely Ill Patients (SOAP) study, a prospective, multicenter, observational evaluation of sepsis epidemiology in Europe, use of DA was associated with higher ICU (42.9% vs. 35.7%; $P = .02$) and hospital (49.9% vs. 41.7%; $P = .01$, diminished Kaplan-Meier 30-day survival, log rank, 4.6; $P = .032$) mortality.[21] This study was observational and nonrandomized, and the original database was not designed to evaluate outcomes.

Overall, there appears to be little benefit to using DA over NE. Indeed, a syndrome of DA-resistant septic shock, characterized by a MAP <70 mm Hg despite high dose DA administration[22] has been associated with very high mortality.[23] Thus, while DA is an effective inotrope and vasopressor, it is an inferior agent to NE in the management of the patient with septic shock.

Dobutamine

Dobutamine is a potent inotrope and vasodilator. It is a β₁-adrenergic receptor agonist that increases myocardial contractility and thus stroke volume, cardiac output and myocardial oxygen demand. It also has potent β₂, that is, vasodilatory effects. Dobutamine is less chronotropic than dopamine. In sepsis, dobutamine increases oxygen delivery and consumption. Compared to DA, dobutamine increased gastric mucosal pH (pHi) and improved mucosal perfusion.[24] In an early goal-directed resuscitation protocol that included aggressive resuscitation, dobutamine was associated with a significant reduction in the risk for mortality.[25] However, the direct contribution of dobutamine is unknown and follow-up studies have been unable to reproduce this outcome benefit.[26–28]

In a study comparing the combination of NE and dobutamine to epinephrine (EPI, adrenaline) in septic shock, lactate levels and the lactate/pyruvate (L/P) ratio were increased by use of EPI; lactate levels were decreased and the L/P ratio was unchanged by NE-dobutamine.[29] EPI also decreased pHi and increased the P_{CO_2} gap (tonometer P_{CO_2} – arterial P_{CO_2})—suggesting reduced splanchnic perfusion—while NE-dobutamine normalized both within 6 hours. The clinical significance of these findings is unclear, especially because these differences cleared within 24 hours.

Annane and colleagues[30] performed a multicenter, randomized, double-blind trial comparing EPI to NE plus dobutamine ($n = 169$), titrated to maintain mean blood pressure at 70 mm Hg or more, in 330 patients with septic shock. There was no difference in 28-day mortality ($P = .31$; relative risk, 0.86; 95% CI, 0.65–1.14) or in serious side effects, time to pressor withdrawal, or time to achieve hemodynamic goals.

Thus, there are currently no data to indicate that dobutamine, or any inotrope, improve outcomes in septic shock. In the absence of specific indications, such as low ejection fraction, we do not recommend the routine use of this agent.

Epinephrine (Adrenaline)

EPI has potent β₁-, β₂-, and α₁-adrenergic activity; the offsetting effects of the latter two limit the effect of EPI on BP.

EPI, however, increases myocardial oxygen demand, serum glucose and lactate levels,[31] and appears to have adverse effects on splanchnic blood flow.[29,32-34] The importance of these effects is unknown.

In a prospective, multicentered, double-blind, randomized controlled trial, Myburgh and colleagues compared use of EPI and NE in 280 ICU patients.[35] No difference in time to achieve target MAP or in vasopressor-free days were noted. However, several patients receiving EPI experienced significant but transient tachycardia, increased insulin requirements, and lactic acidosis, and were withdrawn from the study.

A metaanalysis of 14 studies/2811 patients comparing DA to inotropes and vasopressors in septic shock[36] found that NE and NE plus low-dose vasopressin, but not EPI or NE plus dobutamine, were associated with significantly reduced mortality.

In summary, EPI is not currently recommended as a first-line agent but may be a viable second choice.[4]

Phenylephrine

Phenylephrine is an almost pure α_1-adrenergic agonist with moderate potency; thus it is a less-effective vasoconstrictor than NE or EPI but is also far less arrhythmogenic.[37] Phenylephrine is an ineffective agent in sepsis and its use should be considered only when a peripherally administered agent is required until central venous access has been established.

Vail, Wunsch and colleagues conducted a retrospective cohort study examining the use of NE and phenylephrine during 2011, when there was a shortage of NE in the United States, in 26 centers where there was a quarterly drop in NE use by at least 20% from baseline.[38] Among the 27,835 patients that were included in the study, phenylephrine was the most commonly selected alternative vasopressor. Hospital admission during quarters of normal NE use was associated with a lower rate of in-hospital mortality; the absolute risk increase associated with phenylephrine was 3.7% [95% CI, 1.5%–6.0%]; adjusted odds ratio = 1.15 [95% CI, 1.01–1.30]; $P = .03$).

In summary, phenylephrine is less effective than NE in the treatment of hypotension in septic shock and should not be considered a viable alternative if NE is unavailable.

Vasopressin

Arginine-vasopressin is an endogenous peptide hormone that is released in response to decreased intravascular volume and increased plasma osmolality. Vasopressin directly constricts vascular smooth muscle through V_1 receptors. It also increases the responsiveness of the vasculature to catecholamines.[39,40]

Circulating levels and pituitary content of vasopressin appear to decrease in sepsis.[41-43] The addition of vasopressin to NE increases splanchnic blood flow and urinary output.[44] Vasopressin offers theoretical advantages over EPI because it does not significantly increase myocardial oxygen demand and its receptors are relatively unaffected by acidosis.[45]

Early studies demonstrated that the most effective dose of vasopressin in septic patients was 0.04 U/min,[46] a dose that has little or no effect on normotensive patients. The drug was not titrated. After several small early studies suggested that vasopressin (or its analogs) might be valuable in sepsis, Russell and colleagues[47] performed a multicenter randomized double-blind trial of patients with septic shock who were already receiving NE at 5 μg/min or more. In this trial, called VASST (Vasopressin and Septic Shock Trial), 396 patients were randomized to have NE replaced in a blinded fashion by vasopressin (0.01–0.03 U/min) while 382 received NE (5–15 μg/min) administered in a similar fashion. No differences in 28-day mortality, 90-day mortality or organ dysfunction were detected. Heart rate and total NE dose, early in the course of critical care, were lower in the vasopressin group. A subgroup analysis suggested that vasopressin improved 28-day and 90-day survival in patients who required a lower overall dose of NE to achieve MAP targets. This benefit was not observed in more severe sepsis. Baseline vasopressin levels, where measured, were very low (median, 3.2 pmol/L; interquartile range, 1.7–4.9) and increased in the vasopressin group but not in the NE group. Importantly, this study did not directly examine the efficacy of vasopressin alone; rather it examined the effects of vasopressin supplementation of NE as opposed to NE alone. In addition, the study was powered for an expected mortality rate of 60%; actual mortality rate in the control group was significantly lower (39%); thus the study was underpowered. Finally, the dose of vasopressin used in the study (up to 0.03 U/min) may have been inadequate to show a response in the patients with more severe septic shock.

A subsequent retrospective analysis of the VASST database suggested that, relative to NE alone, NE + vasopressin improved survival in patients who also simultaneously received corticosteroids.[48] In patients who received vasopressin, corticosteroids also significantly increased plasma vasopressin levels. The VANISH trial[49] was a factorial (2×2), double-blind, randomized clinical trial in which patients were randomly allocated to vasopressin (titrated up to 0.06 U/min) and hydrocortisone ($n = 101$), vasopressin and placebo ($n = 104$), NE and hydrocortisone ($n = 101$), or NE and placebo ($n = 103$). The primary endpoints of the study looked at kidney injury and renal replacement therapy. There was no statistically significant difference in outcomes and the study was underpowered to show a mortality benefit.

In summary, septic shock depletes vasopressin. Replacement with arginine vasopressin may be catecholamine sparing, particularly in mild to moderate or early disease. A recent small trial of angiotensin II, conducted by the drug's manufacturer, suggested a similar catecholamine sparing effect but additional evaluation will be required.[50]

Catecholamine Overload

Several investigators have suggested that catecholamine administration in sepsis may be detrimental. Dünser and colleagues[51] found that using catecholamines to drive MAP above 70 mm Hg appeared to worsen outcomes. However, a multicenter trial of high versus lower blood pressure targets in sepsis did not confirm these findings.[52] There are pathobiological arguments and circumstantial evidence that raise concern regarding catecholamine use. For example, excessive adrenergic activity can lead to myocardial ischemia, tachyarrhythmias, cardiomyopathy, immunosuppression, increased bacterial growth, thrombogenicity, and hyperglycemia.[53,54] In the VASST, vasopressin use in the less severe shock group was associated with a lower heart rate and a reduced overall mortality.[47] Use of β-blockade in sepsis has been intermittently advocated for decades. In a phase 1 study designed to determine if β-blockade was possible, Morelli et al. randomized 77 patients with pressor-dependent septic shock to receive esmolol (titrating to a HR between 80-94 beats/min) or to continue ongoing therapy.[54] While survival was not a primary endpoint, β-blockade reduced 28-day mortality from 80.5% to 49.4% (absolute risk reduction [ARR] 31%, NNT 3, $P < .001$). Importantly, mortality in the control group was exceptionally high.

Thus, while the suggestion that catecholamines are detrimental is intriguing, it remains an untested hypothesis.

UNCOMMONLY-USED VASOPRESSORS/INOTROPES

Levosimendan

Levosimendan is a calcium sensitizer, augmenting cardiac sensitivity to calcium without increasing intracellular calcium concentration. Levosimendan enhances calcium binding to troponin-C and inhibits ATP-dependent potassium channels; thus it is both an inotrope and a vasodilator. Levosimendan has a half-life of approximately 1 hour but its active metabolite, OR-1896, has a far longer half-life of 80 hours, thus clinical effects may last for up to 10 days. The LeoPARDS trial randomized 515 patients with septic shock to levosimendan or placebo for 24 hours.[55] There was no statistically significant change in the primary outcome variable (daily SOFA score) or in any secondary variable. While not appropriately powered to achieve significance, 28-day mortality was higher in the levosimendan group 34.5% vs. 30.9% and patients randomized to receive levosimendan were also less likely to liberate from mechanical ventilation. Thus, levosimendan use is not recommended in septic shock.

Phosphodiesterase Inhibitors: Milrinone and Enoximone

Phosphodiesterase inhibitors should in theory be of value in treating the cardiomyopathy of critical illness. However, these agents are pulmonary and systemic vasodilators and may worsen systemic hypotension. Some studies suggest they may improve microcirculatory indices in patients with cardiogenic shock.[56] However, efficacy in sepsis is untested and use of these agents cannot be recommended.

AUTHORS' RECOMMENDATIONS

- The current standard of care in septic shock involves the administration of empiric antibiotics, intravenous fluids, and, if unresponsive, vasopressor agents.
- The goal of vasopressor therapy is to restore MAP and restore blood flow to vital organs and the extremities.
- Controversy continues regarding the choice of vasopressor and the method of monitoring the response to therapy. This will continue until adequately powered, multicentered prospective trials are performed.
- NE is currently the vasopressor agent of choice in septic shock. It is a potent vasoconstrictor that maintains cardiac output and restores midline blood flow. It is not metabolically active and is associated with fewer adverse effects than other agents.
- DA offers no advantage over NE in septic shock, it worsens mortality in septic hypovolemic and cardiogenic shock and has various nonhemodynamic effects that may affect neurohormonal and immune function.
- EPI causes an early lactic acidosis secondary to aerobic glycolysis and may reduce splanchnic blood flow. Both are of unknown clinical significance. EPI is currently recommended as a second-line agent in septic shock.
- Dobutamine is a potent inotrope and splanchnic vasodilator, but no clear data exist that dobutamine improves outcome in septic shock.
- Phenylephrine is a weak vasoconstrictor with little inotropic activity. It should not be used to treat septic shock.
- There is an absolute deficiency of vasopressin in septic shock, and combination therapy with catecholamines should be considered, particularly in early and mild to moderately severe septic shock. There are no data to support the use of vasopressin as first-line therapy.
- There are emerging data that β-blocker administration is safe and may improve outcomes in pressor-dependent septic shock.
- The use of levosimendan in septic shock appears to be harmful, and it should not be used.
- There are no data available to recommend the use of phosphodiesterase inhibitors in septic shock and very limited data to support the use of angiotensin II.

REFERENCES

1. Rhodes A, Evans LE, Alhazzani W, et al. Surviving Sepsis Campaign: International Guidelines for Management of Sepsis and Septic Shock: 2016. *Crit Care Med.* 2017;45(3):486-552.
2. Levy MM, Dellinger RP, Townsend SR, et al. The Surviving Sepsis Campaign: results of an international guideline-based performance improvement program targeting severe sepsis. *Crit Care Med.* 2010;38(2):367-374.
3. Kaukonen KM, Bailey M, Suzuki S, Pilcher D, Bellomo R. Mortality related to severe sepsis and septic shock among critically ill patients in Australia and New Zealand, 2000-2012. *JAMA.* 2014;311(13):1308-1316.
4. Angus DC, van der Poll T. Severe sepsis and septic shock. *N Engl J Med.* 2013;369:840-851.

5. Burgdorff AM, Bucher M, Schumann J. Vasoplegia in patients with sepsis and septic shock: pathways and mechanisms. *J Int Med Res*. 2018;46(4):1303-1310.

6. Lambden S, Creagh-Brown BC, Hunt J, Summers C, Forni LG. Definitions and pathophysiology of vasoplegic shock. *Crit Care*. 2018;22(1):174.

7. Abraham MN, Jimenez DM, Fernandes TD, Deutschman CS. Cecal ligation and puncture alters glucocorticoid receptor expression. *Crit Care Med*. 2018;46(8):e797-e804.

8. Marik PE, Mohedin M. The contrasting effects of dopamine and norepinephrine on systemic and splanchnic oxygen utilization in hyperdynamic sepsis. *JAMA*. 1994;272:1354-1357.

9. Ruokonen E, Takala J, Kari A, Saxén H, Mertsola J, Hansen EJ. Regional blood flow and oxygen transport in septic shock. *Crit Care Med*. 1993;21:1296-1303.

10. Hannemann L, Reinhart K, Grenzer O, Meier-Hellmann A, Bredle DL. Comparison of dopamine to dobutamine and norepinephrine for oxygen delivery and uptake in septic shock. *Crit Care Med*. 1995;23:1962-1970.

11. Martin C, Saux P, Eon B, Aknin P, Gouin F. Septic shock: a goal-directed therapy using volume loading, dobutamine and/or norepinephrine. *Acta Anaesthesiol Scand*. 1990;34:413-417.

12. De Backer D, Biston P, Devriendt J, et al. Comparison of dopamine and norepinephrine in the treatment of shock. *N Engl J Med*. 2010;362(9):779-789.

13. Martin C, Viviand X, Leone M, Thirion X. Effect of norepinephrine on the outcome of septic shock. *Crit Care Med*. 2000;28:2758-2765.

14. Goncalves Jr JA, Hydo LJ, Barie PS. Factors influencing outcome of prolonged norepinephrine therapy for shock in critical surgical illness. *Shock*. 1998;10:231-236.

15. Bai X, Yu W, Ji W, et al. Early versus delayed administration of norepinephrine in patients with septic shock. *Crit Care*. 2014;18:532.

16. De Backer D, Aldecoa C, Njimi H, Vincent JL. Dopamine versus norepinephrine in the treatment of septic shock: a meta-analysis*. *Crit Care Med*. 2012;40(3):725-730.

17. Bellomo R, Chapman M, Finfer S, Hickling K, Myburgh J. Low-dose dopamine in patients with early renal dysfunction: a placebo-controlled randomised trial. Australian and New Zealand Intensive Care Society (ANZICS) Clinical Trials Group. *Lancet*. 2000;356:2139-2143.

18. Kellum JA, Decker JM. Use of dopamine in acute renal failure: a meta-analysis. *Crit Care Med*. 2001;29:1526-1531.

19. Van den Berghe G, de Zegher F, Lauwers P. Dopamine suppresses pituitary function in infants and children. *Crit Care Med*. 1994;22:1747-1753.

20. Denton R, Slater R. Just how benign is renal dopamine? *Eur J Anaesthesiol*. 1997;14:347-349.

21. Sakr Y, Reinhart K, Vincent JL, et al. Does dopamine administration in shock influence outcome? Results of the Sepsis Occurrence in Acutely Ill Patients (SOAP) Study. *Crit Care Med*. 2006;34:589-597.

22. Bollaert PE, Bauer P, Audibert G, Lambert H, Larcan A. Effects of epinephrine on hemodynamics and oxygen metabolism in dopamine-resistant septic shock. *Chest*. 1990;98:949-953.

23. Levy B, Dusang B, Annane D, Gibot S, Bollaert PE. Cardiovascular response to dopamine and early prediction of outcome in septic shock: a prospective multiple-center study. *Crit Care Med*. 2005;33:2172-2177.

24. Nevière R, Mathieu D, Chagnon JL, Lebleu N, Wattel F. The contrasting effects of dobutamine and dopamine on gastric mucosal perfusion in septic patients. *Am J Respir Crit Care Med*. 1996;154:1684-1688.

25. Rivers E, Nguyen B, Havstad S, et al. Early goal-directed therapy in the treatment of severe sepsis and septic shock. *N Engl J Med*. 2001;345:1368-1377.

26. ARISE Investigators, ANZICS Clinical Trials Group, Peake SL, et al. Goal-directed resuscitation for patients with early septic shock. *N Engl J Med*. 2014;371:1496-1506.

27. ProCESS Investigators, Yealy DM, Kellum JA, et al. A randomized trial of protocol-based care for early septic shock. *N Engl J Med*. 2014;370:1683-1693.

28. Mouncey PR, Osborn TM, Power GS, et al. Trial of early, goal-directed resuscitation for septic shock. *N Engl J Med*. 2015;372:1301-1311.

29. Levy B, Bollaert PE, Charpentier C, et al. Comparison of norepinephrine and dobutamine to epinephrine for hemodynamics, lactate metabolism, and gastric tonometric variables in septic shock: a prospective, randomized study. *Intensive Care Med*. 1997;23:282-287.

30. Annane D, Vignon P, Renault A, et al. Norepinephrine plus dobutamine versus epinephrine alone for management of septic shock: a randomised trial. *Lancet*. 2007;370(9588):676-684.

31. Day NP, Phu NH, Mai NT, et al. Effects of dopamine and epinephrine infusions on renal hemodynamics in severe malaria and severe sepsis. *Crit Care Med*. 2000;28:1353-1362.

32. Zhou SX, Qiu HB, Huang YZ, Yang Y, Zheng RQ. Effects of norepinephrine, epinephrine, and norepinephrine-dobutamine on systemic and gastric mucosal oxygenation in septic shock. *Acta Pharmacol Sin*. 2002;23:654-658.

33. Meier-Hellmann A, Reinhart K, Bredle DL, Specht M, Spies CD, Hannemann L. Epinephrine impairs splanchnic perfusion in septic shock. *Crit Care Med*. 1997;25:399-404.

34. Martikainen TJ, Tenhunen JJ, Giovannini I, Uusaro A, Ruokonen E. Epinephrine induces tissue perfusion deficit in porcine endotoxin shock: evaluation by regional CO_2 content gradients and lactate-to-pyruvate ratios. *Am J Physiol Gastrointest Liver Physiol*. 2005;288:G586-G592.

35. Myburgh JA, Higgins A, Jovanovska A, et al. A comparison of epinephrine and norepinephrine in critically ill patients. *Intensive Care Med*. 2008;34:2226-2234.

36. Oba Y, Lone NA. Mortality benefit of vasopressor and inotropic agents in septic shock: a Bayesian network meta-analysis of randomized controlled trials. *J Crit Care*. 2014;29(5):706-710.

37. Morelli A, Ertmer C, Rehberg S, et al. Phenylephrine versus norepinephrine for initial hemodynamic support of patients with septic shock: a randomized, controlled trial. *Crit Care*. 2008;12:R143.

38. Vail E, Gershengorn HB, Hua M, Walkey AJ, Rubenfeld G, Wunsch H. Association between US norepinephrine shortage and mortality among patients with septic shock. *JAMA*. 2017;317(14):1433-1442.

39. Holmes CL, Patel BM, Russell JA, Walley KR. Physiology of vasopressin relevant to management of septic shock. *Chest*. 2001;120:989-1002.

40. Barrett BJ, Parfrey PS. Clinical practice: preventing nephropathy induced by contrast medium. *N Engl J Med*. 2006;354:379-386.

41. Buijk SE, Bruining HA. Vasopressin deficiency contributes to the vasodilation of septic shock. *Circulation*. 1998;98:187.

42. Goldsmith SR. Vasopressin deficiency and vasodilation of septic shock. *Circulation*. 1998;97:292-293.

43. Reid IA. Role of vasopressin deficiency in the vasodilation of septic shock. *Circulation*. 1997;95:1108-1110.

44. Patel BM, Chittock DR, Russell JA, Walley KR. Beneficial effects of short-term vasopressin infusion during severe septic shock. *Anesthesiology*. 2002;96:576-582.

45. Ornato JP. Optimal vasopressor drug therapy during resuscitation. *Crit Care*. 2008;12:123.

46. Tsuneyoshi I, Yamada H, Kakihana Y, Nakamura M, Nakano Y, Boyle WA III. Hemodynamic and metabolic effects of low-dose vasopressin infusions in vasodilatory septic shock. *Crit Care Med*. 2001;29:487-493.

47. Russell JA, Walley KR, Singer J, et al. Vasopressin versus norepinephrine infusion in patients with septic shock. *N Engl J Med*. 2008;358:877-887.

48. Russell JA, Walley KR, Gordon AC, et al. Interaction of vasopressin infusion, corticosteroid treatment, and mortality of septic shock. *Crit Care Med*. 2009;37:811-818.

49. Gordon AC, Mason AJ, Thirunavukkarasu N, et al. Effect of early vasopressin vs norepinephrine on kidney failure in patients with septic shock: the VANISH randomized clinical trial. *JAMA*. 2016;316(5):509-518.

50. Chawla LS, Busse L, Brasha-Mitchell E, et al. Intravenous angiotensin II for the treatment of high-output shock (ATHOS trial): a pilot study. *Crit Care*. 2014;18(5):534.

51. Dünser MW, Ruokonen E, Pettilä V, et al. Association of arterial blood pressure and vasopressor load with septic shock mortality: a post hoc analysis of a multicenter trial. *Crit Care*. 2009;13:R181.

52. Asfar P, Meziani F, Hamel JF, et al. High versus low blood-pressure target in patients with septic shock. *N Engl J Med*. 2014;370:1583-1593.

53. Singer M. Catecholamine treatment for shock—equally good or bad? *Lancet*. 2007;25;370(9588):636-637.

54. Morelli A, Ertmer C, Westphal M, et al. Effect of heart rate control with esmolol on hemodynamic and clinical outcomes in patients with septic shock: a randomized clinical trial. *JAMA*. 2013;310:1683-1691.

55. Gordon AC, Santhakumaran S, Al-Beidh F, et al. *Levosimendan to Prevent Acute Organ Dysfunction in Sepsis: The LeoPARDS RCT. Efficacy and Mechanism Evaluation*. Southampton, UK: NIHR Journals Library; 2018.

56. den Uil CA, Lagrand WK, van der Ent M, et al. Conventional hemodynamic resuscitation may fail to optimize tissue perfusion: an observational study on the effects of dobutamine, enoximone, and norepinephrine in patients with acute myocardial infarction complicated by cardiogenic shock. *PLoS One*. 2014;9(8):e103978.

36

Does Monitoring the Microcirculation Make a Difference in Sepsis? Outcome?

Goksel Guven and Can Ince

INTRODUCTION

The microcirculation is the final destination of the systemic circulation and is comprised of microvessels with a diameter of less than 20 μm consisting of arterioles, venules, and capillaries. A capillary is a microvessel between 5 and 8 μm in diameter. A red blood cell (RBC) is approximately 8 μm in diameter and deforms to enter a capillary to flow in single file formation. This feature distinguishes the capillaries from arterioles and venules where more than one RBC can exist side by side in the lumen. The capillaries flow into collecting venules where leukocyte adhesion, rolling and migration can occur in states of inflammation. Blood flow enters the capillaries from the arterioles. These vessels control blood flow by modulating tone in smooth muscle cells surrounding the endothelial cells lining the inner lumen.[1] Under physiological conditions, the microcirculation contains about 10% of circulating blood and plays a vital role in oxygen transport to and carbon dioxide (CO_2) removal from tissues. The microcirculation also plays a key role in inflammation, hemostasis, and substrate and hormonal transport. Finally, capillaries are the primary interface between the circulating blood and the parenchymal cells. For these reasons the microcirculation and its dysfunction plays a central role in critical illness and monitoring its function is essential to a comprehensive evaluation of the cardiovascular system.[2]

HEMODYNAMIC COHERENCE

Conventional hemodynamic monitoring used in routine clinical practice is focused on the macrocirculatory parameters, such as systemic blood pressure, cardiac output and heart rate. It is often assumed that resuscitation of the macrocirculation also corrects microcirculatory abnormalities. Unfortunately, this assumption is often incorrect, and failure to address microcirculatory parameters can result in unrecognized underresuscitation. Indeed, a number of studies in the critically ill have shown that macrocirculatory improvement may occur independently of the microcirculatory blood flow.[3] Inconsistency between microcirculation and macrocirculation has recently been defined as "loss of hemodynamic coherence" and has been shown to be an independent predictor of organ dysfunction and adverse outcome.[4] The disassociation between the macrocirculation and microcirculation reflects both differences in blood rheology and local metabolic, immunological, myogenic, endothelium-induced and neurovascular factors associated with critical illness.[5] Additional mechanisms remain to be determined in order to understand the mechanisms underlying loss of hemodynamic coherence.

In clinical practice, a loss of hemodynamic coherence can occur when microcirculatory resuscitation is accompanied by any one of four main types of microcirculatory alterations (Fig. 36.1). Type 1 alterations are associated with microcirculatory flow heterogeneity, where the stagnated flow in capillaries occurs next to fast-flowing RBCs. The result is functional shunting around underresuscitated microcirculatory units. Sepsis is the foremost example of Type 1 alterations. Type 2 alterations are characterized by a decrease in the number of RBCs in a capillary below a critical limit needed to adequately transport oxygen to tissues. An example would be hemodilution secondary to iatrogenic excess fluid therapy. Type 3 alterations are characterized by a state of microcirculatory stasis caused by venoconstriction from vasoactive medications or increased venous pressure, such as that seen in cardiac tamponade. In type 4 alterations, a reduction in the density of functional capillaries results in an increase in diffusion distance between capillaries and oxygen-requiring tissue cells. Type 4 alterations typically result from edema.[4]

Direct monitoring of alterations in microcirculatory blood flow and vascular density provides unique insight into the underlying pathophysiological mechanisms in patients with loss of hemodynamic coherence. Specifically, monitoring the microcirculation requires specific devices aimed at the bedside measurement of the functional microcirculatory parameters. Since the early 2000s increasing interest in tools for microcirculatory monitoring in both clinical and preclinical practice has led to the development of several imaging techniques that directly or indirectly measure perfusion, oxygenation, and anatomy, separately or in combination.[6]

OXYGEN TRANSPORT AND THE MICROCIRCULATION

Oxygen transport from the capillaries to the mitochondria in cells is determined by RBC movement through the capillaries and diffusion of oxygen from the RBC into cells. RBC movement is complex because RBC supply to capillaries is heterogeneous, dependent on microcirculatory flow rate and local

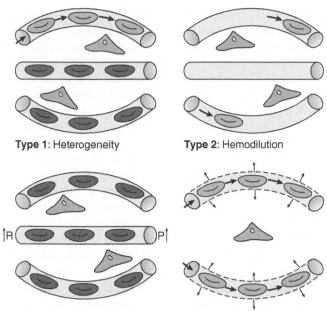

Type 1: Heterogeneity   **Type 2:** Hemodilution

Type 3: Constriction/tamponade   **Type 4:** Edema

Fig. 36.1 Microcirculatory alterations associated with loss of hemodynamic coherence. States of loss of hemodynamic coherence where macrocirculatory resuscitation does not necessarily cause a parallel improvement in perfusion of the microcirculation. Type 1: Heterogeneous red blood cell (RBC) flow where flowing RBCs carry oxygen *(gray RBC)* and stagnant RBC *(dark gray)*; correspondingly, tissue cells receive oxygen *(gray tissue cells)* or not *(blue tissue cells)*. Type 2: A reduction in the oxygen-carrying capacity of the microcirculation due to hemodilution. Type 3: A stagnation in RBC flow in the microcirculation due to arterial vasoconstriction (increased vascular resistance, R) and/or raised venous pressures (P). Type 4: Increased oxygen diffusion distances due to edema. (Modified from Ince C. Hemodynamic coherence and the rationale for monitoring the microcirculation. *Crit Care.* 2015;19 (suppl 3):S8.)

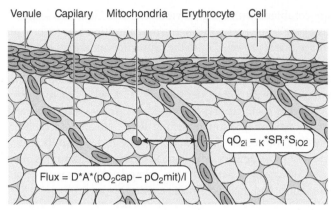

Fig. 36.2 Diffusive and convective mechanism of tissue oxygenation. O_2 flow rate in each capillary and diffusion of O_2 into cell mitochondria are estimated by the equation $[qO_{2i} = \kappa * SR_i * S_iO_2]$ and $[Flux = D*A*(pO_2cap - pO_2mit)/l]$, respectively. *A,* Capillary surface area; *D,* diffusion constant; κ, single RBCs total O_2 carrying capacity at 100% saturation (0.0362 pl O_2/RBC); *l,* length; pO_2cap, capillary O_2 pressure; pO_2mit, mitochondrial O_2 pressure; qO_{2i}, O_2 flow rate of individual capillary; *RBC,* red blood cell; SiO_2, SO_2 in individual capillary; SR_i, red blood cell supply rate.

BOX 36.1   Features of an Ideal Microcirculatory Monitor.

Quantitative and accurate output
Real-time functional information
Safe, efficacious, affective, easy to use at point-of-care
Cost-effective, noninvasive, noncontact
Instant analysis of the images

Data from Fasterholdt I, Krahn M, Kidholm K, et al. Review of early assessment models of innovative medical technologies. *Health Policy* 2017;121(8):870-879.

---

variations in regional oxygen consumption. The variables effecting this process include the RBC supply rate (SR_i) and the oxygen saturation in the individual capillary (S_iO_2). The diffusion of oxygen, in turn, can be estimated by Fick's laws, and is proportionally associated with variables that include capillary surface area, and the difference in partial pressure of oxygen (pO_2) between capillary and mitochondria. Diffusion is also inversely related to the distance from the capillary to the mitochondria (Fig. 36.2). RBC movement and diffusion make similar contributions to O_2 transport.[7] Deterioration in any of these parameters can be corrected by a change in microvascular hemodynamics. Therefore, monitoring these functional parameters in the microcirculation can be used to measure the main determinants of microcirculatory function.[8]

MONITORING THE MICROCIRCULATION

Features of an ideal microcirculatory monitoring technique are detailed in Box 36.1. Structure and the target depth of the investigated tissue and monitored parameters are also important. Laser-based techniques provide a sense of tissue perfusion of large body surfaces and can penetrate into deeper layers of tissue. However, they are not quantitative and do not provide important functional parameters such as RBC velocity, vessel density, or capillary distribution. Conversely, handheld video-microscopes (HVMs) have become the gold standard for clinical microcirculatory imaging because they allow quantification of capillary density, flow heterogeneity, RBC velocity, and single RBC/white blood cell (WBC) imaging. The main limitations of HVMs are the small surfaces (max 0.5 mm penetration) that they can examine. Of these, the sublingual area is the most widely used.

Microscopic observation of a vital tissue requires magnification and illumination. The latter can be accomplished by either trans- or epi-illumination. Trans-illumination, usually used in intravital microscopes in experimental settings, places the light source on the opposite side of the tissue under observation. Conversely, epi-illumination places the light source as well as the magnification lens on the same side of the tissue surface.

NAILFOLD CAPILLAROSCOPY

Nailfold capillaroscopy is a noninvasive imaging technique used to visualize the superficial capillaries within a few millimeters depth of the nail fold. The microscope and magnification lens are combined with a digital video camera. Light backscattered from the tissue passes through a magnification lens to form an image that is projected onto the capturing camera system. Most often this technique visualizes capillary loops characteristic of the nailfold microcirculation. Nailfold capillaroscopy, when combined with other techniques and with micropipettes connected to micropressure devices, provides structural and functional information regarding RBC velocity and capillary pressure. Moreover, the use of fluorescein dye permits assessment of transcapillary diffusion. Nailfold capillaroscopy is often used in assessing patients with scleroderma, Reynaud's phenomenon, and mixed connective tissue disease.[9]

HAND-HELD VIDEO-MICROSCOPES

HVM techniques can be used to directly visualize the microcirculation of all organ surfaces. Because of its accessibility, the sublingual area is the most commonly used target of HVMs, although intraoperative examination of other organ surfaces is feasible.[10–12] HVM analysis of the microcirculation with moving RBCs and WBCs provides unique and direct information regarding the functional activity of the microcirculation.[13] Measurements include capillary RBC flow (mean flow index and proportion of perfused vessel) and the density of perfused capillaries (also referred to as functional capillary density). Blood flow in the microvessels indicates the quality of perfusion and is described as microvascular flow index (MFI).[14] MFI, in turn, is determined by scoring the flow in each microvessel (3 = continuous, 2 = sluggish, 1 = intermittent, 0 = no flow) in each of four quadrants. Predominant flow type defines the MFI score per quadrant and the average of the four quadrants gives the total MFI score. An alternative MFI calculation option is to score all individual vessels and average their scores.[15] The heterogeneity index[16] is calculated as the difference between the highest and lowest MFI divided by mean MFI. It is particularly valuable in sepsis.

RBC velocity is quantitatively calculated with HVMs via space time diagram (STD) analysis (Fig. 36.3). Unfortunately, very fast RBCs, where flow is defined as hyperdynamic, cannot be measured with STD. Moreover, RBCs should be tracked clearly inside the capillary in order to use STD analysis. STD cannot be created for all capillaries and therefore leads to bias.[1] In addition to RBC-based calculations, recently, a new method has been validated using HVMs in monitoring leukocyte kinetics and function.[17]

The density of the vessels is estimated by the proportion of total vessels present in the field of view. The total vessel density (TVD) is calculated as the total length of vessels divided by the total surface area of the field of view as units mm/mm^2. Perfused vessel density (PVD) is estimated as the proportion of perfused vessels divided by the TVD.[1] Direct visualization of these parameters providing quantitative values is the main advantage of HVMs over other microcirculatory monitoring techniques. First generation HVM is based on orthogonal polarization spectral imaging (OPS, see later),[18] second generation, side-stream dark field (SDF)[19] and the third, incident dark field (IDF).[20] HVMs have outperformed OPS imaging,[21] and provided great insight into the microcirculatory basis of the pathophysiology of many disease states in medicine.[22–24]

Orthogonal Polarization Spectral Technique

In OPS imaging, the incident light is polarized and projected through a beam splitter to illuminate the tissue of interest. The penetrated light becomes depolarized after scattering several times within the tissue. The orthogonally polarized analyzer filters the reflected polarized light (surface reflection) allowing only the depolarized light to pass through to

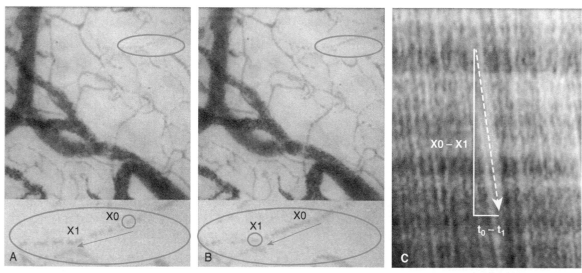

Fig. 36.3 Space time diagram analysis. Incident dark field image of a sublingual microcirculation. **(A)** and **(B)** indicate the same microcirculation image from different time points (1/6 seconds). X0 defines the first localization of the red blood cell, and X1 defines the localization of the same red blood cell (RBC) in 1/6 seconds. **(C)** indicates how the red blood cell velocity is calculated by the space time diagram. t_0 defines the first time point, t_1 defines the last time point. The red blood cell velocity is calculated as the proportion of the distance in a defined time interval.

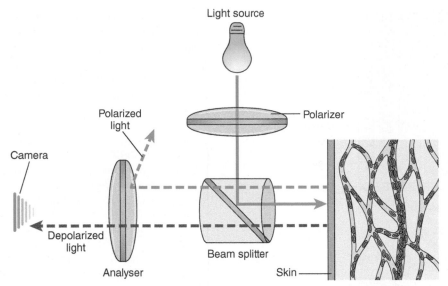

Fig. 36.4 Orthogonal polarized spectral technique.

the camera to generate an image of the microcirculation (Fig. 36.4). By using green light, which is absorbed by hemoglobin (Hb), the technique allows visualization of RBC movement. Thus the technique only visualizes functional blood vessels containing RBCs. A wavelength with 548 nm green light, which is equally absorbed by oxyhemoglobin and deoxyhemoglobin, generates images (black/gray dots) that are independent of Hb oxygenation. This technique can be combined with a hand-held device for bedside imaging in critically ill patients. The OPS technique has been validated with intravital fluorescence and conventional capillary microscopy.[21,25] It has largely been replaced by SDF and IDF, which provide better image quality without requiring high power light sources. Thus, OPS is no longer commercially available.[10,14,26]

Sidestream Dark-Field Technique

The main difference between SDF and OPS lies in the use of dark field imaging via light-emitting diodes (LED) concentrically arranged around a 5× magnification lens located at the tip of the light guide (Fig. 36.5). This approach avoids reflections from the tissue surface, allowing examination of the microcirculation below the organ surface.[20] RBCs can be visualized using green light with a 530 nm wavelength.[19] The use of a rapid, synchronized LED pulse of green light partially eliminates image blurring caused by rapid RBC movement. Thus the SDF technique provides higher quality images and capillary contrast.[19]

Incident Dark Field Technique

The IDF technique uses incident dark field illumination. High power illuminating LEDs with rapid pulse time (2 ms) provide appropriate tissue penetration and allow even more accurate cell tracking by further minimizing motion-induced blurring (Fig. 36.6). An advantage of IDF over OPS and SDF lies in the ability to capture fully digitalized images, eliminating the need to convert images from analog to digital.[27] Secondly, IDF uses a novel stepping motor-assisted quantitative

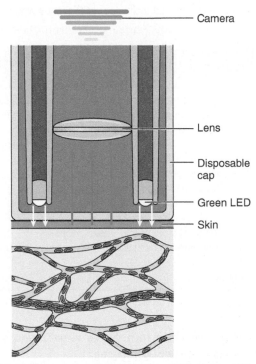

Fig. 36.5 Sidestream dark field technique. *LED*, Light-emitting diode.

focusing mechanism to provide measurement of focal depth,[28] also allowing multiple observations in the same subject without the need to refocus. Thirdly, reducing the weight of the camera from 320 g (SDF) – 500 g (OPS) to 120 g minimizes pressure artifact. Fourthly, the IDF device is integrated and controlled by a computer screen making data acquisition more reliable and controlled. Finally, the new IDF devices have incorporated microscope lenses instead of simple magnification lenses. In summary, improvement of the lens, the use of a high-resolution sensor, and an automatic, and a quantitative focusing mechanism resulted in an increase in contrast and sharpness compared with the

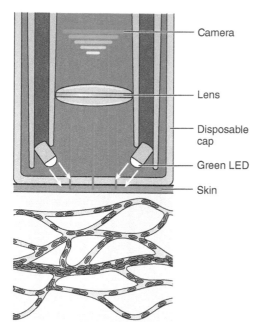

Fig. 36.6 Incident dark field technique. *LED*, Light-emitting diode.

BOX 36.2   **Limitations of Hand-Held Video-Microscopes.**

Movement artifact requiring subject to remain motionless

Pressure artifact constricting microcirculation despite decreasing weight of device[29]

Off-line analysis required for quantitative output (being addressed by novel software)[30]

Training required to optimize scoring metrics[15]

1. illumination (optimal brightness and contrast)
2. duration (minimum 4 seconds per video)
3. focus (optimal image sharpness)
4. content (free of occlusion and vessel loops)
5. stability (adequate stabilization of the video without motion blur)
6. pressure.

SDF technique, which in turn, led to visualization of 30% more microvessels than SDF imaging.[21]

CLINICAL APPLICATION OF HAND-HELD VIDEO-MICROSCOPES

HVM-based microcirculatory assessment represents a promising approach to facilitate the evolution of personalized medicine from randomized trials.[31–33] The technique has proven to be helpful in the management of a number of different types of critically ill patients. Examples include guiding therapy of heart failure patients, timing of withdrawal of cardiac support devices and quantifying the impact of the therapeutic maneuvers on hemodynamics.[24,34–36] In addition, monitoring of microcirculation has shown to be helpful in detection of hemodynamic coherence in patients with sepsis and septic shock.[33,37,38] The accumulated clinical evidence

regarding the use of HVM has led an expert panel to generate a comprehensive consensus article on the assessment of sublingual microcirculation in critically ill patients.[2] In the future, the use of HVMs can be expected to provide clinicians caring for the critically ill with both an important technique for early diagnosis of circulatory inadequacies and a more physiologically-based approach to therapy.

AUTHORS' RECOMMENDATIONS

- Direct visualization of microcirculatory alterations at the bedside is the ideal way of microcirculatory imaging.
- Hand-held video-microscopes are appropriate for direct visualization of microcirculation.
- Further developments of the equipment and techniques are required to overcome the main limitation of video-microscopy. Pressure and movement artifact-free image and new fully automatic analysis software are promising approaches.
- If combined with other monitoring techniques that permit estimation of capillary hematocrit and RBC hemoglobin saturation, evaluation of microcirculatory heterogeneity promises to provide valuable and comprehensive information about shock and resuscitation.

REFERENCES

1. Ince C, Boerma EC, Cecconi M, et al. Second consensus on the assessment of sublingual microcirculation in critically ill patients: results from a task force of the European Society of Intensive Care Medicine. *Intensive Care Med.* 2018;44(3):281-299.
2. De Backer D, Ospina-Tascon G, Salgado D, Favory R, Creteur J, Vincent JL. Monitoring the microcirculation in the critically ill patient: current methods and future approaches. *Intensive Care Med.* 2010;36:1813-1825.
3. Donati A, Domizi R, Damiani E, Adrario E, Pelaia P, Ince C. From macrohemodynamic to the microcirculation. *Crit Care Res Pract.* 2013;2013:892710.
4. Ince C. Hemodynamic coherence and the rationale for monitoring the microcirculation. *Crit Care.* 2015;19(suppl 3):S8.
5. Pries AR, Neuhaus D, Gaehtgens P. Blood viscosity in tube flow: dependence on diameter and hematocrit. *Am J Physiol.* 1992;263:H1770-H1778.
6. De Backer D, Durand A. Monitoring the microcirculation in critically ill patients. *Best Pract Res Clin Anaesthesiol.* 2014;28:441-451.
7. Ince C. The rationale for microcirculatory guided fluid therapy. *Curr Opin Crit Care.* 2014;20:301-308.
8. Sakr Y. Techniques to assess tissue oxygenation in the clinical setting. *Transfus Apher Sci.* 2010;43:79-94.
9. Weekenstroo HH, Cornelissen BM, Bernelot Moens HJ. Green light may improve diagnostic accuracy of nailfold capillaroscopy with a simple digital videomicroscope. *Rheumatol Int.* 2015;35:1069-1071.
10. Mathura KR, Bouma GJ, Ince C. Abnormal microcirculation in brain tumours during surgery. *Lancet.* 2001;358:1698-1699.
11. Dondorp AM, Ince C, Charunwatthana P, et al. Direct in vivo assessment of microcirculatory dysfunction in severe falciparum malaria. *J Infect Dis.* 2008;197:79-84.
12. Uz Z, Ince C, Rassam F, Ergin B, van Lienden KP, van Gulik TM. Assessment of hepatic microvascular flow and density in

patients undergoing preoperative portal vein embolization. *HPB (Oxford)*. 2019;21:187–194.

13. Sallisalmi M, Oksala N, Pettilä V, Tenhunen J. Evaluation of sublingual microcirculatory blood flow in the critically ill. *Acta Anaesthesiol Scand*. 2012;56:298-306.

14. Boerma EC, Mathura KR, van der Voort PH, Spronk PE, Ince C. Quantifying bedside-derived imaging of microcirculatory abnormalities in septic patients: a prospective validation study. *Crit Care*. 2005;9:R601-R606.

15. Massey MJ, Larochelle E, Najarro G, et al. The microcirculation image quality score: development and preliminary evaluation of a proposed approach to grading quality of image acquisition for bedside videomicroscopy. *J Crit Care*. 2013;28:913-917.

16. Trzeciak S, Dellinger RP, Parrillo JE, et al. Early microcirculatory perfusion derangements in patients with severe sepsis and septic shock: relationship to hemodynamics, oxygen transport, and survival. *Ann Emerg Med*. 2007;49:88-98, 98.e1-2.

17. Uz Z, van Gulik TM, Aydemirli MD, et al. Identification and quantification of human microcirculatory leukocytes using handheld video microscopes at the bedside. *J Appl Physiol (1985)*. 2018;124:1550-1557.

18. Slaaf DW, Tangelder GJ, Reneman RS, Jäger K, Bollinger A. A versatile incident illuminator for intravital microscopy. *Int J Microcirc Clin Exp*. 1987;6:391-397.

19. Goedhart PT, Khalilzada M, Bezemer R, Merza J, Ince C. Sidestream Dark Field (SDF) imaging: a novel stroboscopic LED ring-based imaging modality for clinical assessment of the microcirculation. *Opt Express*. 2007;15:15101-15114.

20. Sherman H, Klausner S, Cook WA. Incident dark-field illumination: a new method for microcirculatory study. *Angiology*. 1971;22: 295-303.

21. Mathura KR, Vollebregt KC, Boer K, De Graaff JC, Ubbink DT, Ince C. Comparison of OPS imaging and conventional capillary microscopy to study the human microcirculation. *J Appl Physiol (1985)*. 2001;91:74-78.

22. Bezemer R, Bartels SA, Bakker J, Ince C. Clinical review: Clinical imaging of the sublingual microcirculation in the critically ill—where do we stand? *Crit Care*. 2012;16:224.

23. Donati A, Tibboel D, Ince C. Towards integrative physiological monitoring of the critically ill: from cardiovascular to microcirculatory and cellular function monitoring at the bedside. *Crit Care*. 2013;17(suppl 1):S5.

24. den Uil CA, Caliskan K, Lagrand WK, et al. Dose-dependent benefit of nitroglycerin on microcirculation of patients with severe heart failure. *Intensive Care Med*. 2009;35:1893-1899.

25. Groner W, Winkelman JW, Harris AG, et al. Orthogonal polarization spectral imaging: a new method for study of the microcirculation. *Nat Med*. 1999;5:1209-1212.

26. Biberthaler P, Langer S, Luchting B, Khandoga A, Messmer K. In vivo assessment of colon microcirculation: comparison of the new OPS imaging technique with intravital microscopy. *Eur J Med Res*. 2001;6:525-534.

27. Aykut G, Veenstra G, Scorcella C, Ince C, Boerma C. Cytocam-IDF (incident dark field illumination) imaging for bedside monitoring of the microcirculation. *Intensive Care Med Exp*. 2015;3:40.

28. Weber MA, Diedrich CM, Ince C, Roovers JP. Focal depth measurements of the vaginal wall: a new method to noninvasively quantify vaginal wall thickness in the diagnosis and treatment of vaginal atrophy. *Menopause*. 2016;23:833-838.

29. Balestra GM, Bezemer R, Boerma EC, et al. Improvement of sidestream dark field imaging with an image acquisition stabilizer. *BMC Med Imaging*. 2010;10:15.

30. Arend S, Ince C, Assen M, et al. A software tool to quantify capillary hematocrit and microvascular hemodilution in sublingual incident dark field microscopy video clips. *Critical Care*. 2018;22(suppl 1):115.

31. Ince C. Personalized physiological medicine. *Crit Care*. 2017;21:308.

32. Legrand M, Ait-Oufella H, Ince C. Could resuscitation be based on microcirculation data? Yes. *Intensive Care Med*. 2018;44:944-946.

33. Lima A, Jansen TC, van Bommel J, Ince C, Bakker J. The prognostic value of the subjective assessment of peripheral perfusion in critically ill patients. *Crit Care Med*. 2009;37:934-938.

34. Erol-Yilmaz A, Atasever B, Mathura K, et al. Cardiac resynchronization improves microcirculation. *J Card Fail*. 2007;13:95-99.

35. Lauten A, Ferrari M, Goebel B, et al. Microvascular tissue perfusion is impaired in acutely decompensated heart failure and improves following standard treatment. *Eur J Heart Fail*. 2011;13:711-717.

36. Munsterman LD, Elbers PW, Ozdemir A, van Dongen EP, van Iterson M, Ince C. Withdrawing intra-aortic balloon pump support paradoxically improves microvascular flow. *Crit Care*. 2010;14:R161.

37. De Backer D, Donadello K, Sakr Y, et al. Microcirculatory alterations in patients with severe sepsis: impact of time of assessment and relationship with outcome. *Crit Care Med*. 2013;41:791-799.

38. Edul VS, Enrico C, Laviolle B, Vazquez AR, Ince C, Dubin A. Quantitative assessment of the microcirculation in healthy volunteers and in patients with septic shock. *Crit Care Med*. 2012;40:1443-1448.

37

Are We Getting Any Better at Diagnosing Sepsis?

Stephanie Royer Moss and Hallie C. Prescott

Sepsis has long been established as an important cause of morbidity and mortality, contributing to an estimated 5.8 million deaths around the world each year.[1] In the United States, hospitalization for sepsis is more common than myocardial infarction and stroke, and contributes to as many as half of all hospital deaths.[2,3] Moreover, an estimated 14 million patients survive sepsis hospitalization each year and face increased risk for cognitive impairment, physical disability,[4] further health set-backs,[5] and death[6] in the months following sepsis hospitalization. Because of its worldwide burden of morbidity and mortality, sepsis was recently recognized as a global health priority by the World Health Organization.[7]

Despite improved understanding of sepsis pathogenesis over the past few decades, there have been no new targeted therapies for sepsis.[8] As such, efforts to reduce sepsis-related morbidity and mortality focus on improved recognition, faster time-to-treatment,[9] and implementation of standardized care-bundles,[10] as these are broadly recognized as the main levers by which to improve sepsis outcomes.

OUR EVOLVING DEFINITION OF SEPSIS

'Sepsis', from the Greek word sipsi, or "to make rotten", has been used in a medical context dating back to the poems of Homer (~8500 BCE) and the writings of Hippocrates (~CE 400).[11] Conceptually, sepsis is a life-threatening complication of infection that arises when the body's response to infection injures its own tissues and organs (Fig. 37.1).[12] However, the first modern definition of sepsis (from here called Sepsis-1) was not published until 1992, following a 1991 consensus conference involving eight critical care and infectious disease experts.[13] The goal of this conference was to develop both a conceptual and practical framework to define sepsis, in order to standardize sepsis research and improve the dissemination of study findings.

Sepsis-1 defined sepsis as an inflammatory process (systemic inflammatory response syndrome [SIRS]) in response to infection (Fig. 37.2); SIRS was defined as two or more abnormalities of temperature, heart rate, respiratory rate, and white blood cell count (Box 37.1). In addition, sepsis was defined on a spectrum of illness severity, which could progress to severe sepsis (sepsis with organ dysfunction, such as oliguria, altered mental status, or lactic acidosis), and subsequently to septic shock, (sepsis complicated by hypotension not responsive to fluid resuscitation).[13]

In 2001, the second consensus conference including 29 participants from Europe and North America was held to update sepsis definitions (Sepsis-2). The committee acknowledged that SIRS is non-specific, but may also fail to identify patients who are truly septic. As such, the committee expanded the list of relevant signs and symptoms included in SIRS criteria (Box 37.2).[14] However, no changes to the paradigm of sepsis as SIRS in the setting of infection, or the spectrum of sepsis, severe sepsis, and septic shock, were made, owing to insufficient evidence. These conceptual definitions continued to be used for enrollment in sepsis clinical trials and in clinical practice, and most clinicians continued to use the initial 4-component SIRS criteria.

In 2014, a third consensus panel including 19 infectious disease and critical care experts was convened by the US Society of Critical Care Medicine (SCCM) and the European Society of Intensive Care Medicine (ESICM) to reexamine sepsis definitions in light of improved pathophysiologic understanding and ongoing concerns about the existing definitions (Sepsis-3).[12] By 2014, it had been widely accepted that SIRS criteria in the setting of infection was not sufficient for the identification of sepsis, as the positive and negative predictive values of SIRS criteria are low.[15] Some degree of inflammatory response to infection is adaptive and normal, so SIRS criteria may simply reflect a normal response to infection.[12] Also problematic is that SIRS is not specific for sepsis, as other sterile processes lead to the same inflammatory response,[16] reflecting poor discriminant validity.[12] As only two of four SIRS criteria must be met to have a positive result, one study found that up to 90% of intensive care unit patients met criteria.[17] Another study of ward patients found that 50% met SIRS criteria at some point during hospitalization.[18] Conversely, some patients with severe sepsis manifest fewer than 2 SIRS criteria.[12,19]

The first step to improving sepsis recognition was updating the consensus definition based on the expanded knowledge of the pathogenesis of sepsis. Sepsis-1 and Sepsis-2 conceptualized sepsis as an excessive inflammatory response to infection.[13,14] However, dozens of trials testing antiinflammatory agents failed to show benefit in septic patients,[8] and it was subsequently recognized that sepsis involves activation of both pro- and antiinflammatory pathways,[20,21] as well as alterations to multiple nonimmunologic processes, including coagulation, hormonal, and metabolic pathways.[12] Because of this, and ongoing concerns

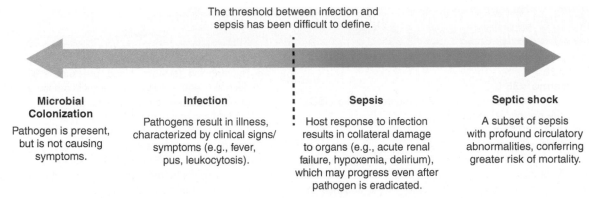

The threshold between infection and sepsis has been difficult to define.

Microbial Colonization
Pathogen is present, but is not causing symptoms.

Infection
Pathogens result in illness, characterized by clinical signs/ symptoms (e.g., fever, pus, leukocytosis).

Sepsis
Host response to infection results in collateral damage to organs (e.g., acute renal failure, hypoxemia, delirium), which may progress even after pathogen is eradicated.

Septic shock
A subset of sepsis with profound circulatory abnormalities, conferring greater risk of mortality.

Fig. 37.1 Spectrum of host response to the presence of a pathogen.

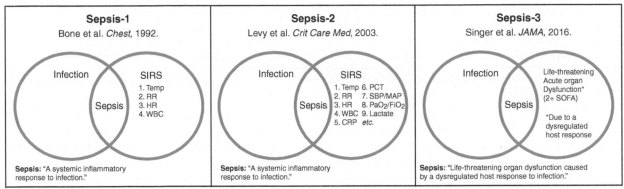

Fig. 37.2 Evolution of modern sepsis definitions. CRP, C-reactive protein; FiO₂, fraction of inspired oxygen; HR, heart rate; MAP, mean arterial pressure; PaO₂, partial pressure of oxygen; PCT, procalcitonin; SBP, systolic blood pressure; SIRS, systemic inflammatory response syndrome; SOFA, sequential organ failure assessment; temp, temperature; RR, respiratory rate; WBC, white blood cell count.

BOX 37.1   Systemic Inflammatory Response Syndrome Criteria.

- Temperature >38°C or <36°C
- Heart rate >90 beats/min
- Respiratory rate >20 breaths/min or $PaCO_2$ <32 mm Hg
- White blood cell count >12,000/mm³ or <4000/mm³ or >10% immature bands

Patients must demonstrate two or more of the above criteria

Data from Bone RC, Balk RA, Cerra FB, et al. Definitions for sepsis and organ failure and guidelines for the use of innovative therapies in sepsis. The ACCP/SCCM Consensus Conference Committee. American College of Chest Physicians/Society of Critical Care Medicine. Chest. 1992;101(6):1644-1655.

---

about SIRS criteria being non-specific, Sepsis-3 redefined sepsis as "life-threatening organ dysfunction caused by a dysregulated host response to infection". Since organ dysfunction is now a critical component of sepsis, the taskforce concluded that severe sepsis was an unnecessary and redundant term.

In addition to updating the definition of sepsis, the task force also sought to identify easily measurable clinical criteria that would identify sepsis and distinguish it from uncomplicated infection in a uniform way that would be readily accessible to researchers and clinicians.[12] The Sepsis-3 taskforce interrogated a large dataset of patients with suspected infection (defined as body fluid cultures sent and antibiotics received) to determine which criteria best identify patients at risk for poor outcomes (in-hospital death or prolonged ICU stay).[12] The Sequential Organ Failure Assessment (SOFA) is a scale for assessing severity of organ dysfunction that is commonly used in clinical trials, and higher scores are associated with increased mortality.[22] Based on their evaluation of a large cohort of infected patients, the taskforce recommended that "life-threatening organ dysfunction" be identified as a SOFA score of 2 or more, where baseline is presumed to be zero in the absence of other clinical information.[12] A SOFA score ≥2 identifies patients with an overall mortality risk of 10% in US cohorts with suspected infection, consistent with the new definition of sepsis as a life-threatening condition.[23]

Finally, in addition to revising the sepsis definition and recommending data-driven criteria for identifying life-threatening organ dysfunction, the taskforce introduced a parsimonious clinical tool – the quick SOFA, or qSOFA – to rapidly identify infected patients on whom additional information should be gathered. qSOFA awards one point each for systolic blood pressure <100 mmHg, respiratory rate >22 breaths/minute, and altered mentation (a Glasgow

---

BOX 37.2   Expanded Systemic Inflammatory Response Syndrome Criteria Used in Sepsis-2 Definition.

- General parameters
  - Fever >38.3°C
  - Hypothermia <36°C
  - Heart rate> 90 beats/min or >2 standard deviation (SD) above the normal value for age
  - Tachypnea >30 bpm
  - Altered mental status
  - Significant edema or positive fluid balance (>20 mL/kg over 24 hours)
  - Hyperglycemia (glucose >110 mg/dL) in the absence of diabetes
- Inflammatory parameters
  - Leukocytosis >12,000/μL
  - Leukopenia <4000/μL
  - Normal white blood cell count with >10% immature forms
  - C reactive protein >2 SD above the normal value
  - Procalcitonin >2 SD above the normal value

- Hemodynamic parameters
  - Hypotension (systolic blood pressure <90 mm Hg or decrease >40 mm Hg, mean arterial pressure <70 mm Hg, or <2 SD below normal value for age)
  - Mixed venous oxygen saturation >70%
  - Cardiac index >3.5 L/min/m^2
- Organ dysfunction parameters
  - Hypoxemia (PaO$_2$/FiO$_2$ <300)
  - Acute oliguria (urine output <0.5 mL/kg/h for 2 hours)
  - Creatinine increase >0.5 mg/dL
  - Coagulation abnormalities (INR >1.5 or aPTT >60 seconds)
  - Ileus (absent bowel sounds)
  - Thrombocytopenia <100,000/μL
  - Hyperbilirubinemia >4 mg/dL
- Tissue perfusion parameters
  - Elevated lactate >3 mmol/L
  - Decreased capillary refill or mottling

Patients must demonstrate *some* of the above criteria

Data from Levy MM, Fink MP, Marshall JC, et al. 2001 SCCM/ESICM/ACCP/ATS/SIS International Sepsis Definitions Conference. *Intensive Care Med.* 2003;29(4):530-538.

Coma Score <15); 2 (out of a possible 3) points on the qSOFA is considered positive. The benefits of qSOFA are that it identifies the very sickest patients (patients with 2+ qSOFA points accounted for 70% of deaths and 70% of prolonged ICU stays in the Seymour, et al., Sepsis-3 validation study),[23] it does not require any laboratory measurements; and it can be calculated within minutes in virtually any healthcare setting.[12] However, because this tool identifies only the sickest subset of septic patients (just 24% of infected patients in Seymour, et al., were qSOFA positive), it is not a screening tool in the traditional sense. It was never intended to rule out sepsis and cannot be used for this purpose.

Overall, Sepsis-3 produced an updated definition of sepsis, better aligned with our current pathophysiological understanding of the syndrome, and put forth clinical criteria to identify patients at highest risk for adverse outcomes. Its strengths are that it is data-driven and provides objective, easily measured criteria to identify infected patients at highest risk of poor outcomes. However, the SOFA score uses lagging indicators of organ dysfunction (e.g. creatinine as opposed to earlier markers of renal injury, such as neutrophil gelatinase-associated lipocalin),[24] and therefore may not identify patients with early organ dysfunction. In addition, the identification of infection and "dysregulated immune function" remain subjective.

NEW SEPSIS DEFINITIONS AND TOOLS IN CLINICAL PRACTICE

Since Sepsis-3 was published, many studies have evaluated its usefulness compared to prior sepsis definitions (Table 37.1). Studies have examined how well qSOFA and SOFA score ≥2 predict mortality across a variety of settings (emergency, ward,

ICU), and in a variety of countries. SOFA and qSOFA consistently outperform SIRS criteria, and all tools perform best in the emergency department (ED), modestly well in the wards, and worst in the ICU. For example, in a prospective evaluation of approximately 900 patients presenting to 30 emergency departments in 4 European countries, both qSOFA and SOFA outperformed SIRS or SIRS plus organ dysfunction at predicting in-hospital mortality. In-hospital mortality was 3% among qSOFA-negative patients versus 24% in qSOFA-positive patients.[25] In a retrospective study of >180,000 ICU patients in Australia and New Zealand, SOFA score outperformed SIRS and qSOFA in predicting in-hospital mortality (AUROC 0.75 vs. 0.59 vs. 0.61, respectively).[26] In a recent study of several sepsis cohorts from low and middle income countries, positive qSOFA was a better predictor of in-hospital mortality than positive SIRS (AUROC 0.70 vs. 0.59).[27] A study of ICU patients in China demonstrated the Sepsis-3 criteria was better able to identify patients with higher 28-day mortality.[28] Similarly, studies of ICU patients out of the Netherlands and South Korea demonstrate that Sepsis-3 criteria identified a patient population at higher risk of death.[29,30]

A recent metaanalysis pooled 23 studies evaluating the prognostic ability of qSOFA versus SIRS in non-ICU patients and found that qSOFA has high specificity (83%) for identifying organ dysfunction and in-hospital mortality, but limited sensitivity (51%).[31] Another meta-analysis of 38 studies evaluating qSOFA in all locations (ED, wards, and ICU) reported a pooled sensitivity of 61% and a specificity of 72% for in-hospital mortality.[32]

While qSOFA is more predictive of poor outcomes than SIRS, it does not perform better than other generic measures of illness severity, such as the Modified or National Early Warning Score.[33] However, with only 3 elements, qSOFA is

TABLE 37.1	Selected Studies Evaluating the Performance of SOFA and qSOFA Criteria.				
Study	Study Design	Region	Number of Patients	Setting	Major Findings
Chen et al., *Crit Care* 2016[56]	Retrospective	China	1,641	1 hospital; ICU, ED, wards	AUROC for in-hospital mortality: 0.655 (qSOFA), 0.661 (CRB-65), $P > 0.05$
Kolditz et al., *Intensive Care Med*, 2016[57]	Retrospective cohort	Germany	9,327	Multicenter wards, ICU	AUROC for 30-day mortality: 0.70 (qSOFA), 0.68 (CRB), $P = 0.42$, 0.77 (CRB-65), $P < 0.001$
Seymour et al., *JAMA* 2016[23]	Retrospective cohort	USA	66,522 non-ICU 7,932 ICU	1 hospital; ED, wards, ICU	AUROC for in-hospital mortality, ICU population: 0.74 (SOFA), 0.75 (LODS), 0.66 (SIRS), 0.64 (qSOFA) $P < 0.05$ all pairwise with SOFA except LODS $P = 0.20$ AUROC for in-hospital mortality, non-ICU population: 0.79 (SOFA), 0.81 (LODS) 0.76 (SIRS), 0.81 (qSOFA) $P < 0.05$ all pairwise with qSOFA except LODS $P = 0.77$
Cheng et al., *Shock* 2017[28]	Retrospective cohort	China	496	6 ICUs	AUROC for 28-day mortality: 0.69 (SOFA), 0.55 (SIRS), $P = 0.008$
Churpek et al., *Am J Respir Crit Care Med* 2017[33]	Observational	United States	30,667	1 ED/wards	AUROC for in-hospital mortality: 0.77 (NEWS), 0.73 (MEWS), 0.69 (qSOFA), 0.65 (SIRS), $P < 0.01$ all pairwise comparisons
Finkelsztein et al., *Crit Care* 2017[58]	Observational	USA	152	1 hospital; wards prior to ICU transfer	AUROC for in-hospital mortality: 0.74 (qSOFA), 0.59 (SIRS), $P = 0.03$
Freund et al., *JAMA* 2017[25]	Prospective cohort	International European	879	30 EDs	AUROC for in-hospital mortality: 0.80 (qSOFA), 0.65 (SIRS and severe sepsis), $P < 0.001$
Raith et al., *JAMA* 2017[26]	Retrospective cohort	Australia/ New Zealand	184,875	182 ICUs	AUROC for in-hospital mortality: 0.753 (SOFA), 0.607 (qSOFA), 0.589 (SIRS), $P < 0.001$
Ranzani et al., *Am J Respir Crit Care Med* 2017[59]	Retrospective cohort	Spain	6,874	2 hospitals; ED, wards, ICU	AUROC for in-hospital mortality: 0.579 (SIRS), 0.697 (qSOFA), 0.716 (CRB), 0.746 (CURB-65), 0.748 (mSOFA), 0.780 (PSI)
Ryoo et al., *Crit Care* 2018[30]	Observational	South Korea	1,028	10 EDs	90-day mortality: 32.1% (Sepsis-3) vs. 23.3% (Sepsis-1), $P < 0.01$
Driessen et al., *Infect Dis* 2018[29]	Prospective cohort	Netherlands	632	1 ICU	ICU mortality: 38.9% (Sepsis-3) vs. 34.0% (Sepsis-2), no statistical analysis performed
Fernando et al., *Ann Int Med* 2018[32]	Systematic review/ meta-analysis	International	385,333	38 studies, ICU, ED, wards	Pooled sensitivity for mortality: 60.8% (qSOFA) vs. 88.1% (SIRS) Pooled specificity for mortality: 72.0% (qSOFA) vs. 25.8% (SIRS)
Rudd et al., *JAMA* 2018[27]	Retrospective secondary analysis of 8 cohort studies and 1 RCT	International (10 LMIC)	6,569	17 hospitals, ICU, ED, wards	AUROC for in-hospital mortality: 0.70 (qSOFA), 0.59 (SIRS), 0.56 (baseline model), $P < 0.001$

Continued

TABLE 37.1   Selected Studies Evaluating the Performance of SOFA and qSOFA Criteria.—cont'd

Study	Study Design	Region	Number of Patients	Setting	Major Findings
Schlapbach et al., *Intensive Care Med* 2018[60]	Retrospective cohort	Australia/ New Zealand	2,594 (pediatric)	ICUs	AUROC for in-hospital mortality: 0.829 (SOFA), 0.727 (SIRS), 0.711 (severe sepsis), 0.739 (qSOFA), $P < 0.001$ all pairwise comparisons with SOFA 0.816 (PELOD-2), $P = 0.97$ compared to SOFA
Song et al., *Crit Care* 2018[31]	Systematic review/ meta-analysis	International	146,551	23 studies, non-ICU	AUROC for in-hospital mortality: 0.74 (qSOFA), 0.71 (SIRS), $P = 0.816$

AUROC, area under the curve of the receiver operating characteristic; *CRB,* confusion, respiratory rate >30 breaths/min, blood pressure <90 mm Hg systolic; *CRB-65,* confusion, respiratory rate >30 breaths/min, blood pressure <90 mm Hg systolic, age >65 years; *CURB-65,* confusion, uremia (blood urea nitrogen >19 mg/dL), respiratory rate >30 breaths/min, blood pressure <90 mm Hg systolic, age >65 years; *ED,* emergency department; *ICU,* intensive care unit; *LMIC,* low- and middle-income countries; *LODS,* logistic organ dysfunction system; *mSOFA,* modified sequential organ failure assessment; *PELOD-2,* pediatric logistic organ dysfunction-2; *qSOFA,* quick sequential organ failure assessment; *SIRS,* systemic inflammatory response syndrome; *SOFA,* sequential organ failure assessment.

less cumbersome to assess than most generic measures of illness severity.

IDENTIFICATION OF SEPSIS IN CLINICAL PRACTICE

Despite our improved understanding of sepsis pathophysiology and new data-driven clinical criteria to identify patients at highest risk for poor outcomes, sepsis identification remains challenging in clinical practice. In standardized vignettes of patients with suspected infection, there is wide disagreement on sepsis diagnosis amongst clinicians (interrater reliability of just 0.29 on a scale of 0–1) despite high self-reported confidence in using sepsis definitions.[34] This poor agreement across clinicians was largely attributed to differences of opinion as to whether organ dysfunction was due to a dysregulated host response versus other mechanisms (e.g., dehydration).[34]

In another study of 2579 patients with presumed sepsis on ICU admission, 30% had only "possible" infection likelihood and 13% had "no" infection likelihood on post-hoc adjudication by multiple clinicians.[35] Of particular concern, the patients who were misdiagnosed as septic had higher mortality than patients who were ultimately confirmed to have infection, highlighting the potential for adverse outcomes with misdiagnosis.

In another study of >105,000 patients treated under New York State's sepsis regulations, there was poor correlation between the patients reported as having sepsis through the QI initiative and those ultimately receiving a sepsis diagnosis at discharge, further underscoring the difficulty of real-time identification.[36]

THE ROLE OF DIAGNOSTIC BIOMARKERS

A key challenge for sepsis identification is the lack of a high-quality biomarker to rule-in or rule-out sepsis, akin to a troponin for acute myocardial infarction—or even biomarkers to rule-in or rule-out specific components of

sepsis, such as infection or a dysregulated host response to infection. Numerous biomarkers of infection and inflammation have been considered, including pro-inflammatory cytokines, complement proteins, coagulation factors, C-reactive protein (CRP), and procalcitonin (PCT).[37] Indeed, a 2010 review identified 178 unique biomarkers for infection and inflammation reported in the literature.[38] However, biomarkers of inflammation are less relevant following the advent of the Sepsis-3 definition and current conceptualization of sepsis as a dysregulated host response (rather than a systemic inflammatory response).

Importantly, few studies have evaluated the performance of biomarkers in the diagnosis of sepsis since the adoption of the Sepsis-3 definition. One German study evaluated the diagnostic value of pentraxin-3 in the intensive care unit and found that it had good diagnostic value throughout the first week of treatment for both sepsis (AUROC 0.82–0.92) and septic shock (AUROC 0.73–0.81).[39] Another study evaluated plasminogen activator inhibitor-1 as a prognostic marker for mortality in patients meeting Sepsis-3 definition, but not for diagnosis.[40]

PCT is the most common biomarker in clinical practice for the identification of infection. PCT is undetectable in health, but is rapidly upregulated by cytokines released in response to bacterial infection.[41] Recent metaanalyses indicate that PCT has good sensitivity (0.67–0.77) and specificity (0.79–0.83) for differentiating infection plus SIRS from noninfectious SIRS.[42,43] However, PCT has not been evaluated for discriminating sepsis using the Sepsis-3 definition.

When considering the utility of PCT in sepsis, it is important to also consider that the presence of a bacterial infection does not necessarily imply sepsis, nor does the absence of bacterial infection preclude sepsis from other infectious sources. Additionally, interpreting PCT is not always straightforward. Renal dysfunction and congestive heart failure can both artificially elevate PCT in the absence of infection.[44]

The Infectious Disease Society of America (IDSA) does not recommend use of procalcitonin for the diagnosis of sepsis.[43]

The Surviving Sepsis Campaign Guidelines recommend that PCT can be used to shorten the duration of antibiotics, but caution that "procalcitonin and all other biomarkers can provide only supportive and supplemental data to clinical assessment" and should not guide decisions independently.[45]

MOLECULAR DIAGNOSTICS

Molecular biomarkers (i.e., biomarkers characterizing gene expression) have been investigated to distinguish infection with SIRS from noninfectious SIRS. Many such biomarkers have been proposed and studies have measured both micro-RNAs and their target proteins.[46]

A molecular host response assay combining four RNA biomarkers, and which was developed in Australia and validated in a small cohort ($n = 345$) in the Netherlands, reported an AUROC of 0.89–0.95 for distinguishing infection plus SIRS from noninfectious SIRS.[47] Another validation study of the same molecular assay, performed in the United States and the Netherlands, reported an AUROC of 0.82–0.89 for distinguishing infection plus SIRS from noninfectious SIRS.[48] A study of this assay in pediatrics similarly reported good discrimination between patients with infection plus SIRS and those who underwent postcardiopulmonary bypass (AUROC 0.99).[49]

One study sought to combine data from the available assays to determine the optimal combination for correctly identifying infection plus SIRS.[50] From five cohorts totaling 663 patient samples, they identified 82 genes that were expressed differentially between infection plus SIRS and nonnfectious SIRS.[50] Their final analysis combined 11 genes that allowed for the correct identification of infection plus SIRS with a mean AUROC of 0.87.[50]

While molecular biomarkers have shown promise in distinguishing infectious from noninfectious SIRS, there is limited data on how such biomarkers fare in distinguishing sepsis based on the current Sepsis-3 definition. However, recently one miRNA (miRNA-122) was studied in patients meeting Sepsis-3 criteria, and was found to discriminate sepsis from infection with an AUROC of 0.760 and to improve the predictive value of the SOFA score for 30-day mortality.[51] Further studies are needed to determine the role of molecular biomarkers in the differentiation of sepsis from infection.

BIOMARKER PANELS

To date, there is no single biomarker with sufficient accuracy to withhold antibiotics from a patient clinically suspected to have sepsis. However, there is a growing body of literature employing a multimarker approach that could provide clinicians with important information regarding the diagnosis and management of sepsis.[37]

There have been several proposals of clinical scores comprised of multiple biomarkers to identify and prognosticate in sepsis. Some of these scores have been comprised of traditional biomarkers of infection, while others have incorporated novel biomarkers. For example, one study found that a combination of PCT, CRP, neutrophils, MIF, suPAR, and sTREM-1 performed better than any individual factor at distinguishing bacterial from nonbacterial causes of systemic inflammation.[52]

Since the publication of Sepsis-3, one multicenter Italian study derived and validated a biomarker panel (PCT, soluble phosphorylase A2 group IIA, presepsin, soluble IL-2a, and sTREM-1) to rule out sepsis with high negative predictive value, 93% in the derivation cohort of 836 patients and 100% in the validation cohort of 158 patients.[53] A recent review of novel biomarkers in sepsis concluded that PCT, presepsin, CD64, suPAR, and sTREM-1 are the best evaluated, but noted that all have important limitations, and further research is needed.[54]

Overall, biomarkers show promise in helping clinicians to distinguish sepsis from noninfectious organ dysfunction. No single biomarker or combination of biomarkers can independently identify patients with sepsis, but biomarkers may improve sepsis diagnosis and guide decisions in ambiguous cases. However, additional studies are needed to confirm the optimal role and implementation of biomarkers in clinical practice. The recent ProACT study[55] found merely providing PCT results to clinicians did not change antibiotic prescribing – suggesting that education on how to incorporate biomarkers into clinical decision making is also needed to change practice.

CONCLUSION

Sepsis-3 has advanced our ability to identify infected patients at high risk for poor outcomes. This is helpful to consistently identify the sickest patients, at high risk for long-term morbidity and mortality to facilitate treatment and research (e.g., enrollment into clinical trials). In contrast to prior modern definitions, the clinical criteria for Sepsis-3 were selected based on interrogation of large datasets, and have subsequently been validated in additional populations.

However, sepsis remains a clinical diagnosis, requiring clinical judgment to identify infection and a dysregulated host response. As such, the diagnosis remains subjective in clinical practice, and recognition is imperfect. Given the many pathways implicated in sepsis, a single biomarker (equivalent to troponin in myocardial infarction) is not likely to be attainable. However, biomarkers may be useful to rule out specific pathogens or specific derangements of the host response, and multicomponent biomarker panels may eventually aid in clinical assessment. The difficulty of sepsis identification is likely to continue since it does not represent a single disease, but rather a heterogeneous syndrome dependent on numerous pathogen and host factors.

AUTHORS' RECOMMENDATIONS
- Sepsis-3 represented a paradigm shift in the definition of sepsis from systemic inflammation in the setting of infection to a dysregulated host immune response to infection leading to organ dysfunction.
- SOFA and qSOFA consistently outperform SIRS criteria in predicting in-hospital mortality; best performance is seen in Emergency Department patients.

- qSOFA is a practical tool and should be utilized to quickly identify patients at highest risk for adverse outcomes on whom additional information should be obtained.
- Given the multiple pathways involved, numerous biomarkers have been proposed for diagnosis and prognostication in sepsis; however, few biomarkers have been evaluated using Sepsis-3 and additional studies are needed.
- No single biomarker can identify sepsis, but there is potential to improve sepsis diagnosis and clinical decision making in combination with other clinical information.
- Despite improved understanding of sepsis pathophysiology, agreement between clinicians remains imperfect.
- Sepsis is a heterogeneous syndrome whose diagnosis continues to require clinical judgment, particularly regarding the presence of a dysregulated immune response.

REFERENCES

1. Fleischmann C, Scherag A, Adhikari NK, et al. Assessment of global incidence and mortality of hospital-treated sepsis. Current estimates and limitations. *Am J Respir Crit Care Med.* 2016;193(3):259-272.
2. Seymour CW, Rea TD, Kahn JM, Walkey AJ, Yealy DM, Angus DC. Severe sepsis in pre-hospital emergency care: analysis of incidence, care, and outcome. *Am J Respir Crit Care Med.* 2012;186(12):1264-1271.
3. Liu V, Escobar GJ, Greene JD, et al. Hospital deaths in patients with sepsis from 2 independent cohorts. *JAMA.* 2014;312(1):90-92.
4. Iwashyna TJ, Cooke CR, Wunsch H, Kahn JM. Population burden of long-term survivorship after severe sepsis in older Americans. *J Am Geriatr Soc.* 2012;60(6):1070-1077.
5. Prescott HC, Angus DC. Enhancing recovery from sepsis: a review. *JAMA.* 2018;319(1):62-75.
6. Prescott HC, Osterholzer JJ, Langa KM, Angus DC, Iwashyna TJ. Late mortality after sepsis: propensity matched cohort study. *BMJ.* 2016;353:i2375.
7. Reinhart K, Daniels R, Kissoon N, Machado FR, Schachter RD, Finfer S. Recognizing sepsis as a global health priority - a WHO resolution. *N Engl J Med.* 2017;377(5):414-417.
8. Cohen J, Vincent JL, Adhikari NK, et al. Sepsis: a roadmap for future research. *Lancet Infect Dis.* 2015;15(5):581-614.
9. Seymour CW, Gesten F, Prescott HC, et al. Time to treatment and mortality during mandated emergency care for sepsis. *N Engl J Med.* 2017;376(23):2235-2244.
10. Miller RR, 3rd, Dong L, Nelson NC, et al. Multicenter implementation of a severe sepsis and septic shock treatment bundle. *Am J Respir Crit Care Med.* 2013;188(1):77-82.
11. Funk DJ, Parrillo JE, Kumar A. Sepsis and septic shock: a history. *Crit Care Clin.* 2009;25(1):83-101, viii.
12. Singer M, Deutschman CS, Seymour CW, et al. The third international consensus definitions for sepsis and septic shock (Sepsis-3). *JAMA.* 2016;315(8):801-810.
13. Bone RC, Balk RA, Cerra FB, et al. Definitions for sepsis and organ failure and guidelines for the use of innovative therapies in sepsis. The ACCP/SCCM Consensus Conference Committee. American College of Chest Physicians/Society of Critical Care Medicine. *Chest.* 1992;101(6):1644-1655.
14. Levy MM, Fink MP, Marshall JC, et al. 2001 SCCM/ESICM/ACCP/ATS/SIS International Sepsis Definitions Conference. *Intensive Care Med.* 2003;29(4):530-538.
15. Lai NA, Kruger P. The predictive ability of a weighted systemic inflammatory response syndrome score for microbiologically confirmed infection in hospitalised patients with suspected sepsis. *Crit Care Resusc.* 2011;13(3):146-150.
16. Vincent JL, Opal SM, Marshall JC, Tracey KJ. Sepsis definitions: time for change. *Lancet.* 2013;381(9868):774-775.
17. Sprung CL, Sakr Y, Vincent JL, et al. An evaluation of systemic inflammatory response syndrome signs in the sepsis occurrence in acutely ill patients (SOAP) study. *Intensive Care Med.* 2006;32(3):421-427.
18. Churpek MM, Zadravecz FJ, Winslow C, Howell MD, Edelson DP. Incidence and prognostic value of the systemic inflammatory response syndrome and organ dysfunctions in ward patients. *Am J Respir Crit Care Med.* 2015;192(8):958-964.
19. Kaukonen KM, Bailey M, Bellomo R. Systemic inflammatory response syndrome criteria for severe sepsis. *N Engl J Med.* 2015;373(9):881.
20. Hotchkiss RS, Monneret G, Payen D. Sepsis-induced immunosuppression: from cellular dysfunctions to immunotherapy. *Nat Rev Immunol.* 2013;13(12):862-874.
21. Hotchkiss RS, Monneret G, Payen D. Immunosuppression in sepsis: a novel understanding of the disorder and a new therapeutic approach. *Lancet Infect Dis.* 2013;13(3):260-268.
22. Vincent JL, de Mendonça A, Cantraine F, et al. Use of the SOFA score to assess the incidence of organ dysfunction/failure in intensive care units: results of a multicenter, prospective study. Working group on "sepsis-related problems" of the European Society of Intensive Care Medicine. *Crit Care Med.* 1998;26(11):1793-1800.
23. Seymour CW, Liu VX, Iwashyna TJ, et al. Assessment of clinical criteria for sepsis: for the third international consensus definitions for sepsis and septic shock (Sepsis-3). *JAMA.* 2016;315(8):762-774.
24. Devarajan P. Neutrophil gelatinase-associated lipocalin: a promising biomarker for human acute kidney injury. *Biomark Med.* 2010;4(2):265-280.
25. Freund Y, Lemachatti N, Krastinova E, et al. Prognostic accuracy of Sepsis-3 criteria for in-hospital mortality among patients with suspected infection presenting to the emergency department. *JAMA.* 2017;317(3):301-308.
26. Raith EP, Udy AA, Bailey M, et al. Prognostic accuracy of the SOFA Score, SIRS Criteria, and qSOFA Score for in-hospital mortality among adults with suspected infection admitted to the intensive care unit. *JAMA.* 2017;317(3):290-300.
27. Rudd KE, Seymour CW, Aluisio AR, et al. Association of the quick sequential (sepsis-related) organ failure assessment (qSOFA) score with excess hospital mortality in adults with suspected infection in low- and middle-income countries. *JAMA.* 2018;319(21):2202-2211.
28. Cheng B, Li Z, Wang J, et al. Comparison of the performance between Sepsis-1 and Sepsis-3 in ICUs in China: a retrospective multicenter study. *Shock.* 2017;48(3):301-306.
29. Driessen RGH, van de Poll MCG, Mol MF, van Mook WNKA, Schnabel RM. The influence of a change in septic shock definitions on intensive care epidemiology and outcome: comparison of sepsis-2 and sepsis-3 definitions. *Infect Dis (Lond).* 2018;50(3):207-213.
30. Ryoo SM, Kang GH, Shin TG, et al. Clinical outcome comparison of patients with septic shock defined by the new sepsis-3 criteria and by previous criteria. *J Thorac Dis.* 2018;10(2):845-853.

31. Song JU, Sin CK, Park HK, Shim SR, Lee J. Performance of the quick Sequential (sepsis-related) Organ Failure Assessment score as a prognostic tool in infected patients outside the intensive care unit: a systematic review and meta-analysis. *Crit Care*. 2018;22(1):28.

32. Fernando SM, Tran A, Taljaard M, et al. Prognostic accuracy of the quick sequential organ failure assessment for mortality in patients with suspected infection: a systematic review and meta-analysis. *Ann Intern Med*. 2018;168(4):266-275.

33. Churpek MM, Snyder A, Han X, et al. Quick sepsis-related organ failure assessment, systemic inflammatory response syndrome, and early warning scores for detecting clinical deterioration in infected patients outside the intensive care unit. *Am J Respir Crit Care Med*. 2017;195(7):906-911.

34. Rhee C, Kadri SS, Danner RL, et al. Diagnosing sepsis is subjective and highly variable: a survey of intensivists using case vignettes. *Crit Care*. 2016;20:89.

35. Klein Klouwenberg PM, Cremer OL, van Vught LA, et al. Likelihood of infection in patients with presumed sepsis at the time of intensive care unit admission: a cohort study. *Crit Care*. 2015;19:319.

36. Prescott HC, Cope TM, Gesten FC, et al. Reporting of sepsis cases for performance measurement versus for reimbursement in New York State. *Crit Care Med*. 2018;46(5):666-673.

37. Faix JD. Biomarkers of sepsis. *Crit Rev Clin Lab Sci*. 2013; 50(1):23-36.

38. Pierrakos C, Vincent JL. Sepsis biomarkers: a review. *Crit Care*. 2010;14(1):R15.

39. Hamed S, Behnes M, Pauly D, et al. Diagnostic value of Pentraxin-3 in patients with sepsis and septic shock in accordance with latest sepsis-3 definitions. *BMC Infect Dis*. 2017;17(1):554.

40. Hoshino K, Kitamura T, Nakamura Y, et al. Usefulness of plasminogen activator inhibitor-1 as a predictive marker of mortality in sepsis. *J Intensive Care*. 2017;5:42.

41. Rhee C. Using procalcitonin to guide antibiotic therapy. *Open Forum Infect Dis*. 2016;4(1):ofw249.

42. Wacker C, Prkno A, Brunkhorst FM, Schlattmann P. Procalcitonin as a diagnostic marker for sepsis: a systematic review and meta-analysis. *Lancet Infect Dis*. 2013;13(5):426-435.

43. Kalil AC, Metersky ML, Klompas M, et al. Management of adults with hospital-acquired and ventilator-associated pneumonia: 2016 clinical practice guidelines by the Infectious Diseases Society of America and the American Thoracic Society. *Clin Infect Dis*. 2016;63(5):e61-e111.

44. Covington EW, Roberts MZ, Dong J. Procalcitonin monitoring as a guide for antimicrobial therapy: a review of current literature. *Pharmacotherapy*. 2018;38(5):569-581.

45. Rhodes A, Evans LE, Alhazzani W, et al. Surviving Sepsis Campaign: international guidelines for management of sepsis and septic shock: 2016. *Intensive Care Med*. 2017;43(3): 304-377.

46. Sandquist M, Wong HR. Biomarkers of sepsis and their potential value in diagnosis, prognosis and treatment. *Expert Rev Clin Immunol*. 2014;10(10):1349-1356.

47. McHugh L, Seldon TA, Brandon RA, et al. A molecular host response assay to discriminate between sepsis and infection-negative systemic inflammation in critically ill patients: discovery and validation in independent cohorts. *PLoS Med*. 2015;12(12):e1001916.

48. Miller RR, III,, Lopansri BK, Burke JP, et al. Validation of a host response assay, septicyte LAB, for discriminating sepsis from SIRS in the ICU. *Am J Respir Crit Care Med*. 2018;198(7):903-913.

49. Zimmerman JJ, Sullivan E, Yager TD, et al. Diagnostic accuracy of a host gene expression signature that discriminates clinical severe sepsis syndrome and infection-negative systemic inflammation among critically ill children. *Crit Care Med*. 2017;45(4):e418-e425.

50. Sweeney TE, Shidham A, Wong HR, Khatri P. A comprehensive time-course-based multicohort analysis of sepsis and sterile inflammation reveals a robust diagnostic gene set. *Sci Transl Med*. 2015;7(287):287ra71.

51. Rahmel T, Schäfer ST, Frey UH, Adamzik M, Peters J. Increased circulating microRNA-122 is a biomarker for discrimination and risk stratification in patients defined by sepsis-3 criteria. *PLoS One*. 2018;13(5):e0197637.

52. Kofoed K, Andersen O, Kronborg G, et al. Use of plasma C-reactive protein, procalcitonin, neutrophils, macrophage migration inhibitory factor, soluble urokinase-type plasminogen activator receptor, and soluble triggering receptor expressed on myeloid cells-1 in combination to diagnose infections: a prospective study. *Crit Care*. 2007;11(2):R38.

53. Mearelli F, Fiotti N, Giansante C, et al. Derivation and validation of a biomarker-based clinical algorithm to rule out sepsis from noninfectious systemic inflammatory response syndrome at emergency department admission: a multicenter prospective study. *Crit Care Med*. 2018;46(9):1421-1429.

54. Larsen FF, Petersen JA. Novel biomarkers for sepsis: A narrative review. *Eur J Intern Med*. 2017;45:46-50.

55. Huang DT, Yealy DM, Filbin MR, et al. Procalcitonin-guided use of antibiotics for lower respiratory tract infection. *N Engl J Med*. 2018;379(3):236-249.

56. Chen YX, Wang JY, Guo SB. Use of CRB-65 and quick Sepsis-related Organ Failure Assessment to predict site of care and mortality in pneumonia patients in the emergency department: a retrospective study. *Crit Care*. 2016;20(1):167.

57. Kolditz M, Scherag A, Rohde G, et al. Comparison of the qSOFA and CRB-65 for risk prediction in patients with community-acquired pneumonia. *Intensive Care Med*. 2016; 42(12):2108-2110.

58. Finkelsztein EJ, Jones DS, Ma KC, et al. Comparison of qSOFA and SIRS for predicting adverse outcomes of patients with suspicion of sepsis outside the intensive care unit. *Crit Care*. 2017;21(1):73.

59. Ranzani OT, Prina E, Menéndez R, et al. New sepsis definition (Sepsis-3) and community-acquired pneumonia mortality. A validation and clinical decision-making study. *Am J Respir Crit Care Med*. 2017;196(10):1287-1297.

60. Schlapbach LJ, Straney L, Bellomo R, MacLaren G, Pilcher D. Prognostic accuracy of age-adapted SOFA, SIRS, PELOD-2, and qSOFA for in-hospital mortality among children with suspected infection admitted to the intensive care unit. *Intensive Care Med*. 2018;44(2):179-188.

38

Do the Surviving Sepsis Campaign Guidelines Work?

Laura Evans and Ariella Pratzer

WHAT ARE BUNDLES?

The development and publication of guidelines seldom lead to changes in clinical behavior and guidelines are rarely integrated into bedside practice in a timely fashion.[1] Used as a tool for implementation and practice change, bundles are a group of evidence-based interventions often based on guidelines that, when instituted together, may provide an impact greater than any single intervention alone.[2] Ideally, a bundle provides a simple and uniform way to implement best practices.

THE NEED FOR BUNDLES IN SEVERE SEPSIS AND SEPTIC SHOCK

Sepsis is the most common cause of intensive care unit (ICU) admission globally. The disorder accounts for 11% of all ICU admissions in high-income countries,[3] and increases to 20% for noncardiac ICUs.[4] There are approximately 750,000 new sepsis cases every year in the United States alone.[5] It is the leading cause of ICU death, with a mortality rate between 18%-35%.[6] It is also the single most expensive condition treated in the United States, with costs exceeding $20 billion annually.[7] Sepsis, like poly-trauma, myocardial infarction, and stroke, is a medical emergency, for which early identification and management improves outcomes. Not surprisingly then, both mortality and healthcare costs associated with sepsis have been shown to be significantly decreased by the timely and coordinated application of a group of evidence-based interventions.[8,9] Thus, sepsis is a syndrome that is particularly amenable to bundle-based management.

Recognizing the global impact of sepsis and the growing evidence for interventions that would improve outcomes, the Surviving Sepsis Campaign (SSC) Guidelines were published initially in 2004, taking into account the best available evidence at that time. Beyond the guidelines, the SSC developed an international collaborative initiative to increase awareness of sepsis and to apply bundles as a means of translating the available evidence into improved patient outcomes on a global scale.

Over the last 14 years, the SSC has progressed in phases with multiple goals: building awareness, educating healthcare professionals, and improving the management of sepsis. Thus, the SSC structured itself into an international practice improvement project, with an in-depth collection of performance data and a goal of reducing sepsis mortality by 25% within five years (2004–09). Since the inception of the SSC, the bundles themselves have been adapted in response to an evolving evidence base and data collected from participants in the SSC effort (Table 38.1).

IS THERE EVIDENCE THAT APPLICATION OF THE SSC BUNDLES IMPROVES OUTCOMES?

While the components of the bundles themselves have generated ample debate since their development, there is little doubt that the SSC bundles have been effective. In fact, the demonstrated association between compliance with bundles and improved survival in sepsis patients has led to the adoption of SSC measures by the National Quality Forum, the New York State Department of Health, and the Centers for Medicare and Medicaid Services.[10,11]

A national educational effort in Spain, based on the SSC guidelines, resulted in a reduction of in-hospital and 28-day mortality from severe sepsis or septic shock by 11% and 14%, respectively.[12]

A large, multicenter study by the Intermountain Healthcare Intensive Medicine Clinical Program, involving 11 hospitals and 18 ICUs, enrolled nearly 4500 patients and conducted a quality improvement study to evaluate the effects of implementation of sepsis bundles (Fig. 38.1).[13] By the end of the study period, bundle compliance was almost 75% and in-hospital mortality rate had fallen below 10%.

A study of over 49,000 patients at 149 hospitals in New York State in 2014-16, found that more rapid completion of the three-hour sepsis bundle was associated with lower risk-adjusted in-hospital mortality.[14] A prospective, observational study of compliance with SCC bundles across 62 countries found overall low compliance (19%), but also found that compliance with the three-hour bundle resulted in a 40% reduction in in-hospital mortality.[15]

The SSC itself has collected data from over 15,000 patients at 165 sites participating in the collaborative. Bundle compliance rates and their association with hospital mortality were examined. Compliance rates with both phases of the bundle improved over the two year campaign. Simultaneously, there was a 7% absolute risk reduction in unadjusted hospital

TABLE 38.1 Surviving Sepsis Campaign Care Bundles.

Original Bundle (2005)	Updated Bundle (2012)	Most Recent Bundle (2018)
Resuscitation bundle (to be completed within the first 6 h) • Serum lactate measured • Blood cultures obtained prior to antibiotic administration • Broad spectrum antibiotics administered within 3 h for ED admissions, 1 h for non-ED admissions • If hypotensive or if lactate ≥4 mmol/L, initial bolus of 20 mL/kg crystalloid (or colloid equivalent) administered. If MAP still <65 mm Hg, vasopressors applied • If hypotension or hyperlactemia persists, CVP >8 mm Hg and ScvO$_2$ of >65% achieved (or MVO$_2$ >65%)	To be completed within the first 3 h • Serum lactate measured • Blood cultures obtained prior to antibiotic administration • Broad spectrum antibiotics administered • 30 mL/kg of crystalloids administered for hypotension or lactate ≥4 mmol/L	To be initiated within the first hour • Serum lactate measured.[a] • Blood cultures obtained prior to antibiotic administration • Broad spectrum antibiotics administered • Administration of 30 mL/kg of crystalloids initiated for hypotension or lactate ≥4 mmol/L • Vasopressors applied for refractory hypotension to maintain MAP ≥65 mm Hg
Management bundle (to be completed within the first 24 h) • Low dose steroids administered for septic shock • Drotrecogin alpha (activated) administered • Glucose control maintained between lower limit of normal and <150 mg/dL • Inspiratory plateau pressures maintained <30 cm water for patients who are mechanically ventilated	To be completed within the first 6 h • Vasopressors applied for refractory hypotension to maintain MAP ≥65 mm Hg • If initial lactate >4 mmol/L or if hypotension persists after volume resuscitation, measure CVP and ScvO$_2$ • Re-measure lactate if initial lactate was elevated	

[a]Remeasure lactate if elevated (does not need to be done in first hour).
Data from Dellinger RP, Levy MM, Townsend SR, et al. Surviving Sepsis Campaign: international guidelines for management of severe sepsis and septic shock: 2012. *Crit Care Med*. 2013;41:580-637; Levy MM, Dellinger RP, Townsend SR, et al. The Surviving Sepsis Campaign: results of an international guideline-based performance improvement program targeting severe sepsis. *Crit Care Med*. 2010;38(2):367-374; Levy MM, Evans LE, Rhodes A. The Surviving Sepsis Campaign Bundle: 2018 update. *Crit Care Med*. 2018;44(6):925-928.

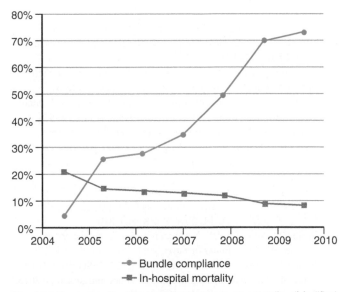

Fig. 38.1 Improving bundle compliance improves mortality. (Modified from Miller RR 3rd, Dong L, Nelson NC, et al. Multicenter implementation of a severe sepsis and septic shock treatment bundle. *Am J Respir Crit Care Med*. 2013;188(1):77-82.)

In 2014, the SSC published the effects of bundle adoption over a 7.5 year period.[8] Analysis of nearly 30,000 patients from three different continents and over 200 hospitals revealed the sustainability of improved outcomes with increasing bundle compliance. Participation in the SSC alone led to an overall decline in mortality. Higher compliance to either resuscitation or management bundles led to improvements in mortality. Continued participation in the SSC led to additional reductions in mortality by 7% per quarter. Additionally, for every 10% increase in bundle use, there were significant decreases in hospital and ICU lengths of stay. Overall, increased compliance with sepsis performance bundles was associated with a 25% relative reduction in mortality.

While there are regional differences in bundle compliance and mortality, improved outcomes when adhering to the SSC bundles are not limited to resource intensive settings. Raymond and colleagues showed that bundle compliance in India reduced mortality from 35% to 21% (unpublished observations),[2] including reductions in intensive care length of stay and ventilator-free days. Similar observations have been seen in China[17] and Brazil.[18] As of 2018, there are more than 50 studies showing that increased bundle compliance leads to improvements in mortality. As a corollary, noncompliance with these bundles was associated with increases in hospital mortality. In fact, a study in the United Kingdom showed that noncompliance with the 6 hour sepsis bundle was associated with a more than two-fold increase in hospital mortality.[19]

mortality over this time period. As the authors noted, by instituting a practice improvement program grounded in evidence-based guidelines, the SSC successfully increased compliance with sepsis bundles, and this change was associated with better patient outcomes.[16]

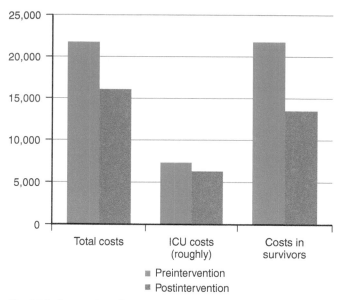

Fig. 38.2 Cost savings from implementation of a SSC bundle. (From Shorr AF, Micek ST, Jackson WL Jr, Kollef MH. Economic implications of an evidence-based sepsis protocol: can we improve outcomes and lower costs? *Crit Care Med.* 2007;35(5):1257-1262.)

Through the bundles, the SSC has successfully created a paradigm shift in the approach to severe sepsis and septic shock. Therein lies the strength of bundles—guidelines that may take years to change clinical behavior can now be distilled into something easily implementable at the bedside. As new evidence becomes available, these bundle elements can continue to be adapted, and the new evidence quickly translated into improved patient care.

AUTHORS' RECOMMENDATIONS
- Sepsis is a medical emergency for which early identification and management improves outcomes.
- The Surviving Sepsis Campaign guidelines and bundles were introduced with the intention of reducing sepsis mortality by 25% over 5 years.
- Numerous studies conducted since their introduction have consistently demonstrated association between compliance with bundles and improved survival in sepsis patients.
- Sepsis guidelines and bundles will continue to be adapted to the most recent evidence, enabling this new evidence to be quickly translated to improved patient care.

IS THERE EVIDENCE THAT THE SSC BUNDLES ARE COST-EFFECTIVE?

Treatment of severe sepsis and septic shock is resource-intensive, with annual costs exceeding $20 billion in the United States alone.[7] Several studies have analyzed the cost effectiveness, from a health care perspective, of compliance with the SSC bundle elements. When implemented, the overall mean cost per patient may increase; however, this may be driven by improved survival leading to increased length of stay.[9] The Incremental Cost-Effectiveness Ratio, a commonly used approach to decision making regarding health interventions, was as low as €4435 per life year gained (LYG) in one such study from Spain.[9] These savings were significantly lower than the frequently used limit of €30,000 per LYG to gauge cost effectiveness of an intervention in that country. Data from the United States showed a reduction of nearly $5000/patient when the SSC bundles were implemented (Fig. 38.2).[20] ICU costs fell by nearly 35%, and there was a simultaneous reduction in hospital length of stay by approximately 5 days. In a subgroup analysis, the cost savings was $8000 per survivor, despite an increase in hospital length of stay.

In a period in which health care spending is being scrutinized, such cost saving measures have important economic implications. Extrapolating the data described earlier, to all patients with severe sepsis and septic shock, consistent adherence to the SSC bundle elements could potentially save $4 billion annually in the United States.

CONCLUSIONS

There is substantial evidence that implementation of the SSC bundles saves lives as well as reduces healthcare spending.

REFERENCES

1. Fischer F, Lange K, Klose K, Greiner W, Kraemer A. Barriers and strategies in guideline implementation—a scoping review. *Healthcare (Basel).* 2016;4(3).
2. Khan P, Divatia JV. Severe sepsis bundles. *Indian J Crit Care Med.* 2010;14(1):8-13.
3. Perner A, Gordon AC, De Backer D, et al. Sepsis: frontiers in diagnosis, resuscitation and antibiotic therapy. *Intensive Care Med.* 2016;42(12):1958-1969.
4. Brun-Buisson C, Doyon F, Carlet J, et al. Incidence, risk factors, and outcome of severe sepsis and septic shock in adults. A multicenter prospective study in intensive care units. French ICU Group for Severe Sepsis. *JAMA.* 1995;274(12):968-974.
5. Institute for Healthcare Improvement. *Sepsis Care Enters New Era.* 2006. Available at: http://www.ihi.org/resources/Pages/ImprovementStories/SepsisCareEntersNewEra.aspx. Accessed September 25, 2018.
6. Singer M, Deutschman CS, Seymour CW, et al. The Third International Consensus Definitions for Sepsis and Septic Shock (Sepsis-3). *JAMA.* 2016;315(8):801-810.
7. Torio CM, Andrews RM. *National inpatient hospital costs: the most expensive conditions by payer, 2011: Statistical Brief #160.* Healthcare Cost and Utilization Project (HCUP) Statistical Briefs. Rockville, MD: Agency for Health Care Policy and Research; 2013.
8. Levy MM, Rhodes A, Phillips GS, et al. Surviving Sepsis Campaign: association between performance metrics and outcomes in a 7.5-year study. *Crit Care Med.* 2015;43(1):3-12.
9. Suarez D, Ferrer R, Artigas A, et al. Cost-effectiveness of the Surviving Sepsis Campaign protocol for severe sepsis: a prospective nation-wide study in Spain. *Intensive Care Med.* 2011;37(3):444-452.
10. Dwyer J. One boy's death moves state to action to prevent others. *New York Times.* December 20, 2012. Available at: http://www.nytimes.com/2012/12/21/nyregion/one-boys-death-moves-state-to-action-to-prevent-others.html. Accessed September 25, 2018.

11. Centers for Medicare & Medicaid Services. *CMS to improve quality of care during hospital inpatient stays.* CMS.gov. August 4, 2014. Available at: https://www.cms.gov/newsroom/fact-sheets/cms-improve-quality-care-during-hospital-inpatient-stays. Accessed September 25, 2018.

12. Ferrer R, Artigas A, Levy MM, et al. Improvement in process of care and outcome after a multicenter severe sepsis educational program in Spain. *JAMA.* 2008;299(19):2294-2303.

13. Miller RR 3rd, Dong L, Nelson NC, et al. Multicenter implementation of a severe sepsis and septic shock treatment bundle. *Am J Respir Crit Care Med.* 2013;188(1):77-82.

14. Seymour CW, Gesten F, Prescott HC, et al. Time to treatment and mortality during mandated emergency care for sepsis. *N Engl J Med.* 2017;376(23):2235-2244.

15. Rhodes A, Phillips G, Beale R, et al. The Surviving Sepsis Campaign bundles and outcome: results from the International Multicentre Prevalence Study on Sepsis (the IMPreSS study). *Intensive Care Med.* 2015;41(9):1620-1628.

16. Levy MM, Dellinger RP, Townsend SR, et al. The Surviving Sepsis Campaign: results of an international guideline-based performance improvement program targeting severe sepsis. *Crit Care Med.* 2010;38(2):367-374.

17. Li ZQ, Xi XM, Luo X, Li J, Jiang L. Implementing surviving sepsis campaign bundles in China: a prospective cohort study. *Chin Med J (Engl).* 2013;126(10):1819-1825.

18. Shiramizo SC, Marra AR, Durão MS, Paes ÂT, Edmond MB, Pavão dos Santos OF. Decreasing mortality in severe sepsis and septic shock patients by implementing a sepsis bundle in a hospital setting. *PLoS One.* 2011;6(11):e26790.

19. Gao F, Melody T, Daniels DF, Giles S, Fox S. The impact of compliance with 6-hour and 24-hour sepsis bundles on hospital mortality in patients with severe sepsis: a prospective observational study. *Crit Care.* 2005;9(6):R764-R770.

20. Shorr AF, Micek ST, Jackson Jr WL, Kollef MH. Economic implications of an evidence-based sepsis protocol: can we improve outcomes and lower costs? *Crit Care Med.* 2007;35(5):1257-1262.

39

Has Outcome in Sepsis Improved?
What Works? What Does Not?

Jean-Louis Vincent

Sepsis, defined as some degree of organ dysfunction attributed to a dysregulated host response in association with severe infection,[1] remains a common condition affecting 1–11% of hospitalized patients[2–4] and about 30% of intensive care unit (ICU) patients.[5,6]

HAVE OUTCOMES FROM SEPSIS IMPROVED?

Recent studies have suggested that outcomes for patients with sepsis have improved over the years.[3,7] As early as 1998, in a review of studies examining patients with septic shock published between 1958 and 1997, Friedman et al. reported a decrease in hospital mortality rates from about 65% to about 42%.[8] In another early study, Martin et al.[9] reported that in-hospital mortality rates for patients with sepsis admitted to a sample of US hospitals decreased from 28% for the period 1979–1984 to 18% for the period 1995–2000. More recently, Stevenson et al.[10] used data from the control arms of randomized clinical trials in patients with sepsis published between 1991 and 2009 and reported a 3% annual decrease in 28-day mortality rates ($P = .009$). The same authors and others have reported similar trends for in-hospital mortality when using administrative hospitalization data in the United States[10–13] and other countries.[14,15] Using data from the Australian and New Zealand Intensive Care Society adult ICU patient database, Kaukonen et al.[16] reported an absolute decrease in the hospital mortality rate of sepsis from 35% in 2000 to 18.4% in 2012; after logistic regression analysis, the odds ratio (OR) for mortality was 0.49 (95% confidence interval [CI] 0.46–0.52) in 2012 with 2000 as reference. In a recent comparison of results from two multicenter observational studies conducted 10 years apart (2002 and 2012) across European ICUs by the same group of investigators, the proportion of patients with sepsis during the ICU stay was slightly higher in the later study (31.9 vs. 29.6%, $P = 0.03$). Multilevel analysis showed that the adjusted odds of ICU mortality in patients with sepsis was lower in 2012 than in 2002 (OR 0.45 [95% CI 0.35–0.59], $P < 0.001$), even though patients in the more recent cohort had higher severity scores.[17]

Taken together, there is therefore some evidence of improved outcomes from sepsis over the last couple of decades (Table 39.1). Nevertheless, the apparent extent of the decrease in mortality should be interpreted with some caution.

Indeed, increased awareness of sepsis, changes in the code definitions used to classify the disorder, and altered reimbursement strategies have likely led to an inclusion of an increased number of patients with less severe disease and, hence, an inherently lower risk of death in studies on sepsis; this effect certainly accounts for some of the reported temporal increase in the number of septic patients—including less severe cases—with the concurrent decrease in mortality.[18–20]

WHAT HAS NOT WORKED?

Over the years, our understanding of the pathophysiology of sepsis has improved to the extent that many of the complex responses to infection and how they interact to cause sepsis are now well detailed and defined.[21] Multiple pathways and molecules have been identified as potential targets for therapeutic intervention; however, despite more than 100 randomized controlled clinical trials of sepsis-modulating therapies, no effective intervention has been identified.[22] Clearly then, this approach to improve survival has not worked. There have been many putative explanations for these apparent "failed" trials, including discrepancies arising when preclinical models and experimental data are translated to the clinical arena; issues with the in vivo efficacy of the intervention under examination; concerns about the dose and timing of the intervention; and problems with clinical trial design, including choice of outcome measures.[22] Perhaps the key problem, though, has been in the selection of patients for these studies. Lack of a clear and specific definition or marker of sepsis has led to the inclusion of very heterogeneous groups of patients. Patients with different degrees of disease severity, different sepsis sources and causative microorganisms, different genetic backgrounds, and different comorbidities and ages have all received the same intervention. Many studies also included multiple centers with an associated variability in standards of care, resource availability, and staff training.[22] Moreover, it has become apparent that patients have different types of immune response—both proinflammatory and antiinflammatory responses are present simultaneously—and the balance between these two forms may determine a patient's response to treatment.[23] This has rarely been taken into consideration when clinical trials are designed. In a trial that includes such heterogeneous groups of patients, a single intervention may

TABLE 39.1   Some of the Published Studies Reporting Trends in Mortality Rates in Sepsis.

First Author (Reference)	Country	Type of Data	Year Span	Change in Mortality Rate
Friedman[8]	Multiple	Systematic review	1958–97	Hospital mortality decreased from 65% to 42%
Martin[9]	USA	Hospital discharge records, ICD codes	1979/1984–95/2000	Hospital mortality decreased from 28% to 18%
van Ruler[58]	Multiple	Control arms of randomized trials of sepsis treatment	1990–2000	Hospital mortality decreased from 44% to 35%
Dombrovskiy[59]	USA	National inpatient database, ICD codes	1995–2002	Hospital case fatality rate decreased from 51% to 45%
Dombrovskiy[60]	USA	ICD codes	1993–2003	Hospital case fatality rate decreased from 46% to 38%
Harrison[14]	UK	National ICU database	1996–2004	Hospital mortality decreased from 48% to 45%
Kumar[11]	USA	National inpatient database, ICD codes	2000–07	Hospital mortality decreased from 39% to 27%
Lagu[12]	USA	National inpatient database, ICD codes	2003–07	Hospital mortality decreased from 37% to 29%
Ani[13]	USA	Administrative database, ICD codes	1999–2008	Hospital mortality decreased from 40% to 28%
Dreiher[61]	Israel	Retrospective multicenter cohort	2002–08	Hospital mortality unchanged (53% vs. 55%)
Stevenson[10]	Multiple	Control arms of randomized trials of sepsis treatment	1991/1995–2006/2009	Hospital mortality decreased from 47% to 29%
Ayala-Ramírez[15]	Spain	Administrative database, ICD codes	2003–11	Hospital mortality decreased from 40% to 32% in males and from 42% to 35% in females, only in patients with severe sepsis
Kaukonen[16]	Australia/New Zealand	Retrospective, multicenter, observational study	2000–12	Hospital mortality decreased from 35% to 18%
Lee[7]	Taiwan	National Health Insurance claims database, ICD codes	2002–12	30-day mortality decreased from 27.8% to 22.8%; annual decrease 0.45%
Vincent[17]	24 European countries	Comparison of two prospective observational studies	2002–12	Adjusted odds of ICU mortality significantly lower in 2012 than 2002 [OR 0.45 (0.35–0.59), $P < 0.001$].
Fleischmann[62]	Germany	Nationwide hospital DRG statistics	2007–13	In-hospital mortality decreased from 27.0% to 24.3%.
Rhee[2]	USA	Retrospective cohort study	2009–14	In-hospital mortality decreased by 3.3%/y [95% CI, −5.6% to −1.0%], $P = .004$ when clinical criteria were used for diagnosis and by 7.0%/y [95% CI, −8.8% to −5.2%], $P < .001$ when ICD codes were used
Meyer[3]	USA	Retrospective cohort study	2010–15	In-hospital mortality decreased from 24.1% to 14.8%.

DRG, Diagnosis-related groups; *ICD,* International Classification of Diseases; *ICU,* intensive care unit.

be of benefit in some but harmful in others so that the overall study outcome may not accurately reflect the true efficacy of the therapeutic agent, had it been tested in a more select population. For example, a patient with a primarily proinflammatory response is unlikely to respond to an agent that further promotes inflammation; thus administration of granulocyte colony-stimulating factor (G-CSF) to all patients with septic shock was not associated with improved outcomes.[24]

Similarly, giving an antiinflammatory agent to a patient who is already immunosuppressed will probably not be of benefit. Indeed, in many of the studies of immunomodulatory agents that showed no overall improvement in outcome, beneficial effects were suggested in certain subgroups.[25–31]

Other specific aspects of patient management have also not been consistently shown to be effective. For example, an early goal-directed therapy protocol reduced mortality in a selected group of patients treated by Rivers et al. at a single center[32] but had no beneficial effects on outcomes in three larger, multicenter studies.[33–35] Similarly, tight blood glucose control improved outcomes in a single center study by Van den Berghe et al. on critically ill surgical patients[36] but not in a more general population of ICU patients.[37]

Single interventions in heterogeneous groups of "septic" patients have therefore clearly not worked. Improving patient characterization so that those patients who are most likely to respond to the intervention(s) in question can be identified and studied is necessary for future clinical trials in sepsis therapeutics.[38]

WHAT HAS WORKED?

Despite the lack of specific sepsis treatments and some problems with diluted data, patient outcomes from sepsis have improved over the years. Therefore if single specific interventions have not been effective, what has worked? It is logical to invoke two major factors in these improved outcomes: (1) the enhanced awareness of sepsis as a possible diagnosis and realization of the importance of early recognition and management[39] and (2) a gradual improvement in the general process of care for these, and indeed all, critically ill patients.[40,41] Taking the former aspect first, early effective antibiotic treatment, infectious source removal, adequate fluid administration, and vasopressor and organ support have all been associated with improved outcomes.[39] Guidelines with recommendations for best patient care that stress the need for rapid institution of these practices have been written by teams of experts,[39] and bundles of care items (including measurement of blood lactate level, early administration of broad-spectrum antibiotics, administration of fluids when hypotension is present, and administration of vasopressors for hypotension that does not readily respond to initial fluid resuscitation) have been developed.[42] Compliance with these bundles has been associated with improved outcomes in different ICU settings,[43–46] although intensivists should not be restricted by specified time limits and all aspects of these bundles should be performed as rapidly as possible. The use of multidisciplinary sepsis response teams ensures that all aspects of management can be performed rapidly and has been associated with improved outcomes.[47] A specially equipped and staffed room or "shock lab" could similarly improve early management in these patients.[48]

In terms of process of care, of the many aspects that have seen gradual change over the years and led, in combination, to improved patient outcomes in all critically ill patients, including those with sepsis, five merit specific discussion. The development of intensive care medicine as a specialty in its own right, and with trained intensivists familiar with the complexities of critical illness, has contributed hugely to the ongoing improved process of care. First, intensivists have generally become less invasive and less aggressive in some aspects of their patient management. They have come to understand that many of the seemingly pathophysiologic effects of sepsis are, in fact, beneficial and should not necessarily be "treated" or

"normalized." The use of interventions that have been associated with poorer outcomes has gradually been reduced and even eliminated. Thus, fewer transfusions are given, patients are fed less, tidal volumes have been reduced, and sedation has been minimized. Second, intensivists have come to appreciate the unique circumstances surrounding each patient and have thus individualized treatment rather than manage all ICU patients in the same way. Conversely, intensivists have standardized critical aspects of care by introducing guidelines and protocols so that key elements are less likely to be forgotten or mismanaged. This dichotomy can, in some circumstances, become problematic. Although protocols can improve the delivery of care when quality is suboptimal, especially when there is a shortage of well-trained staff, they may be too rigid in many centers where care is already optimal and may limit intensivists' ability to account for the importance of individual patient factors; here, checklists may be a better approach.[49] Third, intensivists have realized the importance of multidisciplinary teamwork within the ICU setting, moving from a rather paternal, physician-directed approach to patient management and decision making that is much more inclusive, with input from all members of the ICU team, including nurses, physiotherapists, nutritionists, and pharmacists. Good teamwork can help reduce medical errors and improve job satisfaction, as well as improve patient outcomes.[50,51] One of the key aspects of good teamwork is good communication, and this concept also extends to patients and their relatives. Patients, whenever possible, and next of kin, are now informed more openly of patient progress, treatment options, and likely prognosis. End-of-life decisions in particular are now discussed more candidly and clearly with families, and patients increasingly share in the decision-making process.[52,53] Fourth, realization of the importance of early recognition and management of critical illness has led many hospitals to extend the ICU beyond its physical four-wall structure by creating medical emergency teams or ICU outreach teams. These consist of trained intensivists, nursing staff, or both who can assess and initiate management of patients on the general ward before they deteriorate to the point where they require ICU admission.[54] Critical illness generally starts some time before ICU admission, and the severity of illness could potentially be limited by early intervention, thus improving patient outcomes.[55,56] Fifth, the impact of various aspects of intensive care management on longer term post-ICU physical, cognitive and psychological outcomes is increasingly recognized. Reduced sedation, early mobilization, adequate sleep, improved communication can all help reduce the development of post-ICU syndrome.[57]

CONCLUSION

Sepsis remains a common condition in critically ill patients. Improvements in the process of care for these patients in general, and in early recognition and management of patients with sepsis in particular, have helped improve survival rates, but further progress is needed. Improvements in diagnostic methods will facilitate more rapid diagnosis and thus patient management, and better patient characterization will help select more homogeneous patient groups for clinical trials of new specific sepsis therapies. Early administration of appropriate antibiotics, early source control when needed, rapid resuscitation, and hemodynamic stabilization must remain the key foci of patient management, and dedicated sepsis teams can help achieve these targets.

AUTHORS' RECOMMENDATIONS
- Mortality rates from sepsis have decreased in recent years but likely to a lesser degree than reports suggest.
- There are no specific treatments for sepsis, and management relies on early diagnosis and rapid antiinfective strategies, together with early and complete resuscitation.
- Improvement in the process of care for all critically ill patients is the main reason behind the improved mortality rates in patients with sepsis.

REFERENCES

1. Singer M, Deutschman CS, Seymour CW, et al. The Third International Consensus Definitions for Sepsis and Septic Shock (Sepsis-3). *JAMA*. 2016;315:801-810.
2. Rhee C, Dantes R, Epstein L, et al. Incidence and trends of sepsis in us hospitals using clinical vs claims data. 2009-2014. *JAMA*. 2017;318:1241-1249.
3. Meyer N, Harhay MO, Small DS, et al. Temporal trends in incidence, sepsis-related mortality, and hospital-based acute care after sepsis. *Crit Care Med*. 2018;46:354-360.
4. Knoop ST, Skrede S, Langeland N, Flaatten HK. Epidemiology and impact on all-cause mortality of sepsis in Norwegian hospitals: A national retrospective study. *PLoS One*. 2017; 12:e0187990.
5. Shankar-Hari M, Harrison DA, Rubenfeld GD, Rowan K. Epidemiology of sepsis and septic shock in critical care units: comparison between sepsis-2 and sepsis-3 populations using a national critical care database. *Br J Anaesth*. 2017;119:626-636.
6. Vincent JL, Marshall JC, Namendys-Silva SA, et al. Assessment of the worldwide burden of critical illness: the intensive care over nations (ICON) audit. *Lancet Respir Med*. 2014;2:380-386.
7. Lee CC, Yo MH, Lee MG, et al. Adult sepsis—a nationwide study of trends and outcomes in a population of 23 million people. *J Infect*. 2017;75:409-419.
8. Friedman G, Silva E, Vincent JL. Has the mortality of septic shock changed with time? *Crit Care Med*. 1998;26:2078-2086.
9. Martin GS, Mannino DM, Eaton S, Moss M. The epidemiology of sepsis in the United States from 1979 through 2000. *N Engl J Med*. 2003;348:1546-1554.
10. Stevenson EK, Rubenstein AR, Radin GT, Wiener RS, Walkey AJ. Two decades of mortality trends among patients with severe sepsis: a comparative meta-analysis*. *Crit Care Med*. 2014;42: 625-631.
11. Kumar G, Kumar N, Taneja A, et al. Nationwide trends of severe sepsis in the 21st century (2000-2007). *Chest*. 2011; 140:1223-1231.
12. Lagu T, Rothberg MB, Shieh MS, Pekow PS, Steingrub JS, Lindenauer PK. Hospitalizations, costs, and outcomes of severe sepsis in the United States 2003 to 2007. *Crit Care Med*. 2012;40:754-761.
13. Ani C, Farshidpanah S, Bellinghausen Stewart A, Nguyen HB. Variations in organism-specific severe sepsis mortality in the United States. *Crit Care Med*. 2015;43:65-77.
14. Harrison DA, Welch CA, Eddleston JM. The epidemiology of severe sepsis in England, Wales and Northern Ireland, 1996 to 2004: secondary analysis of a high quality clinical database, the ICNARC Case Mix Programme Database. *Crit Care*. 2006;10:R42.
15. Ayala-Ramírez OH, Domínguez-Berjón MF, Esteban-Vasallo MD. Trends in hospitalizations of patients with sepsis and factors associated with inpatient mortality in the Region of Madrid, 2003-2011. *Eur J Clin Microbiol Infect Dis*. 2013;33: 411-421.
16. Kaukonen KM, Bailey M, Suzuki S, Pilcher D, Bellomo R. Mortality related to severe sepsis and septic shock among critically ill patients in Australia and New Zealand, 2000-2012. *JAMA*. 2014;311:1308-1316.
17. Vincent JL, Lefrant JY, Kotfis K, et al. Comparison of European ICU patients in 2012 (ICON) versus 2002 (SOAP). *Intensive Care Med*. 2018;44:337-344.
18. Lindenauer PK, Lagu T, Shieh MS, Pekow PS, Rothberg MB. Association of diagnostic coding with trends in hospitalizations and mortality of patients with pneumonia, 2003-2009. *JAMA*. 2012;307:1405-1413.
19. Iwashyna TJ, Angus DC. Declining case fatality rates for severe sepsis: good data bring good news with ambiguous implications. *JAMA*. 2014;311:1295-1297.
20. Rhee C, Gohil S, Klompas M. Regulatory mandates for sepsis care—reasons for caution. *N Engl J Med*. 2014;370:1673-1676.
21. Hotchkiss RS, Moldawer LL, Opal SM, Reinhart K, Turnbull IR, Vincent JL. Severe sepsis and septic shock. *Nat Rev Dis Primers*. 2016;2:16045.
22. Marshall JC. Why have clinical trials in sepsis failed? *Trends Mol Med*. 2014;20:195-203.
23. Vincent JL. Assessing cellular responses in sepsis. *EBioMedicine*. 2014;1:10-11.
24. Stephens DP, Thomas JH, Higgins A, et al. Randomized, double-blind, placebo-controlled trial of granulocyte colony-stimulating factor in patients with septic shock. *Crit Care Med*. 2008;36:448-454.
25. Greenman RL, Schein RM, Martin MA, et al. A controlled clinical trial of E5 murine monoclonal IgM antibody to endotoxin in the treatment of gram-negative sepsis. The XOMA Sepsis Study Group. *JAMA*. 1991;266:1097-1102.
26. Dhainaut JF, Tenaillon A, Le Tulzo Y, et al. Platelet-activating factor receptor antagonist BN 52021 in the treatment of severe sepsis: a randomized, double-blind, placebo-controlled, multicenter clinical trial. BN 52021 Sepsis Study Group. *Crit Care Med*. 1994;22:1720-1728.
27. Baudo F, Caimi TM, de Cataldo F, et al. Antithrombin III (ATIII) replacement therapy in patients with sepsis and/or postsurgical complications: a controlled double-blind, randomized, multicenter study. *Intensive Care Med*. 1998;24: 336-342.
28. Ziegler EJ, Fisher Jr CJ, Sprung CL, et al. Treatment of gram-negative bacteremia and septic shock with HA-1A human monoclonal antibody against endotoxin. A randomized, double-blind, placebo-controlled trial. The HA-1A Sepsis Study Group. *N Engl J Med*. 1991;324:429-436.
29. Fisher Jr CJ, Dhainaut JF, Opal SM, et al. Recombinant human interleukin 1 receptor antagonist in the treatment of patients with sepsis syndrome. *JAMA*. 1994;271:1836-1843.

30. Kienast J, Juers M, Wiedermann CJ, et al. Treatment effects of high-dose antithrombin without concomitant heparin in patients with severe sepsis with or without disseminated intravascular coagulation. *J Thromb Haemost*. 2006;4:90-97.

31. Laterre PF, Opal SM, Abraham E, et al. A clinical evaluation committee assessment of recombinant human tissue factor pathway inhibitor (tifacogin) in patients with severe community-acquired pneumonia. *Crit Care*. 2009;13:R36.

32. Rivers E, Nguyen B, Havstad S, et al. Early goal-directed therapy in the treatment of severe sepsis and septic shock. *N Engl J Med*. 2001;345:1368-1377.

33. Yealy DM, Kellum JA, Huang DT, et al. A randomized trial of protocol-based care for early septic shock. *N Engl J Med*. 2014;370:1683-1693.

34. Peake SL, Delaney A, Bailey M, et al. Goal-directed resuscitation for patients with early septic shock. *N Engl J Med*. 2014;371: 1496-1506.

35. Mouncey PR, Osborn TM, Power GS, et al. Trial of early, goal-directed resuscitation for septic shock. *N Engl J Med*. 2015;372:1301-1311.

36. Van den Berghe G, Wouters P, Weekers F, et al. Intensive insulin therapy in critically ill patients. *N Engl J Med*. 2001; 345:1359-1367.

37. Finfer S, Chittock DR, Su SY, et al. Intensive versus conventional glucose control in critically ill patients. *N Engl J Med*. 2009;360: 1283-1297.

38. Grimaldi D, Vincent JL. Clinical trial research in focus: rethinking trials in sepsis. *Lancet Respir Med*. 2017;5: 610-611.

39. Rhodes A, Evans LE, Alhazzani W, et al. Surviving Sepsis Campaign: international guidelines for management of sepsis and septic shock, 2016. *Intensive Care Med*. 2017;43:304-377.

40. Vincent JL, Singer M, Marini JJ, et al. Thirty years of critical care medicine. *Crit Care*. 2010;14:311.

41. Vincent JL. Critical care–where have we been and where are we going? *Crit Care*. 2013;17(suppl 1):S2.

42. Surviving Sepsis Campaign. Bundles. Available at: http://www.survivingsepsis.org/Bundles/Pages/default.aspx. Accessed September 13, 2018.

43. Miller RR III, Dong L, Nelson NC, et al. Multicenter implementation of a severe sepsis and septic shock treatment bundle. *Am J Respir Crit Care Med*. 2013;188:77-82.

44. Prasad PA, Shea ER, Shiboski S, Sullivan MC, Gonzales R, Shimabukuro D. Relationship between a sepsis intervention bundle and in-hospital mortality among hospitalized patients: a retrospective analysis of real-world data. *Anesth Analg*. 2017;125:507-513.

45. van Zanten AR, Brinkman S, Arbous MS, et al. Guideline bundles adherence and mortality in severe sepsis and septic shock. *Crit Care Med*. 2014;42:1890-1898.

46. Levy MM, Rhodes A, Phillips GS, et al. Surviving Sepsis Campaign: association between performance metrics and outcomes in a 7.5-year study. *Intensive Care Med*. 2014;40:1623-1633.

47. Arabi YM, Al-Dorzi HM, Alamry A, et al. The impact of a multifaceted intervention including sepsis electronic alert system and sepsis response team on the outcomes of patients with sepsis and septic shock. *Ann Intensive Care*. 2017;7:57.

48. Piagnerelli M, Van Nuffelen M, Maetens Y, Lheureux P, Vincent JL. A 'shock room' for early management of the acutely ill. *Anaesth Intensive Care*. 2009;37:426-431.

49. Vincent JL. The future of critical care medicine: integration and personalization. *Crit Care Med*. 2016;44(2):386-389.

50. Sexton JB, Berenholtz SM, Goeschel CA, et al. Assessing and improving safety climate in a large cohort of intensive care units. *Crit Care Med*. 2011;39:934-939.

51. Dietz AS, Pronovost PJ, Mendez-Tellez PA, et al. A systematic review of teamwork in the intensive care unit: what do we know about teamwork, team tasks, and improvement strategies? *J Crit Care*. 2014;29:908-914.

52. Akgün KM, Kapo JM, Siegel MD. Critical care at the end of life. *Semin Respir Crit Care Med*. 2015;36:921-933.

53. Curtis JR, Vincent JL. Ethics and end-of-life care for adults in the intensive care unit. *Lancet*. 2010;376:1347-1353.

54. Jones DA, DeVita MA, Bellomo R. Rapid-response teams. *N Engl J Med*. 2011;365:139-146.

55. Beitler JR, Link N, Bails DB, Hurdle K, Chong DH. Reduction in hospital-wide mortality after implementation of a rapid response team: a long-term cohort study. *Crit Care*. 2011;15:R269.

56. Vincent JL, Einav S, Pearse R, et al. Improving detection of patient deterioration in the general hospital ward environment. *Eur J Anaesthesiol*. 2018;35:325-333.

57. Rawal G, Yadav S, Kumar R. Post-intensive care syndrome: an overview. *J Transl Int Med*. 2017;5:90-92.

58. van Ruler O, Schultz MJ, Reitsma JB, Gouma DJ, Boermeester MA. Has mortality from sepsis improved and what to expect from new treatment modalities: review of current insights. *Surg Infect (Larchmt)*. 2009;10:339-348.

59. Dombrovskiy VY, Martin AA, Sunderram J, Paz HL. Facing the challenge: decreasing case fatality rates in severe sepsis despite increasing hospitalizations. *Crit Care Med*. 2005;33:2555-2562.

60. Dombrovskiy VY, Martin AA, Sunderram J, Paz HL. Rapid increase in hospitalization and mortality rates for severe sepsis in the United States: a trend analysis from 1993 to 2003. *Crit Care Med*. 2007;35:1244-1250.

61. Dreiher J, Almog Y, Sprung CL, et al. Temporal trends in patient characteristics and survival of intensive care admissions with sepsis: a multicenter analysis*. *Crit Care Med*. 2012;40:855-860.

62. Fleischmann C, Thomas-Rueddel DO, Hartmann M, et al. Hospital incidence and mortality rates of sepsis. *Dtsch Arztebl Int*. 2016;113:159-166.

40

What Happens to the Autonomic Nervous System in Critical Illness?

Gareth L. Ackland

INTRODUCTION

The term *autonomic dysfunction* is frequently associated with critical illness. Numerous studies have reported a striking association between depressed autonomic activity (usually measured as reduced heart rate variability), disease severity, and outcome.[1,2] More sophisticated interrogation of various components of the autonomic nervous system also reveals that the loss of chemoreflex[3] or baroreflex[4] responses is associated with higher mortality in critically ill patients. However, the debate over the significance of these findings is difficult to disentangle—at least from clinical studies. Moreover, much of the literature that seeks to associate the development of critical illness with autonomic dysfunction is limited by (1) the variety of techniques used to detect alterations in autonomic control, (2) the lack of population norms, (3) variable analysis techniques, and (4) lack of suitable controls and follow-up.[5] Nevertheless, emerging laboratory and trial data suggest that autonomic dysfunction may be a clinically underappreciated driver of established critical illness. Specifically, the argument put forward here is that critical illness occurs as a direct result of autonomic dysfunction, which also serves as an essential biological precursor that primes pathophysiologic responses that subsequently result in multiorgan dysfunction. As a complementary hypothesis, acquired autonomic dysfunction may also portend worse outcomes following disparate triggers of critical illness.

WHAT IS AUTONOMIC DYSFUNCTION?

From a basic biological perspective, autonomic dysfunction should be considered as an uncoupling of cellular and integrative physiologic control.[6] In other words, autonomic dysfunction is characterized by changes in afferent, integrative (central nervous system [CNS]), or efferent components of sympathetic or parasympathetic neural control that are associated with pathologic states. These criteria broaden the potential impact of autonomic dysfunction on our understanding of the pathophysiology of critical illness. Coordinated and self-limiting sympathetic activation, coupled with the maintenance of parasympathetic tone, appears to be associated with a favorable physiologic response to tissue injury and sepsis. The "uncoupling" of these autonomic control mechanisms, and consequent loss of neurally mediated interorgan feedback pathways, is a feature of the multiorgan dysfunction syndrome. In established critical illness, there is a temporally related association between autonomic dysfunction and derangements in immune, metabolic, and bioenergetic mechanisms that appears to be prognostically linked to outcome. From a neuropathologic viewpoint, postmortem samples of tissue obtained from the brains of septic patients show evidence of neuronal death in autonomic centers.[7] At the molecular level, disruption of normal G-protein-coupled receptor (GPCR) recycling[8] is a feature of neurohormonal dysregulation in disease states where biological variability is disrupted. In many respects, core features of established critical illness may be erroneously attributed to conventional clinical explanations rather than to the consequences of autonomic dysfunction alone (Table 40.1).

AT WHAT POINT DOES AUTONOMIC DYSFUNCTION INFLUENCE THE DEVELOPMENT OF CRITICAL ILLNESS?

Many patients who ultimately require critical care have established features of autonomic dysfunction well before the clinical manifestation of critical illness, as a result of various established chronic disease states. The striking observation that several chronic diseases such as cardiac and renal failure confer increased risk for sepsis suggests that an underlying common mechanism contributes to this increased propensity for multiorgan dysfunction.[9] Subclinical changes in autonomic function precede the onset of diabetes and hypertension.[10] Patients with overt or occult heart failure are at particularly high risk of having critical illness, including acquiring infection or sustaining excess postoperative morbidity following cardiac or noncardiac surgery. It has become increasingly apparent that many of the pathophysiologic features of cardiac failure are present in deconditioned patients with poor aerobic capacity and low

TABLE 40.1   Common Symptoms/Signs in Critically Ill Patients Mimicked by Features of Aberrant Autonomic Control.

Symptom of Critical Illness	Conventional Explanation	Alternative "Dysautonomia" Hypothesis
Tachycardia	Agitation[58]/fever[59]	Loss of baroreflex diminution of heart rate Cytokine stimulation of peripheral chemoreceptors
Cardiac ischemia	Underlying or acquired coronary disease[60]/hypercoaguability[61]	Loss of cardioprotective vagal innervation
Loss of inotropic performance	Cardiac ischemic damage	Neurohormonal downregulation of β-adrenoreceptors ± cardiac receptors
Failure to wean	Cardiac failure	All above
Fever of uncertain origin	Undeclared infectious source	Cytokinemia derived from neurohormonal activation of immune cells
Persistently raised inflammatory markers	Undeclared infectious source	Cytokinemia derived from neurohormonal activation of immune cells
Bacterial colonization	Immunosuppression	Adrenergic fuel for microorganism growth

anaerobic threshold yet no formal diagnosis of heart failure.[11] Cardiac failure is characterized by increased sympathetic drive, high levels of circulating catecholamines and cortisol, and withdrawal of parasympathetic activity.[12] Elevated plasma levels of proinflammatory cytokines and deficient immune function are also common features of chronic heart failure.[13] Restoration toward normal autonomic function with conventional or experimental therapies improves cardiac function, as well as reducing excess neurohormonal and inflammatory activation.[13] A growing body of accumulating evidence in both chronic heart failure[14] and critically ill patients indicates that sympatholysis is associated with an apparently counterintuitive improvement in left ventricular function[15] in addition to reductions in left ventricular remodeling and reduced plasma levels of inflammatory cytokines.[16] Loss of vagal activity in chronic heart failure is a predictor of high mortality.[17] Beyond overt cardiovascular disease, patients with extracardiac disease also show features of established autonomic dysfunction. For example, end-stage renal disease[18] and obstructive jaundice[19] are characterized by impaired baroreflex sensitivity and increased levels of plasma atrial natriuretic peptide. Moreover, patients at substantially higher risk of becoming critically ill after major surgery share many of these dysautonomic features, even though only a small fraction of these patients have a clinical diagnosis of cardiac failure as part of their preoperative workup.[20]

AUTONOMIC DYSFUNCTION AT THE VERY ONSET OF CRITICAL ILLNESS

The hallmark of the onset of critical illness is tachycardia, frequently accompanied by tachypnea.[21,22] Sepsis, hypoxia, and acidosis are all major stimuli for driving tachypnea/tachycardia through peripheral chemoreceptor-driven autonomic reflexes.[23] Similarly, sterile inflammation, or danger-associated molecular patterns, may also be an important—although underrecognized—additional driver for this physiologic response.[23] Thus, afferent sensors of the autonomic nervous system are hardwired to detect pathologic changes in oxygen, carbon dioxide, acidosis, glucose, electrolytes, neurohormones, and inflammatory mediators (Fig. 40.1). Experimental models of endotoxin infusion illustrate the speed with which neural afferents detect inflammatory changes, in parallel with the rapid and dramatic pathophysiologic features that can appear in otherwise previously well, healthy individuals.[24,25] Typical pathophysiologic changes in respiratory function—beyond tachypnea—include increased airway resistance and secretions. Discrete activation of the peripheral chemoreflex triggers the release of cortisol and vasopressin, prototypical neurohormones of critical illness. These responses may form part of the protective autonomic response to triggers of critical illness because acute carotid sinus denervation hastens mortality after lethal experimental endotoxemia.[26] Loss of baroreflex control through denervation of the carotid sinus and aortic baroreceptor nerves appears to compromise the compensatory response to hypotension induced by acute sepsis, with lower mean blood pressure, cardiac output, total peripheral resistance, and central venous pressure.[27]

IS AUTONOMIC DYSFUNCTION IN CRITICAL ILLNESS INDUCED BY MODERN CRITICAL CARE STRATEGIES?

By most accounts, many of the therapies used in critically ill patients profoundly alter, if not ablate, central autonomic, baroreflex, and chemoreceptor control. Sedation inhibits parasympathetic neuronal activity while reducing sympathetic drive.[28] Neuromuscular blockade agents inhibit peripheral chemoreceptor sensitivity[29] and conceivably produce immunosuppression through nicotinic receptor blockade.[30] Inotropes dramatically reduce baroreflex control and inhibit parasympathetic activity, as reflected by changes in heart rate variability.[31,32] Furthermore, catecholamines directly fuel infection by promoting bacterial acquisition of normally inaccessible sequestered host iron, which is released by transferrin as a result of catecholamines forming protein complexes with ferric iron.[33]

Perhaps most strikingly, models of enforced bed rest in healthy volunteers are associated with the rapid onset of autonomic dysfunction appearing well before other features of deconditioning. Typically, these changes involve sympathetic activation and parasympathetic withdrawal.[34]

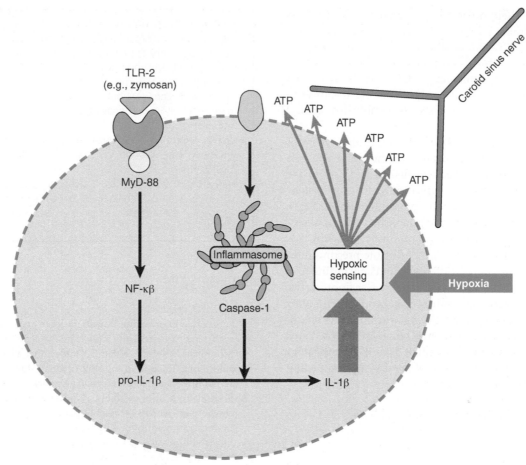

Fig. 40.1 Peripheral autonomic sensing of inflammation by the carotid body chemoreceptors. Hypoxic sensing is transduced by the release of adenosine triphosphate (ATP) as a neurotransmitter at the carotid sinus nerve; ATP is also required for activation of inflammation (NLRP3 inflammasome by the toll-like receptor 2 [TLR-2] agonist zymosan). TLR-2 activation increases production of prointerleukin-1β (pro-IL-1β) in a myeloid differentiation primary response gene 88 (MyD-88), nuclear factor-κB (NF-κB)–dependent fashion. In turn, concomitant NLRP3 activation by extracellular ATP causes caspase-1 upregulation and cleavage of pro-IL-1β, which mimics hypoxia through the induction of hypoxia-inducible factor 1-α (HIF-1α). *IL-1β*, Interleukin 1β.

Decreased activity and/or gradual loss of neurons within the dorsal vagal motor nucleus provides a neurophysiological basis for the progressive decline of exercise capacity in critical illness, because parasympathetic vagal drive determines optimal exercise capacity.[35] The increasingly recognized, though seldom detected, problem of psychological stress induced by the critical care environment reduces baroreflex sensitivity and promotes tachycardia.[36] Experimental models of enforced bed rest demonstrate a mechanistic interaction between dysautonomia and anhedonia (loss of the capacity to experience pleasure),[37] which may relate to depression being a negative prognosticator of outcome in critical illness.[38] Given the current vogue for early physical, occupational, or behavioral therapy,[39] it is tempting to speculate that restoring autonomic control may be an underappreciated feature of the apparent success of this strategy.

CARDIOVASCULAR DYSFUNCTION IN CRITICAL ILLNESS AS A DIRECT RESULT OF AUTONOMIC DYSFUNCTION

Cardiovascular dysfunction, a hallmark of critical illness, frequently prevents successful liberation from mechanical ventilation.[40] The etiology of cardiac injury during critical illness remains unclear and appears unlikely to be merely attributable to coronary artery disease given the strikingly broad demographic associated with abnormal levels of circulating troponin. Excessive sympathetic activity alone leads to accumulation of intracellular calcium, triggering myocardial necrosis.[41] Acute stress, whether it be psychological or hemodynamic in origin, triggers coagulation and endothelial cell dysfunction through sustained increases in sympathetic activity.[42] Together with persistent tachycardia, endothelial dysfunction and a sympathetic-mediated prothrombotic state may explain, in part, elevations in troponin frequently seen in critically ill patients. Catecholamine-associated metabolic dysregulation, typified by "stress" hyperglycemia, may further exacerbate myocardial injury.[43] The carefully targeted use of α-2 agonists[44] and beta blockers[45] may contribute a useful therapeutic role in this context.

In the absence of direct myocardial injury, prolonged sympathetic activation results in β-adrenoreceptor downregulation and desensitization. Circulating inflammatory mediators directly disrupt effective coupling of adrenergic receptors from their downstream signaling kinases.[46] As a result, the pathologic failure to recycle GPCRs may explain the impaired cardiometabolic response to exogenous β-adrenoreceptor stimulation. Several clinical studies have repeatedly shown that increased mortality is associated with the loss of the typical cardiometabolic response to exogenous β-adrenergic agonists in established critical illness.[47]

The parasympathetic limb of the autonomic nervous system also plays an important cardioprotective role through several disparate mechanisms. In addition to the well-recognized hemodynamic effects of increasing diastolic filling time, recent experimental data add important new mechanisms of direct relevance to established critical illness. Activity of a subpopulation of vagal motor neurons tonically inhibit left ventricular contractility.[48] Remote preconditioning is activated by numerous afferent inputs, including pain and transient ischemia in distant organs. Cardioprotective remote ischemic preconditioning is dependent on intact vagal efferent innervations of the myocardium.[49] Some of these cardioprotective effects may further be mediated through a parasympathetic-mediated anti-inflammatory mechanism, at least in the context of myocardial dysfunction triggered by inflammatory myocarditis.[50]

IMMUNE DYSFUNCTION IN CRITICAL ILLNESS AS A RESULT OF AUTONOMIC DYSFUNCTION

Experimental data show that multiple autonomic mechanisms contribute to immunoparesis and immunosuppression, key features of established critical illness. Monocyte deactivation is associated with increased risk of infection and higher mortality, accompanied by β-adrenergic desensitization.[51] Catecholamines exacerbate the hepatic dysfunction observed during sepsis,[52] which may be reversed by targeted beta-blockade.[53] The parasympathetic nervous system, acting through the vagus nerve, can sense inflammation in the periphery and relay this information to the brain, resulting in fever and activation of the hypothalamic-pituitary-adrenal axis and sympathetic activation.[54] Enhancing efferent vagal activity, at least in animal models, attenuates macrophage release of inflammatory cytokines through nicotinic α-7 agonism.[55] Other parasympathetic neurotransmitters[56] and pathways[57] may also contribute to neuroimmunomodulation.

CONCLUSIONS

An abnormal cardiometabolic response to sympathoexcitation is robustly associated with key features of chronic critical illness and paralleled by the loss of parasympathetic activity. Emerging clinical data support these largely experimental concepts. Precedents from the clinical cardiac failure literature suggest that autonomic modulation provides a rational target for preventing/reversing critical illness.

> **AUTHORS' RECOMMENDATIONS**
> - Persistent tachycardia should not automatically be attributed to conventionally thought-of triggers of excess sympathetic activity, such as hypovolemia or pain.
> - Treating dysautonomic features such as hypotension and/or tachycardia without detailed hemodynamic scrutiny may result in inappropriate therapy, including excess fluid administration.
> - Early efforts to minimize prolonged immobility may be beneficial through preventing associated autonomic dysfunction.
> - Targeted treatments to ameliorate tachycardia, using α2 adrenoceptor agonists, such as dexmedetomidine or clonidine, or titratable beta-blockers, such as esmolol, may also be beneficial.

REFERENCES

1. Hoyer D, Friedrich H, Zwiener U, et al. Prognostic impact of autonomic information flow in multiple organ dysfunction syndrome patients. *Int J Cardiol.* 2006;108:359-369.
2. Schmidt H, Müller-Werdan U, Hoffmann T, et al. Attenuated autonomic function in multiple organ dysfunction syndrome across three age groups. *Biomed Tech (Berl).* 2006;51:264-267.
3. Schmidt H, Müller-Werdan U, Nuding S, et al. Impaired chemoreflex sensitivity in adult patients with multiple organ dysfunction syndrome—the potential role of disease severity. *Intensive Care Med.* 2004;30:665-672.
4. Schmidt H, Müller-Werdan U, Hoffmann T, et al. Autonomic dysfunction predicts mortality in patients with multiple organ dysfunction syndrome of different age groups. *Crit Care Med.* 2005;33:1994-2002.
5. Stein PK. Challenges of heart rate variability research in the ICU. *Crit Care Med.* 2013;41:666-667.
6. Godin PJ, Buchman TG. Uncoupling of biological oscillators: a complementary hypothesis concerning the pathogenesis of multiple organ dysfunction syndrome. *Crit Care Med.* 1996; 24:1107-1116.
7. Sharshar T, Gray F, Lorin de la Grandmaison G, et al. Apoptosis of neurons in cardiovascular autonomic centres triggered by inducible nitric oxide synthase after death from septic shock. *Lancet.* 2003;362:1799-1805.
8. Hupfeld CJ, Olefsky JM. Regulation of receptor tyrosine kinase signaling by GRKs and beta-arrestins. *Annu Rev Physiol.* 2007; 69:561-577.
9. Phillips JK. Autonomic dysfunction in heart failure and renal disease. *Front Physiol.* 2012;3:219.
10. Davis JT, Rao F, Naqshbandi D, et al. Autonomic and hemodynamic origins of pre-hypertension: central role of heredity. *J Am Coll Cardiol.* 2012;59:2206-2216.
11. Sultan P, Edwards MR, Gutierrez del Arroyo A, et al. Cardiopulmonary exercise capacity and preoperative markers of inflammation. *Mediators Inflamm.* 2014;2014:727451.
12. Schwartz PJ, De Ferrari GM. Sympathetic-parasympathetic interaction in health and disease: abnormalities and relevance in heart failure. *Heart Fail Rev.* 2011;16:101-107.
13. Maisel AS. Beneficial effects of metoprolol treatment in congestive heart failure. Reversal of sympathetic-induced alterations of immunologic function. *Circulation.* 1994;90:1774-1780.

14. McAlister FA, Wiebe N, Ezekowitz JA, Leung AA, Armstrong PW. Meta-analysis: beta-blocker dose, heart rate reduction, and death in patients with heart failure. *Ann Intern Med.* 2009;150:784-794.

15. Gore DC, Wolfe RR. Hemodynamic and metabolic effects of selective beta1 adrenergic blockade during sepsis. *Surgery.* 2006;139:686-694.

16. Felder RB, Yu Y, Zhang ZH, Wei SG. Pharmacological treatment for heart failure: a view from the brain. *Clin Pharmacol Ther.* 2009;86:216-220.

17. Van Wagoner DR. Chronic vagal nerve stimulation for the treatment of human heart failure: progress in translating a vision into reality. *Eur Heart J.* 2011;32:788-790.

18. Chesterton LJ, McIntyre CW. The assessment of baroreflex sensitivity in patients with chronic kidney disease: implications for vasomotor instability. *Curr Opin Nephrol Hypertens.* 2005; 14:586-591.

19. Song JG, Cao YF, Sun YM, et al. Baroreflex sensitivity is impaired in patients with obstructive jaundice. *Anesthesiology.* 2009; 111:561-565.

20. Abbott TEF, Minto G, Lee AM, et al. Elevated preoperative heart rate is associated with cardiopulmonary and autonomic impairment in high-risk surgical patients. *Br J Anaesth.* 2017;119:87-94.

21. Rangel-Frausto MS, Pittet D, Costigan M, Hwang T, Davis CS, Wenzel RP. The natural history of the systemic inflammatory response syndrome (SIRS). A prospective study. *JAMA.* 1995; 273:117-123.

22. Annane D, Trabold F, Sharshar T, et al. Inappropriate sympathetic activation at onset of septic shock: a spectral analysis approach. *Am J Respir Crit Care Med.* 1999;160:458-465.

23. Ackland GL, Kazymov V, Marina N, Singer M, Gourine AV. Peripheral neural detection of danger-associated and pathogen-associated molecular patterns. *Crit Care Med.* 2013;41:e85-e92.

24. Godin PJ, Fleisher LA, Eidsath A, et al. Experimental human endotoxemia increases cardiac regularity: results from a prospective, randomized, crossover trial. *Crit Care Med.* 1996; 24:1117-1124.

25. Taylor EW, Jordan D, Coote JH. Central control of the cardiovascular and respiratory systems and their interactions in vertebrates. *Physiol Rev.* 1999;79:855-916.

26. Tang GJ, Kou YR, Lin YS. Peripheral neural modulation of endotoxin-induced hyperventilation. *Crit Care Med.* 1998; 26:1558-1563.

27. Koyama S, Terada N, Shiojima Y, Takeuchi T. Baroreflex participation of cardiovascular response to *E. coli* endotoxin. *Jpn J Physiol.* 1986;36:267-275.

28. Bradley BD, Green G, Ramsay T, Seely AJ. Impact of sedation and organ failure on continuous heart and respiratory rate variability monitoring in critically ill patients: a pilot study. *Crit Care Med.* 2013;41:433-444.

29. Eriksson LI, Sato M, Severinghaus JW. Effect of a vecuronium-induced partial neuromuscular block on hypoxic ventilatory response. *Anesthesiology.* 1993;78:693-699.

30. Wang H, Yu M, Ochani M, et al. Nicotinic acetylcholine receptor alpha7 subunit is an essential regulator of inflammation. *Nature.* 2003;421:384-388.

31. Hogue Jr CW, Dávila-Román VG, Stein PK, Feinberg M, Lappas DG, Pérez JE. Alterations in heart rate variability in patients undergoing dobutamine stress echocardiography, including patients with neurocardiogenic hypotension. *Am Heart J.* 1995;130:1203-1209.

32. van de Borne P, Heron S, Nguyen H, et al. Arterial baroreflex control of the sinus node during dobutamine exercise stress testing. *Hypertension.* 1999;33:987-991.

33. Lyte M, Freestone PP, Neal CP, et al. Stimulation of *Staphylococcus epidermidis* growth and biofilm formation by catecholamine inotropes. *Lancet.* 2003;361:130-135.

34. Hughson RL, Yamamoto Y, Maillet A, et al. Altered autonomic regulation of cardiac function during head-up tilt after 28-day head-down bed-rest with counter-measures. *Clin Physiol.* 1994; 14:291-304.

35. Machhada A, Trapp S, Marina N, et al. Vagal determinants of exercise capacity. *Nat Commun.* 2017;8:15097.

36. Truijen J, Davis SC, Stok WJ, et al. Baroreflex sensitivity is higher during acute psychological stress in healthy subjects under β-adrenergic blockade. *Clin Sci (Lond).* 2011;120:161-167.

37. Moffitt JA, Grippo AJ, Beltz TG, Johnson AK. Hindlimb unloading elicits anhedonia and sympathovagal imbalance. *J Appl Physiol (1985).* 2008;105:1049-1059.

38. Desai SV, Law TJ, Needham DM. Long-term complications of critical care. *Crit Care Med.* 2011;39:371-379.

39. Schweickert WD, Pohlman MC, Pohlman AS, et al. Early physical and occupational therapy in mechanically ventilated, critically ill patients: a randomised controlled trial. *Lancet.* 2009;373:1874-1882.

40. Lara TM, Hajjar LA, de Almeida JP, et al. High levels of B-type natriuretic peptide predict weaning failure from mechanical ventilation in adult patients after cardiac surgery. *Clinics (Sao Paulo).* 2013;68:33-38.

41. Ellison GM, Torella D, Karakikes I, et al. Acute beta-adrenergic overload produces myocyte damage through calcium leakage from the ryanodine receptor 2 but spares cardiac stem cells. *J Biol Chem.* 2007;282:11397-11409.

42. Bruno RM, Ghiadoni L, Seravalle G, Dell'oro R, Taddei S, Grassi G. Sympathetic regulation of vascular function in health and disease. *Front Physiol.* 2012;3:284.

43. Weekers F, Giulietti AP, Michalaki M, et al. Metabolic, endocrine, and immune effects of stress hyperglycemia in a rabbit model of prolonged critical illness. *Endocrinology.* 2003;144:5329-5338.

44. MacLaren R. Immunosedation: a consideration for sepsis. *Crit Care.* 2009;13:191.

45. Morelli A, Ertmer C, Westphal M, et al. Effect of heart rate control with esmolol on hemodynamic and clinical outcomes in patients with septic shock: a randomized clinical trial. *JAMA.* 2013;310:1683-1691.

46. Coggins M, Rosenzweig A. The fire within: cardiac inflammatory signaling in health and disease. *Circ Res.* 2012;110:116-125.

47. Collin S, Sennoun N, Levy B. Cardiovascular and metabolic responses to catecholamine and sepsis prognosis: a ubiquitous phenomenon? *Crit Care.* 2008;12:118.

48. Machhada A, Marina N, Korsak A, Stuckey DJ, Lythgoe MF, Gourine AV. Origins of the vagal drive controlling left ventricular contractility. *J Physiol.* 2016;594:4017-4030.

49. Mastitskaya S, Marina N, Gourine A, et al. Cardioprotection evoked by remote ischaemic preconditioning is critically dependent on the activity of vagal pre-ganglionic neurones. *Cardiovasc Res.* 2012;95:487-494.

50. Leib C, Göser S, Lüthje D, et al. Role of the cholinergic antiinflammatory pathway in murine autoimmune myocarditis. *Circ Res.* 2011;109:130-140.

51. Link A, Selejan S, Maack C, Lenz M, Böhm M. Phosphodiesterase 4 inhibition but not beta-adrenergic stimulation suppresses

tumor necrosis factor-alpha release in peripheral blood mononuclear cells in septic shock. *Crit Care.* 2008;12:R159.

52. Aninat C, Seguin P, Descheemaeker PN, Morel F, Malledant Y, Guillouzo A. Catecholamines induce an inflammatory response in human hepatocytes. *Crit Care Med.* 2008;36:848-854.

53. Ackland GL, Yao ST, Rudiger A, et al. Cardioprotection, attenuated systemic inflammation, and survival benefit of beta1-adrenoceptor blockade in severe sepsis in rats. *Crit Care Med.* 2010;38:388–394.

54. Goehler LE, Gaykema RP, Hansen MK, Anderson K, Maier SF, Watkins LR. Vagal immune-to-brain communication: a visceral chemosensory pathway. *Auton Neurosci.* 2000;85:49–59.

55. Tracey KJ. Understanding immunity requires more than immunology. *Nat Immunol.* 2010;11:561–564.

56. Smalley SG, Barrow PA, Foster N. Immunomodulation of innate immune responses by vasoactive intestinal peptide (VIP): its therapeutic potential in inflammatory disease. *Clin Exp Immunol.* 2009;157:225–234.

57. Cailotto C, Gomez-Pinilla PJ, Costes LM, et al. Neuro-anatomical evidence indicating indirect modulation of macrophages by vagal efferents in the intestine but not in the spleen. *PLoS One.* 2014; 9:e87785.

58. Chevrolet JC, Jolliet P. Clinical review: agitation and delirium in the critically ill-significance and management. *Crit Care.* 2007;11:214.

59. Launey Y, Nesseler N, Mallédant Y, Seguin P. Clinical review: fever in septic ICU patients-friend or foe? *Crit Care.* 2011;15:222.

60. Lim W, Qushmaq I, Devereaux PJ, et al. Elevated cardiac troponin measurements in critically ill patients. *Arch Intern Med.* 2006;166:2446–2454.

61. Alhazzani W, Lim W, Jaeschke RZ, Murad MH, Cade J, Cook DJ. Heparin thromboprophylaxis in medical-surgical critically ill patients: a systematic review and meta-analysis of randomized trials. *Crit Care Med.* 2013;41:2088–2098.

41

Is Persistent Critical Illness a Syndrome of Ongoing Inflammation/Immunosuppression/Catabolism?

McKenzie K. Hollen, Philip A. Efron, and Scott C. Brakenridge

INTRODUCTION

The standard host response to infection can be overly robust and effectually cause an auto-destructive state of systemic inflammatory response syndrome (SIRS) that leads to multiple organ dysfunction (MODS), refractory shock, and fulminant death.[1] Due in part to advances in intensive care and organ support, mortality among critically ill septic patients has declined, especially among those receiving aggressive resuscitation and organ support.[2] For example, very few surgical intensive care unit (ICU) patients with sepsis now die from refractory shock, and mortality in this group has dropped from historical rates of 40%–50% to as low as 13% in those that survive the first 48 hours.[3,4] Instead, a new clinical phenotype, termed chronic critical illness (CCI), has emerged. CCI patients experience extended stays in the ICU, develop persistent, low-grade organ dysfunction, and have poor long-term survival rates.[3] CCI patients extensively utilize resources, accrue significant personal and hospital financial burdens, and are frequently discharged to long-term acute care facilities (LTAC) or skilled nursing facilities (SNFs) where they endure further cognitive disabilities, rapid accelerated aging, frailty, and sepsis recidivism requiring rehospitalization.[1] CCI is characterized by a number of immunosuppressive and inflammatory phenotypes. These patients often exhibit:

- persistent inflammation (elevated C-reactive proteins, interleukin-6 [IL-6], and interleukin-8 [IL-8])
- myeloid derived suppressor cell (MDSC) expansion
- immunosuppression (latent viral reactivation and increased secondary infections), and
- protein catabolism with muscle wasting.[1]

Researchers and physicians have investigated mechanisms that might drive these clinical abnormalities. The combination has been termed the persistent inflammation immunosuppression and catabolism syndrome (PICS). It is hoped that this formulation will lead to the identification of mechanistic causes for increased late morbidity and mortality in patients with sepsis and will uncover testable approaches to therapy (Fig. 41.1).[1]

EVIDENCE THAT PERSISTENT CRITICAL ILLNESS IS A SYNDROME OF ONGOING INFLAMMATION, IMMUNOSUPPRESSION, AND CATABOLISM

Three clinical trajectories have emerged following sepsis (Fig. 41.2). A 3-year prospective observational cohort study evaluated surgical ICU (SICU) patients with sepsis for the development of CCI ($\geq$14 days of intensive care unit resource utilization with persistent organ dysfunction).[4] Of the patients studied, only 6% that survived the first 48 hours died within 14 days. Forty-six percent of patients experienced rapid recovery (that is, recovery within 14 days). However, a striking 49% survived but failed to recover with the 14-day window, thus meeting our criteria for CCI. Of the patients who developed CCI, >60% died within six months.[1,4] The patients with CCI that died within this time frame exhibited the following characteristics:

1. persistent inflammation as evidenced by elevated plasma concentrations of cytokines and
2. elevated immunosuppressive proteins, i.e., soluble programmed death ligand 1(sPD-L1) and IL-10.[4]

Seventy percent of RAP patients were discharged to their home or rehabilitation facilities. Of CCI patients who survived to discharge, nearly two thirds were discharged to LTACs, SNFs, inpatient hospitals, or hospice.[4] According to a number of developed health-related quality of life, physical function and performance indices (EuroQol-5D, the Short Physical Performance Battery, and the ECOG/WHO/Zubrod Scale), long-term follow-up demonstrated that CCI patients reported poorer quality of life and greater functional incapacities compared to patients who experienced rapid recovery.[4]

Additionally, PICS has been observed in critical illness arising from disorders other than sepsis. A retrospective cohort study determined that severe acute pancreatitis patients with prolonged ICU stays were associated with a high morbidity of PICS and reported poorer long-term quality of life.[5] A study addressing long-term mortality in burn survivors demonstrated that, when compared to matched controls, survival from the acute phase of burn injury was associated

Three clinical trajectories

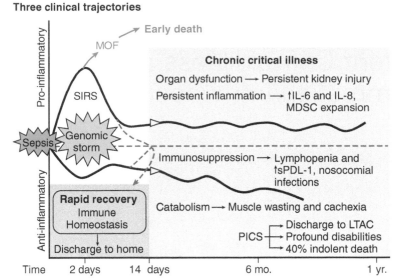

Fig. 41.1 Proposed hypothesis for persistent inflammation, immunosuppression, and catabolism syndrome (PICS). *LTAC,* long-term acute care facilities; *MDSC,* myeloid-derived suppressor cell; *SIRS,* systemic inflammatory response syndrome; *sPDL-1,* soluble programmed death ligand-1. (Redrawn from Hawkins RB, Raymond SL, Stortz JA, et al. Chronic critical illness and the persistent inflammation, immunosuppression, and catabolism syndrome. *Front Immunol.* 2018;9:1511.)

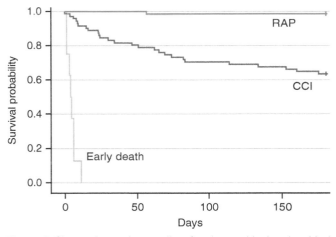

Fig. 41.2 Six-month sepsis mortality of patients with chronic critical illness (CCI) (*n* = 71) and those who experienced rapid recovery (RAP) (*n* = 66). (Redrawn from Stortz JA, Mira JC, Raymond SL, et al. Benchmarking clinical outcomes and the immunocatabolic phenotype of chronic critical illness after sepsis in surgical intensive care unit patients. *J Trauma Acute Care Surg.* 2018;84[2]:342-349.)

with an increased incidence of cognitive disabilities and greater long-term mortality.[6] In addition, severe burn patients demonstrated a sustained elevation of serum cytokines that persisted for up to 3 years.[7] These patients also experienced systemic and skeletal muscle hypermetabolism that was associated with insulin resistance, oxidative stress, cytosolic protein degradation, and mitochondrial stress—hypothesized to be contributors of muscle catabolism postburn.[8]

In summary, an increase in survival from these high acuity insults has unmasked a new phenotype—that of PICS. It is believed that these patients enter a cyclic and persistent but chronically manageable syndrome of organ dysfunction.

This new phenotype is associated with a high likelihood of discharge to long-term care facilities, poor functional outcomes, and high post-ICU discharge mortality rates.[9]

THE SELF-PERPETUATING CYCLE OF PICS

Recent data permit the construction of a model that explains the development of CCI. Accumulating data suggest that CCI is a product of three concurrent, interacting cycles being driven by, and also contributing to the perpetuation of both systemic and local end-organ inflammation (Fig. 41.3), muscle wasting, emergency myelopoiesis and organ injury.[1]

Subsequent to source control and antimicrobial coverage, it is thought that PICS is propagated by sustained release of alarmins and danger-associated molecular pattern (DAMP) molecule signaling from damaged organs. This contributes to a self-perpetuating cycle of "pathophysiologic alterations" driven by chronic low-grade inflammation (elevated serum concentration of interleukin-6), dysfunctional emergency myelopoiesis, catabolism (maladaptive metabolic changes in lipid, carbohydrate, and protein metabolism), compromised host immunity (lymphocyte dysfunction and decreased function of antigen presenting cells), and continued organ injury.[1]

INFLAMMATION/IMMUNOSUPPRESSION

Biopsy-driven studies in CCI patients with burn injury demonstrate defective mitochondrial biogenesis and myocyte necrosis associated with leukocyte infiltration.[10] These findings suggest that persistent inflammation causes mitochondrial and skeletal muscle injury, releasing breakdown products

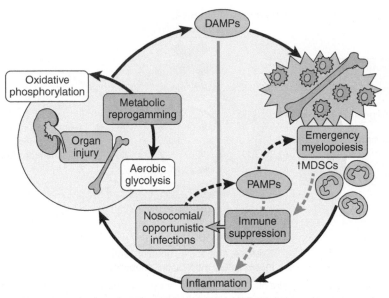

Fig. 41.3 The self-perpetuating cycle of immune dyscrasia, organ injury, dysfunctional metabolic adaptations, and myelodysplasia driving chronic critical illness (CCI). (Redrawn from Hawkins RB, Raymond SL, Stortz JA, et al. Chronic critical illness and the persistent inflammation, immunosuppression, and catabolism syndrome. *Front Immunol.* 2018;9:1511.)

(alarmins) that exacerbate inflammation and continue the vicious cycle. Alarmins, endogenous molecules that signal cell and tissue damage, are of particular interest in the perpetration of persistent inflammation. Two different types are recognized by the pattern-recognition receptors on immune and parenchymal cells that modulate inflammation: exogenous pathogen-associated molecular patterns (PAMPs) of microbial origin and DAMPs from injured organs and inflammatory cells.[11] PAMPs involved in the initiation of sepsis arise from the inciting infection while additional PAMPs that are involved in the pathogenesis of CCI likely arise from nosocomial infections and latent virus reactivation.[12] In burn injury, a number of DAMPs are released from skeletal muscle. These include mitochondrial DAMPs (mitoDAMPs) such as mitochondrial DNA (mtDNA), HMGB1, and transcription factor A, mitochondrial (TFAM) that stimulate the release of additional breakdown products that add to ongoing inflammation.[1] It is also thought that the kidney and skeletal muscle wasting contribute to the expansion of endogenous DAMPs.[1] PAMPs and DAMPs can bind to multiple receptors, including toll-like receptors (TLRs), nucleotide-binding oligomerization domain (NOD)-like receptors (NLRs), and can complement retinoic acid-inducible gene (RIG)-like receptors and mannose-binding lectin or scavenger receptors.[13,14] PAMPs and DAMPs can activate multiple signaling pathways in a variety of cell types.[13,14]

Current paradigms describing the immune response following high acuity events like severe trauma, sepsis, burns, and pancreatitis postulate that inflammation cooccurs with antiinflammation and immunosuppression (Fig. 41.4).[4,9,13,15,16] Immunosuppression in CCI would explain the subclinical reactivation of latent viruses and the high incidence of secondary bacterial infections. During PICS, both myeloid and lymphoid cells are recruited and both pro- and anti-inflammatory

cytokines, reactive oxygen species, and reactive nitrogen species proliferate in conjunction with increased T-cell apoptosis (due in part to the upregulation of PD-L1 and inadequate L-arginine) and tissue wasting.[17,18] The host's immune system develops multiple innate immune deficiencies such as myeloid derived stem cell (MDSC) expansion, increased T-regulatory cells (T_{regs}) and M2 macrophages, T-cell exhaustion, and decreased dendritic cell function.[18] Evidence of a state of immunosuppression includes increased circulating levels of immunosuppressive mediators such as IL-10 and TGF-B, as well as an increased expression of T-cell inhibitory ligands such as PD-L1, and decreased expression of the major histocompatibility complex (e.g., HLA-DR) by monocytes and antigen presenting cells.[2,12,16,18]

EMERGENCY MYELOPOIESIS

Sepsis and other major insults induce an expansion of myeloid lineage cells.[19,20] This acute response likely represents an adaptive, evolutionarily-conserved acute response to injury or infection. However, among patients with prolonged critical illness, the response appears to become chronic and detrimental. This "emergency myelopoiesis" occurs at the expense of lymphopoiesis and erythropoiesis, promoting lymphopenia and anemia. Additionally, cytokines and chemokines are released in conjunction with adrenergic stimulation. These mediators promote the release of myeloid populations from bone marrow and secondary lymphoid tissues.[1,21,22] Most hematopoietic stem cells (HSCs) are relatively quiescent, participating in routine immune and hematologic homeostasis. In response to stress, HSCs are upregulated as part of the normal physiologic innate immune response and enter the cell cycle to differentiate and become active. This process,

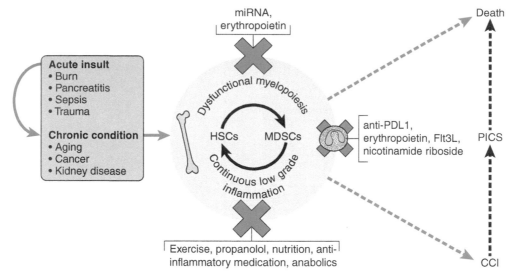

Fig. 41.4 Depiction of Myelodysplasia of persistent inflammation, immunosuppression and catabolism syndrome. *CCI,* chronic critical illness; *HSC,* hematopoietic stem cell; *MDSC,* myeloid derived suppressor cell. (Redrawn from Efron PA, Mohr AM, Bihorac A, et al. Persistent inflammation, immunosuppression, and catabolism and the development of chronic critical illness after surgery. *Surgery.* 2018;164[2]:178-184.)

"emergency myelopoiesis," repopulates innate immune effector cells after acute insult; however, the preferential differentiation of myeloid cells occurs at the expense of lymphopoiesis and erythropoiesis, placing patients at increased risks of anemia and secondary infections following acute physiologic insult.[9]

Additionally, emergency myelopoiesis is modulated by various redundant pathways incorporating growth factors, cytokines and mesenchymal cells, and this process blocks the differentiation of immature myeloid cells into mature innate immune effector cells. Consequently, a heterogeneous population of myeloid-derived suppressor cells expands. MDSCs have the capability to affect nearly every cell involved in host innate and adaptive immunity.[9] Though the distinct roles of MDSCs are still widely unknown, they are believed to emerge as part of the physiologic response to sepsis and trauma to help decrease inflammation through immunosuppression, without eliminating all protective innate immunity.[9,23,24] The persistence of this population of cells has been clinically associated with poor outcomes in sepsis patients.[19,25] One of the characteristic functions of MDSCS appears to be the suppression of the function and proliferation of T lymphocytes. MDSCs also secrete antiinflammatory cytokines, IL-10 and TGF-β, which polarize differentiating macrophages into type II macrophages, in turn, upregulating T$_{regs}$. Additionally, MDSCs deplete L-arginine via arginase 1 and inducible nitric oxide synthase (iNOS), which consequently antagonizes clonal expansion, impairs intracellular signaling, and induces T-cell apoptosis. MDSCs produce reactive oxygen species, which, in conjunction with the nitric oxide byproducts of iNOS, produce peroxynitrites that nitrosylate cell surface proteins on lymphocytes and decrease T-cell responsiveness and alter IL-2 signaling.[9,26] MDSCs have been shown to persistently increase in circulation after clinical sepsis or septic shock in the SICU, and their appearance is a biomarker for nosocomial infections, prolonged hospital stays, increased mortality, and poor functional status at discharge.[19]

ORGAN INJURY

Additionally, many organs are damaged by critical illness, but the kidney is thought to be particularly vulnerable in CCI.[1] A retrospective analysis validated acute kidney injury (AKI; as defined by RIFLE or KDIGO criteria) as a predictor of mortality and adverse outcomes in surgical sepsis, and determined the kidney to be the most frequently injured organ in sepsis.[27] The strong associations between sepsis and AKI/chronic kidney disease (CKD) implement the critical importance of the kidney in long-term outcomes and survival following sepsis and critical illness.[1] The kidney is host to a number of immune cells (dendritic cells (DC), macrophages, and lymphocytes) and expresses a large number TLRs.[28] During CCI, immunosuppressive MDSCs and DAMPs infiltrate the kidney and expose renal dendritic cells and lymph nodes to antigens and pathogens that are continuously processed by the nephrons.[29] Importantly, the kidneys filter the entire blood volume more than 30 times per day effectively exposing renal DCs and lymph nodes to these DAMPs and pathogenic antigens more than any other organ.[28–30]

CATABOLISM IN CCI

Skeletal muscle constitutes the largest protein reservoir in the body and, in cancer and other chronic inflammatory diseases, is subject to catabolism with lean muscle wasting.[9] This depletion is also evident in CCI. Historically, cachexia in ICU patients has been attributed to a normal macro-endocrine and cytokine driven stress response.[10,31] Biopsy-driven studies on CCI have shown the increase in breakdown products, relative to synthesis products, that result in a net catabolic state.[32]

Despite early administration of enteral nutrition, persistent catabolism and sarcopenia have been observed in critically-ill patients, and cross-sectional area reduction of the rectus femoris muscle was associated with multiple organ failure and inflammation.[32] Recent studies have demonstrated that patients who develop CCI following sepsis have decreased levels of albumin and insulin-like growth factor-binding protein 3 and elevated urinary 3-methylhistidine to creatinine ratios, suggestive of a persistent catabolic state.[4,26]

Long-term, prospective follow-up studies on CCI have demonstrated a correlation between loss of lean muscle mass and functional disabilities, breakdown of myofibrillar protein, decreased protein synthesis, increased mitochondrial dysfunction, and the increased release of potential pro-inflammatory degradation products.[1,32,33] These changes are thought to produce systemic inflammatory responses and release DAMPs and exogenous alarmins during skeletal muscle damage or wasting, as previously described. It is likely that dysfunctions in substrate utilization further complicate the cycle of reciprocal catabolism and inflammation.[9] The complexity of this disease will undoubtedly require a multifactorial approach to treatment that includes, but is not limited to supplemented nutrition and physical exercise.

TREATMENT AND THERAPY

Considering that PICS is a complex pathophysiological response to a pro-inflammatory insult on the host's immunity, there is likely no monotherapeutic solution to address all aspects of the persistent inflammation, immunosuppression, and catabolism. However, because the underlying PICS pathophysiology is characteristic of a myelodysplastic disease, immunomodulation therapies should be incorporated to counter the chronic and acute responses to trauma and sepsis.[9] Propranolol and oxandrolone have been show to benefit pediatric burn patients; however, more studies are needed to study the effects with adult CCI patients.

AUTHORS' RECOMMENDATIONS

- A growing number of ICU patients are plagued by chronic critical illness
- CCI is thought to be initiated by alarmin-triggered genomic storm, persistent organ dysfunction, and skeletal muscle wasting
- Pro-inflammatory expansion of myeloid derived suppressor cells occurs in conjunction with immunosuppression
- Adequate nutrition and physical rehabilitation are insufficient to treat persistent catabolism and muscle wasting because substrate utilization is likely involved in this catabolic state
- Future immunopathology research may be directed toward inflammation, immune stimulation, epigenetic modifications, and stem cell administration.[34]
- Propranolol and oxandrolone have been shown to benefit pediatric burn patients; however, more studies are needed to study the effects with adult CCI patients.

REFERENCES

1. Hawkins RB, Raymond SL, Stortz JA, et al. Chronic critical illness and the persistent inflammation, immunosuppression, and catabolism syndrome. *Front Immunol.* 2018;9: 1511.
2. Stevenson EK, Rubenstein AR, Radin GT, Wiener RS, Walkey AJ. Two decades of mortality trends among patients with severe sepsis. *Crit Care Med.* 2014;42(3):625-631.
3. Mira JC, Brakenridge SC, Moldawer LL, Moore FA. Persistent inflammation, immunosuppression and catabolism syndrome (PICS). *Crit Care Clin.* 2017;33(2):245-258.
4. Stortz JA, Mira JC, Raymond SL, et al. Benchmarking clinical outcomes and the immunocatabolic phenotype of chronic critical illness after sepsis in surgical intensive care unit patients. *J Trauma Acute Care Surg.* 2018;84(2): 342-349.
5. Yang N, Li B, Ye B, et al. The long-term quality of life in patients with persistent inflammation-immunosuppression and catabolism syndrome after severe acute pancreatitis: A retrospective cohort study. *J Crit Care.* 2017;42:101-106.
6. Mason SA, Nathens AB, Byrne JP, et al. Increased rate of long-term mortality among burn survivors. *Ann Surg.* 2019; 269(6):1192-1199.
7. Jeschke MG, Gauglitz GG, Kulp GA, et al. Long-term persistence of the pathophysiologic response to severe burn injury. *PLoS One.* 2011;6(7):e21245.
8. Ogunbileje JO, Porter C, Herndon DN, et al. Hypermetabolism and hypercatabolism of skeletal muscle accompany mitochondrial stress following severe burn trauma. *Am J Physiol Endocrinol Metab.* 2016;311(2):E436-E448.
9. Efron PA, Mohr AM, Bihorac A, et al. Persistent inflammation, immunosuppression, and catabolism and the development of chronic critical illness after surgery. *Surgery.* 2018;164(2): 178-184.
10. Jeschke MG, Chinkes DL, Finnerty CC, et al. Pathophysiologic response to severe burn injury. *Ann Surg.* 2008;248(3): 387-401.
11. Kang JW, Kim SJ, Cho HI, Lee SM. DAMPs activating innate immune responses in sepsis. *Ageing Res Rev.* 2015;24(Pt A): 54-65.
12. Stortz JA, Raymond SL, Mira JC, Moldawer LL, Mohr AM, Efron PA. Murine models of sepsis and trauma: can we bridge the gap? *ILAR J.* 2017;58(1):90-105.
13. Stortz JA, Murphy TJ, Raymond SL, et al. Evidence for persistent immune suppression in patients who develop chronic critical illness after sepsis. *Shock.* 2018;49(3): 249-258.
14. Santos CD, Hussain SNA, Mathur S, et al. Mechanisms of chronic muscle wasting and dysfunction after an intensive care unit stay. A pilot study. *Am J Respir Crit Care Med.* 2016;194(7):821-830.
15. Xiao W, Mindrinos MN. A genomic storm in critically injured humans. *J Exp Med.* 2011;208(13):2581-2590.
16. Cheung AM, Tansey CM, Tomlinson G, et al. Two-year outcomes, health care use, and costs of survivors of acute respiratory distress syndrome. *Am J Respir Crit Care Med.* 2006;174(5):538-544.
17. Shindo Y, Unsinger J, Burnham C-A, Green JM, Hotchkiss RS. Interleukin-7 and anti–programmed cell death 1 antibody have differing effects to reverse sepsis-induced immunosuppression. *Shock.* 2015;43(4):334-343.

18. Hotchkiss RS, Moldawer LL. Parallels between cancer and infectious disease. *N Engl J Med*. 2014;371(4):380-383.

19. Mathias B, Delmas AL, Ozrazgat-Baslanti T, et al. Human myeloid-derived suppressor cells are associated with chronic immune suppression after severe sepsis/septic shock. *Ann Surg*. 2017;265(4):827-834.

20. Guirgis FW, Brakenridge S, Sutchu S, et al. The long-term burden of severe sepsis and septic shock. *J Trauma Acute Care Surg*. 2016;81(3):525-532.

21. Cosentino M, Marino F, Maestroni GJ. Sympathoadrenergic modulation of hematopoiesis: a review of available evidence and of therapeutic perspectives. *Front Cell Neurosci*. 2015;9:302.

22. Hasan S, Mosier MJ, Szilagyi A, Gamelli RL, Muthumalaiappan K. Discrete β-adrenergic mechanisms regulate early and late erythropoiesis in erythropoietin-resistant anemia. *Surgery*. 2017;162(4):901-916.

23. Cuenca AG, Delano MJ, Kelly-Scumpia KM, et al. A paradoxical role for myeloid-derived suppressor cells in sepsis and trauma. *Mol Med*. 2011;17:281-292.

24. Goldszmid RS, Dzutsev A, Trinchieri G. Host immune response to infection and cancer: unexpected commonalities. *Cell Host Microbe*. 2014;15(3):295-305.

25. Uhel F, Azzaoui I, Grégoire M, et al. Early expansion of circulating granulocytic myeloid-derived suppressor cells predicts development of nosocomial infections in patients with sepsis. *Am J Respir Crit Care Med*. 2017; 196(3):315-327.

26. Mira JC, Gentile LF, Mathias BJ, et al. Sepsis pathophysiology, chronic critical illness, and persistent inflammation-immunosuppression and catabolism syndrome. *Crit Care Med*. 2017;45(2):253-262.

27. White LE, Hassoun HT, Bihorac A, et al. Acute kidney injury is surprisingly common and a powerful predictor of mortality in surgical sepsis. *J Trauma Acute Care Surg*. 2013;75(3): 432-438.

28. Kurts C, Panzer U, Anders H-J, Rees AJ. The immune system and kidney disease: basic concepts and clinical implications. *Nat Rev Immunol*. 2013;13(10):738-753.

29. Tryggvason K, Wartiovaara J. How does the kidney filter plasma? *Physiology*. 2005;20(2):96-101.

30. Mulay SR, Kulkarni OP, Rupanagudi KV, et al. Calcium oxalate crystals induce renal inflammation by NLRP3-mediated IL-1β secretion. *J Clin Invest*. 2012;123(1):236-246.

31. Yoshida T, Delafontaine P. Mechanisms of cachexia in chronic disease states. *Am J Med Sci*. 2015;350(4):250-256.

32. Puthucheary Z, Harridge S, Hart N. Skeletal muscle dysfunction in critical care: Wasting, weakness, and rehabilitation strategies. *Crit Care Med*. 2010;38(10 Suppl):S676-S682.

33. Batt J, Santos CCD, Cameron JI, Herridge MS. Intensive care unit–acquired weakness. *Am J Respir Crit Care Med*. 2013;187(3):238-246.

34. van der Poll T, van de Veerdonk FL. The immunopathology of sepsis and potential therapeutic targets. *Nat Rev Immunol*. 2017;17:407-420.

42

How Do I Optimize Antibiotic Use in Critical Illness?

Cheston B. Cunha and Steven M. Opal

Septic patients in the intensive care unit (ICU) represent some of the sickest patients in the hospital, and optimal initial antibiotic selection is paramount to their survival. In this patient population, the key is to select an empiric regimen that not only maximizes antibiotic effect but also limits the development of resistance.[1,2] Within each antibiotic class are drugs that may have a high or low resistance potential. The precise mechanism by which the difference arises is unknown. "Low resistance potential" antibiotics are antimicrobials that rarely induce resistance among bacteria even when used frequently and for extended periods of time. In addition to selecting antibiotics that have a low resistance potential, consideration should be given toward selecting an agent with favorable pharmacokinetics (PK) and pharmacodynamics (PD).[3] Essentially, infected patients should be treated urgently with the highest tolerable/nontoxic antimicrobial dose of a drug with low resistance potential to maximize microbial killing while minimizing the risk of selecting out drug-resistant mutants.[4–7]

ANTIBIOTIC PHARMACOKINETIC AND PHARMACODYNAMIC CONSIDERATIONS TO MINIMIZE RESISTANCE AND OPTIMIZE EFFECTIVENESS

PK defines the fate of an antibiotic within the body (i.e., absorption, volume of distribution [V_d], blood and tissue levels, hepatic metabolism/excretion, and renal excretion). Antibiotic PK describes the effects of the antibiotic on both the host and the infecting microorganism. Both parameters are essential to consider in choosing an antimicrobial regimen for critically ill patients with serious infections. The inhibitory/bactericidal effect of antibiotics can be categorized as demonstrating concentration-dependent killing, time-dependent killing, or a combination of both and depends on the antibiotic and the targeted pathogen. Concentration-dependent killing kinetics describes the increased bacterial killing that occurs as antibiotic concentrations increase

above the minimal inhibitory concentration (MIC) and are expressed as the maximum serum antibiotic concentration (C_{max}) to the MIC ratio (C_{max}/MIC).[8,9] The fluoroquinolones—aminoglycosides, metronidazole, and daptomycin—all exhibit concentration-dependent killing. When selecting these antibiotics, the dose must be maximized for optimal effect. The higher the dose used, the more potent the antibiotic killing. Achieving a high concentration is particularly important when selecting an antibiotic with a relatively wide toxic-to-therapeutic ratio (i.e., aminoglycosides), making once daily dosing highly desirable. There are two benefits to this dosing strategy. Giving a high dose of the antibiotic only once per day generates a very high, but rapidly cleared, peak serum concentration, providing optimal and rapid bacterial killing. As the drug concentration subsequently falls, tissue levels rapidly diminish, preventing accumulation and decreasing the risk of toxicity.[10] Adding to the optimized killing provided by the single daily peak level is the prolonged post-antibiotic effect (PAE) characteristic of aminoglycosides. The PAE extends antimicrobial capacity well after the serum concentrations have fallen below the MIC for the pathogenic microorganism (up to 8–12 hours).

Antibiotics that display time-dependent killing kinetics include β-lactams, carbapenems, macrolides, and linezolid. In these compounds, an increase in the serum concentration above four to five times MIC does not increase killing. Thus the key to antimicrobial activity lies in keeping the blood level close to this point for as long as possible—the time of drug concentration above MIC for the dosing period (T > MIC).[8] Therefore, even when antibiotics that demonstrate time-dependent killing are used, there is little downside with high doses of the drug, particularly in critically ill patients with infection.[9] The killing kinetics of other antimicrobials may have more complex PD that better fit an integration of the time over MIC, expressed as the area under the concentration curve over the MIC ($AUC_{0–24}$:MIC).[10–12]

Some antimicrobials, such as doxycycline or vancomycin, exhibit kinetics that are dependent on time and concentration, reflecting the MIC of the pathogen.[13] When gram-positive cocci with an MIC <1 μg/mL are exposed to vancomycin, the drug functions with time-dependent killing kinetics. However, when the MIC is >1 μg/mL, the kinetics are dependent on concentration. The aminoglycosides and quinolones also demonstrate this duality with some pathogens (i.e., concentration-dependent kinetics [C_{max}/MIC ratio]) as well as AUC_{0-24}/MIC ratio[14] (Table 42.1).

PK principles dictate the concentration and distribution of each antibiotic in serum and body fluids over time. The overall concentrations of a drug in the serum are affected by the antibiotic's peak serum concentrations, V_d, serum half-life ($t_{1/2}$), protein binding, and renal or hepatic function. Peak serum concentration, protein binding, and V_d will directly determine the tissue concentrations of an antibiotic in the tissue where the pathogen resides[8,10–12,15] (Table 42.2). Critically ill patients with high fever often have increased cardiac output and kidney blood flow, which increase clearance rates of many antibiotics.[16] Additionally, sepsis-induced increased vascular permeability within the microcirculation expands the apparent V_d, further lowering blood levels of antimicrobial agents.[17] These pathophysiologic events can conspire to result in lower than expected effective blood levels in these severely ill patients. Therapeutic drug monitoring, if available, can avoid possible suboptimal drug dosing resulting in subtherapeutic blood levels at the critical moment when bactericidal activity is most needed.[18]

For the most part, antibiotics that exhibit time-dependent killing are bacteriostatic, whereas those with concentration-dependent kinetics are bactericidal. Exceptions to this are the penicillins, carbapenems, and monobactams, which are bactericidal despite relying on time-dependent kinetics[19] (Tables 42.3 and 42.4). Furthermore, certain antibiotics may exhibit both types of killing kinetics depending on how they are used; for example, doxycycline, which uses time-dependent kinetics and is usually bacteriostatic, is bactericidal at high concentrations, a characteristic usually reserved for concentration-dependent antibiotics.[13] In addition to these factors, antibiotics that exhibit concentration-dependent kinetics tend to have prolonged PAE, but there are some antibiotics that are time-dependent (e.g., doxycycline) and also have a PAE.[8,15]

ANTIBIOTIC SUSCEPTIBILITY TESTING AND RESISTANCE

A discussion on maximizing the dosing of antimicrobials would not be complete without consideration of antibiotic resistance. Resistant organisms are becoming increasingly prevalent worldwide and pose a significant problem for clinicians and ICUs. Despite this fact, there is no international agreement on the definitions of the terms "resistant" or "susceptible".[20,21] The breakpoints used in susceptibility testing are based on achievable serum concentrations using the recommended doses of antibiotics for bloodstream infections. Interpretation of susceptibility reports on non-bloodstream isolates must be carefully performed. Infections are difficult to treat when the chosen antibiotic does not adequately penetrate the target tissues (e.g., the prostate or the central nervous system). The clinician must extrapolate likely tissue concentrations at the infection site from achievable serum concentration. Failure to consider this issue may result in clinical failure to eradicate infection despite laboratory reports indicating that the organism in question is susceptible.[22] It is critical to remember that with certain organisms (e.g., methicillin-resistant *Staphylococcus aureus* [MRSA]), in vitro susceptibility testing does not predict in vivo clinical effectiveness.[23] The source of

TABLE 42.1 Antibiotic Dosing: Pharmacokinetic/Pharmacodynamic Considerations.

Antibiotic PK/PD Parameters	Optimal Dosing Strategies
Concentration-Dependent Antibiotics (C_{max}:MIC)	
• Quinolones • Aminoglycosides • Vancomycin if MIC ≥ 1 μg/mL • Tigecycline • Colistin • Doxycycline	Use highest effective dose (without toxicity)
Time-Dependent Antibiotics (T > MIC)	
• PCN concentrations > MIC for 70% of the dosing interval • β-Lactam concentrations > MIC for 60% of the dosing interval • Carbapenems concentrations > MIC for 40% of the dosing interval	
Vancomycin if MIC ≤ 1 μg/mL	Use high doses (which increase serum concentrations and increase T > MIC for more of the dosing interval)
Other Antibiotics (C_{max}:MIC/T > MIC and/or AUC_{0-24}/MIC)	
Quinolones >125 (effective) >250 (more effective)	Use highest effective dose (without toxicity)

AUC, area under the concentration curve; C_{max}, peak serum concentrations; *MIC*, minimal inhibitory concentration; *PAE*, post-antibiotic effect; *PCN*, penicillin; *PD*, pharmacodynamic; *PK*, pharmacokinetic; *T*, time.

Adapted from Roberts JA, Pharm B, Lipman J. Pharmacokinetic issues for antibiotics in the critically ill patient. *Crit Care Med.* 2009;37:840-851; Roberts JA, Lipman J. Optimizing use of beta-lactam antibiotics in the critically ill. *Semin Respir Crit Care Med.* 2007;28:579-585; Roberts JA, Pharm B, Kruger P, et al. Antibiotic resistance—what's dosing got to do with it? *Crit Care Med.* 2008;36:2433-2440.

TABLE 42.2 Antibiotics: Relevant Pharmacokinetic Characteristics in the Intensive Care Unit.

Antibiotic PK Parameters	Sepsis ↑ with Capillary Permeability[a] (Intravascular → Interstitial Fluid Shifts)	Suggested Dosing Recommendations
Water-Soluble Antibiotics (Low V_d Water Soluble)		
• Renally eliminated • High serum concentrations • Limited tissue penetration	• ↑V_d → ↓ serum concentrations	• ↑ Dose of hydrophilic antibiotic • Change to a lipid-soluble antibiotic
Lipid-Soluble Antibiotics (High V_d → Lipid Soluble)		
• Hepatically eliminated • High tissue penetration • Good serum concentration		• No change in V_d → no change in serum or tissue concentrations • No change needed

[a]Also with mechanical ventilation, burns, and hypoalbuminemia.

PK, pharmacokinetics; *Vd*, volume of distribution.

Adapted from Roberts JA, Pharm B, Lipman J. Pharmacokinetic issues for antibiotics in the critically ill patient. *Crit Care Med*. 2009;37:840-851.

TABLE 42.3 Inherent Resistance Potential of Selected Antibiotics.

High Resistance Potential Antibiotics	Usual Resistant Organisms for Each Antibiotic	Preferred Low Resistance Potential Antibiotic Alternatives
Aminoglycosides		
Gentamicin/ tobramycin	*P. aeruginosa*	Amikacin
Cephalosporins		
Ceftazidime	*P. aeruginosa*	Cefepime
Tetracyclines		
Tetracycline	*S. pneumoniae* *S. aureus*	Doxycycline or minocycline
Quinolones		
Ciprofloxacin	*S. pneumoniae*	Levofloxacin or moxifloxacin
Ciprofloxacin	*P. aeruginosa*	Levofloxacin
Glycopeptides		
Vancomycin	MSSA MRSA	Linezolid or daptomycin or Minocycline
Carbapenems		
Imipenem	*P. aeruginosa*	Meropenem or doripenem
Macrolides		
Azithromycin	*S. pneumonia*	No other macrolide Alternatives include doxycycline, levofloxacin, or moxifloxacin
Dihydrofolate Reductase Inhibitors		
TMP-SMX	*S. pneumonia*	Doxycycline

MRSA, methicillin-resistant *S. aureus*; *MSSA*, methicillin-sensitive *S. aureus*; *TMP-SMX*, trimethoprim-sulfamethoxazole.

discordance may lie in patient physiology that differs from in vitro conditions (e.g., the media used for testing).[24,25] Local acidosis and hypoxia may also decrease the activity of some antibiotics.[26]

Another major issue with antibiotic resistance detection is the prolonged time delay in obtaining in vitro susceptibility results from the microbiology laboratory. Clinicians routinely wait up to 24–48 hours after infection is confirmed to determine if their empiric antibiotic selection is active against the pathogen. Innovations in laboratory genomics and microfluidics promise to reduce that wait time down to less than 1 hour in the near future.[27,28]

Even without these confounding factors, inherent differences between in vitro susceptibility and in vivo efficacy must be considered. As an example, treating MRSA with trimethoprim-sulfamethoxazole (TMP-SMX), doxycycline, or clindamycin, which are often reported as effective on in vitro testing, may not be successful.[23,24] Instead, anti-MRSA antibiotics such as minocycline, linezolid, daptomycin, or vancomycin, with proven clinical effectiveness against MRSA, provide a greater chance of eradicating the infection. *Listeria monocytogenes* appears susceptible to cephalosporins, but clinical experience indicates that this β-lactam class of antibiotics does not work in vivo for meningitis, for example (Box 42.1).

Resistance potential (high vs. low) is an inherent property of an antibiotic (Box 42.2). With high resistance potential antibiotics (e.g., macrolides, TMP-SMX, ampicillin), loss of efficacy is also a function of frequency and duration of use. Low resistance potential antibiotics (e.g., doxycycline, ceftriaxone, amikacin) are less affected by extensive/prolonged use. All other factors being equal, resistance is more likely to develop when tissue concentrations are subtherapeutic in difficult-to-penetrate tissue spaces (e.g., chronic prostatitis, abscesses, and biofilm-associated device infections). Relative resistance, such as that seen with antibiotics like aminoglycosides, may be overcome if antibiotic tissue concentrations are higher than the organism's MIC (Table 42.3). It is always beneficial to use the highest nontoxic dose possible to treat serious infections in ICU patients.

TABLE 42.4 Empiric Antibiotic Coverage for Common Intensive Care Unit Infections.

Infection Type/Site	Usual Pathogen at Site	Usual Nonpathogens at Site	Preferred Empiric Therapy with Low Resistance Potential Antibiotics	Penicillin Allergy
CVC-Associated Bacteremia[a]				
	MSSA MRSA CoNS GNBs (aerobic) VSE	B. fragilis Non-group D streptococci	Meropenem plus either vancomycin (if MRSA likely) or linezolid (if VRE likely)	Meropenem plus either vancomycin (if MRSA likely) or linezolid (if VRE likely)
Intra-Abdominal Sepsis				
Cholecystitis/ cholangitis	E. coli K. pneumoniae VSE	B. fragilis	Levofloxacin or moxifloxacin	Levofloxacin or moxifloxacin
Peritonitis/ colon perforation	B. fragilis GNBs (aerobic)	Non-group D streptococci	Ertapenem or piperacillin/tazobactam or moxifloxacin or tigecycline	Ertapenem or moxifloxacin or tigecycline
VAP/NP	P. aeruginosa GNBs (aerobic)	B. fragilis MSSA/MRSA VSE/VRE Burkholderia cepacia A. baumannii S. maltophilia	Meropenem or doripenem or levofloxacin (750 mg) or cefepime	Meropenem or doripenem or levofloxacin (750 mg)
Urosepsis				
Community acquired	GNBs (aerobic) VSE	B. fragilis MSSA/MRSA	Piperacillin/tazobactam or meropenem	Meropenem
Nosocomial	P. aeruginosa GNBs (aerobic)	B. fragilis MSSA/MRSA	Piperacillin/tazobactam or meropenem	Meropenem
Skin and Soft Tissue Infections				
Cellulitis	Group A, B, C, G streptococci	MSSA/MRSA	Ceftriaxone or cefazolin	Vancomycin or clindamycin
Abscess	MSSA/MRSA	Group A, B, C, G streptococci	Ceftaroline or minocycline or Vancomycin or linezolid	Vancomycin or linezolid or minocycline

[a]Remove/replace CVC as soon as possible.

CoNS, coagulase negative staphylococci; *CVC*, central venous catheter; *GNBs*, gram-negative bacilli; *ICU*, intensive care unit; *MRSA*, methicillin-resistant *S. aureus*; *MSSA*, methicillin-sensitive *S. aureus*; *NP*, nosocomial pneumonia; *VAP*, ventilator-associated pneumonia; *VRE*, vancomycin-resistant enterococci; *VSE*, vancomycin-sensitive enterococci.

Adapted from Cunha BA, ed. *Antibiotic Essentials*, 12th ed. Sudbury, MA: Jones & Bartlett; 2013:17-151.

SPECIFIC ANTIBIOTIC CLASSES

β-Lactams

β-Lactam antibiotics use time-dependent killing and are bactericidal. Although they exert a short but measurable PAE on gram-positive organisms, they have no PAE when used against gram-negative organisms. Maximum bacterial killing occurs when drug concentrations are five times the MIC of the target organism, but no additional benefit is conferred by raising concentrations above this level.[24,25] Thus the goal should be to maintain a serum concentration greater than the MIC for the longest duration possible—at least 60% (penicillins) to 70% (cephalosporins) of the dosing interval. Strategies to achieve this PD effect include increasing the dosing frequency, giving β-lactams with a long serum half-life, or giving the drug as a continuous infusion.[23,24,26-28] Ultimately, when β-lactams are used in the ICU, combining higher doses with increased frequency of administrations will maximize antibiotic effect without increasing the risk of developing resistance.[24,25] Among cephalosporins, cefepime has good activity against *Pseudomonas aeruginosa*. This drug is typically used for systemic *P. aeruginosa* infections and febrile neutropenia as monotherapy or in combination with an aminoglycoside (e.g., amikacin). In extended spectrum β-lactamase–producing organisms, multidrug-resistant organisms (MDROs; with MICs = 4–8 μg/mL), and *P. aeruginosa* infection, a "high dose" of cefepime should be used.[29-31]

BOX 42.1 Difficulty With the Interpretation of Antibiotic Susceptibility Testing Data.

1. The cultured isolate is *not* necessarily the pathogen (e.g., skin colonizers, colonizers of body/fluid secretions).
2. Treating "colonizers" from fluid/body secretions from nonsterile sites often misses the true pathogens at the site of infection.
3. An antibiotic selected based on the cultured "colonizer" is often misleading.
4. Selection of an antibiotic based on susceptibility testing does not guarantee antibiotic effectiveness.
5. Isolates reported to be "resistant" are not always resistant; in fact such isolates are often nonsusceptible or only relatively resistant (i.e., easily susceptible with high-dose therapy).

   In vitro susceptibility vs. In vivo effectiveness
1. Interpretation (breakpoints of resistance) not universally agreed upon (United States of America [Clinical Laboratory Standards Institute] vs. Europe [European Committee on Antimicrobial Susceptibility Testing]).
2. In vitro susceptibility not always predictive of in vivo effectiveness.
   Examples:
   - MRSA reported as "susceptible" to doxycycline and TMP-SMX may not be clinically effective.
   - MRSA reported as "susceptible" in vitro to quinolones or cephalosporins (except ceftaroline) are not effective in vivo.
   - *Klebsiella pneumoniae* reported as "susceptible" in vitro to TMP-SMX is not effective in vivo.
   - Streptococci (Groups A–D) reported as "susceptible" in vitro to aminoglycosides are not effective in vivo.
   - *Listeria monocytogenes* appears susceptible in vitro but is not effective in vivo.
3. Nonsusceptible isolates in vitro may be susceptible in vivo with full/high doses if the MIC can be exceeded.

MIC, minimal inhibitory concentration; *MRSA*, methicillin-resistant *S. aureus*; *TMP-SMX*, trimethoprim-sulfamethoxazole.
Adapted from Cunha BA, ed. *Antibiotic Essentials*, 12th ed. Sudbury, MA: Jones & Bartlett; 2013: 2-10.

BOX 42.2 Effective Approaches to Minimize Resistance.

1. Avoid "covering" colonizers that rarely, if ever, cause infection at the infection site being treated.
2. Select a low resistance potential antibiotic effective against the usual site-determined pathogens.
3. Always consider the penetration potential of the antibiotic selected to be sure of therapeutic concentrations at the site of infection.
4. Use a loading dose or high dose for the first 3 days to eliminate selecting out potentially resistant mutants.
5. Use the shortest effective duration of therapy, taking into account host factors, inoculation size, and pathogen virulence.

   Ineffective Approaches to Minimize Resistance
6. Switching from broad-spectrum to narrow-spectrum antibiotics is less relevant if using appropriate low resistance potential antibiotics.
7. Combination therapy does not prevent resistance.
8. Antibiotic "cycling" does not prevent resistance.
9. De-escalation decreases unnecessary/excessive antibiotic use, but does not, per se, decrease resistance.
10. Decreasing "antibiotic tonnage" or volume decreases costs and *Clostridium difficile* rates, but not resistance.
11. Avoid prolonged/low-dose antibiotic therapy.

Adapted from Cunha BA. Antibiotic resistance: effective control strategies. *Lancet* 357:1307-1308 and 1101, 2001; Roberts JA, Pharm B, Kruger P, et al. Antibiotic resistance—what's dosing got to do with it? *Crit Care Med.* 2008;36:2433-2440.

Carbapenems

Structurally similar to β-lactam antibiotics, carbapenems also rely on time-dependent killing. Concentrations should be targeted to remain at five times the MIC for more than 40% or longer of the dosing interval, which can best be achieved by using high doses or long-acting agents (e.g., ertapenem for susceptible organisms).[24,25,32,33]

Quinolones

As described previously, the fluoroquinolones exhibit both time- and concentration-dependent killing. AUC_{0-24}/MIC ratios directly correlate with clinical outcomes; that is, an AUC_{0-24}/MIC ratio of >125 is usually considered predictive of efficacy in gram-negative infections. However, using the highest doses of quinolones to achieve an AUC_{0-24}/MIC ratio of >250 may be superior and will help reduce the development of resistance.[24] This dosing strategy also confers the benefits of maximizing the C_{max}/MIC ratio.[34–36]

Vancomycin

The PD of vancomycin varies depending on the MICs of the staphylococcal pathogen causing the infection. In cases in which the MICs are >1, vancomycin acts in a concentration-dependent killing manner, whereas in the setting of MICs of <1, its kinetics demonstrates time-dependent killing. Because concerns about the nephrotoxicity of vancomycin are largely unfounded, care should be taken to utilize the highest possible dose to maximize efficacy. Using inadequate doses of vancomycin has been associated with resistance development; therefore, a preferred dosing strategy would be to use high-dose vancomycin (e.g., 60 mg/kg intravenously [IV] every 24 hours [q24h]), with doses appropriately adjusted for kidney function.[23]

Linezolid

Linezolid demonstrates bacteriostatic activity against staphylococci and enterococci but exhibits bactericidal activity against non-Group D streptococci. Linezolid exhibits time-dependent killing kinetics. Despite its bacteriostatic activity against staphylococci, linezolid can be successfully used to treat acute bacterial endocarditis when compared with bactericidal agents.[23] Dosing of linezolid does not need to be adjusted for renal/hepatic dysfunction.

Daptomycin

Daptomycin exhibits concentration-dependent killing and is bactericidal with dual PD characteristics (i.e., C_{max}/MIC

as well as AUC_{0-24}/MIC ratio). It also has a prolonged PAE. Dosing of daptomycin depends on the site of infection. Lower doses are needed for skin and soft tissue infections, whereas larger doses are required to treat bacteremia.[23] Relative or complete resistance may be present when patients with prior exposure to vancomycin are treated for staphylococcal infection, reflecting thickening of the cell wall.[9] In cases in which relatively resistant organisms are suspected, high-dose daptomycin (10–12 mg/kg IV q24h) has been successfully used.[37,38] Daptomycin should be avoided in cases of pneumonia because the calcium present in surfactant inactivates the antibiotic.

Tigecycline

Tigecycline, a derivative of minocycline that is structurally similar to the tetracyclines, exhibits time-dependent killing. Concerns in the literature about the potential therapeutic failures of tigecycline relate to treating organisms that are innately resistant to tigecycline (e.g., *P. aeruginosa*) or to inadequate dosing. When tigecycline is administered, a loading dose, typically twice the maintenance dose, should be given; however, the optimal tigecycline dosing strategy has not yet been determined. Given the high V_d of the drug (8 L/kg), the initial dose may not be sufficient to achieve therapeutic serum concentrations. A higher loading dose may be necessary when treating relatively resistant gram-negative bacilli.[39,40] The half-life of tigecycline is so long ($t_{1/2}$ = 42 hours) that after the initial loading dose of tigecycline, the maintenance dose (half of the loading dose) should instead be dosed every 24 hours.[39]

Aminoglycosides

Aminoglycosides demonstrate concentration-dependent killing kinetics. Amikacin, the aminoglycoside with the highest anti-*P. aeruginosa* activity, achieves much higher serum/MIC ratios than other aminoglycosides and is preferred in the critically ill. This drug may be used as monotherapy for gram-negative bacteremia and used as part of combination therapy to either increase coverage (e.g., tigecycline plus amikacin) or for possible synergy (e.g., levofloxacin plus amikacin). One-time daily dosing optimizes amikacin PK/PD advantages and limits the risk of nephrotoxicity and ototoxicity.[41–43]

Colistin

Colistin is primarily used for serious infection due to MDRO *Acinetobacter* sp. or *P. aeruginosa* resistant to other antibiotics. Acquired resistance to colistin is rare, but many common gram-negative microorganisms are intrinsically resistant (*Proteus, Morganella, Serratia, Burkholderia* spp.). The limiting factor with colistin use is the potential for nephrotoxicity. Recent studies suggest that colistin, when properly dosed, is less nephrotoxic than was once thought.[44] Colistin should be given with a loading dose and then given in a maintenance dose of 1.7 mg/kg (IV) every 8 hours. Renal function should be monitored because renal failure may increase the serum half-life from 3.5 hours up to as long as 48–72 hours.[45,46]

Colistin should be considered the drug of last resort. It is the only antibiotic active against MDRO *Acinetobacter* spp. and *P. aeruginosa*.

CONCLUSION

When selecting an empiric antibiotic for the ICU patient, clinicians must take into account the spectrum of activity, delivery of the drug to the site where the pathogen is located, resistance potential, optimized dosing based on PK/PD, and duration of treatment needed to eradicate the infection. The goal should be to use the highest dose of an antibiotic but avoid toxicity in situations in which there is relative resistance (e.g., penicillin-resistant pneumococci). It is important to resist the temptation to treat isolates that represent colonization rather than true infection because this increases the risk of developing antibiotic resistance.[4] Empiric antibiotic therapy should be reserved for patients with true infection and not used in patients with infectious mimics or otherwise unexplained fever or leukocytosis (Table 42.4).

Ultimately, when using antibiotics in the ICU setting, it is critical to select an agent with a low resistance potential and give the drug at the highest dose without causing toxicity for the shortest amount of time necessary to cure the infection (Boxes 42.3 and 42.4). In this way, clinicians will gain maximum benefit from antimicrobials with the fewest adverse effects.

BOX 42.3   Summary of Optimal Empiric Antibiotic use in the Intensive Care Unit.

1. Base empiric coverage on likely pathogens at the infection site (lungs, not respiratory secretion isolates)
2. Avoid "covering" only cultured organism (colonization) from nonsterile sites
   - Respiratory secretions in intubated patients
   - Urine in patients with Foley catheters
   - Wounds with a nonpurulent discharge
3. Select antibiotic with high degree activity (and low resistance potential) against the usual pathogens at infection site
   - VAP/NP: *P. aeruginosa* and aerobic GNBs (not MSSA/MRSA)
   - Urosepsis: aerobic GNBs and enterococci (not MSSA/MRSA or *B. fragilis*)
   - Intra-abdominal sepsis: *B. fragilis* and aerobic GNBs (not MSSA/MRSA)
4. Minimize resistance by preferentially using low resistance potential (vs. high resistance potential) antibiotics with a spectrum appropriate for the infection site
5. Use full dose/highest dose (nontoxic) possible to maximize effectiveness and minimize the emergence of resistant organisms
6. Use strict infection control precautions to minimize spread of MDROs in ICU and hospital

---

GNBs, gram-negative bacilli; ICU, intensive care unit; MDRO, multidrug-resistant organism; MRSA, methicillin-resistant S. aureus; MSSA, methicillin-sensitive *S. aureus*; NP, nosocomial pneumonia; VAP, ventilator-associated pneumonia.

BOX 42.4 Consequences of Suboptimal Antibiotic Therapy.

1. Therapeutic failure

   Consequences
   - Wasted resources (drug costs of unsuccessful therapy)
   - Cost of re-treatment with another effective antibiotic (sometimes more expensive/toxic)
   - Costs of tests and consultants to evaluate and or re-treat therapeutic failure
   - Covering/chasing colonizers often means missing or not optimally treating the pathogens at the infection site
   - ↑ Length of stay
   - Legal implications of therapeutic failure

2. Antibiotic resistance

   Causes
   - Failure to select low resistance potential antibiotics (vs. high resistance potential antibiotics)
   - Failure to use full/highest tolerable dosing without toxicity (vs. low dose/prolonged treatment duration)
   - Failure to penetrate the target site of infection in therapeutic concentration results in subtherapeutic concentrations at the infection site → therapeutic failure/resistance
   - All other things being equal, subtherapeutic/low antibiotic concentrations likely to promote resistance

   Consequences
   - Cost of cohorting MDRO patients (impairs patient flow/bed utilization)
   - Risk of spread of MDROs within the ICU, hospital, and community
   - Compromised hospital reputation and or public image

ICU, intensive care unit; *MDRO,* multidrug-resistant organism.

AUTHORS' RECOMMENDATIONS

- When selecting an empiric antibiotic for the septic ICU patient, clinicians must take into account the spectrum of activity, delivery of the drug to the site where the pathogen is located, resistance potential, optimized dosing based on PK/PD, and duration of treatment needed to eradicate the infection.
- The goal should be to use the highest dose of an antibiotic, yet avoid toxicity.
- Antibiotics should not be administered to treat isolates that represent colonization rather than true infection or infectious mimics such as unexplained fever or leukocytosis.
- The selected agent should be administered for the shortest duration necessary to cure the infection.

REFERENCES

1. Vincent JL, Opal SM, Marshall JC, Tracey KJ. Sepsis definitions: time for change. *Lancet.* 2013;381:774-775.
2. Dellinger RP, Levy MM, Rodes A, et al. Surviving Sepsis Campaign: international guidelines for management of severe sepsis and septic shock: 2012. *Crit Care Med.* 2013;41:580-637.
3. Hurford A, Morris AM, Fisman DN, Wu J. Linking antimicrobial prescribing to antimicrobial resistance in the ICU: before and after an antimicrobial stewardship program. *Epidemics.* 2012; 4:203-210.
4. Cunha CB, Varughese CA, Mylonakis E. Antimicrobial stewardship programs (ASPs): the devil is in the details. *Virulence.* 2013;4: 147-149.
5. Rimawi RH, Mazer MA, Siraj DS, Gooch M, Cook PP. Impact of regular collaboration between infectious diseases and critical care practitioners on antimicrobial utilization and patient outcome. *Crit Care Med.* 2013;41:2099-2107.
6. Njoku JA, Hermsen ED. Antimicrobial stewardship in the intensive care unit: a focus of potential pitfalls. *J Pharm Pract.* 2010;23:50-60.
7. Amer MR, Akhras NS, Mahmood WA, Al-Jazairi AS. Antimicrobial stewardship program implementation in a medical intensive care unit at a tertiary care hospital in Saudi Arabia. *Ann Saudi Med.* 2013;33:547-554.
8. Roberts JA, Pharm B, Lipman J. Pharmacokinetic issues for antibiotics in the critically ill patient. *Crit Care Med.* 2009;37:840-851.
9. Cunha BA. Vancomycin revisited: a reappraisal of clinical use. *Crit Care Clin.* 2008;24:393-420.
10. Drusano GL. Antimicrobial pharmacodynamics: critical interactions of "bug and drug." *Nat Rev Microbiol.* 2004;2:289-300.
11. Owens Jr RC, Shorr AF. Rational dosing of antimicrobial agents: pharmacokinetic and pharmacodynamic strategies. *Am J Health Syst Pharm.* 2009;66:S23-S30.
12. Winterboer TM, Lecci KA, Olsen KM. Continuing education: alternative approaches to optimizing antimicrobial pharmacodynamics in critically ill patients. *J Pharm Pract.* 2010;23:6-18.
13. Cunha BA, Domenico P, Cunha CB. Pharmacodynamics of doxycycline. *Clin Microbiol Infect.* 2000;6:270-273.
14. Bailey TC, Little JR, Littenberg B, Reichley RM, Dunagan WC. A meta-analysis of extended-interval dosing versus multiple daily dosing of aminoglycosides. *Clin Infect Dis.* 1997;24:786-795.
15. Ambrose PG, Owens Jr RC, Quintiliani R, et al. Antibiotic use in the critical care unit. *Crit Care Clin.* 1998;14:283-308.
16. Jacobs A, Taccone FS, Roberts JA, et al. Beta-lactam dosage regimens in septic patients with augmented renal clearance. *Antimicrob Agents Chemother.* 2018;62(9).
17. Opal SM, van der Poll T. Endothelial barrier dysfunction in septic shock. *J Intern Med.* 2015;277:277-293.
18. Rello J, van Engelen TRS, Alp E, et al. Towards precision medicine in sepsis: A position paper from the European Society of Clinical Microbiology and Infectious Diseases. *Clin Microbiol Infect.* 2018 [Epub ahead of print].
19. Goff DA, Nicolau DP. When pharmacodynamics trump costs: an antimicrobial stewardship program's approach to selecting optimal antimicrobial agents. *Clin Ther.* 2013;35:766-771.
20. Kahlmeter G. Defining antibiotic resistance-towards international harmonization. *Ups J Med Sci.* 2014;119:78-86.
21. Turnidge J, Paterson DL. Setting and revising antibacterial susceptibility breakpoints. *Clin Microbiol Infect.* 2007;20:391-408.
22. Lodise TP, Butterfield J. Use of pharmacodynamic principles to inform β-lactam dosing: "S" does not always mean success. *J Hosp Med.* 2011;6:S16-S23.
23. Cunha BA. Minocycline versus doxycycline for meticillin-resistant Staphylococcus aureus (MRSA): in vitro susceptibility versus in vivo effectiveness. *Int J Antimicrob Agents.* 2010;35: 517-518.
24. Domenico P, O'Leary R, Cunha BA. Differential effects of bismuth and salicylate salts on the antibiotic susceptibility of Pseudomonas aeruginosa. *Eur J Clin Microbiol Infect Dis.* 1992;11:170-175.

25. Cunha BA. Problems arising in antimicrobial therapy due to false susceptibility testing. *J Chemother*. 1997;1:25-35.

26. Cunha BA, ed. *Antibiotic Essentials*. 12th ed. Sudbury, MA: Jones & Bartlett; 2013.

27. Van Belkum A, Dunne Jr WM. Next-generation antimicrobial susceptibility testing. *J Clin Microbiol*. 2013;51(7):2018-2024.

28. Baltekin O, Boucharin A, Tano E, et al. Antimicrobial susceptibility testing in less than 30 min using single-cell imaging. *Proc Natl Acad Sci U S A*. 2017;114(34):9170-9175.

29. Roberts JA, Pharm B, Kruger P, Paterson DL, Lipman J. Antibiotic resistance—What's dosing got to do with it? *Crit Care Med*. 2008; 36:2433-2440.

30. Roberts JA, Lipman J. Optimizing use of beta-lactam antibiotics in the critically ill. *Semin Respir Crit Care Med*. 2007;28: 579-585.

31. McKinnon PS, Paladino JA, Schentag JJ. Evaluation of area under the inhibitory curve (AUIC) and time above the minimum inhibitory concentration (T>MIC) as predictors of outcome for cefepime and ceftazidime in serious bacterial infections. *Int J Antimicrob Agents*. 2008;31:345-351.

32. Roberts JA, Paratz J, Paratz E, Krueger WA, Lipman J. Continuous infusion of beta- lactam antibiotics in severe infections: a review of its role. *Int J Antimicrob Agents*. 2007;30:11-18.

33. Roberts JA, Boots R, Rickard CM, et al. Is continuous infusion ceftriaxone better than once-a-day dosing in intensive care? A randomized controlled pilot study. *J Antimicrob Chemother*. 2006;59:285-291.

34. Altshuler J, Aitken SL, Guervil D, Esaian D, Papadopoulos J, Arias CA. Treatment of extended-spectrum beta-lactamase Enterobacteriaceae with cefepime: the dose matters, too. *Clin Infect Dis*. 2013;57:915-916.

35. Tamma PD, Girdwood SCT, Gopaul R, et al. The use of cefepime for treating AmpC β-lactamase-producing Enterobacteriaceae. *Clin Infect Dis*. 2013;57:781-788.

36. Yahave D, Paul M, Fraser A, Sarid N, Leibovici L. (2007). Efficacy and safety of cefepime: a systematic review and meta-analysis. *Lancet Infect Dis*. 2007;7:338-348.

37. Ogutlu A, Guclu E, Karabay O, Utku AC, Tuna N, Yahyaoglu M. Effects of Carbapenem consumption on the prevalence of Acinetobacter infection in intensive care unit patients. *Ann Clin Microbiol Antimicrob*. 2014;13:7.

38. Palmore TN, Henderson DK. Carbapenem-resistant Enterobacteriaceae: a call for cultural change. *Ann Intern Med*. 2014; 160:567-569.

39. Noreddin AM, Elkhatib WF. Levofloxacin in the treatment of community-acquired pneumonia. *Expert Rev Anti Infect Ther*. 2010;8:505-514.

40. Gous A, Lipman J, Scibante J, et al. Fluid shifts have no influence on ciprofloxacin pharmacokinetics in intensive care patients with intra-abdominal sepsis. *Int J Antimicrob Agents*. 2005; 26:50-55.

41. Zelenitsky SA, Ariano RE. Support for higher ciprofloxacin AUC$_{24}$/MIC targets in treating Enterobacteriaceae bloodstream infection. *J Antimicrob Chemother*. 2010;65:1725-1732.

42. Cunha BA, Eisenstein LE, Hamid NS. Pacemaker-induced Staphylococcus aureus mitral valve acute bacterial endocarditis complicated by persistent bacteremia from a coronary stent: cure with prolonged/high-dose daptomycin without toxicity. *Heart Lung*, 2006;35:207-211.

43. Cunha BA, Mickail N, Eisenstein LE. Faecalis vancomycin-sensitive enterococcal bacteremia unresponsive to a vancomycin tolerant strain successfully treated with high-dose daptomycin. *Heart Lung*. 2007;36:456-461.

44. Cunha BA. Once-daily tigecycline therapy of multidrug-resistant and non-multidrug-resistant gram-negative bacteremias. *J Chemother*. 2007;19:232-233.

45. Cunha BA. Pharmacokinetic considerations regarding tigecycline for multidrug-resistant (MDR) *Klebsiella pneumoniae* or MDR Acinetobacter baumannii urosepsis. *J Clin Microbiol*. 2009; 47:1613.

46. Layeux B, Taccone FS, Fagnoul D, Vincent JL, Jacobs F. Amikacin monotherapy for sepsis caused by panresistant Pseudomonas aeruginosa. *Antimicrob Agents Chemother*. 2010; 54:4939-4941.

43

How Do I Identify Pathologic Organisms in the 21st Century?

Tjitske S.R. van Engelen and Tom van der Poll

INTRODUCTION

Traditional or classical diagnostics in infectious disease rely on the identification and characterization of the pathogen. For more than a century, it has been generally accepted that blood stream infections should be diagnosed by culturing the patient's blood.[1] If executed correctly, blood cultures are valuable but the technique is time-limited, usually requiring 12–72 hours. New molecular-based techniques may advance the field of infectious diagnostics.[2] Rapid diagnostic tests no longer rely solely on positive blood cultures but can be performed using culture-independent methods on blood or other easy-to-obtain samples such as feces or urine. Both pathogen-targeted and host-targeted diagnostics have been developed to provide more rapid and more accurate information on causative pathogens in intensive care unit (ICU) settings.

One of the most common causes of critical illness is sepsis,[3] and a fundamental intervention in sepsis treatment is the early administration of antimicrobial therapy.[4] Indeed, delays in antimicrobial administration are associated with a decrease in survival.[5,6] The causative pathogen is often unknown when the physician needs to choose an antimicrobial treatment. Empiric broad-spectrum antibiotics are potentially life-saving and improve disease-free survival, and are therefore liberally administered.[4] However, overuse of these agents contributes to the current threat of antimicrobial resistance[7] and can also alter the host microbiome in a detrimental manner.[8] There is an urgent need to identify pathogens and test for susceptibility to antimicrobial treatment and resistance mechanisms as early as possible. This approach will not only improve antibiotic stewardship but will also contribute to an increased use of antimicrobials with lesser detrimental side effects. Early identification of causative pathogens is the key to direct therapy early in the course of disease and is likely to improve healthcare outcomes in critical illness.

This chapter provides an overview of how pathologic bacteria are identified in the 21st century. The focus is on culture-dependent and independent pathogen-targeted methods and host-targeted molecular diagnostics.

PATHOGEN-TARGETED DIAGNOSTICS

Classical diagnostics in infectious disease require a positive culture, followed by specification and identification of the pathogen and antimicrobial susceptibility testing (AST). Several diagnostic methods are available that can provide results more rapidly than these conventional methods. Novel approaches include fluorescent in situ hybridization (FISH), mass spectrometry and automated polymerase chain reaction (PCR)-based systems. Some can also detect resistance markers or test antimicrobial susceptibility more rapidly. Culture-independent methods where pathogens are detected directly in whole blood, thereby avoiding the 2-days wait, are highly anticipated and several promising assays are already available.[2]

Culture-Dependent Methods

For rapid microorganism detection in signal positive blood cultures, hybridization, nucleic acid amplification, and post-amplification methods that lead to quicker identification of the causative pathogen than classical diagnostics are available.[9] Despite the fact that the turnaround time from test to result is significantly reduced, these diagnostic tests are described as rapid because of their quick processing after blood cultures turn positive, that is, after amplification of the number of organisms in a sample. These novel culture-dependent tests are a valuable addition but are not yet available for point-of-care testing because the time to initiating appropriate treatment is longer than the 6 hours recommended for sepsis.[4] A summary of the assays on signal positive blood cultures can be found in Table 43.1.

In contrast, FISH does not depend on amplification of the pathogen material. The technique uses fluorescent probes to detect organism-specific deoxyribonucleic acid (DNA) sequences. Amplification methods can be limited due to contamination by human DNA or debris from dead microorganisms.[9] New commercial examples of FISH are *Quick*FISH, a peptide nucleic acid-FISH developed by AdvanDx, and the Accelerate Pheno System, the only CE marked and FDA approved platform for in vitro use for rapid identification and phenotypic AST.[10,11] *Quick*FISH can provide a report within 30 minutes using four specific assays: to distinguish *Staphylococcus aureus* from coagulase-negative staphylococci, to identify *Enterococcus* species, a gram-negative assay that includes *Escherichia coli*, *Klebsiella pneumonia*, and *Pseudomonas aeruginosa*, and rapid identification of methicillin-resistant *S. aureus* (MRSA). The latter has been combined with the *mecA* *Xpress*FISH probe for MRSA identification from signal positive

TABLE 43.1   Summary of Assays on Signal Positive Blood Cultures Discussed in This Chapter.

Principle	Technology	Turnaround Time (h)	Hands-On Time (h)	Targets
FISH	AdvanDx *Quick*FISH	<30 min	<5 min	GN—3 (*Escherichia. coli*, *Klebsiella pneumonia*, *Psuedomonas aeruginosa*) GP—2 (CoNS, *Staphylococcus aureus*) Enterococcal—*Enterococcus faecalis*, *En. faecium* or other enterococcus FP—3 (*Candida albicans*, *C. parapsilosis*, *C. glabrata*)
	Accelerate Pheno System	ID 90 min, AST ~7 h	2 min	GN—8 (4 species), GP—6 (4 species), 2 *Candida* spp. (*C. albicans*, *C. glabrata*) AST–MIC
MALDI-TOF MS	Bruker Sepsityper	30 min	5 min	Database dependent
Real-time PCR	Cepheid GeneXpert Xpert MRSA/SA	62 min	<1 min	MSSA, MRSA (*mecA/C*)
	BD MAX System	2 h	<1 min	MSSA, MRSA (*mecA/C*, MREJ)
PCR and Microarray	Luminex nanosphere VERIGENE	2.5 h	10 min	1) GP—13 (9 species), *mecA*, vanA/B 2) GN—9 (5 species), CTX-M, IMP, KPC, NDM, OXA, VIM
	BioMeriéux Biofire FilmArray®	1 h	2 min	GP -8 (5 species), GN—11 (9 species), 5 *Candida* spp. *mecA*, vanA/B, KPC
	GenMark DX ePlex	1.5 h	<2 min	GN—21 (17 species), CTX-M, KPC, NDM, OXA, VIM, IMP + pan-GP, pan-*Candida* GP—20 (13 species), *mecA/C*, vanA/B + pan-GN, pan-*Candida* FP—16 (13 species)
	Curetis Unyvero	4 h	<2 min	GP—11 (9 species), GN—15 (14 species), FP 8, Mycobacterial spp., 16 resistance genes
	Master Diagnóstica Sepsis Flow Chip	3 h	Not reported	GP—7, GN—10, *C. albicans*, 20 resistance genes

AST, antimicrobial susceptibility testing; *CoNS*, coagulase-negative staphylococci; *FISH*, fluorescent in situ hybridization; *FP*, fungal panel; *GN*, gram-negative; *GP*, gram-positive; *MALDI-TOF MS*, matrix-assisted laser desorption ionization time of flight mass spectrometry; *MIC*, minimum inhibitory concentration; *MRSA*, methicillin-resistant *S. aureus*; *MSSA*, methicillin-susceptible *S. aureus*; *PCR*, polymerase chain reaction.
Modified from Poole S, Kidd SP, Saeed K. A review of novel technologies and techniques associated with identification of bloodstream infection etiologies and rapid antimicrobial genotypic and quantitative phenotypic determination. *Expert Rev Mol Diagn.* 2018;18(6):543-555; Sinha M, Jupe J, Mack H, et al. Emerging technologies for molecular diagnosis of sepsis. *Clin Microbiol Rev.* 2018;31(2).

blood cultures within 2 hours.[12] Charnot-Katsikas et al.[13] compared the workflow of species identification and AST to standard care in 232 blood cultures.[13] The overall sensitivity was 95.6% for the identification of organisms, with a specificity of 99.5%. Regarding antimicrobial susceptibility, the overall agreement was 95.1%. The Accelerate Pheno System decreased the time to identification by 23.47 hours and the time to susceptibility by 41.86 hours compared with those for the

standard-of-care.[14] Also when specifically used for identification and AST for multi-drug resistant gram-negative bacteria, the Accelerate Pheno System appears an accurate, sensitive, and easy-to-use test.[15]

The implementation of matrix-assisted laser desorption ionization time of flight mass spectrometry (MALDI-TOF MS) for detection of bacteria and fungi in patients' samples has had a major impact on clinical microbiology. Identification of microbes using MALDI-TOF MS is based on comparing a mass spectrometry protein profile obtained from a pathogen with a catalog of profiles from characterized pathogens. The performance of MALDI-TOF MS depends on the purity and quantity of the microorganism. Bacterial enrichment and purification procedures are typically required from positive blood cultures, which contain non-microbial material that may affect MALDI-TOF MS identification and AST. Nonetheless, the sensitivity of direct blood culture MALDI-TOF MS analysis has been reported in the range of 80–90%.[16,17] Sepsityper is a sample processing kit that enables standardized sample preparation procedure for direct analysis of signal positive blood cultures. When compared with standard subculture and phenotypic identification methods, Sepsityper produces a genus/species concordance with standard procedures of 94.7–100%/94.7–100% for gram-negative and 91.7–93.3%/70–73.1% for gram-positive microorganisms.[18,19]

Several diagnostic tests entail PCR of a signal positive blood culture. Pathogen specific assays commonly involve genus/species detection that oftentimes are limited in their number of targets. Broad-range assays usually amplify conserved 16S/18S ribosomal RNA. Multiplex assays are preferable for diagnostic use because these diminish time to result and enable the detection of resistance genes. Cepheid GeneXpert, Xpert, combines nucleic acid extraction and amplification that can be extended to suit clinical needs. This product has the ability to detect pathogens within 1 hour.[20] The Xpert MRSA/SA PCR assay can be performed on a signal positive blood culture following a Gram stain with minimal hands-on time (less than 5 minutes). The test targets the *Spa*, *SSSmec* cassette, and *mecA* genes with a sensitivity and specificity of 100%/98.6% for *S. aureus* and 98.3%/99.4% for MRSA, respectively, and is a valuable tool for initial antibiotic choice and/or de-escalation in areas with a high MRSA prevalence.[9] Similarly, the BD MAX System is a fully integrated and automated PCR platform with reported sensitivity and specificity of 100%/100% for *S. aureus*, 97.9%/98.1% for MRSA, and 99.0%/95.8% for coagulase-negative staphylococci, respectively.[21,22]

Post-nucleic acid amplification detection of pathogens can be done using microarray and sequencing approaches. Assays in this category include Luminex nanosphere VERIGENE, BioMeriéux Biofire FilmArray, GenMark DX - ePlex, Curetis Unyvero, and Sepsis Flow Chip.[9] The Luminex nanosphere VERIGENE combines automated nucleic acid extraction and PCR amplification followed by hybridization to nanogrid arrays with gold nanoparticle detection.[23] The turnaround time of VERIGENE is quick, with approximately 10 minutes of hands-on time followed by a 2.5-hour automated run. The assay requires a Gram stain to select the appropriate reagents and is not fully automated; therefore, it needs to be used in a laboratory. The assay can identify common resistance genes with relatively high accuracy. In one study, VERIGENE reduced the length of ICU stay and 30-day mortality.[24] Another investigation reported unaltered length of stay and mortality when using the gram-positive VERIGENE platform, but time to initiation of adequate antimicrobial therapy was reduced.[25] Biofire FilmArray makes use

of syndromic panels that do not require a Gram stain and that, therefore, could be used as a point-of-care test in which extraction, PCR amplification, and array hybridization occur within a sealed pouch.[26] The run time is 1 hour and requires less than 5 minutes of assay pouch preparation. The targets on the blood culture panel include 6 gram-positive pathogens, 10 gram-negative bacteria, and 5 *Candida* species, as well as *mecA*, *vanA/B*, and *KPC* resistance genes.[26] This assay has been validated in several investigations that have reported high sensitivity (89.4–91.6%) and specificity (100%).[27–31] Although at present the panel is somewhat limited, Biofire FilmArray is a promising tool for pathogen detection. GenMark DX-ePlex assay is a fully automated one-step cartridge assay that requires only inoculation and placement in the control module.[32] Separate options are available for signal positive blood cultures after Gram staining (for gram-positive bacteria, gram-negative bacteria, and fungi). The gram-negative assay has 21 targets, 6 resistance genes, a pan-gram-positive, and a pan-*Candida* target; the gram-positive assay has 20 targets, 4 resistance genes, a pan-gram-negative, and a pan-*Candida* target; the fungal assay has 16 targets.[32] The inclusion of "pan-targets" may be helpful in the case of a misread Gram stain or polymicrobial infection. Curetis Unyvero can be used without a Gram stain and contains a cartridge that targets 10 gram-positive bacteria, 15 gram-negative bacteria, 8 fungi, and 16 resistance genes.[33] Clinical data with this assay await publication in the scientific literature. The Sepsis Flow Chip assay comprises a multiplex PCR and an automated reverse hybridization to a DNA array that is designed to identify 7 gram-positives, 10 gram-negatives, *Candida albicans*, and 20 resistance genes.[34] The first evaluation of this assay suggests a high sensitivity and specificity.[35]

Culture-Independent Methods

The overall sensitivity of "gold standard" blood cultures is suboptimal, with positivity of only 30–40% in sepsis.[36] This low sensitivity can be caused by false-negative results due to ongoing antimicrobial therapy, long time to positivity, low numbers of circulating microorganisms, the presence of uncultivable pathogens, and inadequate blood sampling.[37] Direct pathogen detection from whole blood could dramatically decrease time to identification. Nucleic acid amplification technologies have been developed that might circumvent the need for bacterial growth. While these novel assays in theory are valuable diagnostic tools in sepsis, their real-life value in clinical practice needs to be demonstrated. A summary of the assays on whole blood can be found in Table 43.2.

The best studied broad-range PCR assay is the Roche LightCycler SeptiFast system that has been approved for use in Europe.[38] This multiplex PCR assay can detect 25 common blood pathogens and its clinical use; since its introduction, its impact on health-care outcomes has been studied extensively.[39] A metaanalysis encompassing 41 studies reported an overall sensitivity and specificity of 68% (95% confidence interval [CI] 63–73) and 86% (95% CI 84–89), respectively, when compared with blood culture results.[40] Overall sensitivity (75%, 95% CI [65–83] and specificity (92%, 95% CI

TABLE 43.2   Summary of Assays on Whole Blood Discussed in This Chapter.

Principle	Technology	Turnaround Time (h)	Hands-on Time (h)	Targets
PCR and Microarray	Roche LightCycler SeptiFast	6 h	Not reported	GP—6 (4 species), GN—10 (10 species), FP—6 (6 species). Optional *mecA*.
	Molzym SepsiTest	Bacteremia/fungemia 4 h; ID ~4 h	Bacteremia/ fungemia 75 min; ID 70 min	>345 bacteria and 13 fungi; highly expandable
PCR and ESI-MS	Abbott Iridica Plex platform	6 h	30 min	780 bacteria and *Candida*; highly expandable
RT-qPCR and machine learning	Immunexpress SeptiCyte LAB	4-6 h	<5 min	All pathogens, using machine learning and 4 RNA biomarkers of the host response
T2MR nanodiagnostics	T2 Biosystems T2Bacteria and T2Candida	3 h	2 min	T2Bacteria (6 species: *Escherichia coli, Klebsiella pneumoniae, Psuedomonas aeruginosa, Acinetobacter baumannii, Staphylococcus aureus, Enterococcus faecium*) and T2Candida (5 species: *Candida. albicans, C. parasilosis, C. krusei, C. tropicalis, C. glabrata*)

ESI-MS, electrospray ionization mass spectrometry; *FP*, fungal panel; *GN*, gram-negative; *GP*, gram-positive; *PCR*, polymerase chain reaction; *RNA*, ribonucleic acid; *RT-qPCR*, reverse transcription-quantitative PCR; *T2MR*, T2 magnetic resonance.
Modified from Poole S, Kidd SP, Saeed K. A review of novel technologies and techniques associated with identification of bloodstream infection etiologies and rapid antimicrobial genotypic and quantitative phenotypic determination. *Expert Rev Mol Diagn.* 2018;18(6):543-555; Sinha M, Jupe J, Mack H, et al. Emerging technologies for molecular diagnosis of sepsis. *Clin Microbiol Rev.* 2018;31(2).

[90–95] were slightly better in another metaanalyses that only included studies published in scientific journals.[41] Importantly, up to 35% of positive results generated by SeptiFast are not supported by microbiologic or clinical findings and SeptiFast may not detect culture-positive organisms in 20–30% cases.[42] Notably, SeptiFast was the subject of a Health Technology Assessment study in the United Kingdom. The reported sensitivity (50%) in this assessment was much lower than that in previous studies.[43] This broad test may assist in decision-making in patients suspected of having sepsis who are culture-negative but SeptiFast-positive; in contrast, a negative SeptiFast test is unlikely to influence decisions on antimicrobial therapy, considering its low sensitivity.

SepsiTest (Molzym) is a broad-based pathogen identification test for whole blood that can detect more than 345 bacteria and 13 fungi.[44] SepsiTest is available in Europe, but it is not yet approved for clinical use in the United States. It can detect bacteremia and fungemia in less than 4 hours by a PCR targeting 16S and 18S ribosomal RNA; species identification (by sequencing) takes an additional 4–6 hours. SepsiTest has a high specificity (varying between 85% and 96% across studies), while its sensitivity ranges between 11% and 87%.[45–50] The potential value of SepsiTest in clinical practice requires further study.

The Iridica Plex platform (Abbott) represents the broadest detection assay, detecting 780 bacteria and *Candida* species, using multiplexed PCR amplification and electrospray ionization mass spectrometry.[51] Although the spectrum of detection is wide, the sensitivity and specificity of Iridica varied strongly between studies (from 45% to 83% and 69% to 94%, respectively).[52–56]

T2 magnetic resonance (T2MR) nanodiagnostics can detect diverse targets, including cells and nucleic acids, within complex matrices such as blood.[57] This technology (from T2 Biosystems) has been used for the development of two diagnostic panels that detect bacteria and fungi, respectively, directly in blood samples without the need for isolating organisms.[58] These T2Bacteria and T2Candida panels are incorporated in a fully automated process that uses standard K_2 EDTA vacutainer collection tubes and an instrument platform to detect amplified DNA from microbes. T2Bacteria detects *Enterococcus faecium, S. aureus, K. pneumoniae, Acinetobacter baumannii, P. aeruginosa,* and *E. coli*; T2Candida provides positive/negative results for *C. albicans/C. tropicalis, C. glabrata/C. krusei,* and *C. parapsilosis*. T2Candida sensitivity and specificity for candidaemia are around 90% and 98%, respectively. T2 Candida also performed well in predicting the outcomes of empirical antifungal therapy for suspected candidiasis and may shorten times to appropriate antifungal therapy.[57] The first clinical data on T2Bacteria indicate a sensitivity and specificity of 89% and 98%, respectively, among patients with bacteremia or fulfilling criteria for infection.[59] T2MR diagnostics are promising tools for detecting bloodstream infections by bacteria and *Candida*. Further confirmation in real-life clinical investigation is needed.

HOST-TARGETED DIAGNOSTICS

Complementary to pathogen-targeted diagnostics and of high potential are host-targeted diagnostics for the identification of causative pathogens. In sepsis, infection leads to a dysregulated host response, but less severe infections also trigger specific biological pathways that can be linked to invading pathogens.[60] While a large number of host response biomarkers for sepsis have been identified, either for discrimination between infection and noninfectious causes of critical illness or for prognostication,[61] the Surviving Sepsis Campaign guidelines include only a minor role for one biomarker in clinical practice, i.e., procalcitonin (PCT),[4] underlining the current status of biomarkers in sepsis. PCT can distinguish between sepsis and a systemic inflammatory response syndrome of noninfectious origin with a pooled sensitivity of 0.77 (95% CI 0.72–0.81) and a specificity of 0.79 (95% CI, 0.74–0.84).[62] PCT has no value for the identification of specific pathogens, but it may be a useful tool in antibiotic stewardship. In a prospective, randomized, controlled, open-label intervention trial in 15 ICUs in the Netherlands, PCT-guided antibiotic discontinuation was compared with standard-of-care using a nonbinding advice when PCT levels decreased.[63] In the PCT-guided group, duration of treatment and the daily defined doses were reduced in patients with a presumed bacterial infection, which was associated with a decreased mortality.[63] However, other studies in critically ill patients did not find improved antibiotic utilization or other clinical outcomes,[64,65] and in a recent study conducted in 14 US hospitals, the provision of PCT assay results, along with instructions on their interpretation, to physicians did not result in less use of antibiotics than did usual care among patients presented to the emergency room with suspected lower respiratory tract infection.[66] Hence, current data on the use of PCT for antibiotic stewardship in patients with suspected sepsis are not consistent.

Systems biology focuses on complex interactions in biological systems using a holistic approach. These novel host-targeted diagnostics characterize and quantify molecules of genomic, epigenetic, transcriptomic, proteomic, and metabolomics pathways.[61] Most studies published to date reported on the ability of the blood leukocyte transcriptome to discriminate between infection and noninfectious acute disease, while some described distinct RNA profiles in infections caused by different causative pathogens.[61,67] SeptiCyte LAB (from Immunexpress) is the first RNA-based clinical diagnostic tool derived from whole blood that is approved for assisting in the differentiation of infection-positive (sepsis) from infection-negative systemic inflammation in critically ill patients on their first day of ICU admission.[68] SeptiCyte LAB is a four-gene classifier that combines CEACAM4, LAMP1, PLA2G7, and PLAC8 to produce a summary area under the receiver operating characteristic curve (area under the concentration curve [AUC]) of ≥0.82 to differentiate sepsis from noninfectious systemic inflammatory response syndrome.[69,70] Other host RNA biomarkers that can distinguish between infection and noninfectious inflammation include the Sepsis MetaScore, an 11-gene biomarker derived from a large number of

independent cohorts,[71] and, for patients admitted to the ICU with acute respiratory or abdominal symptoms, the FAIM3/PLAC8 ratio can be used for the diagnosis of community-acquired pneumonia,[72] and the 3-gene (NLRP1, IDNK, PLAC8) sNIP score for the diagnosis of abdominal sepsis.[73]

Several studies have pointed to the potential of systems biology for pathogen identification. Blood leukocyte RNA profiling was used to classify the etiology of suspected community-acquired acute respiratory tract infections into bacterial, viral, or noninfectious in adults presenting to the emergency department.[74] The overall precision of gene expression classifiers was 87%, outperforming PCT, which could assign patients as having bacterial or nonbacterial acute respiratory tract infection with 78% accuracy.[74] Likewise, the blood leukocyte transcriptome from hospitalized patients with lower respiratory tract infections was superior to PCT in differentiating between bacteria and viruses.[75] RNA profiling of blood leukocytes of adult ICU patients with influenza A pneumonia, bacterial pneumonia, and noninfectious respiratory disease defined a 29-gene classifier of viral infection that distinguished viral from bacterial infection and noninfectious disease; this classifier could not differentiate bacterial infection from noninfectious disease.[76] A seven-gene classifier derived from a multicohort analysis was able to discriminate bacterial from viral infections.[77] This classifier was validated in 30 independent cohorts and integrated with the Sepsis MetaScore in an antibiotics decision model with a sensitivity and specificity for bacterial infections of 94.0% and 59.8%, respectively.[77] In children, host leukocyte RNA classifiers have been used to assist in the discrimination between viral and bacterial causes of acute infections.[78,79] A 35-gene set was able to divide infections based on broad groups of causative pathogens in children, with different signatures for infections caused by the influenza A virus, E. coli, or Streptococcus pneumoniae.[78] A 70-gene classifier could discriminate between distinct viral pathogens (respiratory syncytial virus, human rhinovirus, and influenza) with 95% accuracy in children.[80] A 38-gene signature distinguishing bacterial from viral infection was identified in febrile children presenting to the hospital, which was reduced to a two-transcript signature (FAM89A and IFI44L) by removing highly correlated mRNA levels.[81]

Besides transcriptomics, proteomics and metabolomics have been used for the discovery of host response biomarkers that may aid in infection diagnosis, although reports are more scarce.[61] A recent proteomics study entailing measurements of 600 proteins in 765 patients presenting to the emergency department with fever identified a three-protein signature (tumor necrosis factor-related apoptosis-inducing ligand 1, chemokine [C-X-C motif] ligand 10, and C-reactive protein) that distinguished bacteria from viruses, and infectious (bacterial and viral) from noninfectious disease with an AUC of 0.94 (95% CI 0.92–0.96).[82] The three-protein signature was strongest in segregating bacterial from viral etiologies in lower respiratory tract infections and fever with an unknown source. A metabolomics study analyzed 186 metabolites encompassing six analyte classes (acylcarnitines, amino acids, biogenic amines, glycerophospholipids, sphingolipids, and carbohydrates) to identify two markers (acylcarnitine C10:1 and glycerophospholipid PCaaC32:0) that may be helpful for differentiation of infectious (higher levels) from noninfectious systemic inflammation.[83] Another investigation reported altered serum concentrations of most acylcarnitines, glycerophospholipids, and sphingolipids in sepsis compared with noninfectious critical illness, and a regression model combining the sphingolipid SM C22:3 and the glycerophospholipid lysoPCaC24:0 was discovered for sepsis diagnosis with a sensitivity of 0.84 and specificity of 0.86.[84]

FUTURE PERSPECTIVES

Innovations in sample preparation and detection methods may revolutionize diagnostics for pathogen detection. However, while novel technologies may accurately identify the causative pathogen, the impact of these approaches on clinical outcomes and health-care costs requires further investigation. Implementation of novel molecular-based diagnostics in routine clinical care on a large scale has not yet occurred. Even with existing diagnostic tools, improving current logistics and infrastructure could enhance the flow of information from patient to microbiology to provider. By considering local resistance rates, antibiotic prescribing patterns, laboratory staffing, and means of communication, cost-neutral benefits can be realized without the use of new high-tech diagnostics.[85] Molecular tests of the future should have limited (or no) hands-on time and should involve fully automated machines that do not require trained laboratory personnel. It is even possible that integration of pathogen-targeted and host-targeted assays may further improve the molecular diagnostics of sepsis.

AUTHORS' RECOMMENDATIONS
- Pathogen detection tests should be rapid (identification of the pathogen in less than 3 hours), use low volumes of easy-to-obtain body specimens (e.g., blood or urine), and depend on fully automated machines that do not require specialized laboratory personnel.
- These tests should have a high sensitivity and specificity and provide immediate information on antimicrobial resistance, thereby allowing quick initiation of targeted antibiotic treatment.
- Future tests may integrate pathogen-targeted and host-targeted diagnostics, the latter utilizing "omics" approaches (e.g., transcriptomics, proteomics, metabolomics) to provide information about pathogen-specific immune responses.

REFERENCES

1. Pulvertaft R. Bacterial blood cultures. *Lancet*. 1930;215(5563):821-822.
2. Kothari A, Morgan M, Haake DA. Emerging technologies for rapid identification of bloodstream pathogens. *Clin Infect Dis*. 2014;59(2):272-278.
3. Singer M, Deutschman CS, Seymour CW, et al. The Third International Consensus definitions for sepsis and septic shock (Sepsis-3). *JAMA*. 2016;315(8):801-810.
4. Rhodes A, Evans LE, Alhazzani W, et al. Surviving Sepsis Campaign: International guidelines for management of sepsis and septic shock: 2016. *Intensive Care Med*. 2017;43(3):304-377.
5. Kumar A, Roberts D, Wood KE, et al. Duration of hypotension before initiation of effective antimicrobial therapy is the critical determinant of survival in human septic shock. *Crit Care Med*. 2006;34(6):1589-1596.
6. Seymour CW, Gesten F, Prescott HC, et al. Time to treatment and mortality during mandated emergency care for sepsis. *N Engl J Med*. 2017;376(23):2235-2244.
7. World Health Organization. *Report by the Secretariat A70/12. Antimicrobial Resistance*. Geneva: World Health Organization; 2017 22-31 May 2017.
8. Blaser MJ. Antibiotic use and its consequences for the normal microbiome. *Science*. 2016;352(6285):544-545.
9. Poole S, Kidd SP, Saeed K. A review of novel technologies and techniques associated with identification of bloodstream infection etiologies and rapid antimicrobial genotypic and quantitative phenotypic determination. *Expert Rev Mol Diagn*. 2018;18(6):543-555.
10. OpGen. AdvanDx. *QuickFISH®*. Available from: http://www.opgen.com/pathogenid/quickfish-products/. Accessed September 21, 2018.
11. Accelerate Diagnostics. *Accelerate PhenoTest™ BC Kit*. Available from: http://acceleratediagnostics.com/products/accelerate-phenotest-bc/. Accessed September 21, 2018.
12. Salimnia H, Fairfax MR, Lephart P, et al. An international, prospective, multicenter evaluation of the combination of AdvanDx Staphylococcus QuickFISH BC with mecA XpressFISH for detection of methicillin-resistant Staphylococcus aureus isolates from positive blood cultures. *J Clin Microbiol*. 2014;52(11):3928-3932.
13. Charnot-Katsikas A, Tesic V, Love N, et al. Use of the Accelerate Pheno system for identification and antimicrobial susceptibility testing of pathogens in positive blood cultures and impact on time to results and workflow. *J Clin Microbiol*. 2018;56(1):pii: e01166-17.
14. Pancholi P, Carroll KC, Buchan BW, et al. Multicenter evaluation of the Accelerate PhenoTest BC kit for rapid identification and phenotypic antimicrobial susceptibility testing using morphokinetic cellular analysis. *J Clin Microbiol*. 2018;56(4):pii: e01329-17.
15. Pantel A, Monier J, Lavigne JP. Performance of the Accelerate Pheno system for identification and antimicrobial susceptibility testing of a panel of multidrug-resistant Gram-negative bacilli directly from positive blood cultures. *J Antimicrob Chemother*. 2018;73(6):1546-1552.
16. Fiori B, D'Inzeo T, Di Florio V, et al. Performance of two resin-containing blood culture media in detection of bloodstream infections and in direct matrix-assisted laser desorption ionization-time of flight mass spectrometry (MALDI-TOF MS) broth assays for isolate identification: clinical comparison of the BacT/Alert Plus and Bactec Plus systems. *J Clin Microbiol*. 2014;52(10):3558-3567.
17. Konnerth S, Rademacher G, Suerbaum S, Ziesing S, Sedlacek L, Vonberg RP et al. Identification of pathogens from blood culture bottles in spiked and clinical samples using matrix-assisted laser desorption ionization time-of-flight mass-spectrometry analysis. *BMC Res Notes*. 2014;7:405.

18. Morgenthaler NG, Kostrzewa M. Rapid identification of pathogens in positive blood culture of patients with sepsis: review and meta-analysis of the performance of the sepsityper kit. *Int J Microbiol*. 2015;2015:827416.

19. Bruker. *MBT Sepsityper IVD Kit*. Available from: https://www.bruker.com/products/mass-spectrometry-and-separations/ivd-ce-certified-maldi-biotyper/mbt-sepsityper-ivd-kit.html. Accessed September 21, 2018.

20. Cepheid. *Xpert® MRSA/SA BC*. Available from: http://www.cepheid.com/us/cepheid-solutions/clinical-ivd-tests/health-care-associated-infections/xpert-mrsa-sa-bc. Accessed September 21, 2018.

21. BD. *BD MAX™ MRSA XT with eXTended Detection Technology*. Available from: https://www.bd.com/en-uk/products/molecular-diagnostics/molecular-systems/max-system/max-mrsa-xt-with-extended-detection-technology. Accessed September 21, 2018.

22. Lee J, Park YJ, Park DJ, Park KG, Lee HK. Evaluation of BD MAX Staph SR assay for differentiating between staphylococcus aureus and coagulase-negative staphylococci and determining methicillin resistance directly from positive blood cultures. *Ann Lab Med*. 2017;37(1):39-44.

23. Luminex. *The VERIGENE® System*. Available from: https://www.luminexcorp.com/the-verigene-system/. Accessed September 21, 2018.

24. Walker T, Dumadag S, Lee CJ, et al. Clinical impact of laboratory implementation of Verigene BC-GN microarray-based assay for detection of gram-negative bacteria in positive blood cultures. *J Clin Microbiol*. 2016;54(7):1789-1796.

25. Beal SG, Thomas C, Dhiman N, et al. Antibiotic utilization improvement with the Nanosphere Verigene Gram-Positive Blood Culture assay. *Proc (Bayl Univ Med Cent)*. 2015;28(2):139-143.

26. bioMérieux. *BioFire ® FilmArray ® Blood Culture Identification Panel*. Available from: https://www.biofiredx.com/products/the-filmarray-panels/#blood-culture. Accessed September 21, 2018.

27. Blaschke AJ, Heyrend C, Byington CL, et al. Rapid identification of pathogens from positive blood cultures by multiplex polymerase chain reaction using the FilmArray system. *Diagn Microbiol Infect Dis*. 2012;74(4):349-355.

28. Altun O, Almuhayawi M, Ullberg M, Ozenci V. Clinical evaluation of the FilmArray blood culture identification panel in identification of bacteria and yeasts from positive blood culture bottles. *J Clin Microbiol*. 2013;51(12):4130-4136.

29. Zheng X, Polanco W, Carter D, Shulman S. Rapid identification of pathogens from pediatric blood cultures by use of the FilmArray blood culture identification panel. *J Clin Microbiol*. 2014;52(12):4368-4371.

30. Banerjee R, Teng CB, Cunningham SA, et al. Randomized trial of rapid multiplex polymerase chain reaction-based blood culture identification and susceptibility testing. *Clin Infect Dis*. 2015;61(7):1071-1080.

31. Paolucci M, Foschi C, Tamburini MV, Ambretti S, Lazzarotto T, Landini MP. Comparison between MALDI-TOF MS and FilmArray Blood Culture Identification panel for rapid identification of yeast from positive blood culture. *J Microbiol Methods*. 2014;104:92-93.

32. GenMark. *ePlex Blood Culture Identification (BCID) panels*. Available from: https://www.genmarkdx.com/int/solutions/panels/eplex-panels/blood-culture-identification-panels/. Accessed September 21, 2018.

33. Curetis. *Unyvero BCU blood culture application*. Available from: http://www.unyvero.com/en/applications/blood-culture.html. Accessed September 21, 2018.

34. Master Diagnóstica. *Sepsis Flow Chip*. Available from: http://www.masterdiagnostica.com/en-gb/products/moleculardiagnostickits/dnaflowtechnology/sepsisflowchip.aspx. Accessed September 21, 2018.

35. Galiana A, Coy J, Gimeno A, et al. Evaluation of the Sepsis Flow Chip assay for the diagnosis of blood infections. *PLoS One*. 2017;12(5):e0177627.

36. Dellinger RP, Levy MM, Carlet JM, et al. Surviving Sepsis Campaign: international guidelines for management of severe sepsis and septic shock: 2008. *Crit Care Med*. 2008;36(1):296-327.

37. Rello J, van Engelen TSR, Alp E, et al. Towards precision medicine in sepsis: a position paper from the European Society of Clinical Microbiology and Infectious Diseases. *Clin Microbiol Infect*. 2018. doi:10.1016/j.cmi.2018.03.011. [Epub ahead of print.]

38. Roche. *LightCycler® SeptiFast Test*. Available from: https://www.roche.co.uk/home/products/diagnostics/product-database-diagnostics/lightcycler_septifast-test-mgrade.html. Accessed September 21, 2018.

39. Korber F, Zeller I, Grünstäudl M, et al. SeptiFast versus blood culture in clinical routine - A report on 3 years experience. *Wien Klin Wochenschr*. 2017;129(11-12):427-434.

40. Dark P, Blackwood B, Gates S, et al. Accuracy of LightCycler((R)) SeptiFast for the detection and identification of pathogens in the blood of patients with suspected sepsis: a systematic review and meta-analysis. *Intensive Care Med*. 2015;41(1):21-33.

41. Chang SS, Hsieh WH, Liu TS, et al. Multiplex PCR system for rapid detection of pathogens in patients with presumed sepsis - a systemic review and meta-analysis. *PLoS One*. 2013;8(5):e62323.

42. Sinha M, Jupe J, Mack H, Coleman TP, Lawrence SM, Fraley SI. Emerging technologies for molecular diagnosis of sepsis. *Clin Microbiol Rev*. 2018;31(2): pii: e00089-17.

43. Warhurst G, Dunn G, Chadwick P, et al. Rapid detection of health-care-associated bloodstream infection in critical care using multipathogen real-time polymerase chain reaction technology: a diagnostic accuracy study and systematic review. *Health Technol Assess*. 2015;19(35):1-142.

44. Molzym. *Molecular Diagnostics - SepsiTest TM*. Available from: https://www.sepsitest.com/products/molecular-diagnosis/whole-blood.html. Accessed September 21, 2018.

45. Leitner E, Kessler HH, Spindelboeck W, et al. Comparison of two molecular assays with conventional blood culture for diagnosis of sepsis. *J Microbiol Methods*. 2013;92(3):253-255.

46. Loonen AJ, de Jager CP, Tosserams J, et al. Biomarkers and molecular analysis to improve bloodstream infection diagnostics in an emergency care unit. *PLoS One*. 2014;9(1):e87315.

47. Kühn C, Disqué C, Mühl H, Orszag P, Stiesch M, Haverich A. Evaluation of commercial universal rRNA gene PCR plus sequencing tests for identification of bacteria and fungi associated with infectious endocarditis. *J Clin Microbiol*. 2011;49(8):2919-2923.

48. Wellinghausen N, Kochem AJ, Disqué C, et al. Diagnosis of bacteremia in whole-blood samples by use of a commercial universal 16S rRNA gene-based PCR and sequence analysis. *J Clin Microbiol*. 2009;47(9):2759-2765.

49. Nieman AE, Savelkoul PHM, Beishuizen A, et al. A prospective multicenter evaluation of direct molecular detection of blood

stream infection from a clinical perspective. *BMC Infect Dis.* 2016;16:314.

50. Orszag P, Disqué C, Keim S, et al. Monitoring of patients supported by extracorporeal membrane oxygenation for systemic infections by broad-range rRNA gene PCR amplification and sequence analysis. *J Clin Microbiol.* 2014;52(1):307-311.

51. Abbott. *Iridica Plex ID platform.* Available from: https://www.molecular.abbott/int/en/home. Accessed September 21, 2018.

52. Desmet S, Maertens J, Bueselinck K, Lagrou K. Broad-range PCR coupled with electrospray ionization time of flight mass spectrometry for detection of bacteremia and fungemia in patients with neutropenic fever. *J Clin Microbiol.* 2016;54(10):2513-2520.

53. Metzgar D, Frinder MW, Rothman RE, et al. The IRIDICA BAC BSI Assay: Rapid, sensitive and culture-independent identification of bacteria and candida in blood. *PLoS One.* 2016;11(7):e0158186.

54. Jordana-Lluch E, Giménez M, Quesada MD, et al. Evaluation of the broad-range PCR/ESI-MS technology in blood specimens for the molecular diagnosis of bloodstream infections. *PLoS One.* 2015;10(10):e0140865.

55. Vincent JL, Brealey D, Libert N, et al. Rapid diagnosis of infection in the critically ill, a multicenter study of molecular detection in bloodstream infections, pneumonia, and sterile site infections. *Crit Care Med.* 2015;43(11):2283-2291.

56. Bacconi A, Richmond GS, Baroldi MA, et al. Improved sensitivity for molecular detection of bacterial and Candida infections in blood. *J Clin Microbiol.* 2014;52(9):3164-3174.

57. Clancy CJ, Nguyen MH. T2 magnetic resonance for the diagnosis of bloodstream infections: charting a path forward. *J Antimicrob Chemother.* 2018;73(suppl_4):iv2-iv5.

58. T2 Biosystems. *T2Dx® T2Bacteria® & T2Candida® Panel.* Available from: https://www.t2biosystems.com/. Accessed September 21, 2018.

59. De Angelis G, Posteraro B, De Carolis E, et al. T2Bacteria magnetic resonance assay for the rapid detection of ESKAPEc pathogens directly in whole blood. *J Antimicrob Chemother.* 2018;73(suppl 4):iv20-iv6.

60. van der Poll T, van de Veerdonk FL, Scicluna BP, Netea MG. The immunopathology of sepsis and potential therapeutic targets. *Nat Rev Immunol.* 2017;17(7):407-420.

61. van Engelen TSR, Wiersinga WJ, Scicluna BP, van der Poll T. Biomarkers in sepsis. *Crit Care Clin.* 2018;34(1):139-152.

62. Wacker C, Prkno A, Brunkhorst FM, Schlattmann P. Procalcitonin as a diagnostic marker for sepsis: a systematic review and meta-analysis. *Lancet Infect Dis.* 2013;13(5):426-435.

63. de Jong E, van Oers JA, Beishuizen A, et al. Efficacy and safety of procalcitonin guidance in reducing the duration of antibiotic treatment in critically ill patients: a randomised, controlled, open-label trial. *Lancet Infect Dis.* 2016;16(7):819-827.

64. Shehabi Y, Sterba M, Garrett PM, et al. Procalcitonin algorithm in critically ill adults with undifferentiated infection or suspected sepsis. A randomized controlled trial. *Am J Respir Crit Care Med.* 2014;190(10):1102-1110.

65. Chu DC, Mehta AB, Walkey AJ. Practice patterns and outcomes associated with procalcitonin use in critically ill patients with sepsis. *Clin Infect Dis.* 2017;64(11):1509-1515.

66. Huang DT, Yealy DM, Filbin MR, et al. Procalcitonin-guided use of antibiotics for lower respiratory tract infection. *N Engl J Med.* 2018;379(3):236-249.

67. Holcomb ZE, Tsalik EL, Woods CW, McClain MT. Host-based peripheral blood gene expression analysis for diagnosis of infectious diseases. *J Clin Microbiol.* 2017;55(2):360-368.

68. Immunexpress. *SeptiCyte™.* Available from: http://www.immunexpress.com/about-septicyte/. Accessed September 21, 2018.

69. McHugh L, Seldon TA, Brandon RA, et al. A molecular host response assay to discriminate between sepsis and infection-negative systemic inflammation in critically ill patients: discovery and validation in independent cohorts. *PLoS Med.* 2015;12(12):e1001916.

70. Miller III RR, Lopansri BK, Burke JP, et al. Validation of a host response assay, Septicyte LAB, for discriminating sepsis from SIRS in the ICU. *Am J Respir Crit Care Med.* 2018;198(7):903-913. [Epub ahead of print.]

71. Sweeney TE, Shidham A, Wong HR, Khatri P. A comprehensive time-course-based multicohort analysis of sepsis and sterile inflammation reveals a robust diagnostic gene set. *Sci Transl Med.* 2015;7(287):287ra71.

72. Scicluna BP, Klein Klouwenberg PM, van Vught LA, et al. A molecular biomarker to diagnose community-acquired pneumonia on intensive care unit admission. *Am J Respir Crit Care Med.* 2015;192(7):826-835.

73. Scicluna BP, Wiewel MA, van Vught LA, et al. Molecular biomarker to assist in diagnosing abdominal sepsis upon ICU admission. *Am J Respir Crit Care Med.* 2018;197(8):1070-1073.

74. Tsalik EL, Henao R, Nichols M, et al. Host gene expression classifiers diagnose acute respiratory illness etiology. *Sci Transl Med.* 2016;8(322):322ra11.

75. Suarez NM, Bunsow E, Falsey AR, Walsh EE, Mejias A, Ramilo O. Superiority of transcriptional profiling over procalcitonin for distinguishing bacterial from viral lower respiratory tract infections in hospitalized adults. *J Infect Dis.* 2015;212(2):213-222.

76. Parnell GP, McLean AS, Booth DR, et al. A distinct influenza infection signature in the blood transcriptome of patients with severe community-acquired pneumonia. *Crit Care.* 2012;16(4):R157.

77. Sweeney TE, Wong HR, Khatri P. Robust classification of bacterial and viral infections via integrated host gene expression diagnostics. *Sci Transl Med.* 2016;8(346):346ra91.

78. Ramilo O, Allman W, Chung W, et al. Gene expression patterns in blood leukocytes discriminate patients with acute infections. *Blood.* 2007;109(5):2066-2077.

79. Hu X, Yu J, Crosby SD, Storch GA. Gene expression profiles in febrile children with defined viral and bacterial infection. *Proc Natl Acad Sci U S A.* 2013;110(31):12792-12797.

80. Mejias A, Dimo B, Suarez NM, et al. Whole blood gene expression profiles to assess pathogenesis and disease severity in infants with respiratory syncytial virus infection. *PLoS Med.* 2013;10(11):e1001549.

81. Herberg JA, Kaforou M, Wright VJ, et al. Diagnostic test accuracy of a 2-transcript host RNA signature for discriminating bacterial vs viral infection in febrile children. *JAMA.* 2016;316(8):835-845.

82. Oved K, Cohen A, Boico O, et al. A novel host-proteome signature for distinguishing between acute bacterial and viral infections. *PLoS One.* 2015;10(3):e0120012.

83. Schmerler D, Neugebauer S, Ludewig K, Bremer-Streck S, Brunkhorst FM, Kiehntopf M. Targeted metabolomics for discrimination of systemic inflammatory disorders in critically ill patients. *J Lipid Res.* 2012;53(7):1369-1375.

84. Neugebauer S, Giamarellos-Bourboulis EJ, Pelekanou A, et al. Metabolite profiles in sepsis: developing prognostic tools based on the type of infection. *Crit Care Med.* 2016;44(9):1649-1662.

85. Banerjee R, Özenci V, Patel R. Individualized approaches are needed for optimized blood cultures. *Clin Infect Dis.* 2016;63(10):1332-1339.

44

How Do I Diagnose and Manage Catheter-Related Bloodstream Infections?

Michael Scully

INTRODUCTION

Since Werner Forssmann first successfully catheterized the right atrium in 1929,[1] central venous access has become an essential component in the management of critically ill patients. Central access is performed to administer vasopressors, parenteral nutrition, and fluids, perform blood sampling and advanced hemodynamic monitoring, and provide renal replacement therapy. Long-term vascular device placement is frequently established for therapeutic reasons in patient groups who are at high risk of developing critical illness, such as for chemotherapy in patients with hematological and oncological malignancies and cases of chronic renal failure requiring access for long-term dialysis. However, central venous catheterization is associated with mechanical, thrombotic, and infectious complications, and given their iatrogenic etiology, intensive efforts have been undertaken by health-care systems to reduce their incidence. Successful control depends on a thorough understanding of the pathophysiology, early recognition, treatment, and crucially, institutional and national adoption of preventative measures supported by surveillance and education.

DEFINITIONS

A catheter-related bloodstream infection (CRBSI) is defined as a bloodstream infection that develops in the presence of a vascular access devices such as short or long-term central venous catheters (CVC), peripheral catheters, or arterial lines in the absence of an alternative attributable source.[1,2] Definitive confirmation is achieved by isolating the organism by quantitative culture of the catheter tip. A central line is defined as a catheter where the tip comes to lie in a great vein, and the majority of CRBSIs are associated with these devices. For surveillance purposes, the National Healthcare Safety Network (NHSN) in the United States has defined these latter infections as central line-associated bloodstream infections (CLASBIs); they are defined as infections in a patient with a central line in situ or infection within 48 hours of a CVC removal in the absence of any other source of sepsis.[2]

A number of different potential portals of infection have been identified.[3–5] The breech in the integrity of the skin surface at the site of catheter placement provides a tract that can permit bacteria, especially skin commensals, to migrate alongside the device to infect the extraluminal surface, with the potential for intraluminal migration. Safdar and Maki[4] have reported that, in a single-center study from the intensive care unit (ICU) of a large tertiary university hospital of >1200 catheters, this was the dominant mechanism by which a CRBSI was acquired, being implicated in almost half the cases. Therefore, strategies aimed at reducing the burden of skin colonization or extending the subcutaneous passage from skin puncture site to the point of vessel entry may be efficacious in reducing the CRBSI risk. In this regard, bathing patients daily with chlorhexidine-impregnated washcloths initially appeared to be efficacious,[6] but further studies have yielded conflicting results and have not confirmed a reduction in CRBSIs.[7,8] The apparent reduction in CRBSIs in the early studies appear related to a reduction in false-positive blood cultures.[9]

In situations where longer-term line placement can be anticipated, such as hemodialysis or chemotherapy administration, the risk of infection through this portal may be reduced by tunneling or implanting the device. Tunneling is the process where a subcutaneous tract, typically about 10 cm in length, is created between the point of skin insertion and the device entry point into the vessel.[1,4,5]

An alternative portal by which infection is acquired is via the catheter hubs, which can become colonized if health-care staff has breeches in hand hygiene practices. Infection via this route will directly enter the catheter's luminal surface. This is reportedly a more common mechanism beyond 10 days after catheter placement. Less commonly, the catheter may also become secondarily infected, either endogenously by metastatic hematogenous seeding of infection from another source or very rarely by the administration of a contaminated infusate.[2–4]

INCIDENCE AND EPIDEMIOLOGY

The incidence of a catheter-related infection is typically expressed as the incidence density or incidence rate, and it is the number of infections over the time that the catheter is in situ. This is usually expressed as the number/1000 catheter days, and is calculated as:

$$\text{CRBSI rate/1000 catheter days} = \text{Number of CVC infections} \times 1000/\text{Number of CVC days}$$

There is evidence that meticulous adherence to best practice in infection control measures from the time of catheter placement and throughout the period that the device is in situ can dramatically reduce the incidence rate. In 2006, Maki et al.[10] reported that in the United States, the incidence of infection in short-term central catheters was 2.7/1000 catheters days and that overall there were 250,000 CRBSIs, with over 80,000 occurring in the critical care areas. In the same era, Pronovost et al.[11] published a practice intervention (discussed later) aimed at reducing the CRBSI incidence. These interventions were subsequently widely adopted, and there is evidence that they have led to a significant improvement in CRBSI rates. Data published in 2018 by the NHSN indicate that the current CRBSI rate in the United States has almost halved in the last decade.[12] It is estimated that approximately 30% of hospitalized patients with CVCs in the United States are located in the critical care area, and that now 30,000 CRBSIs occur annually in this patient cohort, with an incidence rate of 0.8/1000 catheter days. This is comparable with data collected during 2007–2012 from 43 countries by the International Nosocomial Infection Control Consortium, which reported an incident rate of 4.9/1000 catheter days from comparable ICUs.[13] In Europe, surveillance of CRBSIs is under the aegis of the European Centre for Disease Prevention and Control (ECDC). In 2015, for 11 participating countries, the incident rate for ICU-acquired CLASBIs varied from 1.4 infections/1000 catheter days in Luxembourg to 8.0/1000 catheter days in Slovakia (average across all countries 3.2/1000 catheter days).[14] This marked heterogeneity is supported by an international questionnaire of intensive care practitioners in 95 countries. The survey demonstrated marked variation in practices related to the control of CRBSIs and the potential scope for improvement.[15]

CRBSIs have important consequences. Maki et al.[10] reported that based on US data, CRBSIs are associated with an additional 10–20 days in hospital and have reportedly an attributable mortality of 12%–25%. The average additional cost required to treat a CRBSI was in excess of US$70,000. Despite the improvements made, CRBSIs are still associated with substantial morbidity and mortality and continue to impose a substantial added financial burden on healthcare costs.[13]

Risk factors associated with CRBSIs can be grouped according to patient, catheter, operator, personnel, and environmental factors.[1,4,5,10] Severity and duration of illness, immune suppression, malignancy, burns, chronic hepatic and renal dysfunction, and failed source control have been associated with the increased risk. As migration of microorganisms along the catheter underlies the pathogenesis of the majority of CRBSIs, the material's composition can influence the degree of risk. Impregnating the catheter with an antibacterial agent can attenuate the infection risk (discussed later). The choice of technique to secure the device may also modify the risk as well as the type of dressing used. As one of the mechanisms of infection involves colonization of the catheter hubs, the infection risk increases with increased number of lumens. Selecting a catheter with the minimum number of lumens appropriate to the device's purpose is appropriate. Furthermore, the risk of hub contamination can be attenuated by close adherence to infection control measures by staff accessing the catheter for the duration of the device's placement. Hub decontamination and strict hand hygiene will reduce the infective risk by this mechanism. Femoral placement been associated with the highest risk of infection due to the high burden of bacterial colonization at this site, with an intermediate risk in the neck and lowest risk at the subclavian site; however, this has recently been challenged.[16] A metaanalysis published by Marik et al.[16] reported that in more recent studies, an increased risk of CRBSI in the femoral site was not seen when compared with subclavian or internal jugular positions. This may be a reflection of the adoption of improved hygiene practices. Operator skill and experience and especially adherence to strict infection control practices are fundamental to minimizing the infection risk. Finally, the risk posed to an individual patient is modified by the ecology of the local flora in the critical care environment. Critical care units where there are high levels of multi-drug resistant organisms, which suffer from overcrowding, staff shortages, and deficits of isolation facilities, and which lack robust antimicrobial stewardship programs present an added risk to patients acquiring nosocomial infections including CRBSIs.[3]

MICROBIOLOGY

Gran-positive organisms are implicated in the majority of CRBSIs followed by gram-negative infections and yeasts. The US data compiled by the NHSN indicated the attributed infecting organisms as follows: 34.1% coagulase-negative *Staphylococci*, 16% *Enterococci*, 9.9% *S. aureus*, 5.8% *Klebsiella*, 3.9% *Enterobacter*, 3.1% *Pseudomonas*, 2.7% *E. Coli*, 2.2% *Acenitobacter*, 11.8% *Candida*, and miscellaneous infections accounting for the remaining 10.5%.[1]

Gram-positive organisms are particularly likely to occur in hemodialysis patients, while gram-negative infections are associated with a malignancy diagnosis and placement of the device in the femoral site. Line placement at this site and total parenteral nutrition delivery are also risk factors for *Candida* infections.[1,4,10]

DIAGNOSIS

The diagnosis of CRBSIs can be challenging but must be suspected in any patient who manifests typical clinical markers of an inflammatory illness while a CVC is in situ.[17] However, clinicians must remain alert to the possibility that an alternative source of infection is not overlooked and not simply ascribed to the CVC. Indeed, it has been reported that in febrile neutropenic patients who undergo catheter removal because of suspected CRBSI, the catheter is only subsequently confirmed as the source of sepsis on microbiological culture in as few as 20% of cases.[18] In the ECDC surveillance data, CRBSIs were confirmed as the cause of bloodstream infections (BSIs) in only 43% cases, although the cause was not determined in a further 21.5%, some of whom may have missed CRBSIs.[14] Of the remaining approximately 35% cases, the BSIs were secondary to another source, principally respiratory, gastrointestinal, and renal infections. This illustrates the importance of thoroughly evaluating every suspected case of CRBSI for alternative sources of infection.[14]

The catheter site should be evaluated for redness, induration, pus, and discharge at the skin puncture (exit site infection).[17] Soiled dressings may be an early indicator of infection. The inability to draw blood from all ports of the catheter has been identified as a risk factor because it likely indicates thrombosis of a lumen, with the potential this could become a nidus for infection.

The simultaneous acquisition of paired samples for blood cultures is mandatory.[1,3,10] One set should be via the lumen of the CVC, with another sample acquired from a peripheral vein. There is data that with multilumen devices, the diagnostic accuracy can be enhanced by sampling all the lumens of the central catheter in addition to the peripheral sample.[18] If peripheral access is not possible due to tissue edema or poor peripheral venous access, sampling from additional ports on the catheter may be an alternative. Meticulous attention must be paid to antisepsis during blood culture sampling, both from the catheter and peripheral vein, to avoid contamination from commensal organisms. At least 20 mL of blood should be drawn. Growths >15 colony-forming units (CFU)/catheter segment by semiquantitative or $>10^2$ CFU by quantitative (sonication) measurement are considered significant.[17]

Infection is highly likely if the same organism is obtained from the paired peripheral and CVC sampled blood cultures, with a three-fold greater colony count in the sample from the device.[1,3] Also, in CRBSI, the concentration of the organism in the device is believed to be many multiples of that in the bloodstream, with concentrations of >1000 CFU cultures. This is termed the differential time to positivity (DTTP). A DTTP of >120 minutes is considered significant. Using a diagnostic strategy incorporating DTTP may increase the diagnostic specificity cultures and reduce the incidence of unnecessary catheter removal. However, considerable caution should be exercised and a local infectious disease specialist should be consulted prior to this approach.[1,3,19]

Where a catheter is removed from a patient suspected of having a CRBSI, the distal 5-cm tip must be sent for culture. A quantitative growth of >15 CFUs, with the same organisms from the peripheral blood cultures, is also diagnostic.

Biomarkers for early line infection have been studied. In a study of pediatric line infection, presepsin proved valuable as an early marker.[20] Acridine orange is a fluorescent dye that stains bacteria orange and normal tissues yellow to green under acidic conditions. It has been used in conjunction with fluorescence in situ hybridization (FISH) to establish the presence of early CRBSI in patients with hematological malignancies.[19] Real-time polymerase chain reaction (PCR) has been evaluated as a diagnostic tool for the early diagnosis of *S. aureus* infection.[21] However, further research is required to define the potential role of these approaches in establishing an earlier CRBSI than is currently possible in most cases.

TREATMENT

The standard principles of the management of sepsis apply to a suspected or confirmed CRBSI[22,23]: prompt acquisition of appropriate samples for microbiological culture (at a minimum two sets of blood cultures, with simultaneously acquired peripheral and CVC samples) coupled with administration of broad-spectrum antibiotics based on knowledge of the local microbiological flora in accordance with local prescription guidelines. Narrow-spectrum therapy should be invoked once the results of cultures and sensitivities become known; supportive treatment of the circulation should be performed with fluid and vasopressors as appropriate. For the majority of CVCs placed for short-term access in the critical care, a suspected or confirmed CRBSI should prompt immediate consideration for removal of the device to achieve source control. If on-going venous access is required following removal of the infected device, a new catheter should be placed at a new site. Exchange of a new catheter over a guidewire is not appropriate, apart from exceptional circumstances where there may be serious concerns about mechanical complications of a new CVC insertion. Local spread of infection producing septic thrombophlebitis and metastatic spread to the heart valves and eye must be considered. These complications have significant implications for the duration of antibiotic treatment. Therapy should be administered in consultation with local infectious disease specialists.

In the absence of distant infection spread, the duration of antibiotic treatment is determined by the pathogen once it has been identified. Where the signs of sepsis have resolved within 72 hours following the initiation of antibiotics and removal of the catheter, the recommended duration of antibiotics is as follows[1,22,23]:

Coagulase-negative *Staphylococci*: 5–7 days

Enterococci: 7–14 days

Gram-negative bacilli: 7–14 days

S. aureus: 14 days in the absence of endocarditis or other evidence of metastatic involvement, such as osteomyelitis, discitis, or epidural abscess. In these cases, 4–6 weeks of treatment may be required in conjunction with surgical debridement of infected tissue.

Candida: 14 days from the date of the last negative blood culture and in the absence of retinitis.

In selected cases, preservation of the catheter may be attempted by a technique called "antibiotic lock" therapy.[1,23] This approach is typically undertaken in patients with long-term access devices (such as tunneled catheters for dialysis) and should be prescribed in consultation with infectious disease specialists. Following identification and sensitivity of the pathogen, supratherapeutic concentrations of appropriate antibiotics are instilled to fill each lumen of the catheter for a 24–48-hour period before being replenished. Systemic antibiotics are simultaneously administered, and treatment is continued for 10–14 days. This approach is conventionally used to treat infection caused by coagulase-negative *Staphylococci*, *Enterococci*, and gram-negative bacilli (with the important exception of *Pseudomonas*). Care must be taken that the patient is not inadvertently exposed to toxic antibiotic concentrations. It is recommended that treatment success is confirmed by negative blood cultures drawn via the salvaged catheter 1 week after the completion of treatment. This approach is not considered appropriate for infection with *S. aureus*, *Mycobacteria*, *Pseudomonas*, or *Candida*. Irrespective of the pathogen, the catheter should be removed if signs of metastatic infection, systemic shock, or new organ failure ascribed to the catheter infection develop.

PREVENTION

The experience over the past decade has shown that a protocolized program of meticulous adherence to infection control measures[11] can be highly successful in reducing the incidence of CRBSIs at an institutional level.[24–27] There is evidence that this approach, when supported by an education program, can be successfully adopted into institutions in different countries leading to sustained reductions in CRBSIs.[28] Professional health-care bodies in several countries have endorsed this approach and produced guidelines at national level. The common elements of this approach have been summarized by Shah et al.[1]

Personnel:
   Experienced operator/trainee closely supervised.
   Operator to don cap, face mask, sterile gown, and sterile drape after performing hand hygiene.
   All personnel in attendance in addition to the operator to wear cap and face mask.
Site:
   Selection of subclavian site over the internal jugular and femoral vein.
Device:
   Select a catheter with the minimum number of lumens appropriate to the role.
   Select a catheter impregnated with chlorhexidine/silver sulfadiazine or minocycline-rifampicin if otherwise optimal compliance with best infection control practices fails to reduce the CRBSI incident rate.
   Consider peripheral central catheter if feasible.
Technique:
   Use >0.5% chlorhexidine solution for skin antisepsis (caution with neonates) and allow to dry appropriately.
   Whole body drape during insertion.
   If sterile technique compromised during insertion, replace catheter as soon as possible.
   Do not administer prophylactic antibiotics during insertion.
Post-insertion Care:
   All health-care personnel to perform meticulous hand hygiene prior to performing any procedure involving the catheter.
   Observe the insertion site closely on a daily basis.

If insertion site is oozing, apply gauze dressing and change every 2 days. Otherwise, place a semipermeable dressing and change every 7 days. For both dressing types, replace it if wet/soiled.
   Do not change the catheter routinely (e.g. every 7 days).

The evidence supporting these recommendations has been evaluated in a series of systematic reviews published by the Cochrane Library.[29–32] The specific areas evaluated were skin antisepsis, the types of catheter used (impregnated vs. nonimpregnated), antibiotic lock in long-term tunneled access for hemodialysis patients, and type of dressings. The reader is referred to these texts for a more detailed discussion, but in summary, skin antisepsis with a chlorhexidine containing solution (>0.5%) led overall to a 36% reduction in the incidence of CRBSIs compared with povidone-iodine solutions. The issue of impregnated vs. nonimpregnated catheters and the magnitude of the potential benefit of impregnation is complex. Most of the evaluated studies compared minocycline-rifampicin and chlorhexidine silver-sulfadiazine catheters in studies with either standard peripheral venous catheter (PVC) devices or in head-to-head comparisons. However, other agents used to impregnate catheters which were studied included heparin, silver-platinum carbon, benzalkonium, 5-fluorouracil, and miconazole-rifampicin. Definitive conclusions have been difficult to make owing to the heterogeneous nature of study design, patient cohorts, and end-points. The main benefit appears to be in ICU patients followed by hematology/oncology and dialysis patients, with lesser efficacy in general ward patients. Minocycline-rifampicin appeared to reduce site colonization and CRBSI, and its performance is broadly superior to other forms of impregnation, which in turn are superior to standard PVC catheters. However, there appears little evidence of reduced all-cause sepsis or mortality between impregnated and nonimpregnated catheters. Also, there is currently little data on the emergence of antimicrobial resistance in association with the use of these types of catheters. Therefore, it does seem prudent that currently the use of impregnated devices be restricted to higher risk environments, such as the ICU and hematology patients. There is limited evidence to support prophylactic antibiotic lock therapy in hemodialysis patients. Chlorhexidine-impregnated dressings reduce site colonization. Sutureless devices may be beneficial in reducing CRBSI, but the current evidence does not support their routine use.

ARTERIAL LINES AND PERIPHERALLY INSERTED CENTRAL CATHETER LINES

Arterial lines are possibly an under-appreciated source of CRBSIs. Although perceived as comparatively lower risk of infection than venous access catheter infection, in systematic review and metaanalysis, O'Horo et al.[33] found that arterial line infection had an incident rate of 0.7 infections/1000 catheter days, especially with femoral site placement compared with the radial artery.[33] Peripherally inserted central catheter (PICC) lines have gained increasing popularity and have supplanted the placement of conventional venous access in many institutions. However, although associated with low rates of infection in the outpatient setting, there is limited data that these devices are associated with reduced CRBSI rate compared with more conventional CVCs.[34] In summary, it behooves health-care staff to treat these lines with the same level of fastidiousness in terms of hygiene and infection control as CVCs.

CONCLUSIONS

Despite considerable advances that have been made, CRBSIs remain a persistent challenge in health care. The mainstay of success in reducing the incidence of CRBSIs is through institutional governance of adherence to strict hygiene practices, supported by an education program and audited compliance.

AUTHOR'S RECOMMENDATIONS

- CRBSIs are a common and life-threatening complication of critical care.
- The prevalence of CRBSIs is decreasing worldwide due to widespread adoption of "bundles" of simple interventions with meticulous attention to sterility.
- Surveillance at local, regional, and national levels is the key to success.
- Maintaining a low level CRBSI is now an internationally recognized indicator of quality.
- Reduction of CRBSIs leads to shortened hospital stays and cost savings and may improve outcomes in critically ill patients.
- Antibiotic-impregnated catheters may reduce the incidence of CRBSIs in critical care, but there is little data to support their use elsewhere in the hospital.
- Although CRBSIs most commonly involve CVCs, clinicians should always consider arterial lines/PICC lines as potential sources of infection.

REFERENCES

1. Shah H, Bosch W, Thompson KM, Hellinger WC. Intravascular catheter-related bloodstream infection. *Neurohospitalist*. 2013;3(3):144-151.
2. Horan TC, Andrus M, Dudeck MA. CDC/NHSN surveillance definitions of health care-associated infections and criteria for specific types of infections in the acute care setting. *Am J Infect Control*. 2008;36(5):309-332.
3. Gahlot R, Nigam C, Kumar V, Yadav G, Anupurba S. Catheter-related bloodstream infections. *Int J Crit Illn Inj Sci*. 2014;4(2):162-167.
4. Safdar N, Maki DG. The pathogenesis of catheter-related bloodstream infection with noncuffed short-term central venous catheters. *Intensive Care Med*. 2004;30(1):62-67.
5. Safdar N, Kluger DM, Maki DG. A review of risk factors for catheter-related bloodstream infection caused by percutaneously inserted, noncuffed central venous catheters: implications for preventive strategies. *Medicine (Baltimore)*. 2002;81(6):466-479.
6. Climo MW, Yokoe DS, Warren DK, et al. Effect of daily chlorhexidine bathing on hospital-acquired infection. *N Engl J Med*. 2013;368(6):533-542.
7. Noto MJ, Domenico HJ, Byrne DW, et al. Chlorhexidine bathing and health care-associated infections: a randomized clinical trial. *JAMA*. 2015;313(4):369-378.
8. Kengen R, Thoonen E, Daveson K, et al. Chlorhexidine washing in intensive care does not reduce bloodstream infections, blood culture contamination and drug-resistant microorganism acquisition: an interrupted time series analysis. *Crit Care Resusc*. 2018;20(3):231-240.
9. Pittet D, Angus DC. Daily chlorhexidine bathing for critically ill patients: a note of caution. *JAMA*. 2015;313(4):365-366.
10. Maki DG, Kluger DM, Crnich CJ. The risk of bloodstream infection in adults with different intravascular devices: a systematic review of 200 published prospective studies. *Mayo Clin Proc*. 2006;81(9):1159-1171.
11. Pronovost P, Needham D, Berenholtz S, et al. An intervention to decrease catheter-related bloodstream infections in the ICU. *N Engl J Med*. 2006;355(26):2725-2732.
12. Centers for Disease Control and Prevention. *Healthcare-associated infections: HAI Data*. 2018. Available at https://www.cdc.gov/hai/surveillance/index.html. Accessed November 13, 2018.
13. Rosenthal VD, Maki DG, Mehta Y, et al. International Nosocomial Infection Control Consortium (INICC) report, data summary of 43 countries for 2007-2012. Device-associated module. *Am J Infect Control*. 2014;42(9):942-956.
14. European Centre for Disease Prevention and Control. *Annual Epidemiological Report for 2015: Healthcare-associated infections in intensive care units*. 2017. Available at https://ecdc.europa.eu/sites/portal/files/documents/AER_for_2015-healthcare-associated-infections_0.pdf. Accessed November 13, 2018.
15. Valencia C, Hammami N, Agodi A, et al. Poor adherence to guidelines for preventing central line-associated bloodstream infections (CLABSI): results of a worldwide survey. *Antimicrob Resist Infect Control*. 2016;5:49.
16. Marik PE, Flemmer M, Harrison W. The risk of catheter-related bloodstream infection with femoral venous catheters as compared to subclavian and internal jugular venous catheters: a systematic review of the literature and meta-analysis. *Crit Care Med*. 2012;40(8):2479-2485.
17. Mermel LA, Allon M, Bouza E, et al. Clinical practice guidelines for the diagnosis and management of intravascular catheter-related infection: 2009 Update by the Infectious Diseases Society of America. *Clin Infect Dis*. 2009;49(1):1-45.
18. Guembe M, Rodríguez-Créixems M, Sánchez-Carrillo C, Pérez-Parra A, Martin-Rabadán P, Bouza E. How many lumens should be cultured in the conservative diagnosis of catheter-related bloodstream infections? *Clin Infect Dis*. 2010;50(12):1575-1579.
19. Krause R, Auner HW, Gorkiewicz G, et al. Detection of catheter-related bloodstream infections by the differential-time-to-positivity method and gram stain-acridine orange leukocyte cytospin test in neutropenic patients after hematopoietic stem cell transplantation. *J Clin Microbiol*. 2004;42(10):4835-4837.
20. Tanır Basaranoglu S, Karadag-Oncel E, Aykac K, et al. Presepsin: A new marker of catheter related blood stream infections in pediatric patients. *J Infect Chemother*. 2018;24(1):25-30.
21. Zboromyrska Y, De la Calle C, Soto M, et al. Rapid diagnosis of staphylococcal catheter-related bacteraemia in direct blood samples by real-time PCR. *PLoS One*. 2016;11(8):e0161684.

22. Haddadin Y, Regunath H. *Central line associated blood stream infections (CLABSI). StatPearls [Website].* Treasure Island, FL: StatPearls Publishing; 2018.

23. Beekmann SE, Henderson DK. Infections caused by percutaneous intravascular devices. In: Mandell GL, Bennett JE, Dolin R, eds. *Principles and Practice of Infectious Disease.* 6th ed. Philadelphia, PA: Elsevier; 2005:3347-3361.

24. Walz JM, Ellison RT III, Mack DA, et al. The bundle "plus": the effect of a multidisciplinary team approach to eradicate central line-associated bloodstream infections. *Anesth Analg.* 2015;120(4):868-876.

25. Lin KY, Cheng A, Chang YC, et al. Central line-associated bloodstream infections among critically-ill patients in the era of bundle care. *J Microbiol Immunol Infect.* 2017;50(3):339-348.

26. Shimoyama Y, Umegaki O, Agui T, Kadono N, Komasawa N, Minami T. An educational program for decreasing catheter-related bloodstream infections in intensive care units: a pre- and post-intervention observational study. *JA Clin Rep.* 2017;3(1):23.

27. Ista E, van der Hoven B, Kornelisse RF, et al. Effectiveness of insertion and maintenance bundles to prevent central-line-associated bloodstream infections in critically ill patients of all ages: a systematic review and meta-analysis. *Lancet Infect Dis.* 2016;16(6):724-734.

28. Hsin HT, Hsu MS, Shieh JS. The long-term effect of bundle care for catheter-related blood stream infection: 5-year follow-up. *Postgrad Med J.* 2017;93(1097):133-137.

29. Lai NM, Lai NA, O'Riordan E, Chaiyakunapruk N, Taylor JE, Tan K. Skin antisepsis for reducing central venous catheter-related infections. *Cochrane Database Syst Rev.* 2016;7:CD010140.

30. Lai NM, Chaiyakunapruk N, Lai NA, O'Riordan E, Pau WS, Saint S. Catheter impregnation, coating or bonding for reducing central venous catheter-related infections in adults. *Cochrane Database Syst Rev.* 2016;3:CD007878.

31. Arechabala MC, Catoni MI, Claro JC, et al. Antimicrobial lock solutions for preventing catheter-related infections in haemodialysis. *Cochrane Database Syst Rev.* 2018;4:CD010597.

32. Ullman AJ, Cooke ML, Mitchell M, et al. Dressings and securement devices for central venous catheters (CVC). *Cochrane Database Syst Rev.* 2015;10:CD010367.

33. O'Horo JC, Maki DG, Krupp AE, Safdar N. Arterial catheters as a source of bloodstream infection: a systematic review and meta-analysis. *Crit Care Med.* 2014;42(6):1334-1339.

34. Safdar N, Maki DG. Risk of catheter-related bloodstream infection with peripherally inserted central venous catheters used in hospitalized patients. *Chest.* 2005;128(2):489-495.

45

How Do I Manage Central Nervous System Infections (Meningitis/Encephalitis)?

Amy C. Walker, David Foster Gaieski, and Nicholas J. Johnson

INTRODUCTION

Central nervous system (CNS) infections lead to significant mortality and disability and can be challenging to diagnose and treat in the intensive care unit (ICU). This chapter will review the evidence supporting the critical care management of CNS infections, including bacterial meningitis, viral meningitis and encephalitis, CNS abscess, and uncommon infections.

BACTERIAL MENINGITIS

Epidemiology and Microbiology

Bacterial meningitis affects approximately 1.38 in 100,000 people in the United States.[1] In the immunocompetent adult, community-acquired bacterial meningitis is most commonly caused by *Streptococcus pneumoniae*, *Neisseria meningitidis*, and *Listeria monocytogenes*.[2] Patients who have undergone neurosurgical procedures or recent instrumentation are at risk for other health care-associated pathogens, such as *Staphylococcus aureus*, *Pseudomonas aeruginosa*, and other gram-negative rods.

Diagnosis

Bacterial meningitis is a neurological emergency. Prompt diagnosis and initiation of treatment are imperative, as delay in treatment has been associated with increased morbidity and mortality.[3] Approximately 95% patients with meningitis will present with at least two of the following four symptoms: fever, neck stiffness, headache, and change in mental status.[4] Diagnosis is made on cerebrospinal fluid (CSF) sampling, typically via lumbar puncture, with CSF culture as the gold standard. Classic CSF findings of bacterial meningitis include CSF pleocytosis with neutrophil predominance (>80%), elevated protein levels, and decreased glucose levels (Table 45.1). CSF polymerase chain reaction (PCR), lactate concentration, and serum C-reactive protein may be helpful as adjunct tests.[5]

While brain imaging has a limited role in the diagnosis of bacterial meningitis, guidelines recommend that patients with any of the following should undergo neuroimaging prior to lumbar puncture: focal neurological deficit, new onset seizure (within 1 week), moderate to severe altered mental status, immunocompromised state, history of CNS disease (stroke, focal infection, or mass lesion), or papilledema.[2]

Treatment

Airway management, respiratory support, and hemodynamic optimization are priorities for patients with severe bacterial meningitis as they may develop depressed mental status leading to loss of airway reflexes and hemodynamic collapse, thus resulting in septic shock.

Antimicrobial Therapy

Delays in antibiotic administration have been associated with significant increases in mortality.[3] Empiric treatment for community-acquired bacterial meningitis should include a third-generation cephalosporin plus vancomycin. Ampicillin should be added for adults aged >50 years to cover *L. monocytogenes*. Once a positive Gram stain or culture is obtained, antimicrobial therapy may be tailored to the specific causative agent and should take into account regional antimicrobial resistance patterns as well as in vitro susceptibility testing. Duration of antibiotics is variable and depends on the causative organism. Patients with suspected nosocomial meningitis should receive empiric coverage for *P. aeruginosa* and multidrug-resistant gram-negative rods, usually with a fourth-generation cephalosporin or carbapenem, and vancomycin for methicillin-resistant *S. aureus* (MRSA). Fungal coverage should also be considered.

Corticosteroids

Dexamethasone has been found to decrease overall mortality in patients with meningitis due to *S. pneumoniae* and decrease sensorineural hearing loss due to *S. pneumoniae* or *N. meningitidis*.[6] In a metaanalysis of 18 randomized, controlled trials of corticosteroids in the treatment of acute bacterial meningitis the following was determined: (1) there was a protective effect of corticosteroids on severe hearing loss among children; and (2) there was a 10% absolute reduction in mortality among adults.[7] Consequently, guidelines recommend the use of dexamethasone (0.15 mg/kg every 6 hours for 2–4 days) in adults with suspected or proven pneumococcal meningitis.[8,9] Given that CSF culture is generally unavailable at the time of diagnosis, dexamethasone should be initiated for all patients with suspected bacterial meningitis

TABLE 45.1 Cerebrospinal Fluid Characteristics in Central Nervous System Infections.

Characteristic	Normal	Viral	Bacterial	Fungal
WBC (cells/mm³)	<5	10–2,000	100–10,000	200–500
Predominant WBC subset	Monocytes[41]	Lymphocyte	Neutrophil	Lymphocyte
CSF:Serum Glucose	>0.6–0.75	>0.6–0.75	<0.4	<0.8
Protein (g/L)	<0.5	0.5–0.9	>0.5	>0.5
Opening pressure	<20 cm H_2O	<20 cm H_2O	20–50 cm H_2O	>20 cm H_2O

CSF, cerebrospinal fluid; *WBC,* white blood cell.

and may be stopped later if patients are found to have an alternative pathogen or diagnosis.

Temperature Management

Studies evaluating the use of acetaminophen to treat fever demonstrated no difference in outcomes.[5] One randomized controlled trial has been performed to evaluate the effect of therapeutic hypothermia in severe bacterial meningitis; however, the study was stopped early due to increased mortality in the hypothermia group.[10]

Prophylaxis

All close contacts of patients with meningococcal meningitis should receive prophylactic antibiotics in the form of either a single dose of oral ciprofloxacin or intramuscular ceftriaxone, or oral rifampin for 2 days.[11]

Complications
Intracranial Hypertension

Intracranial hypertension and brain herniation are the most common causes of death in meningitis.[12] The pathophysiologic mechanism may involve the following factors: (1) inflammation and disruption of the blood-brain barrier secondarily resulting in brain edema; (2) impaired autoregulation; and (3) hydrocephalus secondary to impaired CSF absorption.[12]

Several studies suggest that reduction in intracranial pressure may yield improved outcomes in patients with severe bacterial meningitis and depressed consciousness.[13–16] A single prospective study demonstrated that aggressive intracranial pressure management among patients with severe bacterial meningitis and impaired consciousness resulted in lower mortality and favorable neurologic outcome when compared with historical controls.[13] Another observational study demonstrated that CSF drainage via lumbar drain to target intracranial pressure (ICP) <15 cm H_2O was associated with decreased mortality.[14] In a randomized, controlled trial in children with CNS infection and depressed consciousness, a strategy targeting cerebral perfusion pressure led to a 20% decrease in absolute mortality at 90 days compared with a strategy aimed at reducing ICP.[17]

ICP monitoring should be considered for patients with bacterial meningitis and altered level of consciousness and/or markedly elevated CSF opening pressure. It is reasonable to apply routine care for intracranial hypertension, including head elevation, neutral head positioning to facilitate cerebral venous drainage, targeting eucapnia and normothermia, hyperosmolar therapy, and CSF drainage. More aggressive therapies, such as barbiturate coma and neuromuscular blockade, are experimental and should be reserved for severe, refractory cases. In rare cases, decompressive craniectomy has been used in patients with refractory intracranial hypertension with good neurologic outcome.[15,18]

Stroke

Cerebral infarction is a common complication with one observational study estimating incidence as high 25%.[19] It is thought to be mediated by inflammatory vasculitis and has not been associated with atherosclerotic risk factors.[20]

Seizures

Seizures are a common complication of meningitis, affecting up to 27% of patients.[21] Seizure activity during an initial episode of meningitis has been associated with higher mortality and future development of epilepsy in patients who survive.[21] Antiepileptic medications are indicated for patients who develop seizures, but routine seizure prophylaxis for all patients with meningitis is not recommended. Nonconvulsive seizure or status epilepticus should be considered in patients with depressed mental status or those receiving heavy sedation; continuous electroencephalogram should be applied if there is concern.

Outcomes

Despite advances in ICU care, morbidity and mortality remain high for bacterial meningitis. Mortality for adults with bacterial meningitis from 1998 to 2007 was estimated to be 16.4% and increased linearly with age.[1] Long-term neurological sequelae including neurological deficits, seizures, hearing loss, and cognitive impairment may occur in >30% survivors.[4]

VIRAL CENTRAL NERVOUS SYSTEM INFECTION

Epidemiology and Microbiology

Viral CNS infections have an annual incidence ranging from 0.26 to 17 cases per 100,000 depending on the age and vaccination status of the population.[22] Enteroviruses are the most common cause of viral CNS infection (nearly 60%),

TABLE 45.2 Common and Important Viral Causes of Central Nervous System Infections.

Virus Genus (Species)	Risk Factor	Diagnosis	Treatment
Picornaviruses (enteroviruses, Coxsackie virus, echoviruses, parechoviruses)	Young age, immunosuppression, fecal-oral transmission	CSF PCR	Intravenous immunoglobulin, Consider pleconaril
Herpesviruses (HSV, VZV, CMV, EBV, HHV 6 & 7)	Previous infection; immunosuppression	CSF PCR	HSV meningitis: acyclovir 10 mg/kg IV VZV meningitis: acyclovir 15 mg/kg IV CMV: ganciclovir 5 mg/kg and foscarnet 90 mg/kg
Arboviruses (West Nile, La Crosse, Toscana, tick borne encephalitis, Japanese encephalitis, Dengue)	Arthropod exposure	CSF PCR or IgM	Supportive care
Lyssavirus (Rabies)	Animal bite	Hair follicle RNA or antigen	Rabies vaccination, Rabies immune globulin, "Milwaukee protocol"

CMV, cytomegalovirus; CSF, cerebrospinal fluid; EBV, Epstein-Barr virus; HHV, human herpes virus; HSV, herpes simplex virus; IgM, immunoglobulin M; PCR, polymerase chain reaction; RNA, ribonucleic acid; VZV, varicella zoster virus.

followed by arbovirus and herpes virus, such as herpes simplex virus (HSV) and varicella zoster virus (VZV).[23] Arbovirus infections, La Crosse and West Nile being the most common in the United States, typically occur in summer and autumn months.[24] Additional important viral CNS infections are listed in Table 45.2.

Diagnosis

The classic clinical presentation of viral CNS infection is a febrile illness followed by the development of nuchal rigidity and headache.[23,25] Other symptoms include photophobia, nausea, and vomiting. Some infections may present more subtly with findings such as behavioral or personality changes, hallucinations, bizarre behavior, focal neurologic deficits, or seizures.[23,25,26]

The diagnosis of viral CNS infection hinges upon CSF sampling (Table 45.1). CSF PCRs are available for numerous viruses including enteroviruses, HSV-2, and human immunodeficiency virus (HIV).[27]

Treatment

Treatment for most cases of viral meningitis and encephalitis is supportive. Acyclovir is the recommended agent for HSV and VZV CNS infection; however, no high-quality randomized trials supporting its use in herpesvirus CNS infection exist.[22]

Two therapies have been studied for enterovirus infection: intravenous immunoglobulin (IVIG) and pleconaril. IVIG has been shown to reduce viral titers in neonates with systemic enterovirus infection and agammaglobulinemic adults with CNS infection.[28,29] Pleconaril blocks enteroviral attachment to cells and inhibits viral uncoating, but no clinical benefit has been shown.[7,30]

A number of treatments for West Nile have been investigated, but none have demonstrated efficacy.[27] Rabies

mortality is best prevented through exposure prevention, pre-exposure vaccination, and post-exposure prophylaxis with a combination of rabies immune globulin and vaccination.[8,9,31] The "Milwaukee protocol" is a controversial intensive care strategy that was developed for a patient who survived a bat bite despite not having received post-exposure prophylaxis and presenting with encephalitis.[32]

Outcomes and Complications

Most cases of viral CNS infections are self-limited and result in no lasting neurologic deficits. Among patients with HSV encephalitis, age and neurologic examination at the time of diagnosis are strong predictors of outcome.[22,23] The majority of patients with West Nile Virus infection recover fully, though neurologic sequelae have been described.[27] Nearly 10% of patients with neuroinvasive West Nile disease die, with advanced age conferring the greatest risk for death. Rabies encephalitis is nearly always fatal in unimmunized patients.

Complications of viral meningitis and encephalitis include hyponatremia, most often due to syndrome of inappropriate antidiuretic hormone secretion, cerebral edema, and seizures.[23] Given its affinity for the temporal lobes, HSV infection is associated with an especially high incidence of seizures. Prophylactic antiepileptic drugs are not routinely recommended.

CENTRAL NERVOUS SYSTEM ABSCESS

Brain Abscess

Brain abscess is a focal encapsulated infection within the brain parenchyma, usually caused by bacterial infection; it may be also caused by fungi, mycobacteria, protozoa, or helminths. Most patients with brain abscess have a predisposing condition including contiguous infection (otitis, mastoiditis, sinusitis, meningitis, or odontogenic infection), metastatic infection from hematogenous spread, recent neurosurgical procedure, or trauma,[33–35] although some are cryptogenic.[34]

Streptococcus and staphylococcus species are the most common causative microorganisms, followed by gram-negative enteric bacteria.[33–35] Brain abscess in patients with HIV may be due to toxoplasmosis, nocardia, or *Mycobacterium tuberculosis*, whereas patients with neutropenia, hematologic malignancy, and stem cell transplant tend to be at higher risk of fungal abscesses.[33,36]

Computed tomography (CT) head with contrast or magnetic resonance imaging (MRI) is recommended for diagnosis. MRI is preferred as it is more sensitive for small abscesses and has the ability to characterize the age of an abscess and differentiate between abscesses and brain metastases; however, it may be less readily available than CT.[33,37]

Optimal management of brain abscess involves a multimodal approach: (1) antimicrobial therapy; (2) surgical drainage of the abscess; and (3) treatment of the predisposing condition, if present. A third-generation cephalosporin, such as ceftriaxone, plus metronidazole is reasonable for most patients, with addition of vancomycin if there is concern for MRSA. A fourth-generation cephalosporin or carbapenem may be substituted in postoperative patients or patients at risk of infection from *P. aeruginosa* or other resistant nosocomial organisms.[35,37] Patients should receive approximately 6–8 weeks of intravenous antibiotics, though this may vary, depending on the organism and source. Pyrimethamine and sulfadiazine should be considered for empiric treatment of *Toxoplasma gondii* in HIV-infected patients; amphotericin should be considered to cover fungal infection in neutropenic patients.

Neurosurgical consultation should be obtained. Nonoperative management may be reasonable in patients with an abscess measuring <2.5 cm in size who are otherwise well. Higher risk features include infratentorial abscess, mass effect, close proximity to ventricles, and hydrocephalus, all of which require urgent drainage.[35]

Since 2000, the estimated mortality of brain abscess has been approximately 10%.[34] Potential complications include seizures, hydrocephalus, and intraventricular rupture, which is associated with poor outcome.[35] Multiloculated abscesses and those <1 mm from the ventricle are at highest risk of rupture and should be treated with early surgical intervention.[33,35]

Epidural Abscess

Spinal epidural abscess is a pyogenic infection between dura mater and vertebral bodies. Incidence has increased in the last several decades, likely due to increased incidence of injection drug usage, long-term vascular access, and spinal instrumentation.[38] Patients may present with back pain, fever, and/or neurological deficit such as weakness, numbness, or incontinence. If left untreated, patients may develop complete spinal cord injury and paralysis. Diagnosis is made by MRI or CT myelogram. Blood cultures should be obtained prior to starting empiric antibiotics. In patients with a normal neurological exam and stable spine, it may be reasonable to attempt nonoperative management with antibiotics and close monitoring. In this subset of patients, CT-guided aspiration may be considered if blood cultures do not identify a causative pathogen for the guidance of antibiotic management. Patients with acute neurological deficit should be treated with emergent operative intervention.

Cranial Subdural Empyema

Subdural empyema is a pyogenic encapsulated infection in the intracranial subdural space, frequently associated with contiguous infection, trauma, or recent instrumentation. Clinical presentation usually includes rapid onset of fever, headache, and possibly altered mental status, focal neurologic deficits, or seizures due to meningeal irritation and inflammation. Diagnosis may be made through CT with contrast or MRI, though MRI is more sensitive, particularly for empyema in the posterior fossa. Similar to the workup of brain abscess described earlier, it is not recommended to obtain CSF sample as (1) the infection is usually contained and not contiguous with the subarachnoid space; and (2) the patient may be at increased risk of herniation due to mass effect. Management consists of blood cultures, empiric antibiotics, and surgical drainage.[37]

CENTRAL NERVOUS SYSTEM INFECTIONS IN THE IMMUNOCOMPROMISED HOST AND GLOBAL TRAVELER

A number of less common CNS infections may develop in hosts with compromised immune systems[39] (Table 45.3). Patients with HIV infection, especially those with low concentrations of CD4 lymphocytes, are at risk for infection by *T. gondii*, *Cryptococcus neoformans*, *M. tuberculosis*, lymphocytic choriomeningitis virus, and various other opportunistic pathogens. Solid organ transplantation, stem cell transplantation, and neutropenia place patients at higher risk for CNS viral, bacterial, and fungal infections, including infections by *Aspergillus spp.* and zygomycetes as well as by the filamentous bacterium *Nocardia spp.* Asplenia increases the risk for infection by encapsulated organisms, including *S. pneumoniae* and *N. meningitidis*, which are common causes of bacterial meningitis.

Among patients returning from global travel, clinicians must consider pathogens endemic to the regions traveled. The "meningitis belt" in sub-Saharan African region, which spans 26 countries extending from Senegal to Ethiopia, has a markedly high incidence of bacterial meningitis (primarily caused by *N. meningitidis*) with major epidemics reaching infection rates of 1000 cases per 100,000 persons.[40] A number of other infections that affect the CNS are described in Table 45.4.

TABLE 45.3   Selected Central Nervous System Infections in Immunocompromised Hosts.

	Pathogen	Risk Factors	Recommended Treatment
Bacteria	*Mycobacterium tuberculosis*	Immunocompromised, HIV, stem cell transplant	Isoniazid, rifampin, pyrazinamide, ethambutol, glucocorticoids (if no HIV infection)
	Nocardia spp.	Immunocompromised, HIV, stem cell transplant	Trimethoprim-sulfamethoxazole, amikacin plus imipenem, ceftriaxone, or linezolid
Fungi	*Aspergillus spp.*	Immunocompromised, neutropenia, malignancy	Voriconazole or liposomal amphotericin
	Candida spp.	Immunocompromised, neurosurgery, IV drug use	Liposomal amphotericin or voriconazole
	Cryptococcus neoformans	HIV, T-cell deficiency	Amphotericin + flucytosine
	Zygomycetes	Immunocompromised, diabetes	Liposomal amphotericin
Viruses	HSV & VZV	HIV, immunocompromised	Acyclovir
	CMV	HIV, stem cell transplant, chemotherapy	Ganciclovir
	EBV	HIV, stem cell transplant	Ganciclovir
	HHV-6	Stem cell transplant	Ganciclovir
	JC virus	HIV, stem cell transplant	Cidofovir, IL-2, interferon, cytarabine
Parasites	*Toxoplasma gondii*	HIV, malignancy, stem cell transplant, immunocompromise	Pyrimethamine + sulfadiazine

CMV, cytomegalovirus; *EBV*, Epstein-Barr virus; *HHV*, human herpes virus; *HIV*, human immunodeficiency virus; *HSV*, herpes simplex virus; *IL*, interleukin; *IV*, intravenous; *JC* virus, John Cunningham virus; *VZV*, varicella zoster virus.

TABLE 45.4   Selected Central Nervous System Infections in Global Travelers.

Disease (Organism)	Endemic Regions	Clinical Manifestations	Recommended Treatment
Ebola virus (*filovirus*)	West & Central Africa	Headache, altered mental status, meningitis, weakness, rarely stroke or seizures	Isolation Supportive care
Zika virus (*flavivirus*)	South America, Central America, the Caribbean, Africa, Southeast Asia, and the western Pacific	Congenital Zika virus syndrome, myelitis, meningoencephalitis	Prevention, Supportive care, IVIG
Cerebral malaria (*Plasmodium falciparum or vivax*)	Africa, Latin America, Asia, Eastern Europe, and the South Pacific	Severe anemia, seizures, coma, cerebral edema	IV artesunate or quinine
Japanese encephalitis (*flavirivus*)	Asia, norther Australia, western Pacific	Fever, headache, vomiting, focal neurologic deficits, acute flaccid paralysis	Supportive care

IV, intravenous; *IVIG*, intravenous immunoglobulin.

AUTHORS' RECOMMENDATIONS

- CNS infections can be challenging to diagnose and treat in the ICU and are associated with high mortality and morbidity.
- When caring for patients with bacterial meningitis, ICU clinicians should be aware of the importance of early antimicrobial therapy and key complications, such as intracranial hypertension and seizures.
- While an uncommon reason for ICU admission, selected viral CNS infections often present subtly; treatment is largely supportive.
- The treatment for CNS abscesses is often surgical, and presentation depends on the neuroanatomic location and degree of mass effect.
- In the returning traveler or immunocompromised host, a myriad of exotic CNS infections should be considered based on travel location and host characteristics.

REFERENCES

1. Thigpen MC, Whitney CG, Messonnier NE, et al. Bacterial meningitis in the United States, 1998–2007. *N Engl J Med.* 2011;364(21):2016-2025.
2. Tunkel AR, Hartman BJ, Kaplan SL, et al. Practice guidelines for the management of bacterial meningitis. *Clin Infect Dis.* 2004;39:1267-1284.
3. Proulx N, Fréchette D, Toye B, Chan J, Kravcik S. Delays in the administration of antibiotics are associated with mortality from adult acute bacterial meningitis. *QJM.* 2005;98(4):291-298.
4. van de Beek D, de Gans J, Spanjaard L, Weisfelt M, Reitsma JB, Vermeulen M. Clinical features and prognostic factors in adults with bacterial meningitis. *N Engl J Med.* 2004;351(18):1849-1859.
5. van de Beek D, Cabellos C, Dzupova O, et al. ESCMID guideline: diagnosis and treatment of acute bacterial meningitis. *Clin Microbiol Infect.* 2016;22:S37-S62.
6. Brouwer MC, McIntyre P, Prasad K, van de Beek D. Corticosteroids for acute bacterial meningitis. *Cochrane Database Syst Rev.* 2015;9:CD004405.
7. Desmond RA, Accortt NA, Talley L, Villano SA, Soong SJ, Whitley RJ. Enteroviral meningitis: natural history and outcome of pleconaril therapy. *Antimicrob Agents Chemother.* 2006;50(7):2409-2414.
8. Wilde H, Hemachudha T. Prophylaxis against rabies. *N Engl J Med.* 2005;352(15):1608-1610; author reply: 1608-1610.
9. Moran GJ, Talan DA, Mower W, et al. Appropriateness of rabies postexposure prophylaxis treatment for animal exposures. Emergency ID Net Study Group. *JAMA.* 2000;284(8):1001-1007.
10. Mourvillier B, Tubach F, van de Beek D, et al. Induced hypothermia in severe bacterial meningitis. *JAMA.* 2013;310(20):2174-2183.
11. Lucas MJ, Brouwer MC, van de Beek D. Neurological sequelae of bacterial meningitis. *J Infect.* 2016;73(1):18-27.
12. Tariq A, Aguilar-Salinas P, Hanel RA, Naval N, Chmayssani M. The role of ICP monitoring in meningitis. *Neurosurg Focus.* 2017;43(5):E7.
13. Glimåker M, Johansson B, Halldorsdottir H, et al. Neuro-intensive treatment targeting intracranial hypertension improves outcome in severe bacterial meningitis: an intervention-control study. *PLoS One.* 2014;9(3):22-24.
14. Abulhasan YB, Al-Jehani H, Valiquette MA, et al. Lumbar drainage for the treatment of severe bacterial meningitis. *Neurocrit Care.* 2013;19(2):199-205.
15. Baussart B, Cheisson G, Compain M, et al. Multimodal cerebral monitoring and decompressive surgery for the treatment of severe bacterial meningitis with increased intracranial pressure. *Acta Anaesthesiol Scand.* 2006;50(6):762-765.
16. Lindvall P, Ahlm C, Ericsson M, Gothefors L, Naredi S, Koskinen LO. Reducing intracranial pressure may increase survival among patients with bacterial meningitis. *Clin Infect Dis.* 2004;38(3):384-390.
17. Kumar R, Singhi S, Singhi P, Jayashree M, Bansal A, Bhatti A. Randomized controlled trial comparing cerebral perfusion pressure-targeted therapy versus intracranial pressure-targeted therapy for raised intracranial pressure due to acute CNS infections in children. *Crit Care Med.* 2014;42(8):1775-1787.
18. Perin A, Nascimben E, Longatti P. Decompressive craniectomy in a case of intractable intracranial hypertension due to pneumococcal meningitis. *Acta Neurochir (Wien).* 2008;150(8):837-842; discussion: 842.
19. Schut ES, Lucas MJ, Brouwer MC, Vergouwen MD, van der Ende A, van de Beek D. Cerebral infarction in adults with bacterial meningitis. *Neurocrit Care.* 2012;16(3):421-427.
20. Bodilsen J, Dalager-Pedersen M, Schønheyder HC, Nielsen H. Stroke in community-acquired bacterial meningitis: a Danish population-based study. *Int J Infect Dis.* 2014;20:18-22.
21. Wang KW, Chang WN, Chang HW, Chuang YC, Tsai NW, Wang HC. The significance of seizures and other predictive factors during the acute illness for the long-term outcome after bacterial meningitis. *Seizure.* 2005;14(8):586-592.
22. McGill F, Griffiths MJ, Solomon T. Viral meningitis: current issues in diagnosis and treatment. *Curr Opin Infect Dis.* 2017;30(2):248-256.
23. Irani DN. Aseptic meningitis and viral myelitis. *Neurol Clin.* 2008;26(3):635-655, vii-viii.
24. Cleton N, Koopmans M, Reimerink J, Godeke GJ, Reusken C. Come fly with me: review of clinically important arboviruses for global travelers. *J Clin Virol.* 2012;55(3):191-203.
25. Lee BE, Chawla R, Langley JM, et al. Paediatric Investigators Collaborative Network on Infections in Canada (PICNIC) study of aseptic meningitis. *BMC Infect Dis.* 2006;6:68.
26. Attia J, Hatala R, Cook DJ, Wong JG. The rational clinical examination. Does this adult patient have acute meningitis? *JAMA.* 1999;282(2):175-181.
27. Petersen LR, Brault AC, Nasci RS. West Nile virus: review of the literature. *JAMA.* 2013;310(3):308-315.
28. Abzug MJ, Keyserling HL, Lee ML, Levin MJ, Rotbart HA. Neonatal enterovirus infection: virology, serology, and effects of intravenous immune globulin. *Clin Infect Dis.* 1995;20(5):1201-1206.
29. Webster AD, Rotbart HA, Warner T, Rudge P, Hyman N. Diagnosis of enterovirus brain disease in hypogammaglobulinemic patients by polymerase chain reaction. *Clin Infect Dis.* 1993;17(4):657-661.
30. Abzug MJ, Cloud G, Bradley J, et al. Double blind placebo-controlled trial of pleconaril in infants with enterovirus meningitis. *Pediatr Infect Dis J.* 2003;22(4):335-341.
31. Crowcroft NS, Thampi N. The prevention and management of rabies. *BMJ.* 2015;350:g7827.
32. Willoughby Jr RE, Tieves KS, Hoffman GM, et al. Survival after treatment of rabies with induction of coma. *N Engl J Med.* 2005;352(24):2508-2514.
33. Brouwer MC, van de Beek D. Epidemiology, diagnosis, and treatment of brain abscesses. *Curr Opin Infect Dis.* 2017;30(1):129-134.
34. Brouwer MC, Coutinho JM, van de Beek D. Clinical characteristics and outcome of brain abscess: systematic review and meta-analysis. *Neurology.* 2014;82(9):806-813.
35. Patel K, Clifford DB. Bacterial brain abscess. *Neurohospitalist.* 2014;4(4):196-204.
36. Sonneville R, Magalhaes E, Meyfroidt G. Central nervous system infections in immunocompromised patients. *Curr Opin Crit Care.* 2017;23(2):128-133.
37. Beckham JD, Tyler KL. Neuro-intensive care of patients with acute CNS infections. *Neurotherapeutics.* 2012;9(1):124-138.
38. Arko L 4th, Quach E, Nguyen V, Chang D, Sukul V, Kim BS. Medical and surgical management of spinal epidural abscess: a systematic review. *Neurosurg Focus.* 2014;37(2):E4.
39. Schmidt-Hieber M, Zweigner J, Uharek L, Blau IW, Thiel E. Central nervous system infections in immunocompromised patients – update on diagnostics and therapy. *Leuk Lymphoma.* 2009;50(1):24-36.
40. Reid S, Thompson H, Thakur KT. Nervous system infections and the global traveler. *Semin Neurol.* 2018;38(2):247-262.
41. Seehusen DA, Reeves MM, Fomin DA. Cerebrospinal fluid analysis. *Am Fam Physician.* 2003;68(6):1103-1108.

46

How Can Biomarkers Be Used to Differentiate Between Infection and Non-Infectious Causes of Inflammation?

Alexandra Binnie, Joel Lage, and Claudia C. Dos Santos

Systemic inflammation may reflect infection. Appropriate therapy includes supportive care and use of antimicrobial agents. Indeed, early initiation of antibiotics is of key importance in the management of sepsis.[1–3] However, inflammation may also arise from noninfectious causes, including pancreatitis, cardiac ischemia, bowel perforation, vasculitis, and pulmonary embolism. Current clinical practice is to initiate empiric antibiotic therapy prior to identification of an infectious agent based on treatment guidelines and knowledge of the local microbiome.[2] Unfortunately, confirmation of infection may take several days. Errors in antibiotic choice can lead to significant increases in mortality,[4] whereas overuse of antibiotics fosters bacterial resistance.[5] Therefore, a method to differentiate between inflammation due to infection and inflammation due to other causes is particularly valuable.

Two biomarkers have been widely studied in the diagnosis of infectious inflammation—C-reactive protein (CRP) and procalcitonin (PCT). Each has found varying success in the clinical context, with some centers relying heavily on these markers and others eschewing their use almost entirely. In this chapter, we present the evidence for their use in the diagnosis of infection and management of antibiotic therapy in the intensive care unit (ICU) context.

C-REACTIVE PROTEIN

Structure and Function

Named for its ability to precipitate the C-polysaccharide of *Streptococcus pneumoniae*, CRP was the first acute-phase protein to be described.[6] It was subsequently identified in the serum of patients with a wide variety of infectious diseases.[7] CRP is an exquisitely sensitive marker of systemic inflammation, infection, and tissue damage, and a central component of the nonspecific acute-phase response.[8]

CRP binds to phosphocholine, a constituent of bacterial and fungal polysaccharides, as well as to components of damaged cell membranes in a calcium-dependent manner.[9] It is principally produced by hepatocytes, and its expression is strongly stimulated by interleukin (IL)-6, a pro-inflammatory cytokine.[10] When bound to phosphocholine, CRP is recognized by C1q, thereby activating the classical complement pathway.[11,12] CRP has a multitude of downstream effects, both pro-inflammatory and anti-inflammatory; it stimulates phagocytosis and binds to immunoglobulin Fcγ

receptors as well as increases the release of anti-inflammatory cytokine IL-10. Conversely, it downregulates the pro-inflammatory cytokine interferon-γ.[13] CRP plays an active role in the immune response to infection and polymorphisms have been shown to increase susceptibility and mortality in invasive pneumococcal disease.[14]

C-Reactive Protein Dynamics

CRP is a nonspecific marker of inflammation. In response to an acute-phase stimulus, serum CRP concentrations rise very quickly, doubling every 6 hours. The plasma half-life of CRP is around 19 hours and peak levels are detected approximately 48 hours after a single stimulus.[8] In healthy adults, the median concentration of CRP is <1 mg/L,[15] but it may increase to >500 mg/L in the context of inflammation.[13,16] When the acute-phase stimulus is past, CRP levels return to normal within 3–7 days[17]; however, patients with sepsis show persistently high CRP levels for at least 7 days and likely longer.[18] In addition to infection, other causes of CRP elevation include pancreatitis, trauma, burns, rheumatologic disease, pericarditis, inflammatory bowel disease, solid tumors, and hematologic malignancy.[16] However, extremely elevated CRP levels (>350 mg/L) are associated with infection in >90% of patients.[16]

C-Reactive Protein as a Marker of Infection

CRP has been widely studied as a marker of bacterial infection in the ICU patient population. It is elevated in patients with infection relative to those with noninfectious systemic inflammation, even when adjusted for severity of illness.[19–21] Ideal cutoffs for diagnosis of infection are in the range of 50–100 mg/L.[19] Sensitivity and specificity estimates vary, but a 2004 metaanalysis provided a pooled sensitivity of 75% and specificity of 67% for the diagnosis of bacterial infection relative to noninfectious inflammation.[22] In the pediatric population, ideal cutoffs are typically lower (20–40 mg/L).[22]

CRP levels tend to be lower in systemic viral and fungal infections than in systemic bacterial infection.[22,23] In the context of viral infection, interferon-α may inhibit CRP production from hepatocytes.[24] However, there is often overlap in CRP levels between patients with bacterial and nonbacterial infections, making them difficult to distinguish. A metaanalysis of CRP in community-acquired pneumonia showed widely varying sensitivity and specificity estimates with significant heterogeneity.[25] Similarly, a metaanalysis of patients with fever of unknown origin failed to show utility for CRP in identifying patients with bacterial vs. nonbacterial infection.[23] However, CRP may have greater utility in distinguishing between bacterial and nonbacterial illness in the critically ill population than in the general hospital population. In a study of 16 ICU patients with H1N1 influenza and 9 ICU patients with bacterial pneumonia, CRP levels were much lower in the H1N1 population (mean, 118 mg/L vs. 363 mg/L).[26] In this study, a CRP cutoff of >200 mg/L identified patients with bacterial pneumonia with 100% sensitivity and 87.5% specificity. Similarly, a cohort study of 76 patients with presumed severe acute respiratory syndrome (SARS) revealed average CRP levels of only 39 mg/L in this population.[27]

Limited data is available for CRP in the context of fungal infection. A single-center study of immunocompromised patients showed that CRP levels were elevated in the context of invasive fungal infections (range, 112–269 mg/L), albeit to a lesser degree than in patients with bacteremia (range, 160–387 mg/L).[28] Another study of post-surgical patients at high risk of fungal infection showed that a CRP cutoff of 100 mg/L was helpful in distinguishing bacterial from fungal infection with a sensitivity of 82% and specificity of 53%.[29] Thus, high CRP levels favor bacterial over fungal causes of infection, but further work is required to clarify appropriate cutoffs as well as to determine sensitivity and specificity.

The utility of CRP as an infection marker increases when combined with other markers. Póvoa et al.[30] reported a prospective observational study of 112 ICU patients in which CRP ≥87 mg/L and temperature ≥38.2 had a specificity of 100% (and sensitivity of 50%) for infectious causes of inflammation. In a separate study, an "infection probability score" incorporating CRP >60 mg/L along with fever, tachycardia, elevated white blood cell count, tachypnea, and elevated sequential organ failure assessment (SOFA) score showed nearly 90% sensitivity and specificity in diagnosing infection in ICU patients.[31]

C-Reactive Protein as a Marker of Postoperative Infection

CRP has also shown utility in the diagnosis of postoperative infections, particularly in patients undergoing major abdominal surgery. CRP levels always rise postoperatively, peaking around postoperative day 3 (POD3).[32,33] However, persistently high CRP levels after POD3 are suggestive of infection. Retrospective studies have shown that elevated postoperative CRP levels (>190 mg/L on POD3 or >140 mg/L on POD4 or POD5) have a sensitivity of 66%–82% and a specificity of 77%–86% for infection.[34–36] Prospective studies have generally confirmed these results; a prospective study of 151 mixed surgical patients showed that CRP >100 mg/L on POD5 had a sensitivity of 69% and specificity of 64% for infection,[33] while a separate study of 50 patients showed that CRP >130 mg/L on POD4 had a sensitivity and specificity of 80% for anastomotic leak. A large prospective study is currently underway with 500 patients, which should provide more clarity on this issue.[37]

C-Reactive Protein as a Marker of Nosocomial Infections

Daily CRP measurements have been studied as a strategy for early detection of nosocomial infections in the ICU. In a prospective observational study, Póvoa et al.[38] evaluated daily CRP measurements in 63 ICU patients with documented ICU-acquired infection ($n = 35$) vs. successful ICU discharge without infection ($n = 28$). In patients with ICU-acquired infection, both temperature and CRP levels increased significantly in 5 days leading up to diagnosis ($P < .001$). Absolute CRP >87 mg/L and daily CRP variation >41 mg/L were both characteristic of infection. When combined, they showed a sensitivity of 92% and specificity of 82% for ICU-acquired infection.[38]

C-Reactive Protein as a Marker of Treatment Success and Failure

CRP can also be used to monitor antibiotic therapy in the critically ill population. Schmit and Vincent[39] conducted a prospective observational study of 50 ICU patients with community-acquired or nosocomial infection: 24 had a favorable response to antibiotics, 18 required a change in antibiotics (as determined by the treating physician), and 8 required a procedure to control the infection.[39] Mean CRP levels rose from Day 0 (initiation of antibiotics) to Day 1 in all groups; however, patients with a favorable response to antibiotics showed a rapid decrease after Day 1 compared with patients requiring a change in antibiotics. An increase in CRP of ≥22 mg/L in the first 48 hours of therapy was associated with ineffective antibiotic therapy with a sensitivity of 77% and specificity of 67%.[39] Treating physicians were not blinded to CRP levels, so rises in CRP may have contributed to the decision to change antibiotics in some patients. A separate cohort study of 68 patients with ventilator-associated pneumonia showed that CRP levels declined significantly within 96 hours of initiating adequate antibiotic therapy but not in patients receiving inadequate antibiotic therapy.[40] A decline of at least 20% in CRP at 96 hours had a sensitivity of 77% and specificity of 87% for effective antibiotic therapy.[40] Finally, amongst hospitalized patients with severe community-acquired pneumonia, appropriate antibiotic therapy was associated with a >60% decrease in CRP by Day 3 of antibiotic therapy and >90% decrease by Day 7.[41] Thus adequate antibiotic therapy is generally associated with significant decreases in CRP by Day 3 or 4 of therapy; however, this effect may be more pronounced in non-ICU patients than in ICU patients.

PROCALCITONIN

Structure and Function

PCT is the 116 amino acid precursor of the calcium-regulating peptide calcitonin. Under normal conditions, the CALC-1 gene is transcribed into PCT in the thyroid C-cells and then cleaved to form calcitonin. PCT is virtually undetectable in the serum of healthy individuals (<0.05 ng/L).[42] In the context of infection, however, CALC-1 expression is upregulated in various tissues including the neuroendocrine cells of the liver and lung,[43] adipocytes,[44] and macrophages.[45] These tissues lack the ability to cleave PCT into calcitonin, leading to a rapid rise in serum PCT levels.[42]

Expression of PCT in nonthryoid tissues is stimulated by bacterial lipopolysaccharides (endotoxin) as well as inflammatory cytokines, IL-6 and IL-1. Conversely, the viral mediator interferon-γ has an inhibitory effect on PCT expression.[44] However, PCT is not entirely specific to bacterial infection. Noninfectious causes of PCT elevation include neuroendocrine malignancies, such as small cell lung cancer, C-cell carcinoma of the thyroid gland, and neuroendocrine tumors of the gastrointestinal tract.[46] Additional causes include acute illnesses such as cardiac arrest,[47] pancreatitis,[48] rhabdomyolysis,[49] and trauma.[50] Finally, PCT levels increase postoperatively, particularly in patients undergoing intestinal surgery.[51] PCT elevations in patients with noninfectious inflammation, however, are typically lower than in those with bacterial infection.[52]

Procalcitonin Dynamics

In the context of bacterial infection, PCT rise has a rapid onset of 2–4 hours and a half-life of 22–26 hours.[42] Peak PCT levels occur 24–48 hours after the onset of symptoms.[52] Clearance of PCT is also comparatively rapid: PCT levels fall to <50% by Day 4 of ICU admission and to near-normal levels by Day 7 even in septic patients. PCT clearance is slightly delayed (30%–50%) in the context of significant renal failure.[53] In patients without renal failure, delayed clearance of PCT is suggestive of treatment failure.[54]

Procalcitonin as a Biomarker of Infection in the ICU

Numerous studies have examined the utility of PCT as a marker of infection in ICU patients. A recent metaanalysis of data from 30 studies determined a pooled sensitivity of 77% and specificity of 79% in distinguishing infection from noninfectious systemic inflammation.[55] Across all studies, prevalence of infection averaged 60% (range, 34%–88%) and PCT cutoff averaged 1.1 ng/mL. A subanalysis comparing surgical and trauma patients with medical patients showed that PCT was slightly more accurate in surgical and trauma patients than in medical patients.[55]

A separate metaanalysis examined PCT as a marker of bacteremia in hospitalized patients.[56] Amongst ICU patients ($n = 399$), the sensitivity and specificity of PCT for bacteremia vs. noninfectious inflammation was 89% and 68%, respectively. The authors calculated the optimal PCT cutoff to be 0.5 ng/mL. Of note, the lowest sensitivity was among immunocompromised patients at only 66% (with a specificity of 78%).[56]

PCT also shows good diagnostic accuracy in distinguishing bacterial from viral infection. A metaanalysis of two pediatric studies and an adult meningitis study indicated that PCT had a sensitivity of 92% and specificity of 73% for diagnosing bacterial vs. viral infection (cutoff range, 0.5–5 ng/mL).[22] Studies of patients with life-threatening viral illnesses, including SARS and influenza H1N1, have also confirmed low levels of PCT in these populations.[57] A cohort study of H1N1 patients ($n = 16$) documented PCT levels of 0.2–5.9 ng/mL in these patients compared with 8.2–81.5 ng/mL in a comparator group with severe community-acquired bacterial pneumonia ($n = 9$).[26]

PCT is also effective in distinguishing bacterial infections from invasive fungal infections. A retrospective study of PCT levels in patients with bacteremia and fungemia showed that PCT >1.6 ng/mL had a sensitivity of 77% and specificity of 96% for distinguishing patients with gram-negative bacteremia from those with fungemia.[58] A separate study of immunocompromised patients showed significantly higher PCT levels in 21 patients with bacteremia (quartile range, 2.6–7.1 ng/mL) than in 13 patients with fungemia (quartile range, 0.1–0.5 ng/mL). The authors noted that a low PCT <0.5 ng/mL combined with a moderately elevated CRP <300 mg/L was 85% specific and 81% sensitive for fungemia in this population. Thus, elevated CRP levels in the context of a low PCT level should prompt consideration of nonbacterial infection.

Procalcitonin as a Marker of Postoperative Infection

PCT can be used to identify patients with postoperative infections. A prospective study of 205 patients undergoing elective colorectal surgery reported that a PCT level >0.31 ng/mL on POD4 was 100% sensitive and 72% specific for major anastomotic leak requiring reoperation.[59] This was confirmed in a multicenter observational trial (PREDICS: Procalcitonin reveals early dehiscence in colorectal surgery) that included 504 patients undergoing elective surgery for malignancy. In this study a PCT >2.7 ng/mL on POD3 was 59.3% sensitive and 91.7% specific for anastomotic leak.[60] Patients with other complications (e.g., bleeding, local wound infection, and cardiac problems) showed more modest elevations in PCT (median, 1.0 ng/mL).[60]

In cardiac surgery patients, elevated PCT levels are also indicative of postoperative infection. In a cohort of 100 cardiac surgery patients, PCT >1.5 ng/mL on POD 3 showed a sensitivity of 93% and specificity of 80% in diagnosing infectious complications, including postoperative pneumonia, mediastinitis, and bacteremia.[61]

In neurosurgical patients PCT levels do not increase routinely postoperatively, whereas CRP and white blood cell counts do.[62] Serum PCT levels have not proven useful in diagnosing postoperative infections in neurosurgical patients.[63] However, cerebrospinal fluid (CSF) PCT levels may be helpful. A case series of patients with bacterial, viral, and post-neurosurgical meningitis showed that PCT >0.9 ng/mL in CSF was 93% sensitive and 67% specific for meningitis. Although the post-neurosurgical meningitis group was small, all 10 patients had CSF PCT levels >0.9 ng/mL.[64] Unfortunately, the study did not include neurosurgical patients without meningitis. A recent study from China examined

93 neurosurgical patients suspected of post-surgical infection. CSF PCT averaged 0.35 ng/mL (range, 0.13–2.74 ng/mL) in noninfected patients, whereas CSF PCT averaged 0.76 ng/mL (range, 0.24–4.67 ng/mL) in infected patients. The authors did not calculate sensitivity and specificity, but the area under the receiver operating curve for CSF PCT was 0.80 (95% confidence interval = 0.71–0.90), and the authors recommended a cutoff of 0.425 ng/mL.[65]

Procalcitonin as a Marker of Nosocomial Infection in the ICU

PCT has not been widely studied in the context of ICU-acquired infections. In one study of 49 trauma patients admitted to the ICU, average PCT level on the day prior to infection diagnosis was 0.85 ng/mL, rising to 2.1 ng/mL on the day of diagnosis.[18] In the same cohort CRP showed almost no correlation with infection diagnosis, averaging 153 mg/L on the day prior to diagnosis and rising to 174 mg/L on the day of diagnosis.[18]

Procalcitonin as a Marker of Treatment Success or Failure

The PRORATA trial (use of PCT to reduce patients' exposure to antibiotics in ICU) was a multicenter, prospective, parallel-group, open-label trial that studied the benefits of PCT-guided antibiotic treatment. Patients in the PCT group were subjected to two interventions: a PCT-guided threshold for initiation of antibiotics and a PCT-guided threshold for discontinuation of antibiotics.[66] At the onset of infectious symptoms, antibiotic initiation was encouraged for patients with PCT levels ≥0.5 ng/mL but not below this threshold. After antibiotics were initiated, daily PCT levels were measured and discontinuation of antibiotics was encouraged if the PCT level dropped below 0.25 ng/mL or if it was <0.5 ng/mL and at least 80% decreased from peak.[66] These two interventions resulted in a significant decrease in antibiotic usage (812 vs. 653 days of antibiotic exposure per 1000 inpatient days) without any corresponding increase in mortality or ICU length of stay.[66]

A follow-up study from 15 ICUs in the Netherlands followed a similar format and again showed a reduction in antibiotic use with no increase in mortality or length of ICU stay.[67] It also demonstrated cost savings associated with fewer days of antibiotics; however, this was counterbalanced by the costs of daily PCT measurements. The authors calculated that a PCT assay cost of <4€ per sample would achieve overall cost savings in their study centers.[67] A third multicenter trial from Germany showed a more modest reduction in antibiotic usage (823 vs. 862 days of antibiotic exposure per 1000 ICU days); however, PCT testing was only performed on Days 1, 4, 7, 10, and 14 of antibiotic therapy.[68] The treating physicians overruled the algorithm in >50% of cases, casting doubts on the practicality of this protocol. Once again, there were no significant differences between the groups in terms of mortality or ICU length of stay.[68] Thus PCT-guided antibiotic prescribing shows promise in the reduction of unnecessary antibiotic use but may require daily PCT testing to be efficacious.

CONCLUSION

Both CRP and PCT are helpful biomarkers to distinguish infection from noninfectious systemic inflammation in ICU patients. Metaanalyses suggest similar sensitivities for both markers in the diagnosis of infection (75% for CRP vs. 77% for PCT), while PCT has a slightly higher specificity (67% for CRP vs. 79% for PCT). Cutoffs are in the range of 50–100 mg/L for CRP and 0.5–1.0 ng/mL for PCT. Extremely elevated CRP (>350 mg/L) or PCT levels (>5 ng/mL) should always prompt suspicion of bacterial etiology.

PCT may also help distinguish bacterial infections from invasive viral and fungal infections. Patients with severe viral illnesses, such as H1N1 and SARS, show low PCT levels, as do patients with invasive fungemia. Further studies are required to determine appropriate cutoffs.

In hospitalized patients, CRP and PCT can be used to help diagnose postoperative and nosocomial infections. Once again, PCT shows greater utility due to its greater specificity and faster clearance. Elevated PCT levels after POD3 are suggestive of postoperative infection, particularly anastomotic leak. In the neurosurgical population, CSF PCT levels may also be a helpful marker of postoperative meningitis.

Finally, both CRP and PCT can be used to monitor the efficacy of antibiotic therapy in ICU patients. In the context of appropriate antibiotic therapy CRP levels decline starting on Day 2 of treatment. Failure to show a decline in CRP levels is suggestive of treatment failure. PCT-guided antibiotic treatment protocols have been effective in reducing unnecessary antibiotic use by reducing antibiotic initiation and encouraging early discontinuation. Daily PCT levels may be required for these protocols to significantly affect physician behavior.

Distinguishing infectious from noninfectious inflammation in critically ill patients can be challenging. CRP and PCT are helpful adjuncts to other clinical parameters. Both are relatively inexpensive and widely available, thus ensuring their use for the foreseeable future. Understanding how to interpret these markers correctly is important for clinicians.

AUTHORS' RECOMMENDATIONS

- Both CRP and PCT are helpful in distinguishing infectious from noninfectious causes of systemic inflammation in ICU patients.
- CRP has a sensitivity of 75% and specificity of 65% for infection using a cutoff of 50–100 mg/L.
- PCT has a sensitivity of 77% and specificity of 79% for infection using a cutoff of 0.5–1.0 ng/mL.
- PCT is also useful in distinguishing bacterial infection from systemic viral and fungal infections, although ideal cut-offs remain to be determined.
- CRP and PCT levels decrease within 1–3 days after initiation of appropriate antibiotic therapy. Failure to show a decrease in CRP or PCT levels in this timeframe is suggestive of treatment failure.
- PCT-guided antibiotic treatment protocols can be used to guide antibiotic initiation and discontinuation, thereby reducing unnecessary use of antibiotics in the ICU.

REFERENCES

1. Singer M, Deutschman CS, Seymour CW, et al. The Third International Consensus definitions for sepsis and septic shock (Sepsis-3). *JAMA*. 2016;315(8):801-810.
2. Rhodes A, Evans LE, Alhazzani W, et al. Surviving Sepsis Campaign: international guidelines for management of sepsis and septic shock: 2016. *Intensive Care Med*. 2017;43(3):304-377.
3. Funk DJ, Kumar A. Antimicrobial therapy for life-threatening infections: speed is life. *Crit Care Clin*. 2011;27(1):53-76.
4. Ibrahim EH, Sherman G, Ward S, Fraser VJ, Kollef MH. The influence of inadequate antimicrobial treatment of bloodstream infections on patient outcomes in the ICU setting. *Chest*. 2000;118(1):146-155.
5. Laxminarayan R, Duse A, Wattal C, et al. Antibiotic resistance-the need for global solutions. *Lancet Infect Dis*. 2013;13(12):1057-1098.
6. Tillett WS, Francis T. Serological reactions in pneumonia with a non-protein somatic fraction of pneumococcus. *J Exp Med*. 1930;52(4):561-571.
7. MacLeod CM, Avery OT. The occurrence during acute infections of a protein not normally present in the blood: III. Immunological properties of the c-reactive protein and its differentiation from normal blood proteins. *J Exp Med*. 1941;73(2):191-200.
8. Pepys MB, Hirschfield GM. C-reactive protein: a critical update. *J Clin Invest*. 2003;111(12):1805-1812.
9. Volanakis JE. Human C-reactive protein: expression, structure, and function. *Mol Immunol*. 2001;38(2-3):189-197.
10. Mantovani A, Garlanda C, Doni A, Bottazzi B. Pentraxins in innate immunity: from C-reactive protein to the long pentraxin PTX3. *J Clin Immunol*. 2008;28(1):1-13.
11. Thompson D, Pepys MB, Wood SP. The physiological structure of human C-reactive protein and its complex with phosphocholine. *Structure*. 1999;7(2):169-177.
12. Suresh MV, Singh SK, Ferguson Jr DA, Agrawal A. Role of the property of C-reactive protein to activate the classical pathway of complement in protecting mice from pneumococcal infection. *J Immunol*. 2006;176(7):4369-4374.
13. Black S, Kushner I, Samols D. C-reactive protein. *J Biol Chem*. 2004;279(47):48487-48490.
14. Eklund C, Huttunen R, Syrjänen J, Laine J, Vuento R, Hurme M. Polymorphism of the C-reactive protein gene is associated with mortality in bacteraemia. *Scand J Infect Dis*. 2006;38(11-12):1069-1073.
15. Imhof A, Fröhlich M, Loewel H, et al. Distributions of C-reactive protein measured by high-sensitivity assays in apparently healthy men and women from different populations in Europe. *Clin Chem*. 2003;49(4):669-672.
16. Landry A, Docherty P, Ouellette S, Cartier LJ. Causes and outcomes of markedly elevated C-reactive protein levels. *Can Fam Physician*. 2017;63(6):e316-e323.
17. Young B, Gleeson M, Cripps AW. C-reactive protein: a critical review. *Pathology*. 1991;23(2):118-124.
18. Castelli GP, Pognani C, Cita M, Stuani A, Sgarbi L, Paladini R. Procalcitonin, C-reactive protein, white blood cells and SOFA score in ICU: diagnosis and monitoring of sepsis. *Minerva Anestesiol*. 2006;72(1-2):69-80.
19. Póvoa P. C-reactive protein: a valuable marker of sepsis. *Intensive Care Med*. 2002;28(3):235-243.
20. Sierra R, Rello J, Bailén MA, et al. C-reactive protein used as an early indicator of infection in patients with systemic inflammatory response syndrome. *Intensive Care Med*. 2004;30(11):2038-2045.
21. Castelli GP, Pognani C, Meisner M, Stuani A, Bellomi D, Sgarbi L. Procalcitonin and C-reactive protein during systemic inflammatory response syndrome, sepsis and organ dysfunction. *Crit Care*. 2004;8 (4):R234-R242.
22. Simon L, Gauvin F, Amre DK, Saint-Louis P, Lacroix J. Serum procalcitonin and C-reactive protein levels as markers of bacterial infection: a systematic review and meta-analysis. *Clin Infect Dis*. 2004;39(2):206-217.
23. Hu L, Shi Q, Shi M, Liu R, Wang C. Diagnostic value of PCT and CRP for detecting serious bacterial infections in patients with fever of unknown origin: a systematic review and meta-analysis. *Appl Immunohistochem Mol Morphol*. 2017;25(8):e61-e69.
24. Enocsson H, Sjöwall C, Skogh T, Eloranta ML, Rönnblom L, Wetterö J. Interferon-alpha mediates suppression of C-reactive protein: explanation for muted C-reactive protein response in lupus flares? *Arthritis Rheum*. 2009;60(12):3755-3760.
25. van der Meer V, Neven AK, van den Broek PJ, Assendelft WJ. Diagnostic value of C reactive protein in infections of the lower respiratory tract: systematic review. *BMJ*. 2005;331(7507):26.
26. Ingram PR, Inglis T, Moxon D, Speers D. Procalcitonin and C-reactive protein in severe 2009 H1N1 influenza infection. *Intensive Care Med*. 2010;36(3):528-532.
27. Wang JT, Sheng WH, Fang CT, et al. Clinical manifestations, laboratory findings, and treatment outcomes of SARS patients. *Emerg Infect Dis*. 2004;10(5):818-824.
28. Marková M, Brodská H, Malíčková K, et al. Substantially elevated C-reactive protein (CRP), together with low levels of procalcitonin (PCT), contributes to diagnosis of fungal infection in immunocompromised patients. *Support Care Cancer*. 2013;21(10):2733-2742.
29. Martini A, Gottin L, Menestrina N, et al. Procalcitonin levels in surgical patients at risk of candidemia. *J Infect*. 2010;60(6):425-430.
30. Póvoa P, Coelho L, Almeida E, et al. C-reactive protein as a marker of infection in critically ill patients. *Clin Microbiol Infect*. 2005;11(2):101-108.
31. Peres Bota D, Mélot C, Lopes Ferreira F, Vincent JL. Infection Probability Score (IPS): a method to help assess the probability of infection in critically ill patients. *Crit Care Med*. 2003;31(11):2579-2584.
32. Meyer ZC, Schreinemakers JM, Mulder PG, de Waal RA, Ermens AA, van der Laan L. The role of C-reactive protein and the SOFA score as parameter for clinical decision making in surgical patients during the intensive care unit course. *PLoS One*. 2013;8(2):e55964.
33. Santonocito C, De Loecker I, Donadello K, et al. C-reactive protein kinetics after major surgery. *Anesth Analg*. 2014;119(3):624-629.
34. Warschkow R, Tarantino I, Torzewski M, Näf F, Lange J, Steffen T. Diagnostic accuracy of C-reactive protein and white blood cell counts in the early detection of inflammatory complications after open resection of colorectal cancer: a retrospective study of 1,187 patients. *Int J Colorectal Dis*. 2011;26(11):1405-1413.
35. Kørner H, Nielsen HJ, Søreide JA, Nedrebø BS, Søreide K, Knapp JC. Diagnostic accuracy of C-reactive protein for intraabdominal infections after colorectal resections. *J Gastrointest Surg*. 2009;13(9):1599-1606.
36. Welsch T, Müller SA, Ulrich A, et al. C-reactive protein as early predictor for infectious postoperative complications in rectal surgery. *Int J Colorectal Dis*. 2007;22(12):1499-1507.

37. U.S. National Library of Medicine. Inflammatory markers after colorectal surgery (IMACORS). ClinicalTrials.gov (website). 2017. Available at: https://clinicaltrials.gov/ct2/show/ NCT01510314. Accessed September 5, 2018.

38. Póvoa P, Coelho L, Almeida E, et al. Early identification of intensive care unit-acquired infections with daily monitoring of C-reactive protein: a prospective observational study. *Crit Care*. 2006;10(2):R63.

39. Schmit X, Vincent JL. The time course of blood C-reactive protein concentrations in relation to the response to initial antimicrobial therapy in patients with sepsis. *Infection*. 2008;36(3):213-219.

40. Lisboa T, Seligman R, Diaz E, Rodriguez A, Teixeira PJ, Rello J. C-reactive protein correlates with bacterial load and appropriate antibiotic therapy in suspected ventilator-associated pneumonia. *Crit Care Med*. 2008;36(1):166–171.

41. Bruns AH, Oosterheert JJ, Hak E, Hoepelman AI. Usefulness of consecutive C-reactive protein measurements in follow-up of severe community-acquired pneumonia. *Eur Respir J*. 2008;32(3):726-732.

42. Davies J. Procalcitonin. *J Clin Pathol*. 2015;68(9):675-679.

43. Russwurm S, Stonans I, Stonane E, et al. Procalcitonin and CGRP-1 mrna expression in various human tissues. *Shock*. 2001;16:109-112.

44. Linscheid P, Seboek D, Nylen ES, et al. In vitro and in vivo calcitonin I gene expression in parenchymal cells: a novel product of human adipose tissue. *Endocrinology*. 2003;144(12):5578-5584.

45. Linscheid P, Seboek D, Schaer DJ, Zulewski H, Keller U, Müller B. Expression and secretion of procalcitonin and calcitonin gene-related peptide by adherent monocytes and by macrophage-activated adipocytes. *Crit Care Med*. 2004;32(8):1715-1721.

46. Durnaś B, Wątek M, Wollny T, et al. Utility of blood procalcitonin concentration in the management of cancer patients with infections. *Onco Targets Ther*. 2016;9:469-475.

47. Annborn M, Dankiewicz J, Erlinge D, et al. Procalcitonin after cardiac arrest - an indicator of severity of illness, ischemia-reperfusion injury and outcome. *Resuscitation*. 2013;84(6):782-787.

48. Mofidi R, Suttie SA, Patil PV, Ogston S, Parks RW. The value of procalcitonin at predicting the severity of acute pancreatitis and development of infected pancreatic necrosis: systematic review. *Surgery*. 2009;146(1):72-81.

49. Jaffe AS, Vasile VC, Milone M, Saenger AK, Olson KN, Apple FS. Diseased skeletal muscle: a noncardiac source of increased circulating concentrations of cardiac troponin T. *J Am Coll Cardiol*. 2011;58(17):1819-1824.

50. Mimoz O, Benoist JF, Edouard AR, Assicot M, Bohuon C, Samii K. Procalcitonin and C-reactive protein during the early posttraumatic systemic inflammatory response syndrome. *Intensive Care Med*. 1998;24(2):185-188.

51. Meisner M, Tschaikowsky K, Hutzler A, Schick C, Schüttler J. Postoperative plasma concentrations of procalcitonin after different types of surgery. *Intensive Care Med*. 1998;24(7):680-684.

52. Meisner M. Update on procalcitonin measurements. *Ann Lab Med*. 2014;34(4):263-273.

53. Meisner M, Lohs T, Huettemann E, Schmidt J, Hueller M, Reinhart K. The plasma elimination rate and urinary secretion of procalcitonin in patients with normal and impaired renal function. *Eur J Anaesthesiol*. 2001;18(2):79-87.

54. Ryu JA, Yang JH, Lee D, et al. Clinical usefulness of procalcitonin and C-reactive protein as outcome predictors in critically ill patients with severe sepsis and septic shock. *PLoS One*. 2015;10(9):e0138150.

55. Wacker C, Prkno A, Brunkhorst FM, Schlattmann P. Procalcitonin as a diagnostic marker for sepsis: a systematic review and meta-analysis. *Lancet Infect Dis*. 2013;13(5):426-435.

56. Hoeboer SH, van der Geest PJ, Nieboer D, Groeneveld AB. The diagnostic accuracy of procalcitonin for bacteraemia: a systematic review and meta-analysis. *Clin Microbiol Infect*. 2015;21(5):474-481.

57. Gilbert DN. Use of plasma procalcitonin levels as an adjunct to clinical microbiology. *J Clin Microbiol*. 2010;48(7):2325-2329.

58. Leli C, Ferranti M, Moretti A, Al Dhahab ZS, Cenci E, Mencacci A. Procalcitonin levels in gram-positive, gram-negative, and fungal bloodstream infections. *Dis Markers*. 2015;2015:701480.

59. Garcia-Granero A, Frasson M, Flor-Lorente B, et al. Procalcitonin and C-reactive protein as early predictors of anastomotic leak in colorectal surgery. *Dis Colon Rectum*. 2013;56(4):475-483.

60. Giaccaglia V, Salvi PF, Antonelli MS, et al. Procalcitonin reveals early dehiscence in colorectal surgery: the PREDICS Study. *Ann Surg*. 2016;263(5):967-972.

61. Jebali MA, Hausfater P, Abbes Z, Aouni Z, Riou B, Ferjani M. Assessment of the accuracy of procalcitonin to diagnose postoperative infection after cardiac surgery. *Anesthesiology*. 2007;107(2):232-238.

62. Laifer G, Wasner M, Sendi P, et al. Dynamics of serum procalcitonin in patients after major neurosurgery. *Clin Microbiol Infect*. 2005;11(8):679-681.

63. Rotman LE, Agee BS, Chagoya G, Davis MC, Markert JM. Clinical utility of serum procalcitonin level and infection in the neurosurgical intensive care unit. *World Neurosurg*. 2018;112:e368-e374.

64. Alons IM, Verheul RJ, Kuipers I, et al. Procalcitonin in cerebrospinal fluid in meningitis: a prospective diagnostic study. *Brain Behav*. 2016;6(11):e00545.

65. Yu Y, Li HJ. Diagnostic and prognostic value of procalcitonin for early intracranial infection after craniotomy. *Braz J Med Biol Res*. 2017;50(5):e6021.

66. Bouadma L, Luyt CE, Tubach F, et al. Use of procalcitonin to reduce patients' exposure to antibiotics in intensive care units (PRORATA trial): a multicentre randomised controlled trial. *Lancet*. 2010;375(9713):463-474.

67. de Jong E, van Oers JA, Beishuizen A, et al. Efficacy and safety of procalcitonin guidance in reducing the duration of antibiotic treatment in critically ill patients: a randomised, controlled, open-label trial. *Lancet Infect Dis*. 2016;16(7): 819-827.

68. Bloos F, Trips E, Nierhaus A, et al. Effect of sodium selenite administration and procalcitonin-guided therapy on mortality in patients with severe sepsis or septic shock: a randomized clinical trial. *JAMA Intern Med*. 2016;176(9):1266-1276.

47

What Is Ventilator-Associated Pneumonia? How Do I Diagnose It? How Do I Treat It?

Eman Ansari and Michael Klompas

INTRODUCTION

Ventilator-associated pneumonia (VAP) causes significant morbidity and mortality in the intensive care unit (ICU). VAP is defined as pneumonia that develops more than 48 hours following endotracheal intubation. It is associated with prolonged hospital stays and significant costs.[1] The estimated incidence of VAP varies widely and depends on how it is measured. In 2012, US hospitals reported VAP rates of 0.9 events per 1000 ventilator-days in medical ICUs and 2.0 events per 1000 ventilator-days in surgical ICUs.[2] An independent audit by the Centers for Medicare and Medicaid Services (CMS), however, found VAP rates of about 10% within selected populations.[3] Evidence-based understandings of risk factors, accurate diagnosis, and appropriate management are discussed in this chapter.

PATHOGENESIS

Risk factors for VAP can be divided into three categories: host factors, hospital and unit factors, and pathogen-related factors.

Host Factors

Microaspiration of oropharyngeal and gastrointestinal organisms is the predominant route of infection[4] (Box 47.1).

Hospital and Unit Factors

Patients become colonized with hospital pathogens (e.g., *Staphylococcus aureus, Pseudomonas aeruginosa,* and other gram-negative bacilli [GNBs]) within 48 hours of admission.[15] Accurate and frequently updated knowledge of local pathogens and their susceptibility profiles is essential to inform empiric antimicrobial treatment strategies.

Pathogen-Related Factors

In addition to hospital-acquired pathogens, patients' baseline flora may also cause VAP, especially within the first few days after admission to the hospital. The number and virulence of the pathogens aspirated contribute to the risk of developing pneumonia. Aerobic GNBs (e.g., *P. aeruginosa*) and gram-positive cocci (e.g., *S. aureus*) remain the most common organisms causing VAP, while other bacteria, including anaerobes,[16] fungi, and parasites are rare, unless the patient is immunocompromised.[17,18] There is increasing appreciation that a significant fraction of VAPs may be caused by respiratory viruses.[19,20] Multidrug-resistant (MDR) organisms are major concerns for patients with VAP.[21] Prior antibiotic exposure and duration of health-care exposure factors are independent determinants of risk for acquiring MDR organisms (Box 47.2).

DIAGNOSIS

The 2016 IDSA/ATS (Infectious Diseases Society of America and the American Thoracic Society) guidelines recommend suspecting VAP in a patient with new or progressive pulmonary infiltrate *plus* new onset of at least two or three of the following factors: fever, purulent sputum, leukocytosis, and decline in oxygenation.[1,22] However, VAP is a notoriously difficult condition to diagnose. The constellation of fever, purulent sputum, leukocytosis, and a new infiltrate is only 69% sensitive and 75% specific for pneumonia compared with postmortem pathologic findings.[23] Neither clinical signs nor radiographs alone are reliable diagnostic tools for VAP.[24,25] The difficulty of diagnosing VAP compels humility and a readiness to revise one's diagnosis depending on each patient's clinical trajectory. Patients that rapidly improve after endotracheal suctioning, pulmonary toilet, diuretics, or recruitment procedures most likely do not have VAP and do not require antibiotics.

Screening Tests (Initial Detection)
Clinical Evidence of VAP

Patients with VAP can exhibit a gradual or sudden onset of symptoms and signs that include fever, tachypnea, increased secretions, purulent sputum, hemoptysis, and/or worsening hypoxia.[26] On auscultation, their breath sounds may reveal rhonchi, crackles, or wheezing, or may be diminished at the site of pulmonary consolidation. Their measured ventilatory parameters may show declining compliance in the form of increased inspiratory pressure, decreased tidal volume, or increased respiratory rate, depending on the patient's ventilator mode. Impaired oxygenation is a sine qua non of pneumonia in ventilated patients. It is therefore helpful to assess serial ventilator settings to look for a rise in fraction of inspired oxygen (FiO_2) or positive end-expiratory pressure (PEEP) to support a diagnosis of VAP. Patients with minimal and stable ventilator settings most likely do not have VAP or have mild pneumonias at best; positive pulmonary cultures in this population are more likely to represent colonization rather than infection.[27]

Laboratory Evidence of VAP

Patients with new-onset VAP may have leukocytosis or, occasionally, leukopenia. If a blood gas analysis is obtained, patients may have hypoxemia or hypercarbia secondary to impaired alveolar gas exchange. Evidence for the role of procalcitonin and C-reactive protein (CRP) in establishing the diagnosis of VAP remains weak.[28] However, serial procalcitonin monitoring may help clinicians to shorten duration of treatment[29] (see Chapter 46).

Imaging

Chest imaging is an integral component in the diagnosis of VAP. A chest radiograph (CXR) may show either a new or an expanding alveolar infiltrate in one or multiple lobes, air bronchograms, pleural effusion, cavitation, pneumatoceles, or pneumothorax. Portable chest radiographs can both overcall and undercall the presence of pneumonia. If clinical signs for VAP are ambiguous, consider computed tomography (CT), as this can help affirm or refute a diagnosis of VAP, particularly if a contrast study is possible. CT can help reveal the presence of an infiltrate not clearly seen on portable CXR and differentiate among atelectasis, pulmonary edema, and consolidation. CT can also be useful in patients who are failing to respond to antibiotic therapy. CT in these cases may reveal a pyogenic complication such as lung abscess or empyema that may require drainage.

Microbiologic Tests (Confirmation)

Current guidelines strongly advise microbiologic sampling whenever VAP is suspected. Both lower respiratory tract specimens and blood cultures must be obtained. Positive cultures can inform the best choice of antibiotic. Negative cultures in a patient who is clinically improving can support a decision to stop antibiotics. Culture data are also necessary at the unit and hospital level to establish the local distribution of pathogens associated with VAP and their susceptibility patterns. These are vital pieces of data to inform future decision making around empiric antibiotic choices for possible VAP. Diagnostic samples should be obtained before antibiotics are started or changed in order to maximize yield.

Respiratory Tract Sampling

There are several methods to obtain a respiratory sample. These methods vary in accuracy, cost, complexity, and risk for complications. Even though both the US and European guidelines recommend lower respiratory tract sampling, the US guidelines favor noninvasive sampling with semi-quantitative cultures to diagnose VAP,[1] while the European guidelines favor invasive sampling with quantitative cultures.[30] The European guidelines favor invasive methods on the basis of a single French study that found that invasive sampling may decrease antibiotic utilization.[31] The US preference for noninvasive sampling is based on a meta-analysis of randomized controlled trials (including the French study) that show no differences in mortality, length of stay, or antibiotic changes with invasive vs. noninvasive sampling.[32] As such, they prefer noninvasive sampling because invasive sampling is more difficult, higher cost, and carries some risks.

A. **Invasive respiratory sampling:** invasive samples of the lower respiratory tract may be less prone to contamination by upper airway organisms compared with noninvasive methods. Invasive methods include:

i. Bronchoscopy, which allows one to inspect the airways for signs of infection and for any other pathology that is possibly contributing to the patient's presentation. It requires a skilled physician and has risks for barotrauma and hypoxemia. Two main types of studies are available—bronchoalveolar lavage (BAL) and protected specimen brush (PSB).

ii. Nonbronchoscopic methods, which include bronchial washings and mini-BAL. These methods can be done by nurses and respiratory therapists and can be safely accomplished in patients who cannot tolerate bronchoscopic procedures. In mini-BAL, a catheter is blindly advanced through an endotracheal tube (ETT) until resistance is encountered; BAL is then performed per standard technique similar to bronchoscopic BAL. In addition to the risks known to BAL, this method carries a higher risk of endobronchial perforation, and the BAL sample is less likely to be a deep alveolar one compared with a bronchoscopic sample.

B. **Noninvasive respiratory sampling:** this includes endotracheal aspirates without instillation of saline into the lungs. This method has multiple advantages, including low cost and low risk of complications, and can be done by nonphysicians with limited training. Even though it is least likely to sample the alveoli, alveolar and airway pathogens are often similar in patients with pneumonia.

Processing of Respiratory Samples

All respiratory samples are sent for microscopic analyses and cultures.

Microscopic Analysis

Microscopic analysis includes cytospin, differential cell count, and Gram stain. The presence of intracellular bacteria is rare but highly suggestive of VAP. The absence of a predominance of neutrophils (<50%) makes VAP unlikely.[33]

Cultures

Respiratory cultures and blood cultures are an integral part of diagnosing VAP but clinicians need to appreciate their limitations. The sensitivity of pulmonary culture ranges from 48% to 75% and the positive predictive values range from 60% to 81% relative to histology depending on sampling method.[1] False positives are typically due to contamination of specimens with organisms colonizing the oropharynx or endotracheal tube. False negatives are typically due to prior exposure to antibiotics or failure to sample the exact segment of lung in which the pneumonia lies. Culture thus provides one more piece of data for clinicians to integrate along with everything else they know about their patient in order to make a decision such as their clinical signs, radiographic findings, clinical response to antibiotics, clinical response to noninfectious treatments (e.g., diuretics), competing diagnoses, etc.

a. Quantitative cultures: some laboratories are able to quantify culture yield. Different thresholds have been suggested

as diagnostic of VAP, depending on sampling method (e.g., $\geq 10^5$ colony-forming units (CFU)/mL for endotracheal aspirates, $>10^4$ CFU/mL for BAL, and $>10^3$ CFU for PSB) but these thresholds ought to be treated as guides rather than hard and fast cut-offs because pneumonia, like any other infectious condition, exists upon a continuum, and sampling technique, laboratory handling, and prior exposure to antibiotics impact yields.

b. Semiquantitative cultures: moderate or heavy bacterial growth in a patient with compatible signs is consistent but not diagnostic of VAP. No bacteria or light growth make VAP less likely.

c. Qualitative cultures: VAP is diagnosed based on a positive culture but no quantification is provided. This method is considered the most sensitive but least specific method to diagnose VAP.

Respiratory Viruses

There is increasing appreciation that substantial number of nosocomial pneumonias may be caused by respiratory viruses. Consider obtaining a respiratory virus PCR (polymerase chain reaction) panel, particularly during respiratory virus season.

DIFFERENTIAL DIAGNOSIS

All the cardinal signs associated with VAP are nonspecific and can also be seen in entities like acute respiratory distress syndrome (ARDS), aspiration pneumonia, cryptogenic organizing pneumonia, pulmonary embolism, vasculitis, pulmonary hemorrhage, pulmonary contusion, infiltrative tumors, and complications of blood transfusion (e.g., transfusion-related acute lung injury or TRALI), medications, or radiation. Lung biopsy may be necessary to differentiate between some of these conditions and ought to be considered in a patient with a progressive pulmonary syndrome that does not respond to antibiotics.

TREATMENT OF VAP

Once the diagnosis of VAP is suspected and respiratory samples and blood cultures have been sent, antibiotics should be started immediately in patients with shock or rapidly progressive hypoxemia because delays in this population are associated with increased mortality.[34,35] If the patient is clinically stable, however, consider watchful waiting alone while gathering more data to support or refute a diagnosis of pneumonia. Helpful data can include sequential vital signs and laboratory parameters such as leukocytes and biomarkers, culture results, and the patient's response to non-VAP therapies (such as deep suctioning to relieve mucous plugs, diuresis, and recruitment maneuvers).

MDR is defined as acquired nonsusceptibility to at least one agent in three different antimicrobial classes. Extensive drug-resistant (XDR) and pandrug-resistant (PDR) bacteria are defined as bacteria resistant to all but two antimicrobial classes, and to all antimicrobial agents, respectively.[36] When patients suffer from XDR or PDR, consultation with an infectious disease (ID) specialist is prudent to help select an appropriate antibiotic regimen.

Empiric Therapy

Empiric treatment for VAP should include coverage of *S. aureus* and GNB, especially *P. aeruginosa*, because the majority of VAPs are caused by these pathogens. Once there is a decision to treat, the choice and number of antibiotics should depend on host factors (e.g., ARDS, renal replacement therapy, septic shock), recent antibiotic exposures, prior pulmonary and nonpulmonary culture results, comorbidities (specifically renal function), hospital- and unit-specific predominant pathogens and their susceptibility patterns, Gram stain result if one was available, and other risk factors for acquiring drug-resistant bacteria (see Box 47.1). In addition, availability of an antibiotic, its cost, side-effect profile, and possible interactions with other medications are important considerations. If VAP is suspected in a patient already on antibiotics, it is generally advisable to change the class of antibiotics in case the patient has acquired a resistant organism.

Patients with VAP and **no risk factors** for MDR pathogens (see Box 47.2), can be treated with any single agent that is likely to cover >90% of *S. aureus* and *P. aeruginosa* in the clinician's institution. Possible options include piperacillin–tazobactam, cefepime, levofloxacin, or imipenem.

Patients **with risk factors** for MDRs should receive **two antibiotics** to target GNBs, specifically to *P. aeruginosa,* and a **third agent** to target methicillin-resistant *S. aureus* (MRSA). Combination gram-negative therapy to target MDR GNBs usually includes a spectrum beta-lactam *plus* either a fluoroquinolone, aminoglycoside, polymyxin, or aztreonam. MRSA can be treated with either linezolid or vancomycin.

Important Antimicrobial Considerations

- Aminoglycosides are not recommended as monotherapy given poor lung penetration and high risk for ear and kidney toxicity.
- If aminoglycosides must be used, then once-daily dosing is preferred for patients with normal renal function. Drug-level monitoring (a single peak level at 8–12 hours after the first dose followed by a trough level 30 minutes before the next planned dose and repeated at least weekly) is important to minimize nephrotoxicity.
- If *Legionella* is suspected, adding a fluoroquinolone is recommended as the second antipseudomonal agent.
- Fluoroquinolones are generally well tolerated but they can prolong the QT interval, potentiate risk for *Clostridium difficile*, and have been associated with neurotoxicity and tendinitis.
- Polymyxins are used in highly resistant GNBs in consultation with ID.

- Aerosolized aminoglycosides or polymyxins can be used as adjunctive therapy in patients who are failing to respond to intravenous treatment alone. Correctly administering aerosolized medications, however, is difficult and could require sedating and even paralyzing the patient to facilitate laminar airflow. Some case series report that up to 10% of patients who receive aerosolized medicines develop cardiorespiratory complications.[37] Expert societies recommend caution before using aerosolized antibiotics.[38]
- Methicillin-sensitive *S. aureus* (MSSA) should be treated with nafcillin, oxacillin, flucloxacillin, or cefazolin.
- Linezolid and vancomycin are associated with similar clinical outcomes for MRSA pneumonia. The choice of agent should therefore be informed by other considerations such as dosing convenience, renal function, blood cell counts, use of selective serotonin reuptake inhibitors (SSRIs), vascular access, and cost.
- The combination of piperacillin–tazobactam and vancomycin should used with caution due to increased risk of kidney injury.[39]
- In patients with history of penicillin or cephalosporin allergy, a thorough history for the type of reaction is important. Most patients with penicillin allergies can tolerate cephalosporins. Consultation with allergy for skin testing, simple graded challenge, and consideration for aztreonam may be necessary.
- In patients with renal insufficiency, most antibiotic doses will need to be adjusted and antibiotic levels measured, especially with aminoglycosides and vancomycin. Imipenem and cefepime have been associated with seizures in patients with underlying seizure disorders.[40]
- Infusions of beta-lactams have been associated with higher survival rates compared with intermittent dosing in critically ill patients with sepsis.[41] Prolonged infusions may also facilitate treating patients with higher minimum inhibitory concentrations (MICs).

De-Escalation of Antimocrobial Therapy

Following 48–72 hours of susceptibility pattern-guided empiric intravenous antibiotic therapy, culture results and clinical response should be reviewed. Antibiotic coverage should be continued, narrowed, or discontinued.

De-escalation is an important step in the management of VAP in order to minimize potential toxicity from antibiotics, risk of superinfection with other nosocomial pathogens like MRSA, or *Pseudomonas*, development of *C. difficile* infection, and promotion of selective pressure for more resistant bacteria.

In patients who are improving clinically on antibiotic therapy, antibiotics should be tailored to bacterial susceptibility results. For clinically improving patients with negative cultures at 48–72 hours, empiric treatment can be discontinued. For patients who are not improving after 48–72 hours of treatment, infection with resistant organisms, pyogenic complications of VAP, comorbidities impacting response to VAP treatments, and alternative diagnoses should all be considered. A CT scan and BAL are recommended.

Duration of Therapy

Both US and European guidelines recommend 7 days as the default duration of therapy for VAP for all pathogens, including *P. aeruginosa* and *S. aureus*.[1] Longer courses are associated with higher antibiotic toxicity, risk of superinfection, and selection of more resistant pathogens, with no significant added benefit.[42] Serial procalcitonin level monitoring can help clinicians to discontinue antibiotics safely after even <7 days of therapy.[28,29,43–45] A drop in the procalcitonin level by ≥80% from its peak value or to ≤0.5 g/L suggests it is safe to stop antibiotics in a patient that is clinically improving. Exceptions that warrant longer antibiotic courses include patients with pyogenic complications, persistent bacteremia, metastatic infections, and other complications. Consultation with an ID specialist is recommended. Once a patient is extubated and stable from a cardiopulmonary standpoint, parenteral antibiotics can be converted to oral formulations if an oral equivalent exists.

PREVENTION

Every effort to minimize the risk of VAP and its associated morbidity and mortality should be undertaken. Strategies to prevent VAP include avoiding intubation when possible (use noninvasive ventilation and/or high-flow nasal cannula instead); minimizing duration of intubation by implementing level-of-sedation goals and paired daily spontaneous awakening and breathing trials; limiting the use of neuromuscular blocking agents and antacids; and reducing the risk of aspiration by elevating the head of the bed.[46]

VENTILATOR-ASSOCIATED EVENT DEFINITIONS

The Centers for Disease Control and Prevention (CDC) developed ventilator-associated event (VAE) surveillance definitions in 2013. Their intent was to expand the breadth of surveillance (and thus the focus of prevention) beyond pneumonia alone while including other common and morbid complications in ventilated patients (such as pulmonary edema, ARDS, and atelectasis). VAE definitions were also designed to be more objective than traditional VAP definitions and amenable to automated surveillance using electronic health data.[47] The first VAE tier is ventilator-associated condition (VAC), which identifies patients with ≥2 days of sustained respiratory deteriorations (measured by increased PEEP and/or FiO_2) following at least 2 days of stability. Infection-related VAC (IVAC) is the second tier, where VAC patients develop fever or leukocytosis or leukopenia, and are started on one or more antibiotics that continue for ≥4 days. And finally, possible VAP (PVAP) is present in patients with IVAC who have microbial evidence of respiratory infection on Gram stain or culture.

AUTHORS' RECOMMENDATIONS

- Ventilator-associated pneumonia (VAP) is a difficult diagnosis. Consider VAP in patients with new or progressive pulmonary infiltrates *plus* new onset of at least two of the following factors: fever, purulent sputum, leukocytosis, and decline in oxygenation.
- A microbial respiratory tract sample and blood cultures are integral aspects of accurate diagnoses and can inform the type and duration of antimicrobial therapy.
- We recommend noninvasive lower respiratory tract sampling with semiquantitative cultures to confirm VAP diagnosis. Consider testing for respiratory viruses as well.
- Immediate treatment is recommended in unstable patients with shock or rapidly progressive respiratory failure following the acquisition of microbial respiratory and blood samples.
- We recommend watchful waiting in stable patients while letting cultures mature; carefully monitor the patient's clinical trajectory and be ready to intervene if the patient deteriorates.
- Empiric treatment for VAP should include coverage for *Staphylococcus aureus* and *Pseudomonas aeruginosa*. In patients with risk factors for antibiotic resistance, choose antibiotics that cover the drug-resistant pathogens that are most common in one's own institution.
- De-escalation of therapy to cover identified pathogens should take place as soon as culture results are available. If cultures are negative at 48–72 hours, re-evaluate the diagnosis. If another diagnosis now seems more likely, then stop antibiotics. If VAP still seems like the most likely diagnosis, then consider narrowing antibiotics.
- Treatment with intravenous antibiotics should not exceed 7 days without thoughtful re-evaluation of the individual patient's trajectory and need for an extended course.

REFERENCES

1. Kalil AC, Metersky ML, Klompas M, et al. Management of adults with hospital-acquired and ventilator-associated pneumonia: 2016 clinical practice guidelines by the Infectious Diseases Society of America and the American Thoracic Society. *Clin Infect Dis.* 2016;63(5):e61-e111.
2. Dudeck MA, Weiner LM, Allen-Bridson K, et al. National Healthcare Safety Network (NHSN) report, data summary for 2012, Device-associated module. *Am J Infect Control.* 2013;41(12):1148-1166.
3. Metersky ML, Wang Y, Klompas M, Eckenrode S, Bakullari A, Eldridge N. Trend in ventilator-associated pneumonia rates between 2005 and 2013. *JAMA.* 2016;316(22):2427-2429.
4. Scheld WM. Developments in the pathogenesis, diagnosis and treatment of nosocomial pneumonia. *Surg Gynecol Obstet.* 1991;172(Suppl):42-53.
5. Ranjan N, Chaudhary U, Chaudhry D, Ranjan KP. Ventilator-associated pneumonia in a tertiary care intensive care unit: analysis of incidence, risk factors and mortality. *Indian J Crit Care Med.* 2014;18(4):200-204.
6. Nakaviroj S, Cherdrungsi R, Chaiwat O. Incidence and risk factors for ventilator-associated pneumonia in the surgical

intensive care unit, Siriraj Hospital. *J Med Assoc Thai.* 2014; 97(Suppl 1):S61-S68.

7. Craven DE, Kunches LM, Kilinsky V, Lichtenberg DA, Make BJ, McCabe WR. Risk factors for pneumonia and fatality in patients receiving continuous mechanical ventilation. *Am Rev Respir Dis.* 1986;133(5):792-796.

8. Celis R, Torres A, Gatell JM, Almela M, Rodríguez-Roisin R, Agustí-Vidal A. Nosocomial pneumonia. A multivariate analysis of risk and prognosis. *Chest.* 1988;93(2):318-324.

9. Kollef MH. Ventilator-associated pneumonia. A multivariate analysis. *JAMA.* 1993;270(16):1965-1970.

10. Lewis SC, Li L, Murphy MV, Klompas M; CDC Prevention Epicenters. Risk factors for ventilator-associated events: a case-control multivariable analysis. *Crit Care Med.* 2014;42(8):1839-1848.

11. Wałaszek M, Kosiarska A, Gniadek A, et al. The risk factors for hospital-acquired pneumonia in the Intensive Care Unit. *Przegl Epidemiol.* 2016;70(1):15-20, 107-110.

12. Eom CS, Jeon CY, Lim JW, Cho EG, Park SM, Lee KS. Use of acid-suppressive drugs and risk of pneumonia: a systematic review and meta-analysis. *CMAJ.* 2011;183(3):310-319.

13. Huang HB, Jiang W, Wang CY, Qin HY, Du B. Stress ulcer prophylaxis in intensive care unit patients receiving enteral nutrition: a systematic review and meta-analysis. *Crit Care.* 2018;22(1):20.

14. Sopena N, Heras E, Casas I, et al. Risk factors for hospital-acquired pneumonia outside the intensive care unit: a case-control study. *Am J Infect Control.* 2014;42(1):38-42.

15. Garrouste-Orgeas M, Chevret S, Arlet G, et al. Oropharyngeal or gastric colonization and nosocomial pneumonia in adult intensive care unit patients. A prospective study based on genomic DNA analysis. *Am J Respir Crit Care Med.* 1997;156(5):1647-1655.

16. Marik PE, Careau P. The role of anaerobes in patients with ventilator-associated pneumonia and aspiration pneumonia: a prospective study. *Chest.* 1999;115(1):178-183.

17. Jones RN. Microbial etiologies of hospital-acquired bacterial pneumonia and ventilator-associated bacterial pneumonia. *Clin Infect Dis.* 2010;51(Suppl 1):S81-S87.

18. Sievert DM, Ricks P, Edwards JR, et al. Antimicrobial-resistant pathogens associated with healthcare-associated infections: summary of data reported to the National Healthcare Safety Network at the Centers for Disease Control and Prevention, 2009-2010. *Infect Control Hosp Epidemiol.* 2013;34(1):1-14.

19. Loubet P, Voiriot G, Houhou-Fidouh N, et al. Impact of respiratory viruses in hospital-acquired pneumonia in the intensive care unit: a single-center retrospective study. *J Clin Virol.* 2017;91:52-57.

20. van Someren Gréve F, Juffermans NP, Bos LDJ, et al. Respiratory viruses in invasively ventilated critically ill patients—a prospective multicenter observational study. *Crit Care Med.* 2018;46(1):29-36.

21. Weiner LM, Webb AK, Limbago B, et al. Antimicrobial-resistant pathogens associated with healthcare-associated infections: summary of data reported to the National Healthcare Safety Network at the Centers for Disease Control and Prevention, 2011-2014. *Infect Control Hosp Epidemiol.* 2016;37(11):1288-1301.

22. Klompas M. Does this patient have ventilator-associated pneumonia? *JAMA.* 2007;297(14):1583-1593.

23. Fàbregas N, Ewig S, Torres A, et al. Clinical diagnosis of ventilator associated pneumonia revisited: comparative validation using immediate post-mortem lung biopsies. *Thorax.* 1999;54(10): 867-873.

24. Fagon JY, Chastre J, Hance AJ, Domart Y, Trouillet JL, Gibert C. Evaluation of clinical judgment in the identification and treatment of nosocomial pneumonia in ventilated patients. *Chest.* 1993;103(2):547-553.

25. Torres A, el-Ebiary M, Padró L, et al. Validation of different techniques for the diagnosis of ventilator-associated pneumonia. Comparison with immediate postmortem pulmonary biopsy. *Am J Respir Crit Care Med.* 1994;149(2 Pt 1):324-331.

26. Meduri GU. Diagnosis and differential diagnosis of ventilator-associated pneumonia. *Clin Chest Med.* 1995;16(1):61-93.

27. Klompas M, Li L, Menchaca JT, Gruber S. Ultra-short-course antibiotics for patients with suspected ventilator-associated pneumonia but minimal and stable ventilator settings. *Clin Infect Dis.* 2017;64(7):870-876.

28. Luyt CE, Combes A, Reynaud C, et al. Usefulness of procalcitonin for the diagnosis of ventilator-associated pneumonia. *Intensive Care Med.* 2008;34(8):1434-1440.

29. Stolz D, Smyrnios N, Eggimann P, et al. Procalcitonin for reduced antibiotic exposure in ventilator-associated pneumonia: a randomised study. *Eur Respir J.* 2009;34(6):1364-1375.

30. Torres A, Niederman MS, Chastre J, et al. International ERS/ESICM/ESCMID/ALAT guidelines for the management of hospital-acquired pneumonia and ventilator-associated pneumonia: Guidelines for the management of hospital-acquired pneumonia (HAP)/ventilator-associated pneumonia (VAP) of the European Respiratory Society (ERS), European Society of Intensive Care Medicine (ESICM), European Society of Clinical Microbiology and Infectious Diseases (ESCMID) and Asociación Latinoamericana del Tórax (ALAT). *Eur Respir J.* 2017;50(3):pii: 1700582.

31. Fagon JY, Chastre J, Wolff M, et al. Invasive and noninvasive strategies for management of suspected ventilator-associated pneumonia. A randomized trial. *Ann Intern Med.* 2000;132(8):621-630.

32. Berton DC, Kalil AC, Teixeira PJ. Quantitative versus qualitative cultures of respiratory secretions for clinical outcomes in patients with ventilator-associated pneumonia. *Cochrane Database Syst Rev.* 2012;1:CD006482.

33. Kirtland SH, Corley DE, Winterbauer RH, et al. The diagnosis of ventilator-associated pneumonia: a comparison of histologic, microbiologic, and clinical criteria. *Chest.* 1997;112(2):445-457.

34. Kuti EL, Patel AA, Coleman CI. Impact of inappropriate antibiotic therapy on mortality in patients with ventilator-associated pneumonia and blood stream infection: a meta-analysis. *J Crit Care.* 2008;23(1):91-100.

35. Muscedere JG, Shorr AF, Jiang X, Day A, Heyland DK; Canadian Critical Care Trials Group. The adequacy of timely empiric antibiotic therapy for ventilator-associated pneumonia: an important determinant of outcome. *J Crit Care.* 2012;27(3):322.e7-e14.

36. Magiorakos AP, Srinivasan A, Carey RB, et al. Multidrug-resistant, extensively drug-resistant and pandrug-resistant bacteria: an international expert proposal for interim standard definitions for acquired resistance. *Clin Microbiol Infect.* 2012; 18(3):268-281.

37. Solé-Lleonart C, Rouby JJ, Blot S, et al. Nebulization of antiinfective agents in invasively mechanically ventilated adults: a systematic review and meta-analysis. *Anesthesiology.* 2017;126(5):890-908.

38. Rello J, Solé-Lleonart C, Rouby JJ, et al. Use of nebulized antimicrobials for the treatment of respiratory infections in invasively mechanically ventilated adults: a position paper from the

European Society of Clinical Microbiology and Infectious Diseases. *Clin Microbiol Infect.* 2017;23(9):629-639.

39. Luther MK, Timbrook TT, Caffrey AR, Dosa D, Lodise TP, LaPlante KL. Vancomycin plus piperacillin-tazobactam and acute kidney injury in adults: a systematic review and meta-analysis. *Crit Care Med.* 2018;46(1):12-20.

40. Sutter R, Rüegg S, Tschudin-Sutter S. Seizures as adverse events of antibiotic drugs: a systematic review. *Neurology.* 2015;85(15):1332-1341.

41. Vardakas KZ, Voulgaris GL, Maliaros A, Samonis G, Falagas ME. Prolonged versus short-term intravenous infusion of antipseudomonal beta-lactams for patients with sepsis: a systematic review and meta-analysis of randomised trials. *Lancet Infect Dis.* 2018;18(1):108-120.

42. Pugh R, Grant C, Cooke RP, Dempsey G. Short-course versus prolonged-course antibiotic therapy for hospital-acquired pneumonia in critically ill adults. *Cochrane Database Syst Rev.* 2015;8:CD007577.

43. Schuetz P, Wirz Y, Sager R, et al. Procalcitonin to initiate or discontinue antibiotics in acute respiratory tract infections. *Cochrane Database Syst Rev.* 2017;10:CD007498.

44. Bouadma L, Luyt CE, Tubach F, et al. Use of procalcitonin to reduce patients' exposure to antibiotics in intensive care units (PRORATA trial): a multicentre randomised controlled trial. *Lancet.* 2010;375(9713):463-474.

45. de Jong E, van Oers JA, Beishuizen A, et al. Efficacy and safety of procalcitonin guidance in reducing the duration of antibiotic treatment in critically ill patients: a randomised, controlled, open-label trial. *Lancet Infect Dis.* 2016;16(7):819-827.

46. Klompas M, Branson R, Eichenwald EC, et al. Strategies to prevent ventilator-associated pneumonia in acute care hospitals: 2014 update. *Infect Control Hosp Epidemiol.* 2014;35(Suppl 2):S133-S154.

47. Klompas M. Complications of mechanical ventilation—the CDC's new surveillance paradigm. *N Engl J Med.* 2013;368(16):1472-1475.

48

What Is the Role of Invasive Hemodynamic Monitoring in Critical Care?

Daniel De Backer

INTRODUCTION

Hemodynamic monitoring provides important information about the approach to the patient in acute circulatory failure. The strength of monitoring lies not in the direct impact on outcome,[1] but rather in directing clinical management. Indeed, accurate hemodynamic data provide important information on (1) the patient's condition, (2) therapeutic choices, and (3) the effects of these choices. Current trends favor the use of minimally invasive[2] (e.g., calibrated pulse wave analysis and esophageal Doppler) or noninvasive approaches (e.g., bioreactance and bioimpedance techniques, noninvasive pulse contour methods, echocardiography) but invasive hemodynamic monitoring techniques (e.g., pulmonary artery catheter and transpulmonary thermodilution) are still widely used.[3] The information provided by noninvasive techniques is often limited to cardiac output and stroke volume variations, while more invasive techniques provide more information, such as intravascular pressures and cardiac volumes. The reliability of the various techniques in severely ill patients is variable and often inversely proportional to invasiveness. Accordingly, the choice of the hemodynamic technique should not be guided solely on the basis of its invasiveness, but should also take into account accuracy of the approach and, most importantly, the potential value of the added information. The choice of the hemodynamic monitoring device should thus be individualized.

Perhaps the most important change in the hemodynamic evaluation of the critically ill patients is the ever-increasing reliance on echocardiography.[4] Echocardiography is now recommended in the initial hours for the classification of shock[5,6] and observational studies suggest that its use, alone or in combination with other tools, is associated with a better outcome.[7] However, echocardiography is discontinuous, even if it can be easily repeated. In addition, hemodynamic evaluation using echocardiography requires skills that go well beyond the basic level.[8] Accordingly, echocardiography is often used in combination with other tools providing online, hemodynamic measurements.

The main indications for hemodynamic monitoring are the identification of the type of shock[6] and therapeutic guidance. Another important indication is cardiopulmonary evaluation of the patient with respiratory failure. In this chapter, we discuss the use of invasive techniques for hemodynamic monitoring.

INVASIVE OR NONINVASIVE ARTERIAL PRESSURE MONITORING?

Arterial pressure is a key determinant of organ perfusion and is routinely measured in critically ill patients, either noninvasively or invasively. Noninvasive measurements can reliably be used in less severely ill patients but are unfortunately less reliable in patients with shock, when accuracy of measurements is most important.[9] For example, an overestimate of 5–10 mm Hg will have minimal impact on patient management if real mean arterial pressure (MAP) is 80 mm Hg, but could have important consequences if MAP is 55 mm Hg. Hence invasive arterial pressure monitoring is recommended in patients with circulatory failure.[5]

CENTRAL VENOUS PRESSURE AND CENTRAL VENOUS OXYGEN SATURATION

Central venous access is often used in the care of critically ill patients, especially when in shock, and the measurements of central venous pressure (CVP) and oxygen saturation can provide important information on the hemodynamic state.

Although CVP measurements reflect cardiac function and volume status, they are also influenced by intrathoracic pressure. A high CVP may reflect impaired cardiac function (biventricular or right heart), hypervolemia, or tamponade. A low CVP usually suggests hypovolemia but can be misleading in patients with isolated left heart dysfunction. Importantly, the measured CVP is also affected by intrathoracic pressures and may overestimate the true CVP (transmural CVP) in patients being mechanically ventilated. This interaction may limit the ability of CVP to evaluate preload responsiveness and even cardiac function. Nevertheless, CVP reflects the backpressure of the venous system and hence the driving force for tissue edema. CVP provides important information on the hemodynamic state of the patient: even though its interpretation is not always easy, it remains an important variable to measure.[10]

Measurement of central venous oxygen saturation ($ScvO_2$) provides information on the adequacy of oxygen transport, and hence cardiac output. A low $ScvO_2$ suggests a low or inadequate cardiac output, anemia, hypoxemia, agitation, or a combination of all factors.

In patients with septic shock, hemodynamic optimization, based on these variables, has been suggested. While an initial trial of early goal directed therapy (EGDT), based on CVP and $ScvO_2$, was associated with a marked reduction in mortality,[11] these findings were not confirmed in three large-scale international trials.[12–14] Several factors may explain these conflicting results.[15] At study entry, $ScvO_2$ was close to 50% in both groups in the original EGDT trial, while the value was approaching goal (70%) on randomization into the three recent trials. If the main variable being corrected is already within target values, one would expect the intervention to have minimal impact. In the ARISE (Australasian Resuscitation in Sepsis Evaluation) trial, 78% of the patients had reached the $ScvO_2$ goal at randomization; additional interventions only increased $ScvO_2$ to 82%.[13] Furthermore, the inclusion rate was much lower in the three recent trials (1 and 0.5 patients per center per month vs. 8 patients per center per month in the original single-center EGDT trial). Thus, there may have been some selection bias toward less severely ill patients in the more recent studies; indeed, this finding might explain the low mortality observed in the recent trials. Indeed, 50% of the included patients did not require administration of vasopressors during their entire stay[12] and 18% were even not admitted to the intensive care unit (ICU).[16] Finally, the "standard of care" has evolved dramatically since the original EGDT study; thus, use of the most impactful interventions were probably not restricted to the intervention groups. In aggregate, the conclusions from these trials are that protocolized EGDT does not offer survival benefit in all patients with septic shock, but that hemodynamic optimization based on $ScvO_2$ may still be justified in the most severe patients presenting with an altered $ScvO_2$.[15]

THE PULMONARY ARTERY CATHETER

The invasive pulmonary artery (PA) catheter has the advantage of providing quasi-continuous information on cardiovascular status. The PA catheter measures three types of variables: intravascular pressures, cardiac output, and mixed-venous blood gases.

Measurements of PA pressure are particularly indicated in cases of right ventricular (RV) dysfunction, where evaluation of RV afterload is crucial for diagnosis and for therapy.[17]

Echocardiography can also provide an estimate of PA pressure. None of the noninvasive techniques can determine PA pressure at bedside. The measurement of PA pressure is less important in disorders that have minimal impact on RV function. The PA occlusion pressure is useful in the identification of left ventricular (LV) dysfunction and can aid in fluid management. It provides information on lung hydrostatic pressure, and thus on the risk of developing pulmonary edema. PA occlusion pressure is not a measurement of true capillary pressure, which is always higher; thus, an elevated PA occlusion pressure is always informative.

Measurement of cardiac output is important for diagnosing the type of shock and evaluating the effect of therapies.[5] Thermodilution cardiac output is measured intermittently by injection of cold bolus or automatically in a semicontinuous fashion. Importantly, most monitors average several sequential cardiac output measurements; rapid changes may be difficult to detect. Thermodilution cardiac output may be unreliable in the presence of severe tricuspid regurgitation or intracardiac shunt. At high cardiac output values, the precision of semicontinuous cardiac output measurements is lower than that of classical thermodilution,[18] Finally, each hemodynamic evaluation should be accompanied by measurement of mixed venous oxygen saturation (SvO_2), which enables the interpretation of the cardiac output by considering oxygen transport in relation to oxygen consumption. Although related, SvO_2 may differ from $ScvO_2$; whereas SvO_2 represents the venous blood collected from all parts of the body, $ScvO_2$ represents only the blood drained from the upper part of the body.

Observational trials have demonstrated that use of a PA catheter allows for more accurate determination of the hemodynamic state than clinical evaluation and is associated with significant changes in therapy that may improve outcome.[19] A series of randomized studies, however, failed to demonstrate outcome benefit from the use of PA catheters in ICU patients. Perioperative hemodynamic optimization using the PA catheter was associated with decreased complication rates[25] and improved survival.[26]

The full value of a PA catheter may only be realized if the data are obtained and interpreted properly.[27,28] The importance of these concerns is highlighted by the lack of decision algorithm use in most trials involving a PA catheter in critically ill patients. Similarly, the addition of echocardiographic data does not necessarily improve data interpretation by practitioners,[29] suggesting that the fault lies with data evaluation and not with technique.[30] Furthermore, the patients included in trials evaluating PA catheters were highly selected. In the Fluids and Catheters Treatment Trial (FACTT), a large number of patients were disqualified from participation because they had a PA catheter at the time of randomization, suggesting that the sickest patients were not included.[31] A report on excluded patients with cardiogenic shock found that those with a PA catheter prior to randomization had significantly higher mortality rates than patients included in the trial.[32] Thus, the results of the study may be biased.[33] Nonetheless, publication of negative trials (and the wide availability of alternatives) was followed by a decrease in the use of PA catheters.[34] Recent data appear to suggest that PA catheter use is increasing again,[35,36] particularly in patients with cardiogenic shock and RV dysfunction.

In summary, use of PA catheters is indicated in some situations, in particular in patients with RV dysfunction.[37] Unfortunately, the decline in PA catheter use presents an educational challenge as fewer intensivists are learing how to place , manipulate and interpret the data from a PA catheter.

TRANSPULMONARY THERMODILUTION AND PULSE WAVE ANALYSIS

A commonly used alternative to the PA catheter is transpulmonary thermodilution (TPTD) coupled with pulse wave analysis. These minimally invasive techniques still require placement of arterial and central venous lines. TPTD is used not only for the calibration of pulse-wave-derived continuous cardiac output measurement but also for volumetric measurements.

Stroke volume can be estimated from an arterial pressure waveform. Calibration with TPTD is used to capture differences in arterial compliance and vascular tone from one patient to another, and from one time to another in a given patient.[38,39] The accuracy of pulse wave analysis is highly dependent on the delay between the two calibrations. Any change in vascular tone can significantly alter the precision of these devices[40] and should prompt recalibration. Newer devices that use autocalibration permit reliable measurements to be made even in patients with septic shock[18] but lack the additional cardiac function and volumetric measurements.

TPTD requires the use of a modified arterial catheter equipped with a thermistor. This catheter is inserted in the femoral artery. The thermodilution curve is determined using a proprietary algorithm. Cardiac output is derived from the area under the curve. TPTD is slightly less sensitive to valvular regurgitation than right-sided thermodilution.

The main advantage of TPTD is that it also allows the measurement of extravascular lung water (EVLW) and of cardiac chamber volume (global end-diastolic volume index [GEDVI]), an index of preload. Volumetric indices perform better than pressures in patients with raised intrathoracic or intra-abdominal pressures or with decreased LV compliance. EVLWI reflects the degree of pulmonary edema, whatever its cause, and is associated with prognosis.[41] Both indices are useful in establishing diagnosis and to aid in fluid management. Given the additional value of volumetric measurements, TPTD should be considered an integral part of hemodynamic assessment.

Cardiac function index (CFI) is a derived parameter calculated as cardiac index divided by GEDVI. In patients with cardiogenic shock, CFI reflects LV ejection fraction,[42,43] provided that RV function is maintained.[43] CFI can be substituted for a PA catheter to identify myocardial depression in septic patients.[42]

Complications related to hemodynamic monitoring with TPTD are relatively minor and are related to arterial and central venous catheterization (local bleeding and infections).[44]

HEMODYNAMIC OPTIMIZATION WITH THE PULMONARY ARTERY CATHETER OR TRANSPULMONARY THERMODILUTION

Several trials have evaluated the impact of hemodynamic optimization on outcome.[26,45-48]

Perioperative optimization using a PA catheter resulted in decreased perioperative complications[25] and improved survival rate.[26] TPTD has also been used for this purpose, with a resultant decrease in perioperative complications.[45,49]

In other conditions, it has been more difficult to determine if the use of TPTD affects outcome. In patients with cardiogenic shock after cardiac arrest, hemodynamic monitoring with TPTD was associated with higher fluid intake in the first 24 hours and resulted in a lower incidence of acute kidney injury compared with CVP and arterial pressure monitoring.[48] In patients with Takotsubo cardiomyopathy related to subarachnoid hemorrhage, a CFI below 4.2/min was predictive of an impaired ejection fraction and an impaired 3-month neurologic outcome.[46] Patients with poor neurologic outcome also had high EVLWI values. In a randomized trial, these authors further reported that targeted hemodynamic resuscitation using TPTD indices was associated with better long-term neurologic outcome.[47]

It is difficult to determine if hemodynamic management with the PA catheter is preferable to management using transpulmonary thermodilution. In a small randomized trial that directly compared the two techniques, pressure-guided resuscitation was superior to volumetric variables, resulting in shorter duration of mechanical ventilation in shock patients with impaired cardiac function, but not in patients with preserved cardiac function. Survival rates in both groups were unaffected.[50]

Given the absence of major differences in outcome between the different monitoring techniques, the choice of the hemodynamic device should be based on severity of illness and the value of the measured variables to a patient's specific condition. We suggest a decision algorithm (Fig. 48.1) based on published review articles.[2,3,37] The starting point is evaluation of the hemodynamic state with echocardiography for identification of the type of shock and of RV function. In the absence of significant comorbidities and if the patient rapidly improves after initial resuscitation, basic hemodynamic monitoring with arterial and central venous lines, along with measurements of lactate, $ScvO_2$, and PCO_2 (partial pressure of carbon dioxide) gradients, may be sufficient. Noninvasive cardiac output measurement may have value by providing continuous evaluation of flow. In complex cases with associated comorbidities, in patients with acute respiratory distress syndrome (ARDS) or cardiac dysfunction

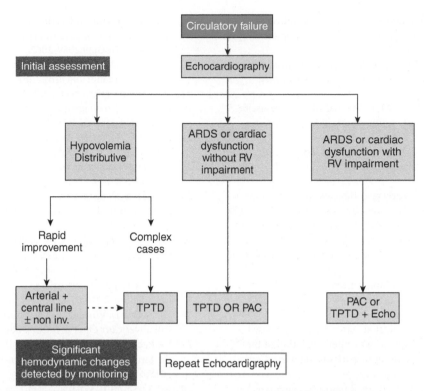

Fig. 48.1 Suggested Decision Algorithm for the Selection of Hemodynamic Monitoring Techniques. The algorithm is inspired from published review articles.[2,3,37] In addition to the measurements of arterial pressure and CVP (central venous pressure), lactate, ScvO$_2$ (central venous oxygen saturation), and PCO$_2$ (partial pressure of carbon dioxide) gradients are suggested at each hemodynamic assessment. *ARDS,* acute respiratory distress syndrome; *Echo,* echocardiography; *PAC,* pulmonary artery catheter; *RV,* right ventricular; *TPTD,* transpulmonary thermodilution.

without RV impairment, or in cases where the patient deteriorates after initial resuscitation, a TPTD system associated with pulse contour analysis provides cardiac volumes and extravascular lung water. In cases of RV dysfunction, the PA catheter is preferred. If the team is inexperienced with the use of the PA catheter, coupling TPTD with echocardiography may be an alternative.

AUTHORS' RECOMMENDATIONS
- Hemodynamic evaluation is often required in critically ill patients. The PA catheter and TPTD can be used for this purpose.
- Beyond perioperative optimization, no large-scale trial has demonstrated improved outcome with either the PA catheter or TPTD.
- Basic hemodynamic monitoring may be sufficient in simple cases, but invasive hemodynamic monitoring is often needed in complex cases.

REFERENCES

1. Ospina-Tascón GA, Cordioli RL, Vincent JL. What type of monitoring has been shown to improve outcomes in acutely ill patients? *Intensive Care Med.* 2008;34:800-820.

2. Teboul JL, Saugel B, Cecconi M, et al. Less invasive hemodynamic monitoring in critically ill patients. *Intensive Care Med.* 2016;42:1350-1359.

3. De Backer D, Bakker J, Cecconi M, et al. Alternatives to the Swan-Ganz catheter. *Intensive Care Med.* 2018;44:730-741.

4. De Backer D, Cholley BP, Slama M, et al. *Hemodynamic Monitoring Using Echocardiography in the Critically Ill.* New York, NY: Springer; 2011:1-311.

5. Cecconi M, De Backer D, Antonelli M, et al. Consensus on circulatory shock and hemodynamic monitoring. Task Force of the European Society of Intensive Care Medicine. *Intensive Care Med.* 2014;40:1795-1815.

6. Vincent JL, De Backer D. Circulatory shock. *N Engl J Med.* 2013;369:1726-1734.

7. Feng M, McSparron JI, Kien DT, et al. Transthoracic echocardiography and mortality in sepsis: analysis of the MIMIC-III database. *Intensive Care Med.* 2018;44:884-892.

8. Expert Round Table on Echocardiography in ICU. International consensus statement on training standards for advanced critical care echocardiography. *Intensive Care Med.* 2014;40:654-666.

9. Monnet X, Picard F, Lidzborski E, et al. The estimation of cardiac output by the Nexfin device is of poor reliability for tracking the effects of a fluid challenge. *Crit Care.* 2012;16:R212.

10. De Backer D, Vincent JL. Should we measure the central venous pressure to guide fluid management? Ten answers to 10 questions. *Crit Care.* 2018;22:43.

11. Rivers E, Nguyen B, Havstadt S, et al. Early goal-directed therapy in the treatment of severe sepsis and septic shock. *N Engl J Med.* 2001;345:1368-1377.

12. Yealy DM, Kellum JA, Huang DT, et al. A randomized trial of protocol-based care for early septic shock. *N Engl J Med.* 2014;370:1683-1693.

13. Peake SL, Delaney A, Bailey M, et al. Goal-directed resuscitation for patients with early septic shock. *N Engl J Med.* 2014;371:1496-1506.

14. Mouncey PR, Osborn TM, Power GS, et al. Trial of early, goal-directed resuscitation for septic shock. *N Engl J Med.* 2015;372:1301-1311.

15. De Backer D, Vincent JL. Early goal-directed therapy: do we have a definitive answer? *Intensive Care Med.* 2016;42:1048-1050.

16. Angus DC, Barnato AE, Bell D, et al. A systematic review and meta-analysis of early goal-directed therapy for septic shock: the ARISE, ProCESS and ProMISe Investigators. *Intensive Care Med.* 2015;41:1549-1560.

17. Ventetuolo CE, Klinger JR. Management of acute right ventricular failure in the intensive care unit. *Ann Am Thorac Soc.* 2014;11:811-822.

18. De Backer D, Marx G, Tan A, et al. Arterial pressure-based cardiac output monitoring: a multicenter validation of the third-generation software in septic patients. *Intensive Care Med.* 2011;37:233-240.

19. Mimoz O, Rauss A, Rekik N, Brun-Buisson C, Lemaire F, Brochard L. Pulmonary artery catheterization in critically ill patients: a prospective analysis of outcome changes associated with catheter-prompted changes in therapy. *Crit Care Med* 1994;22:573-579.

20. Wheeler AP, Bernard GR, Thompson BT, et al. Pulmonary-artery versus central venous catheter to guide treatment of acute lung injury. *N Engl J Med.* 2006;354:2213-2224.

21. Richard C, Warszawski J, Anguel N, et al. Early use of the pulmonary artery catheter and outcomes in patients with shock and acute respiratory distress syndrome: a randomized controlled trial. *JAMA.* 2003;290:2713-2720.

22. Sandham JD, Hull RD, Brant RF, et al. A randomized, controlled trial of the use of pulmonary-artery catheters in high-risk surgical patients. *N Engl J Med.* 2003;348:5-14.

23. Binanay C, Califf RM, Hasselblad V, et al. Evaluation study of congestive heart failure and pulmonary artery catheterization effectiveness: the ESCAPE trial. *JAMA.* 2005;294:1625-1633.

24. Rajaram SS, Desai NK, Kalra A, et al. Pulmonary artery catheters for adult patients in intensive care. *Cochrane Database Syst Rev.* 2013;2:CD003408.

25. Pölönen P, Ruokonen E, Hippeläinen M, Pöyhönen M, Takala J. A prospective, randomized study of goal-oriented hemodynamic therapy in cardiac surgical patients. *Anesth Analg.* 2000;90:1052-1059.

26. Wilson J, Woods I, Fawcett J, et al. Reducing the risk of major elective surgery: randomised controlled trial of preoperative optimisation of oxygen delivery. *BMJ.* 1999;318:1099-1103.

27. Gnaegi A, Feihl F, Perret C. Intensive care physicians' insufficient knowledge of right-heart catheterization at the bedside: time to act? *Crit Care Med.* 1997;25:213-220.

28. Iberti TJ, Fischer EP, Leibowitz AB, Panacek EA, Silverstein JH, Albertson TE. A multicenter study of physicians' knowledge of the pulmonary artery catheter. Pulmonary Artery Catheter Study Group. *JAMA.* 1990;264:2928-2932.

29. Jain M, Canham M, Upadhyay D, Corbridge T. Variability in interventions with pulmonary artery catheter data. *Intensive Care Med.* 2003;29:2059-2062.

30. De Backer D. Hemodynamic assessment: the technique or the physician at fault? *Intensive Care Med.* 2003;29:1865-1867.

31. Wiedemann HP, Wheeler AP, Bernard GR, et al. Comparison of two fluid-management strategies in acute lung injury. *N Engl J Med.* 2006;354:2564-2575.

32. Allen LA, Rogers JG, Warnica JW, et al. High mortality without ESCAPE: the registry of heart failure patients receiving pulmonary artery catheters without randomization. *J Card Fail.* 2008;14:661-669.

33. De Backer D, Schortgen F. Physicians declining patient enrollment in clinical trials: what are the implications? *Intensive Care Med.* 2014;40:117-119.

34. Koo KK, Sun JC, Zhou Q, et al. Pulmonary artery catheters: evolving rates and reasons for use. *Crit Care Med.* 2011;39:1613-1618.

35. Pandey A, Khera R, Kumar N, Golwala H, Girotra S, Fonarow GC. Use of pulmonary artery catheterization in US patients with heart failure, 2001-2012. *JAMA Intern Med.* 2016;176:129-132.

36. De Backer D, Vincent JL. The pulmonary artery catheter: is it still alive? *Curr Opin Crit Care.* 2018;24:204-208.

37. De Backer D, Hajjar LA, Pinsky MR. Is there still a place for the Swan–Ganz catheter? We are not sure. *Intensive Care Med.* 2018;44:960-962.

38. van Lieshout JJ, Wesseling KH. Continuous cardiac output by pulse contour analysis? *Br J Anaesth.* 2001;86:467-469.

39. Michard F. Pulse contour analysis: fairy tale or new reality? *Crit Care Med.* 2007;35:1791-1792.

40. Hamzaoui O, Monnet X, Richard C, Osman D, Chemla D, Teboul JL. Effects of changes in vascular tone on the agreement between pulse contour and transpulmonary thermodilution cardiac output measurements within an up to 6-hour calibration-free period. *Crit Care Med.* 2008;36:434-440.

41. Jozwiak M, Silva S, Persichini R, et al. Extravascular lung water is an independent prognostic factor in patients with acute respiratory distress syndrome. *Crit Care Med.* 2013;42:472-480.

42. Ritter S, Rudiger A, Maggiorini M. Transpulmonary thermodilution-derived cardiac function index identifies cardiac dysfunction in acute heart failure and septic patients: an observational study. *Crit Care.* 2009;13(4):R133.

43. Perny J, Kimmoun A, Perez P, Levy B. Evaluation of cardiac function index as measured by transpulmonary thermodilution as an indicator of left ventricular ejection fraction in cardiogenic shock. *Biomed Res Int.* 2014;2014:598029.

44. Belda FJ, Aguilar G, Teboul JL, et al. Complications related to less-invasive haemodynamic monitoring. *Br J Anaesth.* 2011;106:482-486.

45. Goepfert MS, Reuter DA, Akyol D, Lamm P, Kilger E, Goetz AE. Goal-directed fluid management reduces vasopressor and catecholamine use in cardiac surgery patients. *Intensive Care Med.* 2007;33:96-103.

46. Mutoh T, Kazumata K, Terasaka S, Taki Y, Suzuki A, Ishikawa T. Impact of transpulmonary thermodilution-based cardiac contractility and extravascular lung water measurements on clinical outcome of patients with Takotsubo cardiomyopathy after subarachnoid hemorrhage: a retrospective observational study. *Crit Care.* 2014;18:482.

47. Mutoh T, Kazumata K, Terasaka S, Taki Y, Suzuki A, Ishikawa T. Early intensive versus minimally invasive approach to postoperative hemodynamic management after subarachnoid hemorrhage. *Stroke.* 2014;45:1280-1284.

48. Adler C, Reuter H, Seck C, Hellmich M, Zobel C. Fluid therapy and acute kidney injury in cardiogenic shock after cardiac arrest. *Resuscitation.* 2013;84:194-199.

49. Salzwedel C, Puig J, Carstens A, et al. Perioperative goal-directed hemodynamic therapy based on radial arterial pulse pressure variation and continuous cardiac index trending reduces postoperative complications after major abdominal surgery: a multi-center, prospective, randomized study. *Crit Care.* 2013;17:R191.

50. Trof RJ, Beishuizen A, Cornet AD, de Wit RJ, Girbes AR, Groeneveld AB. Volume-limited versus pressure-limited hemodynamic management in septic and nonseptic shock. *Crit Care Med.* 2012;40:1177-1185.

49

Does the Use of Echocardiography Aid in the Management of the Critically Ill?

Jennifer Cruz and Steven M. Hollenberg

INTRODUCTION

Successful management of the critically ill relies on the ability to identify life-threatening causes of hemodynamic deterioration rapidly and accurately. Echocardiography is a reliable, safe, and noninvasive imaging modality capable of accurately accelerating time to diagnosis in critically ill patients with undifferentiated hemodynamic instability.[1–3] Evidence supporting its utility in the intensive care unit (ICU) is so compelling that basic echocardiography is now a core competency for critical care physicians.[3,4]

Echocardiography by intensivists in critically ill patients is divided into two different applications: focused echocardiography and advanced echocardiography.[2,4] Focused echocardiography has been well validated and allows clinicians to quickly diagnose and exclude potential cardiopulmonary causes of hemodynamic instability. Advanced echocardiography is more involved and entails assessment of cardiac structure and function and also hemodynamics. Neither application is equivalent to full echocardiography performed by certified full-time echocardiographic technicians and interpreted by cardiologists. Full studies assess cardiac structure and function by combining two-dimensional, M-mode, Doppler and strain imaging in different views. The authors discourage the use of the term "bedside echocardiography" as imprecise and potentially misleading; the comprehensiveness of an echocardiographic study should be dictated by the clinical issues and urgency, not the location at which the study is performed.

Training requirements differ among different echocardiographic studies. A basic level of training in focused echocardiography can be achieved by noncardiologists after a 12-hour training program that has been shown to provide trainees with the skills capable of improving patient care.[5,6] Competency in advanced echocardiography requires trainees to perform and interpret a minimum of 100 full studies.[3] Cardiologists are required to spend 6 full months and to perform a minimum of 150 full studies and interpret a minimum of 300 studies in order to read independently (Level II Competence); advanced certification for cardiology (Level III) generally requires an additional 12 months.[7]

The purpose of this chapter is to highlight evidence-based applications of echocardiography. Comprehensive discussion of technique, application, and potential shortcomings of focused echocardiography and advanced echocardiography is beyond the scope of this chapter, but can be found in echocardiography textbooks. Understanding the strengths and limitations of focused echocardiography and advanced echocardiography is the foundation of successful application of this diagnostic modality in the management of critically ill patients.

FOCUSED ECHOCARDIOGRAPHY AND ADVANCED ECHOCARDIOGRAPHY ARE USEFUL IN THE EVALUATION OF UNDIFFERENTIATED SHOCK

Focused echocardiography accurately expedites identification and exclusion of certain potential causes of cardiopulmonary and hemodynamic deterioration.[8,9] Advanced echocardiography can be added to help clinicians define the etiology of undifferentiated shock.[9] Etiologies of hemodynamic instability readily identified by focused echocardiography and advanced echocardiography can be broken down by shock classification and are shown in Fig. 49.1.

Obstructive Shock

Cardiac tamponade, massive pulmonary embolism (PE), and left ventricular outflow tract (LVOT) obstruction are life-threatening cardiopulmonary causes of obstructive shock that can be identified by focused echocardiography.

Cardiac Tamponade

Cardiac tamponade is defined as accumulation of pericardial fluid that impedes normal chamber filling, leading to decreased cardiac output (CO) and obstructive shock. Cardiac tamponade is a life-threatening, time-sensitive clinical diagnosis that can be confirmed by focused echocardiography and advanced echocardiography.

Focused echocardiography has been shown to rapidly identify the presence of and accurately quantify the size of pericardial effusions using two-dimensional (2D) echocardiography.[10] Right ventricular (RV) diastolic collapse is a specific sign of tamponade, and the absence of chamber collapse has >90% negative predictive value for cardiac tamponade.[11]

Evaluation of respiratory variation of mitral and tricuspid inflow velocities (the echocardiographic equivalent of pulsus

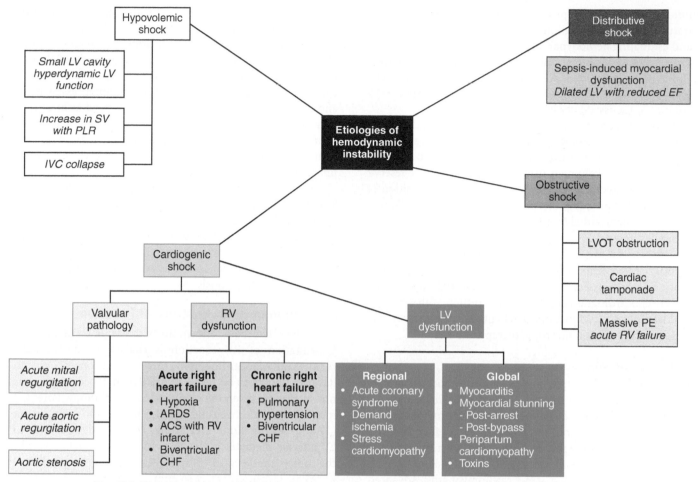

Fig. 49.1 Etiologies of Hemodynamic Instability and their Diagnosis by Echocardiography. *ACS,* acute coronary syndrome; *ARDS,* acute respiratory distress syndrome; *CHF,* congestive heart failure; *IVC,* inferior vena cava; *LV,* left ventricle; *LVOT,* left ventricular outflow tract; *PE,* pulmonary embolism; *PLR,* passive leg raising; *RV,* right ventricle; *SV,* stroke volume.

paradoxus) is an advanced technique that utilizes pulsed-wave Doppler echocardiography. Respiratory variation of transvalvular velocities (for mitral inflow >25%, for tricuspid inflow >40%)[12] is suggestive of hemodynamic compromise.[11,13]

Pulmonary Embolism

A meta-analysis of 22 different studies demonstrated that a variety of echocardiographic signs are highly specific for acute right heart strain and therefore can be used to rule in PE under the correct clinical circumstances.[14] Visualization of thrombus in the right atrium or ventricle documents PE in transit with a specificity of 99%. McConnell's sign (a distinct echocardiographic finding of systolic hypokinesis of the RV mid-free wall with RV apical sparing, felt to be due to RV apical tethering to an often hyperdynamic LV [left ventricular] apex), has a specificity of 97%, and RV:LV ratio >1, and a specificity of 86% for PE. This study suggests that in time-sensitive and life-threatening circumstances, echocardiographic demonstration of RV strain may suggest PE with sufficient specificity to warrant treatment.

Left Ventricular Outflow Tract Obstruction

Early recognition of LVOT obstruction as a cause of hypotension is crucial since therapy differs from other causes of cardiogenic shock. Dynamic LVOT obstruction is usually associated with hypertrophic cardiomyopathy (HCM) but may rarely occur with stress cardiomyopathy. It is important to distinguish hypotension driven by dynamic LVOT obstruction from hypotension secondary to cardiogenic shock from pump failure because inotropic therapy, often implemented in pump failure, can have adverse hemodynamic consequences in dynamic LVOT obstruction. Focused echocardiography can identify HCM and potentially systolic anterior motion of the mitral valve, and advanced echocardiography with Doppler can identify dynamic LVOT obstruction and quantify the gradient.[15]

Septic Shock

Volume resuscitation is a key principle in the management of septic shock. Since overly aggressive volume resuscitation can be deleterious, balancing adequate with excessive volume resuscitation is essential. Echocardiography can help guide fluid management by providing an assessment of volume status through examination of the inferior vena cava (IVC), and estimating hemodynamic parameters such as right atrial pressure (RAP), systolic pulmonary artery pressure (sPAP), and left atrial pressure (LAP). Echocardiographic assessment of hemodynamics and use of echo to predict response to volume is discussed later in this chapter.

Sepsis-induced myocardial dysfunction is a syndrome of left ventricular or biventricular dilation with decreased contractile function that is usually reversible over 7–10 days.[16,17] Although stroke volume is usually preserved, cardiac reserve can be decreased. The pathophysiology of this condition is multifactorial, probably driven by inflammatory mediators. Preexisting myocardial dysfunction can also influence hemodynamics in sepsis.[17]

The Society of Critical Care Medicine (SCCM) recommends focused echocardiography in patients with sepsis and septic shock to assess fluid responsiveness and suggests focused echocardiography in patients admitted with sepsis to evaluate LV and RV function to help guide volume resuscitation, vasopressor, and inotropic therapy.[2]

Cardiogenic Shock

Focused echocardiography and advanced echocardiography can help the intensivist recognize cardiogenic shock and narrow its broad differential. Echocardiography provides crucial information about overall and regional systolic function, and distinct echocardiographic features may point to a specific diagnosis; for example, the presence of apical ballooning with basal sparing may suggest stress cardiomyopathy. Advanced echocardiography can provide initial hemodynamic data to support the diagnosis of cardiogenic shock such as low CO in conjunction with elevated RAP, sPAP, and diastolic PAP (dPAP), and can assist in tracking hemodynamic changes in response to therapy. Full echocardiography can provide important information about valvular disease and diastolic function, and can rapidly diagnose mechanical causes of shock such as papillary muscle rupture, acute ventricular septal defect, and free wall rupture and tamponade.

FOCUSED ECHOCARDIOGRAPHY AND ADVANCED ECHOCARDIOGRAPHY IN THE EVALUATION OF VENTRICULAR FUNCTION

Evaluation of Left Ventricular Function

Up to one-third of critically ill patients have reduced LV systolic function during their ICU stay and more than 40% of all ICU patients have both systolic and diastolic dysfunction.[18] Thus, the SCCM recommends assessment of LV systolic function in all patients with either preexisting or ICU-acquired cardiac disease.[2] The urgency of that assessment should guide whether focused, advanced, or full echocardiography should be employed.

Identification of reduced systolic function may help narrow the differential of causes of hemodynamic collapse. Additionally, awareness of systolic dysfunction may sensitize clinicians

to the potential for fluid overload with volume resuscitation and help direct their selection of vasoactive therapy.

Focused echocardiography performs a qualitative assessment of LV systolic function and wall motion by visual estimation; this is not only effective and fast, but also reasonably consistent with quantitative echocardiographic assessments and nuclear scanning studies.[2,19,20] Advanced echocardiography may supplement qualitative assessment with more quantitative measures, such as the biplane method of disk summation (modified Simpson's rule), myocardial strain imaging, or speckle tracking.[20]

The American Society of Echocardiography recommends evaluation of regional LV function according to a 17-segment model, which reflects coronary perfusion territories.[20] Although regional wall motion abnormalities strongly suggest the presence of myocardial ischemia, they may also be seen in other conditions such as myocarditis, stress cardiomyopathy, and sarcoidosis.

Evaluation of Right Ventricular Function

RV failure has been shown to increase ICU mortality.[21] Quantitation of RV function is challenging and usually requires full echocardiography; three-dimensional (3D) echo has been shown to be more accurate than 2D echo, which is not surprising, given the complicated RV anatomy. Potential measures include tricuspid annular plane systolic excursion (TAPSE), RV fractional area change (FAC), and ratio of RV to LV internal diameter in diastole (RVIDD/ LVIDD).[22] Unlike the other markers, TAPSE is less preload dependent;[23] a TAPSE measurement <16 mm is highly specific for RV dysfunction.[24]

ADVANCED ECHOCARDIOGRAPHY IN THE ASSESSMENT OF HEMODYNAMICS

Advanced echocardiography is attractive for hemodynamic monitoring because it offers a quick and noninvasive method of obtaining hemodynamic data. This information may help clinicians distinguish various etiologies of shock, guide management, and monitor hemodynamic changes in response to therapy.

Volume Responsiveness: Predicting Fluid Responsiveness

In critically ill patients, such as those with septic or hypovolemic shock, aggressive volume resuscitation is the cornerstone of guideline-directed therapy. However, studies have shown that overly aggressive resuscitation can lead to unfavorable outcomes.[25] Clinical assessment and prediction of fluid responsiveness is particularly challenging in the ICU; imperfect methods of measurement melded with patient factors, such as heart failure, mechanical ventilation, intraabdominal hypertension, and body habitus complicate this important assessment.

Passive leg raising (PLR) quickly mobilizes approximately 300 mL of blood from lower extremities, increasing preload without changing intravascular volume.[2] PLR has been well validated in predicting response of CO to volume expansion in patients with acute circulatory failure, but must be performed correctly, with real-time monitoring of CO.[26] In spontaneously breathing patients, the stroke volume, obtained by multiplying the velocity–time integral (VTI) and aortic cross-sectional area, if increased by more than 9–15% during PLR, is highly predictive of fluid responsiveness.[26,27]

In mechanically ventilated patients, fluid responsiveness can be assessed by evaluating changes in IVC diameter during respiration. Studies have demonstrated that a 15% change in IVC diameter between inspiration and expiration in mechanically ventilated patients accurately separates responders from nonresponders.[28] It is important to note that this method assumes that RV and LV function are both normal and is most accurate in volume-control mode in the absence of ventilator dyssynchrony.

Right Atrial Pressure

RAP is correlated with central venous pressure, and can give clinicians a sense of volume status, help guide fluid resuscitation, and help delineate hypovolemic and distributive shock from cardiogenic shock. Advanced echocardiography can provide an estimation of RAP by measurement of IVC diameter and collapsibility.[29]

The following IVC measurements are used to estimate RAP:[30]

- IVC <2.1 cm with >50% collapse during sniff = RAP 0–5 mm Hg
- IVC >2.1 cm collapse >50% during sniff = RAP 5–10 mm Hg
- IVC >2.1 cm collapse <50% during sniff = 10–20 mm Hg
  However, these estimates are not accurate in mechanically ventilated patients.

Left Atrial Pressure and Diastolic Function

Studies have shown that 48% of patients admitted with sepsis had some evidence of diastolic dysfunction and that diastolic dysfunction was associated with increased mortality.[31] Focused echocardiography and advanced echocardiography allow the intensivist to measure LAP noninvasively with good concordance when compared with the gold standard of invasive hemodynamic monitoring.[32,33]

Echocardiographic evaluation of LAP may also be useful in assessing readiness for liberation from mechanical ventilation. An increase in LAP during a spontaneous breathing trial has been shown to indicate load-related heart failure and to predict liberation failure.[34,35]

Evaluation of diastolic function and LAP by full echocardiography utilizes 2D echocardiography and Doppler echocardiography to obtain four distinct variables that are subsequently applied to an algorithm to determine diastolic function in patients with a normal ejection fraction (EF): annular e′ velocity (septal′ and lateral e′), average E/′, LAVI (left atrial volume index), and peak TR (tricuspid regurgitation) velocity.[37] In patients with reduced EF, the E/A ratio is added to the assessment. Based on these measurements, the

clinician can identify the presence of diastolic dysfunction, grade the severity of diastolic dysfunction, and determine whether LAP is elevated or normal.

Several notable limitations of this algorithm may render diastolic function indeterminate. These conditions include basal segmental wall motion abnormalities, rhythm abnormalities such as tachycardia, prolonged atrioventricular conduction, atrial fibrillation, or ventricular pacing, and valvular heart disease.

It is important to recognize that these definitions were developed and validated to define measurable abnormalities in LV filling that allow for characterization of heart failure with a preserved EF. In the ICU, especially in situations with life-threatening and rapid hemodynamic decompensation, these definitions, and indeed the entire concept of diastolic dysfunction, may not be applicable.

However, a body of evidence supports the use of decreased annular velocity (e′ <8 cm/s) and increased E/e′ ratio (>14 cm/s) to define a group of patients with septic shock with high filling pressures who might be prone to fluid overload with unduly aggressive fluid resuscitation.[37]

Systolic Pulmonary Artery Pressure

The sPAP is equivalent to the RV systolic pressure in the absence of pulmonary stenosis, and is a useful hemodynamic measurement obtainable by advanced echocardiography. In patients with TR, the systolic pulmonary artery pressure can be calculated by estimating the pressure gradient between the RA and RV using the modified Bernoulli equation ($P = 4V^2$, where V is the TR velocity), and adding estimated RA pressure.[38] Although application of this technique has been well validated in estimating sPAP, its precision is debatable; one study demonstrated that echocardiography-derived sPAP differed $> \pm 10$ mm Hg from sPAP measured invasively: a majority of values underestimated sPAP.[38,39] These data imply that sPAP may be most useful in guiding and monitoring hemodynamic responses to therapy.

Cardiac Output

The CO is equal to stroke volume (SV) multiplied by heart rate and therefore can be derived by measuring aortic outflow tract diameter and velocity via pulsed-wave Doppler.[24] LVOT cross-sectional area is assumed to be circular and calculated as $r^2 \times \pi/4$. The cross-sectional area is then multiplied by the VTI, which is obtained by pulsed-wave Doppler through the LVOT, to derive stroke volume.[20]

One prospective study demonstrated that in mechanically ventilated patients, estimation of CO by transthoracic echocardiography (TTE) is accurate and precise when compared with CO measured by thermodilution using a pulmonary artery catheter, although median left ventricular ejection fraction (LVEF) was 58%, and patients with valvular disease and arrhythmia were excluded.[40]

Technical expertise is required to obtain accurate results, and critically ill patients can be difficult to image. A meta-analysis of 24 studies comparing echocardiography and thermodilution suggested that given the high percentage of error, echocardiography is not interchangeable with thermodilution.[41] Advanced echocardiography is most useful in tracking changes in CO with therapy; estimation of CO by advanced echocardiography should be performed and interpreted judiciously.

FOCUSED ECHOCARDIOGRAPHY AND ADVANCED ECHOCARDIOGRAPHY IN VALVULAR DISEASE

Various pathologies can precipitate valvular dysfunction and lead to hemodynamic instability. Endocarditis can lead to septic shock and acute valvular dysfunction. Inferior myocardial infarction can cause rupture of the posterior papillary muscle, leading to acute mitral regurgitation with pulmonary edema and cardiogenic shock. The hemodynamic consequences of significant valvular disease may dramatically impact the management of critically ill patients. Patients with severe aortic stenosis are preload dependent and are also sensitive to volume overload. Patients with prosthetic and mechanical valves are susceptible to valve thrombosis and endocarditis, and timely identification of such pathologies is crucial to management strategies and outcomes.

Although it is clear that echocardiography is extremely valuable for evaluation and management of patients with valvular heart disease, it is less clear that focused echocardiography or advanced echocardiography should be used in preference to full echocardiography. The studies are technically demanding and require high precision in both performance and interpretation.

Acute Mitral Regurgitation

Acute severe mitral regurgitation (MR) can cause cardiopulmonary instability with acute respiratory failure and cardiogenic shock. A murmur may not be present due to rapid equalization of pressures or may be hard to hear in patients with pulmonary edema.

One would expect acute severe MR would be easily identified by focused echocardiography using color Doppler imaging, but unfortunately, this is not always the case. In acute severe MR, the MR jet velocity across the mitral valve can be low due to low driving pressure from hypotension and high LAP. The color Doppler jet is usually markedly eccentric, which may also lead to underestimation of the severity of MR by less experienced operators.[42] Transesophageal echocardiography is better than TTE at characterizing the anatomy in acute MR, but not superior in assessing hemodynamics.

Acute Aortic Regurgitation

Severe acute aortic regurgitation (AR) usually presents with sudden cardiovascular collapse and pulmonary edema. Cardiopulmonary collapse is driven mainly by inability to increase forward stroke volume in an LV that has not had time to dilate. Pulmonary edema secondary to acute AR results from sudden rise in left ventricular end-diastolic pressure (LVEDP), which causes elevation of LAP and pulmonary wedge pressures.

The diagnosis of acute severe AR by focused echocardiography may be challenging, particularly with color Doppler. The use of color Doppler relies on a pressure gradient between the aorta and LV, and because of rapid equalization of the end-diastolic aortic and LV pressures along with shorter diastolic filling time due to tachycardia and/or early mitral valve closure, the regurgitant jet may be eccentric and unimpressive.[42]

Full echocardiography can be more revealing. M-mode can be used to identify early closure of the mitral valve (MV), which can suggest the presence of acute severe AR. The density of the continuous wave Doppler (CWD) signal reflects the volume of regurgitation. Measurement of pressure half-time using CWD can estimate severity of AR; a steep slope is indicative of rapid equalization of pressures between the aorta and LV during diastole. Holodiastolic flow reversal in the aorta indicates at least moderate chronic AR, although in acute severe AR, this may not occur due to rapid equilibrating of pressure between the aorta and LV. Furthermore, normal individuals can have brief, early diastolic flow reversal, and so the duration and location of flow reversal is important.

Aortic Stenosis

Severe aortic stenosis (AS) can lead to poor forward flow and hypotension and can cause pulmonary edema, leading to acute hypoxemic respiratory failure. Patients with severe AS are very sensitive to changes in cardiac loading.

The echocardiographic diagnosis of AS is technically challenging. Current imaging guidelines emphasize that diagnosis should be made using an integrative approach that includes clinical assessment of symptoms, blood pressure during the examination, transvalvular velocity/gradient, aortic valve area (AVA), valve morphology, flow rate, and LV morphology and function.[43]

Focused echocardiography can be used as a screening modality to raise suspicion of a severe AS diagnosis. Two-dimensional focused echocardiography can assess the morphology of the aortic valve (AV). Thickening and calcification of the AV cusps and reduced motion suggests calcific AS. Doming of a pliable AV points to congenital AS. Fused commissures raise suspicion for rheumatic AS. Any of these morphologic features, in the appropriate clinical context, should prompt more sophisticated assessment of the aortic valve.

Full echocardiography uses AVA, the mean transvalvular pressure gradient across the aortic valve, and peak jet velocity to evaluate the severity of AS. The AVA is calculated using the continuity equation: LVOT area × LVOT velocity equals AV area × AV jet velocity. An AVA <1.0 cm² is considered severe. Peak jet velocity is measured using CWD in multiple acoustic windows and increases with increasing AS severity; peak velocity ≥ 4.0 m/s is considered severe. Accurate measurements depend on precise LVOT measurement, parallel alignment of the ultrasound beam with blood flow, and accurate tracing of velocity curves. Measurement of LVOT diameter is the greatest source of potential error, given this measurement is squared in the continuity equation and has a reported measurement variability of 5–8%. In addition, application of the continuity equation assumes the LVOT is circular when really it is somewhat elliptical, underestimating LVOT cross-sectional area and ultimately AVA. Peak velocity and mean gradient are flow dependent; therefore, in low CO states, transvalvular flow may be reduced, resulting in underestimation.

CONCLUSION

Focused echocardiography and advanced echocardiography are well-validated noninvasive diagnostic modalities that empower intensivists to rapidly and accurately identify causes of acute cardiovascular collapse, predict response to volume, assess hemodynamics, and monitor hemodynamic changes to therapy in the critically ill. Like every diagnostic modality, focused echocardiography and advanced echocardiography have fundamental strengths and weaknesses better understanding of their advantages and limitations promotes successful application of echocardiography and minimizes misinterpretation of data.

Despite the challenges of imaging in the ICU, evidence supporting the use of echocardiography in the diagnosis and management of critically ill patients with life-threatening hemodynamic instability is so robust that training in focused echocardiography has been assimilated into the critical care curriculum. Advanced echocardiography, in particular the potential to provide noninvasive hemodynamic monitoring, is an attractive skill whose acquisition requires effort and dedication but can reward that effort with improved patient management.

AUTHORS' RECOMMENDATIONS

- Focused echocardiography and advanced echocardiography are reliable, safe, and noninvasive imaging modalities capable of accurately accelerating time to diagnosis in critically ill patients with undifferentiated hemodynamic instability.
- In addition to rapid identification of causes of acute cardiovascular collapse, focused echocardiography and advanced echocardiography provide physicians with a noninvasive means to predict response to volume, assess hemodynamics, and monitor hemodynamic changes to therapy in the critically ill.
- The term "bedside echocardiography" is an imprecise and potentially misleading term as the comprehensiveness of an echocardiographic study should be dictated by the clinical issues and urgency, not the locations at which the study is performed.
- Like every diagnostic modality, focused echocardiography and advanced echocardiography have fundamental strengths and weaknesses better understanding of their advantages and limitations promotes successful application of echocardiography and minimizes misinterpretation of data.
- Proficiency in focused echocardiography and advanced echocardiography is a rewarding skill that offers an opportunity for improved patient management.

REFERENCES

1. Labovitz AJ, Noble VE, Bierig M, et al. Focused cardiac ultrasound in the emergent setting: a consensus statement of the American Society of Echocardiography and American College of Emergency Physicians. *J Am Soc Echocardiogr*. 2010;23(12):1225-1230.
2. Levitov A, Frankel HL, Blaivas M, et al. Guidelines for the appropriate use of bedside general and cardiac ultrasonography in the evaluation of critically ill patients—part II: cardiac ultrasonography. *Crit Care Med*. 2016;44(6):1206-1227.
3. ICU ERToEi. International consensus statement on training standards for advanced critical care echocardiography. *Intensive Care Med*. 2014;40(5):654-666.
4. Mayo PH, Beaulieu Y, Doelken P, et al. American College of Chest Physicians/La Societe de Reanimation de Langue Francaise statement on competence in critical care ultrasonography. *Chest*. 2009;135(4):1050-1060.
5. Vignon P, Mücke F, Bellec F, et al. Basic critical care echocardiography: validation of a curriculum dedicated to noncardiologist residents. *Crit Care Med*. 2011;39(4):636-642.
6. Vignon P, Dugard A, Abraham J, et al. Focused training for goal-oriented hand-held echocardiography performed by noncardiologist residents in the intensive care unit. *Intensive Care Med*. 2007;33(10):1795-1799.
7. Ryan T, Berlacher K, Lindner JR, Mankad SV, Rose GA, Wang A. COCATS 4 Task Force 5: training in echocardiography. *J Am Coll Cardiol*. 2015;65(17):1786-1799.
8. Zanobetti M, Scorpiniti M, Gigli C, et al. Point-of-care ultrasonography for evaluation of acute dyspnea in the ED. *Chest*. 2017; 151(6):1295-1301.
9. Shokoohi H, Boniface KS, Zaragoza M, Pourmand A, Earls JP. Point-of-care ultrasound leads to diagnostic shifts in patients with undifferentiated hypotension. *Am J Emerg Med*. 2017;35(12):1984. e1983-1984. e1987.
10. Luo H, Chen M, Trento A, et al. Usefulness of a hand-carried cardiac ultrasound device for bedside examination of pericardial effusion in patients after cardiac surgery. *Am J Cardiol*. 2004;94(3):406-407.
11. Mercé J, Sagristà-Sauleda J, Permanyer-Miralda G, Evangelista A, Soler-Soler J. Correlation between clinical and Doppler echocardiographic findings in patients with moderate and large pericardial effusion: implications for the diagnosis of cardiac tamponade. *Am Heart J*. 1999;138(4 Pt 1):759-764.
12. Adler Y, Charron P, Imazio M, et al. 2015 ESC Guidelines for the diagnosis and management of pericardial diseases: The Task Force for the Diagnosis and Management of Pericardial Diseases of the European Society of Cardiology (ESC) Endorsed by The European Association for Cardio-Thoracic Surgery (EACTS). *Eur Heart J*. 2015;36(42):2921-2964.
13. Leeman DE, Levine MJ, Come PC. Doppler echocardiography in cardiac tamponade: exaggerated respiratory variation in transvalvular blood flow velocity integrals. *J Am Coll Cardiol*. 1988;11(3):572-578.
14. Fields JM, Davis J, Girson L, et al. Transthoracic echocardiography for diagnosing pulmonary embolism: a systematic review and meta-analysis. *J Am Soc Echocardiogr*. 2017;30(7):714-723. e714.
15. Nagueh SF, Bierig SM, Budoff MJ, et al. American Society of Echocardiography clinical recommendations for multimodality cardiovascular imaging of patients with hypertrophic cardiomyopathy: endorsed by the American Society of Nuclear Cardiology, Society for Cardiovascular Magnetic Resonance,

and Society of Cardiovascular Computed Tomography. *J Am Soc Echocardiogr*. 2011;24(5):473-498.

16. Zanotti-Cavazzoni SL, Hollenberg SM. Cardiac dysfunction in severe sepsis and septic shock. *Curr Opin Crit Care*. 2009;15(5):392-397.

17. Ehrman RR, Sullivan AN, Favot MJ, et al. Pathophysiology, echocardiographic evaluation, biomarker findings, and prognostic implications of septic cardiomyopathy: a review of the literature. *Crit Care*. 2018;22(1):112.

18. Vieillard-Baron A, Caille V, Charron C, Belliard G, Page B, Jardin F. Actual incidence of global left ventricular hypokinesia in adult septic shock. *Crit Care Med*. 2008;36(6):1701-1706.

19. Picard MH, Popp RL, Weyman AE. Assessment of left ventricular function by echocardiography: a technique in evolution. *J Am Soc Echocardiogr*. 2008;21(1):14-21.

20. Lang RM, Badano LP, Mor-Avi V, et al. Recommendations for cardiac chamber quantification by echocardiography in adults: an update from the American Society of Echocardiography and the European Association of Cardiovascular Imaging. *J Am Soc Echocardiogr*. 2015;28(1):1-39. e14.

21. Piazza G, Goldhaber SZ. The acutely decompensated right ventricle: pathways for diagnosis and management. *Chest*. 2005;128(3):1836-1852.

22. Rudski LG, Lai WW, Afilalo J, et al. Guidelines for the echocardiographic assessment of the right heart in adults: a report from the American Society of Echocardiography endorsed by the European Association of Echocardiography, a registered branch of the European Association of Cardiology, and the Canadian Society of Echocardiography. *J Am Soc Echocardiogr*. 2010;23(7): 685-713; quiz 786-688.

23. Forfia PR, Fisher MR, Mathai SC, et al. Tricuspid annular displacement predicts survival in pulmonary hypertension. *Am J Respir Crit Care Med*. 2006;174(9):1034-1041.

24. Porter TR, Shillcutt SK, Adams MS, et al. Guidelines for the use of echocardiography as a monitor for therapeutic intervention in adults: a report from the American Society of Echocardiography. *J Am Soc Echocardiogr*. 2015;28(1):40-56.

25. Boyd JH, Forbes J, Nakada TA, Walley KR, Russell JA. Fluid resuscitation in septic shock: a positive fluid balance and elevated central venous pressure are associated with increased mortality. *Crit Care Med*. 2011;39(2):259-265.

26. Monnet X, Marik P, Teboul JL. Passive leg raising for predicting fluid responsiveness: a systematic review and meta-analysis. *Intensive Care Med*. 2016;42(12):1935-1947.

27. Cavallaro F, Sandroni C, Marano C, et al. Diagnostic accuracy of passive leg raising for prediction of fluid responsiveness in adults: systematic review and meta-analysis of clinical studies. *Intensive Care Med*. 2010;36(9):1475-1483.

28. Barbier C, Loubières Y, Schmit C, et al. Respiratory changes in inferior vena cava diameter are helpful in predicting fluid responsiveness in ventilated septic patients. *Intensive Care Med*. 2004;30(9):1740-1746.

29. Kircher BJ, Himelman RB, Schiller NB. Noninvasive estimation of right atrial pressure from the inspiratory collapse of the inferior vena cava. *Am J Cardiol*. 1990;66(4):493-496.

30. Lang RM, Bierig M, Devereux RB, et al. Recommendations for chamber quantification: a report from the American Society of Echocardiography's Guidelines and Standards Committee and the Chamber Quantification Writing Group, developed in conjunction with the European Association of Echocardiography, a branch of the European Society of Cardiology. *J Am Soc Echocardiogr*. 2005;18(12):1440-1463.

31. Sanfilippo F, Corredor C, Arcadipane A, et al. Tissue Doppler assessment of diastolic function and relationship with mortality in critically ill septic patients: a systematic review and meta-analysis. *Br J Anaesth*. 2017;119(4):583-594.

32. Ommen SR, Nishimura RA, Appleton CP, et al. Clinical utility of Doppler echocardiography and tissue Doppler imaging in the estimation of left ventricular filling pressures: a comparative simultaneous Doppler-catheterization study. *Circulation*. 2000;102(15):1788-1794.

33. Kasner M, Westermann D, Steendijk P, et al. Utility of Doppler echocardiography and tissue Doppler imaging in the estimation of diastolic function in heart failure with normal ejection fraction: a comparative Doppler-conductance catheterization study. *Circulation*. 2007;116(6):637-647.

34. Lamia B, Maizel J, Ochagavia A, et al. Echocardiographic diagnosis of pulmonary artery occlusion pressure elevation during weaning from mechanical ventilation. *Crit Care Med*. 2009; 37(5):1696-1701.

35. Moschietto S, Doyen D, Grech L, Dellamonica J, Hyvernat H, Bernardin G. Transthoracic echocardiography with Doppler tissue imaging predicts weaning failure from mechanical ventilation: evolution of the left ventricle relaxation rate during a spontaneous breathing trial is the key factor in weaning outcome. *Crit Care*. 2012;16(3):R81.

36. Nagueh SF, Smiseth OA, Appleton CP, et al. Recommendations for the evaluation of left ventricular diastolic function by echocardiography: an update from the American Society of Echocardiography and the European Association of Cardiovascular Imaging. *J Am Soc Echocardiogr*. 2016;29(4):277-314.

37. Greenstein YY, Mayo PH. Evaluation of left ventricular diastolic function by the intensivist. *Chest*. 2018;153(3): 723-732.

38. Milan A, Magnino C, Veglio F. Echocardiographic indexes for the non-invasive evaluation of pulmonary hemodynamics. *J Am Soc Echocardiogr*. 2010;23(3):225-239; quiz 332-224.

39. Fisher MR, Forfia PR, Chamera E, et al. Accuracy of Doppler echocardiography in the hemodynamic assessment of pulmonary hypertension. *Am J Respir Crit Care Med*. 2009; 179(7):615-621.

40. Mercado P, Maizel J, Beyls C, et al. Transthoracic echocardiography: an accurate and precise method for estimating cardiac output in the critically ill patient. *Crit Care*. 2017;21(1):136.

41. Wetterslev M, Møller-Sørensen H, Johansen RR, Perner A. Systematic review of cardiac output measurements by echocardiography vs. thermodilution: the techniques are not interchangeable. *Intensive Care Med*. 2016;42(8):1223-1233.

42. Zoghbi WA, Adams D, Bonow RO, et al. Recommendations for noninvasive evaluation of native valvular regurgitation: a report from the American Society of Echocardiography Developed in Collaboration with the Society for Cardiovascular Magnetic Resonance. *J Am Soc Echocardiogr*. 2017;30(4):303-371.

43. Baumgartner H, Hung J, Bermejo J, et al. Recommendations on the echocardiographic assessment of aortic valve stenosis: a focused update from the European Association of Cardiovascular Imaging and the American Society of Echocardiography. *J Am Soc Echocardiogr*. 2017;30(4):372-392.

50

How Do I Manage Hemodynamic Decompensation in a Critically Ill Patient?

Allison Dalton and Michael F. O'Connor

The ability to evaluate and manage a hemodynamically decompensating patient is one of the most important skills the intensivist brings to the bedside. The problem is complicated by two potentially divergent goals:

1. Patients can decompensate from a number of different causes—and which one is operative is often not readily apparent.
2. The recognition that a patient is decompensating usually requires an immediate response, often with insufficient information to identify the underlying causes that ultimately must be corrected.

In general, the need to respond is initiated by a constellation of clinical signs—early hints such as a change in mental status;[1] changes that occur somewhere further along the decompensation spectrum, such as a decrease in urine output; and relatively late signs of hypoperfusion, such as tachycardia or, more ominously, a drop in blood pressure. And, in general, the initial response is most often administration of intravenous (IV) fluids to increase the volume of liquid in the circulation.

ASSESSING VOLUME RESPONSIVENESS

The first response to a hemodynamically unstable patient is usually the administration of IV fluids. While recent literature recommends volume infusion until the mean arterial pressure (MAP) is 65 mm Hg for patients with septic shock, this guideline is not evidence based[2–4] and is provided only as an initial goal, not as a resuscitation end point. Determination of the value of ongoing fluid administration is an important early goal in the management of the hemodynamically unstable patient. Indeed, only about 50% of patients in shock will respond to ongoing volume challenges. Therefore, it is important to determine if a patient will benefit from volume infusion.[5] Correcting a low MAP is almost always inadequate; the presence of hypoperfusion in the presence of a "reasonable" MAP is well-documented. Similarly, evidence strongly suggests that use of a single measurement of central venous pressure (CVP) or pulmonary artery occlusion pressure (PAOP) to guide resuscitation is inadequate. Furthermore, assessment of changes in CVP or PAOP in response to intervention is also problematic.[5–8] These pressures may be proportional to the volume in the right (CVP) or left (PAOP) ventricle at the moment of measurement. However, volume infusion into either chamber alters ventricular compliance, changing the pressure:volume relationship. In addition, neither CVP nor PAOP will help the practitioner determine if volume infusion is improving ventricular emptying (e.g., stroke volume). Similarly, while an initial, single-center study of early goal directed fluid therapy (EGDT) in septic shock touted the value of central venous oxygen saturation (ScvO$_2$) as an endpoint of resuscitation,[9] three recent large, multicenter randomized trials of ScvO$_2$ have not replicated that result.[10–12] Therefore, alternative approaches to assessing volume responsiveness are required. An algorithm for assessing volume responsiveness appears in Fig. 50.1.

Use of Systolic Pressure Variation and Pulse Pressure Variation

Dynamic parameters include systolic pressure variation (SPV) and pulse pressure variation (PPV). Studies suggest that these methods provide highly valuable information regarding volume responsiveness.[7,8,13,14] These methods assess the variation in the blood pressure components in response to the cyclic increases in intrathoracic pressure that are caused by PPV. Increased intrathoracic pressure will increase stroke volume and systolic and pulse pressures in early positive pressure inspiration.[15] This increase is termed delta up (Δup).[15] However, the sustained intrathoracic pressure almost immediately decreases right ventricular (RV) preload and, by increasing transpulmonary pressures, elevates RV afterload, decreasing RV stroke volume.[7] As a result, left ventricular (LV) filling is reduced, and with it LV stroke volume, a decrease termed delta down (Δdown). SPV is defined as the difference between Δup and Δdown within one controlled breath.[15] Several studies indicate that Δdown is a predictor of volume responsiveness.[16,17]

There are limitations in the use of SPV and PPV. An arterial pressure monitoring system that is free of kinks, clots, excess tubing, or stopcocks is required.[18] The patient must be in sinus rhythm.[19] Low tidal volumes (e.g., 6 mL/kg) may lead to falsely low measurements due to small changes in pulmonary and transpleural pressures.[18]

For patients without arterial access or in whom PPV or SVP cannot be accurately measured, plethysmographic waveform variability (PWV) may determine fluid responsiveness.[20] PWV uses the maximal and minimal plethysmographic values divided by the pulse oximeter waveform amplitude during

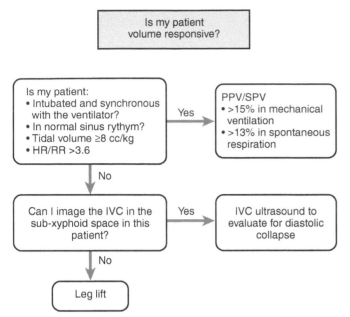

Fig. 50.1 An algorithm for determining volume responsiveness in the shock state: PPV/SPV[7,8,13,14]; IVC ultrasound[23–25]; and leg lift.[26,27] *HR*, heart rate; *IVC*, inferior vena cava; *PPV*, pulse pressure variation; *RR*, respiratory rate; *SPV*, systolic pressure variation.

apnea. Pizov and colleagues found PWV to be comparable to PPV in predicting fluid responsiveness.[20]

Inferior Vena Cava Collapsibility on Ultrasound

Bedside ultrasound of the inferior vena cava (IVC) has been used to assess volume responsiveness. Several studies have touted this noninvasive technique, which measures the effect of the respiratory cycle on the diameter of the IVC.[21–24] In contrast to variables involving the arterial side of the circulation, the IVC does not vasoconstrict in response to volume loss to the same extent. Therefore, this vessel may more directly reflect responses to volume.[25]

Passive Leg Raise

Passive leg raise predicts the volume responsiveness in patients with shock. For this maneuver to be performed, the patient is placed in the supine position and both lower extremities are raised to a 45-degree angle. The passive leg raise is the equivalent of a 300–500 cc fluid challenge.[26,27] While not accurate in predicting fluid responsiveness based upon changes in blood pressure, an increase in cardiac output by ≥10% denotes that fluid will augment cardiac output.[27] Cardiac output may be measured noninvasively using pulse contour analysis, echocardiography, and esophageal Doppler.[27] Continuous pulse oximetry changes may also be used in conjunction with passive leg raise.[27] Importantly, passive leg can be used in patients with cardiac arrhythmias and in patients who are breathing spontaneously.[26]

Mean Systemic Pressure

Mean systemic pressure is the pressure that occurs with temporarily occlusion of circulatory flow after equilibration of venous and arterial pressures.[28] One method of determining mean systemic pressure involves inflating an upper extremity blood pressure cuff 50 mm Hg above systolic pressure and determining the mean pressure 30 seconds after flow stops.[29] This method has been validated against measurements of CVP during inspiratory holds in patients on positive pressure ventilation.[29,30] In recent years, a series of studies have measured the mean systemic pressure in hypotensive patients and shown that this parameter reliably predicts volume responsiveness. If these observations are replicated and instruments that can be used to make this measurement become available in clinical practice, it is possible that determination of the mean systemic pressure may become the gold standard for inferences about volume status and volume responsiveness.[29,30]

INITIAL TREATMENT—ADDRESSING HYPOVOLEMIA/HYPOVOLEMIC SHOCK

An initial bolus of 30 mL/kg of a low-chloride crystalloid solution should be given to patients determined to be fluid responsive. Albumin may be added in patients with septic shock who are receiving large volume resuscitation.[31–33] Ultimately, clinical endpoints (mental status, urine volume), MAP, lactate levels, and mixed/central venous saturations should be used to determine adequacy of resuscitation.[4,5,31]

IDENTIFICATION AND EMERGENT MANAGEMENT OF VASODILATORY SHOCK

Vasodilatory shock manifests as decreased vascular tone, resulting in hypotension and redistribution of blood flow. Because elevated lactate is an independent marker of morbidity and mortality,[34–36] experts recommend normalization of lactate levels as a marker of normalization of tissue perfusion. Jansen et al.[37] incorporated a normalization of lactate algorithm for the management of patients with sepsis. In Jansen's study, protocol-driven normalization of lactate resulted in significant reductions in the ICU length of stay and ICU/hospital mortality in the treatment group.[37] For patients in whom septic shock is suspected, prompt administration of broad-spectrum IV antibiotics improves mortality.[31,38–40] Empirically administered antibiotics should provide coverage for infection with gram-positive, gram-negative, and anaerobic bacteria, and may also include fungal and viral coverage.[38] For patients presenting with septic shock or neutropenia, empiric administration of aminoglycosides reduces mortality.[41–43] Source control aimed at diagnosis of a specific infectious source and subsequent intervention should be performed.

Septic patients who have been adequately volume resuscitated may require therapy with vasoactive drugs to achieve adequate blood pressure and vital organ perfusion. The goal of the addition of vasopressors is not solely to increase MAP to a target of 65 mm Hg but also to obtain acceptable end-organ perfusion. The recommended first-line vasopressor advised for septic shock is norepinephrine.[44] A detailed discussion on the use of vasoactive drugs in septic shock may be found in Chapter 35.

IDENTIFICATION AND EMERGENT MANAGEMENT OF OBSTRUCTIVE SHOCK

Cardiogenic and obstructive shock are important causes of hypotension, and patients who have neither hypovolemic nor vasodilatory shock will need to be evaluated for these. This process can be of pericardial, thoracic, or abdominal origin. Identification of the cause of obstructive shock requires the concurrent or sequential completion of several diagnostic evaluations in short order. These include the inspection of ventilator flow waveforms for the presence of auto-positive end-expiratory pressure (PEEP) or ultrasonography to assess for the presence of tension pneumothorax, measurement of bladder pressures in patients with a tense or distended abdomen to evaluate for abdominal compartment syndrome, and the performance of echocardiography (e.g., FOCUS [focused cardiac ultrasound] examination or FATE [focused assessed transthoracic echocardiography]) to evaluate the patient for cardiogenic shock and tamponade.

Abdominal Compartment Syndrome

Intra-abdominal hypertension is the result of diminished abdominal wall compliance, increased intraluminal contents, increased intra-abdominal contents, or capillary leak/fluid resuscitation. Progression to abdominal compartment syndrome has occurred when intra-abdominal pressure exceeds 25 mm Hg; at this point, the transmitted pressure affects cardiac, pulmonary, and renal functions as well as cerebrospinal fluid pressure.[45,46] The presence of abdominal compartment syndrome should be suspected by a rise in peak airway pressure and is most often diagnosed by measuring bladder pressure.[47] Treatment should follow the guidelines developed by the World Society for Abdominal Compartment Syndrome (detailed in Chapter 75).[47]

Auto-PEEP

Obstructive shock may originate in the thorax. Auto-PEEP is the process by which the respiratory system is unable to return to functional residual capacity at the end of the expiratory phase of ventilation. Auto-PEEP impairs venous return to the heart, increases risk of barotrauma to the lungs, and can increase the patient's work of breathing while impeding their ability to trigger the ventilator.[48] Short respiratory cycles, high minute volumes, and obstructive lung disease predispose a patient to auto-PEEP. It is diagnosed on ventilator waveforms by persistence of flow at end expiration. Management of hemodynamically unstable auto-PEEP requires immediate relief of pressure by disconnecting the patient from the ventilator. Subsequent treatment of auto-PEEP includes decreasing respiratory rate and/or decreasing the I:E ratio to allow for more expiratory time.[49]

Tension Pneumothorax

Tension pneumothorax occurs when air enters the pleural space but is unable to exit, causing increased intrapleural pressure.[48] This increased pressure can shift the mediastinum, compromising ventilation, directly compressing the heart, and, by compressing the vena cava at both the thoracic inlet and at the diaphragm, decreasing venous return. Tension pneumothorax is diagnosed by observing unilateral breath sounds and signs of shock; in the hands of experienced intensivists, thoracic ultrasound may aid in the diagnosis.[50] Management includes needle thoracostomy followed by chest tube placement.

Cardiac Tamponade

Cardiac tamponade is defined as compromise of ventricular filling by an extracardiac collection that ultimately decreases stroke volume. The highly compliant right heart is most susceptible. Causes include blood or exudate from inflammation (pericardial effusion). In some instances (e.g., patients with a right ventricular assist device [RVAD]), mediastinal fluid can compress the great veins of the thorax and obstruct venous return without directly impinging on the pump itself, resulting in tamponade physiology. The condition may present with pulsus paradoxus (drop in systolic blood pressure by >10 mm Hg during inspiration[51]) and electrical alternans (alternation of QRS amplitude and/or axis over subsequent heart beats) and may be accompanied by tachycardia and hypotension. Bedside echocardiography can reveal pericardial effusion and collapse of right-sided cardiac chambers.[52] Prompt needle decompression with or without ultrasound guidance is the definitive treatment of hemodynamically significant pericardial effusions.

IDENTIFICATION AND EMERGENT MANAGEMENT OF CARDIOGENIC SHOCK

Decreased cardiac contractility, increased diastolic stiffness (diastolic dysfunction), increased afterload, valvular abnormalities, and/or abnormal heart rates/rhythms can lead to ventricular dysfunction and cardiogenic shock.[48] Acute myocardial ischemia and infarction are the most common causes of cardiogenic shock arising from the left ventricle.[53] In the modern era, RV infarction is a less frequent and less important cause of cardiogenic shock. Importantly, diastolic dysfunction decreases cardiac output by impairing diastolic filling.

Acute RV shock is most often the result of elevated pulmonary vascular resistance (e.g., pulmonary embolus). Elevated right-sided pressures (including CVP) with low cardiac output and no echocardiographic evidence of LV shock help to identify isolated RV shock. Symptoms are similar to those of cardiac tamponade and constrictive pericarditis; hence, these conditions must be excluded.[48]

Echocardiography is the gold standard in the evaluation of cardiogenic causes of shock. Echocardiography was once limited to cardiologists, but now intensivists and other noncardiologists are trained in basic emergency ultrasound. The FOCUS examination consists of evaluation for presence of pericardial effusion, assessment of global cardiac systolic function, existence of ventricular enlargement, and estimation of intravascular volume.[54]

Identifying right-sided vs. left-sided cardiogenic shock is imperative because treatment strategies differ. Management of patients with LV shock focuses on increasing preload, decreasing afterload and enhancing contractility with vaso-pressors, inotropes, and mechanical support such as intra-aortic balloon counterpulsation or ventricular assist devices.[48] Management of right-sided shock includes maintaining arterial pressure with vasoconstrictors, cardiac contractility with beta-1 agonists, and selective pulmonary vasodilation. Excess fluid infusion may further impair RV function by causing right-to-left intraventricular septal shift, which limits LV filling.[55] Right-sided volume overload may be managed with diuretics, splanchnic vasodilators (e.g., nitroglycerin), or hemofiltration. A complete discussion of cardiogenic shock management can be found in Chapter 52.

In patients with pulmonary embolism, treatment with anticoagulation, thrombolytics, and/or surgical embolectomy can improve underlying right heart failure.[48,56] Right heart shock arising from elevated pulmonary vascular resistance can be treated with pulmonary vasodilation using inspired oxygen, inhaled nitric oxide, or prostaglandin E_1.[48] An algorithm for the evaluation and management of a patient with narrow-pulse pressure shock unresponsive to volume is presented in Fig. 50.2.

CONCLUSION

Unidentified, untreated shock is associated with high morbidity and mortality.[57] Appropriate treatment relies on recognition, initial emergent management, determination of the type of shock present, and ongoing treatment mandated by the specific etiology. New tools have improved both diagnosis and management.

AUTHORS' RECOMMENDATIONS
- When approaching a patient in shock, consider the four classes of shock: hypovolemic, vasodilatory, cardiogenic, and obstructive.
- Dynamic hemodynamic parameters are more accurate than static measurements in the assessment of volume status and fluid responsiveness.
- Echocardiography is a useful tool for assessment of intravascular volume and fluid responsiveness but also for cardiogenic and obstructive causes of shock.

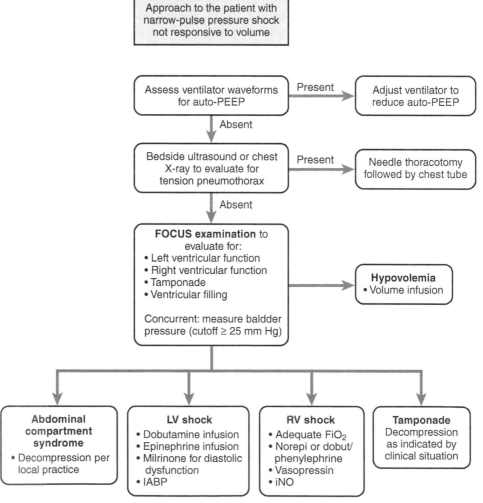

Fig. 50.2 An approach to the patient with narrow-pulse pressure shock: auto-PEEP[49]; tension pneumothorax[50]; FOCUS examination[54]; abdominal compartment syndrome[47]; tamponade[52]; LV shock[48]; RV shock.[48,55,56] *dobut*, dobutamine: *FiO₂*, fraction of inspired oxygen; *FOCUS*, focused cardiac ultrasound; *IABP*, intra-aortic balloon pump; *iNO*, inhaled nitric oxide; *Norepi*, norepinephrine; *PEEP*, positive end-expiratory pressure.

REFERENCES

1. Sprung CL, Peduzzi PN, Shatney CH, et al. Impact of encephalopathy on mortality in the sepsis syndrome. *Crit Care Med.* 1990;18:801-806.

2. Asfar P, Meziani F, Hamel JF, et al. High versus low blood-pressure target in patients with septic shock. *N Engl J Med.* 2014;370:1583-1593.

3. Lehman LW, Saeed M, Talmor D, Mark R, Malhotra A. Method of blood pressure measurement in the ICU. *Crit Care Med.* 2013;41:34-40.

4. Cecconi M, De Backer D, Antonelli M, et al. Consensus on circulatory shock and hemodynamic monitoring. Task force of the European Society of Intensive Care Medicine. *Intensive Care Med.* 2014;40:1795-1815.

5. Marik PE, Baram M, Vahid B. Does the central venous pressure predict fluid responsiveness? A systematic review of the literature and the tale of seven mares. *Chest.* 2008;134:172-178.

6. Osman D, Ridel C, Ray P, et al. Cardiac filling pressures are not appropriate to predict hemodynamic response to volume challenge. *Crit Care Med.* 2007;35(1):64-68.

7. Michard F, Teboul JL. Using heart-lung interactions to assess fluid responsiveness during mechanical ventilation. *Crit Care Med.* 2000;4:282-289.

8. Marik PE, Monnet X, Teboul JL. Hemodynamic parameters to guide fluid therapy. *Ann Intensive Care.* 2011;1:1-9.

9. Rivers E, Nguyen B, Havstad S, et al. Early goal-directed therapy in the treatment of severe sepsis and septic shock. *N Engl J Med.* 2001;345:1368-1377.

10. Mouncey PR, Osborn TM, Power GS, et al. Trial of early, goal-directed resuscitation for septic shock. *N Engl J Med.* 2015;372:1301-1311.

11. Peake SL, Delaney A, Bailey M, et al. Goal-directed resuscitation for patient with early septic shock. *N Engl J Med.* 2014;371:1496-1506.

12. Yealy DM, Kellum JA, Huang DT, et al. A randomized trial of protocol-based care for early septic shock. *N Engl J Med.* 2014;370:1683-1693.

13. Preisman S, Kogan S, Berkenstadt H, Perel A. Predicting fluid responsiveness in patients undergoing cardiac surgery: functional haemodynamic parameters including Respiratory Systolic Variation Test and static preload indicators. *Br J Anaesth.* 2005;95:746-755.

14. Huang CC, Fu JY, Hu HC, et al. Prediction of fluid responsiveness in acute respiratory distress syndrome patients ventilated with low tidal volume and high positive end-expiratory pressure. *Crit Care Med.* 2008;36:2810-2816.

15. Perel A, Pizov R, Gotev S. Systolic blood pressure variation is a sensitive indicator of hypovolemia in ventilated dogs subjected to graded hemorrhage. *Anesthesiology.* 1987;67:498-502.

16. Coriat P, Vrillon M, Perel A, et al. A comparison of systolic blood pressure variations and echocardiographic estimates of end-diastolic left ventricular size in patients after aortic surgery. *Anesth Analg.* 1994;78:46-53.

17. Rooke GA, Schwid HA, Shapira Y. The effect of graded hemorrhage and intravascular volume replacement on systolic pressure variation in humans during mechanical and spontaneous ventilation. *Anesth Analg.* 1995;80:925-932.

18. Michard F. Changes in arterial pressure during mechanical ventilation. *Anesthesiology.* 2005;103:419-428.

19. Michard F, Teboul JL. Predicting fluid responsiveness in ICU patients: a critical analysis of the evidence. *Chest.* 2002;121:2000-2008.

20. Pizov R, Eden A, Bystritski D, Kalina E, Tamir A, Gelman S. Hypotension during gradual blood loss: waveform variables response and absence of tachycardia. *Br J Anaesth.* 2012;109:911-918.

21. Au SM, Vieillard-Baron A. Bedside echocardiography in critically ill patients: a true hemodynamic monitoring tool. *J Clin Monit Comput.* 2012;26:355-360.

22. Royce CF, Canty DJ, Faris J, Haji DL, Veltman M, Royse A. Core review: physician-performed ultrasound: the time has come for routine use in acute care medicine. *Anesth Analg.* 2012;115:1007-1028.

23. Muller L, Bobbia X, Toumi M, et al. Respiratory variations of inferior vena cava diameter to predict fluid responsiveness in spontaneously breathing patients with acute circulatory failure: need for a cautious use. *Crit Care.* 2012;16:R188.

24. Zhang Z, Xu X, Ye S, Xu L. Ultrasonographic measurement of the respiratory variation in the inferior vena cava diameter is predictive of fluid responsiveness in critically ill patients: systemic review and meta-analysis. *Ultrasound Med Biol.* 2014;40:845-853.

25. Dipti A, Soucy Z, Surana A, Chandra S. Role of inferior vena cava diameter in assessment of volume status: a meta-analysis. *Am J Emerg Med.* 2012;30:1414-1419.e1

26. Monnet X, Rienzo M, Osman D, et al. Passive leg raising predicts fluid responsiveness in the critically ill. *Crit Care Med.* 2006;34:1402-1407.

27. Monnet X, Marik PE, Teboul JL. Prediction of fluid responsiveness: an update. *Ann Intensive Care.* 2016;6:111.

28. Rothe CF. Mean circulatory filling pressure: its meaning and measurement. *J Appl Physiol.* 1993;74:499-509.

29. Maas JJ, Pinsky MR, Geerts BF, de Wilde RB, Jansen JR. Estimation of mean systemic filling pressure in postoperative cardiac surgery patients with three methods. *Intensive Care Med.* 2012;38:1452-1460.

30. Maas JJ, Geerts BF, van den Berg PC, Pinsky MR, Jansen JR. Assessment of venous return curve and mean systemic filling pressure in postoperative cardiac surgery patients. *Crit Care Med.* 2009;37:912-918.

31. Rhodes A, Evans LE, Alhazzani W, et al. Surviving Sepsis Campaign: International Guidelines for Management of Sepsis and Septic Shock: 2016. *Intensive Care Med.* 2017;43:304-377.

32. Caironi P, Tognoni G, Masson S, et al. Albumin replacement in patients with severe sepsis or septic shock. *N Engl J Med.* 2014;370(15):1412-1421.

33. Annane D, Siami S, Jaber S, et al. Effects of fluid resuscitation with colloids and crystalloids on mortality in critically ill patients presenting with hypovolemic shock. *JAMA.* 2013;310(17):1809-1817.

34. Kompanje EJ, Jansen TC, van der Hoven B, Bakker J. The first demonstration of lactic acid in human blood in shock by Johann Joseph Scherer (1814-1869) in January 1843. *Intensive Care Med.* 2007;33:1967-1971.

35. Bakker J. Lactate: may I have your votes please? *Intensive Care Med.* 2001;27:6-11.

36. Mikkelsen ME, Miltiades AN, Gaieski DF, et al. Serum lactate is associated with mortality in severe sepsis independent of organ failure and shock. *Crit Care Med.* 2009;37:1670-1677.

37. Jansen TC, von Bommel J, Schoonderbeek FJ, et al. Early lactate-guided therapy in intensive care unit patients. *Am J Respir Crit Care Med.* 2010;182:752-761.

38. Kumar A, Roberts D, Wood KE, et al. Duration of hypotension before initiation of effective antimicrobial therapy is the

critical determinant of survival in human septic shock. *Crit Care Med.* 2006;34:1589-1596.

39. Morrell M, Fraser VJ, Kollef MH. Delaying the empiric treatment of Candida bloodstream infection until positive blood culture results are obtained: a potential risk factor for hospital mortality. *Antimicrob Agents Chemother.* 2005;49:3640-3645.

40. Seymour C, Gesten F, Prescott HC, et al. Time to treatment and mortality during mandated emergency care for sepsis. *N Engl J Med.* 2017;376:2235-2244.

41. Martínez JA, Cobos-Trigueros N, Soriano A, et al. Influence of empiric therapy with a beta-lactam alone or combined with an aminoglycoside on prognosis of bacteremia due to gram-negative microorganisms. *Antimicrob Agents Chemother.* 2010;54:3590-3596.

42. Kumar A, Safdar N, Kethireddy S, Chateau D. A survival benefit of combination antibiotic therapy for serious infections associated with sepsis and septic shock is contingent only on the risk of death: a meta-analytic/meta-regression study. *Crit Care Med.* 2010;38:1651-1664.

43. Kumar A, Zarychanski R, Light B, et al. Early combination antibiotic therapy yields improved survival compared with monotherapy in septic shock: a propensity-matched analysis. *Crit Care Med.* 2010;38:1773-1785.

44. Russell JA, Walley KR, Singer J, et al. VASST investigators: vasopressin versus norepinephrine infusion in patients with septic shock. *N Engl J Med.* 2008;358:877-887.

45. Schein M, Ivatury R. Intra-abdominal hypertension and the abdominal compartment syndrome. *Br J Surg.* 1998;85:1027-1028.

46. Malbrain ML, De Laet IE, De Waele JJ, Kirkpatrick AW. Abdominal hypertension: definitions, monitoring, interpretation and management. *Best Pract Res Clin Anaesthesiol.* 2013;27:249-270.

47. Kirkpatrick AW, Roberts DJ, de Waele J, et al. Intra-abdominal hypertension and the abdominal compartment syndrome: updated consensus definitions and clinical practice guidelines from the World Society of the Abdominal Compartment Syndrome. *Intensive Care Med.* 2013;39:1190-1206.

48. Hall J, Schmidt G, Wood L. *Principles of Critical Care.* 3rd ed. New York, NY: McGraw-Hill; 2005:249-265.

49. Pepe P, Marini J. Occult positive end-expiratory pressure in mechanically ventilated patients with airflow obstruction: the auto-PEEP effect. *Am Rev Respir Dis.* 1982;126:166-170.

50. Ashton-Cleary DT. Is thoracic ultrasound a viable alternative to conventional imaging in the critical care setting? *Br J Anaesth.* 2013;111:152-160.

51. Bilchick KC, Wise RA. Paradoxical physical findings described by Kussmaul's sign. *Lancet.* 2002;359:1940-1942.

52. Beaulieu Y. Bedside echocardiography in the assessment of the critically ill. *Crit Care Med.* 2007;35:S235-S249.

53. Page DL, Caulfield JB, Kastor JA, DeSanctis RW, Sanders CA. Myocardial changes associated with cardiogenic shock. *N Engl J Med.* 1971;285:133-137.

54. Labovitz A, Noble V, Bierig M, et al. Focused cardiac ultrasound in the emergent setting: a consensus statement of the American Society of Echocardiography and American College of Emergency Physicians. *J Am Soc Echocardiogr.* 2010;23:1225-1230.

55. Jacobs AK, Leopold JA, Bates E, et al. Cardiogenic shock cause by right ventricular infarction: a report from the SHOCK registry. *J Am Coll Cardiol.* 2003;41:1273-1279.

56. Konstantinides S, Geibel A, Heusel G, et al.; Prognosis of Pulmonary Embolism-3 Trial Investigators. Heparin plus alteplase compared with heparin alone in patients with submassive pulmonary embolism. *N Engl J Med.* 2002;347:1143-1150.

57. Kopterides P, Bonovas S, Mavrou I, Kostadima E, Zakynthinos E, Armaganidis A. Venous oxygen saturation and lactate gradient from superior vena cava to pulmonary artery in patients with septic shock. *Shock.* 2009;31:561-567.

51

What Are the Best Tools to Optimize the Circulation?

Garima Gupta and Michael R. Pinsky

INTRODUCTION

Functional hemodynamic monitoring (FHM) is the assessment of hemodynamic variables as they respond to a defined reversible physiologic stressor over time. Classical measurements of hemodynamics, such as pulse oximetry to estimate arterial oxygen saturation, sphygmomanometry to assess systolic and diastolic blood pressures, auscultation to identify heart rate, and urine output as a surrogate for tissue perfusion, all provide the bedside clinician with important information about the patient's cardiopulmonary status. Taken as static measures at one point in time, these variables do not have the ability to identify cardiopulmonary reserve in acutely unstable patients who are still able to compensate for hypovolemia, vasodilatory states, or heart failure but who are at risk for hemodynamic collapse and require guided resuscitation.[1] In this chapter, we discuss FHM techniques and their ability to predict volume responsiveness and assess vasomotor tone at the bedside.

BACKGROUND

The goal of initial resuscitation in any patient with circulatory shock is to restore mean arterial pressure (MAP) to sustain organ perfusion pressure and then blood flow to minimize tissue hypoperfusion and end-organ damage. The cornerstone of resuscitation is intravascular volume expansion in order to restore the pressure gradient for venous return. However, volume expansion will result in increased cardiac output (CO) only if both ventricles are preload dependent.[2] If no test is used to predict volume responsiveness, volume expansion results in increased CO in only half of patients with circulatory shock, resulting in unnecessary fluid overload in the other half.[3]

The most recent consensus guideline from the Surviving Sepsis Campaign recommends an initial fluid bolus of 30 mL/kg for patients with sepsis-induced hypovolemia followed by serial assessments of hemodynamic variables to guide further resuscitation. Dynamic variables are preferred to static variables to predict fluid responsiveness.[4] The landmark paper on early goal directed therapy (EGDT) by Rivers et al. described following static measures such as central venous pressure (CVP) and central venous oxygen saturation ($ScvO_2$) over time to determine successful resuscitation of patients with septic shock.[5] Subsequent large multicenter randomized control trials have failed to show mortality reduction using protocolized quantitative EGDT.[6–8] The average volume of fluid given prior to randomization in the ProCESS (Protocolized Care for Early Septic Shock) and ARISE (Australasian Resuscitation in Sepsis Evaluation) trials was approximately 30 mL/kg, and in the ProMISe (Protocolized Management in Sepsis) trial was approximately 2 liters. The ideal amount of fluid a patient will require is unclear but will clearly be different among patients, owing to the inherent heterogeneity of disease, cardiovascular reserve, and time they present during their disease process for therapy. Dynamic measures of fluid responsiveness are recommended to determine which patients will be likely to increase stroke volume with the administration of fluids, and this rule applies across patients and diseases.

Hemodynamic monitoring will be beneficial in the management of acute circulatory shock only if coupled with a management regimen that has been shown to improve outcome.[9] Presumably, using such monitoring will target restoration of tissue blood flow in a timely manner to prevent organ ischemic injury while avoiding volume overload. FHM has been shown to improve outcomes in a large meta-analysis looking at 13 trials that enrolled 1652 patients. Bednarczyk et al.[10] concluded that the use of dynamic tests of fluid responsiveness to guide resuscitation of critically ill patients resulted in reduced mortality, shorter intensive care unit (ICU) length of stay, and shorter duration of mechanical ventilation. The remainder of this chapter reviews current techniques in FHM.

STATIC MEASURES OF VOLUME RESPONSIVENESS

Hemodynamic monitoring techniques are a fundamental and ubiquitous part of the assessment of most critically ill patients. Goal-directed resuscitation protocols have evolved over the past 20 years but initially focused on targeting threshold CVP as an estimate of right ventricular filling pressure, pulmonary artery occlusion pressure (PAOP) as an estimate of left ventricular filling pressure, and CO to achieve adequate $ScvO_2$.[11] These static measures of cardiac preload were measured using an invasive pulmonary artery catheter (PAC).[12] The central hypothesis was that a low CVP or Ppao would predict volume responsiveness, and an elevation in either value would identify volume nonresponders.[1] Although the landmark trial of Shoemaker et al.[13] showed a mortality benefit, reduced complications, decreased cost, and decreased length of stay in patients randomized to the PAC group by targeting a supranormal CO to achieve a supranormal oxygen delivery (DO_2), several trials have since failed to show benefit and indeed have shown increased harm in critically ill patients with circulatory shock.[14-19] Given that both CVP and $ScvO_2$ values can be obtained from less-invasive internal jugular or subclavian catheters, the generic use of PAC has fallen out of favor in the majority of critically ill patients, although its use in specific patient groups is still recommended.[20]

In addition, it is increasingly evident that while CVP may at times be a marker of right ventricular preload when measured correctly, it is not a marker of preload responsiveness and cannot predict if CO will increase with fluid administration. Indeed, increasing CVP levels during fluid resuscitation should reflect a stopping rule.[21] Most studies in the meta-analysis by Eskesen et al. reported mean/median CVP values of 8–12 mm Hg in both responders and nonresponders. In an analysis of 1148 patient data sets, predictive values were low for all specific CVP values assessed.[22-25] The main explanation for this phenomenon comes from an interpretation of basic cardiovascular physiology and the slope of the cardiac function curve, which depends on cardiac systolic function (Fig. 51.1). The shape of the Frank-Starling curve varies from patient to patient and over time. Furthermore, intrinsic contractility also varies in response to varying loads, making CVP a poor measure of effective right ventricular preload. Finally, as circulatory unstressed volume varies to sustain a CO required to meet metabolic demand, CVP has more to do with right ventricular function than volume status or volume responsiveness. A static value of any measure of preload could correspond to preload dependence as well as preload independence. This is true for all static indicators of cardiac preload, including Ppao, global end-diastolic volume measured via

transpulmonary thermodilution, and even left ventricular end-diastolic dimensions measured by echocardiography.[26] Volume infusion will increase mean systemic pressure if enough volume is infused. However, if the subject is not volume responsive, the pressure gradient for venous return will not change. Thus, non-volume responsive patients will increase CVP more for a given fluid challenge than volume responsive patients.[27] Thus, as listed above, if CVP increases by > 2 mm Hg during fluid administration, it should be taken as a stopping rule and the patient reassessed.[21] Additional limitations in measuring CVP include common technical issues related to precise positioning of the pressure transducer with respect to the right atrium measured at end expiration. Similarly, the Ppao suffers from many possible errors in its measurement and interpretation.[28,29]

DYNAMIC MEASURES OF FLUID RESPONSIVENESS

The Starling mechanism can be used to assess volume responsiveness if the heart is challenged in a dynamic fashion. Such reversible dynamic challenges are referred to as FHM challenges. These principles provide the bedside clinician with tools to answer four main questions:

1. Is the patient in compensated shock?
2. Will the patient be volume responsive?
3. Is the arterial tone increased, normal, or decreased?
4. Is the heart able to sustain flow without high filling pressures?[1]

Compensated Shock

Circulatory shock is associated with tissue hypoperfusion. Many markers have been associated with tissue hypoperfusion, including elevated lactate, decreased urine output, decreased mixed venous and $ScvO_2$, increased venoarterial CO_2 gap, altered sensorium, delayed capillary refill, and metabolic acidosis. Specific autonomic responses to circulatory shock increase circulating catecholamine levels early, causing anxiety, tachycardia, diaphoresis, and peripheral vasoconstriction. Because the circulation defends central blood pressure to maintain adequate perfusion pressure for the brain and heart, hypotension is a late sign of shock and is associated with profound tissue hypoperfusion and failure of intrinsic homeostatic mechanisms. Resuscitation therapy should be targeted to individual patient responsiveness as measured by estimates of organ perfusion adequacy (Fig. 51.2). While no proven resuscitation targets exist, it is prudent to use metabolic measures of tissue wellness to guide resuscitation until better predictive markers are validated.[30,31] The remainder of this chapter focuses on answering the question of volume responsiveness (Fig. 51.3) using FHM techniques (Table 51.1).

Pulse Pressure Variation and Stroke Volume Variation

Patients on the steep portion of the Frank-Starling curve are preload dependent. During the inspiratory phase of a

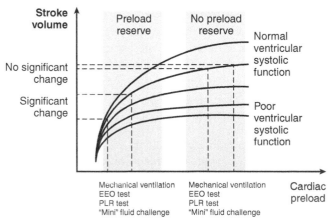

Fig. 51.1 Cardiac Function Curve. When the ventricles function on the steep portion of the cardiac function curve, stroke volume will increase with an increase in cardiac preload whether by end-expiratory occlusion (*EEO*), passive leg raising (*PLR*), or fluid challenge. If the ventricles are functioning on the level portion of the cardiac function curve, they will not be able to increase stroke volume for the same amount of increase in cardiac preload: i.e., they will no longer be fluid responsive.

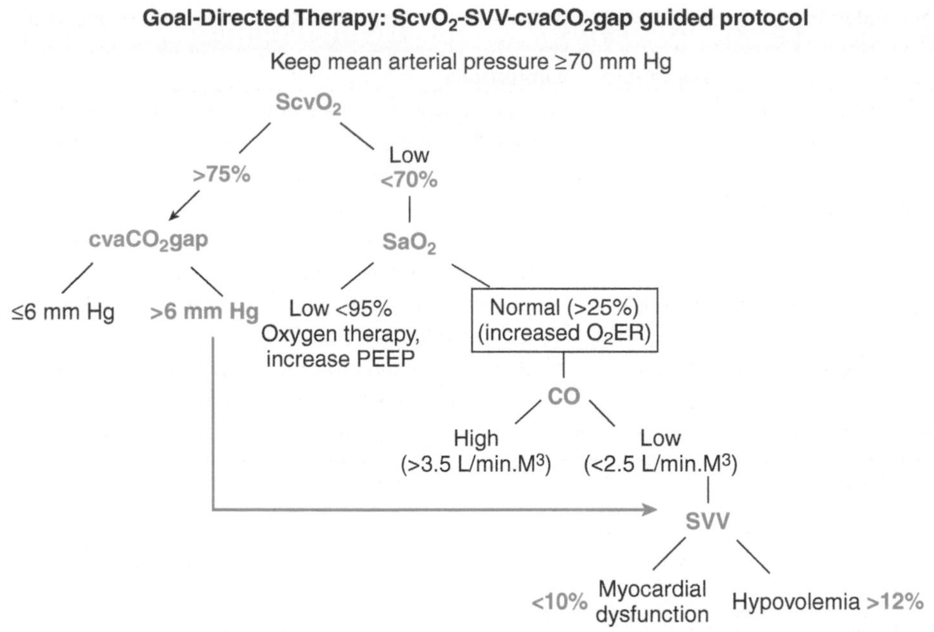

Goal-Directed Therapy: ScvO₂-SVV-cvaCO₂gap guided protocol

Keep mean arterial pressure ≥70 mm Hg

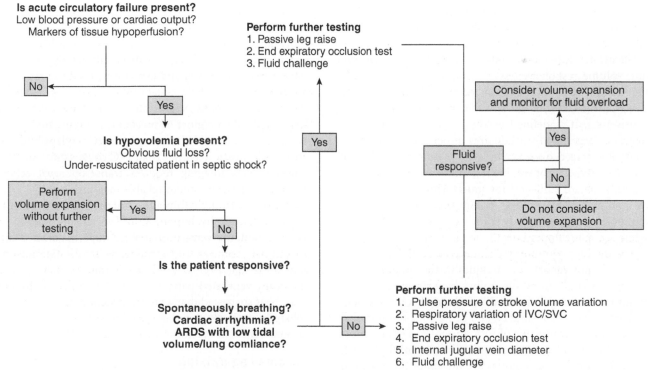

Fig. 51.2 Goal-Directed Therapy Algorithm. Therapeutic options to be considered are presented in the rect-angles. There are gaps for intermediate values, for which several therapeutic options may be considered. *CO,* cardiac output; *cvaCO₂* gap, veno-arterial PCO₂ difference; *PEEP,* positive end-expiratory pressure; *SaO₂,* arterial oxygen saturation; *SvO₂,* mixed venous oxygen saturation; *SVV,* stroke volume variation. (Modified from Vallet et al.[31].)

Fig. 51.3 Evaluating Circulatory Failure. An algorithm for the use of functional hemodynamic monitoring to guide fluid strategies. *ARDS,* acute respiratory distress syndrome; *IVC,* inferior vena cava; *SVC,* superior vena cava. (Modified from Monnet et al.[26].)

TABLE 51.1 Summary of Methods for Functional Hemodynamic Monitoring.

Method	Variable	Threshold	Limitations
PPV or SVV	Pulse pressure or stroke volume	13%	Cannot be used in spontaneously breathing patient, cardiac arrhythmias, low tidal volume/lung compliance. May be false-positive in right heart failure
IVC diameter	Diameter	12%	
IJV diameter	Diameter	18%	
SVC diameter	Diameter	36%	Cannot be used in spontaneously breathing patient, low tidal volume/lung compliance, and requires TEE
PLR	Cardiac output	10%	Requires direct measurement of cardiac output, may be affected by intra-abdominal hypertension
EEO test	Cardiac output	5%	Cannot be used in non-mechanically ventilated patient or in patients who cannot tolerate a 15-second respiratory hold
Ea$_{dyn}$	PPV/SVV	<1%	Cannot be used to predict the change in MAP to inotropes

Ea$_{dyn}$, dynamic arterial elastance; EEO, end-expiratory occlusion; IJV, internal jugular vein; IVC, inferior vena cava; MAP, mean arterial pressure; PLR, passive leg raising; PPV, pulse pressure variation; SVC, superior vena cava; SVV, stroke volume variation; TEE, transesophageal echocardiography.

mechanical ventilation there is an increase in intrathoracic pressure that results in higher right atrial pressures and decreased venous return. This results in decreased right ventricular output and, if both ventricles are fluid responsive, eventual reduction in left ventricular output creating pulse pressure variation (PPV) over the respiratory cycle after 2–3 heart beats. Michard et al.[32] defined volume responsiveness as a 15% increase in cardiac index after a 500 mL volume bolus. Volume responders have a respiratory variation in arterial PPV of >13%, defined as the difference between maximal and minimal pulse pressure over 3–5 positive pressure breaths. Subsequent literature has validated PPV as a method of predicting volume responsiveness.[33,34] Similarly, stroke volume variation (SVV) can also be calculated from the arterial pressure waveforms and is an effective predictor of volume responsiveness. It is defined as the ratio of the difference between the largest and smallest area under the arterial pressure curve averaged over 3–5 breaths. A difference of more than 10% is predictive of volume responsiveness.[35] While arterial waveforms are sufficient for monitoring PPV and SVV, many minimally invasive and noninvasive devices exist to continuously measure hemodynamic variables in the ICU.[36–38]

There are many limitations to the predictive value of PPV and SVV that are commonly encountered in the ICU. PPV and SVV are not validated techniques in the spontaneously breathing patient.[39] Intra-abdominal hypertension, cardiac arrhythmias resulting in a varied R-R interval, low chest wall compliance, open chest surgery, and acute cor pulmonale all decrease the predictive value of PPV and SVV.[1] Perhaps most importantly, low tidal volume ventilation <8 mL/kg, which is currently used as a lung protective mechanical ventilation strategy, decreases the sensitivity but not the specificity of PPV measurement.[40–42] A recent study by Richard et al.[43] applied FHM strategies to guide fluid resuscitation in patients with septic shock, and due primarily to low tidal volume ventilation, only 9% of patients met criteria for PPV-guided fluid therapy.

Respiratory Variation of Vena Caval Diameter

During a positive pressure inspiration in a mechanically ventilated patient, there is increased intrathoracic pressure, causing reduced venous return and increased inferior vena cava (IVC) diameter. During expiration the decreased intrathoracic pressure increases venous return and reduces IVC diameter. A respiratory variation in IVC diameter >12% or IVC collapsibility index >18% has been shown to be predictive of volume responsiveness in mechanically ventilated septic patients.[44–46] These images are easily obtained with transthoracic point-of-care ultrasound at the bedside. The superior vena cava (SVC) is an intrathoracic, rather than intra-abdominal, vessel and can also be used to predict fluid responsiveness. An SVC collapsibility index >36% has been shown to be predictive of fluid responsiveness.[47] In the largest published cohort of mechanically ventilated patients evaluated with echocardiography, SVC collapsibility had greater diagnostic accuracy than IVC collapsibility or PPV[48]; however, SVC imaging requires transesophageal echocardiography (TEE) to obtain reliable measurements.[49]

While cardiac arrhythmias do not preclude the use of IVC or SVC collapsibility, limitations of IVC collapsibility include low tidal volume ventilation <8 mL/kg and elevated intra-abdominal pressures >12 mm Hg. Most investigations have concluded that IVC collapsibility is only predictive in mechanically ventilated patients,[50] but a recent study by Preau et al.[46] has suggested that, with deep standardization, the IVC collapsibility index may be a noninvasive predictor of fluid responsiveness in the nonintubated patient with septic shock.

Passive Leg Raising

The passive leg raising (PLR) maneuver is a reversible fluid challenge that transfers about 300 mL of venous blood from the lower body towards the right heart.[51] It is predictive of whether CO will increase with fluid expansion without the administration of any exogenous fluid. The PLR is performed by placing the patient in a semirecumbent position to a position where the trunk is horizontal and the lower limbs are raised to 45 degrees by adjusting the bed and directly measuring its effects on CO. An increase in CO by 10% with PLR is predictive of preload responsiveness.[26,52,53] A recent meta-analysis by Monnet et al.[54] showed that PLR-induced changes in CO reliably predict fluid responsiveness. Another meta-analysis by Cavallaro et al. showed that PLR can be used regardless of mode of ventilation, low lung compliance, low tidal volume ventilation, or cardiac rhythm.[55,56] Limitations of PLR include intra-abdominal hypertension due to compression of the IVC in the raised leg position; however, this remains a theoretical concern as intra-abdominal pressure has not been measured during PLR.[57,58]

In addition to predicting those patients that will respond to fluid administration, the PLR maneuver can also be used to assess when to stop fluid administration in the patient who is no longer fluid responsive. This avoids fluid overload and provides a simple measure to guide when methods other than fluid administration are needed to treat the hemodynamically unstable patient with circulatory shock.[59]

End-Expiratory Occlusion Test

As described previously, each mechanically ventilated breath decreases cardiac preload by impeding venous return. The end-expiratory occlusion (EEO) test interrupts mechanical ventilation at expiration for 15 seconds to allow cardiac preload to transiently increase, thereby increasing CO. An increase in CO by more that 5% is predictive of fluid responsiveness.[56,60] A 15-second hold is essential to allow the resulting increase in stroke volume, and EEO testing is not accurate in patients whose respiratory activity does not allow a 15-second pause in respiration.

More recently, studies have evaluated the use of transthoracic echocardiography (TTE) to assess CO during EEO testing on apical four- and five-chamber views. Fluid responsiveness was predicted by an increase in the velocity–time integral (VTI) $\geq$5% during EEO testing. The addition of end-inspiratory hold increases the diagnostic threshold to 13%.[61] This test is easy to perform and simply requires an end-expiratory pause while measuring CO. It is also valid in patients with acute respiratory distress syndrome (ARDS), low lung compliance, and cardiac arrhythmias.[62,63]

Jugular Venous Distension

Anytime there is a change in intrathoracic pressure or volume, a similar change also occurs in the extrathoracic veins such as the abdominal IVC and the internal jugular vein (IJV).[64] If PPV is a measure of left ventricular reserve, then IJV distensibility may be used to assess venous return and right ventricular reserve. Guarracino et al.[65] hypothesized that right heart functional status relative to volume responsiveness should be reflected by IVJ diameter variation with respiration. They enrolled 50 septic patients and measured anteroposterior maximal IJV diameter during inspiration and minimal IJV diameter during expiration using M-mode on bedside ultrasound. Ultrasound measurements were taken before and immediately after a 7 mL/kg crystalloid infusion

over 30 minutes. They found that more than 18% IJV distensibility predicted a change in cardiac index >15%, with 80% sensitivity and 95% specificity. The combination of IJV distensibility >9.9% and PPV >12% predicted fluid responsiveness with 100% sensitivity and 95% specificity. While further prospective study is required, IJV distensibility is a potentially simple and reliable measure of fluid responsiveness easily obtained by the bedside clinician.

Echocardiographic Measures of Fluid Responsiveness

As bedside ultrasonography becomes more commonly used in the ICU, both TTE and TEE provide additional methods to evaluate cardiac function. In addition to IVC and SVC diameter mentioned previously, echocardiography allows for measurement of other dynamic parameters of fluid responsiveness in mechanically ventilated patients. Respiratory changes in stroke volume can be measured by Doppler analysis of the VTI with TTE or TEE. Respiratory variation in the maximal ascending aortic velocity or VTI is predictive of fluid responsiveness. A 12% change in maximal flow velocity and a 20% change in aortic VTI have been shown to be predictive of volume responsiveness in patients with septic shock.[66] Left ventricular diastolic area (LVDA) can also be measured using the short-axis view by TEE. Cannesson et al.[67] found that a 16% respiratory variation of LVDA had a 92% sensitivity and 83% specificity for predicting volume responsiveness.

In the spontaneously breathing patient, VTI measurement can be coupled with other forms of dynamic assessment such as PLR. An increase in aortic flow >10% with PLR was predictive of an increase in aortic flow of 15% with volume expansion.[53,68] Thus, echocardiography provides the intensivist skilled in bedside ultrasonography with several methods to differentiate fluid responders from nonresponders in patients with hemodynamic compromise.

Assessment of Vasomotor Tone: Dynamic Arterial Elastance

Arterial compliance and arterial elastance are measures of the relationship between change in volume and change in pressure. Dynamic arterial compliance is defined as the ratio of SVV to PPV. Dynamic arterial elastance (Ea_{dyn}) is the ratio of PPV to SVV and can be used to determine if an increase in CO will result in an increase of arterial pressure.[11,69] Because blood pressure depends directly on left ventricular output and arterial load, Ea_{dyn} is considered to be a functional measure of arterial load. In a hypotensive patient, if Ea_{dyn} is high, then arterial pressure should increase if CO increases. If it is low, then arterial pressure will not be expected to increase proportionally to an increase in CO.[70] In this group of patients, the addition of vasopressors should be added to correct hypotension, sparing the amount of fluids given.[71-73] Not only can Ea_{dyn} be used to predict which patients will benefit from starting vasopressors but it is also a functional marker of arterioventricular coupling that can help to direct vasopressor therapy and de-escalation.

Guinot et al.[74] found that an Ea_{dyn} of <0.94 predicted a MAP decrease of >15% after decreasing norepinephrine dose. Overall, Ea_{dyn} has the potential to be an important tool to individualize fluid administration in volume nonresponders and minimize vasopressor doses in the hemodynamically unstable patient.[75]

AUTHORS' RECOMMENDATIONS

- Resuscitation therapy should be targeted at individual patient responsiveness as measured by estimates of organ perfusion adequacy or recovery.
- If no test is used to predict volume responsiveness, volume expansion results in increased CO in approximately half of patients with circulatory shock, resulting in unnecessary fluid overload in the other half.
- Optimal fluid management improves patient outcome by avoiding both hypovolemia and hypervolemia.
- Commonly used static measures of preload should not be used alone to guide resuscitation therapy.
- Dynamic measure of fluid responsiveness (e.g., PPV, SVV, changes in CO with PLR, Ea_{dyn}) are preferable to static measures of preload in predicting fluid responsiveness.
- Management of high-risk surgery patients and those in septic shock using resuscitation protocols based on dynamic measures improves outcome.

REFERENCES

1. Pinsky MR. Functional hemodynamic monitoring. *Crit Care Clin*. 2015;31(1):89-111.
2. Monnet X, Teboul JL. Assessment of volume responsiveness during mechanical ventilation: recent advances. *Crit Care*. 2013;17(2):217.
3. Michard F, Teboul JL. Predicting fluid responsiveness in ICU patients. a critical analysis of the evidence. *Chest*. 2002;121(6):2000-2008.
4. Rhodes A, Evans LE, Alhazzani W, et al. Surviving Sepsis Campaign: International Guidelines for Management of Sepsis and Septic Shock: 2016. *Crit Care Med*. 2017;45(3):486-552.
5. Rivers E, Nguyen B, Havstad S, et al. Early goal-directed therapy in the treatment of severe sepsis and septic shock. *N Engl J Med*. 2001;345(19):1368-1377.
6. ARISE Investigators; ANZICS Clinical Trials Group; Peake SL, et al. Goal-directed resuscitation for patients with early septic shock. *N Engl J Med*. 2014;371(16):1496-1506.
7. Mouncey PR, Osborn TM, Power GS, et al. Trial of early, goal-directed resuscitation for septic shock. *N Engl J Med*. 2015;372(14):1301-1311.
8. ProCESS Investigators; Yealy DM, Kellum JA, et al. A randomized trial of protocol-based care for early septic shock. *N Engl J Med*. 2014;370(18):1683-1693.
9. Pinsky MR. Choosing sides in predicting fluid responsiveness. *Am J Respir Crit Care Med*. 2017;195(8):973-974.
10. Bednarczyk JM, Fridfinnson JA, Kumar A, et al. Incorporating dynamic assessment of fluid responsiveness into goal-directed therapy: a systematic review and meta-analysis. *Crit Care Med*. 2017;45(9):1538-1545.
11. Suess EM, Pinsky MR. Hemodynamic monitoring for the evaluation and treatment of shock: what is the current state of the art? *Semin Respir Crit Care Med*. 2015;36(6):890-898.
12. Swan HJ, Ganz W, Forrester J, Marcus H, Diamond G, Chonette D. Catheterization of the heart in man with use of a flow-directed balloon-tipped catheter. *N Engl J Med*. 1970;283(9):447-451.
13. Shoemaker WC, Appel PL, Kram HB, Waxman K, Lee TS. Prospective trial of supranormal values of survivors as therapeutic goals in high-risk surgical patients. *Chest*. 1988;94(6):1176-1186.
14. Yu M, Levy MM, Smith P, Takiguchi SA, Miyasaki A, Myers SA. Effect of maximizing oxygen delivery on morbidity and mortality rates in critically ill patients: a prospective, randomized, controlled study. *Crit Care Med*. 1993;21(6):830-838.
15. Tuchschmidt J, Fried J, Astiz M, Rackow E. Elevation of cardiac output and oxygen delivery improves outcome in septic shock. *Chest*. 1992;102(1):216-220.
16. Sandham JD, Hull RD, Brant RF, et al. A randomized, controlled trial of the use of pulmonary-artery catheters in high-risk surgical patients. *N Engl J Med*. 2003;348(1):5-14.
17. Richard C, Warszawski J, Anguel N, et al. Early use of the pulmonary artery catheter and outcomes in patients with shock and acute respiratory distress syndrome: a randomized controlled trial. *JAMA*. 2003;290(20):2713-2720.
18. Binanay C, Califf RM, Hasselblad V, et al. Evaluation study of congestive heart failure and pulmonary artery catheterization effectiveness: the ESCAPE trial. *JAMA*. 2005;294(13):1625-1633.
19. Harvey S, Harrison DA, Singer M, et al. Assessment of the clinical effectiveness of pulmonary artery catheters in management of patients in intensive care (PAC-Man): a randomised controlled trial. *Lancet*. 2005;366(9484):472-477.
20. De Backer D, Hajjar LA, Pinsky MR. Is there still a place for the Swan–Ganz catheter? We are not sure. *Intensive Care Med*. 2018;44(6):960-962.
21. Pinsky MR, Kellum JA, Bellomo R. Central venous pressure is a stopping rule, not a target of fluid resuscitation. *Crit Care Resusc*. 2014;16(4):245-246.
22. Marik PE, Cavallazzi R. Does the central venous pressure predict fluid responsiveness? An updated meta-analysis and a plea for some common sense. *Crit Care Med*. 2013;41(7):1774-1781.
23. Marik PE, Baram M, Vahid B. Does central venous pressure predict fluid responsiveness? A systematic review of the literature and the tale of seven mares. *Chest*. 2008;134(1):172-178.
24. Bentzer P, Griesdale DE, Boyd J, MacLean K, Sirounis D, Ayas NT. Will this hemodynamically unstable patient respond to a bolus of intravenous fluids? *JAMA*. 2016;316(12):1298-1309.
25. Eskesen TG, Wetterslev M, Perner A. Systematic review including re-analyses of 1148 individual data sets of central venous pressure as a predictor of fluid responsiveness. *Intensive Care Med*. 2016;42(3):324-332.
26. Monnet X, Marik PE, Teboul JL. Prediction of fluid responsiveness: an update. *Ann Intensive Care*. 2016;6(1):111.
27. Cecconi M, Aya HD, Geisen M, et al. Changes in the mean systemic filling pressure during a fluid challenge in postsurgical intensive care patients. *Intensive Care Med*. 2013;39(7):1299-1305.
28. Pinsky MR. Pulmonary artery occlusion pressure. *Intensive Care Med*. 2003;29(1):19-22.
29. Richard C, Monnet X, Teboul JL. Pulmonary artery catheter monitoring in 2011. *Curr Opin Crit Care*. 2011;17(3):296-302.
30. De Backer D, Creteur J, Preiser JC, Dubois MJ, Vincent JL. Microvascular blood flow is altered in patients with sepsis. *Am J Respir Crit Care Med*. 2002;166(1):98-104.
31. Vallet B, Pinsky MR, Cecconi M. Resuscitation of patients with septic shock: please "mind the gap"! *Intensive Care Med*. 2013;39(9):1653-1655.

32. Michard F, Boussat S, Chemla D, et al. Relation between respiratory changes in arterial pulse pressure and fluid responsiveness in septic patients with acute circulatory failure. *Am J Respir Crit Care Med*. 2000;162(1):134-138.

33. Marik PE, Cavallazzi R, Vasu T, Hirani A. Dynamic changes in arterial waveform derived variables and fluid responsiveness in mechanically ventilated patients: a systematic review of the literature. *Crit Care Med*. 2009;37(9):2642-2647.

34. Cannesson M, Aboy M, Hofer CK, Rehman M. Pulse pressure variation: where are we today? *J Clin Monit Comput*. 2011;25(1):45-56.

35. Michard F. Changes in arterial pressure during mechanical ventilation. *Anesthesiology*. 2005;103(2):419-428; quiz 449-450.

36. Clement RP, Vos JJ, Scheeren TWL. Minimally invasive cardiac output technologies in the ICU: putting it all together. *Curr Opin Crit Care*. 2017;23(4):302-309.

37. Monnet X, Teboul JL. Minimally invasive monitoring. *Crit Care Clin*. 2015;31(1):25-42.

38. Teboul JL, Saugel B, Cecconi M, et al. Less invasive hemodynamic monitoring in critically ill patients. *Intensive Care Med*. 2016;42(9):1350-1359.

39. Heenen S, De Backer D, Vincent JL. How can the response to volume expansion in patients with spontaneous respiratory movements be predicted? *Crit Care*. 2006;10(4):R102.

40. De Backer D, Heenen S, Piagnerelli M, Koch M, Vincent JL. Pulse pressure variations to predict fluid responsiveness: influence of tidal volume. *Intensive Care Med*. 2005;31(4):517-523.

41. Huang CC, Fu JY, Hu HC, et al. Prediction of fluid responsiveness in acute respiratory distress syndrome patients ventilated with low tidal volume and high positive end-expiratory pressure. *Crit Care Med*. 2008;36(10):2810-2816.

42. Mesquida J, Kim HK, Pinsky MR. Effect of tidal volume, intrathoracic pressure, and cardiac contractility on variations in pulse pressure, stroke volume, and intrathoracic blood volume. *Intensive Care Med*. 2011;37(10):1672-1679.

43. Richard JC, Bayle F, Bourdin G, et al. Preload dependence indices to titrate volume expansion during septic shock: a randomized controlled trial. *Crit Care*. 2015;19:5.

44. Feissel M, Michard F, Faller JP, Teboul JL. The respiratory variation in inferior vena cava diameter as a guide to fluid therapy. *Intensive Care Med*. 2004;30(9):1834-1837.

45. Barbier C, Loubières Y, Schmit C, et al. Respiratory changes in inferior vena cava diameter are helpful in predicting fluid responsiveness in ventilated septic patients. *Intensive Care Med*. 2004;30(9):1740-1746.

46. Preau S, Bortolotti P, Colling D, et al. Diagnostic accuracy of the inferior vena cava collapsibility to predict fluid responsiveness in spontaneously breathing patients with sepsis and acute circulatory failure. *Crit Care Med*. 2017;45(3):e290-e297.

47. Vieillard-Baron A, Chergui K, Rabiller A, et al. Superior vena caval collapsibility as a gauge of volume status in ventilated septic patients. *Intensive Care Med*. 2004;30(9):1734-1739.

48. Vignon P, Repessé X, Bégot E, et al. Comparison of echocardiographic indices used to predict fluid responsiveness in ventilated patients. *Am J Respir Crit Care Med*. 2017;195(8):1022-1032.

49. Jardin F, Vieillard-Baron A. Ultrasonographic examination of the venae cavae. *Intensive Care Med*. 2006;32(2):203-206.

50. Airapetian N, Maizel J, Alyamani O, et al. Does inferior vena cava respiratory variability predict fluid responsiveness in spontaneously breathing patients? *Crit Care*. 2015;19:400.

51. Jabot J, Teboul JL, Richard C, Monnet X. Passive leg raising for predicting fluid responsiveness: importance of the postural change. *Intensive Care Med*. 2009;35(1):85-90.

52. Monnet X, Teboul JL. Passive leg raising. *Intensive Care Med*. 2008;34(4):659-663.

53. Monnet X, Rienzo M, Osman D, et al. Passive leg raising predicts fluid responsiveness in the critically ill. *Crit Care Med*. 2006;34(5):1402-1407.

54. Monnet X, Marik P, Teboul JL. Passive leg raising for predicting fluid responsiveness: a systematic review and meta-analysis. *Intensive Care Med*. 2016;42(12):1935-1947.

55. Cavallaro F, Sandroni C, Marano C, et al. Diagnostic accuracy of passive leg raising for prediction of fluid responsiveness in adults: systematic review and meta-analysis of clinical studies. *Intensive Care Med*. 2010;36(9):1475-1483.

56. Monnet X, Teboul JL. Assessment of fluid responsiveness: recent advances. *Curr Opin Crit Care*. 2018;24(3):190-195.

57. Mahjoub Y, Touzeau J, Airapetian N, et al. The passive leg-raising maneuver cannot accurately predict fluid responsiveness in patients with intra-abdominal hypertension. *Crit Care Med*. 2010;38(9):1824-1829.

58. Malbrain ML, Reuter DA. Assessing fluid responsiveness with the passive leg raising maneuver in patients with increased intra-abdominal pressure: be aware that not all blood returns! *Crit Care Med*. 2010;38(9):1912-1915.

59. Monnet X, Teboul JL. Passive leg raising: five rules, not a drop of fluid! *Crit Care*. 2015;19:18.

60. Monnet X, Osman D, Ridel C, Lamia B, Richard C, Teboul JL. Predicting volume responsiveness by using the end-expiratory occlusion in mechanically ventilated intensive care unit patients. *Crit Care Med*. 2009;37(3):951-956.

61. Jozwiak M, Depret F, Teboul JL, et al. Predicting fluid responsiveness in critically ill patients by using combined end-expiratory and end-inspiratory occlusions with echocardiography. *Crit Care Med*. 2017;45(11):e1131-e1138.

62. Silva S, Jozwiak M, Teboul JL, Persichini R, Richard C, Monnet X. End-expiratory occlusion test predicts preload responsiveness independently of positive end-expiratory pressure during acute respiratory distress syndrome. *Crit Care Med*. 2013;41(7):1692-1701.

63. Monnet X, Bleibtreu A, Ferré A, et al. Passive leg-raising and end-expiratory occlusion tests perform better than pulse pressure variation in patients with low respiratory system compliance. *Crit Care Med*. 2012;40(1):152-157.

64. Constant J. Using internal jugular pulsations as a manometer for right atrial pressure measurements. *Cardiology*. 2000;93(1-2):26-30.

65. Guarracino F, Ferro B, Forfori F, Bertini P, Magliacano L, Pinsky MR. Jugular vein distensibility predicts fluid responsiveness in septic patients. *Crit Care*. 2014;18(6):647.

66. Feissel M, Michard F, Mangin I, Ruyer O, Faller JP, Teboul JL. Respiratory changes in aortic blood velocity as an indicator of fluid responsiveness in ventilated patients with septic shock. *Chest*. 2001;119(3):867-873.

67. Cannesson M, Slieker J, Desebbe O, Farhat F, Bastien O, Lehot JJ. Prediction of fluid responsiveness using respiratory variations in left ventricular stroke area by transoesophageal echocardiographic automated border detection in mechanically ventilated patients. *Crit Care*. 2006;10(6):R171.

68. Lamia B, Ochagavia A, Monnet X, Chemla D, Richard C, Teboul JL. Echocardiographic prediction of volume responsiveness in critically ill patients with spontaneously breathing activity. *Intensive Care Med*. 2007;33(7):1125-1132.

69. Chemla D, Hébert JL, Coirault C, et al. Total arterial compliance estimated by stroke volume-to-aortic pulse

pressure ratio in humans. *Am J Physiol*. 1998;274(2 Pt 2): H500-H505.

70. Monge García MI, Saludes Orduña P, Cecconi M. Understanding arterial load. *Intensive Care Med*. 2016;42(10): 1625-1627.

71. Cecconi M, Monge García MI, Gracia Romero M, et al. The use of pulse pressure variation and stroke volume variation in spontaneously breathing patients to assess dynamic arterial elastance and to predict arterial pressure response to fluid administration. *Anesth Analg*. 2015;120(1):76-84.

72. Monge García MI, Gil Cano A, Gracia Romero M. Dynamic arterial elastance to predict arterial pressure response to volume loading in preload-dependent patients. *Crit Care*. 2011; 15(1):R15.

73. García MI, Romero MG, Cano AG, et al. Dynamic arterial elastance as a predictor of arterial pressure response to fluid administration: a validation study. *Crit Care*. 2014;18(6):626.

74. Guinot PG, Bernard E, Levrard M, Dupont H, Lorne E. Dynamic arterial elastance predicts mean arterial pressure decrease associated with decreasing norepinephrine dosage in septic shock. *Crit Care*. 2015;19:14.

75. Monge García MI, Pinsky MR, Cecconi M. Predicting vasopressor needs using dynamic parameters. *Intensive Care Med*. 2017; 43(12):1841-1843.

52

How Should Cardiogenic Shock Be Managed (Including Assist Devices)?

Matthew R. Biery and Benjamin Kohl

Cardiogenic shock (CS) is defined as an inability of the heart to provide adequate blood flow to maintain the metabolic demands of tissue despite adequate intravascular volume. Despite its inherent vagaries, this definition has, in some form, been used for decades. For practical purposes, CS can be said to exist when a patient exhibits sustained hypotension with evidence of impaired cardiac function. With few exceptions, CS is an emergency that requires prompt diagnosis and appropriate therapy. This chapter reviews how to best diagnose and manage CS in the intensive care unit (ICU).

EPIDEMIOLOGY AND ETIOLOGY

Although there are a plethora of theoretical causes of CS in the ICU (Box 52.1), the most frequent cause of CS in the ICU is acute coronary syndrome (ACS) resulting in acute left ventricular dysfunction.[1,2] Autopsy studies have shown that more than 40% of left ventricular myocardium must be sacrificed for CS to ensue.[3,4] Other common causes of CS, usually as a result of acute myocardial infarction (AMI), include acute mitral regurgitation, cardiac tamponade (from ventricular free-wall rupture), and ventricular septal rupture.[5] Finally, a rare but increasingly recognized cause of CS in the ICU (particularly in the postoperative setting) is stress-induced (takotsubo) cardiomyopathy.[6] CS occurs in 8.6% of patients sustaining ST-elevation myocardial infarction (STEMI) and in roughly 2.5% of patients who have sustained non-ST-elevation myocardial infarction (NSTEMI).[7,8] Rarely, pharmacologic agents have been shown to incite CS. In the Clopidogrel and Metoprolol in Myocardial Infarction Trial (COMMIT), the incidence of CS was 5% in patients receiving early metoprolol (roughly 30% greater than those who did not receive metoprolol).[9] Finally, all of these scenarios incite an acute inflammatory response that augments the initial insult and results in a vicious cycle that, if left untreated, culminates in death (Fig. 52.1).[10] Mortality rates for patients who sustain STEMI *with* CS are approximately 68% over 30 days compared with approximately 10% in those patients who do not have CS.[11–14] Evaluation of mortality trends within the United States reveals that a changing management scheme has decreased the mortality of this disease significantly (60.3% in 1995 vs. 47.9% in 2004).[7] Although this change in mortality is probably multifactorial, it is likely that an increased rate of cardiac catheterization (51.5% in 1995 vs. 74.4% in 2004) and of percutaneous cardiac intervention (27.4% in 1995 vs. 54.4% in 2004) has had a major impact. Of note, during this registry period (that included more than 250,000 patients in more than 750 US hospitals), there was no change in the use of intraaortic balloon pumps (IABPs) (39%) or in immediate coronary artery bypass graft (CABG) surgery (3%). Although prognostication can be difficult in this population, recent evidence suggests that hemodynamic variables in the first 24 hours may be useful.[15]

DIAGNOSIS

Rapid diagnosis of CS is imperative. Hemodynamic criteria consistent with a diagnosis of CS include sustained ($\geq$30 minutes) hypotension with systolic blood pressure less than 90 mm Hg, depressed cardiac index (CI) ($<$2.2 L/min/m^2), and elevated pulmonary artery occlusion pressure (PAOP) ($>$15 mm Hg).[16] These indices suggest that rapid diagnosis of CS should be straightforward if CI is known. However, many patients with CS also have a component of distributive shock, which lowers their systemic vascular resistance (SVR) and normalizes their CI.[17] Thus it is necessary that the clinician has a systematic method of diagnosing CS.

In the absence of more objective data, a critically ill patient in shock usually has hypovolemia, sepsis, pulmonary embolism, or myocardial ischemia. Risk factors for CS include age $>$70 years, systolic blood pressure (SBP) $<$120 mm Hg, heart rate $>$120/min or $<$60/min, or a prolonged period since onset of symptoms.[18] Warm extremities usually eliminate a diagnosis of CS from consideration. With impaired myocardial contraction, auscultation of the lungs frequently reveals crackles due to an elevated left ventricular end-diastolic pressure (LVEDP) with exudate filling the pulmonary interstitium. Most physical findings, however, are nonspecific and additional information is often needed. Signs of interstitial edema (often in the absence of physical examination findings) on chest radiographs are suggestive of CS. An electrocardiogram should reveal signs of myocardial ischemia. If CS remains a consideration, cardiac enzymes should be sent.

Echocardiography is the test of choice to diagnose CS. The sensitivity of this modality for CS approaches 100%, with a specificity of roughly 95%.[19,20] With growing use of point-of-care ultrasound (POCUS), the bedside physician, often a

BOX 52.1 Causes of Cardiogenic Shock.

Acute Myocardial Infarction
- Pump failure
- Large infarction
- Smaller infarction with preexisting left ventricular dysfunction
- Infarction extension
- Severe recurrent ischemia
- Mechanical complications
- Acute mitral regurgitation caused by papillary muscle rupture
- Ventricular septal defect
- Free-wall rupture
- Pericardial tamponade
- Right ventricular infarction

Other Conditions
- End-stage cardiomyopathy
- Myocarditis
- Myocardial contusion (blunt cardiac injury)
- Prolonged cardiopulmonary bypass
- Septic shock with myocardial depression
- Aortic stenosis
- Left ventricular outflow tract obstruction
- Obstruction to left ventricular filling (e.g., mitral stenosis)
- Acute aortic insufficiency
- Pulmonary embolism
- Pheochromocytoma

From Topalian et al.[2]

noncardiac provider, can learn to accurately assess and rule out different causes of shock,[21–25] reducing the need to wait for a formal, comprehensive ultrasound and the unacceptable delays that this may entail. A focused examination permits rapid assessment of left or right ventricular dysfunction, valvular regurgitation, pericardial effusion, and ventricular

septal rupture.[19] Rapid availability of an echocardiogram may preclude the need for further invasive monitors because pulmonary artery systolic pressure and PAOP can be estimated by Doppler echocardiography.[26] Precise physiologic parameters are frequently necessary both to diagnose and to manage patients with CS. Invasive monitoring is recommended if there are persistent signs of hypoperfusion despite adequate volume therapy. The American College of Cardiology and American Heart Association (ACC/AHA) gives a class IC (weight of evidence and opinion is in favor of usefulness and efficacy) recommendation for placement of a pulmonary artery catheter (PAC) in patients with CS.[27] PACs can aid in diagnosis and can be helpful with subsequent management, although data showing a mortality benefit are equivocal.[28–30] There are data to suggest that certain calculated indices, such as cardiac power and stroke work index, may have short-term prognostic value.[31] Interpretation of PAC data requires a detailed knowledge of pathophysiology. A quick look at the numbers will rarely yield the diagnosis. Most causes of cardiogenic shock result in elevated central venous and pulmonary arterial pressures (the exception being isolated right ventricular ischemia). For the various causes to be differentiated, a detailed understanding of the various waveforms is necessary.

The central venous pressure (CVP) is a frequently underused physiologic parameter. A plethora of information can be obtained with proper analysis. For the interpretation of the various waves, the scale must be set so that all portions of the wave can be seen (usually a scale with 20–30 mm Hg maximum is optimal). The various components of the CVP can be seen in Fig. 52.2. By breaking the waveform into various cardiac events, it becomes apparent that not all elevated venous pressures are equal. Cardiac tamponade will cause a

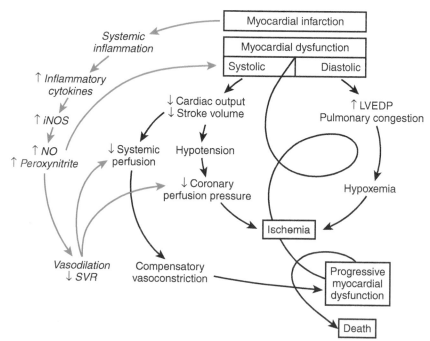

Fig. 52.1 Vicious Cycle of Cardiogenic Shock. *iNOS,* inhaled nitric oxide synthase; *LVEDP,* left ventricular end-diastolic pressure; *NO,* nitric oxide; *SVR,* systemic vascular resistance. (From Antman and Braunwald.[10])

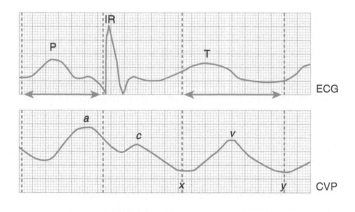

Wave/descent	Cardiac event
a	Ventricular filling (atrial contraction)
c	Tricuspid valve (isovolemic contraction)
v	Atrial filling (ventricular contraction)
x	Atrial relaxation (start of atrial filling)
y	Tricuspid valve opening (rapid ventricular filling)

Fig. 52.2 Components of the Central Venous Pressure (*CVP*) Waveform. *ECG*, electrocardiogram.

monophasic CVP with a very small *x*-descent and often complete loss of the *y*-descent, whereas right ventricular ischemia with tricuspid regurgitation will yield a very large, fused *c-v* wave. Because of the regurgitant flow, there is an inability to differentiate the slightly increased atrial pressure generated from closure of the tricuspid valve and atrial filling during atrial diastole. A complete analysis of CVP waveform is beyond the scope of this chapter, and the reader is referred to other texts.[32,33]

The equivalent CVP for the left side of the heart is the PAOP. Similarly, with correct identification of the waves and translation of the waves into a portion of the cardiac cycle, it becomes possible to identify various disorders.[34–36] Acute mitral regurgitation is associated with very large *v* waves on PAOP. Acute cardiac ischemia often first manifests as left ventricular diastolic dysfunction. This, in turn, leads to a higher left ventricular end-diastolic volume (LVEDV) that causes an elevated LVEDP. Although this culminates in an elevated PAOP, through evaluation of the waveform, an exaggerated *a* wave is consistent with diastolic dysfunction.

MANAGEMENT: AN EVIDENCE-BASED APPROACH

Management of CS should focus on restoring microcirculatory function and optimizing tissue perfusion via improvement of cardiac output (CO). A delay in diagnosis or therapy will directly impact mortality. Management, in most cases, consists of a combined treatment plan of pharmacologic therapy, mechanical therapy, and/or revascularization.

Pharmacologic Therapy

It should be stated at the outset that there have been very few large controlled trials evaluating the efficacy of different vasopressor or inotrope therapies in CS. None of these

studies have confirmed any outcome difference with any particular agent.[37]

Initial treatment for patients with CS should focus on restoration of normal hemodynamics, oxygenation, and delivery, and avoidance of arrhythmia. In patients without significant pulmonary edema, it is reasonable to administer a fluid challenge before vasopressor therapy. If pulmonary edema is present or there is no response to a fluid challenge, pharmacologic therapy should be initiated. Pharmacologic therapy for CS should initially focus on those compounds that have primary inotropic activity.[38,39] Despite having numerous options for therapy, there remains a lack of evidence-based medicine for indicating which drug is superior. A 2018 Cochrane Review was unable to identify data to support the use of one inotrope over others when treating patients in CS or low cardiac output syndrome (LCOS).[40] Drugs to consider as first-line treatment include norepinephrine, milrinone, dobutamine, and epinephrine. The SOAP II (Sepsis Occurrence in Acutely Ill Patients II) trial showed no difference in 28-day mortality between norepinephrine and dopamine when treating patients with generalized shock.[41] In a subanalysis, the 280 patients with CS shock in the dopamine group had an increased 28-day mortality rate.[41] Dopamine was also observed to be more arrhythmogenic, with atrial fibrillation being the most common.[41] In addition, in patients with heart failure, a 2002 meta-analysis showed a trend (not statistically significant) toward increased mortality in patients given adrenergic inotropic agents.[42] Part of the reason for these observations may be that the improved hemodynamics seen with these agents come at a cost of increased myocardial oxygen consumption. One study showed that replacing norepinephrine with vasopressin did not produce significantly different hemodynamic effects.[43] However, a 2017 retrospective study suggested that combining vasopressin with other vasopressors or inotropes was associated with an increase in 30-day hospitalization and mortality.[44] Phosphodiesterase inhibitors (e.g., milrinone) may be considered (particularly with right ventricular dysfunction); however, the resultant decrease in SVR may not be well tolerated by the hemodynamically unstable patient. Finally, levosimendan, a calcium sensitizer that also promotes coronary vasodilation, showed early promise as a novel treatment for CS.[45–47] Levosimendan does not appear to improve outcomes of patients who require hemodynamic support after cardiac surgery.[48–50] In general, the therapeutic goal should be maintenance of normal physiologic parameters (e.g., mean arterial pressure, CI). Although high-dose vasopressors have been associated with poorer survival, this finding may be an epiphenomenon representing only those patients who have greater hemodynamic instability.[51]

Mechanical Therapy

In patients who are unresponsive to conventional pharmacologic therapy, mechanical augmentation of flow may be of benefit.[52] While there are a variety of mechanical devices that augment CO, none have been shown to be superior. The ACCF/AHA

(American College of Cardiology Foundation/American Heart Association) guidelines have recently downgraded the recommendation for use of an IABP for CS from class I ("is recommended") to class IIa ("can be useful").[53] The 2017 Shock II trial showed the use of IABP did not significantly reduce 30-day mortality.[54] A 2015 meta-analysis also failed to show that use of an IABP in CS conferred a mortality benefit.[55] While one randomized trial to evaluate the efficacy of IABP (with or without thrombolysis) in patients with CS was able to show a dramatic decrease in 6-month mortality rate (39% vs. 80%; $P < .05$) in patients with severe shock who received an IABP,[56] subsequent observational studies did not confirmed these findings.[57] Of note, the use of this device is frequently associated with more aggressive therapies such as revascularization.[58]

One of the inherent benefits of IABP counterpulsation devices is that they can be placed at the bedside to augment diastolic pressure and reduce left ventricular afterload (without increasing myocardial oxygen demand). The incidence of major complications (e.g., arterial injury and perforation, limb ischemia, visceral ischemia) with IABP insertion is 2.5–3.0%.[58,59] If an IABP is contraindicated (e.g., severe aortic insufficiency, severe peripheral vascular disease, aortic aneurysm, and dissection) or unavailable, or if the patient is unresponsive, other ventricular assist device (VAD) placement may be considered.[60,61] The most common devices used are the Impella 2.5, Impella 5.0, TandemHeart, and VA ECMO (venoarterial extracorporeal membrane oxygenation). These devices, including institution of ECMO and placement of the CardioWest total artificial heart, have been tried with varying success.[62–64] Newer percutaneous VADs are making this option more feasible in smaller centers.[65] A 2005 investigation randomized patients with CS to IABP or TandemHeart (a percutaneous left ventricular assist device [LVAD]).[66] Although there were no significant differences in 30-day mortality between the two groups, patients in the LVAD subgroup had a significant improvement in hemodynamics, renal function, and clearance of serum lactate compared with the IABP cohort. A multicenter randomized trial comparing TandemHeart with IABP in 42 patients with CS revealed similar improvements in hemodynamics with the LVAD without a statistically significant difference in 30-day mortality.[67] A small pilot study showed superior hemodynamics at 30 minutes when using the Impella 2.5 over the IABP; however, it failed to demonstrate any difference at 4 hours with the same outcomes.[68] When comparing the secondary endpoints such as lactic acidosis, hemolysis and 30-day mortality, there was no difference.[68] The IMPRESS trial, a randomized controlled study, compared the use of an Impella CP to an IABP in patients with CS and showed no reduction in 30-day mortality.[69]

VA ECMO is also an option in the CS patient. A small retrospective study showed that patients placed on VA ECMO for refractory cardiogenic shock had good survival rates, with good neurologic outcomes, and that it was reasonable and safe to transfer these patients to a higher level of care.[70] What may be most exciting is the use of ECMO in out-of-hospital cardiac arrest patients who are refractory to CPR. There may be a survival benefit in select patients who undergo cannulation in the field, but this obviously needs more investigative attention.[71,72]

Although many of these newer devices appear promising, there will clearly be a limited number of centers that can access the technology. Experience with device placement and hemodynamic management is necessary for optimal benefit. In the National Registry of Myocardial Infarction, IABP use was independently associated with survival in those centers with experience in their use.[73] Finally, many of these devices are placed as a bridge to cardiac transplantation, and resources must be available to continue this often lengthy workup.

Revascularization Therapy

Although management of AMI is beyond the scope of this chapter, a brief synopsis is provided here. Because AMI is frequently the inciting event culminating in CS, reestablishing blood flow to the affected myocardial territory is of utmost importance.[74] It has become evident that prompt revascularization reduces the mortality. One method for reestablishing coronary arterial flow is by the administration of thrombolytic agents. In a randomized trial involving more than 40,000 patients with AMI, the GUSTO-I (Global Utilization of Tissue Plasminogen Activator and Streptokinase for Occluded Coronary Arteries) trial demonstrated a survival advantage with the use of tissue plasminogen activator (tPA) over streptokinase.[75] Since these results have been published, a number of other thrombolytics have been developed; however, randomized trials have been unable to show a difference with respect to CS progression between tPA and these newer agents.[76] Moreover, once CS has been established, no studies have shown an improvement in mortality with the administration of thrombolytic agents. The preferred modality of revascularization remains either percutaneous coronary intervention (PCI) or CABG.[14,38,77–80] Although a facilitated PCI strategy (i.e., planned immediate PCI after fibrinolytic administration) has not been shown to be effective,[81,82] fibrinolytics have a class Ib recommendation (ACCF/AHA) in those situations in which PCI is not attainable for more than 120 minutes, the patient is within 3 hours of his or her infarction, and there are no contraindications.[53,83] The Should We Emergently Revascularize Occluded Coronaries for Cardiogenic Shock (SHOCK) trial emphasized this aspect, showing that early revascularization reduced mortality by 22% in those patients who presented with CS and by 16% in those who had CS subsequent to admission.[76] The question of how and when it is best to achieve reperfusion has been evaluated. The SHOCK trial prospectively randomized 302 patients with CS due to AMI to either emergency revascularization (either CABG or PCI) or medical stabilization.[77] Although 30-day mortality was similar for both groups, there was a significant survival advantage in the early revascularization group at 6 months, 1 year, and 6 years. This trial did not demonstrate an advantage of one revascularization therapy over another. Given these results and others, early revascularization (either with PCI or CABG surgery) therapy is a class I recommendation by the ACC/AHA for patients younger than 75 years with CS complicated by ACS.[7] Although there are few data to support revascularization in the non–ST-segment elevation CS population, the SHOCK registry did find a decrease (albeit not statistically significant) in mortality among those patients who underwent early revascularization.[1]

AUTHORS' RECOMMENDATIONS

Cardiogenic shock requires rapid diagnosis and appropriate therapy to significantly affect mortality. ICU patients often have multisytem organ failure, and differentiating CS from other forms of shock can often be difficult. In patients in whom a diagnosis of CS is being entertained, we recommend the following:

- Maximize oxygen delivery, immediately obtain an electrocardiogram, place invasive monitoring (at least arterial and central venous monitoring) and undertake laboratory (including cardiac enzymes) evaluation.
- Rapid echocardiography not only may confirm the diagnosis but also may aid in management. We recommend that use of POCUS for the bedside physician while waiting for a more comprehensive study. This rapid evaluation will aide in a faster diagnosis and exclusion of life-threatening issues in the patient with shock.
- If echocardiography or a bedside ultrasound is not immediately available and there are no signs of pulmonary edema, we recommend giving an initial intravenous fluid challenge with 500 mL of crystalloid. Repeat fluid challenge may be necessary if there is no increase in blood pressure or right atrial pressure.
- If the patient remains in CS despite adequate intravascular volume, we recommend a primary inotropic agent (e.g., dobutamine) with or without the addition of norepinephrine to maintain mean arterial pressure >60 mm Hg and a cardiac index ≥ 2 L/min/m^2.
- If there is not a dramatic improvement in perfusion within 1 hour, placement of an IABP or other ventricular assist device should be *considered*.
- In patients with electrocardiographic changes suggestive of myocardial ischemia, an immediate search for a culprit vessel should be sought, and early revascularization should be considered.
- It is important to recognize that the treatment of CS often crosses multiple disciplines. Communication among the intensivist, invasive cardiologist, and cardiac surgeon is often necessary to ensure optimal care with optimal timing. As bedside echocardiography becomes more commonplace in ICUs, there is no doubt that intensivists will be diagnosing this entity more frequently and in a more timely manner.

REFERENCES

1. Jacobs AK, French JK, Col J, et al. Cardiogenic shock with non-ST-segment elevation myocardial infarction: a report from the SHOCK Trial Registry. SHould we emergently revascularize Occluded coronaries for Cardiogenic shocK? *J Am Coll Cardiol.* 2000;36:1091-1096.
2. Topalian S, Ginsberg F, Parrillo JE. Cardiogenic shock. *Crit Care Med.* 2008;36:S66-S74.
3. Alonso DR, Scheidt S, Post M, Killip T. Pathophysiology of cardiogenic shock: quantification of myocardial necrosis, clinical, pathologic and electrocardiographic correlations. *Circulation.* 1973;48:588-596.
4. Harnarayan C, Bennett MA, Pentecost BL, Brewer DB. Quantitative study of infarcted myocardium in cardiogenic shock. *Br Heart J.* 1970;32:728-732.
5. Hochman JS, Buller CE, Sleeper LA, et al. Cardiogenic shock complicating acute myocardial infarction—etiologies, management and outcome: a report from the SHOCK Trial Registry. SHould we emergently revascularize Occluded coronaries for Cardiogenic shocK? *J Am Coll Cardiol.* 2000;36:1063-1070.
6. Chockalingam A, Mehra A, Dorairajan S, Dellsperger KC. Acute left ventricular dysfunction in the critically ill. *Chest.* 2010;138(1):198-207.
7. Babaev A, Frederick PD, Pasta DJ, et al. Trends in management and outcomes of patients with acute myocardial infarction complicated by cardiogenic shock. *JAMA.* 2005;294:448-454.
8. Holmes Jr DR, Berger PB, Hochman JS, et al. Cardiogenic shock in patients with acute ischemic syndromes with and without ST-segment elevation. *Circulation.* 1999;100:2067-2073.
9. Chen ZM, Pan HC, Chen YP, et al. Early intravenous then oral metoprolol in 45,852 patients with acute myocardial infarction: randomised placebo-controlled trial. *Lancet.* 2005;366:1622-1632.
10. Antman EM, Braunwald E. Acute myocardial infarction. In: Braunwald ED, Fauci E, Kasper D, eds. *Harrison's Principles of Internal Medicine.* New York: McGraw-Hill; 2001:1395.
11. Mehta SR, Yusuf S, Diaz R, et al. Effect of glucose-insulin-potassium infusion on mortality in patients with acute ST-segment elevation myocardial infarction: the CREATE-ECLA randomized controlled trial. *JAMA.* 2005;293:437-446.
12. Goldberg RJ, Gore JM, Alpert JS, et al. Cardiogenic shock after acute myocardial infarction. Incidence and mortality from a community-wide perspective, 1975 to 1988. *N Engl J Med.* 1991;325:1117-1122.
13. Singh M, White J, Hasdai D, et al. Long-term outcome and its predictors among patients with ST-segment elevation myocardial infarction complicated by shock: insights from the GUSTO-I trial. *J Am Coll Cardiol.* 2007;50:1752-1758.
14. Hochman JS, Sleeper LA, Webb JG, et al. Early revascularization and long-term survival in cardiogenic shock complicating acute myocardial infarction. *JAMA.* 2006;295:2511-2515.
15. Rigamonti F, Graf G, Merlani P, Bendjelid K. The short-term prognosis of cardiogenic shock can be determined using hemodynamic variables: a retrospective cohort study. *Crit Care Med.* 2014;41(11):2484-2491.
16. Hollenberg SM, Kavinsky CJ, Parrillo JE. Cardiogenic shock. *Ann Intern Med.* 1999;131:47-59.
17. Lim N, Dubois MJ, De Backer D, Vincent JL. Do all nonsurvivors of cardiogenic shock die with a low cardiac index? *Chest.* 2003;124:1885-1891.
18. O'Gara PT, Kushner FG, Ascheim DD, et al. 2013 ACCF/AHA guideline for the management of ST-elevation myocardial infarction: a report of the American College of Cardiology Foundation/American Heart Association Task Force on Practice Guidelines. *Circulation.* 2013;127(4):e362-425.
19. Berkowitz MJ, Picard MH, Harkness S, Sanborn TA, Hochman JS, Slater JN. Echocardiographic and angiographic correlations in patients with cardiogenic shock secondary to acute myocardial infarction. *Am J Cardiol.* 2006;98;1004-1008.

20. Joseph MX, Disney PJ, Da Costa R, Hutchison SJ. Transthoracic echocardiography to identify or exclude cardiac cause of shock. *Chest*. 2004;126:1592-1597.

21. Moore CL, Rose GA, Tayal VS, Sullivan DM, Arrowood JA, Kline JA. Determination of left ventricular function by emergency physician echocardiography of hypotensive patients. *Acad Emerg Med*. 2002;9(3):186-193.

22. Randazzo MR, Snoey ER, Levitt MA, Binder K. Accuracy of emergency physician assessment of left ventricular ejection fraction and central venous pressure using echocardiography. *Acad Emerg Med*. 2003;10(9):973-977.

23. Alexander JH, Peterson ED, Chen AY, Harding TM, Adams DB, Kisslo Jr JA. Feasibility of point-of-care echocardiography by internal medicine house staff. *Am Heart J*. 2004;147(3):476-481.

24. Kobal SL, Trento L, Baharami S, et al. Comparison of effectiveness of hand-carried ultrasound to bedside cardiovascular physical examination. *Am J Cardiol*. 2005;96(7):1002-1006.

25. Ghane MR, Gharib MH, Ebrahimi A, et al. Accuracy of rapid ultrasound in shock (RUSH) exam for diagnosis of shock in critically ill patients. *Trauma Mon*. 2015;20(1):e20095.

26. Reynolds HR, Anand SK, Fox JM, et al. Restrictive physiology in cardiogenic shock: observations from echocardiography. *Am Heart J*. 2006;151:890e9-15.

27. Yancy CW, Jessup M, Bozkurt B, et al. 2013 ACCF/AHA guideline for the management of heart failure: executive summary: a report of the American College of Cardiology Foundation/American Heart Association Task Force on practice guidelines. *Circulation*. 2013;128(16):1810-1852.

28. Mimoz O, Rauss A, Rekik N, Brun-Buisson C, Lemaire F, Brochard L. Pulmonary artery catheterization in critically ill patients: a prospective analysis of outcome changes associated with catheter-prompted changes in therapy. *Crit Care Med*. 1994;22:573-579.

29. Porter A, Iakobishvili Z, Haim M, et al. Balloon-floating right heart catheter monitoring for acute coronary syndromes complicated by heart failure: discordance between guidelines and reality. *Cardiology*. 2005;104:186-190.

30. Fincke R, Hochman JS, Lowe AM, et al. Cardiac power is the strongest hemodynamic correlate of mortality in cardiogenic shock: a report from the SHOCK trial registry. *J Am Coll Cardiol*. 2004;44:340-348.

31. Magder S. Central venous pressure: a useful but not so simple measurement. *Crit Care Med*. 2006;34:2224-2227.

32. Magder S. Central venous pressure monitoring. *Curr Opin Crit Care*. 2006;12:219-227.

33. Pinsky MR. Clinical significance of pulmonary artery occlusion pressure. *Intensive Care Med*. 2003;29:175-178.

34. Pinsky MR. Pulmonary artery occlusion pressure. *Intensive Care Med*. 2003;29:19-22.

35. O'Quin R, Marini JJ. Pulmonary artery occlusion pressure: clinical physiology, measurement, and interpretation. *Am Rev Respir Dis*. 1983;128:319-326.

36. Antman EM, Anbe DT, Armstrong PW, et al. ACC/AHA guidelines for the management of patients with ST-elevation myocardial infarction. A report of the American College of Cardiology/American Heart Association Task Force on Practice Guidelines (Committee to Revise the 1999 Guidelines for the Management of Patients with Acute Myocardial Infarction). *Circulation*. 2004;110:e82-e292.

37. De Backer D, Biston P, Devriendt J, et al. Comparison of dopamine and norepinephrine in the treatment of shock. *N Engl J Med*. 2010;362:779-789.

38. Reynolds HR, Hochman JS. Cardiogenic shock: current concepts and improving outcomes. *Circulation*. 2008;117:686-697.

39. Sakr Y, Reinhart K, Vincent JL, et al. Does dopamine administration in shock influence outcome? Results of the Sepsis Occurrence in Acutely Ill Patients (SOAP) Study. *Crit Care Med*. 2006;34:589-597.

40. Schumann J, Henrich EC, Strobl H, et al. Inotropic agents and vasodilator strategies for the treatment of cardiogenic shock or low cardiac output syndrome. *Cochrane Database Syst Rev*. 2018;1:CD009669.

41. De Backer D, Biston P, Devriendt J, et al. Comparison of dopamine and norepinephrine in the treatment of shock. *N Engl J Med*. 2010;362:779-789.

42. Jolly S, Newton G, Horlick E, et al. Effect of vasopressin on hemodynamics in patients with refractory cardiogenic shock complicating acute myocardial infarction. *Am J Cardiol*. 2005;96:1617-1620.

43. García-González MJ, Domínguez-Rodríguez A, Ferrer-Hita JJ. Utility of levosimendan, a new calcium sensitizing agent, in the treatment of cardiogenic shock due to myocardial stunning in patients with ST-elevation myocardial infarction: a series of cases. *J Clin Pharmacol*. 2005;45:704-708.

44. Hootman R, Bentley ML, Sane DC. Adjunct vasopressin in cardiogenic shock is associated with increased mortality. *Circulation*. 2017;136:A14934.

45. Rokyta Jr R, Pechman V. The effects of levosimendan on global haemodynamics in patients with cardiogenic shock. *Neuro Endocrinol Lett*. 2006;27:121-127.

46. Follath F, Cleland JG, Just H, et al. Efficacy and safety of intravenous levosimendan compared with dobutamine in severe low-output heart failure (the LIDO study): a randomised double-blind trial. *Lancet*. 2002;360:196-202.

47. Valente S, Lazzeri C, Vecchio S, et al. Predictors of in-hospital mortality after percutaneous coronary intervention for cardiogenic shock. *Int J Cardiol*. 2007;114:176-182.

48. Landoni G, Lomivorotov VV, Alvaro G, et al. Levosimendan for hemodynamic support after cardiac surgery. *N Engl J Med*. 2017;376(21):2021-2031.

49. Mehta RH, Leimberger JD, van Diepen S, et al. Levosimendan in patients with left ventricular dysfunction undergoing cardiac surgery. *N Engl J Med*. 2017;376(21):2032-2042.

50. Cholley B, Caruba T, Grosjean S, et al. Effect of levosimendan on low cardiac output syndrome in patients with low ejection fraction undergoing coronary artery bypass grafting with cardiopulmonary bypass. *JAMA*. 2017;318(6):548-556.

51. Ohman EM, Nanas J, Stomel RJ, et al. Thrombolysis and counterpulsation to improve survival in myocardial infarction complicated by hypotension and suspected cardiogenic shock or heart failure: results of the TACTICS trial. *J Thromb Thrombolysis*. 2005;19:33-39.

52. Pitsis AA, Visouli AN. Mechanical assistance of the circulation during cardiogenic shock. *Curr Opin Crit Care*. 2011;17(5):425-438.

53. O'Gara PT, Kushner FG, Ascheim DD, et al. ACCF/AHA guideline for the management of ST-elevation myocardial infarction: a report of the American College of Cardiology Foundation/American Heart Association Task Force on Practice Guidelines. *J Am Coll Cardiol*. 2013;61:e78-e140.

54. Thiele H, Zeymer U, Neumann FJ. Intraaortic balloon support for myocardial infarction with cardiogenic shock. *N Engl J Med*. 2012;367(14):1287-1296.

55. Ahmad Y, Sen S, Shun-Shin MJ, et al. Intra-aortic balloon pump therapy for acute myocardial infarction: a meta-analysis. *JAMA Intern Med.* 2015;175(6):931-939.

56. Trost JC, Hillis LD. Intra-aortic balloon counterpulsation. *Am J Cardiol.* 2006;97:1391-1398.

57. Taylor J. ESC guidelines on acute myocardial infarction (STEMI). *Eur Heart J.* 2012;33:2501-2502.

58. Stone GW, Ohman EM, Miller MF, et al. Contemporary utilization and outcomes of intra-aortic balloon counterpulsation in acute myocardial infarction: the benchmark registry. *J Am Coll Cardiol.* 2003;41:1940-1945.

59. Leshnower BG, Gleason TG, O'Hara ML, et al. Safety and efficacy of left ventricular assist device support in postmyocardial infarction cardiogenic shock. *Ann Thorac Surg.* 2006;81:1365-1370; discussion 1370-1371.

60. Tayara W, Starling RC, Yamani MH, Wazni O, Jubran F, Smedira N. Improved survival after acute myocardial infarction complicated by cardiogenic shock with circulatory support and transplantation: comparing aggressive intervention with conservative treatment. *J Heart Lung Transplant.* 2006;25:504-509.

61. Chen YS, Yu HY, Huang SC, et al. Experience and result of extracorporeal membrane oxygenation in treating fulminant myocarditis with shock: what mechanical support should be considered first? *J Heart Lung Transplant.* 2005;24:81-87.

62. Dang NC, Topkara VK, Leacche M, John R, Byrne JG, Naka Y. Left ventricular assist device implantation after acute anterior wall myocardial infarction and cardiogenic shock: a two-center study. *J Thorac Cardiovasc Surg.* 2005;130:693-698.

63. El-Banayosy A, Arusoglu L, Morshuis M, et al. CardioWest total artificial heart: Bad Oeynhausen experience. *Ann Thorac Surg.* 2005;80:548-552.

64. White HD, Assmann SF, Sanborn TA, et al. Comparison of percutaneous coronary intervention and coronary artery bypass grafting after acute myocardial infarction complicated by cardiogenic shock. Results from the Should We Emergently Revascularize Occluded Coronaries for Cardiogenic Shock (SHOCK) trial. *Circulation.* 2005;112:1992-2001.

65. Thiele H, Sick P, Boudriot E, et al. Randomized comparison of intra-aortic balloon support with a percutaneous left ventricular assist device in patients with revascularized acute myocardial infarction complicated by cardiogenic shock. *Eur Heart J.* 2005;26:1276-1283.

66. Burkhoff D, Cohen H, Brunckhorst C, O'Neill WW. A randomized multicenter clinical study to evaluate the safety and efficacy of the TandemHeart percutaneous ventricular assist device versus conventional therapy with intraaortic balloon pumping for treatment of cardiogenic shock. *Am Heart J.* 2006;152:469e1-469e8.

67. Chen EW, Canto JG, Parsons LS, et al. Relation between hospital intra-aortic balloon counterpulsation volume and mortality in acute myocardial infarction complicated by cardiogenic shock. *Circulation.* 2003;108:951-957.

68. Seyfarth M, Sibbing D, Bauer I, et al. A randomized clinical trial to evaluate the safety and efficacy of a percutaneous left ventricular assist device versus intra-aortic balloon pumping for treatment of cardiogenic shock caused by myocardial infarction. *J Am Coll Cardiol.* 2008;52:1584-1588.

69. Ouweneel DM, Eriksen E, Sjauw KD, et al. Percutaneous mechanical circulatory support versus intra-aortic balloon pump in cardiogenic shock after acute myocardial infarction. *J Am Coll Cardiol.* 2017;69(3):278-287.

70. Dini CS, Lazzeri C, Chiostri M, Gensini GF, Valente S. A local network for extracorporeal membrane oxygenation in refractory cardiogenic shock. *Acute Card Care.* 2015;17(4):49-54.

71. Lamhaut L, Hutin A, Puymirat E, et al. A pre-hospital extracorporeal cardio pulmonary resuscitation (ECPR) strategy for treatment of refractory out of hospital cardiac arrest: an observational study and propensity analysis. *Resuscitation.* 2017;117:109-117.

72. Lee JJ, Han SJ, Kim HS, et al. Out-of-hospital cardiac arrest patients treated with cardiopulmonary resuscitation using extracorporeal membrane oxygenation: focus on survival rate and neurologic outcome. *Scand J Trauma Resusc Emerg Med.* 2016;24:74.

73. Bengtson JR, Kaplan AJ, Pieper KS, et al. Prognosis in cardiogenic shock after acute myocardial infarction in the interventional era. *J Am Coll Cardiol.* 1992;20:1482-1489.

74. GUSTO Investigators. An international randomized trial comparing four thrombolytic strategies for acute myocardial infarction. *N Engl J Med.* 1993;329:673-682.

75. Hasdai D, Holmes Jr DR, Topol EJ, et al. Frequency and clinical outcome of cardiogenic shock during acute myocardial infarction among patients receiving reteplase or alteplase. Results from GUSTO-III. *Eur Heart J.* 1999;20:128-135.

76. Hochman JS, Sleeper LA, Webb JG, et al. Early revascularization in acute myocardial infarction complicated by cardiogenic shock. SHOCK Investigators: Should We Emergently Revascularize Occluded Coronaries for Cardiogenic Shock. *N Engl J Med.* 1999;341:625-634.

77. Keeley EC, Boura JA, Grines CL. Primary angioplasty versus intravenous thrombolytic therapy for acute myocardial infarction: a quantitative review of 23 randomised trials. *Lancet.* 2003;361:13-20.

78. Hochman JS, Sleeper LA, White HD, et al. One-year survival following early revascularization for cardiogenic shock. *JAMA.* 2001;285:190-192.

79. Antman EM, Hand M, Armstrong PW, et al. 2007 Focused update of the ACC/AHA 2004 guidelines for the management of patients with ST-elevation myocardial infarction. A report of the American College of Cardiology/American Heart Association Task Force on Practice Guidelines. Developed in collaboration with the Canadian Cardiovascular Society endorsed by the American Academy of Family Physicians: 2007 Writing Group to Review New Evidence and Update the ACC/AHA 2004 Guidelines for the Management of Patients with ST-Elevation Myocardial Infarction, Writing on Behalf of the 2004 Writing Committee. *Circulation.* 2008;117:296-329.

80. Assessment of the Safety and Efficacy of a New Treatment Strategy with Percutaneous Coronary Intervention (ASSENT-4 PCI) Investigators. Primary versus tenecteplase-facilitated percutaneous coronary intervention in patients with ST-segment elevation acute myocardial infarction (ASSENT-4 PCI): randomised trial. *Lancet.* 2006;367:569-578.

81. Cantor WJ, Brunet F, Ziegler CP, Kiss A, Morrison LJ. Immediate angioplasty after thrombolysis: a systematic review. *CMAJ.* 2005;173:1473-1481.

82. Hochman JS. Cardiogenic shock complicating acute myocardial infarction: expanding the paradigm. *Circulation.* 2003;107:2998-3002.

83. Jeger RV, Harkness SM, Ramanathan K, et al. Emergency revascularization in patients with cardiogenic shock on admission: a report from the SHOCK trial and registry. *Eur Heart J.* 2006;27:664-670.

53

How Do I Manage Acute Heart Failure?

Larry X. Nguyen and Benjamin Kohl

Acute heart failure (AHF) refers to a rapid deterioration in cardiac function that is life-threatening and requires prompt recognition and urgent pharmacologic and/or mechanical support. While outpatients who have stable, well-treated congestive heart failure have an estimated 1-year mortality of approximately 9%, patients admitted to the hospital with a diagnosis of AHF have an estimated 1-year mortality of almost 25%.[1-3] Much of the additional mortality likely results from multisystem organ dysfunction that can occur rapidly in inadequately managed individuals. With the progression of failure, the heart becomes an ineffective pump and cannot adequately manage circulating blood volume. Therefore timely and appropriate interventions remain the cornerstone of successful heart failure management.

Technical advances and increased use have extended the application of echocardiography to critically ill patients. Cardiac ultrasonography is particularly valuable in the diagnosis and management of AHF. A review of echocardiography use in critical care can be found in an earlier chapter (see Chapter 49). Bedside ultrasound can also be used to interrogate the pulmonary interstitium to quantify the contribution of pulmonary edema to dyspnea and hypoxia that often accompanies AHF; prospective studies indicate that B-lines on lung ultrasound can aid in diagnosis.[4]

Following diagnosis, the cornerstone of therapy is the mitigation of organ congestion and the maximization of organ perfusion. Because elevation of left-sided filling pressure leads to lung congestion and elevation of right-sided filling pressure leads to liver and renal congestion, alleviating organ congestion requires a reduction of cardiac filling pressures and/or augmentation in cardiac output. Among pharmacologic agents that may accomplish these goals, the three primary therapeutic options are vasodilators, diuretics, and inotropes. Hemofiltration (HF) will be discussed briefly as an alternative in those patients who are nonresponsive to diuretics. Finally, mechanical cardiac augmentation remains an alternative for individuals resistant to pharmacologic therapy and is detailed in the previous chapter (see Chapter 52).

VASODILATORS

Vasodilators are the most potent and most rapidly acting drugs for treating AHF. Vasodilators can reduce both left ventricular end-diastolic pressure and systemic vascular resistance (SVR), decreasing both preload and afterload and increasing cardiac output (CO). The European Society of Cardiology guideline[5] and practical recommendation[6] for the management of AHF recommend vasodilator use with normal to high blood pressure (BP) in acute settings. Table 53.1 details the currently recommended agents' doses and side effects, and Table 53.2 indicates the mechanisms and hemodynamic effects of each drug. Although vasodilators have many favorable effects, extreme care should be taken in patients with low admission BP because a rapid drop in systolic BP has been associated with poor outcomes.[7,8] Importantly, while vasodilator therapy remains a cornerstone of treatment, it has never been shown to reduce mortality or provide any post-hospitalization outcome benefit.

The most commonly used vasodilator drugs for AHF are nitrates. These agents exert their effect via activation of cyclic 3',5'-guanosine monophosphate (cGMP). While nitrates can be very helpful in the acute setting, particularly with regard to symptom management, their use for AHF does not appear to protect against either short-or long-term mortality.[9]

Nitroglycerin, the most widely used nitrate, is a potent and rapid acting venodilator and a mild arterial dilator. Its immediate effects occur through venodilation, causing a reduction in preload and, to a lesser extent, afterload, and an increase in CO. When BP is adequate, nitroglycerin can be administered sublingually while preparing for intravenous treatment. Intravenous nitroglycerin is usually started at approximately 10–20 μg/min and is titrated until symptoms improve, the patient has side effects, or the maximum dose (200 μg/min) is

TABLE 53.1 Recommended Doses and Side Effects of Vasodilators.

Drug	Dose	Major Limitations
Nitroglycerin	Start with 10–20 µg/min, 200 µg/min	Hypotension, headache, tachyphylaxis
Sodium nitroprusside	Start with 0.3 µg/kg/min and increase up to 5 µg/kg/min	Hypotension, isocyanate toxicity, coronary steal, rebound vasoconstriction
Nesiritide	Bolus 2 µg/kg + infusion 0.01 µg/kg/min[a]	Hypotension

[a]Nerisitide can be initiated without bolus.

reached. Tachyphylaxis can develop within 24 hours, leading to an escalation in dose to achieve the desired effect.

Nesiritide is a recombinant form of human B-type natriuretic peptide and has variable effects on the vasculature and circulating blood volume. Like nitrates, nesiritide also increases serum cGMP levels. The vasodilatory effects of nesiritide can reduce SVR, increase CO, and increase sodium urinary excretion. However, when compared with placebo, the Acute Study of Clinical Effectiveness of Nesiritide in Decompensated Heart Failure did not demonstrate a significant difference in either symptom burden or 30-day mortality.[10] Similarly, in the Renal Optimization Strategies Evaluation in Acute Heart Failure (ROSE) trial, nesiritide did not increase urine output relative to a placebo control.[11] Despite these data, nesiritide is approved by the Food and Drug Administration in the United States for relief of dyspnea in patients with AHF. Nesiritide infusions can be started at 0.01 µg/kg/min without the need for a bolus. If hypotension occurs during infusion, the dose should be reduced or discontinued and, after BP is restored, it can be restarted at a 30% lower dose. Nesiritide use is not associated with tachyphylaxis.[12]

Serelaxin is a recombinant form of human relaxin-2 that mediates vasodilation by increasing the production of nitric oxide.[13] The RELAX-AF-2 multicenter trial compared Serelaxin (30 µg/kg/day) with placebo in approximately 6600 patients with AHF. Serelaxin neither reduced 180-day cardiovascular mortality nor improved heart failure through day 5. Additionally, there was no beneficial effect on the secondary endpoints of all-cause mortality at 180 days, combined endpoint of cardiovascular death or rehospitalizations due to heart/renal failure through day 180, or length of initial hospital stay.[14]

Diuretics

Loop diuretics are commonly used to treat heart failure (Table 53.3). The use of diuretics to relieve congestive symptoms is mainly based on extensive observational experience rather than randomized controlled trials. The American College of Cardiology Foundation/American Heart Association (ACC/AHA) heart failure guidelines recommend that patients with volume overload receive loop diuretics.[15] In a multicenter, prospective observational study, furosemide started <60 minutes after the time of arrival in the emergency department was associated with lower in-hospital mortality (REALITY-AHF STUDY).[16] The ACC/AHA recommend that diuresis be delayed in patients with severe hypotension or cardiogenic shock.[15] In these cases, the underlying cause of hemodynamic instability should be treated with inotrope or mechanical circulatory support initiation to ensure adequate perfusion preceding diuretic administration.

Loop diuretics inhibit sodium/potassium/chloride cotransporters at the luminal membrane; they are therefore secreted into tubular lumen by the organic acid transporter (OAT).[17] Intravenous administration of loop diuretics can cause mild venodilation with a decrease in cardiac preload before diuretic response, an action that also contributes to rapid improvement of symptoms.[18]. There are a significant number of patients who exhibit diuretic resistance.[19] The etiology of this phenomenon is multifactorial but renal dysfunction is the most important cause. The dose of agent secreted into the tubular lumen will decrease in patients with

TABLE 53.2 Mechanism of Actions and Hemodynamic Effects in Acute Heart Failure.

Drugs	Mechanisms	HEMODYNAMIC EFFECTS						
		CI/CO	PCWP	MAP	HR	SVR	PVR	CBF
Nitroglycerin	NO-mediated vasodilation (vein > artery)	↑	↓	↓	→	↓	↓	↑
Nitroprusside	NO-mediated vasodilation (vein = artery)	↑	↓	↓	→	↓	↓	↓
Nesiritide	cGMP-mediated vasodilation in both endothelial and vascular smooth muscle cells	↑	↓	↓	→	↓	↓	↑

AHF, acute heart failure; CBF, cerebral blood flow; CI, cardiac index; cGMP, cyclic 3′,5′-guanosine monophosphate; CO, cardiac output; HR, heart rate; MAP, mean atrial pressure; NO, nitric oxide; PCWP, pulmonary capillary wedged pressure; PVR, peripheral vascular resistance; SVR, systemic vascular resistance.

TABLE 53.3   Characteristics of Decongestive Agents.

Modality	Urine Na Excretion	RAA Activation	IV Volume	eGFR	CO	PCWP	RAP	PAP	SVR	PVR	Amount of Urine	Bioavailability
Intravenous diuretic	Hypotonic with plasma (half normal saline)	↑↑↑	↓	→, ↓	↓	↓	↓	↓	↑	↑	Unpredictable	10–100 (%)
Tolvaptan	None[a]	→, ↑	?	→	→	↓	↓	↓	→	→, ↓	Unpredictable	42–80 (%)
Ultrafiltration	Isotonic with plasma	↓	→	→	→, ↑	↓	↓	↓	→	→, ↓	Controllable, adjustable	(–)

[a]Na excretion can be increased when it is combined with loop diuretics.
CO, cardiac output; eGFR, estimated glomerular filtration fraction; IV, intravenous; Na, sodium; PAP, pulmonary artery pressure; PCWP, pulmonary capillary wedge pressure; PVR, pulmonary vascular resistance; RAA, renin angiotensin aldosterone; RAP, right arterial pressure; SVR, systemic vascular resistance.

renal dysfunction and titration of the dose may be required. In addition, loop diuretics compete with other organic acids for access to the OAT receptor. The accumulation of acids in renal impairment may contribute to diuretic resistance.[17]

The dosing of loop diuretics should be individualized. However, it is important to recognize that patients who take loop diuretics as part of a chronic regimen may acutely require higher doses. Diuretics can be administered as either an intravenous bolus or a continuous infusion. There is no evidence to show that either approach is superior.

Vasopressin antagonists, that block vasopressin-2 receptors on the basolateral membrane throughout the entire tubule, induce aquaresis (Table 53.3).[20] In contrast to loop diuretics, water excreted in response to vasopressin antagonists comes from both the extracellular (1/3) and the intracellular (2/3) spaces. Thus, aquaresis could limit neurohormonal activation, hemodynamic changes, and altered renal function.[21] Furthermore, vasopressin antagonists do not need to be secreted into the tubular lumen, perhaps providing an advantage over loop diuretics in patients with renal dysfunction. Loop diuretics can be coadministered with vasopressin antagonists to obtain an additive increase in urine output. Importantly, vasopressin antagonists are also vasodilators.

Although mineralocorticoid receptor antagonists are recommended in patients with New York Heart Association class II to IV who have left ventricular systolic dysfunction, evidence does not support their use in AHF patients.

Hemofiltration

Hemofiltration (HF) is an alternative method for removing excess fluid in patients with AHF (Table 53.3). Several small studies have shown that this approach offers several advantages over diuretics. The isotonic nature of fluid removed by HF increases the volume of fluid that can be removed and eliminates hypokalemia.[22] HF also provides control over the rate at which fluid is removed, preventing depletion of blood volume if interstitial fluid is mobilized slowly. Despite these favorable findings, there is no clear evidence that HF is superior to conventional diuretics.

Inotropes

Inotropic drugs improve short-term outcome in patients with signs and symptoms of hypoperfusion-associated organ dysfunction secondary to severely depressed contractility. Although use of inotropic agents is associated with poor prognosis,[23–25] administration of inotropic agents such as dobutamine, dopamine, milrinone, levosimendan, and norepinephrine can dramatically improve hemodynamic parameters in patients with cardiogenic shock. Inotropic and vasopressor agents should be strongly considered in patients with profound hemodynamic disturbances. Similarly, they should be withdrawn without hesitation at the earliest point possible to avoid side effects.

While low-dose dopamine causes diuresis, renal artery vasodilation, and increased renal blood flow, it does not improve glomerular filtration. Indeed, clinical use of "renal dose" dopamine is no longer acceptable. The ROPA-DOP trial compared 90 hospitalized patients with heart failure with preserved ejection fraction (HFpEF). Patients were randomized into four groups: (1) intravenous bolus furosemide administered every 12 h, (2) continuous infusion furosemide, (3) intermittent bolus furosemide with low-dose dopamine, and (4) continuous infusion furosemide with low-dose dopamine. The primary endpoint was percent change in creatinine from baseline to 72 hours. The study concluded that in patients with HFpEF, low-dose dopamine had no significant impact on renal function, irrespective of diuretic strategy.[26] Similarly, the ROSE trial[11] enrolled patients who were hospitalized with AHF and renal dysfunction (glomerular filtration rate of 15–60 mL/min/1.73 m^2 as estimated by the Modification of Diet in Renal Disease equation) and compared low-dose dopamine (2 μg/kg/min for 72 hours) with low-dose nesiritide (0.005 μg/kg/min for 72 hours). The study was unable to demonstrate significant differences in total urine volume, change in cystatin C, plasma creatinine, weight, or N-terminal pro-brain natriuretic peptide from baseline to 72 hours. These two studies demonstrate that dopamine has no advantage over a loop diuretic or a simple vasodilator.

Evidence does not support the use of dobutamine over other agents for the treatment of AHF. However, dobutamine can increase CO with only a modest increase in heart rate. Most patients respond to doses of 2–20 µg/kg/min,[3] but tachycardia, myocardial ischemia, and arrhythmias appear frequently when doses exceed 15 µg/kg/min. Although tolerance to dobutamine has been observed after 72 hours,[27] the plasma half-life is only 2.4 ± 0.7 minutes,[28] indicating that almost all dobutamine could be eliminated within 15 minutes.

Norepinephrine functions as a potent vasoconstrictor. It acts on all three groups of adrenergic receptors, but while it has a strong affinity for α1 and β1 receptors, it is a much weaker β2 agonist. Therefore it increases peripheral vascular resistance primarily because it causes less intense vasodilation (β2 activity) than other agents such as epinephrine. At high doses, it can cause limb ischemia. Norepinephrine is most often used in conjunction with inotropes like dobutamine to treat patients with cariogenic shock. It is usually started at ≈0.1–0.15 µg/kg/min and titrated until the hemodynamic response becomes favorable.[5]

Milrinone is a phosphodiesterase inhibitor approved for use in the United States, Europe, and Japan. It increases CO by inhibiting cyclic adenosine monophosphate (cAMP) breakdown in cardiomyocytes. In vascular muscle cells, increases in cAMP enhance calcium removal, thereby reducing tone. Milrinone can also decrease pulmonary vascular resistance (PVR). Because of its inotropic and vasodilatory effects, it is usually referred to as an "inodilator." There is no clear evidence that milrinone offers advantages over other agents such as dobutamine. However, its mechanism of action may offer an advantage over β-adrenergic drugs in patients taking β-blockers. Caution is required when milrinone is administered to patients with coronary artery disease because its use has been reported to increase mortality.[29] Low-dose milrinone can be combined with low-dose dobutamine because the different sites of actions may provide a synergistic effect. Milrinone administered by bolus may cause acute severe hypotension. Milrinone is renally cleared and thus should be used cautiously in patients with renal dysfunction.

Levosimendan enhances cardiac troponin C (TnC) sensitivity to intracellular calcium, increasing CO.[30] Because levosimendan detaches from TnC during diastole, it acts during systole and, therefore, does not affect diastolic relaxation. Levosimendan can also activate potassium channels in vascular smooth muscle, leading to a reduction in SVR and PVR.[31] Despite levosimendan's favorable effects on hemodynamics, a large randomized, double-blinded, multicenter trial in patients with AHF (Survival of Patients with Acute Heart Failure in Need of Intravenous Inotropic Support trial) did not demonstrate an improvement in 180-day all-cause mortality compared with dobutamine; however, there was a benefit at 30 days and in patients on β-blockers.[32]

Short-Term Mechanical Cardiac Support

Mechanical cardiac support acts as a bridge to recovery or bridge to decision. Appropriate patients typically have a cardiac index <2.0 L/min/m^2, a systolic arterial pressure <90 mm Hg, a pulmonary capillary wedge pressure >18 mm Hg,

a reduced (<25%) ejection fraction, and are refractory to medical management.[5,15] Examples of short-term mechanical circulatory support include intraaortic balloon pump, percutaneous circulatory assist devices (e.g., Tandem Heart, Impella), and extracorporeal membrane oxygenation. These modalities are discussed in depth in Chapter 52.

AUTHORS' RECOMMENDATIONS
- Early recognition of AFH is essential.
- Treatment should then be tailored to the individual and focus on the cause of AHF.
- Support of patients includes the early use of vasodilators, especially when associated with normal or high BP.
- Diuretics or vasopressin antagonists should be used only when there are clear clinical signs of congestion.
- Inotropes should be restricted to cardiogenic shock in the presence of clear signs of organ dysfunction.
- Mechanical circulatory support can be used when medical management is insufficient to optimize the patient's condition.

REFERENCES

1. Kristensen SL, Jhund PS, Køber L, et al. Comparison of outcomes after hospitalization for worsening heart failure, myocardial infarction, and stroke in patients with heart failure and reduced and preserved ejection fraction. *Eur J Heart Fail.* 2014;17(2):169-176.
2. Targher G, Dauriz M, Laroche C, et al. In-hospital and 1-year mortality associated with diabetes in patients with acute heart failure: results from the ESC-HFA Heart Failure Long-Term Registry. *Eur J Heart Fail.* 2017;19(1):54-65.
3. Chioncel O, Lainscak M, Seferovic PM, et al. Epidemiology and one-year outcomes in patients with chronic heart failure and preserved, mid-range and reduced ejection fraction: an analysis of the ESC Heart Failure Long-Term Registry. *Eur J Heart Fail.* 2017;19(12):1574-1585.
4. Price S, Platz E, Cullen L, et al. Expert consensus document: echocardiography and lung ultrasonography for the assessment and management of acute heart failure. *Nat Rev Cardiol.* 2017; 14(7):427-440.
5. McMurray JJ, Adamopoulos S, Anker SD, et al. ESC Guidelines for the diagnosis and treatment of acute and chronic heart failure 2012: The Task Force for the Diagnosis and Treatment of Acute and Chronic Heart Failure 2012 of the European Society of Cardiology. Developed in collaboration with the Heart Failure Association (HFA) of the ESC. *Eur Heart J.* 2012; 33(14):1787-1847.
6. Mebazaa A, Gheorghiade M, Piña IL, et al. Practical recommendations for prehospital and early in-hospital management of patients presenting with acute heart failure syndromes. *Crit Care Med.* 2008;36(suppl 1):S129-S139.
7. Patel PA, Heizer G, O'Connor CM, et al. Hypotension during hospitalization for acute heart failure is independently associated with 30-day mortality: findings from ASCEND-HF. *Circ Heart Fail.* 2014;7(6):918-925.
8. Voors AA, Davison BA, Felker GM, et al. Early drop in systolic blood pressure and worsening renal function in acute heart

failure: renal results of Pre-RELAX-AHF. *Eur J Heart Fail.* 2011;13(9):961-967.

9. Ho EC, Parker JD, Austin PC, Tu JV, Wang X, Lee DS. Impact of nitrate use on survival in acute heart failure: a propensity-matched analysis. *J Am Heart Assoc.* 2016;5(2):e002531.

10. O'Connor CM, Starling RC, Hernandez AF, et al. Effect of nesiritide in patients with acute decompensated heart failure. *N Engl J Med.* 2011;365(1):32-43.

11. Chen HH, Anstrom KJ, Givertz MM, et al. Low-dose dopamine or low-dose nesiritide in acute heart failure with renal dysfunction: the ROSE acute heart failure randomized trial. *JAMA.* 2013; 310(23):2533-2543.

12. Publication Committee for the VMAC Investigators (Vasodilatation in the Management of Acute CHF). Intravenous nesiritide vs. nitroglycerin for treatment of decompensated congestive heart failure: a randomized controlled trial. *JAMA.* 2002; 287(12):1531-1540.

13. Tousoulis D, Kampoli AM, Tentolouris C, Papageorgiou N, Stefanadis C. The role of nitric oxide on endothelial function. *Curr Vasc Pharmacol.* 2012;10(1):4-18.

14. Teerlink JR, Voors AA, Ponikowski P, et al. Serelaxin in addition to standard therapy in acute heart failure: rationale and design of the RELAX-AHF-2 study. *Eur J Heart Fail.* 2017;19(6): 800-809.

15. Yancy CW, Jessup M, Bozkurt B, et al. 2013 ACCF/AHA guideline for the management of heart failure: executive summary: a report of the American College of Cardiology Foundation/ American heart Association Task Force on practice guidelines. *Circulation.* 2013;128(16):1810-1852.

16. Matsue Y, Damman K, Voors AA, et al. Time-to-furosemide treatment and mortality in patients hospitalized with acute heart failure. *J Am Coll Cardiol.* 2017;69(25):3042-3051.

17. Wilcox CS. New insights into diuretic use in patients with chronic renal disease. *J Am Soc Nephrol.* 2002;13(3):798-805.

18. Dormans TP, Pickkers P, Russel FG, Smits P. Vascular effects of loop diuretics. *Cardiovasc Res.* 1996;32(6):988-997.

19. Metra M, Cotter G, Gheorghiade M, Dei Cas L, Voors AA. The role of the kidney in heart failure. *Eur Heart J.* 2012;33(17): 2135-2142.

20. Costello-Boerrigter LC, Smith WB, Boerrigter G, et al. Vasopressin-2-receptor antagonism augments water excretion without changes in renal hemodynamics or sodium and potassium excretion in human heart failure. *Am J Physiol Renal Physiol.* 2006;290(2):F273-F278.

21. Ambrosy A, Goldsmith SR, Gheorghiade M. Tolvaptan for the treatment of heart failure: a review of the literature. *Expert Opin Pharmacother.* 2011;12(6):961-976.

22. Costanzo MR, Guglin ME, Saltzberg MT, et al. Ultrafiltration versus intravenous diuretics for patients hospitalized for acute decompensated heart failure. *J Am Coll Cardiol.* 2007;49(6):675-683.

23. De Backer D, Biston P, Devriendt J, et al. Comparison of dopamine and norepinephrine in the treatment of shock. *N Engl J Med.* 2010;362(9):779-789.

24. O'Connor CM, Gattis WA, Uretsky BF, et al. Continuous intravenous dobutamine is associated with an increased risk of death in patients with advanced heart failure: insights from the Flolan International Randomized Survival Trial (FIRST). *Am Heart J.* 1999;138(1):78-86.

25. Abraham WT, Adams KF, Fonarow GC, et al. In-hospital mortality in patients with acute decompensated heart failure requiring intravenous vasoactive medications: an analysis from the Acute Decompensated Heart Failure National Registry (ADHERE). *J Am Coll Cardiol.* 2005;46(1):57-64

26. Sharma K, Vaishnav J, Kalathiya R, et al. Randomized evaluation of heart failure with preserved ejection fraction patients with acute heart failure and dopamine: the ROPA-DOP trial. *JACC Heart Fail.* 2018;6(10):859-870.

27. Akhtar N, Mikulic E, Cohn JN, Chaudhry MH. Hemodynamic effect of dobutamine in patients with severe heart failure. *Am J Cardiol.* 1975;36(2):202-205.

28. Leier CV, Unverferth DV. Drugs five years later. Dobutamine. *Ann Intern Med.* 1983;99(4):490-496.

29. Felker G, Gattis W, Gheorghiade M, Leimberger J, Adams K, O'Connor C. 114 Anemia as a predictor of death and rehospitalization in patients with advanced decompensated heart failure: insights from the OPTIME-CHF study. *Eur J Heart Fail Suppl.* 2003;2(1):16.

30. Givertz MM, Andreou C, Conrad CH, Colucci WS. Direct myocardial effects of levosimendan in humans with left ventricular dysfunction: alteration of force-frequency and relaxation-frequency relationships. *Circulation.* 2007;115(10):1218-1224.

31. Slawsky MT, Colucci WS, Gottlieb SS, et al. Acute hemodynamic and clinical effects of levosimendan in patients with severe heart failure. Study Investigators. *Circulation.* 2000;102(18):2222-2227.

32. Mebazaa A, Nieminen MS, Packer M, et al. Levosimendan vs. dobutamine for patients with acute decompensated heart failure: the SURVIVE randomized trial. *JAMA.* 2007;297(17): 1883-1891.

54

How Do I Diagnose and Manage Myocardial Ischemia in the ICU?

Audrey E. Spelde, Kristen Carey Rock, and Emily K. Gordon

INTRODUCTION

Myocardial infarction (MI) is defined as myocardial cell death (necrosis) in the setting of prolonged myocardial ischemia. The intensive care unit (ICU) setting presents a unique set of challenges in the diagnosis and treatment of myocardial ischemia and this entity frequently goes unrecognized. Unfortunately, ischemia in this patient population is associated with particularly adverse outcomes.[1] The goals for the critical care physician are to identify myocardial ischemia early, prior to the onset of irreversible cell injury, and to minimize the extent of necrosis when infarction does occur. This chapter reviews the diagnosis and management of the critically ill patient with myocardial ischemia.

PATHOPHYSIOLOGY

The development of myocardial ischemia was once viewed as an ischemic cascade. The classically described abnormalities start with myocardial oxygen supply–demand mismatch, resulting in conversion to anaerobic cell metabolism, changes in perfusion leading to diastolic dysfunction, regional wall motion abnormalities, and ischemic electrocardiogram (ECG) changes.[2,3] However, the cascade concept has been challenged. The current prevailing view is that these events occur concurrently rather than sequentially.[3] This combination of abnormalities is termed acute coronary syndrome (ACS) and can be clinically identified by the appearance of new diagnostic ST-segment elevation myocardial infarction (STEMI) on ECG, ischemic symptoms with positive cardiac biomarkers but without ST elevation (non-ST-elevation myocardial infarction [NSTEMI]), or ischemic symptoms without positive biomarkers (unstable angina).[4]

There are a number of possible etiologies of myocardial ischemia. All lead to a common pathway of myocardial oxygen supply and demand mismatch. Importantly, while infarction does not occur without ischemia, ischemia can occur without leading to infarction. That said, ischemia arising from any etiology is associated with increased mortality.[5,6]

DEFINITION

MI is classified on the basis of five possible etiologies (Table 54.1).[7,8] While elevation of troponin or an alternate biomarker is necessary for diagnosis, the presence of other criteria differentiates MI from other entities, such as myocardial injury, that may also present with a troponin leak. Importantly, troponin rise in the critically ill population may not indicate coronary artery pathology. Rather, the change may reflect physiologic stress.[9] For example, patients may develop troponin elevations due to catecholamine-induced myocardial injury or direct toxic effects from circulating toxins.[7] The most common nonischemic etiologies of troponin elevation in this population include sepsis, respiratory failure, chronic kidney disease, pulmonary embolism, heart failure, stroke, and atrial fibrillation.[9]

One particularly important entity, myocardial injury after noncardiac surgery (MINS),[5] may be caused by ischemia with or without necrosis. MINS occurs within 30 days of noncardiac surgery and is identified by the presence of a peak troponin T that exceeds 0.03 ng/mL in the absence of a nonischemic etiology for cardiac injury. MINS has prognostic relevance—the occurrence of MINS carries a higher 30-day mortality (9.8 vs. 1.1%) when compared with patients free from MINS, suggesting that this is an important perioperative event with implications for mortality and changes in clinical management.[5] Regardless of the etiology of troponin rise, elevated levels are universally predictive of poor outcome.[6]

EPIDEMIOLOGY

Approximately 780,000 people experience ACS per year in the United States, with 70% of these cases being non-ST-elevation ACS.[4] In the general population, the median age at ACS presentation is 68 years old, with a 3:2 male-to-female prevalence. Compared with the general population, critically ill patients have a significantly higher incidence of positive serum cardiac biomarkers, with estimates ranging up to 60%, depending on the patient subgroup.[9] The higher risk of myocardial ischemia for ICU patients probably reflects factors such as older age, increased intrinsic and extrinsic sympathetic stimulation, hypoxia, vasopressor use, and stimulation of prothrombotic pathways.[10] Notably, flow-limiting coronary artery disease (CAD) is the cause of elevated biomarkers in only 30% of critically ill patients vs. 80% in the general population.[9,11,12]

TABLE 54.1 Universal Definition and Classification of Myocardial Infarction (MI).

Type	Etiology	Definition/Criteria
		The term acute MI should be used when there is evidence of myocardial necrosis in a clinical setting consistent with acute myocardial ischemia. Any one of the following criteria meets the diagnosis of MI:
		Detection of a rise and/or fall of cardiac biomarker values [preferably cardiac troponin] with at least one value above the 99th percentile upper reference limit (URL) and with at least one of the following:
		- Symptoms of ischemia
		- New or presumed new significant ST-T changes or new left bundle branch block
		- Development of new pathological Q waves in the ECG
		- Imaging evidence of new loss of viable myocardium or new regional wall motion abnormality
		- Identification of an intracoronary thrombus by angiography or autopsy
Type 1	Spontaneous myocardial infarction	Related to atherosclerotic plaque rupture, ulceration, fissuring, erosion, or dissection with resulting intraluminal thrombus
Type 2	Secondary to an ischemic imbalance	Condition other than coronary artery disease (CAD) contributes to an imbalance between myocardial oxygen supply and/or demand such as coronary endothelial dysfunction, coronary vasospasm, coronary embolism, tachy-/bradyarrhythmias, anemia, respiratory failure, hypotension and hypertension
Type 3	MI resulting in death when biomarkers are unavailable	Cardiac death with symptoms suggestive of MI and presumed new ischemic electrocardiogram (ECG) changes or new left bundle branch block, but death occurred before biomarkers were obtained or before biomarkers would be increased
Type 4a	MI related to percutaneous coronary intervention (PCI) ≤48 h after index procedure	PCI-related MI is arbitrarily defined by elevation of cardiac troponin (cTn) values (>5 × 99th percentile upper reference limit [URL]) in patients with normal baseline values or a rise of cTn values >20% if baseline values are elevated and are stable or falling. In addition, must also have one of the following: (i) new ischemic ECG changes; (ii) development of pathologic Q waves; (iii) angiographic findings consistent with a procedural flow-limiting complication such as dissection or arterial occlusion; or (iv) imaging demonstration of new loss of viable myocardium or new regional wall motion abnormality
Type 4b	MI related to stent thrombosis	Stent/scaffold thrombosis associated with MI when detected by coronary angiography or autopsy using the same criteria utilized for type 1 MI. Timing of stent/scaffold thrombosis in relation to PCI procedure can be categorized as: acute, 0–24 hours; subacute, >24 hours to 30 days; late, >30 days to 1 year; and very late, >1 year after stent/scaffold implantation
Type 4c	Restenosis associated with PCI	In-stent restenosis or restenosis following balloon angioplasty in the infarct territory. Defined as focal or diffuse restenosis, or a complex lesion associated with a rise and/or fall of cTn values above the 99th percentile URL, applying the same criteria utilized for type 1 MI
Type 5	MI related to coronary artery bypass grafting (CABG) ≤48 h after index procedure	CABG-related MI is arbitrarily defined by elevation of cardiac biomarkers (>10 × 99th percentile URL) in patients with normal baseline troponin values (≤ 99th percentile URL) or a rise of cTn values >20% if baseline values are elevated and are stable or falling. In addition, must also have one of the following: (i) new pathologic Q waves; (ii) angiographic documented new graft or new native coronary artery occlusion; or (iii) imaging evidence of new loss of viable myocardium or new regional wall motion abnormality

Data from Thygesen K, Alpert JS, Jaffe AS, et al. Fourth universal definition of myocardial infarction (2018). *J AM Coll Cardiol*. 2018;72(18): 2231–2264.

DIAGNOSIS

Diagnosis of MI is made by applying the universal definition of MI (see Table 54.1). Thus, diagnosis requires an abnormal cardiac biomarker in the presence of ischemic symptoms, ECG changes, functional changes on imaging, or occlusion seen on coronary angiography.[8]

Nonischemic insults can also cause myocardial injury that leads to necrosis. It is important that these abnormalities not be labeled as MI, but rather as myocardial injury. Elevations in cardiac troponin values can be due to:

1. Primary myocardial ischemia (due to plaque rupture or intracoronary thrombus)
2. A supply–demand imbalance leading to myocardial ischemia (such as arrhythmias, aortic dissection, pulmonary embolism, coronary spasm, or severe anemia)
3. Insults unrelated to myocardial ischemia (such as cardiac contusion, ablation, pacing, myocarditis)

4. Multifactorial insults (such as in critical illness and sepsis, heart failure, stress cardiomyopathy, stroke, and renal failure).[7,8]

Given the varied etiologies of myocardial ischemia in the critically ill, determining the cause and a plan of action may be challenging.[4,7,8]

CLINICAL PRESENTATION

ICU patients may have atypical or absent symptoms of ischemia due to sedation or analgesia. Presenting signs may include palpitations, hypotension, arrhythmia, or cardiac arrest.[10] ECG and echo wall motion abnormalities may only be identified by routine surveillance or when prompted by clinical suspicion, and biomarkers may be elevated due to multifactorial causes.[13] Use of the classical approach for detecting MI—clinical signs and symptoms, 2-lead ECG monitoring, 12-lead ECG on demand, and cardiac enzymes as prompted by suspicion of ischemia—will lead to a significant proportion (up to 80%) of missed diagnoses when applied in the ICU.[1,13] Therefore, the intensivist must have a higher level of suspicion and a lower threshold for testing.

Electrocardiogram

The first test to evaluate when MI is suspected is the ECG. It is reasonable to obtain a baseline 12-lead ECG for most patients being admitted to the ICU for future comparison. In addition to diagnosing active ischemia, the ECG can also uncover prior MI. Providers should have a low threshold for repeating 12-lead ECG if an initial recording was nondiagnostic, as dynamic changes may be captured at different time periods.[4,7]

One of the earliest ECG signs of ischemia is T-wave and ST-segment changes. Changes in the ST-T wave interval, degree of ST-segment shifts or Q waves provide information regarding infarct distribution and prognosis, and assist with therapeutic planning (Box 54.1). Other ECG signs may be present that are also associated with myocardial ischemia, including arrhythmia, conduction delays (particularly left bundle branch block), and loss of precordial R-wave amplitude.[4]

BOX 54.1 ECG Manifestations of Active Myocardial Ischemia (in Absence of Left Ventricular Hypertrophy and Bundle Branch Block).

ST Elevation
New ST elevation at the J point in two contiguous leads with cut-points as follows:
- ≥1 mm in all leads other than leads V_2–V_3
- ≥2 mm in men ≥40 years in leads V_2–V_3
- ≥2.5 mm in men <40 years in leads V_2–V_3
- ≥1.5 mm in women in leads V_2–V_3

ST-Depression and T-Wave Changes
New horizontal or downsloping ST depression ≥0.5 mm in two contiguous leads and/or T- wave inversion ≥1 mm in two contiguous leads with prominent R wave or R/S ratio >1

From Thygesen K, Alpert JS, Jaffe AS, et al. Fourth universal definition of myocardial infarction (2018). *J AM Coll Cardiol.* 2018;72(18):2231–2264.

However, there are important limitations to the ECG, including disagreement on ECG findings amongst physicians and a significant false-positive rate with automated ECG interpretation software.[13] Additionally, many conditions may affect the ST segment such as pericarditis, hypertrophy, early repolarization patterns, intracranial processes, and hypothermia,[4] and 12-lead ECG does not adequately display the posterior, lateral, and apical walls.[14]

Biomarkers
Cardiac Troponin

Cardiac troponin (cTn) has become the biomarker of choice for diagnosis of MI, as it is the most sensitive marker for myocardial injury and necrosis.[7] Troponin, a regulatory protein made of three subunits, controls the calcium-mediated interaction of actin and myosin in the contraction of striated muscle. The three subunits are troponin C, found in cardiac and skeletal muscle, and two subunits that are specific to cardiac muscle: troponin I and troponin T. The exact mechanism of release of these intracellular proteins is not well characterized. Troponin is detectable in the blood 3–6 hours following myocardial necrosis using conventional assays (Table 54.2). Concentrations remain elevated for up to 10 days, helping to capture late diagnosis. In addition to a high degree of sensitivity and specificity, troponin is also a powerful predictor of prognosis.[15] Indeed, dynamic changes in cTn levels are a critical part of the acute MI diagnosis, particularly in the setting of chronic disease states associated with steadily elevated cTn concentrations.[16]

Despite its high specificity, determining the clinical cause of cTn elevation can be challenging. In particular, cTn concentrations can be elevated in the critically ill even in the absence of ischemia. Additionally, some argue that the universal upper reference limit (URL) lacks specificity in the critically ill, and that a variable cutoff should be utilized in this population.[10]

CK-MB

Creatine kinase (CK) is an enzyme made up of two subunits, B (brain type) or M (muscle type). Isoenzyme expression varies by tissue type, with the CK-MB subtype being most abundant in myocardial tissue. If a cTn assay is not available, CK-MB is the best alternative biomarker and the same criteria of greater than 99th percentile of the URL is used, also taking into account sex-specific values.[7,8]

TABLE 54.2 Time Course of Biomarker Response in Myocardial Infarction.

Marker	Onset	Peak	Duration
Troponin	3–12 h	18–24 h	10 days
Creatine kinase (total and MB)	3–12 h	18–24 h	36–48 h
Lactate dehydrogenase	6–12 h	24–48 h	6–8 days
Myoglobin	1–4 h	6–7 h	24 h

From Chacko S, Haseeb S, Glover BM, Wallbridge D, Harper A. The role of biomarkers in the diagnosis and risk stratification of acute coronary syndrome. *Future Sci OA.* 2018;4:FSO251.

High-Sensitivity Cardiac Troponin

The use of high-sensitivity cardiac troponin (hs-cTn) assays is becoming routine. This biomarker provides increased diagnostic accuracy at presentation, reduces the "troponin-blind" (less than 3 hours) interval, and shortens the time interval to the second troponin measurement.[17-19] In the critically ill, highly sensitive assays can be useful for early detection of acute MI. As a result, earlier intervention in patients with low tolerance for additional physiologic stress becomes possible. However, while the sensitivity of hs-cTn is high, specificity is low and additional blood sampling is advised.[17] Identification of a variable cutoff may be required before hs-cTn assays can replace conventional cTn measurements in the critically ill.[10] Current diagnostic guidelines accommodate all troponin assays, including high sensitivity, conventional, and point of care.[8]

Imaging

Ischemia leads to myocardial dysfunction, cell death, and healing by fibrosis. These processes can be detected by a variety of imaging modalities, most commonly echocardiography and cardiac magnetic resonance (CMR) imaging. Measurable imaging parameters include perfusion, myocyte viability, wall thickness, myocardial function, and fibrosis.

Echocardiography is the most commonly used diagnostic imaging test in acute myocardial dysfunction. This technique can detect changes almost immediately after the onset of ischemia, when >20% transmural thickness is affected.[20] The modality can easily be applied to even the most unstable patient due to its portability.[8] Abnormal regional motion or thickening on imaging can have many causes, examples include: prior infarction, acute ischemia, stunning, hibernation, and nonischemic conditions such as cardiomyopathy or infiltrative diseases. Therefore, these conditions must be excluded or changes in function must be observed in the setting of other features of acute MI.[8]

MANAGEMENT

ICU patients that are suffering from a type 1 MI should be treated much like any other patient presenting with a type 1 MI: perfusion should be restored as quickly as possible. Risk for bleeding must be considered, especially in surgical patients. A large number of critically ill patients may present with demand ischemia or type II MI, given their often concomitant hypermetabolic states and multiorgan dysfunction. These patients should be managed with medical therapy rather than reperfusion.

Recommendations for medical treatment of ACS have changed over the years.[21] In the following section, we discuss current evidence and guidelines (Table 54.3).

TABLE 54.3	Summary of Recommendations for Early Hospital Care for NSTE-ACS.
Class I (benefit significantly outweighs risk; intervention indicated and should be done)	• Administer supplemental oxygen only with oxygen saturation <90%, respiratory distress • Aspirin • Sublingual NTG every 5 min × 3 for continued ischemic pain • IV NTG for persistent ischemia, HF, HTN • Initiate oral beta blocker within the first 24 h in the absence of HF, low-output state, risk for cardiogenic shock or any contraindications for beta-blockade • Administer initial therapy with nondihydropyridine CCBs with recurrent ischemia and contraindications to beta-blockers in the absence of LV dysfunction, increased risk of cardiogenic shock, or AV nodal blockade • CCBs are recommended for ischemic symptoms when beta blockers are not successful, are contraindicated or cause unacceptable side effects • Long-acting CCBs and nitrates are recommended for patients with coronary artery spasm • Initiate or continue high-intensity statin therapy in patients with no contraindications
Class IIa (benefit outweighs risk; additional focused studies are needed; intervention is reasonable and can be beneficial)	• It is reasonable to continue beta-blocker therapy in patients with normal LV function with NSTE-ACS • Obtain a fasting lipid profile, preferably within the first 24 h
Class IIb (benefit may outweigh risk; further studies are needed and may be considered; effectiveness is uncertain)	• IV morphine may be reasonable for continued ischemic chest pain despite maximally tolerated antiischemic medications
Class III (risk outweighs benefit; not recommended and may be harmful)	• Nitrates are contraindicated with recent use of phosphodiesterase inhibitor • NSAIDs should not be initiated and should be discontinued during hospitalization • IV beta blockers are potentially harmful when risk factors for shock are present • Immediate-release nifedipine is contraindicated in the absence of a beta blocker

AV, arteriovenous; *CCB,* calcium channel blocker; *HF,* heart failure; *HTN,* hypertension; *IV,* intravenous; *LV,* left ventricle; *NSAIDs,* nonsteroidal anti-inflammatory drugs; *NSTE-ACS,* non-ST-elevation acute coronary syndrome; *NTG,* nitroglycerin.
Data from Amsterdam EA, Wenger NK, Brindis RG, et al. 2014 AHA/ACC guideline for the management of patients with non-ST-elevation acute coronary syndromes: a report of the American College of Cardiology/American Heart Association Task Force on Practice Guidelines. *Circulation.* 2014;130:e3414-e426.[4]

Analgesics

It has been proposed that pain control decreases sympathetic stimulation, reduces afterload, and could reduce arrhythmogenesis. However, a 2018 retrospective study comparing patients with anterior STEMI, half of whom received morphine prior to percutaneous coronary intervention (PCI), failed to demonstrate a difference in major adverse coronary events or in infarct size 1 year post-PCI.[22] A large retrospective observational study of 17,000 NSTEMI patients showed that, after risk adjustment, the use of morphine was associated with an increased odds ratio (OR) of 1.48 for mortality.[23] It has been hypothesized that morphine may cause harm by delaying clopidogrel absorption and may reduce systemic concentrations of clopidogrel, leading to treatment failure.[24] In recent recommendations, the use of morphine has been downgraded due to lack of evidence of clinical benefit and potential masking of symptoms.[25] However, the 2014 NSTEMI AHA guideline states that it may be reasonable to administer morphine for chest pain after maximally tolerated anti-ischemic medications have been attempted.[4]

Nonsteroidal anti-inflammatory drugs (NSAIDs) and cyclooxygenase-2 (COX-2) inhibitors have been associated with increased mortality in ACS and therefore are contraindicated.[26–28]

Oxygen

Oxygen has long been a cornerstone in the treatment of patients with suspected MI. The rationale for its use is that it improves the supply side of the supply–demand ratio. However, supranormal levels of oxygen can cause coronary vasoconstriction and produce reactive oxygen species that can result in reperfusion injury.[29,30] In the AVOID trial, patients with STEMI without hypoxia who received oxygen (8 liters) had greater infarct size, higher levels of creatinine kinase (not troponin), and more frequent recurrent MI and arrhythmias.[31] However, in a 2017 randomized controlled trial (RCT), acute MI patients with oxygen saturations above 90% who received 6 liters of oxygen did not have a detectable difference in 1-year mortality when compared with subjects treated on room air.[32] Guidelines currently suggest use of oxygen only if patient oxygen saturation is less than 90% or in respiratory distress.[33]

Nitrates

Nitrates cause vasodilatation and therefore enhance coronary blood flow. These agents can also resolve vasospasm-mediated ischemia. Despite the strong pathobiologic rationale, administration of nitrates has not been shown to improve clinical outcomes compared with placebo in patients with MI.[34,35] The current NSTEMI AHA guidelines recommend administration of up to three doses of sublinguinal nitroglycerin (NTG). If symptoms fail to improve, a decision about intravenous NTG use should be made.[4] Care should be taken in using this drug in the ICU population. Nitrates are selective venodilators and may have untoward consequences in the presence of hypovolemia.

Beta Blockers and Calcium Channel Blockers

Beta blockers were among the first drugs used to treat acute MI where a mortality benefit could be demonstrated.[36] The physiologic rationale—decreased heart rate, myocardial work, and myocardial oxygen consumption—is sound, but concerns regarding timing of beta-blockade initiation and the subset of patients who will benefit remains problematic.[37] Evidence supports the use of beta blockade in patients post-MI with concomitant systolic dysfunction who are not in cardiogenic shock or decompensated heart failure.[38] However, much of this evidence was prior to the era of revascularization, so the benefit may be attenuated in more modern care.[37] A retrospective study of over 30,000 NSTEMI and STEMI patients suggested that treating patients with beta blockers less than 24 hours after an ischemic event was associated with an increased risk for shock or death.[39] Current ACC NSTEMI and STEMI guidelines recommend beta blockade within 24 hours of MI if there is no evidence of heart failure, shock, or heart block.[4,27]

Calcium channel blockers are not first-line therapy in the treatment of ACS because some evidence suggests a trend toward harm in the absence of vasospasm-mediated coronary ischemia. In the absence of vasospasm, nondihydropyridine calcium channel blockers are recommended only in the setting of recurrent symptoms and only in patients with contraindications to beta blockers, or in the face of beta blockers and/or nitrates failure.[4] This class of medication should be avoided in the settings of left ventricular (LV) dysfunction and decreased arteriovenous (AV) conduction.

Statins

Statins have gained enormous popularity in the short- and long-term management of ACS. It has been postulated that statins reduce plaque vulnerability, which has led them to be recommended for all patients with ACS.[4,27,40] Caution should be taken in the ICU patient, who may have elevated transaminase levels due to other comorbidities and who may be on other drugs which interfere with statin metabolism.[41] Statins are relatively contraindicated if hepatic transaminase levels are three times normal.

ACE Inhibitors and ARBs

Angiotensin-converting enzyme (ACE) inhibitors and angiotensin receptor blockers (ARBs) are usually discussed in the same context as they both act along the renin–angiotensin–aldosterone axis. However, ACE inhibitors have been better studied and are recommended over ARBs. While recommended for all ACS patients unless otherwise contraindicated, ACE inhibitors are strongly recommended following ACS with anterior STEMI, history of heart failure, left ventricular ejection fraction (LVEF) ≤40%, hypertension, diabetes, or stable chronic kidney disease due to long-term effects on LV remodeling.[4,27] Caution should be used in critically ill patients with concern for renal dysfunction.

Inotropes and Vasopressors

Shock may be both a cause or a consequence of ACS. Unfortunately, the use of specific management strategies are not supported by high-quality evidence. Thus, there are no international guidelines for management of cardiogenic shock and no evidence that vasopressors in isolation improve outcomes.[42] A small RCT of patients in cardiogenic shock after MI was terminated before completion when preliminary results suggested a higher incidence of refractory shock in patients treated with epinephrine.[43] Physiologic reasoning may support the use of norepinephrine (increased cardiac index without increased heart rate, increased mixed venous oxygen levels, and reduced lactate levels)[44] or dobutamine (improved hemodynamic and metabolic endpoints),[45] but outcome data are lacking.[46] Mechanical support options are discussed elsewhere.

Coronary Revascularization

There are two distinct options for the management of NSTE-ACS because the optimal timing for angiography has not been identified in these patients. The most 2014 guideline recommended immediate angiography in patients who have refractory angina or hemodynamic or electrical instability.[4] In other cases, deferred angiography may allow for plaque stabilization and safer revascularization at a later time. A 2017 multicenter RCT suggested that patients with acute MI and cardiogenic shock should only have the culprit lesion revascularized rather than undergoing PCI with multivessel interventions.[47]

Antiplatelet Therapy

The ISIS-2 trial demonstrated that aspirin administration in the acute phase of MI was associated with a 23% reduction in cardiovascular mortality in the subsequent 5 weeks.[48] As a result, aspirin has remained a mainstay of STEMI and NSTEMI treatment.[27]

Dual antiplatelet therapy (DAPT), consisting of aspirin and a platelet P2Y12 receptor blocker, is strongly recommended for NSTE-ACS. Substitution of ticagrelor for clopidogrel is less strongly recommended.[4] In those patients treated with an early invasive strategy and DAPT with intermediate/high-risk features (e.g., positive troponins), a glycoprotein (GP) IIb/IIIa inhibitor may be considered as part of initial antiplatelet therapy.[4] This therapy may be continued for ≥12 months for all patients with NSTE-ACS without contraindication.[4]

Anticoagulation

In the setting of a non-PCI-capable hospital, STEMI should be treated with fibrinolysis as well as adjunctive anticoagulant therapy. Recommended anticoagulation regimens include unfractionated heparin (UFH), enoxaparin or fondaparinux. In this patient population, anticoagulation should be continued for a minimum of 48 hours.[27,49]

For patients undergoing primary PCI, both the ACCF/AHA and ESC guidelines recommend bivalirudin over UFH. However, these recommendations were made before the release of the HEAT-PPCI trial, which demonstrated that UFH was associated with a lower incidence of major adverse ischemic events than bivalirudin in the setting of primary PCI. Patients also received an oral antiplatelet agent such as ticagrelor or prasugrel, which are preferred to clopidogrel.[50]

In the setting of NSTE-ACS, anticoagulation is highly recommended for all patients, irrespective of initial treatment strategy (early intervention vs. ischemic strategy). Anticoagulation can be achieved using enoxaparin, bivalirudin, fondaparinux or unfractionated heparin titrated to therapeutic partial thromboplastin time for at least 48 hours or until PCI is performed.[4]

Fibrinolytics

Primary PCI is the currently preferred reperfusion strategy for most patients with acute STEMI. However, if a patient is within 12 hours of the onset of STEMI with no absolute contraindication to fibrinolytic therapy and for whom primary PCI is not an option then fibrinolytic therapy is recommended.[27] Fibrin-specific agents, such as tenecteplase, reteplase, and alteplase,[27] are preferred when available but patients must be evaluated for any absolute contraindications. There is no role for fibrinolytics in the setting of NSTE-ACS.[33]

AUTHORS' RECOMMENDATIONS

- Myocardial ischemia in the ICU setting presents a unique set of challenges in diagnosis and treatment and therefore one should always maintain a high index of suspicion.
- In the setting of both STEMI and NSTEMI, involvement of our cardiology colleagues is vitally important in the decision making and management of these patients in terms of anticoagulation, fibrinolytic therapy, and the need for catheterization.
- Though research for ACS has been robust, the critically ill subset would benefit from targeted trials to optimize treatment strategies and improve mortality.

REFERENCES

1. Ostermann M, Lo J, Toolan M, et al. A prospective study of the impact of serial troponin measurements on the diagnosis of myocardial infarction and hospital and six-month mortality in patients admitted to ICU with non-cardiac diagnoses. *Crit Care*. 2014;18:R62.
2. Nesto RW, Kowalchuk GJ. The ischemic cascade: temporal sequence of hemodynamic, electrocardiographic and symptomatic expressions of ischemia. *Am J Cardiol*. 1987;59:23C-30C.
3. Maznyczka A, Sen S, Cook C, Francis DP. The ischaemic constellation: an alternative to the ischaemic cascade—implications for the validation of new ischaemic tests. *Open Heart*. 2015;2:e000178.
4. Amsterdam EA, Wenger NK, Brindis RG, et al. 2014 AHA/ACC guideline for the management of patients with non-ST-elevation acute coronary syndromes: a report of the American College of Cardiology/American Heart Association Task Force on Practice Guidelines. *Circulation*. 2014;130:e344-e426.

5. Botto F, Alonso-Coello P, Chan MT, et al. Myocardial injury after noncardiac surgery: a large, international, prospective cohort study establishing diagnostic criteria, characteristics, predictors, and 30-day outcomes. *Anesthesiology*. 2014;120: 564-578.

6. Sarkisian L, Saaby L, Poulsen TS, et al. Prognostic impact of myocardial injury related to various cardiac and noncardiac conditions. *Am J Med*. 2016;129:506-514.e1.

7. Thygesen K, Alpert JS, Jaffe AS, et al. Third universal definition of myocardial infarction. *Circulation*. 2012;126: 2020-2035.

8. Thygesen K, Alpert JS, Jaffe AS, et al. Fourth universal definition of myocardial infarction (2018). *J Am Coll Cardiol*. 2018; 72(18):2231-2264.

9. Hamilton MA, Toner A, Cecconi M. Troponin in critically ill patients. *Minerva Anestesiol*. 2012;78:1039-1045.

10. Klouche K, Jonquet O, Cristol JP. The diagnostic challenge of myocardial infarction in critically ill patients: do high-sensitivity troponin measurements add more clarity or more confusion? *Crit Care*. 2014;18:148.

11. Saaby L, Poulsen TS, Hosbond S, et al. Classification of myocardial infarction: frequency and features of type 2 myocardial infarction. *Am J Med*. 2013;126:789-797.

12. López-Cuenca A, Gómez-Molina M, Flores-Blanco PJ, et al. Comparison between type-2 and type-1 myocardial infarction: clinical features, treatment strategies and outcomes. *J Geriatr Cardiol*. 2016;13:15-22.

13. Carroll I, Mount T, Atkinson D. Myocardial infarction in intensive care units: a systematic review of diagnosis and treatment. *J Intensive Care Soc*. 2016;17:314-325.

14. Kumar A, Cannon CP. Acute coronary syndromes: diagnosis and management, part I. *Mayo Clin Proc*. 2009;84:917-938.

15. Chacko S, Haseeb S, Glover BM, Wallbridge D, Harper A. The role of biomarkers in the diagnosis and risk stratification of acute coronary syndrome. *Future Sci OA*. 2018;4:FSO251.

16. Kvisvik B, Mørkrid L, Røsjø H, et al. High-sensitivity troponin T vs. I in acute coronary syndrome: prediction of significant coronary lesions and long-term prognosis. *Clin Chem*. 2017;63: 552-562.

17. Mueller C, Giannitsis E, Möckel M, et al. Rapid rule out of acute myocardial infarction: novel biomarker-based strategies. *Eur Heart J Acute Cardiovasc Care*. 2017;6:218-222.

18. Roffi M, Patrono C, Collet JP, et al. 2015 ESC Guidelines for the management of acute coronary syndromes in patients presenting without persistent ST-segment elevation: Task Force for the Management of Acute Coronary Syndromes in Patients Presenting without Persistent ST-Segment Elevation of the European Society of Cardiology (ESC). *Eur Heart J*. 2016;37: 267-315.

19. Reichlin T, Cullen L, Parsonage WA, et al. Two-hour algorithm for triage toward rule-out and rule-in of acute myocardial infarction using high-sensitivity cardiac troponin T. *Am J Med*. 2015;128:369-379.e4.

20. Stillman AE, Oudkerk M, Bluemke DA, et al. Imaging the myocardial ischemic cascade. *Int J Cardiovasc Imaging*. 2018;34: 1249-1263.

21. de Alencar Neto JN. Morphine, oxygen, nitrates, and mortality reducing pharmacological treatment for acute coronary syndrome: an evidence-based review. *Cureus*. 2018;10:e2114.

22. Bonin M, Mewton N, Roubille F, et al. Effect and safety of morphine use in acute anterior ST-segment elevation myocardial infarction. *J Am Heart Assoc*. 2018;7(4):pii: e006833.

23. Meine TJ, Roe MT, Chen AY, et al. Association of intravenous morphine use and outcomes in acute coronary syndromes: results from the CRUSADE Quality Improvement Initiative. *Am Heart J*. 2005;149:1043-1049.

24. Hobl EL, Stimpfl T, Ebner J, et al. Morphine decreases clopidogrel concentrations and effects: a randomized, double-blind, placebo-controlled trial. *J Am Coll Cardiol*. 2014;63:630-635.

25. Kline KP, Conti CR, Winchester DE. Historical perspective and contemporary management of acute coronary syndromes: from MONA to THROMBINS2. *Postgrad Med*. 2015;127:855-862.

26. Gislason GH, Jacobsen S, Rasmussen JN, et al. Risk of death or reinfarction associated with the use of selective cyclooxygenase-2 inhibitors and nonselective nonsteroidal antiinflammatory drugs after acute myocardial infarction. *Circulation*. 2006; 113:2906-2913.

27. O'Gara PT, Kushner FG, Ascheim DD, et al. 2013 ACCF/AHA guideline for the management of ST-elevation myocardial infarction: a report of the American College of Cardiology Foundation/American Heart Association Task Force on Practice Guidelines. *Circulation*. 2013;127:e362-e425.

28. Zhang N, Chen K, Rha SW, Li G, Liu T. Morphine in the setting of acute myocardial infarction: pros and cons. *Am J Emerg Med*. 2016;34:746-748.

29. Moradkhan R, Sinoway LI. Revisiting the role of oxygen therapy in cardiac patients. *J Am Coll Cardiol*. 2010;56:1013-1016.

30. Zweier JL, Talukder MA. The role of oxidants and free radicals in reperfusion injury. *Cardiovasc Res*. 2006;70:181-190.

31. Stub D, Smith K, Bernard S, et al. Air versus oxygen in ST-segment-elevation myocardial infarction. *Circulation*. 2015;131: 2143-2150.

32. Hofmann R, James SK, Jernberg T, et al. Oxygen therapy in suspected acute myocardial infarction. *N Engl J Med*. 2017;377: 1240-1249.

33. Amsterdam EA, Wenger NK, Brindis RG, et al. 2014 AHA/ACC guideline for the management of patients with non-ST-elevation acute coronary syndromes: executive summary: a report of the American College of Cardiology/American Heart Association Task Force on Practice Guidelines. *Circulation*. 2014;130:2354-2394.

34. ISIS-4: a randomised factorial trial assessing early oral captopril, oral mononitrate, and intravenous magnesium sulphate in 58,050 patients with suspected acute myocardial infarction. ISIS-4 (Fourth International Study of Infarct Survival) Collaborative Group. *Lancet*. 1995;345:669-685.

35. GISSI-3: effects of lisinopril and transdermal glyceryl trinitrate singly and together on 6-week mortality and ventricular function after acute myocardial infarction. Gruppo Italiano per lo Studio della Sopravvivenza nell'infarto Miocardico. *Lancet*. 1994;343:1115-1122.

36. Frishman WH, Furberg CD, Friedewald WT. Beta-adrenergic blockade for survivors of acute myocardial infarction. *N Engl J Med*. 1984;310:830-837.

37. Bangalore S, Makani H, Radford M, et al. Clinical outcomes with beta-blockers for myocardial infarction: a meta-analysis of randomized trials. *Am J Med*. 2014;127:939-953.

38. Dargie HJ. Effect of carvedilol on outcome after myocardial infarction in patients with left-ventricular dysfunction: the CAPRICORN randomised trial. *Lancet*. 2001;357:1385-1390.

39. Kontos MC, Diercks DB, Ho PM, Wang TY, Chen AY, Roe MT. Treatment and outcomes in patients with myocardial infarction treated with acute beta-blocker therapy: results from the American College of Cardiology's NCDR(®). *Am Heart J*. 2011;161:864-870.

40. Stone NJ, Robinson JG, Lichtenstein AH, et al. 2013 ACC/AHA guideline on the treatment of blood cholesterol to reduce atherosclerotic cardiovascular risk in adults: a report of the American College of Cardiology/American Heart Association Task Force on Practice Guidelines. *Circulation.* 2014;129:S1-S45.

41. Gillett Jr RC, Norrell A. Considerations for safe use of statins: liver enzyme abnormalities and muscle toxicity. *Am Fam Physician.* 2011;83:711-716.

42. Nativi-Nicolau J, Selzman CH, Fang JC, Stehlik J. Pharmacologic therapies for acute cardiogenic shock. *Curr Opin Cardiol.* 2014; 29:250-257.

43. Levy B, Clere-Jehl R, Legras A, et al. Epinephrine versus norepinephrine for cardiogenic shock after acute myocardial infarction. *J Am Coll Cardiol.* 2018;72:173-182.

44. Perez P, Kimmoun A, Blime V, Levy B. Increasing mean arterial pressure in cardiogenic shock secondary to myocardial infarction: effects on hemodynamics and tissue oxygenation. *Shock.* 2014; 41:269-274.

45. Levy B, Perez P, Perny J, Thivilier C, Gerard A. Comparison of norepinephrine-dobutamine to epinephrine for hemodynamics, lactate metabolism, and organ function variables in cardiogenic shock. A prospective, randomized pilot study. *Crit Care Med.* 2011;39:450-455.

46. van Diepen S. Norepinephrine as a first-line inopressor in cardiogenic shock: oversimplification or best practice? *J Am Coll Cardiol.* 2018;72:183-186.

47. Thiele H, Akin I, Sandri M, et al. PCI strategies in patients with acute myocardial infarction and cardiogenic shock. *N Engl J Med.* 2017;377:2419-2432.

48. Randomised trial of intravenous streptokinase, oral aspirin, both, or neither among 17,187 cases of suspected acute myocardial infarction: ISIS-2. ISIS-2 (Second International Study of Infarct Survival) Collaborative Group. *Lancet.* 1988; 2:349-360.

49. Silvain J, Beygui F, Barthélémy O, et al. Efficacy and safety of enoxaparin versus unfractionated heparin during percutaneous coronary intervention: systematic review and meta-analysis. *BMJ.* 2012;344:e553.

50. Shahzad A, Khanna V, Kemp I, et al. Comparison of the effects of P2Y12 receptor antagonists on platelet function and clinical outcomes in patients undergoing primary PCI: a substudy of the HEAT-PPCI trial. *EuroIntervention.* 2018;13:1931-1938.

55

How Do I Prevent or Treat Atrial Fibrillation in Postoperative Critically Ill Patients?

Jonathan K. Frogel and Stuart J. Weiss

Supraventricular arrhythmias are the most common rhythm disturbance encountered in postsurgical patients.[1] The incidence of postoperative atrial fibrillation (POAF) may be as high as 50% after cardiac surgery,[2] 40% after pneumonectomy,[3] and 20% after lung resection.[4] In contrast, other postsurgical patients have a lower incidence of new-onset supraventricular arrhythmias approaching 10%.[5]

Patients who develop supraventricular arrhythmias after major noncardiac surgery are at increased risk for stroke and have significantly higher early and late mortality.[5] After cardiac surgery, atrial fibrillation may herald a prolonged intensive care unit (ICU) course,[2] increased risk of stroke, and increased risk of early and late mortality.[6] Cost of care in a patient who has postoperative atrial fibrillation is increased by an average of $10,000.[7] The human and economic toll of this disease entity is substantial.

WHAT ARE THE PATIENT RISK FACTORS AND PERIOPERATIVE CONDITIONS THAT INCREASE THE RISK OF POAF?

Multiple risk factors that predispose patients to atrial fibrillation have been identified (Box 55.1).[8–10] Every 10-year increase in age beyond 30 years is associated with a 75% increase in risk after cardiac surgery.[8] Thus the risk of POAF after cardiac surgery in octogenarians may be greater than 50%.[9] A history of cardiac disease (atrial fibrillation, hypertension, valvular disease, and cardiomyopathy) and chronic pulmonary disease are significant factors that predispose to POAF. In addition, obesity and increased body mass index (BMI) have also been shown to be predictors of POAF.[10] Multiple studies have demonstrated that lifestyle modification aimed at improving cardiorespiratory fitness and goal-directed weight loss reduce the burden of atrial fibrillation in outpatients with atrial fibrillation.[11,12] It is possible that similar interventions prior to surgery may reduce new-onset POAF, although specific data demonstrating such an effect are lacking.

WHAT IS THE PATHOGENESIS OF POAF?

The pathogenesis of atrial fibrillation in the postoperative period is complex and multifactorial. Several preoperative disease processes and conditions predispose to atrial enlargement and fibrosis, which in turn provides the substrate for the development of conduction abnormalities.[13] The inflammatory response induced by surgery is associated with increased release of endogenous catecholamines or administration of exogenous inotropes or vasopressors. These and other factors (Box 55.2) trigger supraventricular arrhythmias by altering atrial refractoriness and conductivity, thereby predisposing to increased automaticity and reentrant rhythms.[14] The type of surgery performed has a marked impact on the incidence of POAF. In patients undergoing intrathoracic or cardiac procedures, direct surgical manipulation or compression of the atria and/or pulmonary veins contributes to the pathogenesis.[15] During cardiac surgery, myocardial ischemia and ventricular dysfunction can lead to atrial dilation and elevation of atrial pressure that further contribute to atrial irritability. Although the data for general surgery patients are not as robust as cardiac surgical patients, minimally invasive laparoscopic techniques may decrease the risk of POAF when compared with open approaches.[15,16] This finding has been taken to imply that attenuation of the perioperative inflammatory and stress responses to surgery may decrease the risk of developing POAF.

WHAT STRATEGIES ARE EFFECTIVE FOR THE PREVENTION OF POAF?

Although atrial fibrillation in postsurgical patients has long been recognized, the search for and implementation of prophylactic strategies to prevent new or recurrent arrhythmias has only gained traction relatively recently. As knowledge of the causative factors and resulting pathophysiology continues to evolve, the pool of potentially beneficial interventions has broadened. Conceptually, prophylactic strategies fall into one of five categories: administration of antiarrhythmic agents, electrolyte repletion or maintenance, atrial pacing (in cardiac surgical patients), modulation of the perioperative inflammatory response, and alterations of surgical technique. In general, the utility of prophylactic strategies has been most thoroughly evaluated in cardiac surgical patients. Therefore, considerations pertaining to specific risk and pathophysiology must be considered before extrapolation to the general surgical population.

BOX 55.1   Risk Factors for Postoperative Atrial Fibrillation.

Epidemiologic
    Genetics
    Advanced age
    Male gender
Medical conditions
    History of atrial fibrillation
    Coronary artery disease
    Valvular heart disease
    Congestive heart failure
    Diabetes mellitus
Potentially modifiable risk factors
    Hypertension
    Obstructive sleep apnea
    Obesity
Perioperative stresses
    Type of surgery
    Pain
    Respiratory insufficiency
    Volume overload
    Use of catecholamine inotropes and pressors
    Electrolyte disturbances

BOX 55.2   Stressors of the Perioperative and Intensive Care Periods.

Induction and emergence of general anesthesia
Hemodynamic shifts
Surgical trauma
Manipulation of the heart and pulmonary veins
Pain
Electrolyte abnormalities (hypokalemia, hypomagnesemia)
Hypervolemia (distension of the atria)
Subtherapeutic levels of antiarrhythmics (i.e., beta blockers)
Administration of catecholamine inotropes
Pulmonary insufficiency (dyspnea, weaning from ventilator)

ANTIARRHYTHMIC AGENTS

Beta Blockers

Considering the inciting role of increased sympathetic tone in the pathogenesis of atrial fibrillation, it is not surprising that beta-blocker administration for postoperative prevention has been extensively examined. Many studies have confirmed the utility of prophylactic beta blockers to limit the occurrence of POAF. A meta-analysis of 27 trials published in 2002 found that beta blockers reduce the risk of new-onset POAF after cardiac surgery by more than 60%.[17] These findings were reaffirmed by the same author in a larger 2004 meta-analysis of 58 studies.[18] The antiarrhythmic benefit was observed when adrenergic beta-antagonists were started before or immediately after surgery and was independent of the agent or dose used. A meta-analysis comprising 33 studies and 4698 subjects demonstrated a significant atrial fibrillation risk reduction in cardiac surgical patients receiving perioperative beta blockers.[19] On the basis of this evidence, the American College of Cardiology Foundation (ACCF)/American Heart Association (AHA) guidelines for patients undergoing coronary artery bypass graft (CABG) surgery recommend that all such patients receive perioperative beta blockers from 24 hours prior to surgery onward.[20]

Following general thoracic (noncardiac) surgery, a meta-analysis of two studies totaling 129 subjects demonstrated that perioperative beta blockade significantly reduced the incidence of POAF but also increased the risk of hypotension and pulmonary edema.[21] Of greater concern, the PeriOperative Ischemia Evaluation (POISE) trial, a large (8351 subjects), randomized controlled trial (RCT) in noncardiac surgical patients found that perioperative beta blockers decreased the incidence of cardiac arrest (3.6 vs. 5.1%) and myocardial infarction (4.2 vs. 5.7%) but increased the risk of perioperative hypotension, bradycardia, stroke (1.0 vs. 0.5%) and all-cause mortality.[22] A post hoc analysis suggested that the increased incidence of clinically significant hypotension, bradycardia, and stroke may contribute to the observed increased mortality in the treatment groups. A meta-analysis of 33 RCTs totaling 12,306 subjects confirmed an increased risk of hypotension, bradycardia, and nonfatal stroke observed in the group receiving beta blockers.[23]

The guidelines from the American Association for Thoracic Surgery (AATS) on the prevention of POAF in patients undergoing noncardiac thoracic surgery recommend continuation of beta blockers in patients already receiving them. They do not, however, recommend initiation in beta-blocker naïve patients.[24] The 2016 European Society of Cardiology (ESC) guidelines for the management of atrial fibrillation assign a class 1 recommendation for beta-blocker administration for POAF prophylaxis in all adult patients undergoing cardiac surgery, not limited to CABG.[25] In summary, all patients undergoing CABG surgery should receive beta blockers. As for patients undergoing noncardiac surgery, those who currently take beta blockers should continue receiving them throughout the perioperative period. However, the risk of initiating new beta-blocker therapy appears to outweigh the prophylactic benefit of administration.

Amiodarone

Amiodarone, one of the most commonly used antiarrhythmic agents in the ICU setting, is frequently the antiarrhythmic of choice in patients with obstructive lung disease or cardiomyopathy. The prophylactic use of amiodarone to prevent POAF has been extensively studied. A meta-analysis comprising 33 studies and 5402 subjects demonstrated a significant reduction in the risk of POAF in amiodarone-treated patients undergoing cardiac surgery.[19] However, the use of amiodarone is not benign; long-term use has been associated with hepatic, pulmonary, and endocrine toxicity. In addition, amiodarone administration can cause hypotension, bradycardia, and heart block. A meta-analysis of 18 trials (3408 patients) performed to assess the safety of amiodarone to prevent POAF after cardiac surgery noted an increased risk of bradycardia and hypotension in the amiodarone-treated group, but no statistically significant differences in heart block, myocardial infarction, stroke, or death.[26] These findings were most apparent in patients treated with high doses (>1 g/day), with intravenous formulations, and in those in whom the drug was initiated in the postoperative period. Both the ACCF/AHA guidelines[20] and ESC guidelines[25] ascribe a class IIa recommendation for amiodarone POAF prophylaxis in cardiac surgical patients. The American College of College of Cardiology (ACC) guidelines recommend consideration of amiodarone prophylaxis for cardiac surgical patients in whom beta blockers are contraindicated.[27] There are insufficient data available to recommend amiodarone prophylaxis for patients undergoing noncardiac surgery.

Sotalol

Sotalol is a class II antiarrhythmic agent that has both beta-antagonist and potassium channel-blocking activity. A review of 11 studies (1609 subjects) found significant reductions in the incidence of POAF in patients undergoing cardiac surgery who received perioperative sotalol.[19] Despite these findings, potentially dangerous side effects (QT prolongation, torsades de pointes, hypotension, and bradycardia) have limited the use of this agent in both cardiac and noncardiac surgical populations.

Calcium Channel Blockers and Digoxin

Few data support the use of other antiarrhythmic drugs for POAF prophylaxis. Early data regarding the use of nondihydropyridine calcium channel antagonists were inconclusive and an early meta-analysis failed to demonstrate benefit.[28] A more promising review of four studies in noncardiac thoracic surgical patients found that calcium channel blockers were effective in POAF prevention.[21] However, a more 2013 RCT failed to demonstrate benefit in this population.[29] Currently, the ACCP, ACC/AHA, and ESC do not recommend calcium channel blockers for POAF prophylaxis.

Digoxin was at one time advocated for POAF prophylaxis. However, the literature does not support its use.[28] In fact one study noted an increased risk of POAF after thoracic surgery in digoxin-treated patients.[21] Although it can be effectively used for rate control of atrial fibrillation, no current guidelines recommend digoxin for POAF prophylaxis.

ELECTROLYTE REPLETION AND MAINTENANCE

Magnesium

Electrolyte derangements and membrane instability are postulated to play important roles in the pathogenesis of atrial fibrillation, particularly in the postoperative setting. The importance of the magnesium depletion that typically occurs during cardiopulmonary bypass and after diuretic administration has been studied in patients after cardiac surgery. In a meta-analysis, 16 trials totaling 2029 patients evaluating the use of prophylactic magnesium administration were identified. Supraventricular arrhythmias occurred significantly less often in patients treated with magnesium compared with

controls (23 vs. 31%).[30] A review of 19 studies and 2988 subjects demonstrated similar reductions in patients treated with supplemental magnesium during or after cardiac surgery.[19] It remains unclear whether avoidance of hypomagnesemia or achievement of supernormal magnesium levels is responsible for the observed benefit. Nonetheless, current guidelines of the ACCP recommend maintenance of serum magnesium levels in the normal range after cardiac surgery and suggest that empirical supplementation be considered in this high-risk population.[31]

ATRIAL PACING

Atrial pacing has been proposed as a strategy to decrease the incidence of atrial fibrillation after cardiac surgery. It is theorized that overdrive suppression of supraventricular foci may retard the development of atrial fibrillation in the immediate postsurgical period. Heterogeneity within the literature examining pacing for atrial fibrillation prophylaxis makes interpretation of the data challenging. Nonetheless, several meta-analyses have been published. In a review of 13 prospective RCTs in which right atrial pacing, left atrial pacing, or biatrial pacing was used, Archbold and Schilling found that the most significant reduction in POAF occurred in patients receiving biatrial pacing (relative risk [RR] 0.46; 95% confidence interval [CI] 0.30–0.71).[32] Pacing protocols varied, but usually were set 10–20 beats above the intrinsic rate for a period ranging from 1 to 5 days. Atrial pacing after cardiac surgery appears to be efficacious in preserving sinus rhythm, but identification of the optimal site and pacing algorithm is limited by the lack of large, well-controlled studies.

Although potentially advantageous, this strategy has not been explored in the noncardiac surgery population. Pacing is limited to patients with implanted pacemakers and those with transvenous or temporary epicardial pacing wires placed after cardiac surgery.

REDUCTION OF PERIOPERATIVE STRESSORS AND MODULATION OF THE INFLAMMATORY RESPONSE TO SURGERY

Given the role that the inflammatory response seems to play in the pathogenesis of POAF, various interventions targeting this response have been used in efforts to reduce risk.

Corticosteroids

A meta-analysis of 50 RCTs of prophylactic steroid administration for patients undergoing cardiac surgery supported a role in reducing postoperative atrial fibrillation in patients receiving steroids (25.1 vs. 35.1% incidence).[33] Conversely, the Dexamethasone in Cardiac Surgery (DECS) study and Steroids In caRdiac Surgery (SIRS) trials failed to demonstrate a beneficial response.[34,35] Given the potential risks of routine administration of corticosteroids (hyperglycemia, increased risk of infection), they are not currently recommended for postoperative atrial fibrillation prophylaxis.

Statins

In addition to their effects on lipid profiles, statins have known anti-inflammatory effects that are thought to contribute to the observed reduction in new-onset atrial fibrillation. A meta-analysis of three RCTs and 16 observational studies comprising 31,725 patients found that the incidence of postoperative atrial fibrillation after cardiac surgery was significantly reduced by statins (odds ratio [OR] 0.67; 95% CI 0.51–0.88).[36] Interestingly, a meta-analysis examining data on patients undergoing either isolated CABG or isolated aortic valve replacement (AVR) demonstrated a reduction in atrial fibrillation in the CABG group but not in the AVR group.[37] Current ACCF/AHA recommendations call for perioperative statins in all patients with CABG, regardless of baseline lipid profile.[20] A large prospective RCT of 1922 patients undergoing elective cardiac surgery failed to demonstrate reduction of POAF in patients receiving statins.[38] On the basis of this and other studies, current ESC guidelines do not recommend statin administration for POAF prophylaxis in cardiac surgical patients.[25]

Perioperative Anesthetic Management

One of the more sweeping initiatives to decrease perioperative stressors and improve outcomes has been implementation of Enhanced Recovery After Surgery (ERAS©) type protocols. The multifaceted "bundled" approach to support less invasive procedures, improved pain management, earlier liberation from mechanical ventilation, goal-directed volume resuscitation, and earlier mobilization has become an international focus of many surgical subspecialties. There is some evidence that such protocols have a positive effect on decreasing the incidence of POAF, in addition to improved patient satisfaction, earlier hospital discharge, and lower health-care costs.[39] The rationale for such a decrease in POAF is most likely multifactorial, including use of anti-inflammatory agents, goal-directed volume resuscitation, aggressive pain management, and reduction in catecholamines to restore vascular tone and hemodynamics.

While it is unlikely that any one single component of ERAS protocols will have a positive effect on decreasing POAF, institution of concerted bundled, programmatic changes in perioperative care may prove to decrease the risk of developing POAF.

Aggressive Pain Management

Epidural analgesia modulates the sympathetic nervous system and the inflammatory response to surgery. There is some evidence that use of epidural analgesia in patients undergoing noncardiac surgery under general anesthesia reduces the risk of POAF. A meta-analysis of 9 studies and 2016 subjects demonstrated a statistically significant reduction in the incidence of atrial fibrillation in patients receiving epidural analgesia for noncardiac surgery when compared with controls (20.1 vs. 25.4%).[40]

Colchicine

Colchicine is a powerful anti-inflammatory drug that inhibits neutrophil activity. The initial COPPS (COlchicine for Prevention of Postcardiotomy Syndrome) trial demonstrated a reduction in POAF in patients receiving the drug 3 days after undergoing cardiac surgery.[41] But the COPPS-2 trial failed to show a statistically significant reduction in early POAF (postoperative days 1–2) and incurred an increased risk of gastrointestinal side effects of the drug.[42] Although current AHA/ACC/Heart Rhythm Society (HRS) guidelines ascribe a class IIb recommendation for the use of colchicine for atrial fibrillation prophylaxis in cardiac surgical patients,[27] the COPPS-2 data suggest that colchicine should not be used for this indication.

Evacuation of Pericardial Blood

In addition to systemic inflammation in response to surgery, a growing body of evidence suggests that retained blood in the pericardium may induce a local, surface inflammatory response and predispose to the development of POAF.[43] Strategies to reduce retained blood, including aggressive postoperative drainage of the space and posterior pericardiectomy may prove effective in reducing POAF.[44]

WHAT IS APPROPRIATE THERAPY FOR POAF IN A HEMODYNAMICALLY STABLE PATIENT: RATE CONTROL OR RHYTHM CONTROL?

The initial approach to the development of POAF in the patient who is not hemodynamically compromised is to initially control the ventricular response rate. After this has been accomplished, electrical or pharmacologic cardioversion may be attempted. Early restoration of sinus rhythm theoretically avoids the need for anticoagulation, improves quality of life, decreases the risk for thromboembolic events, improves hemodynamics, and decreases the incidence of future episodes of atrial fibrillation. However, regardless of how intuitively attractive the concept, the data supporting the advantages of chronic rhythm control over rate control in the outpatient population have failed to demonstrate clear superiority of rhythm control. No studies have definitively shown that rhythm control is superior to rate control or vice versa for the primary outcome measure of mortality in outpatients. These conclusions are based on several large RCTs.

The Atrial Fibrillation Follow-up Investigation of Rhythm Management (AFFIRM) trial was the largest of these studies, enrolling 4060 patients. The mean follow-up in the study was 3.5 years, and no significant mortality difference between the rate control and rhythm control groups was found.[45] However, there was a slightly higher incidence of noncardiovascular death, stroke (7.3 vs. 5.7%), and hospitalization (80 vs. 73%) in the rhythm control group. The author's initial conclusion was that the strategy of rhythm control offered no overall mortality benefit and may have contributed to an increased incidence of noncardiac death. However, reevaluation of the data suggests that remaining in sinus rhythm may confer several advantages, including improved hemodynamics, reduction of thromboembolic events, lower mortality, improved quality of life, and improved exercise tolerance.[46,47] A good discussion supporting the early restoration and maintenance of sinus rhythm was presented by van Gelder and Hemels.[48] A post hoc analysis of the AFFIRM trial, Congestive Heart Failure Survival Trial of Antiarrhythmic Therapy (CHF-STA) trial, and Danish Investigators of Arrhythmia and Mortality on Dofetilide (DIAMOND) trial concluded that restoration of sinus rhythm is a marker for improved survival.[45,49,50] The largest multicenter randomized study of 4060 patients found sinus rhythm to be a predictor of survival, with a 47% reduction in mortality.

The premise that maintenance of sinus rhythm improves outcome remains controversial and awaits further clarification. In addition, a multimodal approach with wider application of angiotensin receptor blockers (ARBs), angiotensin-converting enzyme (ACE) inhibitors, and statins may potentially affect success in restoring and maintaining sinus rhythm.

Postoperative atrial fibrillation should be considered an entity distinct from chronic atrial fibrillation. More than 90% of patients who develop post-CABG atrial fibrillation revert to sinus rhythm within 6–8 weeks.[51] Although not demonstrated in the noncardiac surgical patient population, cardioversion to sinus rhythm after the stressors of the postoperative period have abated seems to be a reasonable but as yet unproven strategy.

Rate Control

Beta blockers, with their ability to modulate the hyperadrenergic tone encountered in the postoperative patient, are considered first-line agents for rate control in the ACC/AHA guidelines section on postoperative atrial fibrillation[27] and the ACCP guidelines on the management of postoperative atrial fibrillation after cardiac surgery (Table 55.1).[31]

Rhythm Control

Despite the self-limited nature of most cases of postoperative atrial fibrillation, the current ACC/AHA guidelines ascribe a class IIa recommendation for pharmacologic or electrical cardioversion in this patient population. The ACCP guidelines recommend the use of amiodarone, particularly for patients with depressed left ventricular function. Antiarrhythmic use for postoperative atrial fibrillation should be continued for 4–6 weeks after surgery.[52]

A randomized trial of rate vs. rhythm control in POAF failed to find a difference in hospital admissions during a 60-day follow-up.[53] Given the absence of superiority of either approach, the ESC currently recommends rhythm control for the improvement of symptoms in the patient with POAF. In the asymptomatic patient, rate control or deferred cardioversion after anticoagulation are recommended.[25]

TABLE 55.1	Common Medication Dosage for Rate Control of Atrial Fibrillation.	
	Intravenous Administration	**Usual Oral Maintenance Dose**
Beta Blockers		
Metoprolol tartrate	2.5–5.0 mg IV bolus over 2 min; up to 3 doses	25–100 mg BID
Metoprolol XL (succinate)	N/A	50–400 mg QD
Atenolol	N/A	25–100 mg QD
Esmolol	500 µg/kg IV bolus over 1 min, then 50–300 µg/kg/min IV	N/A
Propranolol	1 mg IV over 1 min, up to 3 doses at 2-min intervals	10–40 mg TID or QID
Nadolol	N/A	10–240 mg QD
Carvedilol	N/A	3.125–25 mg BID
Bisoprolol	N/A	2.5–10 mg QD
Nondihydropyridine Calcium Channel Antagonists		
Verapamil	0.075–0.15 mg/kg IV bolus over 2 min; may give an additional 10.0 mg after 30 min if no response, then 0.005 mg/kg/min infusion	180–480 mg QD (ER)
Diltiazem	0.25 mg/kg IV bolus over 2 min, then 5–15 mg/h	120–360 mg QD (ER)
Digitalis Glycosides		
Digoxin	0.25 mg IV with repeat dosing to a maximum of 1.5 mg over 24 h	0.125–0.25 mg QD
Others		
Amiodarone[a]	300 mg IV over 1 h, then 10–50 mg/h over 24 h	100–200 mg QD

[a]Multiple dosing schemes exist for the use of amiodarone.
BID, twice daily; *ER*, extended release; *IV*, intravenous; *N/A*, not applicable; *QD*, once daily; *QID*, 4 times a day; *TID*, 3 times a day.
From January CT, Wann LS, Alpert JS, et al. 2014 AHA/ACC/HRS guideline for the management of patients with atrial fibrillation: a report of the American College of Cardiology/American Heart Task Force on practice guidelines and the Heart Rhythm Society. *J Am Coll Cardiol.* 2014;64(21):e1-e76.

ANTICOAGULATION STRATEGY BEFORE RESTORATION OF SINUS RHYTHM: ATRIAL FIBRILLATION FOR LESS THAN 48 HOURS

It is common practice for patients with new onset of atrial fibrillation of less than 48 hours' duration to proceed to cardioversion without the need for transesophageal echocardiography or anticoagulation. There is evidence in the literature that new-onset atrial fibrillation (duration <48 hours) may be associated with an incidence of left atrial thrombus formation of up to 4%.[54] Prospective data after cardioversion of 3143 patients found a 0.7% incidence of thromboembolic complications during a 30-day follow-up period but a significantly higher incidence in patients with increased stroke risk factors.[55] Since 2010, the ESC has recommended consideration of anticoagulation with unfractionated or low-molecular-weight heparin for all patients with new-onset atrial fibrillation undergoing cardioversion.[25] In addition, the

ESC recommends lifelong anticoagulation after cardioversion of new-onset atrial fibrillation for patients at high risk for stroke as assessed by the CHADS2 (Congestive heart failure, Hypertension, Age ≥75 years, Diabetes mellitus, Prior Stroke or TIA or Thromboembolism [doubled]) and CHA2DS2-VASc (Congestive heart failure, Hypertension, Age ≥75 years, Diabetes mellitus, Prior Stroke or TIA or Thromboembolism [doubled], Vascular disease, Age 65 to 74 years, Sex thromboembolic) Risk Stratification Scoring Systems (Table 55.2).[25]

Although these recommendations were based on studies of nonsurgical patients, the guidelines have been applied to the postsurgical patients, as the inflammatory response to surgery induces a hypercoagulable state that may increase the risk for an early thromboembolic event. Therefore, it may be prudent to selectively anticoagulate before cardioversion of high-risk patients with atrial fibrillation of less than 48 hours' duration. However, it is clear that in the postoperative setting, the risk of thrombotic events in the absence of anticoagulation

TABLE 55.2   Comparison of the CHADS2 And CHA2DS2-VASc Risk Stratification Scores for Subjects with Nonvalvular Atrial Fibrillation.

DEFINITION AND SCORES FOR CHADS2 AND CHA2DS2-VASC		STROKE RISK STRATIFICATION WITH THE CHADS2 AND CHA2DS2-VASC SCORES	
Score		Adjusted Stroke Rate (%/year)	
CHADS2 Acronym		**CHADS2 Acronym[a]**	
Congestive HF	1	0	1.9
Hypertension	1	1	2.8
Age ≥75 years	1	2	4.0
Diabetes mellitus	1	3	5.9
Stroke/TIA/TE	2	4	8.5
Maximum score	6	5	12.5
		6	18.2
CHA2 DS2-VASc Acronym		**CHA2 DS2-VASc Acronym[b]**	
Congestive HF	1	0	0
Hypertension	1	1	1.3
Age ≥75 years	2	2	2.2
Diabetes mellitus	1	3	3.2
Stroke/TIA/TE	2	4	4.0
Vascular disease (prior MI, PAD, or aortic plaque)	1	5	6.7
Age 65–74 years	1	6	9.8
Sex category (i.e., female sex)	1	7	9.6
Maximum score	9	8	6.7
		9	15.20

[a] These adjusted-stroke rates are based on data for hospitalized patients with atrial fibrillation and were published by Shepard and colleagues in 2001. Because stroke rates are decreasing, actual stroke rates in contemporary, nonhospitalized cohorts might vary from these estimates.
[b] Adjusted-stroke rate scores are based on data from Lip and colleagues. Actual rates of stroke in contemporary cohorts might vary from these estimates.
CHADS2, Congestive heart failure, Hypertension, Age ≥ 75 years, Diabetes mellitus, Prior Stroke or TIA or Thromboembolism (doubled); CHA2DS2-VASc, Congestive heart failure, Hypertension, Age ≥ 75 years, Diabetes mellitus, Prior Stroke or TIA or Thromboembolism (doubled), Vascular disease, Age 65–74 years, Sex thromboembolic; HF, heart failure; MI, myocardial infarction; PAD, peripheral artery disease; TE, thromboembolism; TIA, transient ischemic attack.
From January CT, Wann LS, Alpert JS, et al. 2014 AHA/ACC/HRS guideline for the management of patients with atrial fibrillation: a report of the American College of Cardiology/American Heart Task Force on practice guidelines and the Heart Rhythm Society. J Am Coll Cardiol. 2014;64(21):e1-e76.

must be weighed against the risk of bleeding from fresh surgical sites after anticoagulation administration.

ANTICOAGULATION STRATEGY BEFORE RESTORATION OF SINUS RHYTHM: ATRIAL FIBRILLATION FOR MORE THAN 48 HOURS

At times, patients enter the ICU with atrial fibrillation for more than 48 hours. In these individuals, anticoagulation before cardioversion is the accepted standard. ACC/AHA, ESC, and ACCP guidelines recommend 3 weeks of anticoagulation before cardioversion of patients with chronic atrial fibrillation.[14,25,27] However, in cases of hemodynamic instability, cardioversion should not be delayed for initiation of anticoagulation. Timing for initiation of anticoagulation therapy (heparin as a bridge to an oral agent) in the postoperative patient must account for the potential for bleeding complications.

Selection of an antithrombotic regimen should balance the risks of harm and potential benefit of avoiding ischemic stroke or other embolic complications. Platelet inhibitors, alone or in combination (aspirin and clopidogrel), are less effective than warfarin in preventing stroke.[14] Administration of a direct thrombin inhibitor (dabigatran) or factor Xa inhibitors (rivaroxaban, apixaban) are gaining wider use for in-hospital and outpatient settings. Although these agents are more convenient, they are more costly and difficult to reverse in cases of bleeding or if the need to perform emergency invasive procedures arises. Data from a European observational study found that a greater international normalized ratio (INR) produced better outcomes. The incidence of thromboembolic events was 0.8% (4 of 530 patients) when the INR was 2.0–2.4 compared with no events when the INR was ≥2.5.[56] In addition, reversal of warfarin anticoagulation has the benefit of being dependably achieved by the administration of vitamin K, plasma, or prothrombin complex concentrate. Timing and choice of anticoagulation strategy are made on an individual case basis with input from the primary stakeholders.

WHAT IS APPROPRIATE MANAGEMENT OF POAF IN A HEMODYNAMICALLY UNSTABLE PATIENT?

In the hemodynamically unstable patient with POAF, immediate electrical cardioversion is the therapy of choice. Synchronized, direct current (DC) using a biphasic defibrillator is most effective for converting unstable POAF to a sinus rhythm.[25] It goes without saying that considerations discussed above for the stable POAF patient do not apply for the patient who is hemodynamically unstable.

SHOULD ANTICOAGULATION BE INSTITUTED OR CONTINUED AFTER ELECTRICAL CARDIOVERSION TO SINUS RHYTHM?

The period after conversion to sinus rhythm is associated with an increased risk of thrombus formation and subsequent embolization. The recurrence of asymptomatic atrial fibrillation ranges from 40 to 60%,[46,57] and other predisposing factors such as atheromatous disease and poor ventricular function also may increase the risk for thromboembolism.[58] Perhaps the most significant factor is the transient decrease in atrial mechanical function that occurs after cardioversion to sinus rhythm.[59] Mechanical dysfunction after cardioversion appears to last 24 hours in patients having atrial fibrillation of less than 2 weeks' duration, 1 week in patients with atrial fibrillation of 2–6 weeks' duration, and 1 month for more prolonged precardioversion atrial fibrillation.[59] To date, there is no pharmacologic intervention to hasten the return of atrial mechanical activity.

Support for continued anticoagulation can be gleaned from the AFFIRM and RACE (RAte Control vs. Electrical cardioversion) trials.[48,60] Anticoagulation during these studies was often discontinued after restoration of sinus rhythm. Ischemic events occurred at equal frequency in both arms of the trials (rate control and rhythm control). Review of the data showed that such complications occurred most often after anticoagulation was terminated early (rhythm group) or when the INR was subtherapeutic (rate control group). Although the patients in these studies had chronic (not acute postoperative) atrial fibrillation, restoration of sinus rhythm in subtherapeutic or nonanticoagulated patients was associated with the increased incidence of thromboembolic events. Furthermore, the literature that provides the basis for these recommendations in general does not distinguish between patients who required electric cardioversion and those who spontaneously or pharmacologically converted to sinus rhythm. It seems prudent that guidelines for electrical and pharmacologic cardioversion be followed in a similar manner.

Current guidelines of the ACCP recommend 4 weeks of anticoagulation for patients who undergo cardioversion after an episode of atrial fibrillation lasting >48 hours. For episodes <48 hours' duration, the ACCP guidelines do not recommend post-cardioversion anticoagulation.[61] Similarly, the ESC guidelines recommend that for atrial fibrillation of >48 hours' duration, postcardioversion oral anticoagulation should be maintained for at least 4 weeks.[25] In addition, the ESC guidelines assign a class IIa recommendation for post-POAF oral anticoagulation in cardiac surgical patients after consideration of bleeding risk, noting that these patients are at double the risk for stroke and mortality compared with postoperative patients who remain in sinus rhythm.[25] The ACC/AHA guidelines add that the decision to initiate postcardioversion anticoagulation for patients with atrial fibrillation of <48 hours' duration should be based on the patients' risk for development of thromboembolism.[27] Although neither the ACCP nor ACC/AHA guidelines specifically address postcardioversion anticoagulation for POAF, it seems prudent to follow these recommendations, provided that the risk for bleeding does not outweigh the risk for a thromboembolic event.

AUTHORS' RECOMMENDATIONS

- The pathogenesis of atrial fibrillation in the postoperative period is complex and multifactorial. The inflammatory response and increased levels of circulating catecholamines induced by surgery trigger supraventricular arrhythmias by altering atrial refractoriness and conductivity, predisposing to automaticity and re-entrant rhythms.
- The type of surgery performed has a significant impact on the incidence of perioperative atrial fibrillation. Direct surgical manipulation or compression of the atria or pulmonary veins is associated with postoperative atrial fibrillation.
- Prophylactic strategies against atrial fibrillation include maintenance of electrolytes, atrial pacing, and administration of antiarrhythmic agents (beta blockers and amiodarone). Other strategies that include a role for anti-inflammatory agents and anesthetic choices have been proposed and are under active investigation.
- β-Adrenergic antagonists and alternative agents (such as amiodarone) are recommended for prophylaxis against atrial fibrillation by the ACC/AHA guidelines. Patients taking beta blockers on an outpatient basis should continue receiving them during the perioperative period. However, the prophylactic use of such agents in patients with low cardiac risk is controversial.
- Beta blockers are recommended for all patients undergoing CABG surgery and should be considered for all patients undergoing cardiac surgery.
- Postoperative atrial fibrillation associated with hemodynamic instability should be treated with biphasic cardioversion at 200 J.
- Postoperative atrial fibrillation is often an acute event with a high conversion rate to sinus rhythm. Rate and rhythm control are both acceptable approaches to managing chronic atrial fibrillation. The premise that maintenance of sinus rhythm improves outcome remains controversial.
- Patients with new onset of atrial fibrillation of >48 hours' duration are at increased risk for thromboembolic events and should receive anticoagulant therapy. Anticoagulation should be temporarily continued after restoration of sinus rhythm because of a transient decrease in atrial mechanical function that increases the risk for thromboembolic events. Potential benefits of anticoagulation must be weighed against the risks for postoperative bleeding.
- After cardioversion, anticoagulation may be considered for patients at high risk for stroke. The decision to initiate anticoagulation in this setting should balance the risk of a thromboembolic event with that of bleeding complications in postsurgical patients.

REFERENCES

1. Seguin P, Signouret T, Laviolle B, Branger B, Mallédant Y. Incidence and risk factors of atrial fibrillation in a surgical intensive care unit. *Crit Care Med.* 2004;32(3):722-726.
2. Creswell LL, Schuessler RB, Rosenbloom M, Cox JL. Hazards of postoperative atrial arrhythmias. *Ann Thorac Surg.* 1993; 56(3):539-549.
3. Harpole DH, Liptay MJ, DeCamp Jr MM, Mentzer SJ, Swanson SJ, Sugarbaker DJ. Prospective analysis of pneumonectomy: risk factors for major morbidity and cardiac dysrhythmias. *Ann Thorac Surg.* 1996;61(3):977-982.
4. Roselli EE, Murthy SC, Rice TW, et al. Atrial fibrillation complicating lung cancer resection. *J Thorac Cardiovasc Surg.* 2005; 130(2):438-444.
5. Brathwaite D, Weissman C. The new onset of atrial arrhythmias following major noncardiothoracic surgery is associated with increased mortality. *Chest.* 1998;114(2):462-468.
6. Mariscalco G, Klersy C, Zanobini M, et al. Atrial fibrillation after isolated coronary surgery affects late survival. *Circulation.* 2008;118(16):1612-1618.
7. Villareal RP, Hariharan R, Liu BC, et al. Postoperative atrial fibrillation and mortality after coronary artery bypass surgery. *J Am Coll Cardiol.* 2004;43(5):742-748.
8. Mathew JP, Fontes ML, Tudor IC, et al. A multicenter risk index for atrial fibrillation after cardiac surgery. *JAMA.* 2004;291(14): 1720-1729.
9. Aranki SF, Shaw DP, Adams DH, et al. Predictors of atrial fibrillation after coronary artery surgery. Current trends and impact on hospital resources. *Circulation.* 1996;94(3):390-397.
10. Zacharias A, Schwann TA, Riordan CJ, Durham SJ, Shah AS, Habib RH. Obesity and risk of new-onset atrial fibrillation after cardiac surgery. *Circulation.* 2005;112(21):3247-3255.
11. Pathak RK, Middeldorp ME, Meredith M, et al. Long-term effect of goal-directed weight management in an atrial fibrillation cohort: a long-term follow-up study. *J Am Coll Cardiol.* 2015;65(20):2159-2169.
12. Pathak RK, Elliot A, Middeldorp ME, et al. Impact of cardiorespiratory fitness on arrhythmia recurrence in obese individuals with atrial fibrillation: the CARDIO-FIT study. *J Am Coll Cardiol.* 2015;66(9):985-986.
13. Fuster V, Rydén LE, Cannom DS, et al. ACC/AHA/ESC 2006 guidelines for the management of patients with atrial fibrillation: a report of the American College of Cardiology/American Heart Association Task Force on Practice Guidelines and the European Society of Cardiology Committee for Practice Guidelines (Writing Committee to Revise the 2001 Guidelines for the Management of Patients With Atrial Fibrillation). *Circulation.* 2006;114(7):e257-e354.
14. Hogue Jr CW, Creswell LL, Gutterman DD, Fleisher LA. Epidemiology, mechanisms, and risks: American College of Chest Physicians guidelines for the prevention and management of postoperative atrial fibrillation after cardiac surgery. *Chest.* 2005;128(Suppl. 2):9S-16S.
15. Siu CW, Tung HM, Chu KW, et al. Prevalence and predictors of new-onset atrial fibrillation after elective surgery for colorectal cancer. *Pacing Clin Electrophysiol.* 2005;28(Suppl. 1): S120-S123.
16. Friscia ME, Zhu J, Kolff JW, et al. Cytokine response is lower after lung volume reduction through bilateral thoracoscopy versus sternotomy. *Ann Thorac Surg.* 2007;83(1):252-256.
17. Crystal E, Connolly SJ, Sleik K, Ginger TJ, Yusuf S. Interventions on prevention of postoperative atrial fibrillation in patients undergoing heart surgery: a meta-analysis. *Circulation.* 2002;106(1):75-80.
18. Crystal E, Garfinkle MS, Connolly SS, Ginger TT, Sleik K, Yusuf SS. Interventions for preventing post-operative atrial fibrillation in patients undergoing heart surgery. *Cochrane Database Syst Rev.* 2004;4:CD003611.
19. Arsenault KA, Yusuf AM, Crystal E, et al. Interventions for preventing post-operative atrial fibrillation in patients undergoing heart surgery. *Cochrane Database Syst Rev.* 2013;1:CD003611.

20. Hillis LD, Smith PK, Anderson JL, et al. 2011 ACCF/AHA Guideline for Coronary Artery Bypass Graft Surgery: executive summary: a report of the American College of Cardiology Foundation/American Heart Association Task Force on Practice Guidelines. *Circulation.* 2011;124(23):2610-2642.

21. Sedrakyan A, Treasure T, Browne J, Krumholz H, Sharpin C, van der Meulen J. Pharmacologic prophylaxis for postoperative atrial tachyarrhythmia in general thoracic surgery: evidence from randomized clinical trials. *J Thorac Cardiovasc Surg.* 2005;129(5):997-1005.

22. POISE Study Group; Devereaux PJ, Yang H, et al. Effects of extended-release metoprolol succinate in patients undergoing non-cardiac surgery (POISE trial): a randomised controlled trial. *Lancet.* 2008;371(9627):1839-1847.

23. Bangalore S, Wetterslev J, Pranesh S, Sawhney S, Gluud C, Messerli FH. Perioperative beta blockers in patients having non-cardiac surgery: a meta-analysis. *Lancet.* 2008;372(9654):1962-1976.

24. Frendl G, Sodickson AC, Chung MK, et al. 2014 AATS guidelines for the prevention and management of perioperative atrial fibrillation and flutter for thoracic surgical procedures. Executive summary. *J Thorac Cardiovasc Surg.* 2014;148(3):772-791.

25. Kirchhof P, Benussi S, Kotecha D, et al. 2016 ESC guidelines for the management of atrial fibrillation developed in collaboration with EACTS. *Eur Heart J.* 2016;37(38):2893-2962.

26. Patel AA, White CM, Gillespie EL, Kluger J, Coleman CI. Safety of amiodarone in the prevention of postoperative atrial fibrillation: a meta-analysis. *Am J Health Syst Pharm.* 2006;63(9):829-837.

27. January CT, Wann LS, Alpert JS, et al. 2014 AHA/ACC/HRS guideline for the management of patients with atrial fibrillation: a report of the American College of Cardiology/American Heart Association Task Force on practice guidelines and the Heart Rhythm Society. *J Am Coll Cardiol.* 2014;64(21):e1-e76.

28. Andrews TC, Reimold SC, Berlin JA, Antman EM. Prevention of supraventricular arrhythmias after coronary artery bypass surgery. A meta-analysis of randomized control trials. *Circulation.* 1991;84(Suppl. 5):III236-III244.

29. Ciszewski P, Tyczka J, Nadolski J, Roszak M, Dyszkiewicz W. Comparative efficacy and usefulness of acebutolol and diltiazem for the prevention of atrial fibrillation during perioperative time in patients undergoing pulmonary resection. *Thorac Cardiovasc Surg.* 2013;61(4):365-372.

30. Shiga T, Wajima Z, Inoue T, Ogawa R. Magnesium prophylaxis for arrhythmias after cardiac surgery: a meta-analysis of randomized controlled trials. *Am J Med.* 2004;117(5):325-333.

31. Martinez EA, Epstein AE, Bass EB; American College of Chest Physicians. Pharmacologic control of ventricular rate: American College of Chest Physicians guidelines for the prevention and management of postoperative atrial fibrillation after cardiac surgery. *Chest.* 2005;128(Suppl. 2):56S-60S.

32. Archbold RA, Schilling RJ. Atrial pacing for the prevention of atrial fibrillation after coronary artery bypass graft surgery: a review of the literature. *Heart.* 2004;90(2):129-133.

33. Ho KM, Tan JA. Benefits and risks of corticosteroid prophylaxis in adult cardiac surgery: a dose-response meta-analysis. *Circulation.* 2009;119(14):1853-1866.

34. Dieleman JM, Nierich AP, Rosseel PM, et al. Intraoperative high-dose dexamethasone for cardiac surgery: a randomized controlled trial. *JAMA.* 2012;308(17):1761-1767.

35. Whitlock RP, Devereaux PJ, Teoh KH, et al. Methylprednisolone in patients undergoing cardiopulmonary bypass (SIRS): a randomised, double-blind, placebo-controlled trial. *Lancet.* 2015;386(10000):1243-1253.

36. Liakopoulos OJ, Choi YH, Haldenwang PL, et al. Impact of preoperative statin therapy on adverse postoperative outcomes in patients undergoing cardiac surgery: a meta-analysis of over 30,000 patients. *Eur Heart J.* 2008;29(12):1548-1559.

37. Kuhn EW, Liakopoulos OJ, Stange S, et al. Meta-analysis of patients taking statins before revascularization and aortic valve surgery. *Ann Thorac Surg.* 2013;96(4):1508-1516.

38. Zheng Z, Jayaram R, Jiang L, et al. Perioperative rosuvastatin in cardiac surgery. *N Engl J Med.* 2016;374(18):1744-1753.

39. Khandhar SJ, Schatz CL, Collins DT, et al. Thoracic enhanced recovery with ambulation after surgery: a 6 year experience. *Eur J Cardiothorac Surg.* 2018;53(6):1192-1198.

40. Pöpping DM, Elia N, Van Aken HK, et al. Impact of epidural analgesia on mortality and morbidity after surgery: systematic review and meta-analysis of randomized controlled trials. *Ann Surg.* 2014;259(6):1056-1067.

41. Imazio M, Brucato A, Ferrazzi P, et al. Colchicine reduces postoperative atrial fibrillation: results of the Colchicine for the Prevention of the Postpericardiotomy Syndrome (COPPS) atrial fibrillation substudy. *Circulation.* 2011;124(21):2290-2295.

42. Imazio M, Brucato A, Ferrazzi P, et al. Colchicine for prevention of postpericardiotomy syndrome and postoperative atrial fibrillation: the COPPS-2 randomized clinical trial. *JAMA.* 2014;312(10):1016-1023.

43. St-Onge S, Perrault LP, Demers P, et al. Pericardial blood as a trigger of postoperative atrial fibrillation after cardiac surgery. *Ann Thorac Surg.* 2018;105(1):321-328.

44. Kaleda VI, McCormack DJ, Shipolini AR. Does posterior pericardiectomy reduce the incidence of atrial fibrillation after coronary artery bypass grafting surgery? *Interact Cardiovasc Thorac Surg.* 2012;14(4):384-389.

45. Corley SD, Epstein AE, DiMarco JP, et al. Relationships between sinus rhythm, treatment, and survival in the Atrial Fibrillation Follow-Up Investigation of Rhythm Management (AFFIRM) Study. *Circulation.* 2004;109(12):1509-1513.

46. Singh SN, Tang XC, Singh BN, et al. Quality of life and exercise performance in patients in sinus rhythm versus persistent atrial fibrillation: a Veterans Affairs Cooperative Studies Program Substudy. *J Am Coll Cardiol.* 2006;48(4):721-730.

47. Chung MK, Shemanski L, Sherman DG, et al. Functional status in rate- versus rhythm-control strategies for atrial fibrillation: results of the Atrial Fibrillation Follow-Up Investigation of Rhythm Management (AFFIRM) Functional Status Substudy. *J Am Coll Cardiol.* 2005;46(10):1891-1899.

48. Van Gelder IC, Hemels ME. The progressive nature of atrial fibrillation: a rationale for early restoration and maintenance of sinus rhythm. *Europace.* 2006;8(11):943-949.

49. Deedwania PC, Singh BN, Ellenbogen K, Fisher S, Fletcher R, Singh SN. Spontaneous conversion and maintenance of sinus rhythm by amiodarone in patients with heart failure and atrial fibrillation: observations from the Veterans Affairs Congestive Heart Failure Survival Trial of Antiarrhythmic Therapy (CHF-STAT). The Department of Veterans Affairs CHF-STAT Investigators. *Circulation.* 1998;98(23):2574-2579.

50. Pedersen OD, Bagger H, Keller N, Marchant B, Køber L, Torp-Pedersen C. Efficacy of dofetilide in the treatment of atrial fibrillation-flutter in patients with reduced left ventricular

function: a Danish investigations of arrhythmia and mortality on dofetilide (diamond) substudy. *Circulation.* 2001;104(3):292-296.

51. Kowey PR, Stebbins D, Igidbashian L, et al. Clinical outcome of patients who develop PAF after CABG surgery. *Pacing Clin Electrophysiol.* 2001;24(2):191-193.

52. Martinez EA, Bass EB, Zimetbaum P; American College of Chest Physicians. Pharmacologic control of rhythm: American College of Chest Physicians guidelines for the prevention and management of postoperative atrial fibrillation after cardiac surgery. *Chest.* 2005;128(Suppl. 2):48S-55S.

53. Gillinov AM, Bagiella E, Moskowitz AJ, et al. Rate control versus rhythm control for atrial fibrillation after cardiac surgery. *N Engl J Med.* 2016;374(20):1911-1921.

54. Kleemann T, Becker T, Strauss M, Schneider S, Seidl K. Prevalence of left atrial thrombus and dense spontaneous echo contrast in patients with short-term atrial fibrillation <48 hours undergoing cardioversion: value of transesophageal echocardiography to guide cardioversion. *J Am Soc Echocardiogr.* 2009;22(12):1403-1408.

55. Airaksinen KE, Grönberg T, Nuotio I, et al. Thromboembolic complications after cardioversion of acute atrial fibrillation: the FinCV (Finnish CardioVersion) study. *J Am Coll Cardiol.* 2013;62(13):1187-1192.

56. Gallagher MM, Hennessy BJ, Edvardsson N, et al. Embolic complications of direct current cardioversion of atrial arrhythmias: association with low intensity of anticoagulation at the time of cardioversion. *J Am Coll Cardiol.* 2002;40(5):926-933.

57. Antonielli E, Pizzuti A, Pálinkás A, et al. Clinical value of left atrial appendage flow for prediction of long-term sinus rhythm maintenance in patients with nonvalvular atrial fibrillation. *J Am Coll Cardiol.* 2002;39(9):1443-1449.

58. Echocardiographic predictors of stroke in patients with atrial fibrillation: a prospective study of 1066 patients from 3 clinical trials. *Arch Intern Med.* 1998;158(12):1316-1320.

59. Manning WJ, Silverman DI, Katz SE, et al. Impaired left atrial mechanical function after cardioversion: relation to the duration of atrial fibrillation. *J Am Coll Cardiol.* 1994;23(7):1535-1540.

60. Wyse DG, Waldo AL, DiMarco JP, et al. A comparison of rate control and rhythm control in patients with atrial fibrillation. *N Engl J Med.* 2002;347(23):1825-1833.

61. Singer DE, Albers GW, Dalen JE, et al. Antithrombotic therapy in atrial fibrillation: American College of Chest Physicians Evidence-Based Clinical Practice Guidelines (8th edition). *Chest.* 2008;133(Suppl. 6):546S-592S.

56

How Do I Rapidly and Correctly Identify Acute Kidney Injury?

Gianluca Villa, Zaccaria Ricci, and Claudio Ronco

INTRODUCTION

Acute kidney injury (AKI) is frequently observed among hospitalized patients. The incidence of AKI ranges from 4 to 20%,[1] and reaches 60% among patients in the intensive care unit (ICU).[2] Patients affected by isolated AKI (i.e., a primary renal disease) do not necessarily require admission in the ICU, whereas AKI in the context of critical illness and multiple organ dysfunction is associated with long ICU and in-hospital length of stay, and often with poorer short- and long-term outcomes relative to isolated AKI and to critical illness without AKI.[3] Although there have been recent advances in our understanding of AKI pathophysiology[4] and some improvements in renal replacement therapy (RRT) technology,[5–7] patients with AKI still suffer from significant morbidity and mortality rates (up to 80%).[8]

The best way to improve AKI outcomes in highly susceptible patients is prevention. However, the occurrence of a kidney insult is not a modifiable risk factor in medical scenarios where the "nephrotoxic event" is not avoidable (e.g., high-risk surgery, use of radiographic contrast media, antimicrobial administration, etc., in any critically ill patient). In these cases, the identification of the expected kidney insult may aid in determining when renal adaptive capability (i.e., the patient's renal functional reserve [RFR]) has been exceeded. This approach allows for appropriate biochemical and clinical follow-up planning. These plans are aimed at timely diagnosis of subclinical and clinical AKI[4,9] and at eventual reduction, and perhaps exclusion, of additional renal insults.

A renal insult that is not clinically evident (i.e., reduction of creatinine clearance without serum creatinine increase), and/or that only temporarily affects kidney function, should not be overlooked, as it leaves a silent "scar" on the renal system ("subclinical AKI"). Early identification of subclinical AKI is of fundamental importance in any strategy designed to prevent the progression of the disease and the occurrence of adverse outcomes in these patients.[10]

AKI is often the final step of a process that failed to prevent (1) significant kidney insults in highly susceptible patients, or (2) the progression of subclinical AKI following a relatively minor kidney insult. The most challenging part of the diagnostic process reflects the heterogeneity of AKI etiologies and AKI severity.[1] Moreover, for many years, the absence of consensus on AKI definitions constituted a major limiting factor in the diagnosis and staging of this syndrome.[2]

Ultimately, AKI diagnosis and timely identification are the mainstays of any therapeutic approach, especially in patients with numerous clinical risk factors or unrecognized susceptibility (i.e., with unidentified subclinical AKI). This chapter describes the utility of biomarkers and the importance of a standardized AKI definition in the accurate and timely identification of the potentially compromised renal status of their patients.

THE IDENTIFICATION OF HIGHLY SUSCEPTIBLE PATIENTS

Several diagnostic and therapeutic medical procedures may cause nephrotoxic effects. The pathophysiologic mechanisms leading to AKI have been identified for most, along with the expected prevalence of postprocedural AKI, the effects of renal dysfunction on patients' outcomes and the economic impact of AKI. Unfortunately, these procedures often are not avoidable, particularly when they are necessary to diagnose and/or treat life-threatening conditions (e.g., surgery, contrast media administration, antimicrobials, etc.). In such cases, the risk of AKI should be carefully considered and an adequate patient follow-up plan to prevent any additional renal insult (i.e., by reducing hypotensive periods and/or dosing antibiotic levels) should be identified.

Several papers have suggested the use of the RFR to predict the risk for postcardiac surgery AKI.[11,12] The RFR is an index of the physiologic capacity of the kidneys to increase their filtration rate after an oral protein load (1–1.2 g/kg). When tested in this manner, normal kidneys can increase the glomerular filtration rate (GFR) by about 50%. Importantly, AKI complicates up to 36% of cardiac surgical procedures and doubles total hospital costs.[13,14] Even minor postoperative changes in serum creatinine have been associated with increased mortality rate.[15] In a longitudinal observational study performed on a cohort of elective cardiac surgical patients with normal resting GFR, Husain-Syed et al.[11] found that reduced preoperative RFR was highly predictive of AKI. In this study, patients with a RFR <15 mL/min/1.73 m² had an 11.8-fold increased risk of developing AKI (95% confidence interval [CI] 4.62 to 29.89 times, $P < .001$). The authors' concluded that the preoperative measurement of RFR helped identify patients who benefited most from preventive measures or planned use of biomarkers to detect early kidney damage.[11] In addition, the RFR is a better marker than serum creatinine of "renal recovery" after AKI.[12] RFR was also a better predictor of insult-induced chronic kidney disease than the serum creatinine.[12] Nonetheless, concerns regarding the clinical use of RFR persist. The oral protein-loading test that is the gold standard for RFR measurement is cumbersome to use for routine screening. Work on developing noninvasive, bedside methods to indirectly measure RFR is underway. One proposed approach is ultrasound measurement of the intraparenchymal renal resistive index variation (IRRIV test) during external abdominal pressure.[16]

BIOCHEMICAL DIAGNOSIS

It is only recently that kidney damage without glomerular function loss has been identified; this "subclinical renal dysfunction" is associated with poor renal and overall outcomes. In particular, biomarker-positive, creatinine-negative patients appear to have a particularly high risk of complications, prolonged in-hospital length of stay, and mortality rate than patients without a biomarker rise.[17,18] Thus, the concept of subclinical AKI challenges the traditional view that kidney dysfunction only becomes clinically relevant when a loss of filtration function becomes apparent.[10] As a result, early identification of subclinical renal dysfunction is recommended to potentially prevent complications and adverse outcomes, particularly among patients with a reduced RFR.

To further elaborate, application of a functional stressor (e.g., hypovolemia) sufficient to reduce GFR ("kidney dysfunction") in a healthy kidney should result in subsequent alterations in serum creatinine and urine output. This "clinical AKI" is diagnosed and classified according to the RIFLE (Risk, Injury, Failure, Loss, End-stage), AKIN (AKI Network), or KDIGO (Kidney Disease: Improving Global Outcomes) classifications. However, application of a *metabolic* stressor (such as iodinated contrast media, nephrotoxic drugs, mediators of systemic inflammation during sepsis, etc.) may result in, *kidney damage*. In the early phase, these cellular alterations may be associated with minimally changed serum creatinine levels and only small reductions in urine output. These alterations may not meet the threshold for diagnosis of AKI; this situation is termed "subclinical AKI." If the stressor insult is maintained for a long period, kidney damage can increase, which may adversely affect nephron function. This condition now becomes clinically evident, and may ultimately be associated with a reduction of GFR.[19] While renal biomarkers have been touted as tools for early prediction of AKI, in the setting of subclinical AKI they may identify the so-called *acute kidney syndrome*, a wide-spectrum diseases encompassing both subclinical *kidney damage* and clinical *kidney dysfunction*.[20] Subclinical AKI biomarkers associated with *kidney damage*[21] have different anatomic origins, kinetics, physiologic functions, and peak times after the onset of renal injury.[18] Indeed, some may also provide information about the underlying etiology and pathophysiologic processes involved in AKI.[18] These biomarker molecules or proteins are primarily produced during an insult to the renal parenchyma and/or are released into the systemic circulation after extrarenal synthesis.[22] The biologic roles of these biomarkers may be enzymatic, adaptive (e.g., inflammatory), and/or structural. Some are low-molecular-weight molecules that are filtered through the glomerular barrier and catabolized in normal tubular epithelium (e.g., cystatin-C [Cys-C]).[23] According to these characteristics, biomarkers for AKI can be stratified as noted in Table 56.1.

Since 2010 a specific interest has risen on IGFBP-7 (insulin-like growth factor-binding protein 7) and TIMP-2 (tissue inhibitor metalloproteinase-2) biomarkers indicative of cell-cycle arrest.[24] Both molecules are involved in G1 cell-cycle arrest during the early phases of cell injury. In experimental models of sepsis[25] or ischemia,[26] renal tubular cells enter a short period of cell-cycle arrest following injury. This process may prevent injured cells from dividing when their DNA may be damaged. Cell-cycle arrest allows time for repair of damage, reducing the possibility of cellular demise and senescence. Markers like TIMP-2 and IGFBP-7 may signal that the renal epithelium has been stressed to a point where function is abolished but may be still able to recover without

TABLE 56.1 Stratification of Biomarkers for Acute Kidney Injury.

Biologic Process	Biomarker
Glomerular filtration	Serum cystatin-C (Cys-C)
Glomerular integrity	Albuminuria, proteinuria
Tubular stress/cell cycle arrest	Insulin-like growth factor-binding protein 7 (IGFBP-7) Tissue inhibitor metalloproteinase-2 (TIMP-2)
Tubular damage	Neutrophil gelatinase-associated lipocalin (NGAL) Kidney injury molecule 1 (KIM-1) N-acetyl-β-D-glucosaminidase (NAG) Liver fatty acid-binding protein (L-FABP)
Intrarenal inflammation	Interleukin-18 (IL-18)

Data from Ostermann M, Joannidis M. Acute kidney injury 2016: diagnosis and diagnostic workup. *Crit Care.* 2016;20(1):1-13.

permanent injury once stressors are removed.[24] In a prospective cohort of 728 critically ill patients (the SAPPHIRE study) Kashani et al.[24] compared the predictive validity of the combination of these proteins to that observed for previously used biomarkers. The area under the receiver operator curve (AUROC) for development of AKI was 0.80 in the validation phase, a value significantly higher than any previous examined biomarkers ($P < .002$). The performance of these cell-cycle arrest biomarkers for AKI was independent of the presence of coexisting severe systemic disorders (e.g., sepsis) or comorbidities (e.g., chronic kidney disease). An observational study on patients undergoing cardiac surgery, Meersch et al.[27] demonstrated a significant correlation with renal recovery (AUROC = 0.79) when compared with existing kidney damage biomarkers. In a single-center trial, Meersch et al.[28] examined the effect of euvolemia/hemodynamic optimization, avoidance of nephrotoxic drugs, and prevention of hyperglycemia in cardiac surgical patients at high risk for renal damage (defined as urinary [TIMP-2]·[IGFBP-7] > 0.3). Relative to standard care, these treatments reduced the incidence and severity of postoperative AKI in high-risk patients.[28,29]

Several studies have examined the role of other biomarkers in detection/differential diagnosis, staging, and follow-up of patients with AKI. As with TIMP-2 and IGFBP-7, most of these studies were performed in patients undergoing cardiac surgery because the onset of the insult is known. In the TRIBE study, high levels of urinary interleukin-18 (IL-18) and urinary and plasma N-acetyl-β-D-glucosaminidase (NGAL) measured just 6 hours after ICU admission in more than 1200 patients, primarily undergoing elective on-pump coronary revascularization identified AKI at least 24 hours before its clinical occurrence (AUROC 0.74, 0.67, and 0.7 respectively).[30,31] Biomarkers predicted the development of clinical AKI as well as the need for RRT in critically ill patients at ICU admission or in the emergency department. Based on these studies, the 10th Acute Dialysis Quality Initiative (ADQI) Consensus Conference[23] concluded that patients at high risk for AKI on ICU admission (according to comorbidities and presence of renal stressors) should be considered for AKI biomarker testing. Biomarkers have also identified additional prognostic factors, such as the severity and duration of AKI, the need for RRT, the delayed or absent recovery of kidney function and mortality.[31]

The combined use of clinical classification and AKI biomarkers may allow for a more accurate etiologic diagnosis.[19] For example, a functional reduction (e.g., decreased urine output) without evidence of kidney damage (biomarkers negative) may suggest a volume-responsive and reversible alteration of kidney function.[32] Isolated kidney dysfunction without evidence of kidney damage may also characterize the early phase of "postrenal" obstructive disease, and may indicate that an underlining condition is reversible.[19] As described, the presence of renal biomarkers in the absence of altered function implies subclinical AKI. Finally, biomarker-positive, creatinine-positive AKI may indicate very intense, potentially irreversible functional and structural damage. In these circumstances, markers of kidney damage and kidney dysfunction could be effectively combined to identify the mechanism of renal dysfunction and the sequence of events during AKI.[19]

Based on the current state of knowledge, AKI staging by using kidney damage biomarkers alone cannot be justified. The ADQI Consensus Conference and KDIGO recommendations, continue to support serum creatinine and urinary output measurement in the diagnosis of AKI.[23] It is possible that the next classification will use AKI biomarkers to enhance staging of renal dysfunction. However, we lack verified cut-off values for these biomarkers. Thus, combined criteria for AKI staging should be further tested and validated.[19]

Data suggest that AKI biomarkers have a role in predicting the need for RRT requirement and may inform the decision to initiate a renal support therapy.[33] Although the integration of AKI biomarkers into clinical decision algorithms might improve our ability to predict the need for RRT, their use in creating and testing biomarkers-based strategies for RRT initiation remains challenging.[34] Additionally, most analyses have been based on single specimen collection, and comparing studies is limited by differences in the timing of collection of blood and urine samples (e.g., ICU admission, nephrology consultation, etc.). Because different biomarkers may have different kinetics following AKI, the timing of specimen collection may significantly affect their predictive value. Moreover, studies have not examined the effect of the time elapsed between biomarkers measurement and RRT initiation. Finally, biomarkers lack accepted values after which RRT should be considered: thus, no recommendations or suggestions can be made regarding use of biomarkers to help the clinician make an early and appropriate decision to initiate RRT.[34]

To avoid misinterpretations of results and improve management of patients with AKI, variables that enhance biomarker sensitivity and specificity (such as chronic kidney disease,[35] albuminuria,[36] or the simultaneous presence of systemic illness[37]) should be considered.

CLINICAL DIAGNOSIS

The definition, diagnosis, and staging of AKI are currently obtained through clinical classifications based on indices aimed at estimation of GFR.[38] These classifications have evolved from the RIFLE criteria in 2004[39] and were detailed in the 2007 AKIN classification.[40] Subsequently KDIGO Acute Kidney Injury Work Group[38] proposed changes to the AKI staging paradigm (Table 56.2). This classification includes both the AKIN and RIFLE criteria, and accounts for changes in creatinine within 48 hours or a decline in the GFR over 7 days.

Maximum change of either serum creatinine and urine output are used to define the stage of AKI. A study of more than 30,000 critically ill patients confirmed the importance of both criteria. In this study, the short- and long-term risk of death or RRT were greater in patients who met both

TABLE 56.2   Comparison Among RIFLE, AKIN, and KDIGO Classifications.

SCR CRITERIA			
RIFLE	AKIN	KDIGO	UOP Criteria
Risk Increase in SCr 1.5-fold from baseline or GFR decrease >25%	**Stage 1** Increase of ≥0.3 mg/dL (≥26.5 μmol/L) or increase to ≥150–200% (1.5- to 2-fold) from baseline	**Stage 1** Increase in SCr 1.5- to 1.9-fold from baseline or ≥0.3 mg/dL (≥26.5 μmol/L)	<0.5 mL/kg/h for >6 h
Injury Increase in SCr 2-fold from baseline or GFR decrease >50%	**Stage 2** Increase to >200–300% (>2- to 3-fold) from baseline	**Stage 2** Increase in SCr 2- to 2.9-fold from baseline	< 0.5 mL/kg/h for >12 h
Failure Increase in SCr 3-fold from baseline, or SCr >4 mg/dL (>354 μmol/L) with an acute increase >0.5 mg/dL (>44 μmol/L) or GFR decrease >75%	**Stage 3** Increase to >300% (>3-fold) from baseline, or ≥4.0 mg/dL (≥354 μmol/L) with an acute increase of at least 0.5 mg/dL (44 μmol/L), or on RRT	**Stage 3** Increase in SCr 3-fold from baseline *or* increase in SCr to ≥4.0 mg/dL (≥353.6 μmol/L) *or* initiation of RRT. In patients <18 years, decrease in estimated GFR to <35 mL/min/1.73 m²	<0.3 mL/kg/h for 24 h or anuria for 12 h
Loss Complete loss of kidney function >4 weeks			
ESRD ESRD >3 months			

AKIN, Acute Kidney Injury Network; *ESRD,* end-stage renal disease; *GFR,* glomerular filtration rate; *KDIGO,* Kidney Disease: Improving Global Outcomes; *RIFLE,* Risk, Injury, Failure, Loss, and End-stage renal disease; *RRT,* renal replacement therapy; *SCr,* serum creatinine; *UOP,* urinary output.

criteria for AKI and when abnormalities persisted for more than 3 days.[41] Unfortunately, the urinary output criterion is often underevaluated, especially in retrospective studies. Electronic alarm systems or "sniffers" have been applied in clinical practice to avoid delayed AKI diagnosis. While intriguing, the role of these electronic alerts has not been unequivocally associated with improved patient outcomes. It is possible that studies using "big data" will validate the importance of the automatic decision support systems for timely AKI diagnosis and classification.[42]

While the definition, diagnosis, and staging of AKI are currently obtained using clinical classification criteria based on serum creatinine and urinary output, several confounding factors may affect the clinical reliability of these markers. First, the concentration of serum creatinine depends on several nonrenal factors, such as age, gender, fluid balance and muscle mass. Creatinine metabolism varies during AKI, and clearance may be altered by treatment with several drugs (e.g., *N*-acetylcysteine).[23] Alterations in their metabolism and nutrition support may effect creatinine production in critically ill patients.[18] Finally, the creatinine half-life may increase from 4 hours to 24–72 hours if the GFR decreases.

Consequently, serum creatinine may take 24–36 hours to rise after a renal insult.[18] The RFR can maintain serum creatinine concentrations within the normal range until at least 50% of nephrons have been lost; this preservation reflects recruitment of undamaged nephrons. Creatinine is freely filtered through the glomerulus and partially secreted in the proximal tubules (10–20% of the urinary excreted load). Thus, creatinine clearance can overestimate GFR. The contribution of tubular creatinine secretion to clearance may be as high as 50% when GFR is reduced and is highly variable among individuals.

In some clinical settings (e.g., decompensated heart failure, uncontrolled diabetes), tubular reabsorption of creatinine can increase.[1] Medications (e.g., diuretics) and the simultaneous presence of tubular damage may reduce the sensitivity and specificity of urinary output for detecting AKI.

Hydration status may profoundly affect both urinary output and serum creatinine concentration in critically ill patients. Fluid loading may dilute the serum creatinine concentration, delaying the diagnosis of AKI[1] or producing an "atypical AKI,"[38] or pseudonormal creatinine. As a result, AKI determination may be delayed or even missed in aggressively hydrated patients.[18,43] These situations may have significant clinical repercussions, making the diagnosis and staging of AKI through these clinical classifications retrospective in nature[23] (Fig. 56.1).

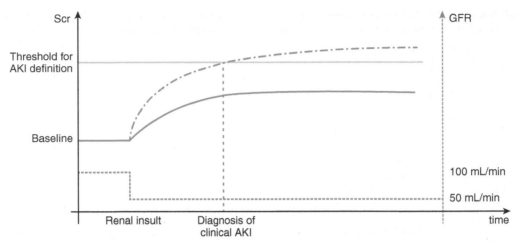

Fig. 56.1 Clinical and subclinical acute kidney injury (*AKI*) diagnosis following an acute decrease of glomerular filtration rate (*GFR*) (*dotted line*) from 100 to 50 mL/min due to a renal insult. The subsequent increase in serum creatinine concentration (*SCr*) requires a specific time lag to reach the threshold value and diagnose AKI (*dot-dashed line*). Therefore, the clinical identification of this syndrome's results are significantly delayed. Moreover, if a patient undergoes fluid resuscitation (*continuous line*), the dilution of SCr may further delay the diagnosis of clinical AKI or may avoid reaching the threshold value to diagnose AKI ("atypical AKI").

CONCLUSION

AKI is a frequently observed condition associated with a poor outcome. Early diagnosis and appropriate treatment may improve outcomes in AKI patients. While the best approach to improved outcomes is the prevention of AKI in highly susceptible patients, kidney insult may be unavoidable. In these cases, factors identifying high susceptibility for AKI should be investigated. Planning for appropriate biochemical and clinical follow-up, aimed at the timely diagnosis of subclinical and clinical AKI, is essential for highly susceptible patients.

Currently, AKI diagnosis is based on the clinical identification of GFR reduction, i.e., kidney dysfunction, via an increase in serum creatinine and/or a decrease in urinary output. However, these parameters are limited by factors that may significantly delay diagnosis. The assessment of RFR has been proposed as a possible (though perhaps impractical) approach to improving our understanding of actual renal function (i.e., before cardiac surgery).

Kidney dysfunction may be functional only or may be associated with anatomic alterations, i.e., kidney damage. Even if clinically undetectable (i.e., subclinical AKI), kidney damage may be associated with poor outcomes, and should be accounted for in clinical practice. Currently, biomarkers of kidney damage are the only indices of this alteration. The literature has shown that biomarkers of kidney damage rise 24–48 hours before clinical diagnosis of AKI; their use has therefore been proposed for early diagnosis of this clinical syndrome. However, while several studies have identified a correlation of biomarkers with renal and nonrenal outcomes, additional research is required to definitively support their role in clinical decision making and their cost-effectiveness.

AUTHORS' RECOMMENDATIONS
- Patients at high risk for developing AKI should be identified in a timely and correct manner.
- The use of biomarkers of kidney damage in high-risk patients can aid in the identification of subclinical AKI.
- Factors that can reduce the sensitivity and specificity of serum creatinine and urinary output in detecting AKI should be considered in clinical practice.
- Consider the use of biomarkers during clinical AKI to determine if kidney dysfunction is associated with kidney damage.

REFERENCES

1. Endre ZH, Pickering JW, Walker RJ. Clearance and beyond: the complementary roles of GFR measurement and injury biomarkers in acute kidney injury (AKI). *Am J Physiol Renal Physiol.* 2011; 301(4):F697-F707.
2. Valette X, du Cheyron D. A critical appraisal of the accuracy of the RIFLE and AKIN classifications in defining "acute kidney insufficiency" in critically ill patients. *J Crit Care.* 2013;28(2): 116-125.
3. Villa G, Ricci Z, Romagnoli S, Ronco C. Multidimensional approach to adequacy of renal replacement therapy in acute kidney injury. *Contrib Nephrol.* 2016;187:94-105.
4. Villa G, Samoni S, De Rosa S, Ronco C. The pathophysiological hypothesis of kidney damage during intra-abdominal hypertension. *Front Physiol.* 2016;7:55.
5. Neri M, Lorenzin A, Brendolan A, et al. Development of the new Kibou® equipment for continuous renal replacement therapy from scratch to the final configuration. *Contrib Nephrol.* 2017; 190:58-70.
6. Neri M, Villa G, Garzotto F, et al. Nomenclature for renal replacement therapy in acute kidney injury: basic principles. *Crit Care.* 2016;20(1):318.

7. Villa G, Neri M, Bellomo R, et al. Nomenclature for renal replacement therapy and blood purification techniques in critically ill patients: practical applications. *Crit Care.* 2016;20(1):283.
8. Thadhani R, Pascual M, Bonventre J. Acute renal failure. *N Engl J Med.* 1996;334(22):1448-1460.
9. Sharma A, Zaragoza JJ, Villa G, et al. Optimizing a kidney stress test to evaluate renal functional reserve. *Clin Nephrol.* 2016;86(7):18-26.
10. Ronco C, Kellum JA, Haase M. Subclinical AKI is still AKI. *Crit Care.* 2012;16(3):313.
11. Husain-Syed F, Ferrari F, Sharma A, et al. Preoperative renal functional reserve predicts risk of acute kidney injury after cardiac operation. *Ann Thorac Surg.* 2018;105(4):1094-1101.
12. Husain-Syed F, Ferrari F, Sharma A, et al. Persistent decrease of renal functional reserve in patients after cardiac surgery-associated acute kidney injury despite clinical recovery. *Nephrol Dial Transplant.* 2019;34(2):308-317.
13. Kuitunen A, Vento A, Suojaranta-Ylinen R, Pettilä V. Acute renal failure after cardiac surgery: evaluation of the RIFLE classification. *Ann Thorac Surg.* 2006;81(2):542-546.
14. Wijeysundera DN, Karkouti K, Dupuis JY, et al. Derivation and validation of a simplified predictive index for renal replacement therapy after cardiac surgery. *JAMA.* 2007;297(16):1801-1809.
15. Hobson CE, Yavas S, Segal MS, et al. Acute kidney injury is associated with increased long-term mortality after cardiothoracic surgery. *Circulation.* 2009;119(18):2444-2453.
16. Samoni S, Nalesso F, Meola M, et al. Intra-parenchymal renal resistive index variation (IRRIV) describes renal functional reserve (RFR): pilot study in healthy volunteers. *Front Physiol.* 2016;7:286.
17. Haase M, Devarajan P, Haase-Fielitz A, et al. The outcome of neutrophil gelatinase-associated lipocalin-positive subclinical acute kidney injury: a multicenter pooled analysis of prospective studies. *J Am Coll Cardiol.* 2011;57(17):1752-1761.
18. Ostermann M, Joannidis M. Acute kidney injury 2016: diagnosis and diagnostic workup. *Crit Care.* 2016;20(1):299.
19. Murray PT, Mehta RL, Shaw A, et al. Potential use of biomarkers in acute kidney injury: report and summary of recommendations from the 10th Acute Dialysis Quality Initiative consensus conference. *Kidney Int.* 2014;85(3):513-521.
20. Ronco C, McCullough PA, Chawla LS. Kidney attack versus heart attack: evolution of classification and diagnostic criteria. *Lancet.* 2013;382(9896):939-940.
21. Ronco C. Kidney attack: overdiagnosis of acute kidney injury or comprehensive definition of acute kidney syndromes? *Blood Purif.* 2013;36(2):65-68.
22. McIlroy DR, Wagener G, Lee HT. Biomarkers of acute kidney injury: an evolving domain. *Anesthesiology.* 2010;112(4):998-1004.
23. McCullough PA, Shaw AD, Haase M, et al. Diagnosis of acute kidney injury using functional and injury biomarkers: workgroup statements from the tenth Acute Dialysis Quality Initiative Consensus Conference. *Contrib Nephrol.* 2013;182:13-29.
24. Kashani K, Al-Khafaji A, Ardiles T, et al. Discovery and validation of cell cycle arrest biomarkers in human acute kidney injury. *Crit Care.* 2013;17(1):R25.
25. Yang QH, Liu DW, Long Y, Liu HZ, Chai WZ, Wang XT. Acute renal failure during sepsis: potential role of cell cycle regulation. *J Infect.* 2009;58(6):459-464.
26. Witzgall R, Brown D, Schwarz C, Bonventre JV. Localization of proliferating cell nuclear antigen, vimentin, c-Fos, and clusterin in the postischemic kidney. Evidence for a heterogenous genetic response among nephron segments, and a large pool of mitotically active and dedifferentiated cells. *J Clin Invest.* 1994;93(5):2175-2188.
27. Meersch M, Schmidt C, Van Aken H, et al. Urinary TIMP-2 and IGFBP7 as early biomarkers of acute kidney injury and renal recovery following cardiac surgery. *PLoS One.* 2014;9(3):e93460.
28. Meersch M, Schmidt C, Hoffmeier A, et al. Prevention of cardiac surgery-associated AKI by implementing the KDIGO guidelines in high risk patients identified by biomarkers: the PrevAKI randomized controlled trial. *Intensive Care Med.* 2017;43(11):1551-1561.
29. Kellum JA. Acute kidney injury: AKI: the myth of inevitability is finally shattered. *Nat Rev Nephrol.* 2017;13(3):140-141.
30. Parikh CR, Coca SG, Thiessen-Philbrook H, et al. Postoperative biomarkers predict acute kidney injury and poor outcomes after adult cardiac surgery. *J Am Soc Nephrol.* 2011;22(9):1748-1757.
31. Parikh CR, Devarajan P, Zappitelli M, et al. Postoperative biomarkers predict acute kidney injury and poor outcomes after pediatric cardiac surgery. *J Am Soc Nephrol.* 2011;22(9):1737-1747.
32. Himmelfarb J, Ikizler TA. Acute kidney injury: changing lexicography, definitions, and epidemiology. *Kidney Int.* 2007;71(10):971-976.
33. Cruz DN, Bagshaw SM, Maisel A, et al. Use of biomarkers to assess prognosis and guide management of patients with acute kidney injury. *Contrib Nephrol.* 2013;182:45-64.
34. Cruz DN, de Geus HR, Bagshaw SM. Biomarker strategies to predict need for renal replacement therapy in acute kidney injury. *Semin Dial.* 2011;24(2):124-131.
35. McIllroy DR, Wagener G, Lee HT. Neutrophil gelatinase-associated lipocalin and acute kidney injury after cardiac surgery: the effect of baseline renal function on diagnostic performance. *Clin J Am Soc Nephrol.* 2010;5(2):211-219.
36. Nejat M, Hill JV, Pickering JW, Edelstein CL, Devarajan P, Endre ZH. Albuminuria increases cystatin C excretion: implications for urinary biomarkers. *Nephrol Dial Transplant.* 2012;27(Suppl. 3):96-103.
37. Doi K, Negishi K, Ishizu T, et al. Evaluation of new acute kidney injury biomarkers in a mixed intensive care unit. *Crit Care Med.* 2011;39(11):2464-2469.
38. Kellum JA, Lameire N, Aspelin P, et al. KDIGO clinical practice guideline for acute kidney injury. *Kidney Int Suppl.* 2012;2(1):1-138.
39. Bellomo R, Ronco C, Kellum JA, Mehta RL, Palevsky P. Acute renal failure—definition, outcome measures, animal models, fluid therapy and information technology needs: the Second International Consensus Conference of the Acute Dialysis Quality Initiative (ADQI) Group. *Crit Care.* 2004;8(4):R204-R212.
40. Mehta RL, Kellum JA, Shah SV, et al. Acute Kidney Injury Network: report of an initiative to improve outcomes in acute kidney injury. *Crit Care.* 2007;11(2):R31.
41. Kellum JA, Sileanu FE, Murugan R, Lucko N, Shaw AD, Clermont G. Classifying AKI by urine output versus serum creatinine level. *J Am Soc Nephrol.* 2015;26(9):2231-2238.
42. Al-Jaghbeer M, Dealmeida D, Bilderback A, Ambrosino R, Kellum JA. Clinical decision support for in-hospital AKI. *J Am Soc Nephrol.* 2018;29(2):654-660.
43. De Rosa S, Samoni S, Ronco C. Creatinine-based definitions: from baseline creatinine to serum creatinine adjustment in intensive care. *Crit Care.* 2016;20:69.

57

What Is the Role of Renal Replacement Therapy in the Intensive Care Unit?

Adeel Rafi Ahmed, Michelle O'Shaughnessy, John O'Regan, and David William Lappin

INTRODUCTION

The aim of this chapter is to review the evidence surrounding the use of renal replacement therapy (RRT) in the intensive care unit (ICU) setting. It examines the conventional indications for emergency RRT and assesses the emerging evidence for both earlier commencement of RRT and the expanded role of RRT in the management of sepsis and the multiple organ dysfunction syndrome (MODS).

What are the Conventional Indications for Initiating Renal Replacement in Acute Kidney Injury?

Expert consensus extrapolated from experience in managing end-stage renal disease (ESRD) has resulted in the formation of conventional indications for initiating RRT in single-organ acute kidney injury (AKI) (Box 57.1). In patients with multiple organ dysfunction syndrome (MODS) and AKI, as seen in the intensive care unit (ICU) setting, no international consensus exists regarding when to initiate RRT.

Intravascular Volume Overload and Pulmonary Edema Refractory to Diuretic Therapy

Fluid overload at AKI diagnosis is associated with increased mortality.[1,2] If initial management with high-dose diuretics has failed, urgent RRT should be implemented. Importantly, diuretics have not been shown to enhance renal recovery or reduce duration of RRT.[3]

Metabolic Acidosis Refractory to Medical Management

Metabolic acidosis results from a combination of chloride-rich fluid resuscitation and the accumulation of lactate, phosphate, and unexcreted metabolic acids. RRT can be highly effective in correcting this abnormality. Continuous renal replacement therapy (CRRT) may be more effective in shortening the duration of treatment than intermittent hemodialysis (IHD).[4] The threshold pH or base deficit at which to initiate RRT has not been established. Since a pH lower than 7.1 is associated with negative inotropic and metabolic effects, in general, one would consider intervening before this level is reached. The BICAR-ICU trial analyzed the treatment of 389 severely acidemic (pH < 7.20, HCO_3^- < 20 mmol/L) critically ill patients with 4.2% sodium bicarbonate. In patients with an AKIN (Acute Kidney Injury Network) score of 2 or 3, treatment reduced 28-day mortality and the need for RRT compared with controls.[5]

Hyperkalemia Refractory to Medical Management

No specific treatment threshold for treatment of hyperkalemia with RRT has been established. In general, myocardial dysfunction is considered unlikely at serum potassium concentrations <6.5 mmol/L. Usually, diuretics do not increase potassium excretion in renal failure. For this reason, the threshold for initiating RRT in AKI might be lower, particularly if the response to emergency treatment (insulin–glucose, inhaled β-agonist, exchange resins) is minimal.[6] IHD is the preferred RRT modality for the rapid correction of hyperkalemia in a hemodynamically stable patient with AKI.[7] CRRT with a high effluent flow rate or dialysate with no or low potassium content can also be used when IHD is not available.

Uremia

Manifestations of "uremia" include encephalopathy, pericarditis, and bleeding diathesis. However, in critically ill patients, both mental status changes and bleeding can be multifactorial, and thus it may be difficult to attribute either solely to renal failure. Once detected, uremic pericarditis requires urgent initiation of RRT because it carries a high risk for intrapericardial hemorrhage and tamponade.

Intoxication With a Dialyzable Drug or Toxin

Extracellular low-molecular-weight toxins with little or no protein binding can be effectively removed by RRT. In general, IHD is preferable to CRRT for this purpose because it clears solute more rapidly. A review of the US Poison Center's "Toxic Exposure Surveillance System" records from 1985 to 2005 identified 19,351 cases where extracorporeal toxin removal was used.[8] Hemoperfusion techniques are used to enhance elimination of toxic levels of lipid-soluble or highly protein-bound substances in cases where endogenous clearance may be inadequate. An important consideration is the platelet-depleting effect of hemoperfusion.

Severe Electrolyte Derangement

AKI can be associated with an array of electrolyte disturbances. In particular, hyperphosphatemia is common in persistent AKI. Rhabdomyolysis and tumor lysis syndrome also cause hyperphosphatemia and can lead to severe hypocalcemia. Dietary phosphate restriction and oral phosphate binders can be considered; however, severe hyperphosphatemia will not correct until native renal function recovers or RRT is started.

Should Renal Replacement Therapy be Initiated in Acute Kidney Injury Before Complications have Developed?

In the absence of an absolute indication, timing the initiation of RRT in critically ill patients with AKI is challenging.[9] There is a general trend to initiate RRT early (Table 57.1) in the ICU setting.[10,11] This trend is primarily driven by observational data.[12–14] However, what constitutes "early" and "late" has varied from study to study. A variety of parameters, including (1) biochemical markers such as blood urea nitrogen (BUN) and creatinine, (2) clinical markers such as urine output and fluid balance, and (3) the time from onset of developing AKI, have been used.[15–18]

Observational Data

The Program to Improve Care in Acute Renal Disease (PICARD) trial was a multicenter observational study of AKI in patients without a history of chronic kidney disease (CKD) compared RRT initiation at a BUN ≤76 mg/dL and ≥76 mg/dL. Initiation at the lower threshold was associated with lower 14- and 28-day mortality.[1,17] In another study, investigators used retrospective data to assess a cohort of 130 septic shock patients who received RRT. Those with a BUN <100 mg/dL at initiation (early RRT) had had significantly lower mortality at 14, 28, and 365 days when compared with patients in whom RRT

was not started until BUN was ≥100 mg/dL (late RRT).[19] Earlier initiation of RRT in patients with postcardiac surgery AKI has been associated with survival benefits in observational studies.[16,18,20] Subgroup analysis of Finnish Acute Kidney Injury study (FINNAKI) compared early RRT with RRT that was delayed until absolute indication(s) were met[21]. Ninety-day mortality was higher in the late RRT group.

Randomized Controlled Trials

Three underpowered randomized controlled trials (RCTs) examined the threshold for/timing of RRT initiation in postcardiopulmonary bypass AKI.[22–24] In the largest of these (106 participants), comparing early vs. late criteria, no significant difference in 28-day mortality was observed.[24] A study from India (208 patients with tropical infections or obstetric complication), similarly, was unable to detect a difference in either mortality or renal recovery.[25] No difference in mortality was detected in a Canadian study involving 101 patients with AKI secondary to hypovolemia or sepsis.[26] Importantly, 25% of the patients assigned to the late group recovered renal function without the need for any dialysis.

The Early Versus Late Initiation of Renal Replacement Therapy In Critically Ill Patients With Acute Kidney Injury (ELAIN) trial was a single-center randomized trial of 231 critically ill patients that compared the effects of early (within 8 hours of fulfilling KDIGO [Kidney Disease: Improving Global Outcomes] stage 2 criteria) RRT to late (within 12 hours of meeting KDIGO stage 3 criteria or meeting an absolute indication) RRT on all-cause 90-day mortality.[27] 94% of the participants were postoperative, 46% of whom were postcardiac surgery. The median difference in time to RRT initiation from randomization between the two interventions was 21 hours. The primary study revealed an absolute reduction in 90-day mortality of 15.4% in the early RRT group (39.3%) compared with the late RRT (54.7%). Early RRT also led to a higher likelihood of dialysis independence, significantly shorter duration of RRT (9 vs. 25 days), and shortening of hospital stay (51 vs. 82 days).

The Initiation Strategies for Renal-Replacement Therapy in the Intensive Care Unit (AKIKI) trial, a multicenter RRT conducted in 31 French ICUs, examined 60-day mortality in 620 critically ill patients randomized to late (meeting absolute criteria) or early (within 6 hours of fulfilling KDIGO stage 3 criteria) RRT[28]. 98% of patients in the early group received RRT, while only 51% in the late group were treated. No significant difference in 60-day mortality was noted. There was no difference in key secondary outcomes, including ventilator- and vasopressor-free days through day 28, ICU length of stay, hospital length of stay, and dialysis dependence at day 60. The number of RRT-free days was greater (19 vs. 17 days) and the occurrence of catheter-related bloodstream infections was lower (5 vs. 10%) in the late group. Importantly, AKIKI was underpowered to detect significant mortality differences.

The Timing of Renal-Replacement Therapy in Patients with Acute Kidney Injury and Sepsis (IDEAL-ICU) trial was a multicenter RCT involving 488 septic patients. The investigators

TABLE 57.1 Early Versus Late RRT Strategy: A Comparison of ELAIN, AKIKI, and IDEAL-ICU Studies.

	ELAIN[27]	AKIKI[28]	IDEAL- ICU[29]
Design	RCT	RCT	RCT
Setting	Single center	Multicenter (31 ICUs)	Multicenter (29 ICUs)
Population	Predominantly postoperative patients: 47% postcardiac surgery	Predominantly medical patients with septic shock	Patients with septic shock
- Inclusion criteria	- KDIGO stage 2 - NGAL >150 mg/mL - Critical illness including at least one of severe sepsis/ vasopressor support/ refractory fluid overload/ SOFA score >2	- KDIGO stage 3 (Cr > 354 µmol/L or anuria for > 12 h or urine output < 0.3 mL/kg/h for 24 hours) - Critical illness (mechanical ventilation or vasopressor)	- Failure stage of RIFLE criteria (: oliguria (urine output <0.3 mL/kg BW/h for ≥24 hours), anuria for ≥12 hours, or a serum Cr level 3 times the baseline level (or ≥4 mg/dL [≥350 µmol/L]) - Septic shock (<48 hours of commencing vasopressor support)
- Exclusion criteria	Preexisting renal disease eGFR <30 mL/min/1.73 m²	Preexisting renal disease CrCl < 30 mL/min/1.73 m²	End-stage renal disease Obstructive nephropathy
- No. of patients	231	620	488
Baseline Characteristics			
- SOFA score (early vs. late)	15.6 vs. 16	10.9 vs. 10.8	12.2 vs. 12.4
- APACHE II score (early vs. late)	30.6 vs. 32.7	Not available (NA)	NA
Intervention—early RRT	<8 h of AKI KDIGO 2	<6 h of AKI KDIGO 3	<12 h of Failure stage of RIFLE
Control—late RRT	<12 h of AKI KDIGO 3 or absolute indication	Absolute indications (urea >40 mg/dL, K⁺ > 6 mmol/L, pH <7.15, acute pulmonary edema, oligouria/anuria >72 h)	>48 h of Failure stage of RIFLE criteria or absolute indications developing
RRT requirement in delayed group (%)	91	51	62
Method of RRT	CVVHDF	Multiple modalities— >50% initially on IHD	Multiple modalities—45% initially on IHD
Primary Outcome			
- Mortality in early vs. late RRT	At 90 days: 39.3 vs. 54.7%	At 60 days: 48.5 vs. 49.7%	At 90 days: 58 vs. 54%
- P value	.03	.79	.38
Secondary Outcome			
- Duration of RRT early vs. late (median days)	9 vs. 25	NA	4 vs. 2
- Ongoing requirement for RRT	At 90 days: 13 vs. 15%	At 60 days: 2 vs. 5%	At 90 days: 2 vs. 3%
Conclusion	Early RRT compared with late initiation of RRT reduced mortality over the first 90 days	No significant difference in mortality between an early and late strategy for the initiation of RRT therapy. A late strategy averted the need for RRT in a large number of patients	No significant difference in 90-day mortality between early and late strategy of RRT among septic shock patients

AKIKI, initiation strategies for renal-replacement therapy in the intensive care unit; *AKI*, acute kidney injury; *BW*, body weight; *Cr*, creatinine; *CVVHDF*, continuous venovenous hemofiltration; *eGFR*, estimated glomerular filtration rate; *ELAIN*, the early versus late initiation of renal replacement therapy in critically ill patients with acute kidney injury; *ICUs*, intensive care units; *IDEAL-ICU*, timing of renal-replacement therapy in patients with acute kidney injury and sepsis; *IHD*, intermittent hemodialysis; *KDIGO*, kidney disease: improving global outcomes; *NGAL*, neutrophil gelatinase-associated lipocalin; *RIFLE*, Risk, Injury, Failure, Loss, and End-stage renal disease; *RRT*, renal replacement therapy; *SOFA*, sequential failure organ assessment.

found no significant difference in 90-day mortality between early RRT (<12 hours of Failure stage of RIFLE criteria, comparative to KDIGO stage 3) and late RRT (> 48 hours of Failure stage of RIFLE criteria).[29]

In the authors' opinion, patients with low physiologic reserve may benefit from initiation of RRT before absolute indications develop.[17,30] There may also be potential benefits in initiating RRT before absolute indications develop in AKI associated with severe burns or in postoperative patients, particularly after cardiac surgery.[27,31] Septic patients may benefit from a relatively delayed strategy of initiating RRT.[28–30] The Acute Dialysis Quality Initiative (ADQI) workgroup on CRRT recommended initiating RRT when metabolic and fluid demands exceed total kidney capacity; however, no specific criteria exist to define excessive demand and low capacity (Box 57.2).[32]

Does CRRT Purify Blood in Sepsis?

Inflammatory mediators can be adsorbed onto the surface of hemofiltration membranes.[33,34] However, this process will remove both proinflammatory and anti-inflammatory cytokines.[34] Current evidence does not support the routine use of high cut-off (HCO) membrane or high effluent flow rate and larger RCTs would be required to elicit any renal or mortality benefits.[35–37]

What is the Role of High Volume Ultrafiltration in Sepsis?

Limited evidence suggested use of very high effluent flow rate (>60 mL/kg/h) to remove inflammatory mediators would be of value in septic patient.[38–40] The IVOIRE study of 137 patients with septic shock-associated AKI receiving high or low flow failed to demonstrate a significant difference in vasopressor requirement and 28-day mortality.[41] In 2017, a recent Cochrane review concluded that there was no mortality benefit with the use of high-volume hemofiltration (HVHF) compared with standard therapy in AKI secondary to septic shock.[37]

Two important studies, the ATN study and the RENAL study[42,43] compared HVHF with standard therapy but were not confined to septic patients. The ATN study found that higher-intensity treatment was not associated with reduced mortality, improved renal recovery, or reduced rate of nonrenal organ failure when compared with less intensive therapy.[42] High-intensity treatment was, however, associated with significantly more hypophosphatemia and in more

---

BOX 57.2   Seventeenth Acute Disease Quality Initiative (ADQI) Consensus on Patient Selection and Timing of Continuous Renal Replacement Therapy (CRRT) (2016).

Consensus statement 1.1: Acute renal replacement therapy (RRT) should be considered when metabolic and fluid demands exceed total kidney capacity.

Consensus statement 1.2: Demand for kidney function is determined by nonrenal comorbidities, the severity of the acute disease, and solute and fluid burden.

Consensus statement 1.3: Total kidney function is measured using a variety of different methods. Changes in kidney function and duration of kidney dysfunction can be anticipated by markers of kidney damage.

Consensus statement 1.4: The demand–capacity imbalance is dynamic and should be evaluated regularly.

Consensus statement 1.5: For patients requiring multiple types of organ support, decisions about initiating or withholding RRT should be considered together with other therapies.

Consensus statement 1.6: Once the decision to initiate RRT has been made, the therapy should be started as soon as possible, typically within less than 3 h.

Consensus statement 2.1: Selection of RRT modality depends on the capability/availability of the technology, its inherited risks, and the current needs of the patient.

Consensus statement 2.2: Continuous types of RRT are recommended in situations where shifts in fluid balance and metabolic fluctuations are poorly tolerated. Intermittent and prolonged intermittent types of RRT have a role in situations where rehabilitation or mobilization is the priority, and fluid and metabolic fluctuations can be tolerated.

Consensus statement 2.3: Availability of technologies is determined by local regulations, local resources, including staff, their training/experience and laboratory support, and financial constraints. The choice of the technologies that should be made available must balance these issues.

Consensus statement 3.1: In situations where other extracorporeal therapies are required, CRRT is recommended and integrated systems are preferred over parallel systems.

Consensus statement 4.1: Transition of modalities should be considered if the demand–capacity imbalance or treatment priorities have changed and can be met better by an alternative technique.

Consensus statement 5.1: RRT should be discontinued if kidney function has recovered sufficiently to reduce the demand–capacity imbalance (current and expected) to acceptable levels or the overall goals of treatment have changed.

Consensus statement 5.2: To determine sustained recovery of kidney function, we recommend monitoring of urine output and serum creatinine (SCr) during RRT.

Consensus statement 5.3: For patients requiring multiple types of organ support, decisions about withdrawing RRT should be considered together with other therapies.

Data from Ostermann M, Joannidis M, Pani A, et al. Patient selection and timing of continuous renal replacement therapy. *Blood Purif.* 2016;42 (3):224-237.

hypotensive episodes requiring vasopressor support. The RENAL study of 1508 patients randomly assigned to high-intensity (40 mL/kg/h) or lower-intensity (25 mL/kg/h) treatment was unable to detect a difference in 90-day mortality, rate of dialysis dependence, or hemodynamic improvement, but was associated with significantly higher rates of hypophosphatemia.[43]

Overall, these studies do not justify the use of high-flow ultrafiltration.

Is Continuous Renal Replacement Therapy Superior to Intermittent Hemodialysis for Sepsis-Associated Acute Kidney Injury?

High-quality data directly comparing CRRT and IHD are lacking due to preferential use of CRRT in hemodynamically unstable patients. There is currently no evidence that CRRT is superior to IHD in terms of mortality or preservation of renal function in critical illness.[44,45]

CRRT is associated with a smaller increase in intracranial pressure (ICP) compared with IHD. Consequently is the preferred option in liver failure awaiting transplantation and acute brain injury, conditions that predispose to cerebral edema.[46–48]

IHD is considered first-line therapy in situations requiring rapid correction of electrolytes (hyperkalemia), urgent fluid removal, and poisoning.

In our practice, CRRT is administered to hemodynamically unstable patients in the ICU with subsequent transitioning to IHD once high dose vasopressor support is no longer required.

Can Ultrafiltration Serve as a Means of Support for Organs Other than the Kidney?

Cardiac Support

The UNLOAD trial, compared early ultrafiltration (UF) with standard diuretic therapy in patients presenting with decompensated heart failure (HF).[49] Early UF produced greater fluid and weight loss at 48 hours with reduced rehospitalization, number of hospital days, and unscheduled clinic visits at the 90-day follow-up. Serum creatinine was similar in both groups.[49] The CARRESS-HF trial compared UF with an approach based on a targeted urine output (UO) of 3–5 L/day,[50] achieved using intravenous diuretics, thiazide-like diuretics (metolazone), inotropic agents, left ventricular assist devices (LVAD), and UF crossover. The stepped pharmacologic therapy was superior to UF in terms of preservation of renal function, lower adverse events, and similar weight loss at 96 hours. A smaller RCT demonstrated a lower rehospitalization rate at 1 year when UF was used as the primary modality to manage decompensated HF.[51]

In light of the above results, we broadly agree with the recommendations of ACC/AHA (American College of Cardiology and American Heart Association) that UF is a reasonable therapeutic modality in refractory HF not responding to medical management.[52]

Lung Support

The FACCT (Fluid and Catheters Treatment Trial) demonstrated that a conservative fluid management strategy may be associated with a reduction in RRT requirements.[53] A few small studies have shown reduced ventilatory requirements and improvement in oxygenation with the use of CRRT in ARDS.[54,55,56] However, a post hoc analysis of the AKIKI trial, investigating early vs. late initiation of RRT in a subgroup of patients with acute respiratory distress syndrome (ARDS) or sepsis and AKI KDIGO 3, was unable to identify a difference in ventilator-free days and 60-day mortality.[57]

In the presence of a positive fluid balance and ARDS, CRRT may be considered to deresuscitate the patient, reduced extravascular lung water and removed extracellular solute (sodium, chloride etc), as an alternative to diuretic therapy.

AUTHORS' RECOMMENDATIONS
- There are no universally accepted criteria for initiating renal replacement therapy in patients with AKI and MODS.
- Widely used indications to initiate CRRT include a BUN higher than 60 mg/dL; uremia defined by pericarditis, platelet dysfunction, and neuropathy; pulmonary edema; hyperkalemia; metabolic acidosis; and intoxication.
- The optimal time to commence CRRT remains a topic of debate. There may be some benefit of initiating early RRT in postoperative patients with AKI, particularly in patients with reduced physiologic reserve. Septic patients with MODS may benefit from a delayed strategy.
- The current evidence base suggests CRRT offers no definite benefits to mortality or preservation of renal function when compared with IHD.
- CRRT may be a better choice than IHD in the hemodynamically unstable patient, liver failure, brain injury, or severe volume excess.
- The current literature does not support the use of high effluent flow rates in CRRT.
- UF is a reasonable therapeutic option in refractory heart failure not responding to medical management.

REFERENCES

1. Bouchard J, Soroko SB, Chertow GM, et al. Fluid accumulation, survival and recovery of kidney function in critically ill patients with acute kidney injury. *Kidney Int.* 2009;76(4):422-427.
2. Vaara ST, Reinikainen M, Wald R, Bagshaw SM, Pettilä V. Timing of RRT based on the presence of conventional indications. *Clin J Am Soc Nephrol.* 2014;9(9):1577-1585.
3. Khwaja A. KDIGO clinical practice guidelines for acute kidney injury. *Nephron Clin Pract.* 2012;120(4):c179-c184.
4. Uchino S, Bellomo R, Ronco C. Intermittent versus continuous renal replacement therapy in the ICU: impact on electrolyte and acid-base balance. *Intensive Care Med.* 2001;27(6):1037-1043.
5. Jaber S, Paugam C, Futier E, et al. Sodium bicarbonate therapy for patients with severe metabolic acidaemia in the intensive care unit (BICAR-ICU): a multicentre, open-label, randomised controlled, phase 3 trial. *Lancet.* 2018;392(10141):31-40.

6. Mahoney BA, Smith WA, Lo DS, Tsoi K, Tonelli M, Clase CM. Emergency interventions for hyperkalaemia. *Cochrane Database Syst Rev.* 2005(2):CD003235.

7. Parham WA, Mehdirad AA, Biermann KM, Fredman CS. Hyperkalemia revisited. *Tex Heart Inst J.* 2006;33(1):40-47.

8. Holubek WJ, Hoffman RS, Goldfarb DS, Nelson LS. Use of hemodialysis and hemoperfusion in poisoned patients. *Kidney Int.* 2008;74(10):1327-1334.

9. Mehta RL. Renal-replacement therapy in the critically ill—does timing matter? *N Engl J Med.* 2016;375(2):175-176.

10. Bagshaw SM, Wald R, Barton J, et al. Clinical factors associated with initiation of renal replacement therapy in critically ill patients with acute kidney injury—a prospective multicenter observational study. *J Crit Care.* 2012;27(3):268-275.

11. Clark E, Wald R, Levin A, et al. Timing the initiation of renal replacement therapy for acute kidney injury in Canadian intensive care units: a multicentre observational study. *Can J Anaesth.* 2012;59(9):861-870.

12. Seabra VF, Balk EM, Liangos O, Sosa MA, Cendoroglo M, Jaber BL. Timing of renal replacement therapy initiation in acute renal failure: a meta-analysis. *Am J Kidney Dis.* 2008;52(2):272-284.

13. Bagshaw SM, Uchino S, Bellomo R, et al. Timing of renal replacement therapy and clinical outcomes in critically ill patients with severe acute kidney injury. *J Crit Care.* 2009;24(1):129-140.

14. do Nascimento GV, Balbi AL, Ponce D, Abrão JM. Early initiation of dialysis: mortality and renal function recovery in acute kidney injury patients. *J Bras Nefrol.* 2012;34(4):337-342.

15. Gettings LG, Reynolds HN, Scalea T. Outcome in post-traumatic acute renal failure when continuous renal replacement therapy is applied early vs. late. *Intensive Care Med.* 1999;25(8):805-813.

16. Elahi MM, Lim MY, Joseph RN, Dhannapuneni RR, Spyt TJ. Early hemofiltration improves survival in post-cardiotomy patients with acute renal failure. *Eur J Cardiothorac Surg.* 2004;26(5):1027-1031.

17. Liu KD, Himmelfarb J, Paganini E, et al. Timing of initiation of dialysis in critically ill patients with acute kidney injury. *Clin J Am Soc Nephrol.* 2006;1(5):915-919.

18. Demirkiliç U, Kuralay E, Yenicesu M, et al. Timing of replacement therapy for acute renal failure after cardiac surgery. *J Card Surg.* 2004;19(1):17-20.

19. Carl DE, Grossman C, Behnke M, Sessler CN, Gehr TW. Effect of timing of dialysis on mortality in critically ill, septic patients with acute renal failure. *Hemodial Int.* 2010;14(1):11-17.

20. Bent P, Tan HK, Bellomo R, et al. Early and intensive continuous hemofiltration for severe renal failure after cardiac surgery. *Ann Thorac Surg.* 2001;71(3):832-837.

21. Vats HS, Dart RA, Okon TR, Liang H, Paganini EP. Does early initiation of continuous renal replacement therapy affect outcome: experience in a tertiary care center. *Ren Fail.* 2011;33(7):698-706.

22. Durmaz I, Yagdi T, Calkavur T, et al. Prophylactic dialysis in patients with renal dysfunction undergoing on-pump coronary artery bypass surgery. *Ann Thorac Surg.* 2003;75(3):859-864.

23. Sugahara S, Suzuki H. Early start on continuous hemodialysis therapy improves survival rate in patients with acute renal failure following coronary bypass surgery. *Hemodial Int.* 2004;8(4):320-325.

24. Bouman CS, Oudemans-Van Straaten HM, Tijssen JG, Zandstra DF, Kesecioglu J. Effects of early high-volume continuous venovenous hemofiltration on survival and recovery of renal function in intensive care patients with acute renal failure: a prospective, randomized trial. *Crit Care Med.* 2002;30(10):2205-2211.

25. Jamale TE, Hase NK, Kulkarni M, et al. Earlier-start versus usual-start dialysis in patients with community-acquired acute kidney injury: a randomized controlled trial. *Am J Kidney Dis.* 2013;62(6):1116-1121.

26. Wald R, Adhikari NK, Smith OM, et al. Comparison of standard and accelerated initiation of renal replacement therapy in acute kidney injury. *Kidney Int.* 2015;88(4):897-904.

27. Zarbock A, Kellum JA, Schmidt C, et al. Effect of early vs. delayed initiation of renal replacement therapy on mortality in critically ill patients with acute kidney injury: the ELAIN randomized clinical trial. *JAMA.* 2016;315(20):2190-2199.

28. Gaudry S, Hajage D, Schortgen F, et al. Initiation strategies for renal-replacement therapy in the intensive care unit. *N Engl J Med.* 2016;375(2):122-133.

29. Barbar SD, Clere-Jehl R, Bourredjem A, et al. Timing of renal-replacement therapy in patients with acute kidney injury and sepsis. *N Engl J Med.* 2018;379(15):1431-1442.

30. Liborio AB, Leite TT, Neves FM, Teles F, Bezerra CT. AKI complications in critically ill patients: association with mortality rates and RRT. *Clin J Am Soc Nephrol.* 2015;10(1):21-28.

31. Chung KK, Lundy JB, Matson JR, et al. Continuous venovenous hemofiltration in severely burned patients with acute kidney injury: a cohort study. *Crit Care.* 2009;13(3):R62.

32. Ostermann M, Joannidis M, Pani A, et al. Patient selection and timing of continuous renal replacement therapy. *Blood Purif.* 2016;42(3):224-237.

33. Kellum JA, Song M, Venkataraman R. Hemoadsorption removes tumor necrosis factor, interleukin-6, and interleukin-10, reduces nuclear factor-kappaB DNA binding, and improves short-term survival in lethal endotoxemia. *Crit Care Med.* 2004;32(3):801-805.

34. De Vriese AS, Colardyn FA, Philippé JJ, Vanholder RC, De Sutter JH, Lameire NH. Cytokine removal during continuous hemofiltration in septic patients. *J Am Soc Nephrol.* 1999;10(4):846-853.

35. Villa G, Chelazzi C, Morettini E, et al. Organ dysfunction during continuous veno-venous high cut-off hemodialysis in patients with septic acute kidney injury: a prospective observational study. *PloS One.* 2017;12(2):e0172039.

36. Villa G, Zaragoza JJ, Sharma A, Neri M, De Gaudio AR, Ronco C. Cytokine removal with high cut-off membrane: review of literature. *Blood Purif.* 2014;38(3-4):167-173.

37. Borthwick EM, Hill CJ, Rabindranath KS, Maxwell AP, McAuley DF, Blackwood B. High-volume haemofiltration for sepsis in adults. *Cochrane Database Syst Rev.* 2017;1:CD008075.

38. Cole L, Bellomo R, Journois D, Davenport P, Baldwin I, Tipping P. High-volume haemofiltration in human septic shock. *Intensive Care Med.* 2001;27(6):978-986.

39. Ghani RA, Zainudin S, Ctkong N, et al. Serum IL-6 and IL-1-ra with sequential organ failure assessment scores in septic patients receiving high-volume haemofiltration and continuous venovenous haemofiltration. *Nephrology (Carlton).* 2006;11(5):386-393.

40. Boussekey N, Chiche A, Faure K, et al. A pilot randomized study comparing high and low volume hemofiltration on vasopressor use in septic shock. *Intensive Care Med.* 2008;34(9):1646-1653.

41. Joannes-Boyau O, Honoré PM, Perez P, et al. High-volume versus standard-volume haemofiltration for septic shock patients with acute kidney injury (IVOIRE study): a multicentre randomized controlled trial. *Intensive Care Med.* 2013;39(9):1535-1546.

42. Palevsky PM, Zhang JH, O'Connor TZ, et al. Intensity of renal support in critically ill patients with acute kidney injury. *N Engl J Med.* 2008;359(1):7-20.

43. Bellomo R, Cass A, Cole L, et al. Intensity of continuous renal-replacement therapy in critically ill patients. *N Engl J Med.* 2009;361(17):1627-1638.

44. Nash DM, Przech S, Wald R, O'Reilly D. Systematic review and meta-analysis of renal replacement therapy modalities for acute kidney injury in the intensive care unit. *J Crit Care.* 2017;41:138-144.

45. Rabindranath K, Adams J, Macleod AM, Muirhead N. Intermittent versus continuous renal replacement therapy for acute renal failure in adults. *Cochrane Database Syst Rev.* 2007;(3):CD003773.

46. Davenport A, Will EJ, Davison AM. Effect of renal replacement therapy on patients with combined acute renal and fulminant hepatic failure. *Kidney Int Suppl.* 1993;41:S245-S251.

47. Davenport A, Will EJ, Davidson AM. Improved cardiovascular stability during continuous modes of renal replacement therapy in critically ill patients with acute hepatic and renal failure. *Crit Care Med.* 1993;21(3):328-338.

48. Davenport A. Renal replacement therapy in the patient with acute brain injury. *Am J Kidney Dis.* 2001;37(3):457-466.

49. Costanzo MR, Guglin ME, Saltzberg MT, et al. Ultrafiltration versus intravenous diuretics for patients hospitalized for acute decompensated heart failure. *J Am Coll Cardiol.* 2007;49(6):675-683.

50. Bart BA, Goldsmith SR, Lee KL, et al. Ultrafiltration in decompensated heart failure with cardiorenal syndrome. *N Engl J Med.* 2012;367(24):2296-2304.

51. Marenzi G, Muratori M, Cosentino ER, et al. Continuous ultrafiltration for congestive heart failure: the CUORE trial. *J Card Fail.* 2014;20(1):9-17.

52. Felker GM, Mentz RJ. Diuretics and ultrafiltration in acute decompensated heart failure. *J Am Coll Cardiol.* 2012;59(24):2145-2153.

53. Wiedemann HP, Wheeler AP, Bernard GR, et al. Comparison of two fluid-management strategies in acute lung injury. *N Engl J Med.* 2006;354(24):2564-2575.

54. Liu KD, Thompson BT, Ancukiewicz M, et al. Acute kidney injury in patients with acute lung injury: impact of fluid accumulation on classification of acute kidney injury and associated outcomes. *Crit Care Med.* 2011;39(12):2665-2671.

55. Han F, Sun R, Ni Y, et al. Early initiation of continuous renal replacement therapy improves clinical outcomes in patients with acute respiratory distress syndrome. *Am J Med Sci.* 2015;349(3):199-205.

56. Garzia F, Todor R, Scalea T. Continuous arteriovenous hemofiltration countercurrent dialysis (CAVH-D) in acute respiratory failure (ARDS). *J Trauma.* 1991;31(9):1277-1284; discussion:1284-1285.

57. Gaudry S, Hajage D, Schortgen F, et al. Timing of renal support and outcome of septic shock and acute respiratory distress syndrome. a post hoc analysis of the AKIKI randomized clinical trial. *Am J Respir Crit Care Med.* 2018;198(1):58-66.

58

What Is the Value of Nondialytic Therapy in Acute Kidney Injury?

Stephen Duff and Patrick T. Murray

INTRODUCTION AND EPIDEMIOLOGY

Acute kidney injury (AKI) is common in hospitalized patients, especially those in the intensive care unit (ICU). The Acute Kidney Injury–Epidemiologic Prospective Investigation (AKI-EPI) study was an international, prospective observational study of AKI incidence and outcomes published in 2015.[1] The trial assessed 1802 patients in 97 centers for AKI as per the Kidney Disease: Improving Global Outcomes (KDIGO) criteria (Table 58.1). Overall, 57.3% (95% confidence interval [CI] 55.0–59.6] of ICU patients experienced AKI. There was an increased risk of death associated with worsening kidney dysfunction for KDIGO (Table 58.1) Stage 2 (odds ratio [OR] 2.945; 95% CI 1.382–6.276; $P = .005$) and KDIGO Stage 3 (OR 6.884; 95% CI 3.876–12.228; $P < .001$). Survivors are at risk of progression to chronic kidney disease or end-stage renal disease. The most common associated etiologies in the AKI-EPI study were sepsis (40.7%), hypovolemia (34.1%), and nephrotoxic medications (14.4%; 95% CI 12.0–17.3). Siew & Davenport[2] found an alarming increase in the rate of AKI and dialysis-requiring AKI in recent decades. Although increased sensitivity of diagnostic criteria contributed to this, large increases were also seen in studies that assessed creatinine-based criteria alone. This trend is particularly concerning considering the high level of associated morbidity and financial costs. In the United States, the estimated increase in inpatient costs of AKI is $5.4 to $24.0 billion.[3] Costs in England were estimated at between £894,193,943 ($1.4 billion USD) and £1,153,732,733 ($1.8 billion USD), accounting for over 1% of the National Health Service budget for 2010–2011.

AKI and its supportive treatment with renal replacement therapy (RRT) are both associated with markedly increased morbidity and mortality. The results of trials of nondialytic therapeutic interventions attempting to ameliorate the course of AKI will be discussed in this chapter.

INTRAVENOUS FLUID TO PREVENT AKI

A widely held belief among clinicians is that AKI frequently results from renal hypoperfusion and that treating the patient with intravenous fluids may improve outcomes. Outside the clear scenario of pure dehydration, fluid (i.e., water and solute) resuscitation remains highly controversial (see Chapter 24). The following section will briefly discuss the current data on various intravenous fluids with respect to kidney injury.

Crystalloids Versus Colloids

Crystalloids are intravenous fluids that combine various minerals and water into an electrochemically balanced solution. Hypotonic crystalloids distribute across the total body water; isotonic crystalloids solutions distribute evenly across the extracellular fluid. Colloids are products that include organic macromolecules, such as albumin, starch, or gelatin, with crystalloids—the goal being to provide a product that will likely remain in the intravascular space. At least theoretically, colloids are an attractive choice for the repletion of blood loss and treatment of relative hypovolemia associated with vasoplegia.

A 2018 Cochrane metaanalysis reviewed 69 studies ($n = 30,020$) in which critically ill patients were administered crystalloids or colloids in either hospital or emergency prehospital settings.[4] The authors found that using colloids (dextrans, starches, plasma, or albumin) (moderate-certainty evidence) or gelatins (low-certainty evidence) versus crystalloids made little or no difference in mortality between groups. However, they found that starches were associated with increased risk of blood transfusion and RRT (moderate-certainty evidence). Colloids are more expensive and are associated with increased risk of allergy compared with crystalloids. Therefore, the use of artificial colloid solutions is not recommended in critical care.[5]

Choice of Crystalloid

Ongoing concerns regarding the potential nephrotoxicity of acquired hyperchloremia has resulted in renewed interest in the composition of crystalloid intravenous fluids, principally between balanced salt solutions (BSS: Hartmann's, lactated Ringer's, and Plasma-lyte 148) and isotonic (NS 0.9%) saline solution. Acquired hyperchloremia is reviewed in detail in Chapter 60 and to a lesser degree in Chapter 59.

The SPLIT trial was a multicenter, cluster randomized, double crossover, feasibility trial based in New Zealand that

TABLE 58.1 Kidney Disease: Improving Global Outcomes Criteria for Acute Kidney Injury.

AKIN Stage	Creatinine Criteria	Urine Output Criteria
Stage 1	SCr 1.5-1.9 x baseline or Scr increase ≥0.3 mg/dL/26.5 µL	Urine volume <5 mL/kg/h for 6 hours
Stage 2	SCr ≥ 2.0-2.9 x baseline SCr ≥3x baseline or Cr Increase 4.0 mg/dL/353.6 µmol/L	Urine volume <5 mL/kg/h for ≥12 hours
Stage 3	Initiation of renal replacement therapy or decrease in eGFR <35 mL/min/1.73 m²	Urine volume <3 mL/kg/h for ≥24 hours or anuria ≥12 hours

AKIN, Acute Kidney Injury Network classification; *eGFR*, estimated glomerular filtration rate.
Modified from Kidney Disease. Improving Global Outcomes (KDIGO) Acute Kidney Injury Work Group. KDIGO clinical practice guideline for acute kidney injury. *Kidney Int Suppl.* 2012;2(1):1–138.

compared 0.9% saline (NS) with Plasma-Lyte 148 in a heterogenous group of ICU patients.[6] There was also no significant difference in the rate of RRT between groups. However, this study was severely limited by both low event rate and relatively low volume of fluid administered (2000 mL median/group).

Two large, randomized controlled trials (RCTs) from the same group subsequently looked at the use of NS versus balanced BSS in emergency medicine patients (SALT-ED)[7] and critically ill patients (SMART).[8] Although the volume of fluid administered intravenously was relatively low, certainly in comparison with perioperative patients, in both studies there was approximately a 1% increase in renal complications, albeit a composite endpoint that necessarily limits the validity of the outcome data.

A 2018 metaanalysis reviewed 19,332 patients randomized to either BSS or NS in six RCTs.[9] There was no significant difference in the primary outcomes of AKI (12% BSS versus 12.7% NS, OR 0.92; 95% CI 0.84–1.01; $P = .1$; $I^2 = 0\%$) or in-hospital mortality (11.5% BSS versus 12.2% NS, OR 0.92; 95% CI 0.85–1.01; $P = .09$; $I^2 = 0\%$). There were also no differences in the secondary outcomes of overall ICU mortality (OR 0.9, 95% CI 0.81–1.01, $P = .08$, $I^2 = 0\%$) or the need for new RRT (OR 0.92, 95% CI 0.67–1.28, $P = 0.65$, $I^2 = 38\%$). It is worth noting that few of these trials reported acquired hyperchloremia or a difference in the plasma sodium and chloride compared between the groups.

The limitations of the metaanalysis include the heterogeneity in study designs, potential exposure of patients to a treatment prior to randomization, inclusion of trials outside ICU, lack of sensitivity analysis, and inclusion of small trials with lower quality. A Trial Sequential Analysis could

be useful to establish how much additional research is necessary to definitively answer the question.[8] A number of ongoing studies are underway that may definitively answer this question.[10,11]

Early Goal-Directed Therapy

Goal-directed fluid resuscitation became part of the standard of care[12] for the management of patients in septic shock following a landmark trial by Rivers et al.,[13] which did not address AKI. Three large, multicenter clinical trials of early goal-directed therapy (EGDT) were subsequently published: the Protocolised Management in Sepsis,[14] Protocolised Care for Early Septic Shock[15] and the Australasian Resuscitation in Sepsis Evaluation[16] study. None of these trials found that fluid resuscitation, beyond initial rehydration, reduced 90-day mortality. A preplanned individual patient metaanalysis found no significant difference in the requirement for RRT between groups: 11% patients in the EGDT versus 10.6% patients in the "usual care" group.[17]

The optimal mean arterial blood pressure target (MAP) to prevent AKI in critical illness is unclear. A multicenter trial ($n = 776$) randomized patients with septic shock to either an MAP of 65–70 mm Hg (low-target) or 80–85 mm Hg (high-target).[18] There was an increased incidence of doubling of serum creatinine: 52% in low-target versus 38.9% in high-target ($P = .02$). There was an elevated need for RRT amongst patients with known hypertension who received a lower blood pressure target: RRT 42.4% in low-target versus 31.7% in high-target ($P = .046$). Further research is required to elucidate the optimal blood pressure management strategy, but most experts agree that patients with hypertension should receive a higher blood pressure target.[19]

Septic AKI is a complex process and of multifactorial etiology that includes dysfunctional inflammation, cellular hibernation, dysregulated blood flow, etc. It is unlikely that AKI can be prevented by simplistic ischemia prevention therapies such as fluid resuscitation and vasopressors.

Fluids and Perioperative Acute Kidney Injury

Observational data have shown a correlation between more positive perioperative fluid balance and AKI risk.[20–22] A landmark study by Nisanevich et al.[23] demonstrated a significant reduction in major and minor complications associated with relative fluid restriction in the perioperative and postoperative period. This was rapidly assimilated by the surgical community personnel who have generated guidelines supporting perioperative fluid restriction despite minimal data.[24]

This approach was not investigated by a high-quality RCT until 2018.[25] The RELIEF Trial ($n = 3000$) compared restrictive versus liberal fluid administration strategies in the setting of major abdominal surgery.[25] The liberal arm and restrictive arm received a median volume of 6.1 L (interquartile range, 5.0–7.4) and 3.7 L (interquartile range, 2.9–4.9; $P < .001$), respectively, in the first 24 hours. The investigators found higher rates of AKI, 8.6% in the restrictive fluid group versus 5.0% in the liberal group ($P < .001$) and RRT

(0.9% versus 0.3%, $P = .048$). Data on weight gain and fluid balance over the 3 days of the surgical stress response were not provided. However, these data are likely to result in less aggressive fluid restriction in the future.

DIURETICS

Loop Diuretics

Loop diuretics are agents administered to control circulating volume, principally in patients with heart failure or fluid overload. They work by venodilation and inhibition of the Na^+/K^+ $2Cl^-$ transporter in the medullary portion of the thick ascending limb of the loop of Henle. Although it is widely believed that diuretics can "convert" an oliguric state to a non oliguric state and stave off RRT, at least for controlling volume, there is no evidence that this approach improves patient outcomes.[26]

Bove et al.[27] undertook metaanalysis of 28 RCTs ($n = 3228$) that looked at intermittent furosemide injection for the treatment or prevention of AKI in critically ill patients. The use of furosemide neither reduced mortality, duration of hospital stay, and need for RRT nor prevented the development of AKI. Large, high-quality RCTs are needed to establish the role of prophylactic intermittent furosemide before recommending its widespread use.

Oliguria in critical illness is multifactorial, and patients are commonly oliguric despite generous fluid resuscitation and apparently normal renal markers. The "furosemide stress test (FST)" is performed to determine whether the kidneys are intact or whether oliguria is a harbinger of AKI. The data for this approach derives from a small study ($n = 77$) by Chawla et al.[28] who administered 1 mg/kg for naïve and 1.5 mg/kg for non-naïve critically ill patients (Fig. 58.1). The urine output response within the first 2 hours postadministration was found to have the best discriminant ability with a receiver operating characteristic curve for progression to AKI Network classification Stage 3 (Table 58.1) of 0.87 ($P = .001$).

A threshold of an output of <200 mL within 2 hours was found to have a sensitivity of 87.1% and specificity 84.1% for progression.

Koyner et al.[29] compared the ability of the FST to predict progression of stage 1 or 2 AKI to Stage 3 with biomarkers including neutrophil gelatinase-associated lipocalin (NGAL), insulin-like growth factor-binding protein 7 (IGFBP-7), and tissue inhibitor of metalloproteinases 2 (TIMP-2). The best performing urinary biomarker for progression was NGAL with an area under the curve (AUC) of 0.7560.08 ($P = .007$). The 2-hour urine output response following FST had a significantly improved ability to predict progression to Stage 3 AKI with an AUC ± standard error of the mean of 0.87 ± 0.09 over any other biomarker ($P < .0001$). The discriminatory performance of the FST was improved by selecting a group of patients with high biomarker levels. AUC for progression to Stage 3 increased to 0.90 ± 0.06 and the AUC for receipt of RRT increased to 0.91 ± 0.08.

McMahon et al.[30] demonstrated that FST can predict delayed graft function post kidney transplant. In a pilot study from Thailand, Lumlertgul et al.[31] demonstrated the feasibility of using FST for identifying high-risk patients for randomization into early versus late RRT. Patients who failed FST were randomized to early (<6 hours) or delayed RRT. Only 6/44 (13.6%) FST-responsive patients ultimately received RRT. Of the 118 FST-nonresponsive patients, 98.3% in the early RRT arm and 75% in the standard RRT arm received RRT. There were no differences in 28-day mortality (62.1% versus 58.3%, $P = .68$), 7-day fluid balance, or RRT dependence at Day 28.

The FST appears to be a promising diagnostic tool, albeit with a limited dataset and likely publication bias.

Natriuretic Peptides

The use of natriuretic peptides for the treatment of established AKI has shown some promising results in small clinical studies but negative results in large-scale clinical trials. In a randomized placebo-controlled trial of 61 patients, Swärd et al.[32] studied the use of atrial natriuretic peptide (ANP) in postoperative cardiac surgery patients with AKI (defined as ≥50% increase in serum creatinine from baseline of <1.8 mg/dL) and showed that ANP use was associated with lower rates of RRT than placebo use.[32] It should be noted, however, that this was a small, probably underpowered study of a specific high-risk patient population in which the degree of AKI was modest.[33] The ANP dose was lower in this study than that in comparable negative multicenter trials.[34] No subsequent studies have replicated this result.

Dopamine

In healthy patients, dopamine increases urine output by stimulating the dopamine (D1, D2, and D4) receptors in the kidney. Dopamine also dilates both the efferent and afferent arterioles and increases renal perfusion.[35] However, these effects are uncertain in patients with AKI. Lauschke et al.[35] performed a Doppler ultrasound study of ICU patients with and without AKI. They found a reduction in renal vascular

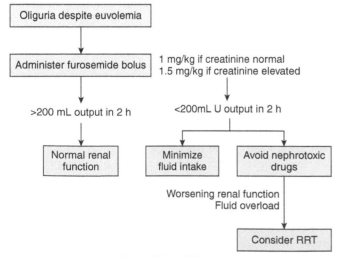

Fig. 58.1 Furosemide Stress Test. *RRT*, renal replacement therapy.

resistance in patients without AKI (median resistive index [RI]/pulsatility index [PI] from 0.70 to 0.65/1.20 to 1.07, $P < .01$) but increased resistance indices in patients with acute renal failure (median RI/PI from 0.77 to 0.81/1.64 to 1.79, $P < .01$).

A low ("renal") dose of dopamine was traditionally believed to have a renoprotective effect, principally as a result of diuresis that follows its administration. The ANZICS Clinical Trials Group performed a randomized, double-blinded, controlled trial that compared a low-dose dopamine infusion (2 μg/kg per minute) with placebo in critically ill patients in 23 different ICUs.[36] There was no difference in the peak serum creatinine, urinary output, RRT requirement, length of ICU stay, or hospital mortality.

De Backer et al.[37] undertook a large multicenter RCT comparing dopamine with norepinephrine as the first-line vasopressor in the treatment of shock. There was no difference in the primary outcome of mortality at 28 days (52.5% in the dopamine group versus 48.5% in the norepinephrine group; $P = .10$). However, the incidence of arrhythmias was significantly higher in the dopamine group (24.1%) than in the norepinephrine group (12.4%; $P < .001$).

Numerous metaanalyses have also shown negative to marginal benefit of dopamine use for renal protection. Friedrich et al.[38] performed a metaanalysis (61 trials with more than 3300 subjects) of the effect of dopamine on renal function, adverse events, or other outcomes. They found that dopamine increased urine output by 24% (95% CI, 14–35%) on Day 1 of use, but there was no identifiable benefit in terms of mortality, development of AKI, or the need for RRT. Following cardiac surgery, the risk for new-onset atrial fibrillation was 74% higher in patients given low-dose dopamine than in controls.[39]

Fenoldopam Mesylate

Fenoldopam mesylate is a benzazepine-derived pure dopaminergic agonist that is approved by the Food and Drug Administration (FDA) for the treatment of severe hypertension. Used intravenously, fenoldopam is a postsynaptic D1 receptor agonist that increases renal blood flow and decreases vascular resistance.[40] Fenoldopam has long been thought to be a superior candidate to low-dose dopamine in preventing and treating AKI because it may increase renal blood flow, perhaps with greater renal medullary vasodilation, without systemic adverse effects of stimulating α- or β-adrenergic receptors.

An Italian multicenter study randomized 667 patients with early AKI following cardiac surgery to either a continuous infusion of fenoldopam or placebo for 4 days.[41] The primary endpoint was the rate of RRT. The trial was stopped early for futility. The investigators found no significant difference: RRT was required in 20% in fenoldopam group and 18% in the placebo group ($P = .47$). The rate of hypotension was significantly greater in the fenoldopam group.

Currently there is no evidence whether low-dose dopamine or fenoldopam has any role in the prevention or treatment of AKI.

Novel Biomarker-Guided Therapy

The diagnosis of AKI remains difficult because of a lack of sensitivity and specificity for conventional markers, such as urea, creatinine, and urinary output. For many years, clinicians have been searching for biomarkers that indicate early kidney injury, with the expectation that some form of intervention or therapy may prevent the need for RRT. The SAPHIRE study, a discovery and then validation project, initially assessed 325 potential biomarkers for diagnosis of early AKI in critically ill patients with at least one KDIGO criterion for AKI.[42] The two best performing biomarkers of AKI were the cell-cycle arrest markers urinary IGFBP-7 and TIMP-2. These progressed to a multicenter validation study ($n = 744$). As IGFBP-7 performed better in surgical patients and TIMP-2 in sepsis, a combination IGFBP-7*TIMP-2 was used. This was found to have an AUC of 0.80 and was commercialized by Astute Medical as the NephroCheck. FDA approval for marketing was secured in 2016 for evaluating the risk of Stage 2 or 3 AKI in critically ill patients within 12 hours of testing.

Although the use of novel biomarkers is encouraging, there are few data to support biomarker-guided therapy, and the cost-benefit ratio has not been established. It is unclear on what basis the SAPHIRE investigators chose the "most promising" biomarkers. Methodology on the analysis of all candidate biomarkers was not provided. An independent study found that the [TIMP-2]·[IGFBP-7] test was affected by comorbidities[43] and a study involving 77 patients found that it did not outperform FST.[41]

Subsequent small interventional clinical studies have assessed whether therapy guided by these biomarkers confers a clinical benefit.[44,45] A single-center trial randomized patients to either a "KDIGO Bundle" of hemodynamic optimization, avoidance of nephrotoxic medications, and prevention of hyperglycemia in patients with a urinary [TIMP-2]·[IGFBP-7] >0.3 scheduled for cardiac surgery.[44] The results showed a significant decrease in KDIGO AKI in the intervention group ($n = 138$) compared with controls ($n = 138$) (55.1% vs. 71.7%; absolute risk reduction 16.6% [95% CI 5.5%–27.9%]; $P = .004$). This trial has some significant limitations including that patients were randomized to a KDIGO care bundle that is recommended as standard of care (Hawthorne effects), the primary outcome is not a patient-centered outcome; there were differences in baseline patient variables, and a large reduction of AKI (65%) was chosen for sample size calculations. It is therefore unclear why this trial required the use of novel biomarkers when a quality improvement study may have been more appropriate.

A similar study in patients after major abdominal surgery did not show any significant difference in the primary outcome of KDIGO AKI in the first 7 days postoperatively (31.7%, 19/60) compared with that in the standard care group (47.5%, 29/61; $P = .076$; OR 1.96; 95% CI 0.93–4.10).

Irrespective of these results, it appears that, while biomarkers may improve and speed up the diagnosis of AKI in perioperative and critical care, in the absence of clear therapeutic interventions, little benefit is likely to arise.

Alkaline Phosphatase

Alkaline phosphatase has been shown to reduce sepsis-associated AKI in animal models.[46] A possible mechanism is the dephosphorylation of bacterial endotoxins. Two small Phase II RCTs showed a reduction in AKI in the groups randomized to alkaline phosphatase.[47]

The STOP-AKI trial was a larger Phase IIa/b, double-blinded, dose-finding RCT ($n = 301$) of recombinant alkaline phosphatase in sepsis-associated AKI. No improvement in daily creatinine clearance or reduction in RRT was reported. It is unclear whether sufficient data exist to progress to a Phase III trial.[48]

CONCLUSION

AKI is known to increase the risk for morbidity and mortality in all patients, particularly in critically ill patients. Numerous therapies have been evaluated for both prevention and treatment. As there are currently no direct therapies, the emphasis remains on prophylaxis.

Rehydration and vasopressor therapy in early sepsis continues to be the mainstay of treatment. Crystalloids are likely safer than colloids; however, the choice of crystalloid fluid remains controversial. The FST appears to be a simple and effective method of identifying patients likely to require RRT. Diuretics and dopamine receptor agonists do not modulate the natural history of AKI. Novel biomarkers may identify AKI at an earlier stage, but without specific therapeutic interventions or treatment strategies, they may not be cost-effective.

ACKNOWLEDGMENTS

We would like to thank Madhav V. Rao and Jay L. Koyner, two of the co-authors of the previous version of this chapter.

AUTHORS' RECOMMENDATIONS

- The morbidity and mortality associated with AKI are significant. Discovery of effective approaches to AKI prevention, early diagnosis, and therapy is imperative, particularly in patients admitted to ICU.
- Intravenous fluid therapy may affect the development of AKI; balanced crystalloids should probably be preferred to isotonic saline. Starch-based colloids should be avoided.
- In the perioperative patient, fluid restriction does not prevent the development of postoperative AKI and may be harmful.
- In sepsis, early antibiotic administration, volume resuscitation, and vasoactive drugs should be used aggressively to maintain renal perfusion in an attempt to prevent or treat AKI.
- The use of diuretics to treat and prevent AKI is not recommended. In many settings, this therapy may increase the likelihood of AKI development. Diuretic-responsive oliguria may be a sign of less severe AKI, but this should not be a treatment goal.

- The FST has a role in identifying whether or not oliguria is consequent of emerging AKI.
- Furosemide has a clear role in the treatment of fluid overload and acute heart failure.
- Neither "renal-dose" dopamine nor fenoldopam should be used for the prevention or treatment of AKI.
- The role of biomarkers in the diagnosis of AKI shows significant promise of questionable value without therapeutic options.

REFERENCES

1. Kellum JA, Sileanu FE, Bihorac A, Hoste EA, Chawla LS. Recovery after acute kidney injury. *Am J Respir Crit Care Med*. 2017; 195(6):784-791.
2. Siew ED, Davenport A. The growth of acute kidney injury: a rising tide or just closer attention to detail? *Kidney Int*. 2015; 87(1):46-61.
3. Silver SA, Chertow GM. The economic consequences of acute kidney injury. *Nephron*. 2017;137(4):297-301.
4. Lewis SR, Pritchard MW, Evans DJ, et al. Colloids versus crystalloids for fluid resuscitation in critically ill people. *Cochrane Database Syst Rev*. 2018;8:CD000567.
5. Kidney disease: improving global outcomes (KDIGO) acute kidney injury work group. KDIGO clinical practice guideline for acute kidney injury. *Kidney Int Suppl*. 2012;2(1):1-138.
6. Young P, Bailey M, Beasley R, et al. Effect of a buffered crystalloid solution vs saline on acute kidney injury among patients in the intensive care unit: the SPLIT randomized clinical trial. *JAMA*. 2015;314(16):1701-1710.
7. Self WH, Semler MW, Wanderer JP, et al. Balanced crystalloids versus saline in noncritically ill adults. *N Engl J Med*. 2018;378:819-828.
8. Semler MW, Self WH, Wanderer JP, et al. Balanced crystalloids versus saline in critically ill adults. *N Engl J Med*. 2018;378: 829-839.
9. Zayed YZM, Aburahma AMY, Barbarawi MO, et al. Balanced crystalloids versus isotonic saline in critically ill patients: systematic review and meta-analysis. *J Intensive Care*. 2018;6:51.
10. Balanced Solution Versus Saline in Intensive Care Study. Available at: https://ClinicalTrials.gov/show/NCT02875873. Accessed February 26, 2019.
11. Comparison of Plasmalyte 148® and Saline for Fluid Resuscitation and Intravenous Fluid Therapy in Critically Ill Adults. Available at: https://ClinicalTrials.gov/show/NCT02721654. Accessed February 26, 2019.
12. Dellinger RP, Carlet JM, Masur H, et al. Surviving Sepsis Campaign guidelines for management of severe sepsis and septic shock. *Crit Care Med*. 2004;32(3):858-873.
13. Rivers E, Nguyen B, Havstad S, et al. Early goal-directed therapy in the treatment of severe sepsis and septic shock. *N Engl J Med*. 2001;345(19):1368-1377.
14. Mouncey PR, Osborn TM, Power GS, et al. Trial of early, goal-directed resuscitation for septic shock. *N Engl J Med*. 2015; 372(14):1301-1311.
15. Yealy DM, Kellum JA, Huang DT, et al. A randomized trial of protocol-based care for early septic shock. *N Engl J Med*. 2014; 370(18):1683-1693.

16. Peake SL, Delaney A, Bailey M, et al. Goal-directed resuscitation for patients with early septic shock. *N Engl J Med.* 2014;371(16): 1496-1506.

17. PRISM Investigators, Rowan KM, Angus DC, et al. Early, goal-directed therapy for septic shock—a patient-level meta-analysis. *N Engl J Med.* 2017;376(23):2223-2234.

18. Asfar P, Meziani F, Hamel JF, et al. High versus low blood-pressure target in patients with septic shock. *N Engl J Med.* 2014;370(17):1583-1593.

19. Rhodes A, Evans LE, Alhazzani W, et al. Surviving Sepsis Campaign: international guidelines for management of sepsis and septic shock: 2016. *Intensive Care Med.* 2017;43(3):304-377.

20. Salahuddin N, Sammani M, Hamdan A, et al. Fluid overload is an independent risk factor for acute kidney injury in critically Ill patients: results of a cohort study. *BMC Nephrol.* 2017; 18(1):45.

21. Haase-Fielitz A, Haase M, Bellomo R, et al. Perioperative hemodynamic instability and fluid overload are associated with increasing acute kidney injury severity and worse outcome after cardiac surgery. *Blood Purif.* 2017;43(4):298-308.

22. Brandstrup B, Tønnesen H, Beier-Holgersen R, et al. Effects of intravenous fluid restriction on postoperative complications: comparison of two perioperative fluid regimens: a randomized assessor-blinded multicenter trial. *Ann Surg.* 2003;238(5):641-648.

23. Nisanevich V, Felsenstein I, Almogy G, Weissman C, Einav S, Matot I. Effect of intraoperative fluid management on outcome after intraabdominal surgery. *Anesthesiology.* 2005;103(1):25-32.

24. Boland MR, Noorani A, Varty K, Coffey JC, Agha R, Walsh SR. Perioperative fluid restriction in major abdominal surgery: systematic review and meta-analysis of randomized, clinical trials. *World J Surg.* 2013;37(6):1193-1202.

25. Myles PS, Bellomo R, Corcoran T, et al. Restrictive versus liberal fluid therapy for major abdominal surgery. *N Engl J Med.* 2018; 378(24):2263-2274.

26. Ho KM, Sheridan DJ. Meta-analysis of frusemide to prevent or treat acute renal failure. *BMJ.* 2006;333(7565):420.

27. Bove T, Belletti A, Putzu A, et al. Intermittent furosemide administration in patients with or at risk for acute kidney injury: meta-analysis of randomized trials. *PLoS One.* 2018;13(4):e0196088.

28. Chawla LS, Davison DL, Brasha-Mitchell E, et al. Development and standardization of a furosemide stress test to predict the severity of acute kidney injury. *Crit Care.* 2013;17(5):R207.

29. Koyner JL, Davison DL, Brasha-Mitchell E, et al. Furosemide stress test and biomarkers for the prediction of AKI severity. *J Am Soc Nephrol.* 2015;26(8):2023-2031.

30. McMahon BA, Koyner JL, Novick T, et al. The prognostic value of the furosemide stress test in predicting delayed graft function following deceased donor kidney transplantation. *Biomarkers.* 2018;23(1):61-69.

31. Lumlertgul N, Peerapornratana S, Trakarnvanich T, et al. Early versus standard initiation of renal replacement therapy in furosemide stress test non-responsive acute kidney injury patients (the FST trial). *Crit Care.* 2018;22(1):101.

32. Swärd K, Valsson F, Odencrants P, Samuelsson O, Ricksten SE. Recombinant human atrial natriuretic peptide in ischemic acute renal failure: a randomized placebo-controlled trial. *Crit Care Med.* 2004;32(6):1310-1315.

33. Allgren RL, Marbury TC, Rahman SN, et al. Anaritide in acute tubular necrosis. Auriculin Anaritide Acute Renal Failure Study Group. *N Engl J Med.* 1997;336(12):828-834.

34. Lewis J, Salem MM, Chertow GM, et al. Atrial natriuretic factor in oliguric acute renal failure. Anaritide Acute Renal Failure Study Group. *Am J Kidney Dis.* 2000;36(4):767-774.

35. Lauschke A, Teichgräber UK, Frei U, Eckardt KU. 'Low-dose' dopamine worsens renal perfusion in patients with acute renal failure. *Kidney Int.* 2006;69(9):1669-1674.

36. Bellomo R, Chapman M, Finfer S, Hickling K, Myburgh J. Low-dose dopamine in patients with early renal dysfunction: a placebo-controlled randomised trial. Australian and New Zealand Intensive Care Society (ANZICS) Clinical Trials Group. *Lancet.* 2000;356(9248):2139-2143.

37. De Backer D, Biston P, Devriendt J, et al. Comparison of dopamine and norepinephrine in the treatment of shock. *N Engl J Med.* 2010;362(9):779-789.

38. Friedrich JO, Adhikari N, Herridge MS, Beyene J. Meta-analysis: low-dose dopamine increases urine output but does not prevent renal dysfunction or death. *Ann Intern Med.* 2005;142(7):510-524.

39. Argalious M, Motta P, Khandwala F, et al. "Renal dose" dopamine is associated with the risk of new-onset atrial fibrillation after cardiac surgery. *Crit Care Med.* 2005;33(6):1327-1332.

40. Morelli A, Ricci Z, Bellomo R, et al. Prophylactic fenoldopam for renal protection in sepsis: a randomized, double-blind, placebo-controlled pilot trial. *Crit Care Med.* 2005;33(11): 2451-2456.

41. Bove T, Zangrillo A, Guarracino F, et al. Effect of fenoldopam on use of renal replacement therapy among patients with acute kidney injury after cardiac surgery: a randomized clinical trial. *JAMA.* 2014;312(21):2244-2253.

42. Kashani K, Al-Khafaji A, Ardiles T, et al. Discovery and validation of cell cycle arrest biomarkers in human acute kidney injury. *Crit Care.* 2013;17(1):R25.

43. Bell M, Larsson A, Venge P, Bellomo R, Mårtensson J. Assessment of cell-cycle arrest biomarkers to predict early and delayed acute kidney injury. *Dis Markers.* 2015;2015:158658.

44. Meersch M, Schmidt C, Hoffmeier A, et al. Prevention of cardiac surgery-associated AKI by implementing the KDIGO guidelines in high risk patients identified by biomarkers: the PrevAKI randomized controlled trial. *Intensive Care Med.* 2017;43(11):1551-1561.

45. Göcze I, Jauch D, Götz M, et al. Biomarker-guided intervention to prevent acute kidney injury after major surgery: the prospective randomized BigpAK study. *Ann Surg.* 2018;267(6):1013-1020.

46. Peters E, Masereeuw R, Pickkers P. The potential of alkaline phosphatase as a treatment for sepsis-associated acute kidney injury. *Nephron Clin Pract.* 2014;127(1-4):144-148.

47. Heemskerk S, Masereeuw R, Moesker O, et al. Alkaline phosphatase treatment improves renal function in severe sepsis or septic shock patients. *Crit Care Med.* 2009;37(2): 417-423, e1.

48. Pickkers P, Mehta RL, Murray PT, et al. Effect of human recombinant alkaline phosphatase on 7-day creatinine clearance in patients with sepsis-associated acute kidney injury: a randomized clinical trial. *JAMA.* 2018;320(19):1998-2009.

59

How Should Acid-Base Disorders Be Diagnosed?

Patrick J. Neligan

INTRODUCTION

Alterations in the hydrogen ion content of blood and extracellular fluid accompany acute illness; analysis of these processes is known as "acid-base balance" or "acid-base chemistry." The presence of acidosis or alkalosis has been, and will remain, one of the most robust biomarkers of illness severity. Each clinician will typically use an arsenal of tools to identify acid-base abnormalities, some of which are quite dated.[1] This chapter will summarize the current thinking about acid-base balance, the diagnostic tools that are available and the clinical relevance of the diagnoses.

SCIENTIFIC BACKGROUND

What Is an Acid? What Is a Base?

The human body is made up principally of water. Water is a highly ionizing solution, on account of its high dielectric constant, so substances with polar bonds will dissociate into their component parts in it. Various salts are dissolved in both intracellular and extracellular water, and these impart an electrical charge that must be balanced. The positive charges and the negative charges must be equal (the law of electrical neutrality). Various definitions of acids and bases exist. Svante Arrhenius (1859–1927) in 1903 defined that, in an aqueous solution, an acid is any substance that delivers a hydrogen ion into the solution.[2] A base is any substance that delivers a hydroxyl ion into the solution. Thus hydrogen chloride (HCl) is an acid and potassium hydroxide (KOH) is a base. In 1923 Brønsted and Lowry proposed an expanded definition. They defined acids as proton donors and bases as proton acceptors. All Arrhenius acids and bases were thus also Brønsted-Lowry acids and bases, but the refined theory accounted for some outlier chemicals, such as carbon dioxide and ammonia.

Acid-Base Balance

The normal hydrogen ion concentration $[H^+]$ of arterial blood is 40 nEq/L. The pH scale, the negative logarithm of the $[H^+]$, was developed by Sorenson in Copenhagen in 1909 and is universally used in medicine and chemistry (Table 59.1). The normal pH of arterial blood is 7.4.

Early in the 20th century, Henderson and Hasselbalch, coined the term "acid-base balance" (ABB) and described extracellular pH in terms of the hydration equation for carbon dioxide. This is known as the Henderson Hasselbalch equation (HHE) (Box 59.1).

Combining the pH scale and the HHE into a tool for clinical practice only became possible with the development of volumetric CO_2 analysis by Van Slyke and others in 1919.[3] This led to 60 years of research and interest in CO_2 and its derivative, bicarbonate, as the principle agents that impact acid-base chemistry.[4] Although it was known in the 1920s that alterations in serum electrolytes impacted ABB, this was not introduced in to clinical practice until the 1970s.[5] Computerization in the early 1980s further enhanced our understanding of ABB and the precision of diagnosis.[6]

Physiologic pH, that is the pH of extracellular fluid, is kept tightly within the window 7.35–7.45 by various homeostatic mechanisms. Conventionally, if the pH is below 7.35, a state of acidosis exists. If the pH is above 7.45, a state of alkalosis exists. Some authors refer to acidemia and alkalemia when referring to low or high blood pH; and the process by which this occurs is known as acidosis and alkalosis. Importantly, pH may be within the normal range despite significant acidosis or alkalosis due to buffering and "compensation."[7]

Strong Ions and Weak Acids

The degree of dissociation of substances, such as salts or proteins, in water determines whether they are strong acids or strong bases. This designation is governed by the ion dissociation constant—pKa. The lower the pKa, the stronger the acid; the higher the pKa, the stronger the base. Lactic acid, pKa of 3.4, is completely dissociated at physiologic pH, and is a strong acid. Lactate is a strong anion; it exists unbound at all ECF pH levels. Sodium, potassium, magnesium and chloride are also strong ions. The difference in charge imparted

TABLE 59.1 Hydrogen Ion Concentration Versus pH.

$[H^+]$ nEq/L	pH
8	7.7
16	7.62
24	7.56
32	7.48
40	7.4
48	7.32
56	7.24
64	7.16
72	7.08
80	7.0
88	6.92

BOX 59.1 The Henderson Hasselbalch Equation.

Equation 1: $pH = 6.1 + \log ([HCO_3^-]/PaCO_2 \times 0.03)$
where 6.1 refers to the pKa of H_2CO_3 and HCO_3^- is in mEq/L and CO_2 is in mm Hg
This can also be expressed as:
Equation 2: $[H^+] = 24 \times PaCO_2/[HCO_3^-]$
So, if the $PaCO_2$ is 40 mm Hg and the HCO_3^- is 24 mEq/L, the pH = 7.4 and the $[H^+]$ is 40 nEq/L
If the $PaCO_2$ is 60 mm Hg and the HCO_3^- is 26 mEq/L, the pH = 7.26 and the $[H^+]$ is 56 nEq/L
If the $PaCO_2$ is 30 mm Hg and the HCO_3^- is 22 mEq/L, the pH = 7.52 and the $[H^+]$ is 32 nEq/L

by strong cations minus strong anions is the strong ion difference (SID); it is typically 40-44 mEq/L.[6]

$$SID = ([Na^+] + [K^+] + [Ca^{2+}] + [Mg^{2+}]) - ([Cl^-] + [\text{Other strong anions: } A^-]) = 40\text{–}44\ mEq$$

Because each strong anion is associated with a hydrogen ion, and each strong cation is associated with a hydroxyl ion, a reduction in the SID is associated with an increase in $[H^+]$ and acidosis. An increase in the SID is associated with a decrease in $[H^+]$ (and an increase in $[OH^-]$), that is, alkalosis. For example, in the equation above, an increase in $[Cl^-]$ relative to the $[\text{cations}^+]$ reduces SID and results in ("hyperchloremic") acidosis. When SID falls and the cause is not apparent within the equation, then acidosis is caused by "unmeasured anions" (UMA), such as ketones or metabolic byproducts that accumulate in acute kidney injury.

Carbonic acid, which has a pKa of 6.4, is incompletely dissociated and is a weak acid. The charge carried by nonvolatile weak acids, such as PO_4^{2-} and albumin, when combined, is known as A_{TOT}.[8] The sum of A_{TOT} and $[HCO_3^-]$ (in mEq/L) is often referred to as "buffer base (BB)," owing to the buffering capabilities of weak acids. BB approximates the SID and is sometimes known as SIDe (effective). A reduction in A_{TOT} is associated with alkalosis.[9]

By convention, acid-base abnormalities associated with changes in SID or A_{TOT} are known as *metabolic* acid-base disorders (Table 59.2). Decreased SID or increased A_{TOT} causes metabolic acidosis. Increased SID or decreased A_{TOT} causes metabolic alkalosis (see Table 59.2).

Carbon Dioxide

Aerobic metabolism results in the production of large quantities of carbon dioxide (CO_2). CO_2 is hydrated by carbonic anhydrase in erythrocytes to carbonic acid. This process liberates the equivalent of 12,500 mEq of H^+ per day. Hydrogen ions bind to histidine residues on deoxyhemoglobin and bicarbonate is actively pumped out of the cell. All carbon dioxide (total CO_2) in the body exists in one of four forms: dissolved carbon dioxide [denoted $CO_2(d)$], carbonic acid (H_2CO_3), bicarbonate ions (HCO_3^-) and carbonate ions (CO_3^{2-}).

$PaCO_2$ is kept constant at approximately 40 mmHg (5.3 kPa) by various homeostatic mechanisms, principally triggering the respiratory center by alterations in cerebrospinal fluid $[H^+]$. A significantly smaller proportion of CO_2 is excreted from the kidney as HCO_3^- as part of a sodium-chloride co-transporter.

By convention, acid-base disorders associated with carbon dioxide handling, usually occurring due to respiratory failure, are known as *respiratory* acid-base disorders. An elevation in $PaCO_2$ associated with pH of <7.35 is known as respiratory acidosis, which may be acute or chronic, depending on the $[HCO_3^-]$ (Table 59.3). Respiratory failure is associated with an increase in total body CO_2 content, reflected principally by an increase in $[HCO_3^-]$. A reduction in $PaCO_2$ associated with pH of >7.45 is known as respiratory alkalosis and is associated with disease processes that increase respiratory drive (see Table 59.2).

To maintain homeostasis, electrical neutrality must be preserved, mass conserved and dissociation equilibria for all partially dissociated compounds must be obeyed.[8] Hence, alterations in SID result in changes in the CO_2/HCO_3^- axis, and vice versa. For example, a fall in SID (metabolic acidosis) results in a reduction of almost equal magnitude in the $[HCO_3^-]$ and a reduction in $PaCO_2$ secondary to increased alveolar ventilation. The opposite occurs when SID increases (metabolic alkalosis). When CO_2/HCO_3^- accumulates in acute respiratory failure (acute respiratory acidosis), SID increases in almost equal magnitude to the increase in $[HCO_3^-]$.

In the next section we will explore the various types of acid-base abnormalities commonly encountered in critical care.

Acid-Base Disorders
Respiratory Alkalosis

The normal partial pressure of carbon dioxide in arterial blood is 40 mm Hg (5.3 kPa). Respiratory alkalosis occurs when there is an acute decrease in $PaCO_2$, due to hyperventilation—self-induced secondary to pain, anxiety or agitation or externally induced due to poorly monitored mechanical ventilation. Acute respiratory alkalosis is characterized by a pH >7.45, a low $PaCO_2$ and a low $[HCO_3^-]$. A simple rule of thumb for this reaction can be seen in Box 59.2.

TABLE 59.2   Classification of Acid-Base Abnormalities.

	Acidosis	Alkalosis
Respiratory	Increased $PACO_2$	Decreased $PACO_2$ $\uparrow SID^+ + \downarrow [Cl^-]$
Metabolic **1. Abnormal SID^+**		
a. **due to water**	Water excess = dilution $\downarrow SID^+ \downarrow [Na+]$	Water deficit = contraction $\uparrow SID^+ \uparrow [Na+]$
b. **due to electrolytes** Chloride (measured)	Chloride excess $\downarrow SID^+ \uparrow [Cl^-]$	Chloride deficit $\uparrow SID^+ + \downarrow [Cl^-]$
Others (unmeasured anions) e.g., lactate, keto acids	$\downarrow SID^+ \downarrow [A^-]$	-
2. Abnormal A_{TOT}		
a. Albumin [Alb]	$\uparrow [Alb^-]$ (intravenous albumin)	$\downarrow [Alb^-]$
b. Phosphate [Pi]	$\uparrow [Pi^-]$	$\downarrow [Pi^-]$

TABLE 59.3   Changes in Bicarbonate and $PaCO_2$ in Acute Hypercarbia.

[H⁺] nEq/L (Approx)	pH	Bicarbonate HCO_3^- mEq/L or mmol/L	PACO₂ IN ACUTE RESPIRATORY FAILURE PaCO₂ mm Hg	PaCO₂ kPa
40	7.4	24	40	5.3
48	7.32	25	50	6.6
56	7.24	26	60	8.0
64	7.16	27	70	9.3
72	7.08	28	80	10.5
80	7.0	29	90	11.8
88	6.92	30	100	13

Note for every 10 mm Hg increase in $PaCO_2$, the H⁺ increases by 8 nEq/L, the pH falls by 0.08 units and the HCO_3^- increases by 1 mEq/L—these data are less accurate below pH 7.1

BOX 59.2   Acute Respiratory Alkalosis.

Acute Respiratory Alkalosis: ΔHCO_3^- mEq/L $= 0.2 \, \Delta PaCO_2$ (in mm Hg)

So, if a patient has a normal baseline $PaCO_2$ (40 mm Hg) and a normal baseline $[HCO_3^-]$ (24 mEq/L), then if the patient hyperventilates to $PaCO_2$ of 30 mm Hg, the $[HCO_3^-]$ falls to 22 mEq/L.

BOX 59.3   Acute Respiratory Acidosis: Relationship Between [H⁺], PH, $PaCO_2$ and HCO_3^-.[7,10]

- ΔH^+ (nEq/L) $= 0.8 \, (\Delta PaCO_2)$
- At pH 7.4 the estimated [H⁺] is 40 nm/L.
- For every 1 nEq/L increase in [H⁺] there is a 0.01 unit fall in pH
- pH falls by 0.08 for every 10 mm Hg (1.3 kPa) rise in $PaCO_2$.
  So, if $PaCO_2$ increases from 40 mm Hg (5.3kPa) to 60 mm Hg (8 kPa), [H⁺] increases to 56 nEq/L and pH falls to 7.24 (see Table 59.3)
- An increase in $PaCO_2$ by 10 mm Hg (1.3 kPa) results in an increase in $[HCO_3^-]$ by 1 mmol/L (1 mEq/L)
  So, in this scenario, a rise in $PaCO_2$ by 20 mm Hg (kPa) to 60 mm Hg (8 kPa) is associated with an increase in $[HCO_3^-]$ to 26 mEq/L (see Table 59.3)

Acute respiratory alkalosis usually accompanies acute metabolic acidosis ("compensation"), where the fall in $PaCO_2$ and $[HCO_3^-]$ can be predicted (see the following section).

Respiratory Acidosis

Respiratory acidosis occurs when there is an acute rise in $PaCO_2$ usually associated with respiratory failure. There is a rapid increase in [H⁺] (Box 59.3).

Compensation for hypercarbia is slow and pH falls rapidly. There is a concomitant increase in the serum bicarbonate $[HCO_3^-]$, reflecting a higher total CO_2 load. Brackett, Cohen and Schwartz, in the mid-1960s elegantly described the relative changes in $[HCO_3^-]$ in response to acute and chronic elevations in $PaCO_2$, providing us with extremely useful "rules of thumb:"[10]

In acute hypercarbia, the bicarbonate concentration of plasma rises slowly—by 1 mEq/L for every 10 mm Hg rise in $PaCO_2$ (see Table 59.3).

In chronic respiratory failure, the total carbon dioxide load in the body increases substantially, reflected by relatively high levels of plasma bicarbonate. There is a concomitant fall in serum chloride, reflecting compensation for elevated levels of carbonic acid.[11]

In chronic respiratory acidosis, there is a significantly higher plasma $[HCO_3^-]$ level (Box 59.4 and Table 59.4), but usually a normal range pH. The calculation in Box 59.4 is a very useful practical tool for clinicians planning mechanical ventilation targeted to normalization of blood gases, for example, during acute exacerbation of COPD. From a baseline total CO_2, $[HCO_3^-]$ can be used to target minute ventilation (see Table 59.4). In ARDS (acute respiratory distress syndrome), there is general consensus amongst intensivists that aggressive mechanical ventilation to normalize pH and $PaCO_2$ is more harmful than "permissive" hypercapnia. Restoration of relatively normal pH in this setting is complex, but is associated with a reduction in SID, strong ion gap (see following section), A_{TOT}.[12]

METABOLIC ACID-BASE ABNORMALITIES

Acute Metabolic Acidosis

Acute metabolic acidosis is caused by an alteration in SID or A_{TOT}. SID falls due to a relative increase in strong anions versus strong cations; strong anion gain or strong cation loss. This is associated with a fall in $[HCO_3^-]$, and various analytic systems use this change to interpret severity and infer cause.[13]

BOX 59.4   Prolonged Respiratory Failure—Relationship Between $PaCO_2$ and Plasma $[HCO_3^-]$.[7]

- An increase in $PaCO_2$ by 10 mm Hg (1.3 kPa) will increase plasma $[HCO_3^-]$ by 3 mmol/L (3 mEq/L)
  So if a patient is chronically hypercarbic, for example to a $PaCO_2$ of 60 mm Hg (8 kPa), the $[HCO_3^-]$ will increase to 30 mEq/L and the pH is expected to be in the normal range (see Table 59.4).

TABLE 59.4   Changes in Bicarbonate and $PaCO_2$ in Chronic Hypercarbia.

Bicarbonate	PACO₂ IN CHRONIC RESPIRATORY FAILURE	
HCO_3^- mEq/L or mmol/L	$PaCO_2$ 10 mm Hg	$PaCO_2$ kPa
24	40	5.3
27	50	6.6
30	60	8.0
33	70	9.3
36	80	10.5
39	90	11.8
42	100	13.0

In metabolic acidosis, anions, mineral or organic, can be gained, as occurs with lactic-, renal-, keto- and hyperchloremic acidosis, or cations can be lost, as occurs with severe diarrhea or renal tubular acidosis. Acute metabolic acidosis is characterized by a pH of <7.35 and a fall in both $PaCO_2$ and $[HCO_3^-]$ below the patients' baseline. For patients without COPD or chronic CO_2 retention, this represents a $PaCO_2$ <40 mm Hg (5.3 kPa) and a $[HCO_3^-]$ below 24 mEq/L (mmol/L); there is a negative base excess (base deficit) whose magnitude represents the net strong anion gain.

TYPES OF METABOLIC ACIDOSIS

Lactic Acidosis

Lactic acid (lactate) is a degradation product of glucose metabolism. It exists as two isoforms, L-lactate, which is produced by the human body and is measured by blood gas analyzers, and D-lactate, which can only be produced by fermentation by bacteria. The formation of L-lactate from pyruvate is catalyzed by lactate dehydrogenase. Lactate is used in isotonic fluids (lactated Ringers' solution and Hartmann's solution); these contain a racemic mixture of both D and L lactate at a concentration of 14 mmol/L each.

Lactate production increases dramatically under anaerobic conditions, such as vigorous exercise, usually interpreted as evidence of increased glycolytic activity. However, in clinical medicine, lactate is often produced under aerobic conditions. Activation of beta-adrenergic receptors in skeletal muscle by stress (increased circulating catecholamines) or exogenous epinephrine infusions increases lactate, resulting in aerobic glycolysis. Lactate is metabolized to pyruvate and then into glucose (gluconeogenesis) in the liver and subsequently to CO_2 and H_2O (the Cori cycle) and HCO_3^-.

The presence of lactic acidosis is an excellent marker of acute critical illness, the magnitude of which often reflects the degree of hyperlactatemia.[14] Hyperlactatemia occurs when the production of lactate in the body is greater than the liver's capacity to clear it: there is a problem of over production or inadequate clearance. Persistence of acidosis associated with hyperlactatemia strongly predicts poor outcomes in acute illness.[15] Rapid clearance (i.e., reduced plasma concentration presumably due to reduced production and increased metabolism) of lactate has been associated with improved outcomes.[16,17]

Serum lactate and arterial pH should be measured early in any critically ill patient. A lactate concentration >2 mEq/L (mmol/L) is clinically significant and a level of 5 mEql/L (mmol/L) in the presence of metabolic acidosis is severe. Isolated hyperlactatemia in the absence of acidosis is of unclear clinical significance.[18] Epinephrine infusions increase serum lactate, diminishing its utility in assessing severity of illness and predicting outcomes.[19]

The presence of evidence of good overall oxygen delivery and normal consumption, as measured by cardiac output monitors and mixed venous oxygen saturation, in lactic acidosis is not reassuring. Indeed, unexplained lactic acidosis may be the only clinical indicator of bowel ischemia.

Hyperlactatemia is now universally recognized as a marker of severity of illness, and is used as a screening tool, for example as a component of the surviving sepsis guidelines.[20] However, misunderstanding of the elements of lactate production and metabolism in stress scenarios may result in inappropriate therapies, such as large volume fluid resuscitation.[21]

Metformin is associated with severe lactic acidosis, a phenomenon that appears more likely when the patient has liver dysfunction, is dehydrated, in heart failure or acute kidney injury or is septic.[22]

D-lactate induced acidosis can occur in patients with short bowel syndrome with bacterial overgrowth.[23] It manifests as a widened anion gap acidosis (see the following section) where no other potential source of metabolic acid is identified. Crucially, point of care blood gas analyzers do not measure D-lactate. However, many labs are able to measure the molecule, and this test should be considered in a high risk patient (e.g., post major abdominal surgery) with unexplained acidosis.

Ketoacidosis

Ketone bodies—acetone (<2%), acetoacetate (20%) and 3-beta-hydroxybutyrate (βOHB) (78%) are normal byproducts of fat metabolism. In situations where fat becomes the primary source of energy (for example in starvation or low carbohydrate diets), ketones can be measured in blood (principally βOHB) and urine (principally acetoacetate). Severe ketosis occurs in a variety of clinical situations, such as prolonged starvation, alcoholism, alcoholic or obesity related steatohepatitis and, most commonly, insulin deficiency (diabetes mellitus). As these are strong anionic compounds, ketones reduce SID, resulting in metabolic acidosis. When this occurs in type-1 diabetes (T1D), it is known as diabetic ketoacidosis (DKA).

DKA may be the first manifestation of T1D, or may result from poor glycemic control or specific stress triggers such as infection, trauma or surgery. Typically there is an imbalance between the relative quantity of insulin and gluconeogenic hormones—cortisol, epinephrine and glucagon. Blood glucose increases—exceeding the renal reabsorption threshold—and induces glycosuria, osmotic diuresis, dehydration and the vicious cycle of activation of stress hormones. There is increased metabolism of fatty acids and, in the absence of insulin or consequent of severe insulin resistance, there is unrestrained oxidation of fatty acids to ketones in the liver. Regardless of the cause, there is usually elevated blood glucose, significant dehydration, and depletion of potassium, phosphate and magnesium.

The diagnosis of DKA is relatively simple—usually there is a clear history of either diabetes or polyuria and polydipsia: the patient presents to the emergency room with hyperglycemia and glycosuria, and, usually, positive urinary ketones. Ketoacidosis is confirmed by performing arterial blood gas analysis.

It is important to measure blood ketones in any patient with unexplained metabolic acidosis. The majority of ketones in the body are in the form of βOHB. These can only be identified by measuring "blood" ketones (reported in mmol/L). Urinary ketone sticks measure only acetoacetate.[24] The absence of ketones in the urine does not eliminate the diagnosis of ketoacidosis (particularly if it is not associated with diabetes).

Acidosis in Acute Kidney Injury (Renal Acidosis)

The kidney excretes water, a variety of metabolic byproducts of protein metabolism and surplus electrolytes (SE), some of which are strong ions. These include chloride, sulfate, formate, urate citric acid cycle metabolites (fumarate, citrate), and phosphate. SEs accumulate in acute kidney injury (AKI) and cause "renal acidosis," due to reduced SID. Early in AKI, hyperchloremia is the principle source of acidosis, and this may occur before a rise in blood urea nitrogen (BUN) and/or creatinine becomes apparent. Subsequently, 50%−60% of acidosis is caused by unmeasured anions and up to 30% is associated with hyperphosphatemia.[25] Currently, no tests are available to clinically identify the unmeasured anions except by a process of exclusion. Hence renal acidosis is usually diagnosed by identifying a widened anion gap, base deficit gap or strong ion gap (see later section), and excluding ketones and lactate.

Continuous renal replacement therapy (CRRT) resolves the acidosis of acute kidney injury by removing strong ions and phosphate.[26] However, metabolic alkalosis manifests as a result of hypoalbuminemia. CRRT is not a recognized treatment for lactic acidosis and lactate clearance by CRRT is poor.[27]

Hyperchloremic Acidosis

Hyperchloremia has been a known cause of metabolic acidosis since the dawn of acid-base chemistry[28] but, due to difficulty in measuring serum Cl$^-$ during most of the 20th century, it was largely ignored until recent decades. Hyperchloremia occurs in AKI, following administration of hyperchloremic (relative to plasma) solutions, particularly 0.9% NaCl,[29] following administration of acetazolamide, in renal tubular acidosis, and when ureters have been re-implanted in the bowel. Hyperchloremia is frequently the cause of the early metabolic acidosis associated with AKI.

Acquired hyperchloremia, associated with reduced SID, consequent of excess chloride administration, is believed to worsen perioperative and critical care outcomes and cause renal injury. Compared with balanced salt solutions (BSS) in a large cohort of surgical patients, patients receiving NS had significantly worse outcomes.[30] These complications included postoperative infections, blood transfusions and kidney injury requiring dialysis. In a relatively large before-and-after cohort study of patients treated in an Australian ICU, the use of chloride-rich fluids was associated with a 3.7% absolute increase in the risk for need in renal replacement therapy relative to balanced salt solution.[31]

Two large randomized controlled trials looked at the use of isotonic saline solution versus BSS in emergency medicine[32] and critically ill patients.[33] Although the volume of fluid administered intravenously was relatively low, certainly in comparison with perioperative patients, in both studies there was approximately a 1% increase in renal complications.

Metabolic Alkalosis

Metabolic alkalosis is associated with increased SID, due to sodium gain, free water loss (contraction alkalosis), chloride loss (chloride "sensitive" alkalosis) or reduced A_{TOT}, principally hypoalbuminemia. The latter is the single most common acid-base chemistry in critical illness.[34] Hypoalbuminemia may mask significant alterations in SID, for example, lactic or renal acidosis.

Hypochloremic metabolic alkalosis may result directly from upper gastrointestinal fluid loss and from administration of chloride-free fluids, such as sodium bicarbonate or sodium citrate. During prolonged respiratory failure, with associated hypercarbia, the body compensates by wasting chloride in the urine—combined respiratory acidosis and hypochloremia alkalosis.[35] A sudden increase in alveolar ventilation may manifest as acute metabolic alkalosis, due to normalization of $PaCO_2$. Loss of water from the body, due to dehydration, polyuria (AKI) or loop diuretic therapy causes an increase in SID and metabolic ("contraction") alkalosis.

Carbonic anhydrase inhibitors such as acetazolamide may be used to treat patients with hypochloremic metabolic alkalosis or respiratory alkalosis by decreasing the serum SID. This effect is explained by the increased renal excretion ratio of sodium to chloride, resulting in an increase in serum chloride.[36]

Analytic Tools Used in Acid-Base Chemistry

This section will consider some of the tools that have evolved over the past 70 years to assist our interpretation of acid-base conundrums. None are entirely accurate, though each has a dedicated group of followers that are not entirely consistent with one another.[37] The approaches can be described as descriptive, based on changes in the Henderson-Hasselbalch equation, semi-quantitative, based on calculations and nomograms, or quantitative, based on physical chemistry.

THE DESCRIPTIVE CO₂-BICARBONATE (BOSTON) APPROACH

Schwartz, Brackett, Relman and colleagues at Tufts University in Boston developed the most popular descriptive approach to acid-base chemistry in the 1960s. Their formulation uses acid-base maps and the mathematical relationship between carbon dioxide tension and serum bicarbonate (or total CO_2), derived from the Henderson-Hasselbalch equation, to classify acid-base disturbances in terms of two independent variables: $PaCO_2$ and $[HCO_3^-]$.[38,10] They described six primary states of acid-base imbalance. For any given acid-base disturbance, an expected HCO_3^- concentration was determined. These were subsequently compiled into a series of mathematical rules (Box 59.5).

BOX 59.5   The Descriptive (CO_2-HCO_3) Approach to Acid-Base.

RESPIRATORY DISORDERS
Acute Respiratory Acidosis
Expected $[HCO_3^-] = 24 + [(\text{measured } PaCO_2 - 40) / 10]$
Chronic Respiratory Acidosis
Expected $[HCO_3^-] = 24 + 4 [(\text{measured } PaCO_2 - 40) / 10]$
Acute Respiratory Alkalosis
Expected $[HCO_3^-] = 24 - 2 [(40 - \text{measured } PaCO_2) / 10]$
Chronic Respiratory Alkalosis
Expected $[HCO_3^-]] = 24 - 5 [(40 - \text{measured } PaCO_2) / 10]$
    (range: +/– 2)

METABOLIC DISORDERS
Metabolic Acidosis
Expected $PaCO_2 = 1.5 \times [HCO_3^-] + 8$ (range: +/– 2)
Metabolic Alkalosis
Expected $PaCO_2 = 0.7 [HCO_3^-] + 20$ (range: +/– 5)

In acute metabolic acidosis, the $[HCO_3^-]$ falls by 1 mEq/L for every 1 mEq/L increase in strong anions. The respiratory center is activated, resulting in a predictable fall in the $PaCO_2$. This response was neatly characterized by Winters, in a pediatric population in 1967, and remains robust.[39] In acute metabolic acidosis, the $PaCO_2$ (in mm Hg) $= 1.5 \times [HCO_3^-]$ plus 8 rule (Box 59.6). Winters also described expected compensation using the base excess approach (see the next section): for every 1 mEq/L reduction in the base excess the $PaCO_2$ is expected to fall by 1 mm Hg—otherwise "compensation" is inadequate (see Box 59.3).

In metabolic alkalosis, in order to restore pH to homeostatic levels, it is necessary to retain carbonic acid and hypoventilation occurs, ultimately resulting in increased $[HCO_3^-]$. The expected $PaCO_2$ equals $0.7 \times [HCO_3^-] + 20$ (in mm Hg) (see Box 59.5). So if a patient has a $[HCO_3^-]$ of 34 mEq/L (mmol/L), then the $PaCO_2$ should be 44 mm Hg.

Using these maps and equations and rules, physicians can determine the nature of most respiratory and metabolic acid-base disturbances in a manner that is usually accurate. Although there is a mathematical relationship in place, alterations in $[H^+]$ and $[HCO_3^-]$ do not reflect cause and effect.

BOX 59.6   Winters' Formula for Prediction of $PaCO_2$ in Metabolic Acidosis.

- $PaCO_2$ (in mm Hg) $= 1.5 \times [HCO_3^-]$ plus 8
  For example, if the $[HCO_3^-]$ is 12 mmol/L (mEq/L), then the expected $PaCO_2$ is $1.5 \times 12 + 8 = 26$ mm Hg.
- $\downarrow PaCO_2$ (in mm Hg) $= \downarrow$ Base Excess (in mEq/L)
  If the base excess (base deficit) is –5 mEq/L, then the $PaCO_2$ should be 35 mm Hg.
  If the $PaCO_2$ is higher than what is predicted in either of these formulas, then compensation is inadequate and there is a concomitant respiratory problem (for example, ketoacidosis in the presence of a respiratory tract infection).

Despite widespread use, the $PaCO_2$-HCO_3^- approach has inherent pitfalls, particularly in relation to the metabolic component. The system neither explains nor accounts for many of the complex acid-base abnormalities seen in perioperative and critically ill patients, such as those with acute acidosis in the setting of hypoalbuminemia, free water deficit or excess, hyperchloremia, hyperphosphatemia, or concurrent metabolic acidosis and alkalosis.

Anion Gap Approach

To address the primary limitation of the Boston approach, the anion gap (AG) was developed by Emmet and Narins in 1975.[5] This is based on the law of electrical neutrality and the fact that for every 1mEq/L fall in SID there is a 1mEq/L fall in $[HCO_3^-]$.

The sum of the difference in charge of the common extracellular ions reveals a "gap" of −12 to −16 mEq/L (anion gap = $(Na^+) - (CL^- + HCO_3^-)$) (Fig. 59.1). The gap reflects the relative charge on albumin and phosphate. If the patient develops a metabolic acidosis and the gap "widens" to, for example −20 mEq/L due to consumption of HCO_3^-, then the acidosis is caused by unmeasured anions—lactate, ketones or "renal" acids. If the gap does not widen, then the anions *are* being measured and the acidosis has been caused by hyperchloremia.

While this approach is useful, it is weakened by the assumptions about what does or does not constitute a "normal gap," and the fact that it ignores electrochemical abnormalities associated with metabolic alkalosis. The majority of critically ill patients are hypoalbuminemic and many are also hypophosphatemic. Consequently, the gap may be normal in the presence of unmeasured anions. Fencl and Figge have provided us with a variant known as the "corrected anion gap (AG_{corr}):"[40]

There are a number of variants of the AG depending on whether or not potassium and lactate are included (Box 59.7).

Another version of the anion gap is the delta anion gap (ΔAG)—an approach that has successfully predicted adverse outcomes in critical illness, where prehospital and postadmission anion gaps were compared.[41] Confusingly, other clinicians utilize the delta-ratio (delta delta Δ/Δ):[42]

$$Delta\ ratio = \Delta AG/\Delta\ [HCO_3^-]$$

Simply, if the anion gap is normal, or unchanged, and the bicarbonate level falls, then the delta ratio will be less than 0.4 and a hyperchloremic acidosis is present. A DR between 1 and 2 is what one would expect from metabolic acidosis due to unmeasured anions or lactate. If the ratio is greater than 2, mixed acid-base abnormalities are present.

The anion gap remains a very simple, useful and reliable screening tool in acute illness and usefully distinguishes metabolic acidosis due to hyperchloremia from acidosis due to UMA. It is also worth noting that modern blood gas analyzers measure a variety of electrolytes, lactate, hemoglobin etc., and calculate and print out the AG. The measured $[Na^+]$ and $[Cl^-]$ on point of care (blood gas) reports is likely more accurate than that reported by a conventional laboratory analysis. This is because the ion selective electrode measurement in the blood gas analyzer is not influenced by alterations in serum protein concentrations, which are frequently reduced in critical illness. Hypoproteinemia results in overestimation of $[Na^+]$ and $[Cl^-]$.[43]

The AG calculation provided by the blood gas machine is likely more accurate than using the standard "labs." It is important that, if a point of care device is being used, for example, to frequently measure serum $[Na^+]$ and titrate therapy, the same machine should be used for all measurements.[44]

The Semi-Quantitative (Base Deficit/ Excess (Copenhagen)) Approach

In metabolic acidosis, the change in the bicarbonate concentration from baseline reflects the total quantity of anions gained. Adherents to the descriptive approach to acid-base refer to this as the "delta" bicarbonate. However, this approach is problematic, as it does not account for the effect of CO_2 metabolism on the $[HCO_3^-]$. In the late 1950s, in Copenhagen, Astrup and Siggaard Anderson, using recently developed CO_2 electrodes, carefully titrated known amounts of acid or base to blood maintained by tonometry at various $PaCO_2$ values and a wide range of hemoglobin concentrations at 37°C. From this they constructed an alignment nomogram that allowed for the determination of a concept

Anion gap

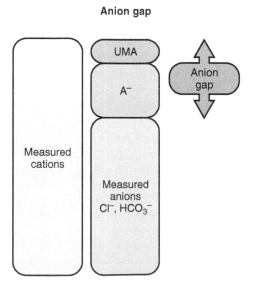

Fig. 59.1 The Anion Gap. A^- represents the charge carried by phosphate and albumin (the calculation is in Box 59.11); *UMA*, unmeasured anions.

known as base excess (BE) from a single measurement of pH, $PaCO_2$ and hemoglobin concentration at 37°C.

The base excess (BE) and its negative counterpart, the base deficit (BD or 1-BE), are used to quantify metabolic alkalosis or metabolic acidosis, independent of the respiratory component. As defined, the BE is the amount of strong acid (strong anion) or base (strong cation) required to return the pH of 1L of fully oxygenated blood to 7.4, assuming that $PaCO_2$ is constant at 40 mm Hg (5.3 kPa) and that the temperature is 37°C. The current convention is to use the *standard base excess* (SBE), which is the BE of extracellular fluid (Box 59.8).[45]

Application of simple mathematical rules allows for use of the BE in each of the common acid-base disturbances (Table 59.5).[46] For example, in acute respiratory acidosis or alkalosis, BE does not change. Conversely, in acute metabolic acidosis, the magnitude of change of the $PaCO_2$ (in millimeters of mercury) is the same as that of the BE (in mmol/L or mEq/L).

The major advantage of the BE approach over the "Boston" approach is that it provides a simple scanning tool that can be instantly identified from a blood gas printout. Consequently, the BD approach remains popular around the world.[45] Because both the Boston and Copenhagen approaches rely on changes in $[HCO_3^-]$ concentrations, they lack the precision to determine the mechanism of the abnormity or identify the presence of multiple simultaneous abnormalities. Consequently, the majority of clinicians who use these "traditional" approaches also utilize the anion gap or one of its derivatives.

Changes in the base excess occur secondary to alterations in the relative concentrations of sodium, chloride, free water, albumin, phosphate and unmeasured anions. A variety of investigators have demonstrated that it is possible to unpack the base excess and isolate the components, thus increasing the precision of the diagnosis.[47] This approach has been labeled the "base excess gap (BEG) (Box 59.9)." The BEG should mirror the strong ion gap (following section) the AG_{corr}. This simplified, but relatively accurate version of the BEG can be easily calculated using mental arithmetic (Box 59.10).[48]

Stewart (Quantitative) Approach

A more accurate reflection of true acid-base status can be derived using the "Stewart" electrochemical approach. This formulation, like the anion gap, is based on the concept of electrical neutrality. This approach looks for a gap between SID (SIDa, apparent) and the combination of A_{TOT} and $[HCO_3^-]$ (SIDe, effective); the difference represents the impact of unmeasured anions (SIG strong ion gap) (Box 59.11 and Fig. 59.2).

The AG_{corr}, BE and SIG approaches are consistent with one another and can be derived from a master equation.[49]

BOX 59.9   Calculating the Base Excess Gap (BEG).[47]

BE-NaW (water and sodium effect) = 0.3 × ([Na+ measured] − 140) mEq/L

BE-Cl (chloride effect) = 102 − [Cl-effective] (mEq/L)

BE-PO4 (phosphate effect) = (0.309 × (pH −0.46) × (0.8- [Phos-measured mmol/L])

BE-Prot (protein effect) = (42 − [Albumin g/L]) × (0.148 × pH−0.818)

BE_{calc} = BE-NaW + BE-Cl + BE-PO4 + BE-Prot

BE_{Gap} = BE_{calc} − BE_{actual} − [lactate mEq/L]

BOX 59.10   Calculation of Simplified Base Excess Gap (BEGs).[48]

BE_{NaCl} = ([Na+]–[Cl−]) − 38

BE_{Alb} = 0.25 (42 − albumin g/L)

BE_{NaCl}- BE_{Alb}= BDE_{calc}

BE actual− BE_{calc} − [lactate] = BE gap = the effect of unmeasured anions or cations.

BE_{NaCl}, base excess for sodium, chloride and free water—this assumes that the normal [Cl−] is 102 mEq/L—this can be adjusted for local lab values; BE_{Alb}, base excess for albumin

---

BOX 59.8   The Standard Base Excess.

- SBE = (HCO_3^- *actual* mEq/L) −24.8 + (16.2×(pH −7.40))
  The value of 16.2 mEq/L approximates all of the nonbicarbonate buffers in ECF (albumin, phosphate and mean ECF hemoglobin).
  So, if the pH is 7.25 and the measured HCO_3^- is 14 mEq/L, then the SBE is 8.4 mEq/L or mmol/L.

TABLE 59.5   Changes in Standard Base Excess in Response to Acute and Chronic Acid-Base Disturbances.

Disturbance	SBE vs. $PaCO_2$
Acute respiratory acidosis	ΔBE = 0
Acute respiratory alkalosis	ΔBE = 0
Chronic respiratory acidosis	ΔBE = 0.4 Δ$PaCO_2$
Metabolic acidosis	Δ$PaCO_2$ = ΔBE
Metabolic alkalosis	Δ$PaCO_2$ = 0.6 ΔBE

BE, base excess; *Δ*, change in value; *$PaCO_2$*, partial pressure of arterial oxygen.

BOX 59.11   The Strong Ion Gap.

The SIDa (apparent SID) = ([Na+]+ [K+]+ [Mg2+]+ [Ca2+]) − [Cl−] mEq/L

The SIDe (effective) is $[HCO_3^-]$ + [charge on albumin] + [charge on PO_4^{2-}]

Weak acids' degree of ionization is pH dependent, so one must calculate for this:

[alb-] = [alb g/l]×(0.123×pH − 0.631)

$[PO_4^{2-}]$ (in mg/dl) = $[PO_4^{2-}]$× (0.309×pH − 0.47)

Strong Ion Gap (**SIG**) = SIDa-SIDe

Strong ion gap

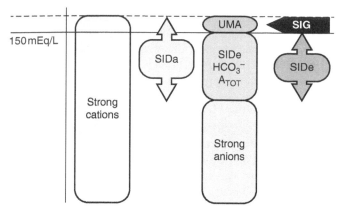

Fig. 59.2 The Strong Ion Gap. *SIDa,* apparent SID; *SIDe,* effective SID; *SIG,* strong ion gap (see Box 59.11); *UMA,* unmeasured anions.

Moreover, now that lactate is routinely reported in blood gas analyzers, the insertion of the lactate concentration (in mEq/L) into the various AG, BEG and SIG calculations should increase their precision.

The weakness of this system is that the SIG does not necessarily represent unmeasured strong anions, merely all anions that are unmeasured. For example, gelatin fluid solutions that carry a negative charge will increase the SIG. Further, SID changes quantitatively in absolute and relative terms when there are changes in plasma water concentration. Fencl[50] addressed this by correcting the chloride concentration for free water (Cl⁻ corr) using the following equation:

$$[Cl^-]corr = [Cl^-]observed \times ([Na^+]normal/[Na^+]observed).$$

This corrected chloride concentration may be then inserted into the SIDa equation above. Likewise, the derived value for unmeasured anions (UMA) should also be corrected for free water using UMA instead of Cl⁻ in the above equation.[50]

Calculation of SIG is cumbersome. The data required are more extensive and thus more expensive than other approaches and there is much confusion about the normal range of SIG. It is unclear, in standard clinical practice, that SIG has any advantage over AGc (which is SIG without calcium, magnesium and phosphate—which usually cancel each other's charges).[51]

Kaplan and Kellum looked at a variety of acid-base measurements in the acute trauma setting. SIG was superior at predicting outcome versus all other measures.[52] Only one (2%) survivor had an SIG greater than 5 mEq/L and only two (7%) nonsurvivors had an SIG less than 5 mEq/L. However, to date, studies of critically ill patients have failed to demonstrate that SIG predicts outcomes. This may be due to the complexity of the various acid-base disturbances that are going on simultaneously and the impact of hypercatabolism on metabolic byproducts. For example, Moviat and colleagues found that unmeasured strong anions were present in 98%,

hyperchloremia was present in 80% and elevated lactate levels were present in 62% of patients.[53]

CONCLUSIONS

All acid-base disorders can be explained in terms of SID, A_{TOT} and $PaCO_2$. Acid-base disturbances may be respiratory, secondary to alterations in CO_2 metabolism, or metabolic, secondary to changes in strong ion or weak acid concentrations in ECF. The majority of clinicians use analytic tools that are more than a half century old, and while these remain useful—providing rules of thumb that for simple acid-base disturbances—they are limited in complex critically ill patients. The modern electrochemical approach utilizes the full battery of standard laboratory tests to aid precision in diagnosis and enhances our understanding of acid-base chemistry. The physical chemistry (Stewart) approach also helps identify the multiple simultaneous acid-base abnormalities found in critically ill patients.

AUTHORS' RECOMMENDATIONS

- Acid-base balance remains a core diagnostic tool in acute medicine and critical care. Although acidosis occurs if the pH falls below 7.35 and alkalosis occurs above pH 7.45, with compensatory maneuvers pH may be in the normal range.
- Only three factors independently affect acid-base balance: $PaCO_2$, SID, and A_{TOT}.
- Respiratory acidosis and alkalosis are caused by hypercarbia and hypocarbia, respectively.
- Acute and chronic respiratory acidosis and alkalosis can be assessed in terms of pH, $PaCO_2$ and HCO_3^-.
- Metabolic acidosis is caused by decreased SID or increased A_{TOT}. Decreased SID results from accumulation of metabolic anions (i.e., chloride, lactate, ketones, and renal acids). Increased A_{TOT} results from hyperphosphatemia.
- Metabolic alkalosis is caused by increased SID or decreased A_{TOT}. The SID increases because of sodium gain, chloride loss, or free water deficit. A_{TOT} decreases in hypoalbuminemia and hypophosphatemia. This condition is particularly common in critical illness.
- The Boston, Copenhagen, and Stewart approaches are widely used to assess acid-base abnormalities. With increasing complexity there is increased precision of diagnosis, but not necessarily prognosis, particularly in critical illness.

REFERENCES

1. Kellum JA. Reunification of acid-base physiology. *Crit Care.* 2005;9:500-507.
2. Fencl V, Leith DE. Stewart's quantitative acid-base chemistry: applications in biology and medicine. *Respir Physiol.* 1993;91:1-16.
3. Van Slyke DD. An apparatus for determination of the gases in blood and other solutions. *Proc Natl Acad Sci U S A.* 1921;7:229-231.

4. Seifter JL. Integration of acid base and electrolyte disorders. *N Engl J Med*. 2014;371:1821-1831.

5. Emmett M, Narins RG. Clinical use of the anion gap. *Medicine (Baltimore)*. 1977;56:38-54.

6. Stewart PA. Modern quantitative acid-base chemistry. *Can J Physiol Pharmacol*. 1983;61:1444-1461.

7. Narins R, Emmett M. Simple and mixed acid-base disorders: A practical approach. *Medicine (Baltimore)*. 1980;59:161-187.

8. Stewart PA. Independent and dependent variables of acid-base control. *Respir Physiol*. 1978;33:9-26.

9. Figge J, Mydosh T, Fencl V. Serum proteins and acid-base equilibria: a follow-up. *J Lab Clin Med*. 1992;120:713-719.

10. Brackett NC, Cohen JJ, Schwartz WB: Carbon dioxide titration curve of normal man. *N Engl J Med*. 1965;272:6-12.

11. Alfaro V, Torras R, Ibanez J, Palacios L. A physical-chemical analysis of the acid-base response to chronic obstructive pulmonary disease. *Can J Physiol Pharmacol*. 1996;74: 1229-1235.

12. Romano TG, Correia MD, Mendes PV, Zampieri FG, Maciel AT, Park M. Metabolic acid-base adaptation triggered by acute persistent hypercapnia in mechanically ventilated patients with acute respiratory distress syndrome. *Rev Bras Ter Intensiva*. 2016;28:19-26.

13. Sirker AA, Rhodes A, Grounds RM, Bennett ED. Acid-base physiology: the 'traditional' and the 'modern' approaches. *Anaesthesia*. 2002;57:348-356.

14. Mikkelsen ME, Miltiades AN, Gaieski DF, et al. Serum lactate is associated with mortality in severe sepsis independent of organ failure and shock. *Crit Care Med*. 2009;37:1670-1677.

15. Arnold RC, Shapiro NI, Jones AE, et al. Multicenter study of early lactate clearance as a determinant of survival in patients with presumed sepsis. *Shock*. 2009; 32:35-39.

16. Jones AE, Shapiro NI, Trzeciak S, Arnold RC, Claremont HA, Kline JA. Lactate clearance vs central venous oxygen saturation as goals of early sepsis therapy: a randomized clinical trial. *JAMA*. 2010;303:739-746.

17. Jansen TC, van Bommel J, Schoonderbeek FJ, et al. Early lactate-guided therapy in intensive care unit patients: a multicenter, open-label, randomized controlled trial. *Am J Respir Crit Care Med*. 2010;182:752-761.

18. Lee SW, Hong YS, Park DW, et al. Lactic acidosis not hyperlactatemia as a predictor of inhospital mortality in septic emergency patients. *Emerg Med J*. 2008;25:659-665.

19. Hartmann C, Radermacher P, Wepler M, Nussbaum B: Non-hemodynamic effects of catecholamines. *Shock*. 2017;48:390-400.

20. Levy MM, Evans LE, Rhodes A: The Surviving Sepsis Campaign Bundle: 2018 update. *Crit Care Med*. 2018;46:997-1000.

21. Garcia-Alvarez M, Marik P, Bellomo R. Stress hyperlactataemia: present understanding and controversy. *Lancet Diabetes Endocrinol*. 2014;2:339-347.

22. DeFronzo R, Fleming GA, Chen K, Bicsak TA. Metformin-associated lactic acidosis: Current perspectives on causes and risk. *Metabolism*. 2016;65:20-29.

23. Kowlgi NG, Chhabra L. D-lactic acidosis: an underrecognized complication of short bowel syndrome. *Gastroenterol Res Pract*. 2015;2015:476215.

24. Brewster S, Curtis L, Poole R. Urine versus blood ketones. *Practical Diab*. 2017;34:13-15.

25. Rocktaeschel J, Morimatsu H, Uchino S, et al. Acid-base status of critically ill patients with acute renal failure: analysis based on Stewart-Figge methodology. *Crit Care*. 2003;7:R60.

26. Rocktäschel J, Morimatsu H, Uchino S, Ronco C, Bellomo R. Impact of continuous veno-venous hemofiltration on acid-base balance. *Int J Artif Organs*. 2003;26:19-25.

27. Cheungpasitporn W, Zand L, Dillon JJ, Qian Q, Leung N. Lactate clearance and metabolic aspects of continuous high-volume hemofiltration. *Clin Kidney J*. 2015;8:374-377.

28. Henderson LH. Blood as a physiochemical system. *J Biol Chem*. 1921;46:411-419.

29. Myles PS, Andrews S, Nicholson J, Lobo DN, Mythen M. Contemporary approaches to perioperative IV fluid therapy. *World J Surg*. 2017;41:2457-2463.

30. Shaw AD, Bagshaw SM, Goldstein SL, et al. Major complications, mortality, and resource utilization after open abdominal surgery: 0.9% saline compared to Plasma-Lyte. *Ann Surg*. 2012;255:821-829.

31. Yunos N. Association between a chloride-liberal vs chloride-restrictive intravenous fluid administration strategy and kidney injury in critically ill adults. *JAMA*. 2012;308: 1566-1572.

32. Self WH, Semler MW, Wanderer JP, et al. Balanced crystalloids versus saline in noncritically ill adults. *N Engl J Med*. 2018; 378:819-828.

33. Semler MW, Self WH, Wanderer JP, et al. Balanced crystalloids versus saline in critically ill adults. *N Engl J Med*. 2018;378:829-839.

34. Figge J, Rossing TH, Fencl V. The role of serum proteins in acid-base equilibria. *J Lab Clin Med*. 1991;117:453-467.

35. Adrogue HJ, Eknoyan G, Suki WK. Diabetic ketoacidosis: role of the kidney in the acid-base homeostasis re-evaluated. *Kidney Int*. 1984;25:591-598.

36. Moviat M, Pickkers P, van der Voort PH, van der Hoeven JG: Acetazolamide-mediated decrease in strong ion difference accounts for the correction of metabolic alkalosis in critically ill patients. *Crit Care*. 2006;10:R14.

37. Kimura S, Shabsigh M, Morimatsu H. Traditional approach versus Stewart approach for acid-base disorders: inconsistent evidence. *SAGE Open Med*. 2018;6:2050312118801255.

38. Schwartz WB, Brackett NC, Cohen JJ. The response of extracellular hydrogen ion concentration to graded degrees of chronic hypercapnia: the physiologic limits of the defense of pH*. *J Clin Invest*. 1965;44:291-301.

39. Albert MS, Dell RB, Winters RW. Quantitative displacement of acid-base equilibrium in metabolic acidosis. *Ann Intern Med*. 1967;66:312-322.

40. Figge J, Jabor A, Kazda A, Fencl V. Anion gap and hypoalbuminemia. *Crit Care Med*. 1998;26:1807-1810.

41. Lipnick MS, Braun AB, Cheung JT, Gibbons FK, Christopher KB. Difference between critical care initiation anion gap and prehospital admission anion gap is predictive of mortality in critical illness. *Crit Care Med*. 2013;41:49-59.

42. Rastegar A. Use of the delta AG/delta bicarbonate ratio in the diagnosis of mixed acid-base disorders. *J Am Soc Nephrol*. 2007;18:2429-2431.

43. Stove V, Slabbinck A, Vanoverschelde L, Hoste E, De PP, Delanghe J. How to solve the underestimated problem of overestimated sodium results in the hypoproteinemic patient. *Crit Care Med*. 2016;44:e83-e88.

44. Weld BA, Morgan TJ, Presneill JJ, Weier S, Cowley D. Plasma sodium measurements by direct ion selective methods in laboratory and point of care may not be clinically interchangeable. *J Clin Monit Comput*. 2017;31:1103-1109.

45. Berend K. Diagnostic use of base excess in acid-base disorders. *N Engl J Med.* 2018;378:1419-1428.

46. Schlichtig R, Grogono AW, Severinghaus JW. Human PaCO2 and standard base excess compensation for acid-base imbalance. *Crit Care Med.* 1998;26:1173-1179.

47. Gilfix BM, Bique M, Magder S: A physical chemical approach to the analysis of acid-base balance in the clinical setting. *J Crit Care.* 1993;8:187-197.

48. Story DA, Morimatsu H, Bellomo R. Strong ions, weak acids and base excess: a simplified Fencl-Stewart approach to clinical acid-base disorders. *Br J Anaesth.* 2004;92:54-60.

49. Wooten EW. Analytic calculation of physiological acid-base parameters in plasma. *J Appl Physiol.* 1999;86:326-334.

50. Fencl V, Jabor A, Kazda A, Figge J. Diagnosis of metabolic acid-base disturbances in critically ill patients. *Am J Respir Crit Care Med.* 2000;162:2246-2251.

51. Antonogiannaki EM, Mitrouska I, Amargianitakis V, Georgopoulos D. Evaluation of acid-base status in patients admitted to ED: physicochemical vs traditional approaches. *Am J Emerg Med.* 2015;33:378-382.

52. Kaplan LJ, Kellum JA. Comparison of acid-base models for prediction of hospital mortality after trauma. *Shock.* 2008;29:662-666.

53. Moviat M, van Haren F, van der Hoeven H. Conventional or physicochemical approach in intensive care unit patients with metabolic acidosis. *Crit Care.* 2003;7:R41-R45.

60

Is Hyperchloremia Harmful?

Ida-Fong Ukor and Keith R. Walley

INTRODUCTION

Hyperchloremia is very common in critically ill patients, most often as a result of fluid resuscitation with 0.9% (normal) saline. Normal saline is anything but normal. Both the sodium and chloride concentrations are 154 mmol/L and the concentrations of other common plasma electrolytes, such as bicarbonate, are zero. While sodium concentration in this solution is mildly elevated compared to plasma, the concentration of chloride is markedly higher than a normal plasma chloride concentration of ~100 mmol/L. Therefore, even modest fluid resuscitation will result in hyperchloremia. Whatever the cause, there is substantial evidence that hyperchloremia has an adverse impact on clinical outcomes; primarily related to kidney injury.

Here we review the normal physiology of chloride handling by the kidney, consider relevant basic research, and review human patient studies of crystalloid fluid resuscitation/replacement and related hyperchloremia, with a particular emphasis on recent large clinical trials and metaanalyses. This leads to an understanding of why hyperchloremia may lead to kidney injury and highlights that the overall adverse effects of hyperchloremia are small but real, and that they are clinically relevant in individual patients.

BRIEF CHLORIDE PHYSIOLOGY

Chloride is the main extracellular anion and therefore plays a major role in acid-base balance, particularly in critically ill patients where extracellular fluid volume is actively managed by fluid administration, diuretics, and renal replacement therapy. Chloride is a Stewart strong ion so it exists in an almost completely dissociated state and therefore has a direct effect on hydrogen ion concentration and blood pH.[1] Chloride plays a major role in production of lower respiratory tract secretions, sweat, and pancreatic secretions.[2] Hydrochloric acid secretion is important in producing an acidic gastric environment. Moreover, chloride transport into the gut is the major osmotic driver of gastrointestinal tract secretions. Decreased concentrations of chloride contribute to smooth muscle cell contraction.[2] Chloride transport into and out of red blood cells in exchange for bicarbonate reduces the change in extracellular pH that occurs with CO_2 loading in the peripheral tissues and unloading in the lungs, while also assisting in oxygen unloading in peripheral tissues.[3] Most relevant to critical illness, chloride concentration is sensed by the kidney and impacts the kidney's glomerular filtration rate (GFR) principally through tubuloglomerular feedback.[4]

Chloride is filtered by the kidney (GFR × 100 mmol/L = approximately 18,000 mmol chloride filtered per day) and all but 100–200 mmol is reabsorbed, primarily in the proximal convoluted tubule (~60%) but also in the ascending limb of the loop of Henle (~25%) and in distal tubules (~5%). Na^+ and Cl^- concentrations in the thick ascending limb are sensed by the macula densa of the juxtaglomerular apparatus, which then regulates sodium, potassium, and chloride reabsorption. When Na^+ and Cl^- concentrations are high in the thick ascending limb, as sensed by the macula densa (for example, when extracellular fluid volume is abundant), renin production by juxtaglomerular cells is low. In addition, high Na^+ and Cl^- concentrations detected by the macula densa decrease afferent glomerular arteriolar blood flow via purinergic vasoconstrictor signaling, decreasing GFR. This phenomenon is termed tubuloglomerular feedback.[4–6] In hypovolemic states the reverse is observed; renin production is high and afferent arterioles are not vasoconstricted. Normal saline resuscitation of hypovolemic states increases Na^+ and Cl^- delivery to the macula densa which then down regulates the renin-angiotensin-aldosterone system and decreases afferent arteriolar flow and GFR by tubuloglomerular feedback. In contrast, fluid resuscitation with balanced crystalloid solutions delivers less chloride to the macula densa, so afferent arteriolar flow and GFR may not be decreased as much (Fig. 60.1). In sepsis, tubuloglomerular feedback is altered and may contribute to decreased GFR.[5]

POTENTIAL MECHANISMS OF HYPERCHLOREMIA'S ADVERSE EFFECTS

The possible mechanisms by which hyperchloremia causes harm in critically ill patients have been investigated in numerous animal and clinical studies. Administration of clinically relevant volumes of normal saline causes a notable rise in Cl^- concentration ($[Cl^-]$) and a concurrent fall in pH.[7] Increases in $[Cl^-]$ in the absence of bicarbonate administration increase the total strong ion contribution, resulting in metabolic acidosis.[1] Hyperchloremic metabolic acidosis, when severe and particularly in the setting of critical illness, may contribute to impaired cardiovascular performance,

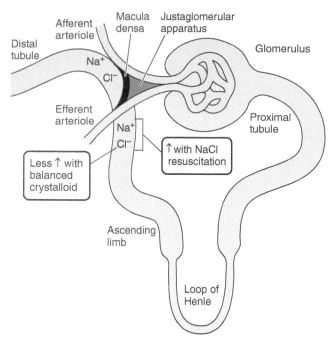

Fig. 60.1 Tubuloglomerular Feedback. In hypovolemic states delivery of Na⁺ and Cl⁻ to the ascending limb is reduced and sensed by macula densa cells of the juxtaglomerular apparatus. Low concentrations result in increased renin production by the juxtaglomerular apparatus. Normal saline resuscitation increases Na⁺ and Cl⁻ delivery to the ascending limb, which is sensed by the macula densa cells. This results in decreased renin production. Importantly, this also results in purinergic signaling from the juxtaglomerular apparatus to the adjacent afferent arteriole to induce vasoconstriction. The result is decreased afferent arteriolar blood flow and glomerular filtration rate—termed tubuloglomerular feedback. Both Na+ and Cl⁻ concentrations play a role in this regulation and the contribution by Cl⁻ can be substantial. When balanced crystalloids are used for resuscitation, less Cl⁻ is delivered resulting in decreased tubuloglomerular feedback resulting in a greater glomerular filtration rate.

vasopressor insensitivity, coagulopathy and possibly impaired immune function.[8-13] Bicarbonate administration does not, however, confer a mortality benefit, suggesting that acidosis is neither the only nor the most important mechanism involved in hyperchloremia's adverse effects. A link between high-chloride fluids and increased inflammatory markers has been noted in some studies.[14-16] A substantial body of evidence suggests that hyperchloremia impairs renal function. Hyperchloremia directly decreases renal perfusion via tubuloglomerular feedback,[6] constricting afferent glomerular vessels, limiting glomerular blood flow and causing a fall in GFR.[17] Indeed, when tested in animal models and in humans, administration of normal saline decreases renal blood flow and glomerular filtration rate,[7,17] although the effect is likely small.[18,19]

RETROSPECTIVE OBSERVATIONAL STUDIES OF HYPERCHLOREMIA

Hyperchloremia is very common in critically ill patients. Indeed, recent studies report hyperchloremia ([Cl⁻] > 100 mmol/L) in at least half of all critically ill patient populations.[20,21]

A number of retrospective observational studies across a variety of patient cohorts suggest that hyperchloremia exerts true negative effects on renal function. While the impact of hyperchloremia on renal function may be transient and reversible in health, in critically ill patients the effect may translate into significant increases in morbidity and mortality.

Recent, moderately powered retrospective studies of cohorts (from n = 240 to n = 6025, Table 60.1) all revealed an increased incidence of acute kidney injury (AKI) and/or mortality in patients receiving high chloride solutions compared to balanced crystalloid solutions.[20-25] Several nonrandomized but controlled before-after studies also reported similar results (see Table 60.1). In two reports of single center before-after trials, Yunos and colleagues found that chloride-liberal resuscitation/replacement resulted in greater AKI and use of renal replacement therapy compared to the use of balanced crystalloid solutions.[26,27] Patients who were hyperchloremic before fluid resuscitation were also at risk and a resuscitation-induced increase in [Cl⁻] >5 mmol/L was also associated with acute kidney injury, even in previously hypochloremic patients.[21] However, the effect sizes observed in these moderately powered non-randomized studies were small so that retrospective studies with n <200 often do not find a statistically significant result-possibly because they are underpowered.

Recent large retrospective cohort studies also support the finding that hyperchloremia is associated with increased acute kidney injury and mortality in a variety of patient groups. McCluskey and colleagues assessed the effects of acute post-operative hyperchloremia ([Cl⁻] > 110 mmol/L) in a surgical population (n = 22,851).[28] These investigators observed a 22% (n = 4995) incidence of acute post-operative hyperchloremia and, on comparison with a propensity matched sample (n = 4266 per group), found that hyperchloremia was associated with a significantly increased 30-day mortality (hyperchloremia mortality 3.0% vs. 1.9%; OR 1.58 [95% CI 1.25–1.98]). Hyperchloremia was also associated with a longer hospital length of stay (7.0 vs. 6.3 days, $p < 0.01$), and an increased likelihood of kidney injury (>25% decrease in creatinine clearance: 12.9% vs. 9.2%, $p < 0.01$).[28] Similar findings were seen in when critically ill patients with septic shock (n = 53,448) who received predominantly normal saline were compared with patients who received predominantly balanced crystalloids.[29] There was a lower post-Day 2 absolute in-hospital mortality on propensity matched cohort analysis (19.6% in balanced crystalloid vs. 22.8% in normal saline patients, relative risk ratio [RR] = 0.86 [95% CI 0.78–0.94], $p = 0.001$), however, no significant difference in the rates of AKI or ICU length of stay were found. It is important to note, as highlighted by these authors, that less than 1% of patients received exclusively balanced fluids. Analyses were therefore performed according the proportion of balanced crystalloid received. Additionally, patients were analyzed by quantiles according to the total volume of fluid they received, with no change in the difference in mortality outcome.[29]

TABLE 60.1   Recent Nonrandomized Studies of Crystalloid Solutions.

	n	Patient Population	Greater AKI / RRT With Hyperchloremia	Greater Mortality With Hyperchloremia	Propensity Matching
Moderate Size Observational					
Zhang 2013[22]	1221	ICU	Yes	Not tested	
Neyra 2015[23]	1940	Sepsis		Yes	
Shaw 2015[24]	3116	SIRS	Not tested	Yes	Yes
Marttinen 2016[20]	445	ICU	Yes	Yes, Not sig.	
Suetrong 2016[21]	240	Sepsis	Yes	Yes, Not sig.	
Shao 2016[25]	6025	ICU	Yes	Yes, Not sig.	
Moderate Size Before-After Design					
Yunos 2012[26]	1533	ICU	Yes	Yes, Not sig.	
Yunos 2015[27]	2994	ICU	Yes	Yes, Not sig.	
Large Observational					
Shaw 2012[36]	926 BCS, 30,994 NS	Abdominal surgery	Yes	Yes	Yes
McCluskey 2013[28]	22,851	Surgical	Yes	Yes	Yes
Raghunathan 2014[29]	53,448	Septic shock	No	Yes	Yes
Shaw 2014[31]	109,836	SIRS	Not tested	Yes	

AKI, acute kidney injury; *RRT*, renal replacement therapy; *BCS*, balanced crystalloid solution; *NS*, normal saline; *SAH*, subarachnoid hemorrhage; *SIRS*, systemic inflammatory response syndrome; *Not sig*, not statistically significant.

The largest reported retrospective analysis included 109,836 predominantly medical patients meeting systemic inflammatory response syndrome (SIRS)[30] criteria who received crystalloid fluid resuscitation over a 72 hour period. Changes in plasma [Cl$^-$], administered chloride load, and intravenous fluid volume were assessed for their association with in-hospital mortality.[31] Baseline hyperchloremia ([Cl$^-$] $\geq$110 mmol/L) and total intravenous chloride load were both associated with increased mortality ($p < 0.001$ for both). Further, investigators found that the greater the increase in [Cl$^-$] from baseline to maximum levels, the higher the mortality rate, even when absolute [Cl$^-$] remained within the normal range. In-hospital mortality was lowest with a 0–10 mmol/L increase in [Cl$^-$] (3.7%), with significantly increasing mortality for each 10 mmol/L increment above this (10–20 mmol/L: 7.2%; 20–30 mmol/L: 9.2%; 20–40 mmol/L: 9.7%; $p < 0.001$ for pairwise comparisons with 0–10 mmol/L group). When weighted for the number of patients in each group, this dose-response relationship showed that mortality increased linearly with increasing peak-baseline [Cl$^-$] ($r^2 = 0.97$). Given the existing evidence supporting an association between high fluid load and increased morbidity and mortality, particularly in critically ill patients,[32–35] the authors performed a volume-adjusted analysis to delineate chloride-specific effects.[31] After separation into predefined volume strata (1500 mL increments), the relationship between increasing volume-adjusted chloride load (above 98 mmol/L) and mortality persisted in all but the group who received the lowest fluid volumes (<1500 mL). Importantly, in this last group there was an inverse relationship between increasing chloride load and mortality, perhaps reflecting a degree of under-resuscitation. On regression analysis, a chloride load $\geq$105 mmol/L was identified as the point beyond which increasing mortality was seen ($R^2 = 0.82$, $p < 0.001$). Adjustment for illness severity using the acute physiology score (APS) did not alter these results (adjusted mortality odds ratio (OR) for [Cl$^-$] <105 mmol/L: 0.888 [95% confidence interval (CI) 0.827–0.957]). Further, larger fluid volumes were also found to be associated with higher in-hospital mortality ($R^2 = 0.97$; $p < 0.001$); however, this was independent of the chloride effect.

CRYSTALLOID CLINICAL TRIALS

Many clinical trials have compared balanced crystalloid solutions to normal saline for resuscitation/replacement in critically ill patients. Comparison of retrospective observational studies to prospectively randomized clinical trials has led to considerable controversy. For example, a large observational clinical study compared balanced crystalloid-treated patients (n = 926) to normal saline-treated patients (n = 30,994) undergoing major open abdominal surgery.[36] Balanced crystalloid-treated patients had lower mortality (2.9%) than normal saline-treated patients (5.6%, $p < 0.001$). Several years later, the results of a reasonably large (n = 2278) prospective cluster-randomized crossover trial were reported.[37] These investigators did not find significant differences in in-hospital mortality (7.6% in the balanced crystalloid group and 8.6% in the saline group) or in the primary outcome of incidence of AKI. Because of these discrepant results, recent adequately powered randomized trials are particularly helpful.

In a cluster randomized clinical trial of balanced crystalloid versus normal saline for fluid administration in critically ill adults, the SMART investigators conducted tested the hypothesis that saline administration results in chloride-induced organ injury and acidosis.[38] The primary outcome was measured over 30 days and was a composite of death, need for new renal replacement therapy, or an elevation of the final creatinine to greater than double the baseline value. Cluster randomization allowed recruitment of all critically ill patients in the participating ICUs. The ICUs were randomized to balanced crystalloid or normal saline and crossed over to the alternative treatment monthly so patients were not individually randomized or consented. The study was able to rapidly recruit over 15,000 patients, approximately half of whom received balanced crystalloid and half normal saline for any fluid administration during their ICU admission. Approximately one third of the patients were mechanically ventilated and one quarter received vasopressors. The median volume of fluid used per patient was just over 1 liter. Thus, the average severity of illness and need for fluid replacement was modest in the overall cohort. Nonetheless, patients who received normal saline had an average increase in plasma chloride of 1–2 mmol/L and approximately a 1 mmol/L reduction in plasma bicarbonate over the first week of ICU admission. The study identified a significant difference in the composite endpoint (p = 0.04) and a trend toward a difference in death (p = 0.06) and use of renal replacement therapy (p = 0.08). Again, in the context of the modest amount of fluid replacement, these differences are impressive. Importantly, the difference in outcomes was greater in patients who received larger volumes of fluid resuscitation/replacement. In a subgroup analysis of patients with sepsis, 30-day mortality was 25.2% in those treated with balanced crystalloid versus 29.4% in those treated with saline (p = 0.02).

At the same time, the same investigators also conducted the SALT-ED trial of balanced crystalloid versus normal saline resuscitation in patients seen in the Emergency Department and subsequently admitted to the hospital to a non-ICU bed (n = 13,347).[39] On a monthly basis, fluid administration was crossed over between balanced crystalloid and normal saline. Again, the volume of fluid administered was just over 1 liter. Similar to the SMART trial, normal saline resuscitation/replacement led to higher chloride and lower bicarbonate concentrations over the first 3 days and a higher incidence of hyperchloremia and acidemia. In this 30-day study there was no difference in the primary outcome of number of days the patients were alive and not in the hospital. Balanced crystalloids, compared to normal saline, resulted in a decrease in major adverse kidney events (p = 0.01). Balanced crystalloids were particularly beneficial in patients with hyperchloremia at presentation ([Cl⁻] > 110 mmol/L) or renal dysfunction (creatinine ≥ 1.5 mg/dL = 133 μmol/L).

CRYSTALLOID TRIALS META-ANALYSES

The SMART and SALT-ED trials are the most recent and statistically powerful trials of low versus high chloride content resuscitation/replacement fluid. Many previous studies have been subjected to metaanalyses with results virtually the same as those in the SMART and SALT-ED trials. In a metaanalysis that predated SMART and SALT-ED, Krajewski et al. focused specifically on the issue of hyperchloremia and included RCTs as well as controlled clinical trials and observational studies.[40] The metaanalysis involved 21 previous studies that included 6253 patients and was designed to compare high-chloride fluids (fluid [Cl⁻] > 111 mmol/L, which was typically normal saline) to low-chloride content fluids (fluid [Cl⁻] ≤ 111 mm/L; typically Ringer's lactate, Hartmann's solution, or Plasma-Lyte). The investigators found a weak but statistically significant relationship between high-chloride content fluid resuscitation/replacement and adverse outcomes. High-chloride fluids did not significantly alter mortality but there was a significant association between high-chloride solutions and acute kidney injury (relative risk 1.64; 95% CI 1.27–2.13, p <0.001). As in all of these trials, high-chloride fluids resulted in hyperchloremia (p <0.001) and metabolic acidosis (p <0.001). An important secondary outcome was that patients resuscitated with high-chloride fluids spent a longer time on mechanical ventilation. A post-hoc sensitivity analysis repeated the statistical analysis after exclusion of three large studies that heavily influenced the overall results. The results were the same. Importantly, these investigators found virtually no heterogeneity in outcomes between studies, suggesting a consistent effect and magnitude observed in all studies.

A more recent metaanalysis involved only six RCTs but included recent trials and, in total, many more patients (n = 19,332)[41] with the vast majority of patients coming from the SMART trial (n =15,802). These investigators found that, compared to patients receiving normal saline, patients administered balanced crystalloid solutions had a small reduction of in-hospital mortality (11.5% versus 12.2 %) and had a confidence interval that just crossed 1 and therefore was not quite statistically significant (OR 0.92, 95% CI 0.85−1.01, p = 0.09). Similarly, the reduction in incidence of AKI had a confidence interval that just crossed 1 (OR 0.92, 95% CI 0.84–1.01, p = 0.10). Low heterogeneity between studies was again observed, indicating that all investigators were observing similar small effects.

Importantly, while this analysis included the pilot SALT trial, it did not include the much more powerful SALT-ED trial because the ED patients who received fluid resuscitation in the SALT-ED trial were defined as "not critically ill" and therefore did not meet inclusion criteria. However, the excluded SALT-ED patients received the same amount of crystalloid solution as patients in the included and dominant SMART trial.

CONCLUSIONS FROM CRYSTALLOID CLINICAL TRIALS

There is remarkable concordance among all of the studies discussed. Principally, when compared to resuscitation with normal saline, administration of balanced crystalloid solutions resulted in a small improvement in mortality. The studies demonstrated a stronger and statistically significant effect of balanced crystalloid solutions on reducing the incidence of acute kidney injury and on the need for renal replacement therapy. Importantly, a dose-response relationship was observed; that is, the improvements in clinical outcomes associated with the use of balanced crystalloid solutions was greater in those patients who received high volumes of fluid resuscitation. This finding provided additional evidence for a mechanistic link between the use of high-chloride solutions and adverse outcomes. Additional large, randomized controlled trials will help provide definitive evidence and guide best practice. The planned follow-up to the recent FISSH pilot randomized controlled trial may well meet this need, and further illuminate the mechanisms behind any harmful sequelae of hyperchloremia.

Because there is little heterogeneity between outcomes in reported clinical studies, there is no doubt that the effect of balanced crystalloid solutions on improved clinical outcomes is small. There is similarly little doubt that balanced crystalloid resuscitation/replacement is superior to high-chloride normal saline resuscitation/replacement although this effect is modest—in the range of a 1% absolute reduction in risk.

COVARIATION WITH NON-ANION GAP METABOLIC ACIDOSIS

The mechanism underlying the adverse effects of normal saline could be hyperchloremia, the induced metabolic acidosis, or another as yet unidentified cause. No evidence has yet emerged to suggest that the mild degree of metabolic acidosis observed in the cited studies results in increased mortality. No adequately powered clinical trial of bicarbonate administration in critically ill patients has shown a mortality benefit, again arguing against an important effect of acidosis. It therefore appears that hyperchloremia is the most likely explanation for the adverse consequences of normal saline resuscitation compared to balanced crystalloid solutions.

DIFFERENCES BETWEEN AVAILABLE BALANCED CRYSTALLOID SOLUTIONS

The most common readily-available balanced crystalloid solutions are Ringer's lactate, Hartman's solution, and Plasmalyte (Table 60.2, Fig. 60.2). The choice of any one of these fluids has not been found to effect clinical outcomes. Theoretical concerns have been raised regarding the use of each solution. However, none have translated into clinical outcome differences. For example, Ringer's lactate and Hartman's solution contain both lactate and potassium. Therefore it could be argued that they would be problematic in patients with elevated lactate or potassium levels. The number of mmol of lactate for one liter of volume resuscitation (28 mEq) distributed across the extracellular fluid volume is low and the normal rate of lactate clearance per minute is high so that this extra lactate load does not appear to alter clinical outcome and typically does not cloud the clinical picture. These arguments are even stronger for potassium. A liter of Ringer's

TABLE 60.2	Composition of Selected Common Crystalloid Solutions in Current Use.				
Component	Normal Range (Plasma)	0.9% NaCl	Compound Sodium Lactate (Hartmann's)	Ringer's Lactate	Plasma-Lyte 148
$[Na^+]$ (mmol/L)	136–145	154	129	130	140
$[Cl^-]$ (mmol/L)	98–106	154	109	109	98
$[K^+]$ (mmol/L)	3.5–5.0	0	5	4	5
$[Ca^{2+}]$ (mmol/L)	2.2–2.6	0	2.5	3	0
$[HCO_3^-]$ l/ substitute source (mEq/L)	24–32	0	29 (lactate)	28 (lactate)	23 (acetate)/ 27(gluconate)
[Glucose] (mmol/L)	3.5–5.5	0	0	0	0
$[Mg^{2+}]$ (mmol/L)	0.8–1.0	0	0	0	1.5
pH	7.35–7.45	4.5–7.0	5.0–7.0	5.0–7.0	4.0–8.0
Osmolarity (theoretical) (mOsm/L)	275–295	308	278	273	295

Modified from Reddy S, Weinberg L, Young P. Crystalloid fluid therapy. *Crit Care*. 2016;20:59.

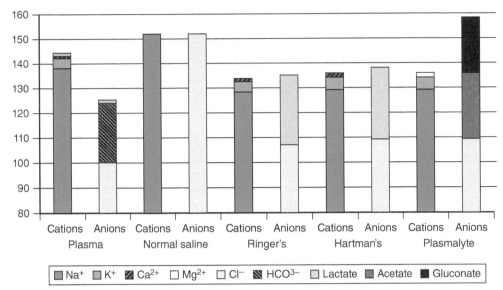

Fig. 60.2 Concentrations of Cations and Anions in Plasma and Resuscitation Fluids. (Note that the y-axis starts at 80 mmol/L since Na⁺ and Cl⁻ make up all of the information below that point.) Normal saline is very different from plasma and all of the balanced crystalloid solutions. All of the balanced crystalloid solutions use strategies to approximately match plasma concentrations.

lactate will deliver 4 mmol of potassium which, distributed across the extracellular fluid volume, is remarkably small, especially when compared to the vast intracellular stores of potassium.

SUMMARY

Hyperchloremia is harmful. It appears to result in an increased incidence of AKI and increased mortality. The effect size is small—in the range of a 1% absolute risk reduction of death—but is certainly important to the one-in-one hundred patient who dies. In addition, changing practice to favor the use of balanced salt solutions over normal saline should be relatively simple and inexpensive—and will be further magnified by the enormous number of patients who receive crystalloid fluid resuscitation/replacement every day.

AUTHORS' RECOMMENDATIONS
- In the absence of other dominant specific issues in an individual patient, fluid resuscitation and replacement in critically ill patients should use a balanced crystalloid solution such as Ringer's lactate, Ringer's acetate, Hartman's solution, or Plasmalyte.
- The routine use of normal saline should be avoided.

REFERENCES

1. Jones NL. A quantitative physicochemical approach to acid-base physiology. *Clin Biochem.* 1990;23(3):189-195.
2. Puljak L, Kilic G. Emerging roles of chloride channels in human diseases. *Biochim Biophys Acta.* 2006;1762(4):404-413.
3. Crandall ED, Bidani A. Effects of red blood cell HCO3(-)/Cl- exchange kinetics on lung CO2 transfer: theory. *J Appl Physiol Respir Environ Exerc Phsiol.* 1981;50(2):265-271.
4. Singh P, Thomson SC. Renal homeostasis and tubuloglomerular feedback. *Curr Opin Nephrol Hypertens.* 2010;19(1):59-64.
5. Street JM, Koritzinsky EH, Bellomo TR, Hu X, Yuen PST, Star RA. The role of adenosine 1a receptor signaling on GFR early after the induction of sepsis. *Am J Physiol Renal Physiol.* 2018;314(5):F788-F797.
6. Blantz RC. Making sense of the sensor: mysteries of the macula densa. *Kidney Int.* 2006;70(5):828-830.
7. Chowdhury AH, Cox EF, Francis ST, Lobo DN. A randomized, controlled, double-blind crossover study on the effects of 2-L infusions of 0.9% saline and plasma-lyte(R) 148 on renal blood flow velocity and renal cortical tissue perfusion in healthy volunteers. *Ann Surg.* 2012;256(1):18-24.
8. Orbegozo D, Su F, Santacruz C, et al. Effects of different crystalloid solutions on hemodynamics, peripheral perfusion, and the microcirculation in experimental abdominal sepsis. *Anesthesiology.* 2016;125(4):744-754.
9. Ho AM, Karmakar MK, Contardi LH, Ng SS, Hewson JR. Excessive use of normal saline in managing traumatized patients in shock: a preventable contributor to acidosis. *J Trauma.* 2001;51(1):173-177.
10. Kellum JA, Song M, Venkataraman R. Effects of hyperchloremic acidosis on arterial pressure and circulating inflammatory molecules in experimental sepsis. *Chest.* 2004;125(1):243-248.
11. Bidani A, Wang CZ, Saggi SJ, Heming TA. Evidence for pH sensitivity of tumor necrosis factor-alpha release by alveolar macrophages. *Lung.* 1998;176(2):111-121.
12. Bellocq A, Suberville S, Philippe C, et al. Low environmental pH is responsible for the induction of nitric-oxide synthase in macrophages. Evidence for involvement of nuclear factor-kappaB activation. *J Biol Chem.* 1998;273(9):5086-5092.
13. Pedoto A, Caruso JE, Nandi J, et al. Acidosis stimulates nitric oxide production and lung damage in rats. *Am J Respir Crit Care Med.* 1999;159(2):397-402.

14. Kellum JA, Song M, Almasri E. Hyperchloremic acidosis increases circulating inflammatory molecules in experimental sepsis. *Chest.* 2006;130(4):962-967.

15. Khan R, Kirschenbaum LA, Larow C, Astiz ME. The effect of resuscitation fluids on neutrophil-endothelial cell interactions in septic shock. *Shock.* 2011;36(5):440-444.

16. Rhee P, Wang D, Ruff P, et al. Human neutrophil activation and increased adhesion by various resuscitation fluids. *Crit Care Med.* 2000;28(1):74-78.

17. Wilcox CS. Regulation of renal blood flow by plasma chloride. *J Clin Invest.* 1983;71(3):726-735.

18. Olivier PY, Beloncle F, Seegers V, et al. Assessment of renal hemodynamic toxicity of fluid challenge with 0.9% NaCl compared to balanced crystalloid (PlasmaLyte®) in a rat model with severe sepsis. *Ann Intensive Care.* 2017;7(1):66.

19. Zhou F, Peng ZY, Bishop JV, Cove ME, Singbartl K, Kellum JA. Effects of fluid resuscitation with 0.9% saline versus a balanced electrolyte solution on acute kidney injury in a rat model of sepsis*. *Crit Care Med.* 2014;42(4):e270-278.

20. Marttinen M, Wilkman E, Petäjä L, Suojaranta-Ylinen R, Pettilä V, Vaara ST. Association of plasma chloride values with acute kidney injury in the critically ill—a prospective observational study. *Acta Anaesthesiol Scand.* 2016;60(6):790-799.

21. Suetrong B, Pisitsak C, Boyd JH, Russell JA, Walley KR. Hyperchloremia and moderate increase in serum chloride are associated with acute kidney injury in severe sepsis and septic shock patients. *Crit Care.* 2016;20(1):315.

22. Zhang Z, Xu X, Fan H, Li D, Deng H. Higher serum chloride concentrations are associated with acute kidney injury in unselected critically ill patients. *BMC Nephrol.* 2013;14:235.

23. Neyra JA, Canepa-Escaro F, Li X, et al. Association of hyperchloremia with hospital mortality in critically ill septic patients. *Crit Care Med.* 2015;43(9):1938-1944.

24. Shaw AD, Schermer CR, Lobo DN, et al. Impact of intravenous fluid composition on outcomes in patients with systemic inflammatory response syndrome. *Crit Care.* 2015;19:334.

25. Shao M, Li G, Sarvottam K, et al. Dyschloremia is a risk factor for the development of acute kidney injury in critically ill patients. *PloS One.* 2016;11(8):e0160322.

26. Yunos NM, Bellomo R, Hegarty C, Story D, Ho L, Bailey M. Association between a chloride-liberal vs. chloride-restrictive intravenous fluid administration strategy and kidney injury in critically ill adults. *JAMA.* 2012;308(15):1566-1572.

27. Yunos NM, Bellomo R, Glassford N, Sutcliffe H, Lam Q, Bailey M. Chloride-liberal vs. chloride-restrictive intravenous fluid administration and acute kidney injury: an extended analysis. *Intensive Care Med.* 2015;41(2):257-264.

28. McCluskey SA, Karkouti K, Wijeysundera D, Minkovich L, Tait G, Beattie WS. Hyperchloremia after noncardiac surgery is independently associated with increased morbidity and mortality: a propensity-matched cohort study. *Anesth Analg.* 2013;117(2):412-421.

29. Raghunathan K, Shaw A, Nathanson B, et al. Association between the choice of IV crystalloid and in-hospital mortality among critically ill adults with sepsis*. *Crit Care Med.* 2014;42(7):1585-1591.

30. Bone RC, Balk RA, Cerra FB, et al. Definitions for sepsis and organ failure and guidelines for the use of innovative therapies in sepsis. The ACCP/SCCM Consensus Conference Committee. American College of Chest Physicians/Society of Critical Care Medicine. *Chest.* 1992;101(6):1644-1655.

31. Shaw AD, Raghunathan K, Peyerl FW, Munson SH, Paluszkiewicz SM, Schermer CR. Association between intravenous chloride load during resuscitation and in-hospital mortality among patients with SIRS. *Intensive Care Med.* 2014;40(12):1897-1905.

32. National Heart, Lung, and Blood Institute Acute Respiratory Distress Syndrome (ARDS) Clinical Trials Network, Wiedemann HP, Wheeler AP, et al. Comparison of two fluid-management strategies in acute lung injury. *N Engl J Med.* 2006;354(24):2564-2575.

33. Boyd JH, Forbes J, Nakada TA, Walley KR, Russell JA. Fluid resuscitation in septic shock: a positive fluid balance and elevated central venous pressure are associated with increased mortality. *Crit Care Med.* 2011;39(2):259-265.

34. RENAL Replacement Therapy Study Investigators, Bellomo R, Cass A, et al. An observational study fluid balance and patient outcomes in the Randomized Evaluation of Normal vs. Augmented Level of Replacement Therapy trial. *Crit Care Med.* 2012;40(6):1753-1760.

35. Schol PB, Terink IM, Lancé MD, Scheepers HC. Liberal or restrictive fluid management during elective surgery: a systematic review and meta-analysis. *J Clin Anesth.* 2016;35:26-39.

36. Shaw AD, Bagshaw SM, Goldstein SL, et al. Major complications, mortality, and resource utilization after open abdominal surgery: 0.9% saline compared to Plasma-Lyte. *Ann Surg.* 2012;255(5):821-829.

37. Young P, Bailey M, Beasley R, et al. Effect of a buffered crystalloid solution vs. saline on acute kidney injury among patients in the intensive care unit: the SPLIT randomized clinical trial. *JAMA.* 2015;314(16):1701-1710.

38. Semler MW, Self WH, Wanderer JP, et al. Balanced crystalloids versus saline in critically ill adults. *N Engl J Med.* 2018;378(9):829-839.

39. Self WH, Semler MW, Wanderer JP, et al. Balanced crystalloids versus saline in noncritically ill adults. *N Engl J Med.* 2018;378(9):819-828.

40. Krajewski ML, Raghunathan K, Paluszkiewicz SM, Schermer CR, Shaw AD. Meta-analysis of high- versus low-chloride content in perioperative and critical care fluid resuscitation. *Br J Surg.* 2015;102(1):24-36.

41. Zayed YZM, Aburahma AMY, Barbarawi MO, et al. Balanced crystalloids versus isotonic saline in critically ill patients: systematic review and meta-analysis. *J Intensive Care.* 2018;6:51.

61

Dysnatremias—What Causes Them and How Should They Be Treated?

Peter Moran, John Bates, and Patrick J. Neligan

INTRODUCTION

Disorders of sodium balance (dysnatremias) are present in up to one-third of intensive care unit (ICU) admissions and are independent risk factors for mortality.[1,2] Sodium is predominantly an extracellular mineral and is evenly distributed across the extracellular fluid (ECF). When plasma sodium $[Na^+]$ is <135 mmol/L or mEq/L (Box 61.1 for definitions), it is referred to as "hyponatremia," that is, low plasma $[Na^+]$ indicates low ECF $[Na^+]$. If plasma $[Na^+]$ exceeds 145 mmol/L, the state is referred to as "hypernatremia." Dysnatremias are manifestations of disorders of water homeostasis caused by diseases that retain or lose electrolytes or add osmotic forces to ECF. Dysnatremias may also be iatrogenic caused by diuretics, intravenous fluids, or hormones. This chapter will initially review normal sodium homeostasis and then look at hyponatremia, its diagnosis and management, and finally hypernatremia and its diagnosis and management.

Homeostatic Mechanisms Relating to Sodium Concentration

Sodium is the most abundant extracellular ion responsible for maintenance of the extracellular volume. There is a dynamic relationship between total body water and extracellular sodium concentration. This water balance is influenced by intakes and outputs, antidiuretic hormone (ADH/vasopressin), renin-angiotensin-aldosterone (RAS), and plasma osmolality. As the sodium cation is excluded from the intracellular space and is the predominant osmotically active substance in the ECF, isolated changes in water volume are generally reflected by inverse changes in the plasma sodium concentration and plasma osmolality. Hyponatremia generally indicates an expansion in free water volume compared with normal. Hypernatremia generally indicates a reduction in free water concentration.

The daily adult requirement for sodium averages 1–2 mmol/kg per day (2–4 g). Normal dietary intake may be two or three times this value. The kidney is the principle site of sodium and water regulation by way of changes in the rates of glomerular filtration and tubular resorption. Approximately 180 L of water and 24,000 mmol of Na^+ are filtered and resorbed by the kidneys each day. This system is controlled by the interaction of various neurohormonal modulators, including the sympathetic nervous system, RAS, atrial natriuretic peptide, and ADH.

When a patient is dehydrated or if circulating volume falls, there is increased firing of osmoreceptors in the anterior hypothalamus. There is increased thirst, reduced baroreceptor activity, and increased release of ADH, which acts in the distal convoluted tubule and collecting ducts via aquaporins to increase water absorption.[3,4]

When circulating volume is increased, stretch-sensitive baroreceptors are activated in the left atrium, carotid sinus, and aortic arch, and there is inhibition of vasopressin secretion.[5] This results in a brisk diuresis of dilute urine.[6]

Diseases or drugs that impact the normal renal or neuroendocrine function impair normal sodium-water homeostasis. For example, congestive heart failure is characterized by adrenergic activation, release of RAS, retention of both salt and water in the renal tubules, and hypervolemia. The administration of angiotensin-converting enzyme inhibitors results in vasodilatation, lowering the blood pressure, diuresis, and natriuresis. In certain physiologic and pathologic states, vasopressin may be released in an unregulated manner. This is known as the syndrome of inappropriate antidiuretic hormone release (SIADH).[7]

HYPONATREMIA

The Patient Has a Low $[Na^+]$—What Does This Mean and What Do I Do?

The hyponatremic patient presents with either an isolated laboratory sample displaying a $[Na^+]$ <135 mmol/L or an array of neurologic symptoms (Box 61.2) where a low $[Na^+]$ is subsequently identified. The latter scenario, a common indication for ICU admission, is a metabolic emergency and requires immediate meticulous medical attention.

Plasma osmolality is governed by contributions from all molecules in the body that cannot easily move between the intravascular and extravascular space. Sodium is the most abundant electrolyte; glucose, urea, plasma proteins, and lipids are also important. Therefore, in hyponatremia, it is imperative that the clinician calculate the plasma osmolality using the calculation in Box 61.3.

There are several ways to classify hyponatremia (see Box 61.2): (1) by the degree of fall of the plasma sodium (mild, moderate, or severe); (2) by the duration of development (acute or chronic); (3) by the plasma osmolality (hypotonic,

BOX 61.1 Commonly Used Chemistry Reference Terms in Clinical Medicine.

The QUANTITY of a substance in the body is expressed in MOLES/MMOLES (mmol).

One mole (1 M) of any substance is its molecular weight expressed in grams and contains 6.023×10^{23} molecules (Avogadro's number). A millimole of a substance is 1/1000 of a mole, or the substance's weight expressed in milligrams.

The CONCENTRATION of a substance in a liquid is expressed as MOLALITY and MOLARITY.

Molality is the number of moles of solute per 1000 g of solvent (e.g., extracellular fluid).

Molality is the number of moles of solute per 1000 g of solvent. It is independent of temperature. Molarity is the number of moles of solute per 1000 mL of solution at a specified temperature. In medicine we use molarity when describing particles in blood—millimoles per liter of solution (millimolar, [mM]) or extracellular fluid. We use millimoles per kilogram of solution (millimolal, [mm]) when describing, for example, intravenous fluids.

The electrical charge or VALENCE of a substance is expressed in MILLI-EQUIVALENTS (mEq/L).

In the case of univalent ions, 1 mEq is equal to 1/1000 of the gram-atomic weight. It is the same as 1 mMol of the ion in question and consists of 6.023×10^{20} particles. For divalent ions, 1 mEq consists of 3.012×10^{20} particles and weighs 1/2000 of the gram-atomic weight. One mMol of divalent ions equals 2 mEq.

The force that controls the flow of water across membranes is OSMOTIC PRESSURE is expressed in MILLI-OSMOLES.

Osmotic pressure is the hydrostatic pressure that must be applied to the solution of greater concentration to prevent water movement across the membrane. One gram molecular weight (i.e., 1 M) of a non-dissociating compound (e.g., glucose, urea) consists of 6.023×10^{23} molecules and is termed 1 osmole (osmol, Osm). For non-dissociating compounds, 1 mM is equivalent to 1 mOsm. Ionized substances tend to dissociate in solution and thereby generate more osmotically active particles.

Osmolarity is the number of osmoles of solute per liter of solvent plus solute. Osmolality is the solute concentration per kilogram of solvent (water). Osmolality is more widely used in clinical practice, as its value is unaffected by the presence of fat and protein in plasma.

BOX 61.2 Classification of Hyponatremia.

1. Serum concentration of sodium
   Mild: 130–135 mmol/L
   Moderate: 125–129 mmol/L
   Severe/profound: <125 mmol/L
2. Duration of development
   Acute hyponatremia <48 h
   Chronic hyponatremia >48 h
3. Plasma osmolality
   Hypotonic hyponatremia, serum osmolality <275 mOsm/L
   Isotonic hyponatremia, serum osmolality >275 mOsm/L
   Pseudohyponatremia
4. Volume status
   Isovolemic hyponatremia
   Hypovolemic hyponatremia
   Hypervolemic hyponatremia

BOX 61.3 Calculation of the Plasma Osmolality.

Plasma osmolality
$$= 2\left(Na^+ + K^+\right) + BUN/2.8 + Glucose/16 \ \text{(in mg/dL)}$$

or in SI units (mmol/L)

$$2\left(Na^+ + K^+\right) + Urea + Glucose$$

One should also request that the lab measure plasma osmolality; the presence of an osmolar gap (measured minus calculated) indicates the presence of unmeasured osmoles in extracellular fluid.

isotonic, hypertonic, or pseudohyponatremia); and (4) by the volume status (isovolemic, hypovolemic, or hypervolemic). We will explore the problem using the osmolality and volume status.

Pseudohyponatremia—When the [Na+] Is Not Really Low at All

The first question is whether the laboratory result is accurate. There is often a discrepancy between the [Na+] reported from the laboratory and that derived from a point-of-care blood gas machine, which is likely more accurate depending on the method used for [Na+] measurement in the laboratory.[8] This is because the ion-selective electrode measurement in the blood gas analyzer is not influenced by alterations in plasma protein concentrations.

Pseudohyponatremia is caused by a displacement of plasma water by elevated concentrations of lipids or proteins. It is a laboratory artefact.[9] Normally, a plasma sample comprises 93% water, which includes all the dissolved electrolytes. The remaining 7% consists of other material, principally protein and fat. If the protein or fat concentration of plasma increases due to, for example, a macroglobulinemia, the laboratory test that uses indirect ion-specific electrodes (ISE) will erroneously calculate a low sodium as it assumes a plasma water content of 93%. Hyperlipidemia occurs in pancreatitis, biliary obstruction, diabetes, and with parenteral nutrition. Pseudohyponatremia is confirmed by checking [Na+] on a device that performs direct ISE, such as blood gas machines. The recognition of pseudohyponatremia is important because therapy for the decreased plasma sodium concentration is not indicated.

True Hyponatremia

Hyponatremia is principally a disorder of relative water excess compared with total body sodium content. If the plasma [Na$^+$] is low, but plasma osmolality is normal or high, it is referred to as hypertonic hyponatremia. If the plasma [Na$^+$] is low relative to extracellular water and plasma osmolality is also low, it is hypotonic hyponatremia (Fig. 61.1). Hypotonic hyponatremia may occur with normal ECF volume (normovolemic hypotonic hyponatremia), increased ECF volume (hypervolemic hypotonic hyponatremia), or low ECF volume (hypovolemic hyponatremia).

Hypertonic Hyponatremia

Hypertonic hyponatremia occurs when decreased plasma [Na$^+$] coexists with an increased serum osmolality (Fig. 61.2). An increase in the concentration of any osmotically active substance, which is confined predominately to the ECF (e.g., glucose, glycerol, mannitol), will result in water movement out of cells along the osmolar gradient. The osmolar load usually evokes an osmotic diuresis, leading to urinary loss of both sodium and water. These losses may, in turn, potentiate both hypertonicity and hyponatremia. Clinically, the most frequent cause of hypertonic hypernatremia is hyperglycemia in uncontrolled or poorly controlled diabetes mellitus. The measured serum sodium concentration decreases approximately 2.4 mmol/L for each 100 mg/dL (5.5 mmol/L) increment of blood glucose.[10] Hypertonic hyponatremia may also be seen in acute kidney injury (AKI) associated with large quantities of retained solute.

Hypotonic Hyponatremia

In hypotonic hyponatremia there is a low [Na$^+$] and low plasma osmolality. This may be associated with normal, increased, or decreased ECF volume (Box 61.4).

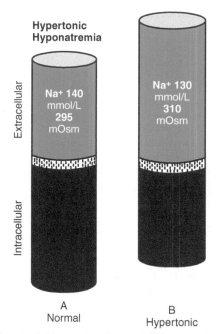

Fig. 61.2 Hypertonic Hypernatremia: panel (A) represents normal fluid distribution between the intracellular and extracellular compartments. Panel (B) represents hypertonic hypernatremia: there is contraction of intracellular fluid volume.

Hypotonic Hyponatremia With Decreased ECF Volume (Hypovolemic)

In situations where the body loses both sodium and water, for example, with the use of thiazide diuretics, the body attempts to defend ECF volume by increasing ADH/vasopressin secretion, resulting in a relative increase in the proportion of water to sodium (Fig. 61.3C).[11] This picture may also be seen in other scenarios where renal handling of sodium is

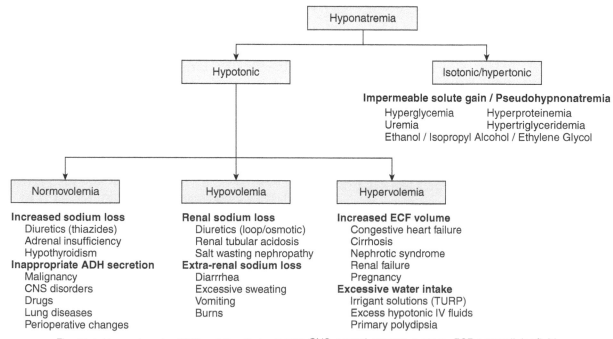

Fig. 61.1 Hyponatremia. *ADH,* antidiuretic hormone; *CNS,* central nervous system; *ECF,* extracellular fluid.

1. Hypovolemic hypotonic hyponatremia (decreased extracellular fluid volume)
   a. Diuretics
   b. Hypoaldosteronism
   c. Vomiting/diarrhea
   d. Sweating
   e. Burns
   f. Tubulopathies—e.g., following chemotherapy
2. Isovolemic hypotonic hyponatremia (normal extracellular fluid volume)
3. Hypervolemic hypotonic hyponatremia (increased extracellular fluid volume)

dysfunctional, consequent of hypoaldosteronism following chemotherapy and with medullary cystic kidney disease.

Salt and water are also lost from the body when there is blood loss (particularly when repleted with hypotonic fluid), vomiting, diarrhea, sweating, burns, and bowel obstruction.

Hypotonic Hyponatremia With Normal ECF Volume (Isovolemic)

When the $[Na^+]$ is low and ECF volume is normal (isovolemic hypotonic hyponatremia [IHH]), there is a problem of neurohormonal control of sodium and water balance (Fig. 61.3B). This may occur, for example, following surgery or in acute critical illness, when there is activation of the RAS-ADH axis, and hypotonic fluids are administered. IHH may also occur as a result of excess sodium loss from sweating (during intense exercise) when hypotonic fluid

(such as water) is taken for fluid replacement. Occasionally one will encounter patients who obsessively drink large amounts of water irrespective of losses ("psychogenic polydipsia"), and this overwhelms the body's homeostatic controls. In addition, the excretion of free water is dependent on adequate solute intake. In patients who are malnourished or with very low solute intake, the ability of the kidney to clear free water is inhibited by the deficiency of these osmoles. Vasopressin plays no role in the development of hyponatremia in these states and urine osmolarity is low.[12] IHH is also associated with hypocortisolism[13] and hypothyroidism.[14]

As ADH/vasopressin is a core control hormone for body water content, and its secretion is responsive to changes in ECF osmolality, increased secretion may result in a water overload syndrome—SIADH (see Fig. 61.2D).

SIADH is caused by either pituitary or ectopic release of vasopressin that is not under homeostatic control. It is commonly associated with small cell lung cancer and occasionally with subarachnoid hemorrhage (Box 61.5).[7] Inappropriate antidiuresis can also occur with increased activity of vasopressin and from mutations in the V2 receptor.[15] SIADH is diagnosed based on clinical and biochemical criteria (see Box 61.5).

Hypotonic Hyponatremia Associated With Increased ECF Volume (Hypervolemic)

In hypervolemic hypotonic hyponatremia, $[Na^+]$ is low (hypotonia) and the ECF volume is increased (Fig. 61.3D). This typically occurs in progressive heart failure due to upregulation of RAS, consequent of reduced renal perfusion and sympathetic activation. Increased baroreceptor activity results in

Hypotonic hyponatremia

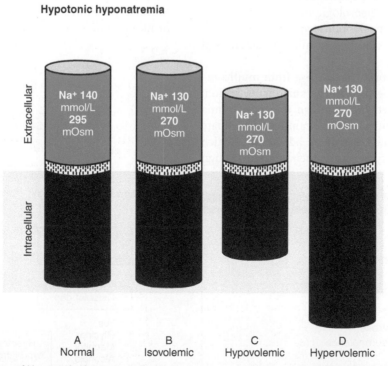

Fig. 61.3 **Types of Hypotonic Hyponatremia.** (A) represents normal fluid and electrolyte balance; (B) is isovolemic hyponatremia; (C) is hypovolemic hyponatremia and (D) is hypervolemic hyponatremia.

BOX 61.5   Diagnosis of Syndrome of Inappropriate Antidiuretic Hormone Release.

- Essential criteria
    - Effective serum osmolarity <275 mOsm/kg
    - Urine osmolality >100 mOsm/kg
    - Clinical euvolemia
    - Urinary sodium >30 mmol/L
    - Absence of adrenal, thyroid, pituitary, or renal insufficiency
    - No recent diuretic use
- Supplemental criteria
    - Serum uric acid <0.24 mmol/L
    - Serum urea <3.6 mmol/L
    - Failure to correct hyponatremia after 0.9% saline infusion
    - Fractional sodium excretion >0.5%
    - Fractional urea excretion >55%
    - Fractional uric acid excretion <12%
    - Correction of hyponatremia through fluid restriction

increased vasopressin secretion. There is sodium and water retention.

Similarly, in liver failure, the hyperdynamic circulation and systemic vasodilation caused by elevated nitric oxide is associated with upregulation of the RAS and vasopressin secretion.

Nephrotic syndrome is associated with urinary protein loss and a fall in plasma oncotic pressure. Neurohormonal activation results in both sodium and water retention to maintain intravascular volume, leading to hyponatremia.[16]

Symptoms and Complications of Hyponatremia

If the blood is hypo-osmolar in relation to the brain, water enters the brain and may cause acute cerebral edema. This may lead to a spectrum of neurologic upsets ranging from confusion to seizures to coma to brain stem herniation. These complications are usually classified as mild, moderate, and severe (Box 61.6).[17]

The symptoms of cerebral edema arise from multicompartment compression effects of intracranial hypertension. Cerebral edema is of particular concern if hyponatremia develops acutely (<48 hours) as the brain has inadequate time to adapt to hypotonia.[18] During adaptation, which takes 24–48 hours,[19] astrocytes restore their volume through

BOX 61.6   Symptoms of Acute Hyponatremia.

1. Mild—nonspecific
2. Moderately severe
    i. Nausea without vomiting
    ii. Confusion
    iii. Headache
3. Severe
    i. Vomiting
    ii. Cardiorespiratory distress
    iii. Abnormal and deep somnolence
    iv. Seizures
    v. Coma (Glasgow coma scale <8)

loss of organic osmolytes, a process that increases the risk posed by rapid correction of hyponatremia.[6]

In nonhypotonic hyponatremia, plasma osmolality is often normal, so there is no risk of cerebral edema. The most common causes of this are hyperglycemia, mannitol, and glycine. Once the effective osmoles are metabolized/removed from the serum, water moves intracellularly and measured sodium levels rise. In hyperglycemia, cerebral edema can occur if serum glucose falls more rapidly than serum sodium rises, as the effective serum osmolarity decreases.[20]

Clinical Assessment of the Patient With Hyponatremia (Fig. 61.4)

The initial diagnostic process should be to determine whether the patient has isotonic/hypertonic hyponatremia or hypotonic hyponatremia. A plasma osmolality should be calculated (see Box 61.3). If osmolality is normal, then the source of additional osmoles is within the formula, either hyperglycemia or uremia. If the calculated osmolality is low (<275 mOsm/kg), a sample should be sent to the laboratory to measure actual osmolality. If measured osmolality is within the normal range, then there is an osmolar gap, and unmeasured osmoles are present. There are few noniatrogenic causes of an osmolar gap; it is usually associated with mannitol or glycine ("TUR-syndrome") and very occasionally with ethanol, methanol, or ethylene glycol poisoning. If the measured and calculated osmolality are both <275 mOsm/Kg, it is hypotonic hyponatremia.

Diagnostic Workup for Hypotonic Hyponatremia (Fig. 61.5)

When hypotonic hyponatremia is suspected, it is essential to check urinary osmolality and urinary [Na$^+$]. Very low urinary osmolality (<100 mOsm/Kg) is associated with water overload syndrome, usually seen in psychiatric patients who drink enormous quantities of water and have defeated the

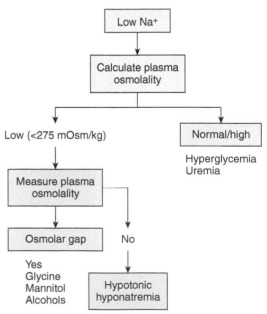

Fig. 61.4 Initial Diagnostic Pathway for Hyponatremia.

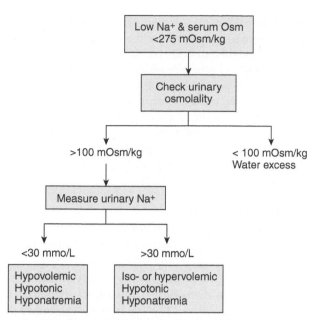

Fig. 61.5 Diagnostic Workup for Hypotonic Hyponatremia.

body's control of sodium.[21] The alternate diagnosis is low solute intake where isotonic fluid loss is replaced by low solute water. It may also be seen in individuals who drink distilled water as a lifestyle choice.

If the urine osmolarity is >100 mOsm/L, then urinary [Na$^+$] measurement can be used to establish the patients' volume status. If the urinary [Na$^+$] is <30 mmol/L, the body is holding onto water and sodium aggressively, and this usually indicates hypovolemia or renal hypoperfusion (low body [Na$^+$] and low body water; see Fig. 61.2).[22] This may occur due to excessive fasting, vomiting, diarrhea, or "third space" fluid loss, as is seen with bowel obstruction. There should be clinical signs of hypovolemia, such as sunken eyes, dry mouth, and so on. If the patient is edematous and the urinary [Na$^+$] is low, then there is a problem with neuroendocrine handling of ECF volume. Further investigations should look for evidence of cirrhosis (hepatic ultrasound and liver function tests), congestive heart failure (beta-natriuretic peptide and echocardiography), and nephrotic syndrome (urinary protein).

If the urinary [Na$^+$] exceeds 30 mmol/L, the patient is either isovolemic or is wasting sodium in the urine. This may be as a result of diuretic (particularly thiazides) therapy, cerebral salt wasting (CSW), secondary adrenal insufficiency, SIADH, or hypothyroidism.[7]

CSW is distinguished from SIADH by the following criteria: in CSW there is polyuria rather than oliguria and the patient tends to be hypovolemic, characterized by increased serum urea, albumin, bicarbonate, and hemoglobin.

Symptom Assessment and Immediate Treatment Indications

The reader should be aware that, although dysnatremias are very common in critical illness, most of the literature

regarding investigation and treatment involves retrospective cohort studies. International guidelines have been produced using "expert" panels who interpret this limited dataset.[17,22] Although the following discussion is based on such guidelines, the foundation evidence is flimsy.

The goal of treating hyponatremia is to reduce the risk of brain injury by stabilizing ECF osmolality while avoiding the risk of excessively rapid correction with associated demyelination. It is generally agreed that acute or severely symptomatic hyponatremia should be managed aggressively within the first hour using hypertonic saline (HTS; 3%) to avoid irreversible damage (Fig. 61.6).[17,22] Evidence for the use of HTS is from small retrospective trials ($n < 100$) or case series. In a case series of seven patients who presented with severe symptomatic hyponatremia, patients treated with variable rates of 3% HTS achieved a mean rise of 2.4 ± 0.5 mmol/L per hour.[23] A 2005 retrospective study of severe symptomatic hyponatremic patients treated with HTS infusions of 250–750 mL of 3% HTS found resolution of symptoms with mean serum sodium rises of 1.6 ± 0.5 mmol/L per hour.[24]

"Expert" opinion suggests the use of repeated boluses of 150 mL of 3% HTS with frequent checking of serum sodium.[17] Discontinuation of hypertonic therapy is suggested once symptoms resolve or when sodium rises by 5 mmol/L.[17] It is unknown whether the use of bolus therapy is more effective than an infusion.[25]

Predicting Sodium Rise

Various formulae such as the Adrogué–Madias formula (Box 61.7) can be used to predict serum sodium rises with treatment but they are not wholly reliable because each patient is different, and the clinician must dynamically change infusion rates in response to changes in [Na$^+$].[26,27]

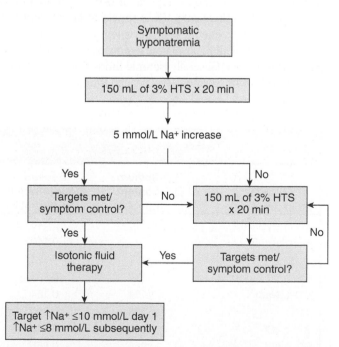

Fig. 61.6 Treatment of Acute Hyponatremia. *HTS,* hypertonic saline.

BOX 61.7　Calculating the Change in [Na⁺] – Adrogué–Madias Formula.

$$\text{Change in serum } Na^+ = \frac{\text{infusate } Na^+ - \text{serum } Na^+}{\text{total body water} + 1}$$

Data from Adrogué HJ, Madias NE. Hyponatremia. *N Engl J Med.* 2000;342(21):1581-1589.

Once there has been a 5 mmol/L rise in plasma sodium and symptoms have resolved, there is general consensus that sodium correction rates should be restricted to <10 mmol/L in the first 24 hours and <8 mmol/L in the subsequent 24-hour period, irrespective of whether or not the patient is symptomatic.[17]

If symptoms persist after a 5 mmol/L rise in sodium or if [Na⁺] exceeds 130 mmol/L, it is possible that the diagnosis is incorrect and that the neurological symptoms are coincidental; further investigations should be considered, for example computed tomography scanning of the brain.

In asymptomatic patients presenting with hyponatremia, the use of HTS is unnecessary, and alternative therapies such as water restriction, diuresis, and isotonic fluids may be considered.

Chronic hyponatremia is associated with increased risk of death, likely coincidental with the underlying diagnosis, such as cirrhosis and heart failure. It is unclear whether treating low [Na⁺] in this setting improves outcomes. The use of vasopressin receptor antagonists (VRA) has been suggested in this setting. Two systematic reviews have performed meta-analysis on 15 and 18 trials where the use of VRAs was compared with placebo.[28,29] Both reviews demonstrated significant increases in plasma [Na⁺], lower urinary osmolality, reduction in blood pressure, and diuresis-associated weight loss. Plasma potassium was stable, and there were no significant complications and no reports of osmotic-related brain injury. Based on these data, VRAs appear to be safe and may be beneficial in euvolemic or hypervolemic hyponatremia.

For patients with hypovolemic hyponatremia, fluid resuscitation is necessary. Generally isotonic fluids (Table 61.1), such as Plasmalyte-148, Normosol-R, Lactated Ringer's / Hartmann's

TABLE 61.1　Sodium Content of Various Intravenous Fluids.

Fluid (infusate)	Sodium Content (mmol/L)	Sodium Concentration (mmol/mL)
Plasmalyte-148	140	0.140
Normosol-R	140	0.140
Hartmann's solution	131	0.131
Lactated Ringer's	130	0.130
0.9% NaCl	154	0.154
1.8%	308	0.380
3% NaCl	513	0.513
5% NaCl	855	0.855

solution, or 0.9% saline (care should be taken to avoid acquired hyperchloremia), can be used at the rate of 0.5–1.0 mL/kg per hour, with careful monitoring of the plasma [Na⁺].

The SIADH is generally treated with fluid restriction for moderate or profound hyponatremia. For patients admitted to intensive care, it may be worthwhile to use low-dose loop diuretic and oral sodium chloride tablets or intravenous isotonic fluid.[17] The use of demeclocycline or lithium to induce nephrogenic diabetes insipidus (DI) is controversial, but likely of little benefit in critical care.[17,22] The US guidelines favor the use of VRAs in SIADH.[22]

Potential Complications

Osmotic Demyelination Syndrome

Osmotic demyelination syndrome (ODS) results from an osmotic / ischemic injury to the pons ("central pontine myelinolysis"), which appears to be exquisitely sensitive to osmotic shifts when dysnatremia, in particular hyponatremia, is precipitously corrected. This syndrome is characterized by dysarthria, dysphagia, development of an initial flaccid quadriparesis that later becomes spastic, and occasionally "locked-in syndrome." Although ODS can cause permanent disability, many patients make a full recovery.[30]

Risk factors for ODS include chronic alcoholism, malnutrition, liver failure, and prolonged diuretic use.[31] The true incidence of the syndrome is unknown. Prevention of this condition relies on conservative rates of sodium correction.[32]

Rapid Overcorrection

So, what does one do if the rate of correction is >10 mmol/L in 24 hours, and ODS is looming?[33] One can either prevent water from being excreted by administering intravenous desmopressin 2 μg,[34] and redosing if necessary at 8-hour intervals, or by administering water in the form of dextrose 5% intravenously at 10 mL/kg per hour.[17]

Severe Hyponatremia Management With Continuous Renal Replacement Therapies

Continuous renal replacement therapy (CRRT) can be used to correct plasma sodium concentration, but with extreme care. Either the replacement fluid or the dialysate sodium concentration can be adjusted to gradually correct the plasma [Na⁺].[35] It is our preference to dilute the replacement fluid with varying amounts of distilled water to achieve this (Table 61.2).[36] This approach should not be performed in circuits that use citrate anticoagulation.

HYPERNATREMIA

The Patient Has a High [Na⁺]—What Does this Mean and What Do I Do?

Hypernatremia is defined as a plasma sodium concentration >145 mmol/L. There is an absolute or relative deficit of free water (Box 61.8, Eq. 1, and Fig. 61.7).[37,38] The incidence of hypernatremia in the general hospital population is 1% and may be as high as 26% in patients admitted to ICUs.[39,40]

TABLE 61.2 Impact of Adding Sterile Water to Hemosol B0 (Baxter).

Target [Na$^+$] mmol/L	H$_2$O Added (mL)	Dialysate Volume (mL)	[K$^+$] (mmol/L)	[HCO$_3^-$] (mmol/L
140	0	5000	4.0	35
136	150	5150	3.9	34
133	250	5250	3.8	33
131	350	5350	3.7	33
127	500	5500	3.6	32
122	750	5750	3.5	30
117	1000	6000	3.3	29

This is the simplest method of reducing the [Na$^+$] of the dialysate bag. We do not advocate for removing fluid from the bag, so the volume of dialysate increases (column 2) in proportion to the volume of water added.

BOX 61.8 Hypernatremia Calculations.

Equation 1: Plasma Sodium Concentration Edelman Equation[38]

$$[Na^+] = \left(\text{Total exchangeable Na} + \text{total exchangeable K}^+\right)/\text{TBW}$$

Equation 2: Electrolyte Free Water Clearance

$$EFWC = \text{Urine volume (in liters)} \times \left(1 - \left(Na^+ \text{ uring} + K^+ \text{ urine}\right)/Na^+ \text{ Plasma}\right)$$

Equation 3: Sodium Balance

$$\left(Na^+ + K^+\right) \text{ infused} - \left(Na^+ + K^+\right) \text{ excreted} > 0$$

Equation 4: Estimating the Free Water Deficit

$$\text{Free water deficit} = TBW \times \left(\text{serum Na}^+ - \text{ideal serum Na}^+\right)/\text{ideal serum Na}^+$$

Equation 5: Equation for Estimating Rate of [Na$^+$] correction

$$\text{Change in serum Na}^+ = \left(\text{Infusate Na}^+ + \text{Infusate K-serum Na}^+\right)/\text{Total body water} + 1$$

TBW, total body water.

Causes of Hypernatremia

Hypernatremia develops as a result of either free water loss or plasma sodium gain, or both (see Fig. 61.7).[37,38] Free water loss may be renal or extrarenal[41] or due to inadequate water intake.[42] Hypernatremia may be hypovolemic (Fig. 61.8B), isovolemic (Fig. 61.8C), or hypervolemic (Fig. 61.8D).

Hypovolemic Hypernatremia

The calculation of the electrolyte free water clearance (EFWC) may be used to differentiate water deficiency from sodium overload (see Box 61.8 Eq. 2). It is the volume of water over time and if the calculation is negative, then the body is losing water from a nonrenal location. In this scenario the kidney is working hard to maintain homeostasis. If plasma sodium is rising and EFWC is positive, water losses are from the kidneys.[38]

Renal causes of hypernatremia include the use of diuretics, particularly loop or osmotic diuretics, and polyuric states, including DI (neurogenic or nephrogenic), hyperglycemia, hypokalemia, hypercalcemia, and in the polyuric phase of AKI and chronic kidney disease.[43–45] Nonrenal causes of pure water loss include open abdomen, using non humidified oxygen, and burns. Sodium and water loss may occur with vomiting, nasogastric drainage, diarrhea, and bowel obstruction.

DI is caused by an absolute deficiency of ADH, usually associated with brain injury—neurogenic DI—(the posterior pituitary gland fails to produce sufficient vasopressin), or renal insensitivity to ADH—nephrogenic DI—usually associated with drugs, principally lithium. DI causes hypovolemic hypernatremia (see Fig. 61.8B). DI is characterized by the production of urine that is largely free from solute.[46]

The diagnosis of DI is based on the presence of polyuria (>40 mL/kg per 24 hours), hypernatremia, and a low urine osmolarity (<200 mOsm/L in central DI and 200–500 mOsm/L in nephrogenic DI).[47] To differentiate between the two causes, desmopressin is administered. A response to desmopressin with a rise in urine osmolarity >600 mOsm/kg confirms central DI.[48]

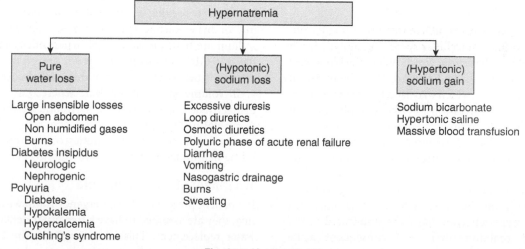

Fig. 61.7 Hypernatremia.

Hypernatremia

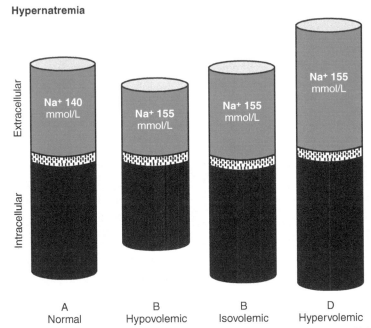

Fig. 61.8 **Types of Hypernatremia.** (A) represents normal fluid and electrolyte balance; (B) is hypovolemic hypernatremia; (C) is isovolemic hypernatremia and (D) is hypervolemic hypernatremia.

Isovolemic or Hypervolemic Hypernatremia

Hypernatremia also accompanies sodium gain and may be isovolemic or hypervolemic (see Figs. 61.8C and D). In the setting of an acute stress response, there is active retention of salt and water. Hence the administration of large quantities of sodium and other electrolytes results in acquired hypernatremia. Over 50% of ICU patients have a positive sodium balance.[41] This results from administration of isotonic and HTS, sodium bicarbonate, blood products, various antibiotics, and dilutants for intravenous infusions.[49] Perioperative patients typically receive relatively large volumes of isotonic crystalloids to treat blood loss. The calculation of the sodium balance can be viewed in Box 61.8 as Eq. 3.[37] Spontaneous or active deresuscitation of patients who have accumulated extracellular crystalloid in the perioperative period and early in critical illness results in more rapid removal of water compared with solute and isovolemic hypernatremia results.[50]

Symptoms and Signs of Hypernatremia

Hypovolemic hypernatremia results in water movement from the intracellular to the extracellular space. Initially the brain shrinks due to volume depletion, which makes the blood vessels vulnerable to rupture. The brain adapts to dehydration by expressing more solute, which may lead to cerebral edema, neurological deficit, or convulsions.[37] Other complications of hypernatremia include muscle weakness,[51] restless legs, lethargy, coma,[52] and delayed weaning from mechanical ventilation.[53] Hypernatremia also effects glycemic control. The hyperosmolar state impairs glucose utilization and insulin-mediated glucose metabolism resulting in hyperglycemia.[54] An association with impaired cardiac function has also been described,[55] and hypernatremia has been implicated in the development of rhabdomyolysis and consequent acute kidney injury.[56]

Currently there are no data to associate ICU-acquired hypernatremia with any specific complications.[57] Although hypernatremia is an independent risk factor for mortality even in patients with mild elevations in serum sodium concentration,[53] this may be a secondary phenomenon.[33]

Assessment and Treatment of Hypernatremia

When initially encountering hypernatremic patients, it is important to ascertain whether the disorder is acute (<48 hours) or chronic (>48 hours). In acute hypernatremia, rapid correction of serum sodium improves both symptoms and prognosis, without an increased risk of cerebral edema.[17] In chronic hypernatremia, rapid correction may result in ODS. The second step in management is determining the cause of hypertonicity (loss of free water, sodium gain, or both).[58]

There is no easy or reliable method of determining volume status in critically ill patients. The presence of significant edema or increased body weight or a cumulative positive fluid balance in the setting of hypernatremia is indicative of isovolemic or hypervolemic hypernatremia. Total body water and sodium are both increased, and hypertonicity likely activates the RAS-ADH axis to prevent water and solute loss.[59] There may be associated disruption of the renal glycocalyx.[59,60]

If volume status is unclear, we recommend checking urinary [Na$^+$]: a low urinary [Na$^+$] indicates hypovolemia.[21] A normal or high urinary [Na+] may reflect isovolemia or hypervolemia, the use of diuretics or a sodium, and water losing nephropathy, such as following AKI (Fig. 61.9).

Treatment of Hypernatremia

If a patient presents to the emergency room with hypernatremia, they are assumed to have a free water deficit and require water replacement. This is accomplished by administering either free water orally or enterally, or relatively hypotonic

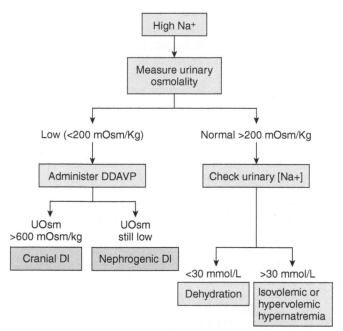

Fig. 61.9 Assessment of Hypernatremia.

TABLE 61.3 Sodium Content of Fluids Used to Treat Hypernatremia.

Fluid (Infusate)	Sodium Content (mmol/L)	Change per Liter in 70 kg Male With Na⁺ 150 mmol/L
Dextrose 5% in water	0	-3.5 mmol Na⁺/L
0.2% NaCl in D5%	34	-2.7 mmol Na⁺/L
0.45% NaCl	77	-1.7 mmol Na⁺/L
Lactated Ringer's	130	-0.5 mEmol Na⁺/L

fluid intravenously (Fig. 61.10). Equations to calculate free water deficit are routinely used to quantify the volume of replacement fluid required to treat the hypernatremic state (see Box 61.8 Eq. 4).[41] Any hypotonic fluid can be used to correct the water deficit, the more hypotonic the fluid the more rapid the correction (Table 61.3). In cases of severe hypernatremia ([Na⁺] >170 mmol/L) associated with dehydration, we recommend initial fluid resuscitation with isotonic fluid such as 0.9% NaCl ([Na⁺] 154 mmol/L or balanced salt solutions ([Na⁺] 140 mmol/L) to prevent over rapid correction.

In either acute or chronic hypernatremia, the goal is to stabilize the extracellular sodium content and prevent

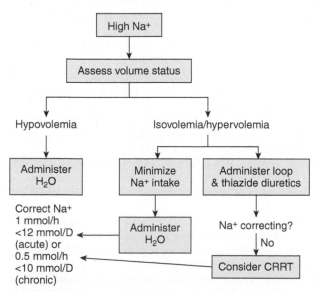

Fig. 61.10 Management of Hypernatremia. *CRRT,* continuous renal replacement therapy.

osmotic-related brain injury; the rate of correction should not exceed 8–12 mmol/L per day.[61] If the problem is of acute (<48 hours) onset, [Na⁺] can be corrected at an initial rate of 1 mmol/L per hour. For chronic or unknown duration hypernatremia, the initial rate should be ≤0.5 mmol/L per hour.[62]

The Adrogué–Madias formula (see Box 61.8 Eq. 5) can be used to determine appropriate infusion rates for the correction of hypernatremia. This has been prospectively validated in both hyponatremia and hypernatremia, but should be used with care due to interpatient variability of response.[63,64]

Acquired hypernatremia in critical illness is usually iatrogenic (with the exception of DI). It is unlikely that active correction of mild to moderate hypernatremia in the euvolemic critically ill patient is beneficial.[57] Many patients, however, are hypernatremic and hypervolemic. Hypervolemia results in pulmonary edema, ileus, poor wound healing, and a variety of compartment syndromes.[50] One must remove both sodium and water as part of a deresuscitation paradigm, which is very challenging. Loop diuretics preferentially remove water and may precipitate and worsen hypernatremia.[65] A variety of different recipes using loop diuretics, sodium restriction, and water or dextrose replacement have been reported and validated.[66–68] However, in severe fluid overload or volume-sensitive states, such as acute respiratory distress syndrome, the use of hypotonic fluid may worsen rather than improve hypervolemia. Where possible medications should be administered enterally or dissolved in dextrose rather than in salt solutions, thiazide diuretics are widely used to facilitate natiuresis in the setting of hypervolemic hypernatremia. Though anecdotally effective, there are currently few data to support this approach.[69]

It is important to note that as the serum albumin is universally low in critically ill patients, it is possible that pseudohypernatremia may be identified as a "free water deficit."[70] Again we recommend that clinicians used point-of-care testing devices to confirm the diagnosis.

CRRT has also been used to control both sodium and water in this setting. While rapid correction is possible using isotonic dialysate for patients with severe hypernatremia, there is a significant risk of ODS. The dialysate can be adjusted using HTS to dynamically control [Na⁺] reduction (Table 61.4).[71]

TABLE 61.4 Impact of 3% NaCl to Hemosol B0 (Baxter).

Target [Na⁺] (mmol/L)	3% NaCl Added	Dialysate Volume (mL)
140	0	5000
145	50	5050
150	100	5100
155	150	5150
160	200	5200
165	250	5250
170	300	5300

This is the simplest method of increasing the [Na⁺] of the dialysate bag. We do not advocate for removing fluid from the bag, so the volume of dialysate increases (column 2) in proportion to the volume of water added. 1 mL 3% NaCl = 0.5 mmol Na⁺/mL. Note that the [K⁺] and [HCO₃⁻] concentrations change very little with this level of dilution.

AUTHORS' RECOMMENDATIONS

- About 30% of patients in ICU present with disorders of sodium [Na⁺] metabolism.
- There is a strong correlation between the sodium concentration [Na⁺] in plasma and ECF volume. A low [Na⁺] (<135 mmol/L), known as hyponatremia, represents a relative excess of free water in ECF compared with [Na⁺]. This may be acute or chronic and may be associated with an array of neurological symptoms or may be asymptomatic.
- Hyponatremia may be associated with normal or increased body water (isovolemic or hypervolemic) or low body water (hypovolemic).
- The SIADH is caused by various cancers and brain injuries and results in renal water retention.
- Acute symptomatic hyponatremia should be treated immediately with HTS (3%) to increase [Na⁺] by 5 mmol/L and control symptoms. The goal of treating hyponatremia is to reduce the risk of brain injury by stabilizing ECF osmolality while avoiding the risk of excessively rapid correction, with associated demyelination. The maximum increase in [Na⁺] should be <10 mmol/L in the first 24 hours (and <8 mmol/L subsequently).
- Hypernatremia is associated with profound dehydration or isovolemic or hypervolemic sodium overload; usually iatrogenic.
- Dehydration is treated by repleting the free water deficit. In acute symptomatic hypernatremia, the goal is to stabilize the balance of sodium and extracellular volume to avoid neurologic injury associated with the condition or over rapid correction.
- We recommend that the clinician correct the [Na⁺] at a rate of 0.5–1 mmol/L per hour depending on whether the disorder is chronic or acute. The maximum rate of correction is 8–12 mmol/L per day. Hypervolemic hypernatremia is treated with hypotonic fluids and loop and thiazide diuretics.
- CRRT may be used to correct both hyponatremia and hypernatremia. In severe cases, extreme care must be taken to avoid over rapid correction, requiring adjustment of the dialysate and/or the replacement fluid.

REFERENCES

1. Upadhyay A, Jaber BL, Madias NE. Epidemiology of hyponatremia. *Semin Nephrol.* 2009;29(3):227-238.
2. Darmon M, Diconne E, Souweine B, et al. Prognostic consequences of borderline dysnatremia: pay attention to minimal serum sodium change. *Crit Care.* 2013;17(1):R12.
3. Norsk P. Influence of low- and high-pressure baroreflexes on vasopressin release in humans. *Acta Endocrinol (Copenh).* 1989; 121(Suppl. 1):3-27.
4. Robertson GL. Thirst and vasopressin function in normal and disordered states of water balance. *J Lab Clin Med.* 1983;101:351-371.
5. Verbalis JG. Disorders of body water homeostasis. *Best Pract Res Clin Endocrinol Metab.* 2003;17(4):471-503.
6. Sterns RH. Disorders of plasma sodium– causes, consequences, and correction. *N Engl J Med.* 2015;372(1):55-65.
7. Schwartz WB, Bennett W, Curelop S, Bartter FC. A syndrome of renal sodium loss and hyponatremia probably resulting from inappropriate secretion of antidiuretic hormone. *Am J Med.* 1957;23(4):529-542.
8. Aw TC, Kiechle FL. Pseudohyponatremia. *Am J Emerg Med.* 1985;3(3):236-239.
9. Dimeski G, Morgan TJ, Presneill JJ, Venkatesh B. Disagreement between ion selective electrode direct and indirect sodium measurements: estimation of the problem in a tertiary referral hospital. *J Crit Care.* 2012;27(3):326.e6-e16.
10. Hillier TA, Abbott RD, Barrett EJ. Hyponatremia: evaluating the correction factor for hyperglycemia. *Am J Med.* 1999;106(4): 399-403.
11. Mann SJ. The silent epidemic of thiazide-induced hyponatremia. *J Clin Hypertens (Greenwich).* 2008;10(6):477-484.
12. Musch W, Xhaet O, Decaux G. Solute loss plays a major role in polydipsia-related hyponatraemia of both water drinkers and beer drinkers. *QJM.* 2003;96(6):421-426.
13. Faustini-Fustini M, Anagni M. Beyond semantics: defining hyponatremia in secondary adrenal insufficiency. *J Endocrinol Invest.* 2006;29(3):267-269.
14. Curtis RH. Hyponatremia in primary myxedema. *Ann Intern Med.* 1956;44(2):376-385.
15. Feldman BJ, Rosenthal SM, Vargas GA, et al. Nephrogenic syndrome of inappropriate antidiuresis. *N Engl J Med.* 2005;352(18):1884-1890.
16. Hurley JK. Symptomatic hyponatremia in nephrotic syndrome. *Am J Dis Child.* 1980;134(2):204-206.
17. Spasovski G, Vanholder R, Allolio B, et al. Clinical practice guidelines on diagnosis and treatment of hyponatremia. *Eur J Endocrinol.* 2014;170(3):G1-G47.
18. Nzerue CM, Baffoe-Bonnie H, You W, Falana B, Dai S. Predictors of outcome in hospitalized patients with severe hyponatremia. *J Natl Med Assoc.* 2003;95(5):335-343.
19. Renneboog B, Musch W, Vandemergel X, Manto MU, Decaux G. Mild chronic hyponatremia is associated with falls, unsteadiness, and attention deficits. *Am J Med.* 2006;119(1): 71.e1-e8.
20. Hoorn EJ, Carlotti AP, Costa LA, et al. Preventing a drop in effective plasma osmolality to minimize the likelihood of cerebral edema during treatment of children with diabetic ketoacidosis. *J Pediatr.* 2007;150(5):467-473.
21. Hoorn EJ, Zietse R. Hyponatremia revisited: translating physiology to practice. *Nephron Physiol.* 2008;108(3):46-59.

22. Verbalis JG, Goldsmith SR, Greenberg A, et al. Diagnosis, evaluation, and treatment of hyponatremia: expert panel recommendations. *Am J Med.* 2013;126(10 Suppl. 1):S1-S42.

23. Ayus JC, Olivero JJ, Frommer JP. Rapid correction of severe hyponatremia with intravenous hypertonic saline solution. *Am J Med.* 1982;72(1):43-48.

24. Hsu YJ, Chiu JS, Lu KC, Chau T, Lin SH. Biochemical and etiological characteristics of acute hyponatremia in the emergency department. *J Emerg Med.* 2005;29(4):369-374.

25. Lee A, Jo YH, Kim K, et al. Efficacy and safety of rapid intermittent correction compared with slow continuous correction with hypertonic saline in patients with moderately severe or severe symptomatic hyponatremia: study protocol for a randomized controlled trial (SALSA trial). *Trials.* 2017;18(1):147.

26. Mohmand HK, Issa D, Ahmad Z, Cappuccio JD, Kouides RW, Sterns RH. Hypertonic saline for hyponatremia: risk of inadvertent overcorrection. *Clin J Am Soc Nephrol.* 2007;2(6):1110-1117.

27. Castello L, Pirisi M, Sainaghi PP, Bartoli E. Quantitative treatment of the hyponatremia of cirrhosis. *Dig Liver Dis.* 2005;37(3):176-180.

28. Rozen-Zvi B, Yahav D, Gheorghiade M, Korzets A, Leibovici L, Gafter U. Vasopressin receptor antagonists for the treatment of hyponatremia: systematic review and meta-analysis. *Am J Kidney Dis.* 2010;56(2):325-337.

29. Zhang X, Zhao M, Du W, et al. Efficacy and safety of vasopressin receptor antagonists for euvolemic or hypervolemic hyponatremia: a meta-analysis. *Medicine (Baltimore).* 2016;95(15):e3310.

30. Louis G, Megarbane B, Lavoué S, et al. Long-term outcome of patients hospitalized in intensive care units with central or extrapontine myelinolysis. *Crit Care Med.* 2012;40(3):970-972.

31. Martin RJ. Central pontine and extrapontine myelinolysis: the osmotic demyelination syndromes. *J Neurol Neurosurg Psychiatry.* 2004;75(Suppl. 3):iii22-iii28.

32. Geoghegan P, Harrison AM, Thongprayoon C, et al. Sodium correction practice and clinical outcomes in profound hyponatremia. *Mayo Clin Proc.* 2015;90(10):1348-1355.

33. Adrogué HJ, Madias NE. The challenge of hyponatremia. *J Am Soc Nephrol.* 2012;23(7):1140-1148.

34. Perianayagam A, Sterns RH, Silver SM, et al. DDAVP is effective in preventing and reversing inadvertent overcorrection of hyponatremia. *Clin J Am Soc Nephrol.* 2008;3(2):331-336.

35. Yessayan L, Yee J, Frinak S, Szamosfalvi B. Continuous renal replacement therapy for the management of acid-base and electrolyte imbalances in acute kidney injury. *Adv Chronic Kidney Dis.* 2016;23(3):203-210.

36. Ostermann M, Dickie H, Tovey L, Treacher D. Management of sodium disorders during continuous haemofiltration. *Crit Care.* 2010;14(3):418.

37. Adrogué HJ, Madias NE. Hypernatremia. *N Engl J Med.* 2000;342(20):1493-1499.

38. Edelman IS, Leibman J, O'Meara MP, Birkenfeld LW. Interrelations between serum sodium concentration, serum osmolarity and total exchangeable sodium, total exchangeable potassium and total body water. *J Clin Invest.* 1958;37(9):1236-1256.

39. Palevsky PM, Bhagrath R, Greenberg A. Hypernatremia in hospitalized patients. *Ann Int Med.* 1996;124(2):197-203.

40. Darmon M, Timsit JF, Francais A, et al. Association between hypernatremia acquired in the ICU and mortality: a cohort study. *Nephrol Dial Transplant.* 2010;25(8):2510-2515.

41. Lindner G, Kneidinger N, Holzinger U, Druml W, Schwarz C. Tonicity balance in patients with hypernatremia acquired in the intensive care unit. *Am J Kidney Dis.* 2009;54(4):674-649.

42. Gennari FJ, Kassirer JP. Osmotic diuresis. *N Engl J Med.* 1974;291(14):714-720.

43. Ares GR, Caceres PS, Ortiz PA. Molecular regulation of NKCC2 in the thick ascending limb. *Am J Physiol Renal Physiol.* 2011;301(6):F1143-F1159.

44. Oster JR, Singer I, Thatte L, Grant-Taylor I, Diego JM. The polyuria of solute diuresis. *Arch Intern Med.* 1997;157:721-729.

45. Feinfeld DA, Danovitch GM. Factors affecting urine volume in chronic renal failure. *Am J Kidney Dis.* 1987;10:231-235.

46. Blevins Jr LS, Wand GS. Diabetes insipidus. *Crit Care Med.* 1992;20(1):69-79.

47. Rose BD. *Clinical Physiology of Acid-base and Electrolyte Disorders.* 5th ed. New York, NY: Mcgraw-Hill; 2001.

48. Aiyagari V, Deibert E, Diringer MN. Hypernatremia in the neurologic intensive care unit: how high is too high? *J Crit Care.* 2006;21:163-172.

49. Kahn T. Hypernatremia with edema. *Arch Intern Med.* 1999;159(1):93-98.

50. Malbrain MLNG, Van Regenmortel N, Saugel B, et al. Principles of fluid management and stewardship in septic shock: it is time to consider the four D's and the four phases of fluid therapy. *Ann Intensive Care.* 2018;8(1):66.

51. Knochel JP. Neuromuscular manifestations of electrolyte disorders. *Am J Med.* 1982;72:521-535.

52. Finberg L, Harrison HE. Hypernatremia in infants; an evaluation of the clinical and biochemical findings accompanying this state. *Pediatrics.* 1955;16:1-14.

53. Funk GC, Lindner G, Druml W, et al. Incidence and prognosis of dysnatremias present on ICU admission. *Intensive Care Med.* 2010;36:304-311.

54. Komjati M, Kastner G, Waldhäusl W, Bratusch-Marrain P. Detrimental effect of hyperosmolality on insulin-stimulated glucose metabolism in adipose and muscle tissue in vitro. *Biochem Med Metab Biol.* 1988;39:312-318.

55. Lenz K, Gössinger H, Laggner A, Druml W, Grimm G, Schneeweiss B. Influence of hypernatremic-hyperosmolar state on hemodynamics of patients with normal and depressed myocardial function. *Crit Care Med.* 1986;14:913-914.

56. Abramovici MI, Singhal PC, Trachtman H. Hypernatremia and rhabdomyolysis. *J Med.* 1992;23:17-28.

57. Quinn JW, Sewell K, Simmons DE. Recommendations for active correction of hypernatremia in volume-resuscitated shock or sepsis patients should be taken with a grain of salt: A systematic review. *SAGE Open Med.* 2018;6:2050312118762043.

58. Buckley MS, Leblanc JM, Cawley MJ. Electrolyte disturbances associated with commonly prescribed medications in the intensive care unit. *Crit Care Med.* 2010;38:S253-S264.

59. Hoorn EJ, Betjes MG, Weigel J, Zietse R. Hypernatraemia in critically ill patients: too little water and too much salt. *Nephrol Dial Transplant.* 2008;23(5):1562-1568.

60. Bhave G, Neilson EG. Volume depletion versus dehydration: how understanding the difference can guide therapy. *Am J Kidney Dis.* 2011;58(2):302-309.

61. Hogan GR, Dodge PR, Gill SR, Master S, Sotos JF. Pathogenesis of seizures occurring during restoration of plasma tonicity to

normal in animals previously chronically hypernatremic. *Pediatrics*. 1969;43:54-64.

62. Kahn A, Brachet E, Blum D. Controlled fall in natremia and risk of seizures in hypertonic dehydration. *Intensive Care Med*. 1979;5:27-31.

63. Adrogué HJ, Madias NE. Aiding fluid prescription for the dysnatremias. *Intensive Care Med*. 1997;23(3):309-316.

64. Lindner G, Funk GC. Hypernatremia in critically ill patients. *J Crit Care*. 2013;28(2):216.e11-e20.

65. Al-Absi A, Gosmanova EO, Wall BM. A clinical approach to the treatment of chronic hypernatremia. *Am J Kidney Dis*. 2012;60(6):1032-1028.

66. Shafiee MA, Bohn D, Hoorn EJ, Halperin ML. How to select optimal maintenance intravenous fluid therapy. *QJM*. 2003;96(8):601-610.

67. van IJzendoorn MCO, Buter H, Kingma WP, Navis GJ, Boerma EC. The development of intensive care unit acquired hypernatremia is not explained by sodium overload of water deficit: a retrospective cohort study on water balance and sodium handling. *Crit Care Res Pract*. 2016;2016:9571583.

68. Nguyen MK, Kurtz I. Correction of hypervolaemic hypernatraemia by inducing negative Na and K balance in excess of negative water balance: a new quantitative approach. *Nephrol Dial Transplant*. 2008;23(7):2223-2227.

69. van IJzendoorn MM, Buter H, Kingma WP, Koopmans M, Navis G, Boerma EC. Hydrochlorothiazide in intensive care unit-acquired hypernatremia: a randomized controlled trial. *J Crit Care*. 2017;38:225-230.

70. Oude Lansink-Hartgring A, Hessels L, Weigel J, et al. Long-term changes in dysnatremia incidence in the ICU: a shift from hyponatremia to hypernatremia. *Ann Intensive Care*. 2016;6(1):22.

71. Paquette F, Goupil R, Madore F, Troyanov S, Bouchard J. Continuous venovenous hemofiltration using customized replacement fluid for acute kidney injury with severe hypernatremia. *Clin Kidney J*. 2016;9(4):540-542.

62

Why Is Lactate Important in Critical Care?

Jan Bakker

INTRODUCTION

In clinical conditions, we characterize circulatory dysfunction by a combination of abnormalities in different systems. Without a particular order of importance, these changes consist of abnormal hemodynamic parameters like blood pressure and heart rate, abnormal tissue perfusion parameters like a cold, discolored sweaty skin, altered mental state and decreased urine production and abnormal metabolic parameters like lactate, arterial pH and base excess. Oxygen demand dictates oxygen delivery and is equal to oxygen consumption under normal conditions. Therefore, a decrease in oxygen consumption during unchanged oxygen demand denotes a state where either the delivery of oxygen to the tissues or the ability of tissues to use oxygen is inadequate to meet the demands for normal tissue function (tissue hypoxia). If uncorrected, this state will result in tissue damage and organ dysfunction. Invariably, in both experimental and clinical conditions, this situation is characterized by a sharp rise in lactate levels. Therefore, increased lactate levels have been seen as a hallmark of circulatory or metabolic dysfunction and have been associated with increased morbidity and mortality in many different clinical conditions.

In this chapter, we review the current states on how abnormal lactate levels arise and lactate measurements can be used to diagnose and treat circulatory dysfunction.

METABOLISM OF LACTATE

Under normal conditions, 1 mmol of glucose is metabolized to 2 mmol of pyruvate generating 2 mmol ATP (glycolysis). In the presence of mitochondria and oxygen, far more energy is produced when pyruvate is subsequently metabolized in the Krebs cycle and via the electron transport chain (oxidative phosphorylation). Glycolysis and oxidative phosphorylation have different kinetics. Where the Krebs cycle is slow and efficient, glycolysis has the ability to increase the speed of ATP generation by two to three orders of magnitude. Therefore, although the net production of ATP from glucose via glycolysis is limited, speeding up the process can greatly increase ATP production either in the presence or absence of oxygen.[1] In such cases, pyruvate will accumulate and lactate levels will rise. Lactate can be converted back to pyruvate when metabolism normalizes.

The enzyme lactate dehydrogenase catalyzes both conversion of pyruvate to lactate and of lactate to pyruvate.[2] However, lactate can also function as an intermediate fuel and be exchanged between tissues (liver, kidneys, muscles) and even cells (astrocytes, neurons) via lactate shuttles.[3] The Cori cycle, the pathway responsible for both hepatic and renal gluconeogenesis, requires oxygen; the interorgan/cellular exchange does not. Thus, lactate shuttles represent an interesting energy transport mechanism.[4] Even exogenous lactate can be used as a fuel in this context.[3]

LACTATE AND ACIDOSIS

Metabolism of glucose results in the production of ATP, water and the lactate anion—the production of H^+ results from the hydrolysis of ATP to ADP.[5] When the Krebs cycle functions normally, the charge associated with H^+ production is balanced by lactate generation and H^+ does not accumulate. Stewart argued that maintenance of acid-base equilibrium was the net result of the dissociation of water that can rapidly correct the presence of lactate.[6] Therefore, a strong relationship between increased lactate levels and arterial pH would not be expected and the terminology "lactic acidosis" is a misnomer that should be called "lactate associated acidosis." Indeed, in clinical practice, only a weak correlation exists between lactate and pH, and only at higher lactate levels (>5 mmol/L) does pH rapidly drop as lactate levels further increase.[2] These high lactate levels are also indicators of more severe circulatory or metabolic dysfunction that likely reflect decreased organ function (liver, kidney); other factors may contribute to the acidosis and thus result in mortality that is unexpectedly higher[7] than might be associated with increased lactate levels arising from other clinical conditions.[8] However, a clinically efficient therapy in the case of lactic acidosis is not available,[9] although clinical studies may be imminent.

LACTATE AND TISSUE HYPOPERFUSION

Oxygen delivery is a function of hemoglobin levels, arterial oxygen saturation and cardiac output (and its distribution). In experimental conditions, decreasing any of these components below a critical level will result in decreased oxygen consumption.[10] This state of delivery-dependent oxygen consumption is a hallmark of tissue hypoxia and further reductions in oxygen delivery will immediately result in sharp lactate increases. The same effect has been observed clinically.[11] Ronco et al.[12] demonstrated the occurrence of this phenomenon when therapy is withdrawn during end-of-life care. In experimental conditions, when the state of supply dependency is corrected, lactate levels return to normal/baseline levels.[13] Clinically, Friedman et al.[14] showed that supply dependency is present in the early phase of septic shock while, in the post resuscitation phase, supply dependency was absent and lactate levels were normal.

In the presence of normal oxygen delivery, abnormal microcirculatory perfusion may still be present[15] and may limit cellular oxygen availability. In sepsis, microcirculatory derangement may lead to insufficient oxygen delivery to the cell, thereby increasing lactate levels.[10] Thus, improving capillary perfusion has been associated with a reduction in lactate levels in some patients with septic shock, independent of changes in systemic hemodynamic variables.[16] Nevertheless, given the abnormal metabolism,[17–19] mitochondrial dysfunction[20] and decreased lactate clearance in sepsis, restoration of microcirculatory perfusion may not correct elevated lactate levels.[21] This situation contrasts with circulatory failure secondary to low cardiac output, where correction of microcirculatory perfusion is associated with normalization of lactate levels.[21] In septic shock and similar conditions, increased lactate levels may not be due to tissue hypoxia.[22] Additional parameters reflecting tissue perfusion and metabolism have been proposed to aid in the diagnosis.[23,24] In addition, the lactate/pyruvate (L/P) ratio has been proposed to aid in the diagnosis of hypoxia-related tissue metabolism.[25] However, the interpretation of .L/P ratios in relation to tissue hypoxia is a complex parameter.[26]

OTHER CAUSES OF INCREASED LACTATE

Increased aerobic glucose metabolism can increase lactate levels in the absence of tissue hypoxia. Most notably, epinephrine administration increases lactate levels by stimulating beta-driven Na/K-linked ATPases.[27] Thus epinephrine use in circulatory failure can improve hemodynamics without correcting elevated lactate levels.[28] In addition, alkalosis (respiratory and metabolic) can increase lactate levels,[29] as can corticosteroids, which increase glucose metabolism and lactate levels.[30] The aerobic production of lactate in tumor cells (the Warburg effect) may result in very high lactate levels in clinically stable patients.[31] Treatment of the tumor is associated with rapid decreases in lactate levels while renewed growth may first become evident when lactate increases.[2]

One of the most energy-requiring processes is the Na^+/K^+ pump system present in every cell. In both experimental and clinical conditions, the pump is related to increased lactate levels even under aerobic conditions.[19,32] Both cytokines and catecholamines increase the activity of the pump and thus increase lactate levels in the absence of tissue hypoxia.[19,32]

Renal replacement therapy eliminates only small amounts of lactate; therefore using lactate-buffered solutions can transiently cause hyperlactataemia.[33] Other putative causes of increased lactate levels not related to tissue hypoxia have been described.[34–36]

CLEARANCE OF LACTATE

Blood lactate levels reflect both production and clearance. Thus, impaired elimination may increase lactate levels. Conditions associated with impaired clearance include liver dysfunction/failure, cardiac surgery and sepsis.[18,37–39]

HOW AND WHERE TO MEASURE LACTATE LEVELS

Lactate levels can be adequately measured using bedside point of care devices[40,41] without unacceptable variability due to the site of the sampling.[42–44] When using lactate measurements to guide therapy, with the aim of decreasing lactate levels in relatively short periods, the same sampling sites and devices should be used whenever possible.

LACTATE MEASUREMENTS IN EMERGENCY CARE

Several studies have shown that prehospital lactate levels are related to outcome parameters and thus may be useful in triage, even in patients whose vital signs are normal.[45,46]

Further, normal vital signs in the Emergency Department may be accompanied by increased lactate levels and be associated with increased mortality.[47] In septic patients with normal vital signs, a lactate level >4.0 mmol/L was associated with a mortality odds ratio of 7.1; The Surviving Sepsis Campaign recommends immediate treatment of these patients.[48]

LACTATE MEASUREMENT IN THE INTENSIVE CARE UNIT

Decreases in elevated lactate levels during treatment are universally associated with improved outcome in critically ill patients and can provide an early and objective evaluation of the response to therapy.[49,50] The area under the lactate vs. time curve (where time spent above 2.0 mmol/L is calculated) is related to organ failure and mortality.[51,52] Therefore, it seems intuitive to normalize lactate levels rapidly in patients admitted with increased lactate levels.

GOAL-DIRECTED THERAPY USING LACTATE LEVELS

Investigations into the use of lactate to initiate and direct treatment are limited. Several recent large scale randomized trials have evaluated the use of early goal-directed therapy but, in contrast to Rivers' initial study,[53] optimization of blood pressure, preload status and tissue perfusion has not provided the expected improvement. Three large randomized studies[54–56] randomizing more than 4000 patients in total were unable to demonstrate a survival advantage. Importantly, high (>5.0 mmol/L) initial lactate levels, whose correction might be associated with a survival benefit,[54] were not used to direct therapy in these studies.

In a randomized trial in the Netherlands Jansen et al.[57] studied 348 patients with a lactate level >3.0 mmol/L. Following measurement of central venous oxygen saturation (ScvO$_2$), therapy was adjusted to optimize oxygen delivery and to reduce oxygen demand in the lactate group. The intervention was designed to decrease lactate by at least 20% every 2 hours over the initial first 8 hours following admission. Therapeutic interventions that both improved ScvO$_2$ and decreased lactate were associated with an improvement in intensive care unit and hospital survival once baseline imbalances were corrected. These findings contrast with a study by Jones et al.[58] who compared the use of either ScvO$_2$- or lactate-guided therapy and were unable to identify an outcome difference. Results obtained by combining the septic shock patients in the Jansen study with other studies using lactate to guide therapy in septic shock demonstrated an association between reduced lactate levels and improved outcome.[59]

HOW TO USE LACTATE IN CLINICAL PRACTICE

Under any circumstances, an increased lactate should warn clinicians that immediate attention is required. The first action should be to create context (Fig. 62.1). If the increased lactate is most likely the result of metabolic derangements or other causes as opposed to decreased tissue perfusion[60] these potential diagnoses should be investigated. When there are signs of impaired tissue perfusion (hypotension, tachycardia, abnormal peripheral perfusion, altered mentation, etc.) ScvO$_2$ should be measured. If the ScvO$_2$ is normal, adding measurements of the delta-PCO$_2$ (difference between central venous and arterial PCO$_2$)[24] or a surrogate of the respiratory quotient (venous-arterial CO$_2$ to arterial-venous O$_2$ content difference ratio)[23] or the venous-arterial CO$_2$ to arterial-venous O$_2$ difference ratio[61] may aid in the diagnosis of tissue hypoperfusion requiring hemodynamic and microcirculatory interventions. Treatment should rapidly decrease or normalization lactate levels. Current evidence suggests that measurements be repeated every 1–2 hours.[50] However, evidence does not support continuing treatment of increased lactate levels via hemodynamic interventions for more that the initial 8 hours. Indeed, in patients with septic shock, increased lactate levels beyond the first 8 hours may be associated with survival.[22] Persistently

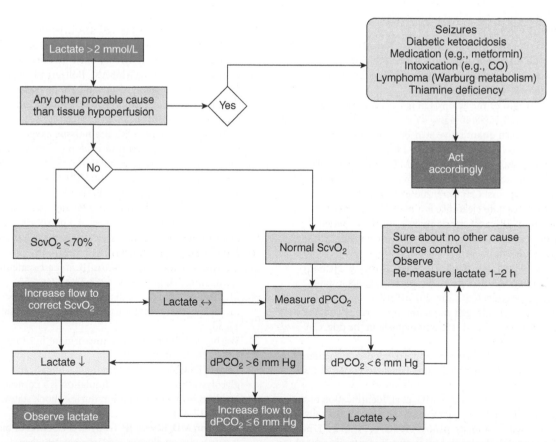

Fig. 62.1 Steps to guide treatment using repeated measurements of lactate using central venous oxygen saturation (ScvO$_2$) and central venous-to-arterial PCO$_2$ difference.

increased lactate levels should signal the clinician to review the diagnosis and assess the adequacy of treatment.

AUTHORS' RECOMMENDATIONS

- When used correctly, lactate levels may aid in diagnosing and treating patients.
- Changes in lactate can provide an early and objective evaluation of the patient's response to therapy.
- Current evidence indicates that increased lactate levels in the presence of other markers of tissue hypoperfusion should lead to immediate hemodynamic optimization designed to improve tissue perfusion.
- Elevated lactate levels in the absence of other markers of tissue hypoperfusion or that persist beyond the first 8 hour of treatment should be interpreted with caution and should lead to reassessment of both diagnosis and the adequacy of the supporting treatment.

REFERENCES

1. Gore DC, Jahoor F, Hibbert JM, DeMaria EJ. Lactic acidosis during sepsis is related to increased pyruvate production, not deficits in tissue oxygen availability. *Ann Surg.* 1996;224(1):97-102.
2. Bakker J, Nijsten MW, Jansen TC. Clinical use of lactate monitoring in critically ill patients. *Ann Intensive Care.* 2013;3(1):12.
3. Leverve XM. Energy metabolism in critically ill patients: lactate is a major oxidizable substrate. *Curr Opin Clin Nutr Metab Care.* 1999;2(2):165-169.
4. Ferguson BS, Rogatzki MJ, Goodwin ML, Kane DA, Rightmire Z, Gladden LB. Lactate metabolism: historical context, prior misinterpretations, and current understanding. *Eur J Appl Physiol.* 2018;118(4):691-728.
5. Zilva JF. The origin of the acidosis in hyperlactataemia. *Ann Clin Biochem.* 1978;15(1):40-43.
6. Stewart PA. Modern quantitative acid-base chemistry. *Can J Physiol Pharmacol.* 1983;61(12):1444-1461.
7. Gunnerson KJ, Saul M, He S, Kellum JA. Lactate versus non-lactate metabolic acidosis: a retrospective outcome evaluation of critically ill patients. *Crit Care.* 2006;10(1):R22.
8. Zhang Z, Xu X. Lactate clearance is a useful biomarker for the prediction of all-cause mortality in critically ill patients: a systematic review and meta-analysis*. *Crit Care Med.* 2014; 42(9):2118-2125.
9. Kimmoun A, Novy E, Auchet T, Ducrocq N, Levy B. Hemodynamic consequences of severe lactic acidosis in shock states: from bench to bedside. *Crit Care.* 2015;19:175.
10. Zhang H, Vincent JL. Oxygen extraction is altered by endotoxin during tamponade-induced stagnant hypoxia in the dog. *Circ Shock.* 1993;40(3):168-176.
11. Bakker J, Vincent JL. The oxygen supply dependency phenomenon is associated with increased blood lactate levels. *J Crit Care.* 1991;6(3):152-159.
12. Ronco JJ, Fenwick JC, Tweeddale MG, et al. Identification of the critical oxygen delivery for anaerobic metabolism in critically ill septic and nonseptic humans. *JAMA.* 1993;270(14):1724-1730.
13. Zhang H, Spapen H, Benlabed M, Vincent JL. Systemic oxygen extraction can be improved during repeated episodes of cardiac tamponade. *J Crit Care.* 1993;8(2):93-99.
14. Friedman G, De Backer D, Shahla M, Vincent JL. Oxygen supply dependency can characterize septic shock. *Intensive Care Med.* 1998;24(2):118-123.
15. Ince C. Hemodynamic coherence and the rationale for monitoring the microcirculation. *Crit Care.* 2015;19(Suppl 3):S8.
16. De Backer D, Creteur J, Dubois MJ, et al. The effects of dobutamine on microcirculatory alterations in patients with septic shock are independent of its systemic effects. *Crit Care Med.* 2006;34(2):403-408.
17. Levy B. Lactate and shock state: the metabolic view. *Curr Opin Crit Care.* 2006;12(4):315-321.
18. Vary TC. Sepsis-induced alterations in pyruvate dehydrogenase complex activity in rat skeletal muscle: effects on plasma lactate. *Shock.* 1996;6(2):89-94.
19. Levy B, Gibot S, Franck P, Cravoisy A, Bollaert PE. Relation between muscle Na+K+ ATPase activity and raised lactate concentrations in septic shock: a prospective study. *Lancet.* 2005;365(9462):871-875.
20. Ruggieri AJ, Levy RJ, Deutschman CS. Mitochondrial dysfunction and resuscitation in sepsis. *Crit Care Clin.* 2010;26(3): 567-575.
21. van Genderen ME, Klijn E, Lima A, et al. Microvascular perfusion as a target for fluid resuscitation in experimental circulatory shock. *Crit Care Med.* 2014;42(2):E96-E105.
22. Hernandez G, Luengo C, Bruhn A, et al. When to stop septic shock resuscitation: clues from a dynamic perfusion monitoring. *Ann Intensive Care.* 2014;4:30.
23. Ospina-Tascón GA, Umaña M, Bermúdez WF, et al. Can venous-to-arterial carbon dioxide differences reflect microcirculatory alterations in patients with septic shock? *Intensive Care Med.* 2016;42(2):211-221.
24. Alegría L, Vera M, Dreyse J, et al. A hypoperfusion context may aid to interpret hyperlactatemia in sepsis-3 septic shock patients: a proof-of-concept study. *Ann Intensive Care.* 2017;7(1):29.
25. Levy B, Sadoune LO, Gelot AM, Bollaert PE, Nabet P, Larcan A. Evolution of lactate/pyruvate and arterial ketone body ratios in the early course of catecholamine-treated septic shock. *Crit Care Med.* 2000;28(1):114-119.
26. Lazaridis C, Andrews CM. Brain tissue oxygenation, lactate-pyruvate ratio, and cerebrovascular pressure reactivity monitoring in severe traumatic brain injury: systematic review and viewpoint. *Neurocrit Care.* 2014;21(2):345-355.
27. Griffith Jr FR, Lockwood JE, Emery FE. Adrenalin lactacidemia: proportionality with dose. *Am J Physiol.* 1939;127(3):415-421.
28. Levy B, Clere-Jehl R, Legras A, et al. Epinephrine versus norepinephrine for cardiogenic shock after acute myocardial infarction. *J Am Coll Cardiol.* 2018;72(2):173-182.
29. Zborowska-Sluis DT, Dossetor JB. Hyperlactatemia of hyperventilation. *J Appl Physiol.* 1967;22(4):746-755.
30. McMahon M, Gerich J, Rizza R. Effects of glucocorticoids on carbohydrate metabolism. *Diabetes Metab Rev.* 1988;4(1): 17-30.
31. Warburg O. On respiratory impairment in cancer cells. *Science.* 1956;124(3215):269-270.
32. Levy B, Desebbe O, Montemont C, Gibot S. Increased aerobic glycolysis through beta-2 stimulation is a common mechanism involved in lactate formation during shock states. *Shock.* 2008; 30(4):417-421.
33. Bollmann MD, Revelly JP, Tappy L, et al. Effect of bicarbonate and lactate buffer on glucose and lactate metabolism during hemodiafiltration in patients with multiple organ failure. *Intensive Care Med.* 2004;30(6):1103-1110.

34. Lalau JD, Lacroix C, Compagnon P, et al. Role of metformin accumulation in metformin-associated lactic acidosis. *Diabetes Care*. 1995;18(6):779-784.

35. Marinella MA. Lactic acidosis associated with propofol. *Chest*. 1996;109(1):292.

36. Claessens YE, Cariou A, Monchi M, et al. Detecting life-threatening lactic acidosis related to nucleoside-analog treatment of human immunodeficiency virus-infected patients, and treatment with L-carnitine. *Crit Care Med*. 2003;31(4):1042-1047.

37. Tapia P, Soto D, Bruhn A, et al. Impairment of exogenous lactate clearance in experimental hyperdynamic septic shock is not related to total liver hypoperfusion. *Crit Care*. 2015; 19:188.

38. Almenoff PL, Leavy J, Weil MH, Goldberg NB, Vega D, Rackow EC. Prolongation of the half-life of lactate after maximal exercise in patients with hepatic dysfunction. *Crit Care Med*. 1989; 17(9):870-873.

39. Mustafa I, Roth H, Hanafiah A, et al. Effect of cardiopulmonary bypass on lactate metabolism. *Intensive Care Med*. 2003;29(8): 1279-1285.

40. Aduen J, Bernstein WK, Khastgir T, et al. The use and clinical importance of a substrate-specific electrode for rapid determination of blood lactate concentrations. *JAMA*. 1994;272(21):1678-1685.

41. Brinkert W, Rommes JH, Bakker J. Lactate measurements in critically ill patients with a hand-held analyser. *Intensive Care Med*. 1999;25(9):966-969.

42. Weil MH, Michaels S, Rackow EC. Comparison of blood lactate concentrations in central venous, pulmonary artery, and arterial blood. *Crit Care Med*. 1987;15(5):489-490.

43. Younger JG, Falk JL, Rothrock SG. Relationship between arterial and peripheral venous lactate levels. *Acad Emerg Med*. 1996; 3(7):730-734.

44. Fauchère JC, Bauschatz AS, Arlettaz R, Zimmermann-Bär U, Bucher HU. Agreement between capillary and arterial lactate in the newborn. *Acta Paediatr*. 2002;91(1):78-81.

45. Jansen TC, van Bommel J, Mulder PG, Rommes JH, Schieveld SJ, Bakker J. The prognostic value of blood lactate levels relative to that of vital signs in the pre-hospital setting: a pilot study. *Crit Care*. 2008;12(6):R160.

46. van Beest PA, Brander L, Jansen SP, Rommes JH, Kuiper MA, Spronk PE. Cumulative lactate and hospital mortality in ICU patients. *Ann Intensive Care*. 2013;3(1):6.

47. Mikkelsen ME, Miltiades AN, Gaieski DF, et al. Serum lactate is associated with mortality in severe sepsis independent of organ failure and shock. *Crit Care Med*. 2009;37(5):1670-1677.

48. Rhodes A, Evans LE, Alhazzani W, et al. Surviving Sepsis Campaign: International Guidelines for Management of Sepsis and Septic Shock: 2016. *Intensive Care Med*. 2017; 43(3):304-377.

49. Vincent JL, Dufaye P, Berré J, Leeman M, Degaute JP, Kahn RJ. Serial lactate determinations during circulatory shock. *Crit Care Med*. 1983;11(6):449-451.

50. Vincent JL, Quintairos ESA, Couto Jr L, Taccone FS. The value of blood lactate kinetics in critically ill patients: a systematic review. *Crit Care*. 2016;20(1):257.

51. Bakker J, Gris P, Coffernils M, Kahn RJ, Vincent JL. Serial blood lactate levels can predict the development of multiple organ failure following septic shock. *Am J Surg*. 1996;171(2):221-226.

52. Jansen TC, van Bommel J, Woodward R, Mulder PG, Bakker J. Association between blood lactate levels, Sequential Organ Failure Assessment subscores, and 28-day mortality during early and late intensive care unit stay: a retrospective observational study. *Crit Care Med*. 2009;37(8):2369-2374.

53. Rivers E, Nguyen B, Havstad S, et al. Early goal-directed therapy in the treatment of severe sepsis and septic shock. *N Engl J Med*. 2001;345(19):1368-1377.

54. ProCESS Investigators, Yealy DM, Kellum JA, et al. A randomized trial of protocol-based care for early septic shock. *N Engl J Med*. 2014;370(18):1683-1693.

55. ARISE Investigators, ANZICS Clinical Trials Group, Peake SL, et al. Goal-directed resuscitation for patients with early septic shock. *N Engl J Med*. 2014;371(16):1496-1506.

56. Mouncey PR, Osborn TM, Power GS, et al. Trial of early, goal-directed resuscitation for septic shock. *N Engl J Med*. 2015; 372(14):1301-1311.

57. Jansen TC, van Bommel J, Schoonderbeek FJ, et al. Early lactate-guided therapy in intensive care unit patients: a multicenter, open-label, randomized controlled trial. *Am J Respir Crit Care Med*. 2010;182(6):752-761.

58. Jones AE, Shapiro NI, Trzeciak S, et al. Lactate clearance vs central venous oxygen saturation as goals of early sepsis therapy: a randomized clinical trial. *JAMA*. 2010;303(8): 739-746.

59. Gu WJ, Zhang Z, Bakker J. Early lactate clearance-guided therapy in patients with sepsis: a meta-analysis with trial sequential analysis of randomized controlled trials. *Intensive Care Med*. 2015;41(10):1862-1863.

60. Jansen TC, van Bommel J, Bakker J. Blood lactate monitoring in critically ill patients: a systematic health technology assessment. *Crit Care Med*. 2009;37(10):2827-2839.

61. Monnet X, Julien F, Ait-Hamou N, et al. Lactate and venoarterial carbon dioxide difference/arterial-venous oxygen difference ratio, but not central venous oxygen saturation, predict increase in oxygen consumption in fluid responders. *Crit Care Med*. 2013;41(6):1412-1420.

63

How Does Critical Illness Alter Metabolism?

Mark E. Nunnally and Greta Piper

Critical illness increases metabolism globally. The body provides and consumes basic substrates taken from its own structures to run at an accelerated metabolic rate, a rate that cannot be sustained indefinitely. Clinicians in the critical care setting are familiar with the long-term consequences of catabolic processes; in patients whose illness is not alleviated, outcomes are poor and mortality is high. These patients contrast with those undergoing an acute stress response that transitions to a later period of recovery and anabolism. Patterns vary, but all critically ill patients experience increased metabolism in a neurologic, hormonal, and immunologic milieu that reprioritizes many physiologic functions to healing. This process is both adaptive and, in prolonged and uncontrolled situations, pathogenic. In the latter state, globally increased metabolism fuels critical illness.

The stress response is a pattern of metabolic changes in injured patients.[1] In this framework the physiology of critical illness is adaptive. Metabolic changes from "normal" are necessary to heal serious injury, and patients may become so ill as to require aggressive therapies. Supporting organ system function continues to be a core element of critical care practice; another is the search for ways to attenuate the process leading to illness, which extends to nutrition, care of endocrine systems, and intervention in immunologic signaling. Many metabolic changes in this syndrome have been described, but the meaning of these changes remains subject to a dearth of clear evidence, a glut of theory, and an absence of consensus. This chapter considers the predictable pattern in response to injury, the interventions that alter this pattern, pathologic deviations from that pattern, and the diagnostic utility of comparing a patient's clinical data with the stress response pattern.

PATHOPHYSIOLOGY AND MECHANISM OF ACTION

Cells metabolize glucose, lactate, amino acids, fatty acids, ketones, and their derivatives. They assemble these components into larger carbohydrates (glycogen), proteins, and triglycerides for energy storage and cellular function. Catabolic processes deconstruct larger molecules and generate energy. Anabolic processes assemble them and store energy. Catabolism is the trademark of critical illness, the hypermetabolic recovery period of "flow" that follows the "ebb" of shock.[2] These two phases are followed by an anabolic recovery phase after the stress response resolves. This recovery phase may persist for weeks to months (Fig. 63.1). Changes affect each organ system and the connections between them. Examples include immune, endocrine, and neurologic changes, such as alterations in circadian rhythms. Available evidence supports the theory that this adaptive response enables tissue healing.

Resting energy expenditure increases in critical illness. Glucose and fatty acids are consumed at accelerated rates. Serum levels of both exceed the normal range. Proteins are catabolized to amino acids, which in turn are converted by the liver to glucose. Patients develop hyperglycemia. Levels of lactate increase because of a metabolic shift and do not necessarily reflect tissue hypoperfusion, as is the case in acute shock. The catabolism of critical illness is not the same as that of starvation. In catabolism, tissue protein is consumed preferentially rather than spared. The liver produces more acute phase reactants, such as C-reactive protein, immunoglobulins, fibrinogen, and haptoglobin, and less of other proteins such as prealbumin, albumin, and transferrin. Muscle tissue provides most of the amino acids for fuel and protein synthesis. Ketosis is rare, because insulin levels still suppress ketogenesis. Additional nutrition cannot stop the loss of body proteins. The intestines maintain glutamine absorption, but conversion to citrulline drops, suggesting nutritional reprioritization.[3] Serum amino acid profiles change in septic patients in concert with their illness trajectory.[4] These findings underscore that nutrients have different effects during critical illness and metabolic priorities are changed. Critically ill patients will not respond to endocrine, nutritional, or metabolic therapies the same way that unstressed patients do.

End-organ cells lose part of their ability to oxidize fuels in the mitochondria.[5] For these cells, metabolism and oxygen utilization decrease, leading to a metabolic "shunt" and organ dysfunction. This bioenergetic failure correlates with illness severity. Recovery is sometimes possible, but resulting organ dysfunctions frequently require additional medical support. Thiamine deficiency, exacerbated by heightened pyruvate dehydrogenase activity and carbohydrate oxidation, may also cause a form of bioenergetic failure.

Endocrine and neurologic axes promote and reflect the change in metabolism. The anterior pituitary releases large

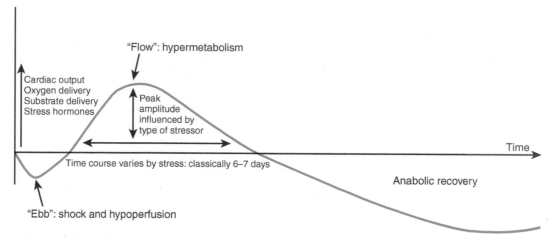

Fig. 63.1 Stress Response Curve, as Described by Cuthbertson. A period of shock may or may not precede the hyperdynamic phase during which nutrient and oxygen delivery are increased to peripheral tissues. For details on organ-specific alterations, see chapter text.

amounts of growth hormone, thyroid-stimulating hormone, luteinizing hormone, and prolactin, but there is peripheral resistance to normal metabolic effects.[6–10] Metabolism and cardiovascular function change as a consequence of elevated levels of catecholamines and vasopressin. Although insulin levels are increased, the anabolic effects of the hormone are attenuated.

Changes in organ systems function characterize the acute phase of critical illness. These findings can sometimes herald a new diagnosis, such as sepsis, and clinicians should recognize the pattern to increase monitoring, consider empiric therapy, and search for illness sources. Only source control can definitively resolve an acute phase response. Failure to do so can lead to chronic dysfunction.

Neurologic

Brain tissue uses a wide variety of metabolic fuel. During acute illnesses, glucose, amino acid, and lactate metabolism increases. Encephalopathy frequently develops, possibly related to the presence of elevated levels of aromatic amino acids and their metabolites.[11–13] Global cerebral function declines, manifested as alterations ranging from delirium to overt coma. Survivors of critical illness may have ongoing cognitive deficits that may be severe in chronic critical illness.[14]

Cardiovascular

Acute illness accelerates oxygen consumption in the periphery. To compensate, cardiac output increases and peripheral vascular tone decreases, augmenting blood flow to peripheral tissues, possibly at the expense of flow to other vascular beds. Oxygen consumption is highest in leukocyte-dense tissues, suggesting oxygen delivery is destined for cells that repair tissue and control infection.[15,16] Capillary beds leak because of alterations in glycocalyx function.[17] The balance between fluid extravasation and reabsorption consequently favors the formation of edema, as plasma proteins accumulate outside vessel walls, pulling fluid and electrolytes with them.

The result of these changes is a hyperdynamic circulation and edema. In some patients, there may be myocardial injury. Damage may lead to a failure to supplement oxygen delivery, which is associated with a high mortality in critical illness lung injury.[18] A hyperdynamic circulation is adaptive, but there is generally no benefit from attempts to enhance normal oxygen delivery with inotropes or blood products.[19,20] Right ventricle-limited circulation may be an exception.[21]

Fluids, Electrolytes, and Nutrition

Tissue edema and intravascular resuscitation increase body water, and patients characteristically gain kilograms in weight. Extracellular and vascular compartments expand,[22–25] but intracellular water is lost. This finding suggests that water shifts from the intracellular space to the extracellular space and back again as edema resolves, which has implications for electrolyte balance.

Insensible water loss and diuretic use produce hypernatremia. At times, renal water retention causes hyponatremia. As the acute response abates, water shifts dilute potassium, magnesium, phosphate, and proteins; as a result, hypokalemia, hypomagnesemia, and hypophosphatemia are common. Hypermetabolism or the refeeding syndrome exacerbates hypophosphatemia.[26,27]

Whole-body glucose delivery increases as a consequence of decreased peripheral uptake[28,29] and increased production. Hepatic gluconeogenesis converts amino acids and glycerol to glucose, even during hyperglycemia.[30,31] Amino acids, freed from peripheral protein stores, are the substrate. Glucose uptake is reduced in many tissues, but hyperglycemia fuels leukocyte demand in injured areas. Hyperglycemia and edema formation deliver glucose to avascular injured areas.

Lipid metabolism increases in the stress response, more so triglyceride hydrolysis and re-esterification, resulting in elevated serum triglycerides.[32,33] Patients with chronic critical illness generally retain most of their fat stores but are severely depleted of protein,[34] which manifest as susceptibility to injuries and inability to heal wounds.

Pulmonary

Pulmonary insufficiency accompanies the acute critical illness. Enhanced oxygen consumption and carbon dioxide production tax the pulmonary system. Tachypnea and type I (oxygenation) and II (ventilation) failure occur. Perivascular fluid flux forces fluids and proteins into alveoli. Inflammatory cell infiltration exacerbates extravasation. Altered immune function and risk for aspiration foment pulmonary infection. Such changes culminate in pulmonary failure, including the acute respiratory distress syndrome (ARDS). Respiratory muscles lose strength and coordination, worsening ventilatory function and secretion clearance. Chronic illness is frequently accompanied by a need for ongoing respiratory support.

Gastrointestinal

Intestinal villi atrophy and the gut swells.[35] Ileus heralds worsening stress. These changes confound attempts to provide enteric nutrition and raise the risk of bowel obstruction. Hepatic metabolic changes include impaired excretion of bilirubin and other metabolites. Chronic illness is marked by problems in nutrient absorption and gastrointestinal motility.[36]

Renal

Peripheral vasodilatation steals blood flow from the kidneys. Reduced perfusion and circulating mediators produce a syndrome of oliguria. Metabolically active tubular cells suspend function and become quiescent until the acute phase initiator has long resolved. The extreme example of this condition is acute kidney injury. With recovery, renal function often returns.[37] Chronic states may impede effective renal recovery, with subsequent changes in distribution and metabolism of drugs, including antibiotics.

Immunologic

Cell-mediated immunity is suppressed during inflammation.[38] Susceptibility to infection increases as systemic inflammatory signals are elevated. Chronic illness is marked by susceptibility to a variety of bacterial, viral, and fungal pathogens,[39–41] many of which are rarely pathologic in healthy patients. Myeloid-derived suppressor cells (MDSCs) play a key role in the pathophysiology of persistent inflammatory, immunosuppressed, catabolic syndrome (PICS). MDSCs suppress T-lymphocyte proliferation as well as Th1 and Th2 cytokine release. Early expansion of MDSCs in sepsis portends early mortality, and persistent MDSC expansion correlates with longer intensive care unit (ICU) stays and increased nosocomial infections.[42]

Endocrine

Cortisol, catecholamines, and glucagon accelerate metabolism and hyperglycemia.[29] Relative cortisol deficiency worsens vasodilatory shock and stalls recovery.[43] Muscle and fat anabolic responses to insulin diminish.[44–47] Changes in endocrine signaling include the euthyroid sick syndrome, disorders of sleep cycles, and altered immunologic function. Eventually, pituitary hypersecretion and altered peripheral sensitivity may give way to endocrine exhaustion.

If critical illness continues unabated, metabolic signaling changes. Adiponectin levels decrease with acute critical illness but then normalize as illness continues,[48] part of changing immune and metabolic signaling. Catabolism continues. Anterior pituitary hormone levels, including thyroid stimulating hormone, growth hormone, and prolactin, decline in a functional state of neuroendocrine exhaustion.

In chronic critical illness, neuroendocrine exhaustion is compounded by widespread bioenergetic mitochondrial failure, organ failure, kwashiorkor-like protein malnutrition, and a stymied immune response. Regular biologic oscillators fail to fluctuate,[49] suggesting that a loss of organ systems interconnectivity is part of the disorder. PICS has been described in trauma patients, pancreatitis, enterocutaneous fistulae, burns, and sepsis.[50–53] Following the initial insult, patients manifest proinflammatory and anti-inflammatory processes. Patients surviving critical illness for 14 or more days with persistent organ dysfunction express classic chronic illness changes. Despite often optimized traditional nutritional support, a smoldering inflammatory state persists, characterized by chronic illness, high levels of inflammatory markers, low albumin and prealbumin, and low lymphocyte count. Patients with PICS have sarcopenia, are prone to recurrent infections, and have poor wound healing.

Recovery from any of these phases entails source control followed by prolonged anabolism. In PICS and chronic states, full recovery may not be possible. Tissue protein stores recover slowly. It takes time to replete proteins, endocrine axes, and immune responses to normal function. Myopathies, neuropathies, and poor wound healing are the most visible manifestations of the slow recovery. While traditional nutritional therapies have focused on the acute phase of illness, future nutritional optimization will probably need to better address the recovery phase.

AVAILABLE DATA

Multiple clinical trials suggest ways in which metabolism in critical illness is mediated and how attempts to interfere with it might help or harm.

Beta blockade can attenuate the loss of muscle mass, as demonstrated in severely burned children.[54] This finding supports the idea that neuroendocrine signaling is related to acute phase metabolism. Endocrine studies support the role of this system in metabolism.

Steroids are supported as adjunctive therapy for refractory septic shock.[55] Reversal of shock is a reproducible outcome in trials of steroid administration,[43,56–59] as is hyperglycemia, but mortality has been unchanged in several key studies.[57,58] This leaves open the question of utility. Unresolved issues include the role of continuous vs. bolus infusion, mineralocorticoid co-administration, and the appropriate selection of patients likely to be relatively steroid deficient or, more importantly, likely to benefit. Other adverse effects of steroids include hypernatremia and neuromuscular weakness.

Circadian rhythms are frequently disrupted in critically ill patients due to artificial lighting, auditory stimulation, and pharmacologic agents, including analgesics and sedatives, vasopressors, inotropes, and beta agonists. These changes also likely reflect abnormalities of normal patterns of physiologic oscillation and organ coordination.[60] Mechanical ventilation and continuous enteral nutrition disrupt normal rhythms of metabolism, including cortisol levels. Melatonin administration to regulate day/night cycles may decrease the need for sedatives, and delirium.[61]

Vitamin C may play a role in circulatory and metabolic abnormalities in sepsis. Because septic patients consume their stores of vitamin C and are unable to generate more, supplementation may be beneficial. Recent data suggest vitamin C administration with hydrocortisone and thiamine may improve recovery from sepsis,[62] although thiamine alone also demonstrates benefit.[63] These dramatic results await replication. Vitamin D receptors are expressed in immune cells, including T cells, activated B cells, and dendritic cells, and regulate antimicrobial peptides. Vitamin D deficiency is common in critically ill patients and is associated with increased infection severity, organ failure, and mortality.[64,65] Supplementation, while relatively safe and inexpensive, requires high doses of vitamin D to normalize levels. Although a randomized trial demonstrated no improvement in overall mortality or length of stay, there was improvement in mortality in severely deficient patients.[66] Vitamin D deficiency is probably a problem in some critically ill patients, but the role of supplementation is unresolved.

The adequate amount of nutrition needed during critical illness is an ongoing conundrum. Nutritional support modestly prevents excessive protein loss, hyperglycemia, or hyperlipidemia, and may improve organ and immune function. The available literature is highly prone to bias. A few findings are consistent. Very high levels of nutrients are associated with worse outcomes, "underfeeding" may be beneficial, and parenteral nutrients do not have the same effects as enteric nutrition.[67] Obese critically ill patients warrant additional consideration.[68] Nutritional topics are treated elsewhere in this text. Controlling the drivers of catabolism (i.e., source control) is likely to have more impact than the provision of nutrition.

Attempts to alter stress metabolism can have adverse consequences. Although administration of anabolic hormones might attenuate loss of lean muscle mass and improve outcomes in critical illness, studies of androgen supplementation show mixed results.[69] In one study, growth hormone supplementation increased mortality.[70] In a surgical population, aggressive insulin therapy improved survival and reduced organ dysfunction when serum glucose was driven to nonstress levels.[71] Subsequent studies failed to replicate these results.[72–75] The original study was criticized for its large proportion of cardiac surgery patients, the restriction of benefit to patients who stayed in the ICU longer, and the aggressive nutrition given to the patients.[76] Given the changes and variability in stress metabolism during critical illness, it is quite conceivable that the goals of insulin therapy should vary with a patient's position on the stress curve such that catabolism is not overly suppressed early and anabolism is supported late.

INTERPRETATION OF DATA

Acute phase metabolism is incompletely characterized, variable, and multifaceted. Attempts to regulate specific elements on the arc of inflammation have been mostly unsuccessful, but available data do provide useful tools for the care of critically ill patients. It is likely that inflammation is mostly adaptive and necessary for survival. The stress response model is a template on which a patient's progress can be mapped. Signs of increased metabolism and neurohormonal stress should prompt a search for a cause, and aggressive, sometimes empiric, therapy. As an example, the triad of encephalopathy, hyperglycemia, and impaired intestinal motility may herald the onset of sepsis. Conversely, signs that stress is abating, such as negative spontaneous fluid balance and hypokalemia, can inform decisions to de-escalate monitoring and therapy, reducing iatrogenic risk. In the future, aminograms, lipograms, and even biograms of endogenous flora may help inform clinicians about these transitions.[77] Given that bacteria outnumber somatic cells and mostly fulfill commensal roles, cultivating and monitoring a healthy resident flora should be the subject of ongoing investigation.

Nutrition goals are incompletely characterized and should be tailored to patient response. Clinicians should decrease the provision of dextrose if it worsens hyperglycemia in a patient. Protein and fat goals, and the best way to provide them, beg further study. Using lactate as a marker for adequate resuscitation may be helpful in early shock, but lactate has a limited effect once the stress response commences. Therapies must be tested in patients with acute, prolonged, and chronic critical illness.[78–80] As a whole, the evidence suggests that preventing the transition to chronic critical illness with aggressive source control is the best available strategy.

SUMMARY

Metabolism increases with critical illness. The pattern of increase and decline is predictable, affects every organ system, and is known as the stress response. Increased oxygen and nutrient delivery underlies the observed physiologic changes. The stress response pattern is a useful tool to guide clinical therapy. The most reliable method of controlling the response is to reverse the conditions that drive it, i.e., source control. Repeated or ongoing sources can lead to chronic pathologic dysfunction.

AUTHORS' RECOMMENDATIONS

- Critical illness increases global metabolism.
- The process of elevated global metabolism can be thought of as an adaptive response to facilitate tissue healing.
- Critically ill patients undergo a predictable pattern of metabolic and physiologic changes in the stress response. After injury (with or without initial shock), metabolism accelerates with gradual (days to week) recovery followed by a longer (weeks to months) period of anabolic recovery of proteins. The response is manifested in every organ system in the body.
- Astute clinicians can exploit their knowledge of the stress response by predicting the pattern, mapping patient physiology to the expected changes, and making diagnostic and therapeutic decisions based on expected trajectory or unexpected variation from the common stress response pattern.
- Prolonged or ongoing injuries lead to chronic dysfunctions that include catabolic depletion of protein and nutrient stores, organ dysfunction, and an inhibited immune response.

REFERENCES

1. Cuthbertson DP. The disturbance of metabolism produced by bony and non-bony injury, with notes on certain abnormal conditions of bone. *Biochem J*. 1930;24:1244-1263.
2. Cuthbertson D, Tilstone WJ. Metabolism during the postinjury period. *Adv Clin Chem*. 1969;12:1-55.
3. Kao C, Hsu J, Bandi V, Jahoor F. Alteration in glutamine metabolism and its conversion to citrulline in sepsis. *Am J Physiol Endocrinol Metab*. 2013;304:E1359-E1364.
4. Hiroso T, Shimizu K, Ogura H, et al. Altered balance of the angiogram in patients with sepsis—the relation to mortality. *Clin Nutr*. 2013;33:179-182.
5. Azevedo LC. Mitochondrial dysfunction during sepsis. *Endocr Metab Immune Disord Drug Targets*. 2010;10:214-223.
6. Van den Berghe G, de Zegher F, Bouillon R. The somatotrophic axis in critical illness: effects of growth hormone secretagogues. *Growth Horm IGF Res*. 1998;8(Suppl. B):153-155.
7. Noel GL, Suh HK, Stone JG, Frantz AG. Human prolactin and growth hormone release during surgery and other conditions of stress. *J Clin Endocrinol Metab*. 1972;35:840-851.
8. Landry DW, Levin HR, Gallant EM, et al. Vasopressin deficiency contributes to the vasodilation of septic shock. *Circulation*. 1997;95:1122-1125.
9. Kakucska I, Romero LI, Clark BD, et al. Suppression of thyrotropin-releasing hormone gene expression by interleukin-1-beta in the rat: implications for nonthyroidal illness. *Neuroendocrinology*. 1994;59:129-137.
10. Bacci V, Schussler GC, Kaplan TB. The relationship between serum triiodothyronine and thyrotropin during systemic illness. *J Clin Endocrinol Metab*. 1982;54:1229-1235.
11. Stevens RD, Pronovost PJ. The spectrum of encephalopathy in critical illness. *Semin Neurol*. 2006;26:440-451.
12. Takezawa J, Taenaka N, Nishijima MK, et al. Amino acids and thiobarbituric acid reactive substances in cerebrospinal fluid and plasma of patients with septic encephalopathy. *Crit Care Med*. 1983;11:876-879.
13. Freund HR, Muggia-Sullam M, Peiser J, Melamed E. Brain neurotransmitter profile is deranged during sepsis and septic encephalopathy in the rat. *J Surg Res*. 1985;38:267-271.
14. Milbrandt EB, Angus DC. Bench-to-bedside review: critical illness-associate cognitive dysfunction—mechanisms, marker, and emerging therapeutics. *Crit Care*. 2006;10:238.
15. Mészáros K, Lang CH, Bagby GJ, Spitzer JJ. Contribution of different organs to increased glucose consumption after endotoxin administration. *J Biol Chem*. 1987;262:10965-10970.
16. Mészáros K, Bojta J, Bautista AP, Lang CH, Spitzer JJ. Glucose utilization by Kupffer cells, endothelial cells, and granulocytes in endotoxemic rat liver. *Am J Physiol*. 1991;260:G7-G12.
17. Woodcock TE, Woodcock TM. Revised Starling equation and the glycocalyx model of transvascular fluid exchange: an improved paradigm for prescribing intravenous fluid therapy. *Br J Anaesth*. 2012;108:384-394.
18. Bajwa EK, Boyce PD, Januzzi JL, Gong MN, Thompson BT, Christiani DC. Biomarker evidence of myocardial cell injury is associated with mortality in acute respiratory distress syndrome. *Crit Care Med*. 2007;25:2484-2490.
19. Hayes MA, Timmins AC, Yau EH, Palazzo M, Hinds CJ, Watson D. Elevation of systemic oxygen delivery in the treatment of critically ill patients. *N Engl J Med*. 1994;330:1717-1722.
20. Shoemaker WC, Appel PL, Kram HB, Waxman K, Lee TS. Prospective trial of supranormal values of survivors as therapeutic goals in high-risk surgical patients. *Chest*. 1988;94:1176-1186.
21. Furian T, Aguiar C, Prado K, et al. Ventricular dysfunction and dilation in severe sepsis and septic shock: relation to endothelial function and mortality. *J Crit Care*. 2012;27:319.e9-319.e15.
22. Moore FD, Dagher FJ, Boyden CM, Lee CJ, Lyons JH. Hemorrhage in normal man: I. distribution and dispersal of saline infusions following acute blood loss: clinical kinetics of blood volume support. *Ann Surg*. 1966;163:485-504.
23. Flexner LB, Gellhorn A, Merrell M. Studies on rates of exchange of substances between the blood and extravascular fluid. I. The exchange of water in the guinea pig. *J Biol Chem*. 1942;144:35-40.
24. Flexner LB, Cowie DB, Vosburgh GJ. Studies on capillary permeability with tracer substances. *Cold Spring Harb Symp Quant Biol*. 1948;13:88-98.
25. Stewart JD, Rourke GM. Intracellular fluid loss in hemorrhage. *J Clin Invest*. 1936;15:697-702.
26. Crook MA, Hally V, Panteli JV. The importance of the refeeding syndrome. *Nutrition*. 2001;17:632-637.
27. Subramanian R, Khardori R. Severe hypophosphatemia. Pathophysiologic implications, clinical presentations, and treatment. *Medicine (Baltimore)*. 2000;79:1-8.
28. Clemens MG, Chaudry IH, Daigneau N, Baue AE. Insulin resistance and depressed gluconeogenic capability during early hyperglycemic sepsis. *J Trauma*. 1984;24:701-708.
29. Lang CH. Beta-adrenergic blockade attenuates insulin resistance induced by tumor necrosis factor. *Am J Physiol*. 1993;264:R984-R991.
30. Jeevanandam M, Young DH, Schiller WR. Glucose turnover, oxidation, and indices of recycling in severely traumatized patients. *J Trauma*. 1990;30:582-589.
31. Shaw JH, Klein S, Wolfe RR. Assessment of alanine, urea and glucose interrelationships in normal subjects and in patients with sepsis with stable isotope tracers. *Surgery*. 1985;97:557-568.
32. Hardardóttir I, Grünfeld C, Feingold KR. Effects of endotoxin and cytokines on lipid metabolism. *Curr Opin Lipidol*. 1994;5:207-215.
33. Robin AP, Askanazi J, Greenwood MR, Carpentier YA, Gump FE, Kinney JM. Lipoprotein lipase activity in surgical patients: influence of trauma and infection. *Surgery*. 1981;90:401-408.

34. Mire JC, Brakenridge SC, Moldawer LL, Moore FA. Persistent inflammation, immunosuppression and catabolism syndrome. *Crit Care Clin*. 2017;33:245-258.

35. Hernandez G, Velasco N, Wainstein C, et al. Gut mucosal atrophy after a short enteral fasting period in critically ill patients. *J Crit Care*. 1999;14:73-77.

36. Greis C, Rasuly Z, Janosi RA, Kordelas L, Beelen DW, Liebregts T. Intestinal T lymphocyte homing is associated with gastric emptying and epithelial barrier function in critically ill: a prospective observational study. *Crit Care*. 2017;21:70.

37. Bagshaw SM, Laupland KB, Doig CJ, et al. Prognosis for long-term survival and renal recovery in critically ill patients with severe acute renal failure: a population-based study. *Crit Care*. 2005;9:R700-R709.

38. Hotchkiss RS, Karl IE. The pathophysiology and treatment of sepsis. *N Engl J Med*. 2003;348:138-150.

39. Van Vught LA, Klein Klouwenberg PM. Spitoni C, et al. Incidence, risk factors, and attributable mortality of secondary infections in the intensive care unit after admission for sepsis. *JAMA*. 2016;315:1469-1479.

40. Limaye AP, Kirby KA, Rubenfeld GD, et al. Cytomegalovirus reactivation in critically ill immunocompetent patients. *JAMA*. 2008;300:413-422.

41. Luyt CE, Combes A, Deback C, et al. Herpes simplex virus lung infection in patients undergoing prolonged mechanical ventilation. *Am J Respir Crit Care Med*. 2007;175:935-942.

42. Mathias B, Delmas AL, Ozrazgat-Baslanti T, et al. Human myeloid-derived suppressor cells are associated with chronic immune suppression after severe sepsis/septic shock. *Ann Surg*. 2017;265:827-834.

43. Annane D, Sébille V, Charpentier C, et al. Effect of treatment with low doses of hydrocortisone and fludrocortisone on mortality in patients with septic shock. *JAMA*. 2002;288:862-871.

44. Vary TC, Drnevich D, Jurasinski C, Brennan Jr WA. Mechanisms regulating skeletal muscle glucose metabolism in sepsis. *Shock*. 1995;3:403-410.

45. Wolfe RR, Durkot MJ, Allsop JR, Burke JF. Glucose metabolism in severely burned patients. *Metabolism*. 1979;28:1031-1039.

46. Shangraw RE, Jahoor F, Miyoshi H, et al. Differentiation between septic and postburn insulin resistance. *Metabolism*. 1989;38:983-989.

47. Virkamäki A, Puhakainen I, Koivisto VA, Vuorinen-Markkola H, Yki-Järvinen H. Mechanisms of hepatic and peripheral insulin resistance during acute infections in humans. *J Clin Endocrinol Metab*. 1992;74:673-679.

48. Marques MB, Langouche L. Endocrine, metabolic and morphologic alterations of adipose tissue during critical illness. *Crit Care Med*. 2013;41:317-325.

49. Godin PJ, Buchman TG. Uncoupling of biological oscillators: a complementary hypothesis concerning the pathogenesis of multiple organ dysfunction syndrome. *Crit Care Med*. 1996;24:1107-1116.

50. Gentile LF, Cuenca AG, Efron PA, et al. Persistent inflammation and immunosuppression: a common syndrome and new horizon for surgical intensive care. *J Trauma Acute Care Surg*. 2012;72:1491-1501.

51. Hu D, Ren J, Wang G, et al. Persistent inflammation-immunosuppression catabolism syndrome, a common manifestation of patients with enterocutaneous fistula in intensive care unit. *J Trauma Acute Care Surg*. 2014;76:725-729.

52. Horiguchi H, Loftus TJ, Hawkins RB, et al. Innate immunity in the persistent inflammation, immunosuppression, and catabolism syndrome and its implications for therapy. *Front Immunol*. 2018;9:595.

53. Moore FA, Phillips SM, McClain CJ, Patel JJ, Martindale RG. Nutrition support for persistent inflammation, immunosuppression, and catabolism syndrome. *Nutr Clin Pract*. 2017;32(suppl 1):121S-127S.

54. Herndon DN, Hart DW, Wolf SE, Chinkes DL, Wolfe RR. Reversal of catabolism by beta-blockade after severe burns. *N Engl J Med*. 2001;345:1223-1229.

55. Rhodes A, Evans LE, Alhazzani W, et al. Surviving Sepsis Campaign: International Guidelines for Management of Sepsis and Septic Shock: 2016. *Intensive Care Med*. 2017;43:304-377.

56. Bone RC, Fisher Jr CJ, Clemmer TP, Slotman GJ, Metz CA, Balk RA. A controlled clinical trial of high-dose methylprednisolone in the treatment of severe sepsis and septic shock. *N Engl J Med*. 1987;317:653-658.

57. Sprung CL, Annane D, Keh D, et al. Hydrocortisone therapy for patients with septic shock. *N Engl J Med*. 2008;358:111-124.

58. Venkatesh B, Finfer S, Cohen J, et al. Adjunctive glucocorticoid therapy in patients with septic shock. *N Engl J Med*. 2018;378:797-808.

59. Annane D, Renault A, Brun-Buisson C, et al. Hydrocortisone plus fludrocortisone for adults with septic shock. *N Engl J Med*. 2018;378:809-818.

60. Chan MC, Spieth PM, Quinn K, Parotto M, Zhang H, Slutsky AS. Circadian rhythms: from basic mechanisms to the intensive care unit. *Crit Care Med*. 2012;40:246-253.

61. Mistraletti G, Umbrello M, Sabbatini G, et al. Melatonin reduces the need for sedation in ICU patients: a randomized controlled trial. *Minerva Anestesiol*. 2015;81:1298-1310.

62. Marik PE, Khangoora V, Rivera R, Hooper MH, Catravas J. Hydrocortisone, vitamin C, and thiamine for the treatment of severe sepsis and septic shock: a retrospective before-after study. *Chest*. 2017;151:1229-1238.

63. Woolum JA, Abner EL, Kelly A, Thompson Bastin ML, Morris PE, Flannery AH. Effect of thiamine administration on lactate clearance and mortality in patients with septic shock. *Crit Care Med*. 2018;46(11):1747-1752.

64. Matthews LR, Ahmed Y, Wilson KL, Griggs DD, Danner OK. Worsening severity of vitamin D deficiency is associated with increased length of stay, surgical intensive care unit cost, and mortality rate in surgical intensive care unit patients. *Am J Surg*. 2012;204:37-43.

65. Braun A, Chang D, Mahadevappa K, et al. Association of low serum 25-hydroxyvitamin D levels and mortality in the critically ill. *Crit Care Med*. 2011;39:671-677.

66. Amrein K, Schnedl C, Holl A, et al. Effect of high-dose vitamin D₃ on hospital length of stay in critically ill patients with vitamin D deficiency: the VITdAL-ICU randomized clinical trial. *JAMA*. 2014;312:1520-1530.

67. Stapleton RD, Jones N, Heyland DK. Feeding critically ill patients: What is the optimal amount of energy? *Crit Care Med*. 2007;35:S535-S540.

68. Dickerson RN. Metabolic support challenges with obesity during critical illness. *Nutrition*. 2018;57:24-31.

69. Herndon DN, Tompkins RG. Support of the metabolic response to burn injury. *Lancet*. 2004;363:1895-1902.

70. Takala J, Ruokonen E, Webster NR, et al. Increased mortality associated with growth hormone treatment in critically ill adults. *N Engl J Med*. 1999;341:785-792.

71. Van den Berghe G, Wouters P, Weekers F, et al. Intensive insulin therapy in critically ill patients. *N Engl J Med*. 2001;345:1359-1367.

72. Van den Berghe G, Wilmer A, Hermans G, et al. Intensive insulin therapy in the medical ICU. *N Engl J Med.* 2006;354: 449-461.

73. Arabi YM, Dabbagh OC, Tamim HM, et al. Intensive versus conventional insulin therapy: a randomized control trial in medical and surgical critically ill patients. *Crit Care Med.* 2008;36:3190-3197.

74. Gandhi GY, Nuttall GA, Abel MD, et al. Intensive intraoperative insulin therapy versus conventional glucose management during cardiac surgery. *Ann Intern Med.* 2007; 146:233-243.

75. NICE-SUGAR Investigators, Finfer S, Chitlock DR, et al. Intensive versus conventional glucose control in critically ill patients. *N Engl J Med.* 2009;360:1283-1297.

76. Nunnally ME. Con: tight perioperative glycemic control: poorly supported and risky. *J Cardiothorac Vasc Anesth.* 2005;19:689-690.

77. Langley RJ, Tsalik EL, van Velkinburgh JC, et al. An integrated clinic-metabolomic model improves prediction of death in sepsis. *Sci Transl Med.* 2013;5:195ra95.

78. Nunnally ME, Neligan P, Deutschman CS. Metabolism in acute and chronic illness. In: Rolandelli RH, Bankhead R, Boullata JI, Compher CW, eds. *Clinical Nutrition: Enteral and Tube Feeding.* 4th ed. Philadelphia, PA: Elsevier; 2008:80-94.

79. Vanhorebeek I, Langouche L, Van den Berghe G. Endocrine aspects of acute and prolonged critical illness. *Nat Clin Pract Endocrinol Metab.* 2006;2:20-31.

80. Van den Berghe G. Neuroendocrine pathobiology of chronic critical illness. *Crit Care Clin.* 2002;18:509-528.

64

How Should Traumatic Brain Injury Be Managed?

Lindsay Raab, W. Andrew Kofke, and Danielle K. Sandsmark

INTRODUCTION

The morbidity and mortality resulting from traumatic brain injury (TBI) stems from the primary brain damage caused by the initial impact as well as from secondary insults that follow. While the primary injury occurs nearly immediately and is largely irreversible, secondary insults include various ischemic, metabolic, and inflammatory disturbances that occur in the vulnerable brain tissue. These insults develop over hours to days following injury. Given the delayed presentation, these insults represent an opportunity for clinical intervention. Recognition and treatment of these evolving processes is critical to ensuring optimal outcome following serious brain injury.

In the following discussion, we outline the evidence supporting various intensive care unit (ICU) practices in the management of serious brain injury to prevent secondary brain damage. We follow and summarize the general format of the Brain Trauma Foundation (BTF) management guidelines.[1] Specific studies that are included were evaluated using the Grading of Recommendations Assessment, Development and Evaluation (GRADE) criteria.

Systemic Blood Pressure and Oxygenation

Background

Both hypotension and hypoxemia contribute to secondary brain injury and influence the outcomes after trauma.[2–4] Due to ethical constraints, it is not possible to perform randomized studies to establish absolute thresholds for oxygenation and blood pressure support. Further, we discuss the available evidence that can provide some guidance to these thresholds.

Evidence

Hypoxemia. Analysis of the prospectively collected Traumatic Coma Data Bank showed that episodes of hypoxemia (partial pressure of oxygen [PaO$_2$] <60 mm Hg or apnea/cyanosis in the field) in the acute period after injury were associated with increased mortality.[2] Studying pre-hospital trauma patients, Stocchetti et al.[3] found that hypoxemia, defined as a peripheral O$_2$ saturation <60%, at the accident scene, was associated with a universally poor prognosis (death or severe disability), as was severe hypotension, defined as systolic blood pressure [SBP] <60 mm Hg. In 3240 patients included in the San Diego County trauma registry, both hypoxemia (PaO$_2$ <110 mm Hg) and extreme hyperoxemia were associated with increased mortality and poorer clinical outcomes in survivors of TBI.[4] Hypoxemia was shown to increase mortality in ICU-treated patients with head injuries.[5]

Hypotension. Poor outcomes have been reported with pre-hospital and in-hospital hypotension.[6] A single episode of hypotension with a SBP <90 mm Hg was associated with increased morbidity and doubled mortality.[2] Marmarou et al.[7] used the Traumatic Coma Data Bank to study 428 patients with severe TBI and found that as the proportion of SBP measurements <80 mm Hg or intracranial pressure (ICP) >20 mm Hg increased, patient outcome worsened. A series of prospective studies by Vassar et al.,[8] evaluating resuscitative fluids pre-hospital admission in hypotensive trauma patients, demonstrated that hyperosmolar fluid resuscitation (7.5% hypertonic saline [HTS] ± Dextran) raised blood pressure more effectively than isotonic solutions, and patients who received hyperosmolar resuscitation had better outcomes than predicted. In the subset of trauma patients with a Glasgow Coma Scale (GCS) score of ≤8, the hyperosmolar treatment group fared significantly better than the isotonic group. However, a follow-up prospective study evaluating pre-hospital resuscitation of hypotensive patients with severe TBI showed no difference in neurological outcome at 6 months in patients resuscitated with hypertonic fluid vs. conventional fluid resuscitation.[9]

Recommendations

Hypoxemia and hypotension are associated with poor outcomes from TBI and should be avoided. GRADE B evidence supports maintaining SBP >90 mm Hg. Similarly, we advise that PaO$_2$ should be maintained >60 mm Hg (8 kPa) and O$_2$ saturation >90%.

Cerebral Perfusion Thresholds

Background

Based on Poiseuille's law describing laminar flow, cerebral blood flow (CBF) is directly related to the cerebral perfusion pressure (CPP, defined as the difference between mean arterial pressure [MAP] and ICP) and inversely related to the cerebral vascular resistance (CVR; CBF = CPP/CVR). Under normal conditions, CBF remains constant despite changes in CPP by constriction and dilation of the cerebral blood vessels, termed cerebral autoregulation. Following brain injury, cerebral autoregulation is often disrupted such that the blood vessel radius either remains constant despite changes in MAP and CPP or varies directly (inversely) with CPP. In both cases, even small changes in CPP can trigger alterations in CBF, blood flow velocity, and ICP, which in turn compromises oxygen and glucose delivery to the brain tissue. Given the lack of tools to directly and continuously measure CBF, CPP has been used as a monitoring parameter reflective of cerebral perfusion.

Evidence

Low CPP (generally defined as <50 mm Hg), typically caused by systemic hypotension (low MAP) or intracranial hypertension (high ICP), is associated with poor clinical outcome as well as poor physiological variables, including jugular venous oxygen saturation (SjvO$_2$), brain O$_2$ saturation, and cerebral microdialysis parameters.[10–13]

Rosner and Daughton[14] originally reported regarding the management of head-injured patients based on CPP thresholds. They studied 34 patients and used various interventions to achieve CPP >70 mm Hg. They concluded that this was associated with a decreased mortality and an improvement in functional outcome over prior cohorts; however, it was unclear if this was solely due to a lower incidence of systemic hypotension.[15] Follow-up studies, however, suggested that there were risks of CPP augmentation. Robertson et al.[16] performed a randomized controlled trial (RCT) of CPP-guided vs. ICP-guided management and found a five-fold increase in the development of acute respiratory distress syndrome (ARDS) in patients managed by CPP, presumably a result of overenthusiastic fluid resuscitation. Contant et al.[17] found a similar incidence of ARDS in their TBI patients managed by CPP. This complication was associated with an increased risk of mortality and poor neurological outcome.

By its very nature, TBI is a heterogeneous disease process with varying cerebral physiologies not only between patients but also between brain regions in a single patient. Thus, it is likely overly simplistic to believe that every individual (or perhaps, every region of the brain) requires the same CPP to maintain adequate perfusion and avoid hyperperfusion and/or ICP changes. To this end, methods to measure individual cerebral autoregulation have been developed. Steiner et al.[18] retrospectively calculated a correlation coefficient defining the relationship between CPP and ICP to determine the CPP at which autoregulation was best preserved. Maintaining the mean CPP near the level of autoregulation was associated with better outcomes than those observed in patients whose CPPs were higher or lower than this calculated value. These data suggest that CPP can be optimized on an individual basis with adjunctive physiological monitoring. However, the efficacy of this approach remains to be tested in large, prospective randomized trials.

Another consideration in optimizing CPP is how the CPP is measured. Lassen[19] originally defined CPP based on "arterial blood pressure measured at the level of the head" using the tragus of the ear as an external landmark. However, there is much heterogeneity in current practice and MAP is often measured at the level of the right atrium.[20] When the head of the bed is elevated, as it should be for the management of head-injured patients, MAP measurements at the level of the right atrium may be higher than those measured at the tragus by up to 18 mm Hg, thereby overestimating CPP.[21] This variability in practice may contribute to difficulty in defining optimal CPP and MAP targets following head injury. In this regard, the Neuroanesthesia Society of Great Britain and Ireland and the Society of British Neurological Surgeons issued a joint position statement advocating for MAP measurement at the level of the tragus in patients with TBI.[22]

Recommendations

We recommend measuring MAP (to calculate CPP) at the level of the tragus. Low CPP, generally defined as <50 mm Hg, should be prevented (GRADE B). Augmentation of CPP, using fluids, should be avoided due to the risk of iatrogenic complications based on GRADE B evidence. Adjunctive physiological monitors to determine the CPP at which autoregulation is optimized may be helpful to individualize care; however, there is currently no evidence to support a recommendation regarding their use.

Intracranial Pressure Thresholds

Background

The bony, rigid skull and vertebral canal contain a fixed volume including the brain parenchyma, cerebrospinal fluid (CSF), and blood, creating a nearly incompressible system. Any increase in the volume of one of these compartments is met first with a compensatory shift in another compartment (for example, CSF shifting down the less rigid spinal column). When compensatory changes are exhausted, the ICP increases dramatically and can cause secondary brain injury due to brain compression, herniation, and cerebral perfusion compromise. However, treatment of ICP must be balanced with the potential side effects of medical and pharmacologic ICP management.

Evidence

There are no prospective randomized studies designed to determine the threshold for initiation of ICP-reducing therapy. Several prospective observational studies reviewed suggest that outcomes improve when ICP is maintained at <20–25 mm Hg and that brain herniation is more likely above these thresholds.[7,23,24] However, in situations without intracranial mass lesions, an ICP >20 mm Hg may be tolerated.[25]

Chestnut et al.[26] first examined outcomes in patients managed with or without ICP-guided treatment. They focused on monitoring ICP, not its treatment. Thus, both arms underwent ICP-reducing therapy that was guided by either an ICP monitor or neurological examination and neuroimaging. In this population, there was no difference in ICU length of stay; 14-day or 6-month mortality in those who had aggressive management to maintain ICP <20 mm Hg compared with patients who were managed based on clinical examination and radiographic imaging alone. The generalizability of these findings has been questioned,[27] but this study raises an important point that ICP monitoring in and of itself may not influence clinical outcomes.

Recommendations

Despite an absence of high-quality evidence, in most cases, an ICP >20–25 mm Hg should be an indication to increase ICP-reducing therapy (GRADE C). This must be tempered with the iatrogenic risks of ICP-lowering therapy. When ICP monitoring is unavailable, management based on clinical examination and imaging is reasonable based on the available evidence.

Seizure Prophylaxis
Background

Post-traumatic seizures (PTS) are classified as early (<7 days after TBI) or late (>7 days after TBI). The incidence of PTS varies from 4 to 25% early and 9 to 42% late in untreated TBI patients.[28] Early PTS may contribute to secondary brain injury by inducing cerebral hypermetabolism, elevated ICP, and hypertension. It has been proposed that early PTS beget late PTS and epilepsy through neuronal kindling. Epilepsy can have a significant impact on the quality of life in TBI survivors.[29]

Evidence

Temkin et al.[30] performed a randomized, placebo controlled trial in 404 patients with severe head trauma who received phenytoin or placebo for 1 year after head injury. They found that patients receiving phenytoin had a decrease in the incidence of seizures in the acute period (<7 days), but no difference in late seizures. The same group found that both valproic acid and phenytoin also decreased seizures in the acute period.[31] The BTF metaanalysis concluded that anticonvulsant prophylaxis with phenytoin, carbamezapine, or valproic acid is indicated in the first 7 days after TBI, but longer treatment is not warranted.[1] The American Academy

of Neurology metaanalysis of eight RCTs arrived at similar conclusions.[32]

Given the potential toxicities and need for drug level monitoring with phenytoin and valproic acid, neurointensivists and neurosurgeons have started using levetiracetam for seizure prophylaxis after TBI.[33] In a retrospective review, Caballero et al.[34] found that seizure activity rates were not different in patients treated with levetiracetam compared with those treated with phenytoin. Levetiracetam therapy was slightly less expensive. Similar results were noted in a recent metaanalysis that included nearly 1200 patients.[35] Larger, prospective studies are needed to determine if levetiracetam is efficacious and cost-effective in preventing acute seizures after TBI.

Recommendations

Seizure prophylaxis is indicated in the first 7 days after TBI (GRADE A). Phenytoin, valproic acid, and carbamezapine are all reasonable antiseizure medications for prophylaxis. In the absence of PTS, treatment should be stopped after 7 days. Levetiracetam may be a reasonable alternative for seizure prophylaxis in patients in whom phenytoin is contraindicated, but further studies are needed. There is no evidence to support antiepileptic administration for >7 days after TBI in the absence of clinical or electrophysiologic seizure activity.

Management of Elevated Intracranial Pressure: Hyperventilation
Background

During hyperventilation carbon dioxide concentrations fall, resulting in constriction of cerebral blood vessels. Vasoconstriction decreases CBF to reduce intravascular volume in the cranial cavity and to lower ICP. In this regard, voluntary hyperventilation may be one of the first clinical signs of elevated ICP as consequent tissue acidosis from high ICP produces compensatory hyperventilation. Similarly, hyperventilation and maintenance of a modestly lower partial pressure of carbon dioxide ($PaCO_2$; 30–35 mm Hg/4–4.5 kPa) is one of the first measures that can be used to lower ICP in the mechanically ventilated patient. Given that hypocarbia triggers intracranial vasoconstriction, the risk of decreased CBF and resultant cerebral ischemia as a consequence of hyperventilation must be considered, though hyperventilation has not been reported to cause brain injury in the absence of TBI.

Evidence

Several studies of CBF suggest that CBF is dangerously low in the acute period after TBI, leading the BTF to advise against aggressive hyperventilation ($PaCO_2$ <25 mm Hg/3.3 kPa) after TBI.[1] Muizelaar et al.[36] performed a prospective, randomized study of hyperventilation in TBI finding a worse functional outcome, though no difference in mortality at

3 and 6 months, but not 12 months, in the hyperventilated patients.

Recommendations

Prolonged prophylactic hyperventilation to $PaCO_2$ of 25–30 mm Hg (3.3–4 kPa) should be avoided in TBI patients (GRADE B) due to risks of cerebral ischemia. It may be justified if accompanied by a monitor of CBF adequacy. It also may be justified as a temporary intervention in emergency and temporary sudden increases in ICP such as with life-threatening herniation syndromes. Hypercarbia ($PaCO_2$ >45 mm Hg/6 kPa) should be avoided, as this can trigger hyperemia, decreased CPP, and potentially trigger a sudden ICP elevation. There is insufficient evidence to determine the effect of hyperventilation on patient outcome after TBI.

Hyperosmolar Therapy

Background

Osmotic agents may lower ICP primarily by drawing free water out of the brain parenchyma and into the systemic vasculature. The simplest way to maintain a modest osmotic gradient is to maintain the serum sodium on the upper range of normal (~145) in the euvolemic patient. When a stronger gradient is needed, mannitol and HTS are the two most commonly used agents.

Evidence

While RCTs are lacking, mannitol and HTS are both effective agents for lowering ICP after TBI. Mannitol was superior to barbiturates in ICP control, maintenance of CPP, and mortality when given as a 20% bolus at 1 g/kg and repeated to maintain ICP <20 mm Hg.[37]

Early studies focused on the use of HTS for resuscitation in trauma patients.[38,39] Shackford et al.[40] were the first to specifically look at HTS infusion and ICP and found that HTS significantly lowered ICP. Several studies reported regarding the efficacy of HTS in decreasing ICP, notably being effective in cases where ICP is refractory to mannitol therapy.[41,42] A trial evaluating equiosmolar doses of mannitol and 3% HTS in the operating room revealed equivalent effect on "brain relaxation," suggesting equivalent ICP reduction with equiosmolar therapy.[43]

Another prospective, randomized study of 20 TBI patients looked at the effect of equivalent volumes of 7.5% HTS and 20% mannitol (2400 mOsm/kg HTS, 1160 mOsm/kg mannitol), showing a lower incidence of treatment failure with HTS.[38] A study using brain tissue oxygen monitoring in TBI found that compared with 0.75 g/kg 20% mannitol, 7.5% HTS boluses were associated with lower ICP and higher CPP and cardiac output.[44] They concluded that in patients with severe TBI and elevated ICP refractory to previous mannitol treatment, 7.5% HTS administered as second-tier therapy is associated with a significant increase of brain oxygenation and improved cerebral and systemic hemodynamics.[44]

Recommendations

Mannitol and HTS are both effective to treat elevated ICP based on GRADE B evidence. While small studies suggest that HTS may result in better ICP control in patients who no longer respond to mannitol therapy, no RCTs have directly compared the two treatments. As such, it is not possible to recommend one agent over the other. Other factors such as volume status and/or kidney function may favor utilization of one agent over another but should be assessed on a case-by-case basis.

Surgical Decompressive Therapy

Background

When severe cerebral edema causes elevated ICP, decompressive craniectomy, a surgical procedure in which a portion of the skull is removed and the dura is opened, can provide definitive management. By opening the rigid cranium, brain swelling can occur outside of the cranial cavity without compromising surrounding structures. The surgical approach varies depending on the site and extent of injury. Hemispheric, bifrontal, or bihemispheric bone flaps may be removed. A durotomy is also performed to provide additional space into which the swelling brain can expand. The use of decompressive craniectomy to control elevated ICP has a history dating to the early 20th century. Only in the 21st century has the procedure started to undergo scrutiny for impact on outcome.

Evidence

In 26 patients who underwent bifrontal craniectomy for the treatment of refractory elevated ICP after severe TBI, surgical intervention was associated with significant reductions in ICP and outcomes were favorable in 69% of patients, a significant improvement over similarly described cohorts.[45] In this regard, Aarabi et al.[46] found that decompressive craniectomy significantly lowered ICP in 85% of patients and was associated with a favorable outcome in 51% of patients at 3 months.

Based on these initial observations, 155 patients with severe, diffuse TBI who had refractory elevated ICP to standard first-line therapies were enrolled in the first RCT of craniectomy following TBI.[47] Patients were randomized to undergo bifrontotemperoparietal craniectomy or standard medical therapy. While decompressive craniectomy did control ICP and result in fewer ICU days, surgical intervention was associated with more unfavorable outcomes (death, vegetative state, or severe disability) than standard medical therapy. However, questions regarding the generalizability of these data remain, particularly given that a large proportion (27%) of patients in the surgical arm had bilateral unreactive pupils at randomization (compared with 12% in the medical management arm), a clinical finding historically associated with very poor outcomes.[48]

Recommendations

Surgical decompressive therapy is an effective measure for the management of persistently elevated ICP. However, there is no evidence that decompression improves clinical outcomes. We recommend that surgical decompressive therapy be considered as a life-saving measure in patients in whom other measures to control ICP have failed and who may have a chance of functional outcome.

Anesthetics, Analgesics, and Sedatives
Background
Pain and agitation after TBI contribute to ICP elevations and increased cerebral metabolic demand. Thus, controlling anxiety, pain, and agitation are important first steps towards controlling ICP after TBI. High-dose barbiturates, benzodiazepines, and propofol decrease metabolic rate in intact brain areas, resulting in decreased CBF and ICP. The use of these medications must be balanced with the need for careful neurological clinical examinations that may be limited in the presence of sedating medications. While the use of sedation is generally easy for the neurointensivist to justify when ICP is an issue, pain can be difficult to quantify in these severely injured patients.

Evidence
There is no prospective randomized data supporting treatment of pain and agitation as a means to prevent elevated ICP. In a single, prospective randomized study comparing propofol with morphine for sedation in TBI patients, propofol use was associated with a trend toward lower ICP that did not reach statistical significance. Post-hoc analysis of patients who received high-dose propofol suggested a better neurologic outcome despite the lack of a difference in ICP, possibly implying a potential neuroprotective effect. Barbiturates have been shown to decrease ICP[23]; however, they are so often complicated by severe hypotension that these risks seem to outweigh any benefits.[1,49]

More recently, dexmedetomidine, an α-2-agonist, has been used to effectively control agitation and allow for serial neurological examinations[50] and has been shown to decrease CBF without affecting the cerebral metabolic rate.[51] When directly compared with propofol, both had similar cerebral physiological effects using multimodal monitoring.[52] Schomer et al.[53] found that dexmedetomidine use resulted in a decreased number of hyperosmolar boluses being needed to control ICP without a significant increase in adverse events (hypotension, bradycardia, or decreased CPP).[53] Similar results were seen in a metaanalysis of dexmedetomidine use in a broader group of neurocritical care patients.[54] However, larger, prospective studies are required to make definitive recommendations regarding dexmedetomidine use in severe TBI.

Recommendations
Propofol is recommended over morphine for sedation in severe TBI with GRADE C evidence. GRADE A evidence suggests that barbiturates should not be given prophylactically for TBI. Barbiturate use is supported in cases of severe refractory intracranial hypertension with GRADE C evidence.

Prophylactic Hypothermia and Therapeutic Normothermia
Background
Fever is common in patients with severe brain injuries and has been associated with poor outcome.[55–57] The mechanisms by which fever worsens outcomes are unclear but likely include potentiation of inflammatory cascades, increased tissue metabolic demand, and excitotoxicity. As such, fever control (induced normothermia) is frequently employed early in the care of brain-injured neurocritical care patients.

Hypothermia (generally defined as cooling to 32°C–33°C, though protocols vary) appears to be neuroprotective in preclinical[58] and single-institution human studies and improves neurological outcomes after cardiac arrest.[59,60] These data suggest that it may be useful in the care of TBI patients.

Evidence
Studies have reported conflicting results regarding the efficacy of prophylactic hypothermia in TBI. The most consistent studies have been those demonstrating the beneficial impact of hypothermia on ICP control.[61] While hypothermia can aid in ICP control, the influence on patient outcome has been less obvious. Despite the preclinical evidence of neuroprotection associated with hypothermia, a randomized, prospective multicenter trial failed to show improvement when TBI patients were treated with induced hypothermia.[62] This study was limited by significant heterogeneity in therapeutic protocols between centers. A follow-up analysis suggested that better outcomes were achieved in high-volume centers.[63] Several metaanalyses concluded that evidence was insufficient to confidently recommend the use of prophylactic hypothermia in TBI.[64–67] In the BTF analysis, although a mortality effect favoring hypothermia was not quite significant, there was a statistically significant 46% increased chance of a good outcome in the hypothermic patients.[68] Further analysis indicated that a minimum duration of 48 hours of induced hypothermia was needed to see a protective effect but was associated with an increased risk for pneumonia. The BTF and American Association of Neurological Surgeons thus issued a level III recommendation for cautious and selective use of moderate hypothermia for TBI.[68]

One proposed limitation of the earlier studies was a relatively late induction of hypothermia. Clifton et al.[69] conducted a prospective, multicenter, RCT of hypothermia vs. normothermia induced 2–5 hours after injury. The study was terminated early due to futility, showing no benefit of hypothermia despite a relatively fast time to cooling. Maekawa et al.[70] reported a prospective, multicenter, RCT of prolonged hypothermia (32°C–34°C for >72 hours) vs. monitored temperature management (35°C–37°C) after TBI but found no improvement in neurological outcome. Similarly, hypothermia did not reduce mortality or improve functional outcome over fever control in children with severe TBI.[71]

These data supported a larger multicenter study. The European Study of Therapeutic Hypothermia (32°C–35°C) for Intracranial Pressure Reduction after Traumatic Brain Injury (the Eurotherm3235 Trial) was a randomized, prospective, multicenter trial of 387 patients with severe TBI and refractory intracranial hypertension.[72] Patients were randomized to hypothermia vs. standard therapies (i.e., hyperosmolar therapy) to control ICP. This study was specifically powered to assess the functional outcome 6 months after injury. While escalation of therapy to control ICP was more commonly required in the control group than in the hypothermia group (54 vs. 44%, respectively), when outcomes were assessed at 6 months, a favorable outcome occurred in 37% of patients in the control group vs. 26% of patients in the hypothermia group ($P = .03$).[72]

Hypothermia may cause additional physiological effects (e.g., immunosuppression, bleeding diathesis, and cardiac arrhythmias) and complications due to related therapies (e.g., induced paralysis and shivering control) that may negate the positive effects of cooler temperature. In this regard, a case series comparing prophylactic hypothermia at 33°C vs. 35°C after severe TBI found equivalent ICP control at the milder hypothermia target with fewer complications, including hypokalemia, infection, ventricular tachycardias, pulmonary embolus, renal failure, and tendency to lower mortality.[73] Fever control (induced normothermia), rather than true hypothermia, with an intravascular cooling catheter similarly controlled ICP in 21 patients with severe TBI.[74] A multicenter RCT, POLAR, of early hypothermia vs. normothermia in TBI wherein patients were cooled to <35°C vs. normothermia for a minimum of 72 hours and up to 7 days failed to demonstrate improved outcomes at 6 months.[75]

Recommendations

In severe TBI there is now GRADE A evidence that induced hypothermia should not be used as a means of ICP control as it does not improve functional outcomes. Therapeutic normothermia (monitored temperature management) using endovascular cooling is supported by GRADE D evidence. Hyperthermia should be avoided.

Brain Oxygen Monitoring
Background

CBF ensures delivery of glucose and oxygen to the brain parenchyma and should be proportional to the metabolic demands of the tissue. Brain oxygen monitors have been used as indirect indicators of adequate CBF.

Oxygen delivery to the brain can be measured both globally (whole brain) and regionally. Jugular bulb catheters use a fiberoptic oximeter to measure the content of oxygen in the jugular veins to measure global brain oxygenation. The jugular venous oxygen concentration is compared with the oxygen content in the arterial system; the difference between the two ($SjvO_2$) serves as a surrogate measure of the balance between CBF and metabolic demand (normal values: 55–69%). Regional oxygenation can be measured using a Clarke-type electrode. Oxygen molecules diffuse from the brain parenchyma into the probe through a diffusible membrane and are reduced at the cathode, creating an electrical current that is proportional to the partial pressure of oxygen in brain tissue ($PbtO_2$) in the sampled region (normal values $PbtO_2$ >20 mm Hg).

Evidence

In the BTF metaanalysis,[1] numerous studies of jugular bulb oxygen monitoring in TBI were reviewed. Worse outcomes were seen in patients who had episodes of $SjvO_2$ of less than 50%, as may occur in tissue ischemia or states of high metabolic demand such as status epilepticus. Episodes of $SjvO_2$ higher than 75%, which may be associated with hyperemia or infarcted, metabolically inactive tissue, were also associated with poor outcomes. These studies suggest that $SjvO_2$ be maintained between 50 and 75%. However, there are no randomized, prospective studies that have tested this hypothesis.

Using a regional brain oxygen monitor, Meixensberger et al.[76] compared 53 patients who received brain oxygen-directed therapy with 40 historical controls who received ICP/CPP-directed therapy. They found that over the whole monitoring period, $PbtO_2$ was higher in the group who received brain oxygen-directed therapy; this was not statistically significant. Spiotta et al.[77] prospectively compared 70 patients with severe TBI who received brain oxygen-directed therapy with 53 patients who received ICP/CPP-directed therapy and found that the former group had improved survival and clinical outcomes at 3 months. In patients who had brain oxygen monitoring and later died, there was a longer mean duration of compromised brain O_2 and a lower rate of response to efforts to increase brain oxygen. Using historical controls, Stiefel et al.[78] compared the impact of a change in local practice to use $PbtO_2$ to guide therapy and reported a significant improvement in outcome. This report was neither prospective nor randomized, and the historical controls had a higher mortality than expected.

Okonkwo et al.[79] performed a phase II (BOOST II), randomized, prospective clinical trial to determine if treatment guided by brain oxygen and ICP monitoring vs. ICP monitoring alone resulted in fewer periods of brain hypoxia. This study showed that a protocol based on brain tissue oxygenation and ICP monitoring reduced the proportion of time with brain tissue hypoxia by 66% after severe TBI and confirmed safety and feasibility of the treatment protocol. This study was not powered for clinical efficacy but showed a trend toward reduced mortality (34% in the ICP only treatment group vs. 25% in the ICP + oxygen monitoring group) and improved recovery compared with therapies based on ICP monitoring alone. BOOST III (NCT03754114) has been funded and will similarly randomize patients to receive targeted interventions based on ICP alone or ICP + brain oxygen monitoring. This study will be powered to assess the impact of brain oxygen monitoring on long-term outcome after TBI.

Not all studies have found an improvement in patient outcome with brain oxygen-directed therapy. Adamides et al.[80] studied 30 patients who underwent brain oxygen monitoring. Twenty patients in whom treatment was aimed at targeting a predefined goal brain oxygenation value (>15 mm Hg) had less cerebral hypoxia during the duration of monitoring but neurologic outcome at 6 months was no different between groups. Martini et al.[81] studied 123 patients who underwent brain tissue oxygen monitoring compared with 506 patients who received ICP-directed therapy. The study found that patients treated based on brain oxygen thresholds had longer lengths of stay in the ICU and a greater utilization of clinical resources without any improvement in survival or neurological outcome at hospital discharge. Notably, patients who received brain oxygen-directed therapy had more severe injury at the time of enrollment as measured by admission GCS and injury severity scores.

While the effect of brain oxygen-guided management on patient outcomes (and whether or not that is even the best endpoint to measure) remains to be determined, $PbtO_2$ or $SjvO_2$ monitoring does provide unique insight into aspects of brain physiology not provided by other monitors. For example, Eriksson et al.[82] found that survivors of severe head injury had significantly higher brain oxygen values than non-survivors; however, there was no difference in ICP and CPP values for the two groups. Thus, brain oxygen monitoring may provide unique physiologic information that can be used in conjunction with other physiologic monitors in the management of these complex patients to optimize their clinical outcomes.

Recommendations

There is now GRADE B evidence to support the use of $PbtO_2$ monitoring as supplements to ICP monitoring in TBI. The evidence to support $SjvO_2$ monitoring is less clear (GRADE C). $SjvO_2$ of less than 50% and $PbtO_2$ <20 mm Hg should be avoided. The extent of time and the depth of the drop in brain oxygen values below these thresholds likely also impact outcome.

Steroids

Background

Corticosteroids have been used extensively to decrease brain edema from brain tumors and inflammatory processes. Therefore, corticosteroids have been examined for their effects on secondary injury due to brain swelling following TBI.

Evidence

Saul et al.[83] first explored the use of high-dose methylprednisolone (5 mg/kg/day) in severe TBI patients but found no difference in outcomes at 6 months. Braakman et al.[84] similarly found no benefit from high-dose dexamethasone given within 6 hours of injury. In 2005, a metaanalysis of 20 studies including over 12,000 patients concluded that there was an increased risk of death associated with the use of corticosteroids[85] and thus their use is not recommended by the BTF.[1]

Recommendations

Corticosteroids should not be given after TBI (Grade A).

Nutrition

Background

Hypermetabolism and nitrogen wasting have long been reported in patients after head injury, resulting in an increase of approximately 140% of the expected metabolic expenditure.[86–88]

Evidence

Among 797 severe TBI patients treated at 22 trauma centers, patients who were not fed within 5 days after TBI had a two-fold increase in mortality.[84] Results were even worse when feeding was delayed for 7 days; mortality in that cohort was increased four-fold. The researchers found that the amount of nutrition during the first 5 days inversely correlated with mortality even after correcting for other factors known to affect mortality after TBI. They were able to calculate that for every 10 kcal/kg decrease in caloric intake was associated with a 30–40% increase in mortality.

A few small studies have compared enteral vs. parenteral nutrition after TBI and have found no substantial differences between feeding methods.[89,90]

Recommendations

There is GRADE B evidence that full enteral or parenteral nutritional support should be implemented at least by Day 5 after injury in patients without the evidence of previous malnutrition.

AUTHORS' RECOMMENDATIONS
- Prevention of secondary brain injury is the primary focus of critical care management after severe TBI.
- Careful attention to maintaining cerebral perfusion and oxygenation is critical to prevent further brain tissue injury from ischemia and hypoxia.
- Hyperosmolar therapy and decompressive hemicraniectomy should be considered for the management of elevated ICP.
- Brain tissue oxygen monitoring, in addition to ICP monitoring, is beneficial for preventing brain tissue hypoxia.
- Seizure prophylaxis should be continued for 7 days after injury only unless there is clinical or electrophysiological evidence of seizure activity.
- Fever control, nutritional support, and appropriate analgesia are likely important for minimizing secondary brain injury.
- Steroids have no role in the management of cerebral edema associated with severe TBI.

REFERENCES

1. Carney N, Totten AM, Hawryluk GWJ, et al. *Guidelines for the Management of Severe Traumatic Brain Injury.* 4th ed. Brain Trauma Foundation. 2016. Available at: https://braintrauma.org/uploads/03/12/Guidelines_for_Management_of_Severe_TBI_4th_Edition.pdf. Accessed December 20, 2018.

2. Chesnut RM, Marshall SB, Piek J, Blunt BA, Klauber MR, Marshall LF. Early and late systemic hypotension as a frequent and fundamental source of cerebral ischemia following severe brain injury in the Traumatic Coma Data Bank. *Acta Neurochir Suppl (Wien)*. 1993;59:121-125.

3. Stocchetti N, Furlan A, Volta F. Hypoxemia and arterial hypotension at the accident scene in head injury. *J Trauma*. 1996;40(5):764-767.

4. Davis DP, Meade W, Sise MJ, et al. Both hypoxemia and extreme hyperoxemia may be detrimental in patients with severe traumatic brain injury. *J Neurotrauma*. 2009;26(12):2217-2223.

5. Jones PA, Andrews PJ, Midgley S, et al. Measuring the burden of secondary insults in head-injured patients during intensive care. *J Neurosurg Anesthesiol*. 1994;6(1):4-14.

6. Manley G, Knudson MM, Morabito D, Damron S, Erickson V, Pitts L. Hypotension, hypoxia, and head injury: frequency, duration, and consequences. *Arch Surg*. 2001;136(10):1118-1123.

7. Marmarou A, Anderson RL, Ward JD, et al. Impact of ICP instability and hypotension on outcome in patients with severe head trauma. *J Neurosurg*. 1991;75(Suppl. 1):S59-S66.

8. Vassar MJ, Fischer RP, O'Brien PE, et al. A multicenter trial for resuscitation of injured patients with 7.5% sodium chloride. The effect of added dextran 70. The multicenter group for the study of hypertonic saline in trauma patients. *Arch Surg*. 1993;128(9):1003-1011, discussion 1011-1013.

9. Cooper DJ, Myles PS, McDermott FT, et al. Prehospital hypertonic saline resuscitation of patients with hypotension and severe traumatic brain injury. *JAMA*. 2004;291(11):1350-1357.

10. Chan KH, Miller JD, Dearden NM, Andrews PJ, Midgley S. The effect of changes in cerebral perfusion pressure upon middle cerebral artery blood flow velocity and jugular bulb venous oxygen saturation after severe brain injury. *J Neurosurg*. 1992;77(1):55-61.

11. Andrews PJ, Sleeman DH, Statham PF, et al. Predicting recovery in patients suffering from traumatic brain injury by using admission variables and physiological data: a comparison between decision tree analysis and logistic regression. *J Neurosurg*. 2002;97(2):326-336.

12. Clifton GL, Miller ER, Choi SC, Levin HS. Fluid thresholds and outcome from severe brain injury. *Crit Care Med*. 2002;30(4):739-745.

13. Nelson DW, Thornquist B, MacCallum RM, et al. Analyses of cerebral microdialysis in patients with traumatic brain injury: relations to intracranial pressure, cerebral perfusion pressure and catheter placement. *BMC Med*. 2011;9(1):21.

14. Rosner MJ, Daughton S. Cerebral perfusion pressure management in head injury. *J Trauma*. 1990;30(8):933-940, discussion 940-941.

15. Chesnut RM. Avoidance of hypotension: conditio sine qua non of successful severe head-injury management. *J Trauma*. 1997;42(Suppl. 5):S4-S9.

16. Robertson CS, Valadka AB, Hannay HJ, et al. Prevention of secondary ischemic insults after severe head injury. *Crit Care Med*. 1999;27(10):2086-2095.

17. Contant CF, Valadka AB, Gopinath SP, Hannay HJ, Robertson CS. Adult respiratory distress syndrome: a complication of induced hypertension after severe head injury. *J Neurosurg*. 2001;95(4):560-568.

18. Steiner LA, Czosnyka M, Piechnik SK, et al. Continuous monitoring of cerebrovascular pressure reactivity allows determination of optimal cerebral perfusion pressure in patients with traumatic brain injury. *Crit Care Med*. 2002;30(4):733-738.

19. Lassen NA. Cerebral blood flow and oxygen consumption in man. *Physiol Rev*. 1959;39(2):183-238.

20. Kosty JA, Leroux PD, Levine J, et al. A comparison of clinical and research practices in measuring cerebral perfusion pressure. *Anesth Analg*. 2013;117(3):694-698.

21. Rosner MJ, Coley IB. Cerebral perfusion pressure, intracranial pressure, and head elevation. *J Neurosurg*. 1986;65(5):636-641.

22. Neuroanaesthesia and Critical Care Society of Great Britain and Ireland, Society of British Neurological Surgeons. Joint position statement by the Councils of the Neuroanaesthesia and Critical Care Society of Great Britain and Ireland (NACCS) and the Society of British Neurological Surgeons (SBNS) with regards to the calculation of cerebral perfusion pressure in the management of traumatic brain injury. NACCS; 2014. Available at: https://www.sbns.org.uk/files/8914/3282/6634/Final_Revised_NACCSGBI__SBNS_statement_Aug_2014.pdf. Accessed December 20, 2018.

23. Eisenberg HM, Frankowski RF, Contant CF, Marshall LF, Walker MD. High-dose barbiturate control of elevated intracranial pressure in patients with severe head injury. *J Neurosurg*. 1988;69(1):15-23.

24. Ratanalert S, Phuenpathom N, Saeheng S, Oearsakul T, Sripairojkul B, Hirunpat S. ICP threshold in CPP management of severe head injury patients. *Surg Neurol*. 2004;61(5):429-434, discussion 434-435.

25. Chambers IR, Treadwell L, Mendelow AD. Determination of threshold levels of cerebral perfusion pressure and intracranial pressure in severe head injury by using receiver operating—characteristic curves: an observational study in 291 patients. *J Neurosurg*. 2001;94(3):412-416.

26. Chesnut RM, Temkin N, Carney N, et al. A trial of intracranial-pressure monitoring in traumatic brain injury. *N Engl J Med*. 2012;367(26):2471-2481.

27. Ropper AH. Brain in a box. *N Engl J Med*. 2012;367(26):2539-2541.

28. Teasell R, Bayona N, Lippert C, Villamere J, Hellings C. Post-traumatic seizure disorder following acquired brain injury. *Brain Inj*. 2007;21(2):201-214.

29. Kolakowsky-Hayner SA, Wright J, Englander J, Duong T, Ladley-O'Brien S. Impact of late post-traumatic seizures on physical health and functioning for individuals with brain injury within the community. *Brain Inj*. 2013;27(5):578-586.

30. Temkin NR, Dikmen SS, Wilensky AJ, Keihm J, Chabal S, Winn HR. A randomized, double-blind study of phenytoin for the prevention of post-traumatic seizures. *N Engl J Med*. 1990;323(8):497-502.

31. Temkin NR, Dikmen SS, Anderson GD, et al. Valproate therapy for prevention of posttraumatic seizures: a randomized trial. *J Neurosurg*. 1999;91(4):593-600.

32. Chang BS, Lowenstein DH, Quality Standards Subcommittee of the American Academy of Neurology. Practice parameter: antiepileptic drug prophylaxis in severe traumatic brain injury: report of the Quality Standards Subcommittee of the American Academy of Neurology. *Neurology*. 2003;60(1):10-16.

33. Kruer RM, Harris LH, Goodwin H, et al. Changing trends in the use of seizure prophylaxis after traumatic brain injury: a shift from phenytoin to levetiracetam. *J Crit Care*. 2013;28(5):883.e9-883.e13.

34. Caballero GC, Hughes DW, Maxwell PR, Green K, Gamboa CD, Barthol CA. Retrospective analysis of levetiracetam compared to phenytoin for seizure prophylaxis in adults with traumatic brain injury. *Hosp Pharm*. 2013;48(9):757-761.

35. Khan NR, VanLandingham MA, Fierst TM, et al. Should levetiracetam or phenytoin be used for posttraumatic seizure prophylaxis? a systematic review of the literature and meta-analysis. *Neurosurgery.* 2016;79(6):775-782.

36. Muizelaar JP, Marmarou A, Ward JD, et al. Adverse effects of prolonged hyperventilation in patients with severe head injury: a randomized clinical trial. *J Neurosurg.* 1991;75(5):731-739.

37. Schwartz ML, Tator CH, Rowed DW, Reid SR, Meguro K, Andrews DF. The University of Toronto head injury treatment study: a prospective, randomized comparison of pentobarbital and mannitol. *Can J Neurol Sci.* 1984;11(4):434-440.

38. Vialet R, Albanèse J, Thomachot L, et al. Isovolume hypertonic solutes (sodium chloride or mannitol) in the treatment of refractory posttraumatic intracranial hypertension: 2 mL/kg 7.5% saline is more effective than 2 mL/kg 20% mannitol. *Crit Care Med.* 2003;31(6):1683-1687.

39. Vassar MJ, Perry CA, Gannaway WL, Holcroft JW. 7.5% sodium chloride/dextran for resuscitation of trauma patients undergoing helicopter transport. *Arch Surg.* 1991;126(9):1065-1072.

40. Shackford SR, Bourguignon PR, Wald SL, Rogers FB, Osler TM, Clark DE. Hypertonic saline resuscitation of patients with head injury: a prospective, randomized clinical trial. *J Trauma.* 1998;44(1):50-58.

41. Horn P, Münch E, Vajkoczy P, et al. Hypertonic saline solution for control of elevated intracranial pressure in patients with exhausted response to mannitol and barbiturates. *Neurol Res.* 1999;21(8):758-764.

42. Suarez JI, Qureshi AI, Bhardwaj A, et al. Treatment of refractory intracranial hypertension with 23.4% saline. *Crit Care Med.* 1998;26(6):1118-1122.

43. Rozet I, Tontisirin N, Muangman S, et al. Effect of equiosmolar solutions of mannitol versus hypertonic saline on intraoperative brain relaxation and electrolyte balance. *Anesthesiology.* 2007;107(5):697-704.

44. Oddo M, Levine JM, Frangos S, et al. Effect of mannitol and hypertonic saline on cerebral oxygenation in patients with severe traumatic brain injury and refractory intracranial hypertension. *J Neurol Neurosurg Psychiatry.* 2009;80(8):916-920.

45. Whitfield PC, Patel H, Hutchinson PJ, et al. Bifrontal decompressive craniectomy in the management of posttraumatic intracranial hypertension. *Br J Neurosurg.* 2001;15(6):500-507.

46. Aarabi B, Hesdorffer DC, Ahn ES, Aresco C, Scalea TM, Eisenberg HM. Outcome following decompressive craniectomy for malignant swelling due to severe head injury. *J Neurosurg.* 2006;104(4):469-479.

47. Cooper DJ, Rosenfeld JV, Murray L, et al. Decompressive craniectomy in diffuse traumatic brain injury. *N Engl J Med.* 2011;364(16):1493-1502.

48. Attia J, Cook DJ. Prognosis in anoxic and traumatic coma. *Crit Care Clin.* 1998;14(3):497-511.

49. Roberts I, Sydenham E. Barbiturates for acute traumatic brain injury. *Cochrane Database Syst Rev.* 2012;12:CD000033.

50. Tang JF, Chen PL, Tang EJ, May TA, Stiver SI. Dexmedetomidine controls agitation and facilitates reliable, serial neurological examinations in a non-intubated patient with traumatic brain injury. *Neurocrit Care.* 2011;15(1):175-181.

51. Wang X, Ji J, Fen L, Wang A. Effects of dexmedetomidine on cerebral blood flow in critically ill patients with or without traumatic brain injury: a prospective controlled trial. *Brain Inj.* 2013;27(13-14):1617-1622.

52. James ML, Olson DM, Graffagnino C. A pilot study of cerebral and haemodynamic physiological changes during sedation with dexmedetomidine or propofol in patients with acute brain injury. *Anaesth Intensive Care.* 2012;40(6):949-957.

53. Schomer KJ, Sebat CM, Adams JY, Duby JJ, Shahlaie K, Louie EL. Dexmedetomidine for refractory intracranial hypertension. *J Intensive Care Med.* 2019;34(1):62-66.

54. Tran A, Blinder H, Hutton B, English SW. A systematic review of Alpha-2 agonists for sedation in mechanically ventilated neurocritical care patients. *Neurocrit Care.* 2018;28(1):12-25.

55. Saxena M, Andrews PJ, Cheng A, Deol K, Hammond N. Modest cooling therapies (35°C to 37.5°C) for traumatic brain injury. *Cochrane Database Syst Rev.* 2014;8:CD006811.

56. Bohman LE, Levine JM. Fever and therapeutic normothermia in severe brain injury: an update. *Curr Opin Crit Care.* 2014;20(2):182-188.

57. Commichau C, Scarmeas N, Mayer SA. Risk factors for fever in the neurologic intensive care unit. *Neurology.* 2003;60(5):837-841.

58. Dietrich WD, Atkins CM, Bramlett HM. Protection in animal models of brain and spinal cord injury with mild to moderate hypothermia. *J Neurotrauma.* 2009;26(3):301-312.

59. Bernard SA, Gray TW, Buist MD, et al. Treatment of comatose survivors of out-of-hospital cardiac arrest with induced hypothermia. *N Engl J Med.* 2002;346(8):557-563.

60. Hypothermia after Cardiac Arrest Study Group. Mild therapeutic hypothermia to improve the neurologic outcome after cardiac arrest. *N Engl J Med.* 2002;346(8):549-556.

61. Jiang JY, Yu M, Zhu C. Effect of long-term mild hypothermia therapy in patients with severe traumatic brain injury: 1-year follow-up review of 87 cases. *J Neurosurg.* 2000;93(4):546-549.

62. Clifton GL, Miller ER, Choi SC, et al. Lack of effect of induction of hypothermia after acute brain injury. *N Engl J Med.* 2001;344(8):556-563.

63. Clifton GL, Choi SC, Miller ER, et al. Intercenter variance in clinical trials of head trauma—experience of the National Acute Brain Injury Study: Hypothermia. *J Neurosurg.* 2001;95(5):751-755.

64. Sydenham E, Roberts I, Alderson P. Hypothermia for traumatic head injury. *Cochrane Database Syst Rev.* 2009;1;CD001048.

65. Alderson P, Gadkary C, Signorini DF. Therapeutic hypothermia for head injury. *Cochrane Database Syst Rev.* 2004;4:001048.

66. Harris OA, Colford Jr JM, Good MC, Matz PG. The role of hypothermia in the management of severe brain injury: a meta-analysis. *Arch Neurol.* 2002;59(7):1077-1083.

67. McIntyre LA, Fergusson DA, Hébert PC, Moher D, Hutchison JS. Prolonged therapeutic hypothermia after traumatic brain injury in adults: a systematic review. *JAMA.* 2003;289(22):2992-2999.

68. Brain Trauma Foundation, American Association of Neurological Surgeons, Congress of Neurological Surgeons. Guidelines for the management of severe traumatic brain injury 3rd Edition. *J Neurotrauma.* 2007;24(Suppl. 1):i-vi.

69. Clifton GL, Valadka A, Zygun D, et al. Very early hypothermia induction in patients with severe brain injury (the National Acute Brain Injury Study: Hypothermia II): a randomised trial. *Lancet Neurol.* 2011;10(2):131-139.

70. Maekawa T, Yamashita S, Nagao S, Hayashi N, Ohashi Y, Brain-Hypothermia Study Group. Prolonged mild therapeutic hypothermia versus fever control with tight hemodynamic monitoring and slow rewarming in patients with severe traumatic brain injury: a randomized controlled trial. *J Neurotrauma.* 2015;32(7):422-429.

71. Adelson PD, Wisniewski SR, Beca J, et al. Comparison of hypothermia and normothermia after severe traumatic brain injury in children (Cool Kids): a phase 3, randomised controlled trial. *Lancet Neurol.* 2013;12(6):546-553.

72. Andrews PJD, Sinclair HL, Rodriguez A, et al. Hypothermia for intracranial hypertension after traumatic brain injury. *N Engl J Med.* 2015;373(25):2403-2412.

73. Tokutomi T, Miyagi T, Takeuchi Y, Karukaya T, Katsuki H, Shigemori M. Effect of 35°C hypothermia on intracranial pressure and clinical outcome in patients with severe traumatic brain injury. *J Trauma.* 2009;66(1):166-173.

74. Puccio AM, Fischer MR, Jankowitz BT, Yonas H, Darby JM, Okonkwo DO. Induced normothermia attenuates intracranial hypertension and reduces fever burden after severe traumatic brain injury. *Neurocrit Care.* 2009;11(1):82-87.

75. Cooper DJ, Nichol AD, Bailey M, et al. Effect of early sustained prophylactic hypothermia on neurologic outcomes among patients with severe traumatic brain injury: the POLAR randomized clinical trial. *JAMA.* 2018;320(21):2211-2220.

76. Meixensberger J, Jaeger M, Väth A, Dings J, Kunze E, Roosen K. Brain tissue oxygen guided treatment supplementing ICP/CPP therapy after traumatic brain injury. *J Neurol Neurosurg Psychiatry.* 2003;74(6):760-764.

77. Spiotta AM, Stiefel MF, Gracias VH, et al. Brain tissue oxygen–directed management and outcome in patients with severe traumatic brain injury. *J Neurosurg.* 2010;113(3):571-580.

78. Bohman LE, Heuer GG, Macyszyn L, et al. Medical Management of Compromised Brain Oxygen in Patients with severe traumatic brain injury. *Neurocrit Care.* 2011;14(3):361-369.

79. Okonkwo DO, Shutter LA, Moore C, et al. Brain oxygen pptimization in severe traumatic brain injury phase-II. *Crit Care Med.* 2017;45(11):1907-1914.

80. Adamides AA, Rosenfeldt FL, Winter CD, et al. Brain tissue lactate elevations predict episodes of intracranial hypertension in patients with traumatic brain injury. *J Am Coll Surg.* 2009;209(4):531-539.

81. Martini RP, Deem S, Yanez ND, et al. Management guided by brain tissue oxygen monitoring and outcome following severe traumatic brain injury. *J Neurosurg.* 2009;111(4):644-649.

82. Eriksson EA, Barletta JF, Figueroa BE, et al. Cerebral perfusion pressure and intracranial pressure are not surrogates for brain tissue oxygenation in traumatic brain injury. *Clin Neurophysiol.* 2012;123(6):1255-1260.

83. Saul TG, Ducker TB, Salcman M, Carro E. Steroids in severe head injury. *J Neurosurg.* 1981;54(5):596-600.

84. Braakman R, Schouten HJ, Blaauw-van Dishoeck M, Minderhoud JM. Megadose steroids in severe head injury. *J Neurosurg.* 1983;58(3):326-330.

85. Alderson P, Roberts I. Corticosteroids for acute traumatic brain injury. *Cochrane Database Syst Rev.* 2005;1:CD000196.

86. Clifton GL, Robertson CS, Grossman RG, Hodge S, Foltz R, Garza C. The metabolic response to severe head injury. *J Neurosurg.* 1984;60(4):687-696.

87. Young B, Ott L, Norton J, et al. Metabolic and nutritional sequelae in the non-steroid treated head injury patient. *Neurosurgery.* 1985;17(5):784-791.

88. Deutschman CS, Konstantinides FN, Raup S, Thienprasit P, Cerra FB. Physiological and metabolic response to isolated closed-head injury. Part 1: Basal metabolic state: correlations of metabolic and physiological parameters with fasting and stressed controls. *J Neurosurg.* 1986;64(1):89-98.

89. Borzotta AP, Pennings J, Papasadero B, et al. Enteral versus parenteral nutrition after severe closed head injury. *J Trauma.* 1994;37(3):459-468.

90. Justo Meirelles CM, de Aguilar-Nascimento JE. Enteral or parenteral nutrition in traumatic brain injury: a prospective randomised trial. *Nutr Hosp.* 2011;26(5):1120-1124.

65

How Should Aneurysmal Subarachnoid Hemorrhage Be Managed?

Rick Gill, David Kung, and Joshua M. Levine

INTRODUCTION

Aneurysmal subarachnoid hemorrhage (SAH), a type of hemorrhagic stroke due to rupture of an intracranial aneurysm, affects approximately 30,000 Americans each year (mean age 55 years) and has a mortality rate of nearly 45%.[1,2] At least 15% of people with SAH die before reaching the hospital. Of those who survive, a substantial proportion is left with significant disability.[3] Prompt diagnosis, treatment, and anticipation of complications may improve outcome. Case fatality rates have been declining and functional outcomes have been improving.[4] These changes in the natural history of SAH may be attributable to early aneurysm repair and aggressive management of medical complications. This chapter reviews major clinical management points and discusses the relevant literature.

EMERGENCY SETTING

In the emergency setting, once the diagnosis of SAH has been established, initial goals are to stabilize the patient's airway, breathing, and circulation. Early referral to a large-volume center with experienced vascular neurosurgeons, neuroendovascular specialists, and dedicated neurointensivists should be considered. Four studies have demonstrated that hospital volume of SAH patients and procedural experience correlate with improved mortality.[5–8]

SUBARACHNOID HEMORRHAGE-RELATED COMPLICATIONS

Rebleeding

Aneurysmal rebleeding is one of the most serious initial threats to the patient. The incidence may be as high as 30%,[9] with the greatest risk (roughly 4%) during the first 24 hours.[10] Rebleeding may account for nearly 20% of all deaths related to aneurysmal SAH and early rebleeding is associated with worse outcome than later rebleeding.[11,12] Temporizing medical measures are used to reduce the risk of rebleeding until the culprit aneurysm is excluded from the circulation through surgical or endovascular means.

Medical Measures

Bed rest does not alter the incidence of rebleeding,[13] but it has become a standard practice. Blood pressure control is widely recommended to reduce the risk of aneurysmal rebleeding. The benefit of blood pressure reduction must be weighed against the risk of precipitating cerebral ischemia.[14] Although there are no prospective studies that demonstrate the efficacy of antihypertensive therapy, retrospective data suggest an association between hypertension and aneurysmal rebleeding.[15,16] Ohkuma et al. found a statistically significant increase in the incidence of prehospitalization rebleeding in patients whose systolic blood pressure was greater than 160 mm Hg.[16] Interpretation of these data is confounded by variable times at which rebleeding was observed and variations in antihypertensive therapies. Because rebleeding may be related to changes in transmural pressure, surges in blood pressure may be more important than absolute levels of blood pressure.[16–18] Therefore, it is reasonable to treat extreme hypertension and to minimize blood pressure lability with a short-acting, intravenous agent that has a predictable dose–response relationship. Premorbid baseline blood pressure should be taken into consideration for setting blood pressure goals, and hypotension should be avoided.[19]

Antifibrinolytics

Antifibrinolytic agents such as tranexamic acid and epsilon-aminocaproic acid have been well studied. Ten prospective randomized studies (1904 participants) have been performed (Table 65.1) and were included in a 2013 Cochrane Review.[20] Summarizing, death and poor outcome (death, vegetative state, or severe disability) were not influenced by treatment.[20–30] It appears that, although antifibrinolytic medications reduce the risk of rebleeding, their benefit is offset by an increased risk of cerebral infarction.[21,28,29] In several of these studies, patients received antifibrinolytic therapy for weeks, well after the risk for rebleeding had declined and the risk of delayed cerebral ischemia (DCI) increased. Two more recent case–control studies and a prospective randomized study using an early surgical aneurysm treatment protocol have shown that an early and short course of epsilon-aminocaproic acid or tranexamic acid before exclusion of the aneurysm from the circulation might reduce the risk of rebleeding without significantly increasing complications.[21,31,32] In one study, patients treated with epsilon-aminocaproic acid had an eightfold increase in deep venous thrombosis without an increase in pulmonary embolism.[31] This nonrandomized study was not adequately powered to

TABLE 65.1 Summary of Randomized Controlled Trials Evaluating Antifibrinolytic Therapy in SAH.

Study, Year	Number of Subjects (Intervention/No Intervention)	Study Design	Intervention	Control	Outcomes
Girvin, 1973	66 (39/27)		Episilon-aminocaproic acid	Standard treatment	No effect on rebleeding, ischemia, or mortality
van Rossum, 1977	51 (26/25)	DB, P	Tranexamic acid	Placebo	No effect on rebleeding or mortality
Chandra, 1978	39 (20/19)	DB, P	Tranexamic acid	Placebo	No effect on rebleeding or mortality
Maurice, 1978	79 (38/41)		Tranexamic acid	Standard treatment	No effect on rebleeding or mortality
Kaste, 1979	64 (32/32)	DB, P	Tranexamic acid	Placebo	No effect on rebleeding or mortality
Fodstad, 1981	59 (30/29)		Tranexamic acid	Standard treatment	No effect on rebleeding, cerebral ischemia, or mortality
Vermeulen, 1984	479 (241/238)	DB, P	Tranexamic acid	Placebo	Decreased rebleeding, increased cerebral ischemia; no effect on outcome or mortality
Tsementzis, 1990	100 (50/50)	DB, P	Tranexamic acid	Placebo	Increased cerebral ischemia; no effect on rebleeding, outcome, or mortality
Roos, 2000	452 (229/223)	DB, P	Tranexamic acid	Placebo	Decreased rebleeding; no effect on ischemia, outcome, or mortality
Hillman, 2002	505 (254/251)		Tranexamic acid	Standard treatment	Decreased rebleeding; no effect on cerebral ischemia, outcome, or mortality
ULTRA[a]	940 (470/470)		Tranexamic acid	Standard treatment	Primary endpoint: functional outcome; secondary endpoints: case fatality, rebleeding rate, complication rates

[a]Ongoing study.
DB, double blind; *P*, placebo; *SAH*, subarachnoid hemorrhage.

determine the effect of antifibrinolytic therapy on overall patient outcome. A Dutch multicenter, randomized, open-label study, Ultra-Early Tranexamic Acid after Subarachnoid Hemorrhage (ULTRA), began enrolling patients in 2013 and is anticipated to complete in early 2020.[33] It is designed to study the effect on functional outcome (blinded endpoint) of early administration of tranexamic acid in patients with moderate- to high-grade aneurysmal SAH for a duration of up to 24 hours. The results of this study might inform whether an early and short course of antifibrinolytic therapy is clinically warranted. Neurocritical Care Society Consensus Guidelines advise that an early and short course of antifibrinolytic therapy should be considered for patients who are at high risk of rebleeding (such as those with high clinical grade) and in whom definitive aneurysm treatment will be delayed.[34] The American Heart Association endorses as reasonable a short course (<72 hours) of tranexamic acid or

epsilon-aminocaproic acid in this situation.[19] Antifibrinolytic agents should be avoided in patients who are at high risk of thromboembolic complications, and patients treated with antifibrinolytic therapy should be monitored for systemic and cerebral thrombotic complications.

Surgical and Endovascular Measures

There are two primary methods for excluding aneurysms from the circulation: (1) surgical, in which a craniotomy is performed and a clip is placed across the aneurysm neck and (2) endovascular, in which detachable coils are placed into the aneurysm by means of catheter-based techniques. On occasion, an endovascular technique known as flow diversion may be used, in which a stent is placed into the parent vessel across the neck of the aneurysm, allowing blood flow to bypass the aneurysm. The 2005 International Subarachnoid Aneurysm Trial (ISAT) was a large prospective trial that compared surgical aneurysm clipping to endovascular aneurysm coiling.[35] In this trial, 2143 of 9559 patients were deemed "good candidates" for either therapy and were randomized to the surgical or endovascular treatment arm. In the short term, endovascular therapy was associated with less disability (15.6 vs. 21.6%) but lower rates of complete aneurysm obliteration (58 vs. 81%) and higher recurrent SAH rates (2.9% per year vs. 0.9% per year). At 1 year, there was no difference in mortality. Long-term follow-up of these patients found low rates of rebleeding from the treated aneurysm in both groups (10 in the coiling group, 3 in the clipped group), which was insignificant by intention-to-treat analysis. At 5 years, the risk of death was significantly lower in the endovascular arm compared with the surgical arm (11 vs. 14%). This advantage was maintained up to 7 years, but in patients who survived there was no difference in good outcome (modified Rankin Scale [mRS] >2).[36] The 2012 Barrow Ruptured Aneurysm Trial aimed at decreasing selection bias by assigning, in alternate fashion, every patient who agreed to participate into a surgical or endovascular treatment group. Worse outcome was seen in the surgical group compared to the endovascular group (mRS >2, 33.7 vs. 23.2%, P = .02).[37] At 3- and 6-year follow-up, there was no difference in poor outcome between surgical clipping and coiling overall. However, patients with posterior circulation aneurysms fared significantly better with endovascular coiling.[38] Metaanalyses of all randomized trials comparing endovascular coiling and surgical clipping suggest a lower rate of poor outcome at 1 year in patients undergoing coiling.[39,40]

Although endovascular therapy is effective in the short term, aneurysm re-canalization remains a significant limitation. In a retrospective analysis, aneurysm recurrence was found in 33.6% of coiled aneurysms within 1 month and up to 2 years after treatment, although the rebleeding rate from aneurysms that recur after coiling is very low.[41,42] Another retrospective review suggested that the use of a high-porosity stent (to retain coils within the aneurysm) was associated with a higher rate of complete aneurysm obliteration but also with increased morbidity and mortality, likely due to the need for dual-antiplatelet therapy.[43] Therefore the use of stents should be avoided if safer alternatives exist.

Whether to clip or to coil an aneurysm is a complex decision that depends on patient factors (age, comorbidities), aneurysm factors (size, shape, location), and availability of local resources and expertise. On the basis of several single-institution retrospective case series and nonrandomized prospective studies, there is evidence that patients with middle cerebral artery (MCA) aneurysms and large (>50 mL) hematomas might benefit from microsurgical clipping,[44–46] whereas older patients, who are seen during the vasospasm period, have poor clinical grade, or have a basilar apex aneurysm might be considered for endovascular therapy.[45,47–49] Ideally, experienced neurosurgeons and interventional neuroradiologists collaboratively make the decision.[40]

Timing

In recent years, there has been a trend toward early aneurysm treatment. Multiple retrospective and prospective studies have established an association between a longer interval to treatment and increased risk of pretreatment hemorrhage. Patients with larger volumes of SAH (modified Fisher grades 3 and 4) have a higher risk of in-hospital rebleeding within 24 hours of the initial hemorrhage (adjusted hazard ratio 4.4).[50] The International Cooperative study on the Timing of Aneurysm Surgery explored early vs. late surgical intervention based on the neurosurgeons' intention to treat.[51] Patients whose surgery was planned for within the first 3 days had an overall mortality rate equal to the patients whose surgery was planned for between days 11 and 32. However, patients in the early surgical group had a significantly better clinical recovery than those whose surgery was delayed (P < .01). The patients with the highest mortality were those whose surgery was planned for days 7 to 10 after ictus, a time when risk of vasospasm and DCI is greatest. On the basis of this study and a more recent systematic review and metaanalysis, early surgery/endovascular therapy is recommended.[52] After the aneurysm is excluded from the circulation, delayed follow-up vascular imaging should be performed, and if there is a significant aneurysmal remnant or aneurysmal growth, then further intervention should be considered.[19]

Hydrocephalus

Acute hydrocephalus (enlargement of the ventricles) occurs in 15–30% of patients with SAH.[53–57] The presence of hydrocephalus correlates with worse radiographic and clinical grades and with an unfavorable prognosis.[53–56] The symptoms associated with hydrocephalus range from no symptoms to signs of intracranial hypertension, such as impairment of upward gaze, sixth nerve palsy, and headache. Hydrocephalus may be "noncommunicating" because of obstruction (by blood) within the ventricular system or "communicating" because of obstruction of cerebrospinal fluid (CSF) reabsorption into the venous system.

If severe, hydrocephalus may impair the level of consciousness and should be treated immediately with CSF diversion. Ventriculostomy is the most common method of treatment; however, in a select group of patients with communicating hydrocephalus, who are not at risk for central or tonsillar herniation, lumbar CSF drainage may be reasonable. Two small, single-institution studies suggested that in appropriately selected patients, lumbar CSF drainage is associated with a reduction in "clinical vasospasm" (i.e., neurological deficits not attributable to other structural or metabolic causes).[58,59] CSF drainage usually leads to an improvement in signs and symptoms.[57,60,61]

Hydrocephalus and the need for CSF diversion are typically temporary. In some patients, hydrocephalus does not resolve, and ongoing CSF diversion with a permanent indwelling shunt is necessary.[62] In a single-center, prospective, randomized controlled trial, extending the duration of weaning external ventricular drainage for more than 24 hours did not affect the need for permanent shunting and was associated with increased length of both intensive care unit (ICU) and hospital stay.[63] There are insufficient data to support routine fenestration of the lamina terminalis to decrease the rate of permanent shunting.[64,65] Data regarding treatment of hydrocephalus in SAH are largely retrospective; optimal management of patients with mild symptoms is unknown.

Seizures

The evidence regarding the incidence, prophylaxis, and treatment of seizures is mostly retrospective. The reported incidence of seizures after SAH varies from 8 to 35%.[66–72] In one retrospective cohort study, most seizures after SAH occurred before hospitalization, and the incidence of in-hospital seizures was 4.1%. These seizures occurred despite prophylaxis with an antiepileptic drug (AED) and occurred at least 1 week after aneurysmal rupture.[66] Risk factors associated with the development of seizures include ruptured MCA aneurysm, intracerebral hemorrhage, thicker cisternal clot, rebleeding, ischemic infarct, and a history of hypertension.[66–69] Two studies demonstrated no difference in outcome between patients who had seizures and those who did not.[66,70] However, a third study found that seizures at the time of hemorrhage were associated with poor outcome.[73]

The incidence of generalized convulsive status epilepticus (GCSE) is 0.2%, but the incidence of nonconvulsive status epilepticus (NCSE) is much higher.[74,75] A prospective study found that 31% of stuporous or comatose SAH patients had NCSE when monitored with continuous electroencephalography (cEEG). The mean onset of NCSE was 18 days after hemorrhage.[75] GCSE and NCSE are associated with worse outcome.[74–76] Therefore it is reasonable to use periodic or cEEG to assess unconscious patients and those who have a change in neurologic examination for seizures.

The benefit of prophylactic AEDs has not been definitively established.[77–79] It is reasonable to use AEDs before aneurysm treatment because of potential catastrophic harm from seizure-related rebleeding (due to a seizure-associated surge in blood pressure). However, there is no evidence to support the long-term use of AEDs in patients without a history of seizure. A retrospective analysis of 353 patients with spontaneous SAH suggested that prophylactic AEDs do not significantly reduce the risk of seizure occurrence.[80] In fact, cumulative phenytoin exposure is associated with a worse cognitive outcome at 3 months.[81] A small single-center randomized study that compared brief (3-days) to extended (until discharge) prophylactic treatment with levetiracetam found that extended prophylaxis was associated with worse functional outcomes and more medication side effects.[82]

Delayed Cerebral Ischemia

DCI (also referred to as *delayed ischemic neurologic deficits* [DIND]) is defined as neurologic deterioration, presumed to be ischemic, that lasts for more than an hour and that cannot be attributed to another cause.[83] DCI accounts for most morbidity and mortality from SAH; therefore its detection and treatment are the major foci of intensive care. Although historically attributed exclusively to cerebral vasospasm (narrowing of the large caliber arteries at the base of the brain), DCI likely has protean causes, including a local inflammatory and hypercoagulable state that results in formation of

microthrombi and microemboli.[84] Consequently, consensus statements recommend that the term *vasospasm* be reserved to describe only radiologic findings of vessel narrowing and not clinical deterioration.[34,81] DCI may present with agitation followed by an indolent decrease in level of consciousness or focal neurologic deficits that vary depending on the affected arterial distribution.[85] Vasospasm and DCI usually begin at postbleed day 3, peak at postbleed days 6–8, and resolve over 2–4 weeks.[85,86] Thickness of cisternal clot has been associated with the risk of vasospasm.[87] Almost one third of patients who survive the initial SAH develop DCI,[51,88] and approximately half of these patients die.[89]

The diagnosis of and the decision to treat DCI due to vasospasm are made with an observed clinical deterioration along with the radiographic finding of vasospasm. For SAH patients who have impaired consciousness and in whom subtle clinical deteriorations are not easily seen, bedside monitoring modalities such as cEEG, transcranial Doppler ultrasound (TCD), and invasive physiologic monitors might serve as surrogates for clinical changes.

Detection

Monitoring for ischemia includes clinical, radiologic, and physiologic assessments. Although by definition, DCI is detected by serial neurologic examination, not all ischemic insults are clinically apparent, especially in comatose patients.

Radiologic monitoring includes methods to assess for cerebral vasospasm and methods that assess cerebral blood flow (CBF) (perfusion). The gold standard for vasospasm detection is invasive digital subtraction angiography (DSA). Risks associated with DSA include hematoma, infection, peripheral thromboembolic events, and stroke. The rate of neurologic complications from DSA in patients with SAH is 1.8%.[90] Noninvasive angiography with computed tomography (CT) or magnetic resonance imaging (MRI) is less sensitive for detecting vasospasm.[91–94] CT angiography (CTA) has a sensitivity of 86–91.6%[91–93] and is better suited to detect vasospasm of proximal arterial segments. CTA has a high negative predictive value (95–99%); therefore it may be used as a screening tool to limit the use of DSA. Magnetic resonance angiography (MRA) has a sensitivity for vasospasm detection of 45.6% compared with conventional angiography.[94]

TCD detects increased cerebral blood flow velocity (CBFV) associated with vasospasm. This noninvasive study may be performed daily at the bedside and is less expensive than many other monitoring tests.[95] TCD is most useful in detecting evidence of vasospasm in the middle cerebral and basilar arteries.[95,96] Compared with DSA, TCD has a high specificity but poor sensitivity (42–67%) for vasospasm detection.[96,97] Several conditions other than cerebral vasospasm increase CBFV, such as increased blood pressure and hyperemia.[98,99] The Lindegaard ratio (hemispheric index), the ratio between the blood flow velocities in the MCA and the ipsilateral extracranial internal carotid artery, may be used to distinguish increased CBFV due to vasospasm from other causes. Lindegaard ratios between 3 and 6 correlate with mild and moderate vasospasm, whereas indices greater than 6 suggest severe vasospasm.[99] Importantly, elevated TCD velocities do not correlate with the development of DCI.[100] No study has shown that TCD monitoring affects outcome after SAH.

Although imaging blood flow may be a more direct way to assess for ischemia than imaging of blood vessels (for vasospasm), it has been less well studied. Methods for blood flow imaging include CT perfusion (CTP), xenon CT (Xe-CT), MR perfusion, and single-photon emission CT. In the ICU, CT-based imaging studies (CTP, Xe-CT) are typically more practical because they involve less time than MRI and nuclear imaging studies and may be done at the bedside with a portable CT scanner. Although Xe-CT is a well-established tool that provides quantitative blood flow information, xenon gas is no longer approved by the US Food and Drug Administration for this use. Therefore Xe-CT blood flow imaging is currently not in clinical use. The literature regarding the utility of CTP consists of multiple small studies, and there are considerably fewer studies on the utility of MR perfusion. Neither CT nor MR perfusion imaging is widely used for detection of DCI, and further study of these modalities is required.

Physiologic monitoring for DCI includes invasive techniques, such as regional brain tissue oxygen monitoring, regional CBF monitoring, and regional biochemical monitoring, and noninvasive techniques, such as quantitative cEEG and near-infrared spectroscopy. Although there is much enthusiasm for regional brain tissue oxygen monitoring and cerebral microdialysis, there is little supportive evidence in this setting.[34] Although traditionally used to detect seizures, cEEG is also becoming a tool for detection of ischemia. Ischemia produces characteristic changes on EEG, namely loss of fast-frequency waves followed by an increase in slow-frequency waves and ultimately suppression of brain waves. Various software analytic tools are available that provide some measure of the relative proportion of fast waves to slow waves; therefore, they might allow cEEG to serve as a continuous, noninvasive ischemia detector. The optimal EEG parameters for DCI detection and the effect on outcome of therapy based on cEEG ischemia monitoring are unknown. The literature consists exclusively of small prospective and retrospective single-center observational studies that used varying definitions of DCI and that included patients with varying severities of SAH. These studies suggest that it might be possible to detect ischemia by cEEG 1–3 days before changes in clinical examination. As with other physiologic monitors, quantitative cEEG is not employed widely and its utility requires further study.

Prevention and Treatment

Table 65.2 summarizes the randomized trials that have been performed on therapies to treat vasospasm and DCI. Therapy consists of medical and endovascular measures.

TABLE 65.2 Summary of Randomized Controlled Trials Evaluating the Prevention of Vasospasm and DINDs in SAH.

Study, Year	Number of Subjects (Intervention/No Intervention)	Study Design	Intervention	Control	Outcomes
Hemodynamic Augmentation					
Lennihan, 2000	82 (41/41)		Hypervolemic therapy	Normovolemic therapy	No difference in symptomatic vasospasm
Egge, 2001	32 (16/16)		Hypervolemic hypertensive hemodilution therapy	Normovolemic therapy	No difference in DIND or TCD vasospasm
HIMALAIA	240 (120/120)		Induced hypertension	Standard therapy without induced hypertension	Primary endpoint: functional outcome Secondary endpoints: adverse effects, CBF measured by perfusion CT
Magnesium Therapy					
van den Bergh, 2005	283 (139/144)	DB, P	Magnesium IV	Placebo	Decreased incidence of DINDs; improved clinical outcome at 3 months
Veyna, 2002	40 (20/20)		Magnesium IV	Standard therapy	Trend toward improved clinical outcome
Wong, 2006	60 (Numbers unknown)	DB	Magnesium IV	Saline	Trend toward decrease in symptomatic vasospasm; decrease TCD vasospasm timeframe; no difference in clinical outcome

Continued

TABLE 65.2   Summary of Randomized Controlled Trials Evaluating the Prevention of Vasospasm and DINDs in SAH.—cont'd

Study, Year	Number of Subjects (Intervention/No Intervention)	Study Design	Intervention	Control	Outcomes
Schmid-Eisaeser, 2006	104 (53/51)		Magnesium IV	Nimodipine IV	Incidence of vasospasm and clinical outcome comparable
Muroi, 2008	58 (31/27)	P	Magnesium IV	Placebo	No difference in DINDs; improved clinical outcome at 3 months
IMASH, 2010	328 (169/159)	DB, P	Magnesium IV	Saline	No difference in clinical outcome at 6 months
MASH-2, 2012	1203 (606/597)	DB, P	Magnesium IV	Saline	No difference in clinical outcome at 3 months
Calcium Channel Blockers					
Allen, 1983	116 (56/60)	DB, P	Nimodipine PO	Placebo	Decreased incidence of DINDs
Philippon, 1986	70 (Numbers unknown)	DB, P	Nimodipine PO	Placebo	No difference in vasospasm; decreased incidence of DINDs; improved mortality
Neil-Dwyer, 1987	75 (Numbers unknown)	DB, P	Nimodipine PO	Placebo	Improved clinical outcome at 3 months
Petruk, 1988	154 (72/82)	DB, P	Nimodipine PO	Placebo	Decreased incidence of DINDs; improved clinical outcome at 3 months
Pickard, 1989	554 (278/276)	DB, P	Nimodipine PO	Placebo	Decreased incidence of DINDs; improved clinical outcome at 3 months
Haley, 1993	906 (449/457)	DB, P	Nicardipine IV	Placebo	Decreased incidence of vasospasm; no difference in clinical outcome
Haley, 1994	365 (184/181)	DB	High-dose nicardipine IV	Low-dose nicardipine IV	Incidence of vasospasm and clinical outcome comparable
Statin Therapy					
Lynch, 2005	39 (19/20)	DB, P	Simvastatin	Placebo	Decreased incidence of vasospasm
Tseng, 2005	80 (40/40)	DB, P	Pravastatin	Placebo	Decreased incidence of vasospasm and DINDs; improved mortality
Tseng, 2006	80 (40/40)	DB, P	Pravastatin	Placebo	Improved clinical outcome at 6 months
Chou, 2008	39 (19/20)	DB, P	Simvastatin	Placebo	No difference in vasospasm or DINDs; trend toward decreased mortality
STASH, 2014	812 (391/421)	DB, P	Simvastatin	Placebo	No difference in short- and long-term outcome
Wong[a]	240 (120/120)	DB	Simvastatin 80 mg	Simvastatin 40 mg	Presence of DIND at 1 month
Other Approach					
Bulters, 2013	71 (35/36)		Intraaortic balloon pump	Hypervolemic therapy	No difference in clinical outcome, mean cardiac output, or CBF

[a]Ongoing study.

CBF, cerebral blood flow; *CT,* computed tomography; *DB,* double blind; *DIND,* delayed ischemic neurologic deficit; *IV,* intravenously; *P,* placebo; *PO,* by mouth; *SAH,* subarachnoid hemorrhage; *TCD,* transcranial Doppler ultrasound.

Hemodynamic Augmentation Strategies

Although induced hypertension, hypervolemia, and hemodilution ("Triple-H therapy") have historically been the mainstays of medical treatment for vasospasm and DCI, this strategy is at best supported by moderate quality evidence. Hypovolemia is associated with worsening vasospasm and DCI and should be avoided[101–103]; however, volume loading is associated with harm. Two randomized controlled trials (RCTs) evaluated the effect of prophylactic hypervolemia on CBF and the incidence of vasospasm.[104,105] Neither study found a significant improvement in CBF, incidence of "symptomatic vasospasm" (now referred to as DCI), or functional outcome in patients receiving hypervolemic therapy compared with those receiving normovolemic therapy.[104,105] Patients receiving hypervolemic therapy had more complications, including bleeding, congestive heart failure, and infection.[105] On the basis of these studies, prophylactic hypervolemia is not recommended, and patients should be maintained in a euvolemic state.

Induced hypertension is widely used and supported only by case series. The HIMALAIA (Hypertension Induction in the Management of AneurysmaL subArachnoid haemorrhage with secondary IschaemiA) trial was a Dutch multicenter, randomized, controlled, single-blinded study on the effect of induced hypertension on functional outcome and CBF in patients with DCI after SAH. This study was stopped prematurely based on a lack of effect on cerebral perfusion and slow recruitment. The study was unable to support the use of induced hypertension and showed a trend towards serious adverse events (risk ratio 2.1, 95% CI 0.9–5.0).[106]

Endovascular Treatments

When neurologic deterioration due to vasospasm is refractory to medical therapy, endovascular treatment should be considered. Transluminal balloon angioplasty mechanically dilates the vasospastic vessels to improve CBF. Although the effect is durable, balloon angioplasty may cause vessel rupture beyond the level of the carotid and M1 segments and does not affect long-term outcome.[107,108] Disruption of aneurysm clips and thrombus formation are other recognized complications of balloon angioplasty.[109–111] Catheter-based intraarterial delivery of vasodilators, including papaverine, verapamil, nicardipine, nimodipine, and milrinone, may be more effective in the treatment of vasospasm in the distal vessels.[112–116] Patients should be monitored for increased intracranial pressure and systemic hypotension during intraarterial vasodilator therapy. RCTs to establish the efficacy of these agents are lacking.

Magnesium

Magnesium is a physiologic antagonist of calcium and has neuroprotective properties. Magnesium modulates calcium channels and relaxes vascular smooth muscles. Hypomagnesemia is associated with vasospasm and should be corrected.[117] Pilot data supporting an association between intravenous magnesium therapy and improved clinical outcomes[118–121] were not corroborated in two multicenter, randomized, placebo-control trials. Both the IMASH (Intravenous Magnesium Sulphate for Aneurysmal Subarachnoid Hemorrhage)[122] and MASH-2 (Magnesium for Aneurysmal Subarachnoid Hemorrhage)[123] studies detected no functional outcome benefit at 6 months and 3 months, respectively, in patients treated with intravenous magnesium infusion compared to placebo groups. Although hypomagnesemia should be avoided, magnesium administration to achieve supranormal levels is not recommended.

Calcium Channel Blockers

Calcium channel blockers may improve outcome after SAH. Five double-blinded, placebo-controlled trials of oral nimodipine demonstrated improved functional outcomes despite no effect on the incidence or severity of vasospasm.[124–128] Two RCTs of intravenous nicardipine demonstrated no effect on 3-month outcome despite a reduction in the incidence of vasospasm.[129,130] A Cochrane Review of 16 trials, involving 3361 patients, found that oral nimodipine alone reduced the risk of poor outcome by 33%. For intravenous nimodipine and other calcium channel blockers, the results were not statistically significant.[131] Patients with SAH should receive oral nimodipine 60 mg every 4 hours for 21 days.[132]

Statins

Statins have pleotropic vascular and neuroprotective effects, which created interest in their use for the treatment of SAH. Several small studies suggested that pravastatin and simvastatin administration was associated with a decreased incidence of vasospasm and DCI and a shorter duration of vasospasm.[133,134] In addition, mortality due to vasospasm and clinical outcomes at 6 months were improved.[135] However, in a well-designed multicenter RCT, 40 mg simvastatin instituted within 96 hours of SAH for up to 21 days was not associated with improved 6-month functional outcome (modified Rankin scale score).[136] Therefore de novo initiation of statin therapy is not recommended; however, continuation of statin therapy in patients with premorbid statin use is reasonable. An ongoing trial comparing the effects of 80 with 40 mg of simvastatin on outcome after SAH is currently underway.[137]

Endothelin 1 Receptor Antagonists

Endothelin 1 (ET1) is a potent mediator of vascular tone that acts upon endothelin receptors A (vasoconstriction and smooth muscle proliferation) and B (vasodilation). Clazosentan is an investigational drug that is a specific ET receptor antagonist which has a much higher affinity for ET-A receptors and only weakly inhibits ET-B, making it a theoretically attractive treatment for vasospasm after SAH. While demonstrating a dose dependent reduction in angiographic vasospasm in the CONSCIOUS-1 trial, subsequent trials looking at patients treated with clipping (CONSCIOUS-2) and coiling (CONSCIOUS-3) did not show an association between clazosentan administration and improved mortality or functional outcome in patients with SAH.[138–140] A metaanalysis demonstrated that clazoentan was associated with an increased risk of anemia, pulmonary edema, and hypotension.[141]

Hyponatremia

Approximately one third of patients with SAH develop hyponatremia.[102,142–144] Hyponatremia is associated with an increased incidence of DCI and is more common in patients with anterior communicating artery aneurysms, higher grade of SAH, and hydrocephalus.[102,142,143] Although hyponatremia may be due to the syndrome of inappropriate secretion of antidiuretic hormone (SIADH), treatment with fluid restriction is detrimental and leads to increased mortality from DCI.[102] Alternatively, hyponatremia may be due to cerebral salt wasting, a form of hypovolemic hyponatremia that is treated with volume replacement and salt.[145] Irrespective of the cause of hyponatremia, oral or intravenous sodium chloride is usually sufficient to correct mild hyponatremia. In patients with vasospasm-related DCI or severe hyponatremia, hypertonic saline may be given.[146] Two small prospective, randomized trials found that fludrocortisone may reduce natriuresis and prevent hyponatremia.[147,148] In patients with SIADH, a prospective trial found that conivaptan, an oral vasopressin receptor agonist, effectively corrects hyponatremia.[149]

Cardiac Dysfunction

Electrocardiographic Abnormalities

Ninety percent of patients with SAH experience cardiac arrhythmias, including supraventricular and ventricular premature complexes, supraventricular and ventricular tachyarrhythmias, and sinoatrial and atrioventricular block. Life-threatening arrhythmias—usually Torsade de Pointes or ventricular flutter/fibrillation—are seen in 3–4% of patients. They occur most commonly in the first 48 hours and are associated with QT prolongation and with hypokalemia. The clinical and radiographic findings of SAH do not correlate with the presence of arrhythmias.[150,151] Patients with QT prolongation are more likely to have increased serum cardiac troponin I.[152] A total of 6–12% of patients have ST-segment elevations or, more commonly, depressions.[151, 152] These abnormalities are associated with neurogenic stunned myocardium (see later) and are not usually due to coronary artery disease or to coronary vasospasm.[153]

Cardiomyopathy

Patients with SAH are susceptible to a reversible cardiomyopathy known as neurogenic stunned myocardium. One purported mechanism is activation of the sympathetic nervous system with consequent catecholamine toxicity.[154] Fifteen percent of patients have global left ventricular dysfunction, and another 13–18% have regional wall motion abnormalities (RWMAs). The RWMAs do not respect coronary arterial vascular distributions but may occur in the distribution of myocardial sympathetic nerve terminals.[155–157] Predictors of neurogenic stunned myocardium include poor clinical grade, temporal proximity to aneurysm rupture, female gender, larger body surface area, larger left ventricular mass index,

elevated serum cardiac troponin I, tachycardia, lower systolic blood pressure, higher doses of phenylephrine, and previous cocaine or amphetamine use.[157,158] RWMAs most commonly affect the mid regions of the anteroseptal, anterior, inferoseptal, and anterolateral left ventricular walls (apical-sparing pattern) or the left ventricular base ("inverted Takotsubo" pattern). The apex occasionally is disproportionately involved ("Takotsubo" pattern). RWMAs are an independent risk factor for DCI, death, and poor functional outcome.[159] Patients may have a range of symptoms from mild heart failure to cardiogenic shock. Treatment is supportive and prognosis is excellent.[157]

Fever

The incidence of fever in patients with SAH is 23–70%.[160–164] Risk factors for developing fever include the presence of intraventricular blood, older age, and poor clinical grade.[160,162,164] Pyrexia has been associated with poor clinical outcome in multiple studies.[162,164,165] In one prospective study, fever was associated with poor outcome independent of the presence of DCI, infection, or disease severity.[165] It remains unclear whether fever is merely a marker of disease severity or is causally related to poor outcome. In one case control study, compared with conventional fever management (with acetaminophen and water-cooled blankets), aggressive temperature control (with a modern servo-controlled temperature-management device) was associated with improved outcomes at 12 months, increased ICU length of stay, increased use of sedatives, and higher rates of tracheostomy.[166] Despite a paucity of evidence, fever control has become standard of care.

Anemia

Anemia, defined as a hemoglobin level less than 10 g/dL, develops in 39–57% of patients with SAH.[167–169] Higher hemoglobin levels have been associated with improved outcomes in two retrospective studies,[170,171] and another study that incorporated positron-emission tomography (PET) found improved oxygen delivery without reduction in global CBF.[172] These benefits must be weighed against the increased rates of medical complications and infections associated with blood transfusion in this population.[168,173] A prospective, single-institution RCT trial compared hemoglobin transfusion thresholds of 10 and 11.5 g/dL and found no significant difference in rates of fever or ventilator days but less cortical infarction in the higher hemoglobin threshold group.[174] Further study is required to define the optimal triggers for red blood cell transfusion in patients with aneurysmal SAH. A multicenter randomized controlled trial is being organized to provide additional information about optimal transfusion thresholds.[175]

CONCLUSION

The goal of critical care management of patients with SAH is to limit further neurologic injury. Prompt diagnosis and treatment of SAH are crucial. Anticipating complications from rebleeding, hydrocephalus, seizures, and DCI is imperative. Further prospective randomized trials are needed to establish the efficacy of new and existing therapies.

AUTHORS' RECOMMENDATIONS

- Rebleeding is the most serious initial threat to the patient with SAH. Aneurysms should be promptly clipped or coiled. Blood pressure should be controlled until the aneurysm is secured. An early and brief course of antifibrinolytic therapy until aneurysm treatment may be considered for patients who are at low risk of thromboembolic events.
- Prophylactic AEDs are reasonable in the acute setting, but there is no evidence supporting their long-term use.
- The maximal risk for DCI occurs between postbleed days 3 and 14. Vasospasm is one cause of DCI. The gold standard for vasospasm detection is conventional cerebral angiography; however, TCD may be used to monitor for vasospasm. The utility of monitoring for DCI with quantitative cEEG, near-infrared spectroscopy, and invasive physiologic probes requires further study.
- Treatment of DCI includes maintenance of euvolemia and induced hypertension. In patients with vasospasm and symptomatic ischemia refractory to medical measures, balloon angioplasty and intraarterial vasodilator administration should be considered.
- Oral nimodipine improves outcome in SAH and should be given to all patients unless contraindicated.
- Hypomagnesemia should be corrected. Supplemental magnesium administration to achieve supranormal levels is not recommended.
- De novo initiation of statin therapy in the setting of acute SAH is not recommended.
- Hyponatremia, anemia, fever, and cardiac dysfunction are common medical complications of SAH.

REFERENCES

1. King JT Jr. Epidemiology of aneurysmal subarachnoid hemorrhage. *Neuroimaging Clin N Am*. 1997;7(4):659-668.
2. Wong GK, Chan MT, Boet R, Poon WS, Gin T. Intravenous magnesium sulfate after aneurysmal subarachnoid hemorrhage: a prospective randomized pilot study. *J Neurosurg Anesthesiol*. 2006;18(2):142-148.
3. Johnston SC, Selvin S, Gress DR. The burden, trends, and demographics of mortality from subarachnoid hemorrhage. *Neurology*. 1998;50(5):1413-1418.
4. Nieuwkamp DJ, Setz LE, Algra A, Linn FH, de Rooij NK, Rinkel GJ. Changes in case fatality of aneurysmal subarachnoid haemorrhage over time, according to age, sex, and region: a meta-analysis. *Lancet Neurol*. 2009;8(7):635-642.
5. Johnston SC. Effect of endovascular services and hospital volume on cerebral aneurysm treatment outcomes. *Stroke*. 2000;31(1):111-117.
6. Bardach NS, Zhao S, Gress DR, Lawton MT, Johnston SC. Association between subarachnoid hemorrhage outcomes and number of cases treated at California hospitals. *Stroke*. 2002; 33(7):1851-1856.
7. Cross DT 3rd, Tirschwell DL, Clark MA, et al. Mortality rates after subarachnoid hemorrhage: variations according to hospital case volume in 18 states. *J Neurosurg*. 2003;99(5):810-817.
8. Berman MF, Solomon RA, Mayer SA, Johnston SC, Yung PP. Impact of hospital-related factors on outcome after treatment of cerebral aneurysms. *Stroke*. 2003;34(9):2200-2207.
9. Winn HR, Richardson AE, Jane JA. The long-term prognosis in untreated cerebral aneurysms: I. The incidence of late hemorrhage in cerebral aneurysm: a 10-year evaluation of 364 patients. *Ann Neurol*. 1977;1(4):358-370.
10. Sundt TM Jr, Whisnant JP. Subarachnoid hemorrhage from intracranial aneurysms. Surgical management and natural history of disease. *N Engl J Med*. 1978;299(3):116-122.
11. Lantigua H, Ortega-Gutierrez S, Schmidt JM, et al. Subarachnoid hemorrhage: who dies, and why? *Crit Care*. 2015; 19(1):309.
12. Cha KC, Kim JH, Kang HI, Moon BG, Lee SJ, Kim JS. Aneurysmal rebleeding: factors associated with clinical outcome in the rebleeding patients. *J Korean Neurosurg Soc*. 2010;47:119-123.
13. Nibbelink DW, Torner JC, Henderson WG. Intracranial aneurysms and subarachnoid hemorrhage—report on a randomized treatment study. IV-A. Regulated bed rest. *Stroke*. 1977;8(2):202-218.
14. Wijdicks EF, Vermeulen M, Murray GD, Hijdra A, van Gijn J. The effects of treating hypertension following aneurysmal subarachnoid hemorrhage. *Clin Neurol Neurosurg*. 1990;92(2): 111-117.
15. Fuji Y, Takeuchi S, Sasaki O, Minakawa T, Koike T, Tanaka R. Ultra-early rebleeding in spontaneous subarachnoid hemorrhage. *J Neurosurg*. 1996;84(1):35-42.
16. Ohkuma H, Tsurutani H, Suzuki S. Incidence and significance of early aneurysmal rebleeding before neurosurgical or neurological management. *Stroke*. 2001;32(5):1176-1180.
17. Stornelli SA, French J. Subarachnoid hemorrhage—factors in prognosis and management. *J Neurosurg*. 1964;21:769-780.
18. Lin QS, Ping-Chen, Lin YX, et al. Systolic blood pressure variability is a novel risk factor for rebleeding in acute subarachnoid hemorrhage: a case-control study. *Medicine (Baltimore)*. 2016;95(11):e3028.
19. Connolly ES Jr, Rabinstein AA, Carhuapoma JR, et al. Guidelines for the management of aneurysmal subarachnoid hemorrhage: a guideline for healthcare professionals from the American Heart Association/American Stroke Association. *Stroke*. 2012;43(6): 1711-1737.
20. Baharoglu M, Germans M, Rinkel G, et al. Antifibrinolytic therapy for aneurysmal subarachnoid haemorrhage. *Cochrane Database Syst Rev*. 2013;8:CD001245.
21. Hillman J, Fridriksson S, Nilsson O, Yu Z, Saveland H, Jakobsson KE. Immediate administration of tranexamic acid and reduced incidence of early rebleeding after aneurysmal subarachnoid hemorrhage: a prospective randomized study. *J Neurosurg*. 2002;97(4):771-778.
22. Girvin JP. The use of antifibrinolytic agents in the preoperative treatment of ruptured intracranial aneurysms. *Trans Am Neurol Assoc*. 1973;98:150-152.
23. Van Rossum J, Wintzen AR, Endtz LJ, Schoen JH, de Jonge H. Effect of tranexamic acid on rebleeding after subarachnoid hemorrhage: a double-blind controlled clinical trial. *Ann Neurol*. 1977;2:238-242.
24. Chandra B. Treatment of subarachnoid hemorrhage from ruptured intracranial aneurysm with tranexamic acid: a double-blind clinical trial. *Ann Neurol*. 1978;3:502-504.

25. Maurice-Williams RS. Prolonged antifibrinolysis: an effective nonsurgical treatment for ruptured intracranial aneurysms? *Brit Med J.* 1978;1:945-947.

26. Kaste M, Ramsay M. Tranexamic acid in subarachnoid hemorrhage. A double-blind study. *Stroke.* 1979;10:519-522.

27. Fodstad H, Forssell A, Liliequist B, Schannong M. Antifibrinolysis with tranexamic acid in aneurysmal subarachnoid hemorrhage: a consecutive controlled clinical trial. *Neurosurgery.* 1981;8:158-165.

28. Vermeulen M, Lindsay KW, Murray GD, et al. Antifibrinolytic treatment in subarachnoid hemorrhage. *N Engl J Med.* 1984;311:432-437.

29. Tsementzis SA, Hitchcock ER, Meyer CH. Benefits and risks of antifibrinolytic therapy in the management of ruptured intracranial aneurysms. A double-blind placebo-controlled study. *Acta Neurochirurgica.* 1990;102:1-10.

30. Roos Y. Antifibrinolytic treatment in aneurysmal subarachnoid haemorrhage: a randomized placebo-controlled trial. STAR Study Group. *Neurology.* 2000;54:77-82.

31. Starke R, Kim G, Fernandez A, et al. Impact of a protocol for acute antifibrinolytic therapy on aneurysm rebleeding after subarachnoid hemorrhage. *Stroke.* 2008;39(9):2617-2621.

32. Harrigan M, Rajneesh K, Ardelt A, Fisher W. Short-term antifibrinolytic therapy before early aneurysm treatment in subarachnoid hemorrhage: effects on rehemorrhage, cerebral ischemia, and hydrocephalus. *Neurosurgery.* 2010;67(4):935-939.

33. Germans M, Post R, Coert B, Rinkel GJ, Vandertop WP, Verbaan D. Ultra-early tranexamic acid after subarachnoid hemorrhage (ULTRA): study protocol for a randomized controlled trial. *Trials.* 2013;14:143.

34. Diringer MN, Cleck TP, Hemphill J 3rd, et al. Critical care management of patients following aneurysmal subarachnoid hemorrhage: recommendations from the Neurocritical Care Society's Multidisciplinary Consensus Conference. *Neurocrit Care.* 2011;15:211-240.

35. Molyneux AJ, Kerr RSC, Yu LM, et al. International subarachnoid aneurysm trial (ISAT) of neurosurgical clipping versus endovascular coiling in 2143 patients with ruptured intracranial aneurysms: a randomised comparison of effects on survival, dependency, seizures, rebleeding, subgroups, and aneurysm occlusion. *Lancet.* 2005;366(9488):809-817.

36. Molyneux AJ, Kerr RS, Birks J, et al. Risk of recurrent subarachnoid haemorrhage, death, or dependence and standardised mortality ratios after clipping or coiling of an intracranial aneurysm in the International Subarachnoid Aneurysm Trial (ISAT): long-term follow-up. *Lancet Neurol.* 2009;8(5):427-433.

37. McDougall CG, Spetzler RF, Zabramski JM, et al. The Barrow Ruptured Aneurysm Trial. *J Neurosurg.* 2012;116:135-144.

38. Spetzler RF, McDougall CG, Zabramski JM, et al. The Barrow Ruptured Aneurysm Trial: 6-year results. *J Neurosurg.* 2015;123(3):609-617.

39. Lanzino G, Murad MH, d'Urso PI, Rabinstein AA. Coil embolization versus clipping for ruptured intracranial aneurysms: a meta-analysis of prospective controlled published studies. *AJNR Am J Neuroradiol.* 2013;34:1764-1768.

40. Li H, Pan R, Wang H, et al. Clipping versus coiling for ruptured intracranial aneurysms: a systematic review and meta-analysis. *Stroke.* 2013;44:29-37.

41. Raymond J, Guilbert F, Weill A, et al. Long-term angiographic recurrences after selective endovascular treatment of aneurysms with detachable coils. *Stroke.* 2003;34:1398-1403.

42. Darflinger R, Thompson LA, Zhang Z, Chao K. Recurrence, retreatment, and rebleed rates of coiled aneurysms with respect to the Raymond–Roy scale: a meta-analysis. *J Neurointerv Surg.* 2016;8(5):507-511.

43. Piotin M, Blanc R, Spelle L, et al. Stent-assisted coiling of intracranial aneurysms: clinical and angiographic results in 216 consecutive aneurysms. *Stroke.* 2010;41(1):110-115.

44. Regli L, Dehdashti AR, Uske A, de Tribolet N. Endovascular coiling compared with surgical clipping for the treatment of unruptured middle cerebral artery aneurysms: an update. *Acta Neurochir Suppl.* 2002;82:41-46.

45. Bracard S, Lebedinsky A, Anxionnat R, et al. Endovascular treatment of Hunt and Hess grade IV and V aneurysms. *Am J Neuroradiol.* 2002;23:953-957.

46. Rinne J, Hernesniemi J, Niskanen M, Vapalahti M. Analysis of 561 patients with 690 middle cerebral artery aneurysms: anatomic and clinical features as correlated to management outcome. *Neurosurgery.* 1996;38:2-11.

47. Proust F, Gérardin E, Derrey S, et al. Interdisciplinary treatment of ruptured cerebral aneurysms in elderly patients. *J Neurosurg.* 2010;112:1200-1207.

48. Brilstra EH, Rinkel GJ, van der Graaf Y, van Rooij WJ, Algra A. Treatment of intracranial aneurysms by embolization with coils: a systematic review. *Stroke.* 1999;30:470-476.

49. Lusseveld E, Brilstra EH, Nijssen PC, et al. Endovascular coiling versus neurosurgical clipping in patients with a ruptured basilar tip aneurysm. *J Neurol Neurosurg Psychiatry.* 2002;73:591-593.

50. van Donkelaar CE, Bakker NA, Veeger NJ, et al. Predictive factors for rebleeding after aneurysmal subarachnoid hemorrhage: rebleeding aneurysmal subarachnoid hemorrhage study. *Stroke.* 2015;46(8):2100-2106.

51. Haley EC Jr, Kassell NF, Torner JC. The International Cooperative Study on the Timing of Aneurysm Surgery. The North American experience. *Stroke.* 1992;23(2):205-214.

52. Yao Z, Hu X, Ma L, You C, He M. Timing of surgery for aneurysmal subarachnoid hemorrhage: a systematic review and meta-analysis. *Int J Surg.* 2017;48:266-274.

53. Mehta V, Holness RO, Connolly K, Walling S, Hall R. Acute hydrocephalus following aneurysmal subarachnoid hemorrhage. *Can J Neurol Sci.* 1996;23:40-45.

54. Suarez-Rivera O. Acute hydrocephalus after subarachnoid hemorrhage. *Surg Neurol.* 1998;49:563-565.

55. Lin CL, Kwan AL, Howng SL. Acute hydrocephalus and chronic hydrocephalus with the need of postoperative shunting after aneurysmal subarachnoid hemorrhage. *Kaohsiung J Med Sci.* 1999;15:137-145.

56. Sheehan JP, Polin RS, Sheehan JM, Baskaya MK, Kassell NF. Factors associated with hydrocephalus after aneurysmal subarachnoid hemorrhage. *Neurosurgery.* 1999;45:1120-1127; discussion: 1127-1128.

57. Hasan D, Vermeulen M, Wijdicks EF, Hijdra A, van Gijn J. Management problems in acute hydrocephalus after subarachnoid hemorrhage. *Stroke.* 1989;20:747-753.

58. Klimo P Jr, Kestle JR, MacDonald JD, Schmidt RH. Marked reduction of cerebral vasospasm with lumbar drainage of cerebrospinal fluid after subarachnoid hemorrhage. *J Neurosurg.* 2004;100:215-224.

59. Kwon OY, Kim YJ, Cho CS, Lee SK, Cho MK. The utility and benefits of external lumbar CSF drainage after endovascular coiling on aneurysmal/subarachnoid hemorrhage. *J Korean Neurosurg Soc.* 2008;43:281-287.

60. Rajshekhar V, Harbaugh RE. Results of routine ventriculostomy with external ventricular drainage for acute hydrocephalus following subarachnoid haemorrhage. *Acta Neurochir.* 1992;115:8-14.

61. Milhorat TH. Acute hydrocephalus after aneurysmal subarachnoid hemorrhage. *Neurosurgery.* 1987;20:15-20.

62. Gruber A, Reinprecht A, Bavinzski G, et al. Chronic shunt-dependent hydrocephalus after early surgical and early endovascular treatment of ruptured intracranial aneurysm. *Neurosurgery.* 1999;44(3):503-509.

63. Klopfenstein JD, Kim LJ, Feiz-Erfan I, et al. Comparison of rapid and gradual weaning from external ventricular drainage in patients with aneurysmal subarachnoid hemorrhage: a prospective randomized trial. *J Neurosurg.* 2004;100:225-229.

64. Komotar RJ, Hahn DK, Kim GH, et al. Efficacy of lamina terminalis fenestration in reducing shunt-dependent hydrocephalus following aneurysmal subarachnoid hemorrhage: a systematic review: clinical article. *J Neurosurg.* 2009;111:147-154.

65. Winkler EA, Burkhardt JK, Rutledge WC, et al. Reduction of shunt dependency rates following aneurysmal subarachnoid hemorrhage by tandem fenestration of the lamina terminalis and membrane of Liliequist during microsurgical aneurysm repair. *J Neurosurg.* 2017;15:1-7.

66. Rhoney DH, Tipps LB, Murry KR, Basham MC, Michael DB, Coplin WM. Anticonvulsant prophylaxis and timing of seizures after aneurysmal subarachnoid hemorrhage. *Neurology.* 2000;55:258-265.

67. Ohman J. Hypertension as a risk factor for epilepsy after aneurysmal subarachnoid hemorrhage and surgery. *Neurosurgery.* 1990;27:578-581.

68. Ukkola V, Heikkinen ER. Epilepsy after operative treatment of ruptured cerebral aneurysms. *Acta Neurochir.* 1990;106:115-118.

69. Hasan D, Schnonck RS, Avezaat CJ, et al. Epileptic seizures after subarachnoid hemorrhage. *Ann Neurol.* 1993;33(3):286-291.

70. Lin CL, Dumont AS, Lieu AS, et al. Characterization of perioperative seizures and epilepsy following aneurysmal subarachnoid hemorrhage. *J Neurosurg.* 2003;99(6):978-985.

71. Cabral RJ, King TT, Scott DF. Epilepsy after two different neurosurgical approaches to the treatment of ruptured intracranial aneurysm. *J Neurol Neurosurg Psychiatry.* 1976;39:1052-1056.

72. Kotila M, Waltimo O. Epilepsy after stroke. *Epilepsia.* 1992; 33:495-498.

73. Butzkueven H, Evans AH, Pitman A, et al. Onset seizures independently predict poor outcome after subarachnoid hemorrhage. *Neurology.* 2000;55(9):1315-1320.

74. Claassen J, Bateman BT, Willey JZ, et al. Generalized convulsive status epilepticus after nontraumatic subarachnoid hemorrhage: the nationwide inpatient sample. *Neurosurgery.* 2007;61(1):60-64; discussion: 64-65.

75. Dennis LJ, Claassen J, Hirsch LJ, Emerson RG, Connolly ES, Mayer SA. Nonconvulsive status epilepticus after subarachnoid hemorrhage. *Neurosurgery.* 2002;51(5):1136-1143; discussion: 1144.

76. Claassen J, Hirsch LJ, Frontera JA, et al. Prognostic significance of continuous EEG monitoring in patients with poor-grade subarachnoid hemorrhage. *Neurocrit Care.* 2006;4(2):103-112.

77. Sbeih I, Tamas LB, O'Laoire SA. Epilepsy after operation for aneurysms. *Neurosurgery.* 1986;19(5):784-788.

78. O'Laoire SA. Epilepsy following neurosurgical intervention. *Acta Neurochir Suppl.* 1990;50:52-54.

79. Shaw MD. Post-operative epilepsy and the efficacy of anticonvulsant therapy. *Acta Neurochir Suppl.* 1990;50:55-57.

80. Panczykowski D, Pease M, Zhao Y, et al. Prophylactic antiepileptics and seizure incidence following subarachnoid hemorrhage: a propensity score–matched analysis. *Stroke.* 2016;47(7):1754-1760

81. Naidech AM, Kreiter KT, Janjua N, et al. Phenytoin exposure is associated with functional and cognitive disability after subarachnoid hemorrhage. *Stroke.* 2005;36(3):583-587.

82. Human T, Diringer MN, Allen M, et al. A randomized trial of brief versus extended seizure prophylaxis after aneurysmal subarachnoid hemorrhage. *Neurocrit Care.* 2018;28(2):169-174.

83. Vergouwen M, Vermeulen M, van Gijn J, et al. Definition of delayed cerebral ischemia after aneurysmal subarachnoid hemorrhage as an outcome event in clinical trials and observational studies: proposal of a multidisciplinary research group. *Stroke.* 2010;41(10):2391-2395.

84. Stein SC, Levine JM, Nagpal S, LeRoux PD. Vasospasm as the sole cause of cerebral ischemia: how strong is the evidence? *Neurosurg Focus.* 2006;21(3):E2.

85. Heros RC, Zervas NT, Varsos V. Cerebral vasospasm after subarachnoid hemorrhage: an update. *Ann Neurol.* 1983;14:599-608.

86. Fisher CM, Roberson GH, Ojemann RG. Cerebral vasospasm with ruptured saccular aneurysm—the clinical manifestations. *Neurosurgery.* 1977;1:245-248.

87. Fisher CM, Kistler JP, Davis JM. Relation of cerebral vasospasm to subarachnoid hemorrhage visualized by computerized tomographic scanning. *Neurosurgery.* 1980;6:1-9.

88. Haley EC Jr, Kassell NF, Apperson-Hansen C, Maile MH, Alves WM. A randomized, double-blind, vehicle-controlled trial of tierilazad mesylate in patients with aneurysmal subarachnoid hemorrhage: a cooperative study in North America. *J Neurosurg.* 1997;86:467-474.

89. Kassell NF, Boarini DJ, Adams HP Jr, et al. Overall management of ruptured aneurysm: comparison of early and late operation. *Neurosurgery.* 1981;9:120-128.

90. Cloft HJ, Joseph GJ, Dion JE. Risk of cerebral angiography in patients with subarachnoid hemorrhage, cerebral aneurysm, and arteriovenous malformation: a meta-analysis. *Stroke.* 1999;30(2):317-320.

91. Otawara Y, Ogasawara K, Ogawa A, Sasaki M, Takahashi K. Evaluation of vasospasm after subarachnoid hemorrhage by use of multi slice computed tomographic angiography. *Neurosurgery.* 2002;51(4):939-942.

92. Anderson GB, Ashforth R, Steinke DE, Findlay JM. CT angiography for the detection of cerebral vasospasm in patients with acute subarachnoid hemorrhage. *Am J Neuroradiol.* 2000;21(6):1011-1015.

93. Chaudhary SR, Ko N, Dillon WP, et al. Prosepctive evaluation of multidetector-row CT angiography for the diagnosis of vasospasm following subarachnoid hemorrhage: a comparison with digital subtraction angiography. *Cerebrovasc Dis.* 2008;25(1–2):144-150.

94. Tamatani S, Sasaki O, Takeuchi S, Fujii Y, Koike T, Tanaka R. Detection of delayed cerebral vasospasm, after rupture of intracranial aneurysms, by magnetic resonance, angiography. *Neurosurgery.* 1997;40(4):748-753.

95. Sloan MA, Alexandrov AV, Tegeler CH, et al. Assessment: transcranial Doppler ultrasonography: report of the Therapeutics and Technology Assessment Subcommittee of the American Academy of Neurology. *Neurology.* 2004;62:1468-1481.

96. Sloan MA, Haley EC Jr, Kassell NF, et al. Sensitivity and specificity of transcranial Doppler ultrasonography in the diagnosis of vasospasm following subarachnoid hemorrhage. *Neurology.* 1989;39:1514-1518.

97. Lysakowski C, Walder B, Costanza M, Ramer M. Transcranial Doppler versus angiography in patients with vasospasm due to a ruptured cerebral aneurysm. *Stroke*. 2001;32:2292-2298.

98. Manno EM, Gress DR, Schwamm LH, Diringer MN, Ogilvy CS. Effects of induced hypertension on transcranial Doppler ultrasound velocities in patients after subarachnoid hemorrhage. *Stroke*. 1998;29:422-428.

99. Lindegaard KF, Nornes H, Bakke SJ, Sorteberg W, Nakstad P. Cerebral vasospasm diagnosis by means of angiography and blood velocity measurements. *Acta Neurochir*. 1989;100(1–2):12-24.

100. Ekelund A, Saveland H, Romner B, Brandt L. Is transcranial Doppler sonography useful in detecting late cerebral ischaemia after aneurysmal subarachnoid haemorrhage? *Br J Neurosurg*. 1996;10(1):19-25.

101. Maroon JC, Nelson PB. Hypovolemia in patients with subarachnoid hemorrhage: therapeutic implications. *Neurosurgery*. 1979;4:223-226.

102. Solomon RA, Post KD, McMurtry JG. Depression of circulating blood volume after subarachnoid hemorrhage: implications for treatment of symptomatic vasospasm. *Neurosurgery*. 1984;15:354-361.

103. Wijdicks EF, Vermeulen M, Hijdra A, van Gijn J. Hyponatremia and cerebral infarction in patients with ruptured intracranial aneurysms: is fluid restriction harmful? *Ann Neurol*. 1985;17:137-140.

104. Lennihan L, Mayer SA, Matthew EF, et al. Effect of hypervolemic therapy on cerebral blood flow after subarachnoid hemorrhage: a randomized control trial. *Stroke*. 2000;31:383-391.

105. Egge A, Waterloo K, Sjøholm H, Solberg T, Ingebrigtsen T, Romner B. Prophylactic hyperdynamic postoperative fluid therapy after aneurysmal subarachnoid hemorrhage: a clinical, prospective, randomized, controlled study. *Neurosurgery*. 2001;49:593-606.

106. Gathier CS, van den Bergh WM, van der Jagt M, et al. Induced hypertension for delayed cerebral ischemia after aneurysmal subarachnoid hemorrhage: a randomized clinical trial. *Stroke*. 2018;49(1):76-83.

107. Polin RS, Coenen VA, Hansen CA, et al. Efficacy of transluminal angioplasty for the management of symptomatic cerebral vasospasm following aneurysmal subarachnoid hemorrhage. *Neurosurg*. 2000;92:284-290.

108. Zwienenberg-Lee M, Hartman J, Rudisill N, Madden L. Effect of prophylactic transluminal balloon angioplasty on cerebral vasospasm and outcome in patients with Fisher grade III subarachnoid hemorrhage: results of a phase II multicenter, randomized, clinical trial. *Stroke*. 2008;39(6):1759-1765.

109. Higashida RT, Halbach VV, Cahan LD, et al. Transluminal angioplasty for treatment of intracranial arterial vasospasm. *J Neurosurg*. 1989;71(5 Pt 1):648-653.

110. Higashida RT, Halbach VV, Dormandy B, Bell JD, Hieshima GB. Endovascular treatment of intracranial aneurysms with a new silicone microballoon device: technical considerations and indications for therapy. *Radiology*. 1990;174(3 Pt 1):687-691.

111. Higashida RT, Halbach VV, Dowd CF, Dormandy B, Bell J, Hieshima GB. Intravascular balloon dilatation therapy for intracranial arterial vasospasm: patient selection, technique, and clinical results. *Neurosurg Rev*. 1992;15:89-95.

112. Kassell NF, Helm G, Simmons N, Phillips CD, Cail WS. Treatment of cerebral vasospasm with intra-arterial papaverine. *J Neurosurg*. 1992;77(6):848-852.

113. Feng L, Fitzsimmons BF, Young WL, et al. Intraarterially administered verapamil as adjunct therapy for cerebral vasospasm: safety and 2-year experience. *Am J Neuroradiol*. 2002;23(8):1284-1290.

114. Badjatia N, Topcuoglu MA, Pryor JC, et al. Preliminary experience with intra-arterial nicardipine as a treatment for cerebral vasospasm. *Am J Neuroradiol*. 2004;25(5):819-826.

115. Biondi A, Ricciardi GK, Puybasset L, et al. Intra-arterial nimodipine for the treatment of symptomatic cerebral vasospasm after aneurismal subarachnoid hemorrhage: preliminary results. *Am J Neuroradiol*. 2004;25(6):1067-1076.

116. Fraticelli AT, Cholley BP, Losser MR, Saint Maurice JP, Payen D. Milrinone for the treatment of cerebral vasospasm after aneurismal subarachnoid hemorrhage. *Stroke*. 2008;39(3):893-898.

117. van den Bergh WM, Algra A, van der Sprenkel JW, Tulleken CA, Rinkel GJ. Hypomagnesemia after aneurysmal subarachnoid hemorrhage. *Neurosurgery*. 2003;52(2):276-281; discussion 281-282.

118. van den Berg WM, Algra A, van Kooten F, et al. Magnesium sulfate in aneurysmal subarachnoid hemorrhage: a randomized controlled trial. *Stroke*. 2005;36(5):1011-1015.

119. Veyna RS, Seyfried D, Burke DG, et al. Magnesium sulfate therapy after aneurysmal subarachnoid hemorrhage. *J Neurosurg*. 2002;96(3):510-514.

120. Schmid-Elsaesser R, Kunz M, Zausinger S, Prueckner S, Briegel J, Steiger HJ. Intravenous magnesium versus nimodipine in the treatment of patients with aneurysmal subarachnoid hemorrhage: a randomized study. *Neurosurgery*. 2006;58(6):1054-1065; discussion 1054-1065.

121. Muroi C, Terzic A, Fortunati M, Yonekawa Y, Keller E. Magnesium sulfate in the management of patients with aneurysmal subarachnoid hemorrhage: a randomized, placebo-controlled, dose-adapted trial. *Surg Neurol*. 2008;69(1):33–39; discussion 39.

122. Wong GK, Poon WS, Chan MT, et al. IMASH Investigators. Intravenous magnesium sulphate for aneurysmal subarachnoid hemorrhage (IMASH): a randomized, double-blinded, placebo-controlled, multicenter phase III trial. *Stroke*. 2010;41(5):921-926.

123. Dorhout Mees SM, Algra A, Vandertop WP, et al. MASH-2 Study Group. Magnesium for aneurysmal subarachnoid hemorrhage (MASH-2): a randomized placebo-controlled trial. *Lancet*. 2012;380(9836):44-49.

124. Allen GS, Ahn HS, Preziosi TJ, et al. Cerebral arterial spasm—a controlled trial of nimodipine in patients with subarachnoid hemorrhage. *N Eng J Med*. 1983;308(11):619-624.

125. Phillippon J, Grob R, Dagreou F, Guggiari M, Rivierez M, Viars P. Prevention of vasospasm in subarachnoid haemorrhage. A controlled study with nimodipine. *Acta Neurochir (Wien)*. 1986;82(3-4):110-114.

126. Neil-Dwyer G, Mee E, Dorrance D, Lowe D. Early intervention with nimodipine in subarachnoid hemorrhage. *Eur Heart J*. 1987;8(Suppl. K):41-47.

127. Petruck KC, West M, Mohr G, et al. Nimodipine treatment in poor-grade aneurysm patients. Results of a multicenter double-blind placebo-controlled trial. *J Neurosurg*. 1988;68(4):505-517.

128. Pickard JD, Murray GD, Illingworth R, et al. Effect of oral nimodipine on cerebral infarction and outcome after subarachnoid haemorrhage: British aneurysm nimodipine trial. *Br Med J*. 1989;298(6674):636-642.

129. Haley EC Jr, Kassell NF, Torner JC. A randomized controlled trial of high-dose intravenous nicardipine in aneurysmal subarachnoid hemorrhage. A report of the Cooperative Aneurysm Study. *J Neurosurg*. 1993;78(4):537-547.

130. Haley EC Jr, Kassell NF, Torner JC, Truskowski LL, Germanson TP. A randomized trial of two doses of nicardipine in aneurysmal subarachnoid hemorrhage. A report of the Cooperative Aneurysm Study. *J Neurosurg*. 1994;80(5):788-796.

131. Dorhout Mees SM, Rinkel GJ, Feigin VL, et al. Calcium antagonists for aneurysmal subarachnoid hemorrhage. *Cochrane Database Syst Rev*. 2007;3:CD000277.

132. Mayberg MR, Batjer HH, Dacey R, et al. Guidelines for the management of aneurysmal subarachnoid hemorrhage. A statement for healthcare professionals from a special writing group of the Stroke Council, American Heart Association. *Circulation*. 1994;90(5):2592-2605.

133. Tseng MY, Czosnyka M, Richards H, Pickard JD, Kirkpatrick PJ. Effects of acute treatment with pravastatin on cerebral vasospasm, autoregulation, and delayed ischemic deficits after aneurysmal subarachnoid hemorrhage: a phase II randomized placebo-controlled trial. *Stroke*. 2005;36(8):1627-1632.

134. Lynch JR, Wang H, McGirt MJ, et al. Simvastatin reduces vasospasm after aneurysmal subarachnoid hemorrhage: results of a pilot randomized clinical trial. *Stroke*. 2005;36(9):2024-2026.

135. Tseng MY, Hutchinson PJ, Czosnyka M, Richards H, Pickard JD, Kirkpatrick PJ. Effects of acute pravastatin treatment on intensity of rescue therapy, length of inpatient stay, and 6-month outcome in patients after aneurysmal subarachnoid hemorrhage. *Stroke*. 2007;38(5):1545-1550.

136. Kirkpatrick PJ, Turner CL, Smith C, Hutchinson PJ, Murray GD, STASH Collaborators. Simvastatin in aneurysmal subarachnoid hemorrhage (STASH): a multicenter randomized phase III trial. *Lancet Neurol*. 2014;13(7):666-675.

137. Wong GK, Liang M, Lee MW, et al. High-dose simvastatin for aneurysmal subarachnoid hemorrhage: a multicenter, randomized, controlled, double-blind clinical trial protocol. *Neurosurgery*. 2013;72(5):840-844.

138. MacDonald RL, Kassell NF, Mayer S, et al. Clazosentan to overcome neurological ischemia and infarction occurring after subarachnoid hemorrhage (CONSCIOUS-1): randomized, double-blind, placebo-controlled phase 2 dose-finding trial. *Stroke*. 2008;39(11):3015-3021.

139. MacDonald RL, Higashida RT, Keller E, et al. Clazosentan, an endothelin receptor antagonist, in patients with aneurysmal subarachnoid haemorrhage undergoing surgical clipping: a randomised, double-blind, placebo-controlled phase 3 trial (CONSCIOUS-2). *Lancet Neurol*. 2011;10(7):618-625.

140. Macdonald RL, Higashida RT, Keller E, et al. Randomized trial of clazosentan in patients with aneurysmal subarachnoid hemorrhage undergoing endovascular coiling. *Stroke*. 2012; 43(6):1463-1469.

141. Vergouwen MD, Algra A, Rinkel GJ. Endothelin receptor antagonists for aneurysmal subarachnoid hemorrhage: a systematic review and meta-analysis update. *Stroke*. 2012; 43(10):2671-2676.

142. Hasan D, Wijdicks EF, Vermeulen M. Hyponatremia is associated with cerebral ischemia in patients with aneurysmal subarachnoid hemorrhage. *Ann Neurol*. 1990;27(1):106-108.

143. Sayama T, Inamura T, Matsushima T, Inoha S, Inoue T, Fukui M. High incidence of hyponatremia in patients with ruptured anterior communicating artery aneurysms. *Neurol Res*. 2000;22(2):151-155.

144. Qureshi AI, Suri MF, Sung GY, et al. Prognostic significance of hypernatremia and hyponatremia among patients with aneurysmal subarachnoid hemorrhage. *Neurosurgery*. 2002;50(4):749-755.

145. Wijdicks EF, Vermeulen M, ten Haaf JA, Hijdra A, Bakker WH, van Gijn J. Volume depletion and natriuresis in patients with a ruptured intracranial aneurysm. *Ann Neurol*. 1985;18(2):211-216.

146. Suarez JI, Qureshi AI, Parekh PD, et al. Administration of hypertonic (3%) sodium chloride/acetate in hyponatremic patients with symptomatic vasospasm following subarachnoid hemorrhage. *J Neurosurg Anesthesiol*. 1999;11(3):178-184.

147. Hasan D, Lindsay KW, Wijdicks EF, et al. Effect of fludrocortisone acetate in patients with subarachnoid hemorrhage. *Stroke*. 1989;20(9):1156-1161.

148. Mori T, Katayama Y, Kawamata T, Hirayama T. Improved efficiency of hypervolemic therapy with inhibition of natriuresis by fludrocortisone in patients with aneurysmal subarachnoid hemorrhage. *J Neurosurg*. 1999;91(6):947-952.

149. Ghali JK, Koren MJ, Taylor JR, et al. Efficacy and safety of oral conivaptan: a V1A/V2 vasopressin receptor antagonist, assessed in a randomized, placebo-controlled trial in patients with euvolemic or hypervolemic hyponatremia. *J Clin Endocrinol Metab*. 2006;91(6):2142-2152.

150. Andreoli A, di Pasquale G, Pinelli G, Grazi P, Tognetti F, Testa C. Subarachnoid hemorrhage: frequency and severity of cardiac arrhythmias. A survey of 70 cases studied in the acute phase. *Stroke*. 1987;18(3):558-564.

151. Di Pasquale G, Pinelli G, Andreoli A, Manini G, Grazi P, Tognetti F. Holter detection of cardiac arrhythmias in intracranial subarachnoid hemorrhage. *Am J Cardiol*. 1987;59(6):596-600.

152. Sommargren CE, Zaroff JG, Banki N, Drew BJ. Electrocardiographic repolarization abnormalities in subarachnoid hemorrhage. *J Electrocardiol*. 2002;35 (Suppl):257-262.

153. Kono T, Morita H, Kuroiwa T, Onaka H, Takatsuka H, Fujiwara A. Left ventricular wall motion abnormalities in patients with subarachnoid hemorrhage: neurogenic stunned myocardium. *J Am Coll Cardiol*. 1994;24(3):636-640.

154. Lambert G, Naredi S, Edén E, Rydenhag B, Friberg PE. Monoamine metabolism and sympathetic nervous activation following subarachnoid haemorrhage: influence of gender and hydrocephalus. *Brain Res Bull*. 2002;58(1):77-82.

155. Zaroff JG, Rordorf GA, Ogilvy CS, Picard MH. Regional patterns of left ventricular systolic dysfunction after subarachnoid hemorrhage: evidence for neurally mediated cardiac injury. *J Am Soc Echocardiogr*. 2000;13(8):774-779.

156. Kothavale A, Banki NM, Kopelnik A, et al. Predictors of left ventricular regional wall motion abnormalities after subarachnoid hemorrhage. *Neurocrit Care*. 2006;4(3):199-205.

157. Banki N, Kopelnik A, Tung P, et al. Prospective analysis of prevalence, distribution, and rate of recovery of left ventricular systolic dysfunction in patients with subarachnoid hemorrhage. *J Neurosurg*. 2006;105(1):15-20.

158. Tung P, Kopelnik A, Banki N, et al. Predictors of neurocardiogenic injury after subarachnoid hemorrhage. *Stroke*. 2004; 35(2):548-551.

159. van der Bilt I, Hasan D, van den Brink R, et al. Cardiac dysfunction after aneurysmal subarachnoid hemorrhage: relationship with outcome. *Neurology*. 2014;82(4):351-358.

160. Fernandez A, Schmidt JM, Claassen J, et al. Fever after subarachnoid hemorrhage: risk factors and impact on outcome. *Neurology*. 2007;68:1013-1019.

161. Dorhout Mees SM, Luitse MJ, van den Bergh WM, Rinkel GJ. Fever after aneurysmal subarachnoid hemorrhage: relation with extent of hydrocephalus and amount of extravasated blood. *Stroke*. 2008;39:2141-2143.

162. Kilpatrick MM, Lowry DW, Firlik AD, Yonas H, Marion DW. Hyperthermia in the neurosurgical intensive care unit. *Neurosurgery*. 2000;47:850-855.

163. Badjatia N. Fever control in the neuro-ICU: why, who and when? *Curr Opin Crit Care*. 2009;15(2):79-82.

164. Zhang G, Zhang JH, Qin X. Fever increased in-hospital mortality after subarachnoid hemorrhage. *Acta Neurochir Suppl*. 2011;110(Pt 1):239-243.

165. Oliveira–Filho J, Ezzeddine MA, Segal AZ, et al. Fever in subarachnoid hemorrhage: relationship to vasospasm and outcome. *Neurology*. 2001;56(10):1299-1304.

166. Badjatia N, Fernandez L, Schmidt JM, et al. Impact of induced normothermia on outcome after subarachnoid hemorrhage: a case-control study. *Neurosurgery*. 2010;66(4):696-700.

167. Sampson TR, Dhar R, Diringer MN. Factors associated with the development of anemia after subarachnoid hemorrhage. *Neurocrit Care*. 2010;12(1):4-9.

168. Kramer AH, Gurka MJ, Nathan B, Dumont AS, Kassell NF, Bleck TP. Complications associated with anemia and blood transfusion in patients with aneurysmal subarachnoid hemorrhage. *Crit Care Med*. 2008;36(7):2070-2075.

169. Giller CA, Wills MJ, Giller AM, Samson D. Distribution of hematocrit values after aneurysmal subarachnoid hemorrhage. *J Neuroimaging*. 1998;8(3):169-170.

170. Naidech AM, Drescher J, Ault ML, Shaibani A, Batjer HH, Alberts MJ. Higher hemoglobin is associated with less cerebral infarction, poor outcome, and death after subarachnoid hemorrhage. *Neurosurgery*. 2006;59(4):775-779.

171. Naidech AM, Jovanovic B, Wartenberg KE, et al. Higher hemoglobin is associated with improved outcome after subarachnoid hemorrhage. *Crit Care Med*. 2007;35(10):2383-2389.

172. Dhar R, Zazulia AR, Videen TO, Zipfel GJ, Derdeyn CP, Diringer MN. Red blood cell transfusion increases cerebral oxygen delivery in anemic patients with subarachnoid hemorrhage. *Stroke*. 2009;40(9):3039-3044.

173. Levine J, Kofke A, Cen L, et al. Red blood cell transfusion is associated with infection and extracerebral complications after subarachnoid hemorrhage. *Neurosurgery*. 2010;66(2):312-318.

174. Naidech AM, Shaibani A, Garg RK, et al. Prospective, randomized trial of higher goal hemoglobin after subarachnoid hemorrhage. *Neurocrit Care*. 2010;13(3):313-320.

175. English SW, Fergusson D, Chassé M, et al. Aneurysmal SubArachnoid Hemorrhage-Red Blood Cell Transfusion and Outcome (SAHaRA): a pilot randomised controlled trial protocol. *BMJ Open*. 2016;6(12):e012623.

66

How Should Acute Ischemic Stroke Be Managed in the Intensive Care Unit?

Yunis Mayasi and Robert David Stevens

EPIDEMIOLOGY AND TRIAGE

Cerebrovascular disease is one of the leading causes of death and disability worldwide, with an incidence of more than 800,000 cases per year and an estimated health care cost of $37 billion in the United States alone.[1] Approximately 85% of strokes are ischemic,[1] and the treatment of acute ischemic stroke (AIS) has undergone major advances in the past several years. Delivery of care in a medical facility with expertise in stroke care leads to better outcomes, irrespective of acute stroke therapy received. This might be related to advanced capabilities to prevent secondary brain injury, treat comorbid conditions, and to prevent or treat stroke-related complications.[2] To enhance patient identification and triage to the appropriate level of care, the American Heart Association has designated medical centers as Stroke-Ready, Primary Stroke Center and Comprehensive Stroke Center.[3] Comprehensive Stroke Centers have expertise in endovascular and neurosurgical stroke therapy as well as neurointensive care.[3]

CLASSIFICATION

Several classification systems have been proposed, the most commonly used is the Trial of ORG10172 in Acute Stroke Treatment (TOAST)[4] that is based on the presumed etiological mechanisms, which in turn are linked to distinct diagnostic evaluations and treatment plans. The TOAST classification system describes five major stroke subtypes including large vessel atherosclerotic disease (LAA), small vessel occlusion (SVO), cardioembolic (CE), other determined cause, and incomplete evaluation.[4] Using this system, a model was developed and validated to predict the most likely stroke subtype given the diagnostic evaluation.[5] Different vascular territories typically segregate with specific stroke subtypes, for example internal carotid artery (ICA) territory strokes are commonly due to LAA, vertebrobasilar territory are associated with SVO, whereas CE strokes are common in the superior cerebellar artery (SCA) distribution.[4]

INITIAL EVALUATION AND TREATMENT

The initial evaluation of a patient presenting acutely with a suspected ischemic stroke should include a thorough physical examination and scoring according to the National Institues of Health Stroke Score/Scale (NIHSS), measurement of vital signs, a blood glucose level, a computed tomography (CT) scan of the head to rule out intracerebral hemorrhage, and head and neck vascular imaging to identify larger arterial occlusion which might be treatable with endovascular intervention. Evaluation of the stroke patient should include a comprehensive assessment of modifiable risks including smoking, hypertension, dyslipidemia and diabetes mellitus. Also, an evaluation of cardiac rhythm and function is essential.[6] The standard treatment of ischemic stroke up to 4.5 hours following symptom onset is the administration of the thrombolytic drug tissue plasminogen activator (tPA).[7,8] The efficacy of tPA is reduced in patients with large arterial occlusions, and if patient selection criteria are met, these patients may benefit from mechanical thrombectomy.[9,10] This treatment modality has been conclusively validated starting in 2015 when five studies demonstrated improved outcomes in strokes caused by large arterial occlusions (Table 66.1).[11–15] As with thrombolytic therapy, the efficacy of endovascular therapy is time-dependent and most recently the time window for intervention was extended, which led to an increase in patient eligibility for such a treatment. The DAWN trial showed a striking increase in the probability of favorable outcomes among those patients having large vessel occlusion with a favorable imaging profile on CT perfusion.[16,17] In addition, the multicenter DEFUSE-3 trial conducted in patients 6–16 hours after onset of symptoms who had an infarct volume less than 70 mL with an ischemic penumbra of 15 mL or more found that endovascular therapy is superior to medical therapy, even in patients up to 90 years of age.[18]

ADMISSION TO THE INTENSIVE CARE UNIT

Structured medical optimization in a specialized environment is widely regarded as beneficial for patients with AIS, and there is extensive evidence supporting the association between admission to dedicated stroke units and improved survival and functional outcome.[19] Far less is known or understood about the impact of intensive car unit (ICU) admission, and evidence-based or consensus criteria for admission of ischemic stroke patients to an ICU are therefore lacking. After tPA administration or mechanical thrombectomy,

TABLE 66.1   Summary of Endovascular Stroke Therapy Trials.

Trial	NIHSS Criteria	Time Window	Recanalization Success	Clinical Outcome	Symptomatic Hemorrhage
MR-CLEAN	>2	<6 h	TICI 2B-3, 58.7%	Greater neurologic recovery at 90 days OR =1.67 (1.21–2.30)	7.7%
EXTEND-IA	0–42	<4.5 h	TIMI 2-3, 89%	Greater neurologic recovery –3 days (P = .002) –90 days (P = .006)	0%
ESCAPE	>5	<12 h	TICI 2B-3, 72.4%	Favorable shift in the modified Rankin scale –90 days (P <.001) –NNT of 2.6	3.6%
SWIFTPRIME	8–29	<6 h	TICI 2B-3, 88%	Favorable shift in the modified Rankin scale –90 days (P <.001) –NNT of 2.6	3%
REVASCAT	>5	<8 h	TICI 2B-3, 65.7%	Favorable shift in modified Rankin scale scores –90 days (OR 1.7 [1.05–2.8]) –NNT of 6.4	1.9%
DAWN	GrpA/B >10 Grp C >20	6-24 h	TICI 2B-3, 84%	Favorable shift in utility-weighted modified Rankin scale –90 days (5.5 compared to 3.4 in medical Grp) –NNT of 2.7	6%
DEFUSE-3	≥6	6-16 h	TICI 2B-3, 76%	EST: Favorable shift in modified Rankin scale scores –90 days (OR 2.77; P <.001) –NNT of 3.6	7%

TICI, thrombolysis in cerebral infarction; *TIMI*, thrombolysis in myocardial infarction.

it is recommended that patients are admitted to a step-down unit or ICU for at least 24 hours for frequent monitoring of the neurological examination and optimization of cardiopulmonary physiology.[3] Reports indicate that the provision of specialized neurological intensive care may be associated with improved outcomes and decreased length of stay and health care cost in patients with stroke.[20,21]

It is estimated that approximately 20% of ischemic stroke patients require an ICU admission.[22] Critical care is needed to detect, prevent, recognize and treat complications of stroke which for convenience may be classified as neurologic and systemic.[23] Neurologic complications include consequences of cerebral revascularization, hemorrhagic transformation, seizures, brain swelling and herniation. Systemic complications include hypertensive crisis, metabolic decompensation, hyperthermia, sepsis, venous thromboembolism as well as cardiac and respiratory failure.

INTRACRANIAL PRESSURE MONITORING OF STROKE PATIENTS

It has been proposed that patients with large cerebral infarctions might benefit from invasive monitoring of ICP because changes in ICP waveforms or absolute values might provide an early signal of impending clinical deterioration. This hypothesis is controversial. Given the compartmentalized nature of brain structures, ICP readings are necessarily regional and may overlook significant changes occurring in noncontiguous tissues. In nonintubated awake patients who are at risk for malignant MCA syndrome, it has been shown that clinical deterioration may precede sustained elevations in ICP.[38] Alternatively, ICP monitors might be of greater value in intubated patients receiving sedation, in whom clinical assessment is more challenging. Optimizing cerebral perfusion pressure (CPP) is generally thought to be beneficial, yet optimal targets for CPP have not been identified. Static imaging studies such as CT scan could be utilized to verify effects of focal mass effects, but the correlation between CT findings and ICP is poor.[38] Studies are evaluating several noninvasive modalities of ICP measurement including optic nerve sheath diameter and pupillometry.[39]

Seizures

Seizures occur in 2–8% of patients presenting with AIS.[40] Although isolated clinical seizures may be managed on the general neurology ward, generalized status epilepticus, convulsive or nonconvulsive, is an indication for critical care management including continuous electroencephalogram monitoring, hemodynamic and pulmonary monitoring, and stepwise antiepileptic drug escalation. It has been shown that nonconvulsive seizures are present in 30% of patients presenting with AIS who have an unexplained depression in consciousness. Cortical infarction, embolic causes of AIS, and hemorrhagic conversion are associated with a higher risk of seizures in this setting.[40,41]

Complications of Mechanical Thrombectomy

Parenchymal hemorrhage after mechanical thrombectomy is common, seen in up to 43% of patients. Petechial hemorrhages, hyperdensities within the infarct bed not associated with mass effect, are generally benign, however larger parenchymal bleeds, seen as homogenous hyperdensities with mass effect, are associated with worse outcomes.[35] Significant elevations in blood pressure increase the risk of postprocedural hemorrhage, likely caused by the loss of cerebral autoregulation. Several imaging biomarkers were developed to aid in identifying at-risk patients. The early cerebral vein sign (ECV) was shown not only to be associated with higher risk of postprocedural hemorrhage but also with worse 90 day outcomes.[42] In addition, the spot sign, which is a sign of continued contrast extravasation observed in CT angiography is associated with higher risk of recurrent hemorrhage.[43] The early identification of high risk patients can help with the early implementation of a treatment plan that includes strict blood pressure management.[42]

Cerebral hyperperfusion syndrome (CHS), or cerebral reperfusion injury, is a relatively infrequent syndrome that was described after repair of high-grade carotid artery stenosis, but has also been reported in cases of mechanical thrombectomy.[44,45] The pathophysiology of CHS is not entirely elucidated yet aberrant cerebral autoregulation is believed to play a role, wherein, in the absence of an appropriate vasoconstriction response there is an unopposed increase in cerebral blood volume. The presenting symptoms and signs include headache, seizures, cerebral edema and/or hemorrhage.[45] Diagnosis is made with imaging studies including MRI, single photon emission computed tomography (SPECT), magnetic resonance perfusion imaging and transcranial Doppler studies (TCDs).[45] The cornerstone of management of CHS following mechanical thrombectomy is carefully titrated blood pressure control with the aim of avoiding pressure spikes which have been linked to worse outcome. In this setting, vasodilator medications are detrimental and alternative blood pressure lowering strategies, e.g., cardioselective calcium channel medications or beta blockers or clonidine, should be considered, in addition to other measures to treat cerebral edema, seizures and headache.[45]

NEUROLOGIC COMPLICATIONS

Malignant Middle Cerebral Artery Syndrome

Malignant middle cerebral artery (MCA) syndrome is a rapid deterioration in neurological function seen in a subset of patients who have occlusion of the ICA or proximal MCA. In these patients the size of the infarction and associated edema and mass effect can lead to transtentorial herniation and death unless promptly recognized and treated (Fig. 66.1). Malignant

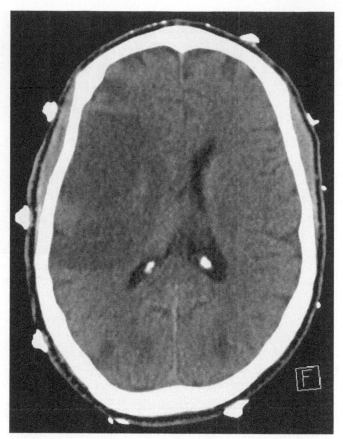

Fig. 66.1 Noncontrast computed tomography (CT) scan of the head showing a right malignant middle cerebral artery (MCA) ischemic stroke with surrounding edema and midline shift.

MCA syndrome is seen in up to 10% of supratentorial ischemic strokes in the ICA or proximal MCA territory and is associated with a mortality of up to 80%.[24] The development of cerebral edema begins in the first 24 hours and reaches a maximum 3–5 days after symptom onset, during which patients must be monitored in the ICU.[24] The most common clinical presentation is a decline in the level of consciousness, worsening of lateralized deficits and pupillary changes progressing to a full-blown transtentorial herniation syndrome in the absence of therapeutic intervention.[25,26] Factors associated with malignant MCA syndrome include younger age, female gender, carotid occlusion, and an incomplete circle of Willis.[27] The risk of malignant MCA syndrome is directly linked to the size of the cerebral infarction, thus an infarct volume greater than 145 cm³ on CT or MRI is widely used as a predictive marker, although other imaging criteria are being developed such as optic nerve sheath diameter.[28]

The initial medical management of malignant MCA syndrome is aimed at mitigating cerebral edema and intracranial pressure via osmolar therapy, controlled mechanical ventilation, and metabolic suppression with propofol or pentobarbital. Surgical decompressive hemicraniectomy has been associated with significantly reduced disability and mortality in selected patients, when compared to medical management alone. This was demonstrated in four clinical trials: Decompressive Craniectomy in Malignant Middle

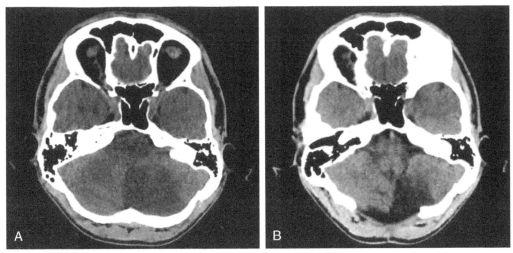

Fig. 66.2 Noncontrast computed tomography (CT) scan of the head with an acute ischemic infarct of the left cerebellar hemisphere. **(A)** There is mass effect and effacement of the fourth ventricle. **(B)** After suboccipital decompressive hemicraniectomy.

Cerebral Artery Infarcts (DECIMAL), Decompressive Surgery for the Treatment of Malignant Infarction of the Middle Cerebral Artery (DESTINY), Hemicraniectomy after Middle Cerebral Artery Infarction with Life-threatening Edema trial (HAMLET), and Decompressive Surgery for the Treatment of Malignant Infarction of the Middle Cerebral Artery (DESTINY II).[29–32] Collectively, these trials show that decompressive craniectomy accomplished at or before 48 hours, in patients younger than 60 years of age, is associated with a 50% absolute reduction of death and a nearly twofold increased probability of achieving favorable outcome defined as modified Rankin Scale of three or less.[29–32] Other measures that have been considered in patients with malignant MCA syndrome include invasive monitoring of intracranial pressure (ICP), or even invasive multimodality monitoring; however the value of such approaches is unclear (see further sections).[33]

Hemorrhagic Transformation

Hemorrhagic transformation (HT) occurs in 0.6% of all AIS patients, in 5% of patients who received tPA, and in 10% of patients who underwent endovascular therapy.[8,34] HT can be classified into hemorrhagic infarction (HI) or parenchymal hemorrhage (PH). HI is seen as heterogeneous nonconfluent hyperdensities within the infarcted tissue, as compared to confluent homogenous bleed with mass effect in PH.[35] Factors associated with hemorrhagic transformation include higher NIHSS, larger infarct volumes and age.[36] Significant HT is consistently associated with worse outcomes. A CT scan of the head should be obtained with any clinical deterioration and is the gold standard in diagnosing HT. Spontaneous HT is managed conservatively by optimizing modifiable risks including elevated blood pressure, hyperglycemia as well as intubation and mechanical ventilation if indicated. As for significant HT related to tPA, reversal of tPA should be

instituted acutely with cryoprecipitate or fibrinogen, and transfusion of plasma and platelets. In addition, surgical decompression might be necessary in selected cases, for example, clinically symptomatic lobar hemorrhages or hemorrhages in the posterior fossa.

Posterior Fossa Infarction

Infarction involving the cerebellum and brainstem are of particular concern given the small posterior fossa size, with edema formation leading to very rapid neurologic decline due to compression of major brainstem centers and/or obliteration of the fourth ventricle causing acute obstructive hydrocephalus (Fig. 66.2).[37] Very close monitoring of such patients in the ICU is essential to enable early detection of neurological changes. Medical management is similar to supratentorial malignant cerebral infarction. Given the risk of clinical deterioration, consultation with neurosurgery should be sought early. Operative management includes either decompressive suboccipital craniectomy or placement of an external ventricular drain for hydrocephalus, or in some instances both.[37]

OTHER COMPLICATIONS IN THE STROKE PATIENT

Infection

Infections occur in up to a third of stroke patients, with pneumonia being the most common occurring in approximately 10% of AIS. Irrespective of the type, infection is strongly linked to decreased survival and higher rates of long-term disability, as well as longer lengths of stay and higher health care costs. Models have been constructed to predict the likelihood of infection in this population, with higher risk associated with increased age, male gender, more severe strokes, dysphagia and presence of an indwelling catheter. Prophylactic or preventive administration of antibiotics has not been shown to modify outcomes.[46] Sepsis has been noted to occur at higher rates in the critically ill neurologic patients compared to general ICU patients, possibly caused by the immunologic suppression associated with severe brain injury.[47] The more severe the stroke, the more likely the patient is to develop sepsis (e.g., NIHSS >10).[46] The most common infection in this setting is pneumonia; early detection and treatment is crucial. As with all cases of sepsis, early antibiotic and carefully titrated fluid resuscitation and vasopressors is generally recommended in the stroke population.[48]

Angiodema

Angioedema is seen in 1–3% of stroke patients receiving tPA, typically within 30–120 minutes of the infusion.[49] This complication is believed to reflect plasmin-induced activation of the complement and kinin systems. Treatment is directed at maintenance of the airway with urgent intubation if the airway is compromised, and diphenhydramine, methylprednisolone and nebulized epinephrine are recommended.[49]

Acute Respiratory Distress Syndrome

The acute respiratory distress syndrome (ARDS) has been observed in up to one third of patients presenting with severe cerebrovascular or traumatic brain injury.[50] This syndrome is less frequent than AIS, but does occur in up to 4% of this population and is linked to higher mortality. Factors associated with development of ARDS in stroke include all source sepsis, decompressive hemicraniectomy and following tPA.[51,52] The management of ARDS should involve treating the inciting process (e.g., pneumonia), and different levels of pulmonary support (including lung protective ventilation) depending on the severity of lung injury.[51,52] It should be noted that major randomized trials conducted in ARDS patients excluded those with an underlying neurologic diagnosis, and consideration should be given to the impact of elevated levels of arterial carbon dioxide and cerebral blood flow.

CRITICAL CARE OF THE STROKE PATIENT

Airway Management and Mechanical Ventilation

To prevent secondary injury and possible extension of the infarct, an important priority in the management of patients with stroke is to detect and correct hypoxemia; however, specific criteria or targets for oxygenation, supplemental oxygen therapy, intubation and mechanical ventilation have not been validated.[23] Compromise of the airway and respiratory function is common in patients with ischemic stroke and is believed to reflect a combination of neurological and pulmonary factors. Neurologic factors include a depressed level of consciousness and oropharyngeal dysfunction with increased aspiration risk. Stroke patients in particular are at significant risk of airway compromise owing to dyssynchrony

or weakness of the swallowing and cough reflexes and paresis of bulbar muscles. Pulmonary factors include respiratory insufficiency most commonly caused by pneumonia, decompensation of heart failure, and pulmonary embolism. Stroke patients who require intubation acutely or during the course of admission have worse prognosis although it is unclear that studies reporting this association were able to completely adjust for confounders.[53–55]

Indications for endotracheal intubation in stroke patients include decreased level of arousal, inability to protect the airway, aspiration, seizures and status epilepticus. In stroke patients without increased intracranial pressure, mechanical ventilation settings should be as with any other critically ill patient with the goal of correcting or preventing hypoxemia and maintaining normocapnia. Successful weaning and extubation of stroke patients is predicted by smaller sized infarcts, NIHSS below 15, as well as absence of dysarthria prior to intubation.[56] In intubated stroke patients undergoing mechanical ventilation, a tracheostomy is recommended when prolonged ventilation is expected. After an initial trail demonstrating safety,[57] an ongoing study in stroke patients, the Stroke-related Early Tracheostomy vs. Prolonged Orotracheal Intubation in Neurocritical Care Trial II (SETPOINT II, clinical trial identifier NCT02377167), is evaluating the outcome benefits of early tracheostomy (1–3 days) compared to standard practice.

Blood Pressure Management

Cerebral pressure autoregulation (CA), the ability to maintain a constant and adequate cerebral blood flow (CBF) across a wide range of arterial pressures (MAP), is severely compromised in the setting of brain ischemia and infarction. In fact, it has been shown that CA remains abnormal for about a month after the ictus.[58,59] The degree of dysregulation of CA in stroke has been linked to worse outcomes, higher rates of hemorrhagic transformation as well as the development of brain edema; overzealous attempts by clinicians to lower the blood pressure might lead to relative hypoperfusion and clinical deterioration.[58,59] Evidence from the International Stroke Trial (IST) suggests that there is a U-shaped relationship between admission blood pressure and mortality, with mortality rates increasing by up to 4 and 18% with every 10 mm Hg above or below 150 mm Hg, respectively.[60] It follows that optimal control of blood pressure is a fundamental principle in the management of acute stroke. Management of blood pressure in AIS patients depends in part on whether they are candidates for reperfusion therapy (tPA or mechanical thrombectomy). In candidates for reperfusion therapy, strict blood pressure targets must be attained prior to the intervention; however, persistently elevated blood pressures lead to delays in intervention, with each additional minute accounting for the loss of 1.9 million neurons.[61] Guidelines recommend a blood pressure below 185/105 mm Hg in candidates for tPA. Intravenous boluses of labetalol or infusions of nicardipine or labetalol are recommended.[62]

In patients undergoing mechanical thrombectomy, evidence or guidelines are limited regarding optimal blood pressure management targets. As with all AIS patients, an association between high blood pressures and worse outcomes has been reported in this group.[63,64] A recent survey of the StrokeNet group investigating institutional practice demonstrated that blood pressure goals typically are established on a case-by-case basis with higher pressures permitted if recanalization was not attained.[65] Different institutions have different blood pressure parameters in patients successfully recanalized, and irrespective of the institutional blood pressure parameters, continuous intravenous nicardipine was the most commonly used agent.[65]

In AIS patients who are not candidates for reperfusion, current guidelines recommend maintaining blood pressure below 220/120 or 200/100 mm Hg with end organ damage, and not to start prestroke antihypertensive therapy in the acute setting because it might lead to decreased perfusion.[66] Several randomized trials are underway to evaluate optimal blood pressure parameters in this setting including the Enhanced Control of Hypertension and Thrombolysis Stroke Study (ENCHANTED, clinicaltrials.gov identifier NCT01422616), and the blood pressure in acute stroke collaboration, stage-3.[59,67–69] As for the pharmacologic agents used to treat hypertension, continuously infused intravenous medications are preferred so as to minimize major fluctuations in blood pressure. Calcium channel blockers and beta blockers are equivalently effective at achieving targeted blood pressure control.[70–72]

Symptomatic hypotension is uncommon in the acute stroke population, but may indicate a critical underlying condition such as myocardial ischemia or infarction, aortic dissection, post-tPA bleeding, and septic shock. These patients should undergo a timely and thorough workup including serum hemoglobin, troponin, urinalysis, echocardiography and, when needed, CT angiography of the chest.

Therapeutically induced hypertension could increase cerebral blood flow and this theoretically could result in hyperperfusion and hemorrhagic stroke transformation. Pilot studies suggest that blood pressure augmentation with vasoactive medications is safe, but a clear impact on outcomes has not been documented.[73]

Fluid Management

In AIS, periodic assessment of effective intravascular volume status is essential to avoid hypo- and hypervolemic states. Stroke patients on admission are commonly dehydrated owing to decreased oral intake caused by dysphagia, aphasia leading to difficult communication, and altered mental status. Intravenous resuscitation with isotonic fluids is recommended, since hypotonic fluids are believed to worsen underlying cerebral edema in this patient population.[23] In addition, there is no known benefit in using albumin over crystalloids in brain injured patients.[74] Regarding hyperosmolar solutions (mannitol, hypertonic saline), these might represent effective temporizing measures in patients who have smaller stroke volumes and are awake, while their impact in larger and malignant infarction syndromes is unclear.[75]

Management of Nutrition

Malnutrition is a common comorbid condition in patients presenting with AIS, and this problem is frequently perpetuated during hospitalization, with 65% of patients being underfed at 10 days.[76] Malnutrition is associated with higher mortality and worse functional outcomes, and hence it is an important factor to evaluate. Patients in the ICU are at risk of malnutrition owing to deficient swallowing function, concurrent mechanical ventilation, and fasting status maintained for procedures and tests. In nonintubated patients there is often a restriction of oral intake owing to legitimate concerns for aspiration. Patients should be evaluated for swallowing function and monitored on daily basis for dehydration with caloric intake calculated. In patients who fail swallowing assessments, naso- or oro-gastric tube feeding should be started, and a percutaneuos endoscopic gastrostomy tube (PEG-tube) considered when the swallowing impairment is predicted to persist after the acute phase.[77]

Glycemic Management

Hyperglycemia, whether as a consequence of uncontrolled diabetes mellitus or owing to a generalized stress response, is detrimental in AIS and has been associated with cellular acidosis, impaired neural repair, decreased rates of recanalization, and increased rates of hemorrhagic transformation.[78–81] Hypoglycemia is also detrimental because it leads to reduced substrate delivery in cerebral tissues already compromised by lack of perfusion. Consequently blood glucose should be kept between 140 and 180 mg/dL, using insulin infusion if necessary. An ongoing study, the SHINE trial (clinicaltrials.gov identifier NCT01369069), is underway to evaluate the optimal blood glucose levels in this patient population.[78–81]

Temperature Management

Fever is common in AIS, occurring in up to 50% of patients, and has been independently linked to worse functional outcomes.[82] There is a 2.2-fold increase in the relative risk of poor outcomes with every 1°C increase in body temperature.[83] Fever in stroke patients might be related to noninfectious inflammatory mechanisms, but it should be worked up meticulously and systematically, with potential sources of infection treated accordingly. Temperature control is recommended with antipyretic agents and, if persistent, with cooling devices. Although it has been demonstrated that therapeutic hypothermia is safe in AIS even in those receiving tPA,[84,85] to date there is no evidence of clinical benefit. Ongoing clinical trials are evaluating the efficacy of strict temperature management in the acute phase of ischemic stroke (e.g., ClinicalTrials.gov Identifier: NCT01833312).

AUTHORS' RECOMMENDATIONS

- The management of AIS has evolved significantly in recent years and currently is centered on achieving timely cerebral reperfusion using intravenous tPA and mechanical thrombectomy.
- tPA is recommended within 4.5 hours of symptom onset in eligible patients, whereas mechanical thrombectomy should be considered in patients who have a proximal circle of Willis occlusion.
- Decompressive craniectomy for malignant cerebral infarction is lifesaving and has been associated with higher levels of functional independence in patients less than 60 years
- Suboccipital decompressive craniectomy for space-occupying cerebellar infarction is recommended to treat hydrocephalus and reduce brainstem compression.
- There is strong evidence linking admission to a dedicated stroke unit with improved survival and functional outcome.
- The impact of critical care management, although less well studied, is likely also to be significant because it enables early detection and treatment of life-threatening neurologic (hemorrhagic transformation, malignant cerebral infarction seizures) and systemic complications (pneumonia, respiratory failure, venous thromboembolism and cardiac failure).

REFERENCES

1. Benjamin EJ, Blaha MJ, Chiuve SE, et al. Heart disease and stroke statistics-2017 update: a report from the American heart association. *Circulation*. 2017;135:e146-e603.
2. Mayasi Y, Helenius J, Goddeau Jr RP, Moonis M, Henninger N. Time to presentation is associated with clinical outcome in hemispheric stroke patients deemed ineligible for recanalization therapy. *J Stroke Cerebrovasc Dis*. 2016;25:2373-2379.
3. Silva GS, Schwamm LH. Review of stroke center effectiveness and other get with the guidelines data. *Curr Atheroscler Rep*. 2013;15:350.
4. Chung JW, Park SH, Kim N, et al. Trial of org 10172 in acute stroke treatment (toast) classification and vascular territory of ischemic stroke lesions diagnosed by diffusion-weighted imaging. *J Am Heart Assoc*. 2014;3(4):pii: e001119.
5. Arsava EM, Ballabio E, Benner T, et al. The causative classification of stroke system: an international reliability and optimization study. *Neurology*. 2010;75:1277-1284.
6. Khatri P. Evaluation and management of acute ischemic stroke. *Continuum (Minneap, Minn.)*. 2014;20:283-295.
7. Hacke W, Kaste M, Bluhmki E, et al. Thrombolysis with alteplase 3 to 4.5 hours after acute ischemic stroke. *N Engl J Med*. 2008;359:1317-1329.
8. National Institute of Neurological Disorders and Stroke rt-PA Stroke Study Group. Tissue plasminogen activator for acute ischemic stroke. *N Engl J Med*. 1995;333:1581-1587.
9. Smith WS, Lev MH, English JD, et al. Significance of large vessel intracranial occlusion causing acute ischemic stroke and tia. *Stroke*. 2009;40:3834-3840.
10. Bhatia R, Hill MD, Shobha N, et al. Low rates of acute recanalization with intravenous recombinant tissue plasminogen activator in ischemic stroke: real-world experience and a call for action. *Stroke*. 2010;41:2254-2258.
11. Berkhemer OA, Fransen PS, Beumer D, et al. A randomized trial of intraarterial treatment for acute ischemic stroke. *N Engl J Med*. 2015;372:11-20.
12. Campbell BC, Mitchell PJ, Kleinig TJ, et al. Endovascular therapy for ischemic stroke with perfusion-imaging selection. *N Engl J Med*. 2015;372:1009-1018.
13. Goyal M, Demchuk AM, Menon BK, et al. Randomized assessment of rapid endovascular treatment of ischemic stroke. *N Engl J Med*. 2015;372:1019-1030.
14. Saver JL, Goyal M, Bonafe A, et al. Stent-retriever thrombectomy after intravenous t-pa vs. T-pa alone in stroke. *N Engl J Med*. 2015;372:2285-2295.
15. Goyal M, Menon BK, van Zwam WH, et al. Endovascular thrombectomy after large-vessel ischaemic stroke: a meta-analysis of individual patient data from five randomised trials. *Lancet*. 2016;387:1723-1731.
16. Tudor G, Jovin RN. Dawn trial. *NCT02142283*. 2017;2017.
17. Nogueira RG, Jadhav AP, Haussen DC, et al. Thrombectomy 6 to 24 hours after stroke with a mismatch between deficit and infarct. *N Engl J Med*. 2018;378:11-21.
18. Albers GW, Marks MP, Kemp S, et al. Thrombectomy for stroke at 6 to 16 hours with selection by perfusion imaging. *N Engl J Med*. 2018;378:708-718.
19. Stroke Unit Trialists' Collaboration. Organised inpatient (stroke unit) care for stroke. *Cochrane Database Syst Rev*. 2013;(9): CD000197.
20. Suarez JI. Outcome in neurocritical care: advances in monitoring and treatment and effect of a specialized neurocritical care team. *Crit Care Med*. 2006;34:S232-238.
21. Suarez JI, Zaidat OO, Suri MF, et al. Length of stay and mortality in neurocritically ill patients: impact of a specialized neurocritical care team. *Crit Care Med*. 2004;32:2311-2317.
22. Coplin WM. Critical care management of acute ischemic stroke. *Continuum (Minneap, Minn.)*. 2012;18:547-559.
23. Powers WJ, Rabinstein AA, Ackerson T, et al. 2018 guidelines for the early management of patients with acute ischemic stroke: a guideline for healthcare professionals from the american heart association/american stroke association. *Stroke*. 2018; 49:e46-e110.
24. Qureshi AI, Suarez JI, Yahia AM, et al. Timing of neurologic deterioration in massive middle cerebral artery infarction: a multicenter review. *Crit Care Med*. 2003;31:272-277.
25. Hacke W, Schwab S, Horn M, Spranger M, De Georgia M, von Kummer R. 'Malignant' middle cerebral artery territory infarction: clinical course and prognostic signs. *Arch Neurol*. 1996; 53:309-315.
26. Berrouschot J, Sterker M, Bettin S, Köster J, Schneider D. Mortality of space-occupying ('malignant') middle cerebral artery infarction under conservative intensive care. *Intensive Care Med*. 1998;24:620-623.
27. Jaramillo A, Góngora-Rivera F, Labreuche J, Hauw JJ, Amarenco P. Predictors for malignant middle cerebral artery infarctions: a postmortem analysis. *Neurology*. 2006;66:815-820.
28. Albert AF, Kirkman MA. Clinical and radiological predictors of malignant middle cerebral artery infarction development and outcomes. *J Stroke Cerebrovasc Dis*. 2017;26:2671-2679.
29. Vahedi K, Vicaut E, Mateo J, et al. Sequential-design, multicenter, randomized, controlled trial of early decompressive craniectomy in malignant middle cerebral artery infarction (decimal trial). *Stroke*. 2007;38:2506-2517.
30. Hofmeijer J, Kappelle LJ, Algra A, et al. Surgical decompression for space-occupying cerebral infarction (the hemicraniectomy

after middle cerebral artery infarction with life-threatening edema trial [hamlet]): a multicentre, open, randomised trial. *Lancet Neurol.* 2009;8:326-333.

31. Jüttler E, Schwab S, Schmiedek P, et al. Decompressive surgery for the treatment of malignant infarction of the middle cerebral artery (destiny): a randomized, controlled trial. *Stroke.* 2007;38:2518-2525.

32. Jüttler E, Unterberg A, Woitzik J, et al. Hemicraniectomy in older patients with extensive middle-cerebral-artery stroke. *N Engl J Med.* 2014;370:1091-1100.

33. Hofmeijer J, van der Worp HB, Kappelle LJ. Treatment of space-occupying cerebral infarction. *Crit Care Med.* 2003;31:617-625.

34. Furlan A, Higashida R, Wechsler L, et al. Intra-arterial prourokinase for acute ischemic stroke. The proact ii study: a randomized controlled trial. Prolyse in acute cerebral thromboembolism. *JAMA.* 1999;282:2003-2011.

35. Zhang J, Yang Y, Sun H, Xing Y. Hemorrhagic transformation after cerebral infarction: current concepts and challenges. *Ann Transl Med.* 2014;2:81.

36. Intracerebral hemorrhage after intravenous t-pa therapy for ischemic stroke. The ninds t-pa stroke study group. *Stroke.* 1997;28:2109-2118.

37. Jensen MB, St Louis EK. Management of acute cerebellar stroke. *Arch Neurol.* 2005;62:537-544.

38. Schwab S, Aschoff A, Spranger M, Albert F, Hacke W. The value of intracranial pressure monitoring in acute hemispheric stroke. *Neurology.* 1996;47:393-398.

39. Khan MN, Shallwani H, Khan MU, Shamim MS. Noninvasive monitoring intracranial pressure - a review of available modalities. *Surg Neurol Int.* 2017;8:51.

40. Bladin CF, Alexandrov AV, Bellavance A, et al. Seizures after stroke: a prospective multicenter study. *Arch Neurol.* 2000;57:1617-1622.

41. Beghi E, D'Alessandro R, Beretta S, et al. Incidence and predictors of acute symptomatic seizures after stroke. *Neurology.* 2011;77:1785-1793.

42. Cartmell SCD, Ball RL, Kaimal R, et al. Early cerebral vein after endovascular ischemic stroke treatment predicts symptomatic reperfusion hemorrhage. *Stroke.* 2018;49:1741-1746.

43. Wada R, Aviv RI, Fox AJ, et al. Ct angiography "spot sign" predicts hematoma expansion in acute intracerebral hemorrhage. *Stroke.* 2007;38:1257-1262.

44. Hashimoto T, Matsumoto S, Ando M, Chihara H, Tsujimoto A, Hatano T. Cerebral hyperperfusion syndrome after endovascular reperfusion therapy in a patient with acute internal carotid artery and middle cerebral artery occlusions. *World Neurosurg.* 2018;110:145-151.

45. Farooq MU, Goshgarian C, Min J, Gorelick PB. Pathophysiology and management of reperfusion injury and hyperperfusion syndrome after carotid endarterectomy and carotid artery stenting. *Exp Transl Stroke Med.* 2016;8:7.

46. Westendorp WF, Vermeij JD, Hilkens NA, et al. Development and internal validation of a prediction rule for post-stroke infection and post-stroke pneumonia in acute stroke patients. *Eur Stroke J.* 2018;3:136-144.

47. Chamorro A, Urra X, Planas AM. Infection after acute ischemic stroke: a manifestation of brain-induced immunodepression. *Stroke.* 2007;38:1097-1103.

48. Berger B, Gumbinger C, Steiner T, Sykora M. Epidemiologic features, risk factors, and outcome of sepsis in stroke patients treated on a neurologic intensive care unit. *J Crit Care.* 2014;29:241-248.

49. Ottomeyer C, Hennerici MG, Szabo K. Raising awareness of orolingual angioedema as a complication of thrombolysis in acute stroke patients. *Cerebrovasc Dis.* 2009;27:307-308.

50. Hoesch RE, Lin E, Young M, et al. Acute lung injury in critical neurological illness. *Crit. Care Med.* 2012;40:587-593.

51. Rincon F, Maltenfort M, Dey S, et al. The prevalence and impact of mortality of the acute respiratory distress syndrome on admissions of patients with ischemic stroke in the united states. *J Intensive Care Med.* 2014;29:357-364.

52. Davies SW, Leonard KL, Falls Jr RK, et al. Lung protective ventilation (ardsnet) versus airway pressure release ventilation: ventilatory management in a combined model of acute lung and brain injury. *J Trauma Acute Care Surg.* 2015;78:240-249; discussion 249-251.

53. Bushnell CD, Phillips-Bute BG, Laskowitz DT, Lynch JR, Chilukuri V, Borel CO. Survival and outcome after endotracheal intubation for acute stroke. *Neurology.* 1999;52:1374-1381.

54. Pinheiro de Oliveira R, Hetzel MP, dos Anjos Silva M, Dallegrave D, Friedman G. Mechanical ventilation with high tidal volume induces inflammation in patients without lung disease. *Crit Care.* 2010;14:R39.

55. Stevens RD, Puybasset L. The brain-lung-brain axis. *Intensive Care Med.* 2011;37:1054-1056.

56. Lioutas VA, Hanafy KA, Kumar S. Predictors of extubation success in acute ischemic stroke patients. *J Neurol Sci.* 2016;368:191-194.

57. Bösel J, Schiller P, Hook Y, et al. Stroke-related early tracheostomy versus prolonged orotracheal intubation in neurocritical care trial (setpoint): a randomized pilot trial. *Stroke.* 2013;44:21-28.

58. Castro P, Azevedo E, Sorond F. Cerebral autoregulation in stroke. *Curr Atheroscler Rep.* 2018;20:37.

59. Appiah KO, Minhas JS, Robinson TG. Managing high blood pressure during acute ischemic stroke and intracerebral hemorrhage. *Curr Opin Neurol.* 2018;31:8-13.

60. Leonardi-Bee J, Bath PM, Phillips SJ, Sandercock PA. Blood pressure and clinical outcomes in the international stroke trial. *Stroke.* 2002;33:1315-1320.

61. Saver JL. Time is brain—quantified. *Stroke.* 2006;37:263-266.

62. Martin-Schild S, Hallevi H, Albright KC, et al. Aggressive blood pressure-lowering treatment before intravenous tissue plasminogen activator therapy in acute ischemic stroke. *Arch Neurol.* 2008;65:1174-1178.

63. Maïer B, Gory B, Taylor G, et al. Mortality and disability according to baseline blood pressure in acute ischemic stroke patients treated by thrombectomy: a collaborative pooled analysis. *J Am Heart Assoc.* 2017;6(10):pii: e006484.

64. Maier IL, Tsogkas I, Behme D, et al. High systolic blood pressure after successful endovascular treatment affects early functional outcome in acute ischemic stroke. *Cerebrovasc Dis.* 2018;45:18-25.

65. Mistry EA, Mayer SA, Khatri P. Blood pressure management after mechanical thrombectomy for acute ischemic stroke: a survey of the strokenet sites. *J Stroke Cerebrovasc Dis.* 2018;27(9):2474-2478.

66. Gąsecki D, Coca A, Cunha P, et al. Blood pressure in acute ischemic stroke: Challenges in trial interpretation and clinical management: position of the esh working group on hypertension and the brain. *J Hypertens.* 2018;36:1212-1221.

67. Woodhouse LJ, Manning L, Potter JF, et al. Continuing or temporarily stopping prestroke antihypertensive medication in acute stroke: an individual patient data meta-analysis. *Hypertension.* 2017;69:933-941.

68. Sandset EC, Sanossian N, Woodhouse LJ, et al. Protocol for a prospective collaborative systematic review and meta-analysis of individual patient data from randomized controlled trials of vasoactive drugs in acute stroke: the blood pressure in acute stroke collaboration, stage-3. *Int J Stroke*. 2018;13(7):759-765.

69. Lobanova I, Qureshi AI. Blood pressure goals in acute stroke-how low do you go? *Curr Hypertens Rep*. 2018;20:28.

70. Hecht JP, Richards PG. Continuous-infusion labetalol vs nicardipine for hypertension management in stroke patients. *J Stroke Cerebrovasc Dis*. 2018;27:460-465.

71. Allison TA, Bowman S, Gulbis B, Hartman H, Schepcoff S, Lee K. Comparison of clevidipine and nicardipine for acute blood pressure reduction in patients with stroke. *J Intensive Care Med*. 2017. doi:10.1177/0885066617724340. [Epub ahead of print].

72. Rosenfeldt Z, Conklen K, Jones B, Ferrill D, Deshpande M, Siddiqui FM. Comparison of nicardipine with clevidipine in the management of hypertension in acute cerebrovascular diseases. *J Stroke Cerebrovasc Dis*. 2018;27:2067-2073.

73. Hillis AE, Ulatowski JA, Barker PB, et al. A pilot randomized trial of induced blood pressure elevation: effects on function and focal perfusion in acute and subacute stroke. *Cerebrovasc Dis*. 2003;16:236-246.

74. Ginsberg MD, Palesch YY, Hill MD, et al. High-dose albumin treatment for acute ischaemic stroke (alias) part 2: a randomised, double-blind, phase 3, placebo-controlled trial. *Lancet Neurol*. 2013;12:1049-1058.

75. Ong CJ, Keyrouz SG, Diringer MN. The role of osmotic therapy in hemispheric stroke. *Neurocrit Care*. 2015;23:285-291.

76. Mosselman MJ, Kruitwagen CL, Schuurmans MJ, Hafsteinsdóttir TB. Malnutrition and risk of malnutrition in patients with stroke: prevalence during hospital stay. *J Neurosci Nurs*. 2013;45:194-204.

77. Crary MA, Humphrey JL, Carnaby-Mann G, Sambandam R, Miller L, Silliman S. Dysphagia, nutrition, and hydration in ischemic stroke patients at admission and discharge from acute care. *Dysphagia*. 2013;28:69-76.

78. Baker L, Juneja R, Bruno A. Management of hyperglycemia in acute ischemic stroke. *Curr Treat Options Neurol*. 2011;13:616-628.

79. Bruno A, Durkalski VL, Hall CE, et al. The stroke hyperglycemia insulin network effort (shine) trial protocol: a randomized, blinded, efficacy trial of standard vs. Intensive hyperglycemia management in acute stroke. *Int J Stroke*. 2014;9:246-251.

80. Ribo M, Molina C, Montaner J, et al. Acute hyperglycemia state is associated with lower tpa-induced recanalization rates in stroke patients. *Stroke*. 2005;36:1705-1709.

81. Weir CJ, Murray GD, Dyker AG, Lees KR. Is hyperglycaemia an independent predictor of poor outcome after acute stroke? Results of a long-term follow up study. *BMJ*. 1997;314:1303-1306.

82. Azzimondi G, Bassein L, Nonino F, et al. Fever in acute stroke worsens prognosis. A prospective study. *Stroke*. 1995;26:2040-2043.

83. Reith J, Jørgensen HS, Pedersen PM, et al. Body temperature in acute stroke: relation to stroke severity, infarct size, mortality, and outcome. *Lancet*. 1996;347:422-425.

84. De Georgia MA, Krieger DW, Abou-Chebl A, et al. Cooling for acute ischemic brain damage (cool aid): a feasibility trial of endovascular cooling. *Neurology*. 2004;63:312-317.

85. Lyden PD, Hemmen TM, Grotta J, Rapp K, Raman R. Endovascular therapeutic hypothermia for acute ischemic stroke: Ictus 2/3 protocol. *Int J Stroke*. 2014;9:117-125.

67

How Should Status Epilepticus Be Managed?

Jessica Falco-Walter and Thomas P. Bleck

Status epilepticus (SE) is a medical emergency that requires prompt recognition and treatment to prevent serious morbidity and mortality. This chapter discusses the epidemiology, classification, etiologies, management, pathophysiology and prognosis of SE. Evidence-based consensus guidelines and randomized trials are discussed as much as possible. Unfortunately, for the treatment of later stages of SE, there is currently a lack of good data, and this is discussed as well.

EPIDEMIOLOGY

SE is the most severe form of epilepsy and has an annual incidence of 10–41 per 100,000 people.[1] Mortality rates are high: 24–26% in adults and 3–6% in children, with an overall mortality rate of approximately 20%,[2,3] with only approximately half of patients returning to their prior baseline.[4] The longer convulsive SE persists, the higher the mortality;[4] thus the importance of rapid and effective treatment. The evidence for aggressive treatment for nonconvulsive SE is less clear, and many advocate a less aggressive approach than outlined below (which should be applied to convulsive SE).[5]

CLASSIFICATION

The International League Against Epilepsy (ILAE) redefined SE in 2015. It was previously defined as seizures lasting at least 5 minutes and did not account for different types of SE.[6] The 5-minute timing was based predominantly on animal data as well as the fact that most seizures that persist past this time will not abort spontaneously. The current definition of SE is: ongoing seizure activity caused by failure of mechanisms responsible for seizure termination or initiation of mechanisms provoking ongoing seizures causing prolonged seizures after timepoint t1, which can have long-term consequences after timepoint t2, with the values for t1 and t2 differing for different forms of SE[7] (Fig. 67.1). To define the forms of SE there are four axes, and a patient should be defined in as many of these as possible. These axes are: (1) semiology, (2) etiology, (3) electroencephalography (EEG) correlates, and (4) age. Semiology (Axes I) is the most important, and is a clinical definition defined by whether there is motor activity (and if so what type) and impairment of consciousness (or whether consciousness is preserved).

Regarding the motor activity it is defined as: (1) convulsive (tonic-clonic), (2) myoclonic, (3) focal, (4) tonic, or (5) hyperkinetic. In focal seizures/status the epileptiform activity is coming from a focal brain region and produces focal symptoms (e.g., unilateral twitching of a part of a limb, abnormal smell, visual abnormality in a specific portion of the visual field, etc.). While in convulsive SE consciousness is always altered, in focal SE consciousness may be preserved.

Etiology (Axes II) is defined as known and unknown, with the following subcategories under known: (1) acute (e.g., stroke, intoxication, infection, encephalitis), (2) remote (e.g., posttraumatic, postencephalopathic, poststroke), (3) progressive (e.g., brain tumor, progressive myoclonic encephalopathies, dementias), and (4) SE in defined electroclinical syndromes.[7] Different types of SE should be managed differently, and while currently the majority of the literature focuses solely on convulsive SE, these axes provide a framework for research going forward, with EEG playing a major role in non-convulsive SE (NCSE).

When attempting to determine if a patient is in SE, for those having generalized shaking this is usually clear, and treatment should commence immediately. While there are mimics such as psychogenic nonepileptic seizures, this is a diagnosis that is best clarified by EEG monitoring unless features are atypical because delayed treatment can be fatal. Diagnosing NCSE is much more difficult and can only reliably be performed with EEG. NCSE should be considered part of the differential in any patient with altered mental status, particularly of unknown cause. Patients with NCSE may present with a variety of symptoms, including agitation, aggression, confusion, psychosis, or coma. Motor findings may be minimal or absent. Findings to look for include subtle muscle twitching, nystagmus, and eye deviation. A variety of other disorders may present with similar symptoms and signs; however when a patient is not responding to treatment, it is paramount to consider NCSE in the differential.

Besides being defined by type and duration (as described previously), SE may be defined by its response to treatment according to stages: initial (stage I), established (stage II), refractory (stage III), and superrefractory (stage IV) (Fig. 67.2). While these are defined by response to treatment and not time, they do correspond to SE that persists for subsequently longer and longer periods of time at each stage.

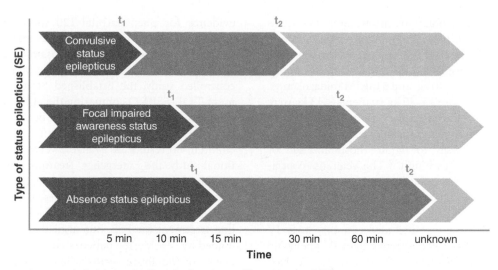

t_1 = onset of status epilepticus for the above different types of SE.

t_2 = point at which permanent intracerebral damage occurs if seizure activity continues to persistt.

Fig. 67.1 Types of SE and time points at which the type of seizure they describe becomes SE and time points at which permanent neuronal injury occurs.

Seizure
- A transient occurrence of signs and/or symptoms caused by abnormal excessive or synchronous neuronal activity in the brain (usually <2 min in duration)

Initial status epilepticus
- Persistent seizure activity for a prolonged period of time (t_1), which varies depending upon the type of status epilepticus (see chart with ILAE definitions of the different types of status epilepticus)

Established status epilepticus
- Persistent seizures after treatment with a benzodiazepine (ex. lorazepam)

Refractory status epilepticus
- Continued seizures after treatment with a benzodiazepine (1st line treatment) as well as a second line agent (ex. levetiracetam, valproic acid, fosphenytoin)

Super refractory status epilepticus
- Continued seizure despite treatment with a benzodiazepine (1st line), 2nd line agent, and an infusion of an anesthetic agent (3rd line agent)

Fig. 67.2 Definitions of seizure and types of SE: initial, established, refractory, and superrefractory.

ETIOLOGIES OF STATUS EPILEPTICUS

Prolonged SE is most often due to encephalitis, massive strokes, or large brain tumors in adults.[8] While these are the most common, nearly any insult to the brain can cause seizures or SE, from metabolic insults (e.g., hypoglycemia, hyponatremia) to hypoxia, global ischemia (e.g., cardiac arrest), ingested toxins or medications (e.g., bupropion), withdrawal (from alcohol, benzodiazepines, and other toxins), meningitis or encephalitis (infectious or autoimmune), sepsis, stroke (hemorrhagic > ischemic), traumatic brain injury, eclampsia, etc. In children, the most common causes are: fever, low AED levels, electrolyte imbalances, inborn errors of metabolism, ingestions, CNS infections, bacteremia,

and structural abnormalities (cortical malformations, trauma, stroke/hemorrhage, tumors, arteriovenous malformations, and hydrocephalus).[9] While SE is common in patients with epilepsy, up to 50% of SE occurs in patients with no prior history of seizures.[10] The underlying etiology and the duration of SE prior to treatment are the most important factors effecting the efficacy of drug therapy.

MANAGEMENT OF STATUS EPILEPTICUS

Initial Treatment

After stabilization of the patient, if seizures persist for more than 5 minutes, then intramuscular (IM) midazolam has been shown to be as effective as obtaining intravenous (IV) access and giving IV lorazepam.[11] The Rapid Anticonvulsant Medication Prior to Arrival Trial (RAMPART) showed this by having paramedics in the field give 10 mg IM midazolam vs. 4 mg IV lorazepam for all patients >40 kg, and 5 mg IM midazolam vs. 2 mg IV lorazepam for those 13–40 kg (patients <13 kg were excluded). On arrival to the emergency room, those who had received IM midazolam were significantly less likely to still be seizing and were less likely to require hospitalization or admission to an intensive care unit.[12] The Veterans Association (VA) Cooperative Trial, published in 1998, compared IV lorazepam 0.1 mg/kg, IV diazepam 0.15 mg/kg followed by phenytoin, IV phenobarbital 15 mg/kg, and IV phenytoin 18 mg/kg (midazolam was not included). In this study IV lorazepam 0.1 mg/kg was more effective than IV phenytoin alone, and equivalent to IV phenobarbital as well as IV diazepam followed by phenytoin. This study did not give lorazepam in 4-mg increments and also did not limit the maximum dose of lorazepam to 8 mg (as the RAMPART study did).[13] From these studies, it is recommended by the Neurocritical Care Society (NCS) that first line treatment is: IM midazolam (10 mg if >40 kg, 5 mg if 13–40 kg), or IV lorazepam (0.1 mg/kg/dose, max 4 mg/dose should be given, may repeat once) or IV midazolam (0.15–0.2 mg/kg/dose, max 10 mg/dose should be given, may repeat once). Diazepam has not performed as well as lorazepam to abort seizures,[14] and has Class IIa, level a evidence, vs. lorazepam and midazolam have Class I, level a evidence.

Simultaneous or even prior (if timing allows) to starting treatment, electrocardiogram (ECG) and labs (electrolytes, hematology, coags/toxicology screen and AED levels if appropriate) should be obtained to look for treatable causes. If a reversible cause is found (e.g., hypoglycemia in a diabetic), this should be treated emergently to prevent further seizures and avoid the need for further anticonvulsant therapy. If seizures persist despite benzodiazepine therapy, the patient is considered in established SE (ESE). Approximately 40% of patients with generalized convulsive SE will be refractory to first line treatment and meet criteria for ESE[13] (Fig. 67.3).

Established Status Epilepticus Treatment

The NCS and the American Epilepsy Society (AES) published clinical practice guidelines most recently in 2012 and 2016, respectively. Unfortunately, there are not yet any class 1, head-to-head, blinded comparisons of different agents for ESE. The American Epilepsy Society recommends administering IV fosphenytoin (20 mg phenytoin equivalents (PE)/kg, max dose of 1500 mg PE), IV valproic acid (40 mg/kg, max: 3000 mg) or IV levetiracetam (60 mg/kg, max 4500 mg), and if none of those three are available, then IV phenobarbital (15 mg/kg). The NCS cites Class IIb, level a evidence for use of IV valproic acid (20–40 mg/kg IV, may give additional 20 mg/kg), Class IIB, level B evidence for IV fosphenytoin (20 mg PE/kg, may give additional 5 mg PE/kg) and midazolam as a continuous infusion, and Class IIb, level C

evidence for phenobarbital (20 mg/kg IV, may give an additional 5–10 mg/kg) and levetiracetam (1000–3000 mg IV). They also discuss dosing for lacosamide and topiramate—although do not recommend these. A recent randomized controlled study, the Established Status Epilepticus Treatment Trial (ESETT) comparing the efficacy of fosphenytoin, levetiracetam, and valproic acid in both adults and children has completed enrollment for adults, but is still enrolling children; no results are available yet.[15] In children, an additional study, the Emergency Treatment with Levetiracetam or Phenytoin in status epilepticus in children (EcLiPSE), is also ongoing.[16] When results of these studies are available we may have more clear recommendations on a preferred first line treatment for ESE, but until then agent choice is best guided by considering patient's comorbidities as well as side effects of the above agents when choosing which agent to administer.

Refractory and Super-Refractory Status Epilepticus Treatment

There is no clear evidence to guide treatment for seizures that continue at this phase, and both the NCS and AES recommended additional agents that were not yet given from the choices discussed for treatment of ESE or moving directly to anesthetic doses of one of the following agents: midazolam, propofol, pentobarbital, or thiopental, with continuous EEG monitoring to evaluate for continued subclinical seizures. If anesthetic agents are chosen the patient will require mechanical ventilation, cardiovascular monitoring, and may need vasopressor agents, owing to vasodilatation and cardiopulmonary depression. Of these agents, midazolam seems to be the safest, with the lowest rate of cardiovascular and metabolic complications; barbiturates are associated with the most complications; propofol causes more hypotension and, rarely may cause metabolic acidosis, rhabdomyolysis, kidney and heart failure.[17] Emergence from anesthesia is significantly quicker with propofol than midazolam, which is quicker than barbiturates. Many alternative agents have been used, with anecdotal success, for refractory SE treatment. These include: ketamine, corticosteroids, inhaled anesthetics, immunomodulation (IVIG or plasma exchange), ketogenic diet, vagus nerve stimulation, hypothermia, electroconvulsive therapy, transcranial magnetic stimulation, and intracranial surgery.[18]

Pathophysiology

Continuous seizures, as occur in SE, cause an increase in cerebral oxygen demand. Blood pressure and cardiac output increase, resulting in increased cerebral blood flow, thereby increasing cerebral blood volume and intracranial pressure. As seizures persist cerebral hypoxia develops. Systemic complications include: hypotension, metabolic acidosis, hyperthermia, rhabdomyolysis, and hypoglycemia. Permanent damage to brain cells occurs after varying amounts of time for different types of SE (after time point t2 as discussed

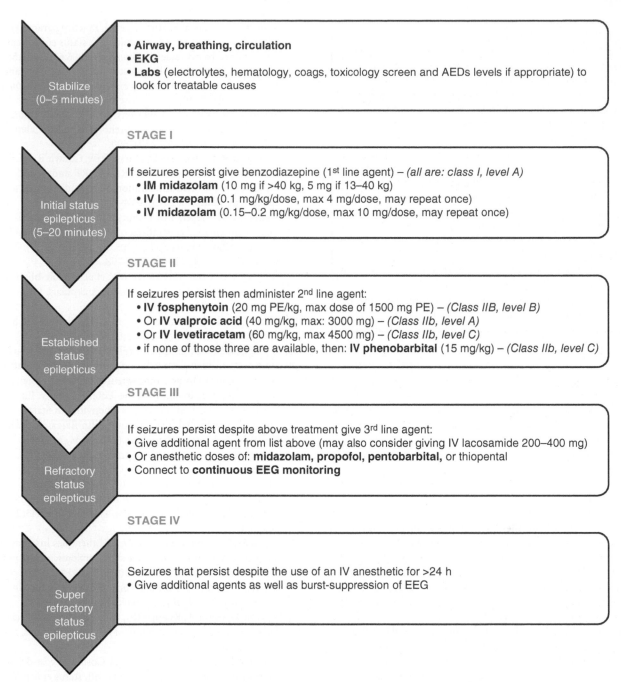

Stabilize (0–5 minutes)
- **Airway, breathing, circulation**
- **EKG**
- **Labs** (electrolytes, hematology, coags, toxicology screen and AEDs levels if appropriate) to look for treatable causes

STAGE I

Initial status epilepticus (5–20 minutes)

If seizures persist give benzodiazepine (1st line agent) – *(all are: class I, level A)*
- **IM midazolam** (10 mg if >40 kg, 5 mg if 13–40 kg)
- **IV lorazepam** (0.1 mg/kg/dose, max 4 mg/dose, may repeat once)
- **IV midazolam** (0.15–0.2 mg/kg/dose, max 10 mg/dose, may repeat once)

STAGE II

Established status epilepticus

If seizures persist then administer 2nd line agent:
- **IV fosphenytoin** (20 mg PE/kg, max dose of 1500 mg PE) – *(Class IIB, level B)*
- Or **IV valproic acid** (40 mg/kg, max: 3000 mg) – *(Class IIb, level A)*
- Or **IV levetiracetam** (60 mg/kg, max 4500 mg) – *(Class IIb, level C)*
- if none of those three are available, then: **IV phenobarbital** (15 mg/kg) – *(Class IIb, level C)*

STAGE III

Refractory status epilepticus

If seizures persist despite above treatment give 3rd line agent:
- Give additional agent from list above (may also consider giving IV lacosamide 200–400 mg)
- Or anesthetic doses of: **midazolam, propofol, pentobarbital,** or thiopental
- Connect to **continuous EEG monitoring**

STAGE IV

Super refractory status epilepticus

Seizures that persist despite the use of an IV anesthetic for >24 h
- Give additional agents as well as burst-suppression of EEG

Fig. 67.3 Recommended Medical Management of SE as it Progresses from Stage I to IV.

previously), and for convulsive SE this is believed to be after approximately 30 minutes (these data are derived from animal studies).

Additionally, resistance develops to medications the longer the seizures persist. This may be caused by internalization of GABA$_A$ receptors (inhibitory), or increased numbers of NMDA and AMPA receptors (both excitatory) along the synaptic membrane, or both. Inflammatory cytokines may cause upregulation of drug-efflux transporters such as P-glycoprotein—but no data have shown

that these mechanisms effect the efficacy of antiseizure medications.[19]

Prognosis

The sooner SE is treated, the better the outcome. Studies have shown that earlier treatment is associated with more rapid cessation of seizures, fewer medications, and lower morbidity and mortality.[4,20] Given the high cost of refractory SE, earlier treatment also likely reduces overall medical costs.[21]

REFERENCES

1. Shorvon S. *Status Epilepticus: Its Clinical Features and Treatment in Children and Adults.* Cambridge, UK: Cambridge University Press; 1994:27.
2. Jallon P. Mortality in patients with epilepsy. *Curr Opin Neurol.* 2004;17:141-146.
3. Logroscino G, Hesdorffer DC, Cascino G, et al. Mortality after a first episode of status epilepticus in the United States and Europe. *Epilepsia.* 2005;46:46-48.
4. Legriel S, Azoulay E, Resche-Rigon M, et al. Functional outcome after convulsive status epilepticus. *Crit Care Med.* 2010;38: 2295-2303.
5. Wasim M, Husain AM. Non-convulsive seizure control in the intensive care unit. *Curr Treat Options Neurol.* 2015;17:340.
6. Working Group on Status Epilepticus. Treatment of convulsive status epilepticus. *JAMA.* 1993;270(7):854-859.
7. Trinka E, Cock H, Rossetti AO, et al. A definition and classification of status epilepticus—Report of the ILAE Task Force on Classification of Status Epilepticus. *Epilepsia.* 2015;56:1515-1523.
8. Abend NS, Bearden D, Helbig I, et al. Status epilepticus and refractory status epilepticus management. *Semin Pediatr Neurol.* 2014;21:263-274.
9. Riviello Jr JJ, Ashwal S, Hirtz D, et al. Practice parameter: Diagnostic assessment of the child with status epilepticus (an evidence-based review). *Neurology.* 2006;67:1542-1550.
10. Neligan A, Shorvon SD. Prognostic factors, morbidity and mortality in tonic clonic status epilepticus: a review. *Epilepsy Res.* 2011;93(1):1-10.
11. Silbergleit R, Durkalski V, Lowenstein D, et al. Intramuscular versus intravenous therapy for prehospital status epilepticus. *N Engl J Med.* 2012;366(7):591-600.
12. Silbergleit R, Lowenstein D, Durkalski V, Conwit R; NETT Investigators. Lessons from the RAMPART study—and which is the best route of administration of benzodiazepines in status epilepticus. *Epilepsia.* 2013;54:74-77.
13. Treiman DM, Meyers PD, Walton NY, et al. A comparison of four treatments for generalized convulsive status epilepticus. Veterans Affairs Status Epilepticus Cooperative Study Group. *N Engl J Med.* 1998;339(12):792-798.
14. Leppik IE, Derivan AT, Homan RW, et al. Double-blind study of lorazepam and diazepam in status epilepticus. *JAMA.* 1983; 249(11):1452-1454.
15. Bleck T, Cock H, Chamberlain J, et al. The Established Status Epilepticus Trial. *Epilepsia.* 2013;54:89-92.
16. A pragmatic randomized controlled trial of intravenous levetiracetam *versus* intravenous phenytoin in terminating acute, prolonged tonic clonic seizures including convulsive status epilepticus in children, the 'EcLiPSE' Study: Emergency Treatment with Levetiracetam or Phenytoin in Status Epilepticus. National Institute for Health Research (NHS). NIHR HTA Reference Number: 12/127/134. Available at: http://www.nets.nihr.ac.uk/projects/hta/12127134. Accessed October 11, 2018.
17. Claassen J, Hirsch LJ, Emerson RG, Mayer SA. Treatment of refractory status epilepticus with pentobarbital, propofol, or midazolam: a systematic review. *Epilepsia.* 2002;43(2): 146-153.
18. Ferlisi M, Shorvon S. The outcome of therapies in refractory and super-refractory convulsive status epilepticus and recommendations for therapy. *Brain.* 2012;135:2314-2328.
19. Löscher W. Molecular mechanisms of drug resistance in status epilepticus. *Epilepsia.* 2009;50(Suppl. 8):19-21.
20. Madžar D, Geyer A, Knappe RU, et al. Association of seizure duration and outcome in refractory status epilepticus. *J Neurol.* 2016;263:485-491.
21. Kortland LM, Alfter A, Bähr O, et al. Costs and cost-driving factors for acute treatment of adults with status epilepticus: a multicenter cohort study from Germany. *Epilepsia.* 2016;57(12): 2056-2066.

68

When and How Should I Feed the Critically Ill Patient?

Patrick J. Neligan

INTRODUCTION

Anorexia is a near-universal accompaniment to acute illness. Prolonged fasting is harmful, due to rapid loss of lean body mass and depletion of physiologic reserves. The majority of critically ill patients are unable to meet their caloric and nutritional needs. There is a correlation between adequacy of critical care nutrition and outcomes,[1] particularly for high-risk, low body mass index (BMI) patients.[2] Consequently, some form of dietary support is necessary. Critical illness is a multiphasic dysnutritional state that probably requires patient-specific assessment and therapy. Debate persists regarding the timing, content, and goals of exogenous feeding of the critically ill. This chapter reviews recent literature on early nutrition in the intensive care unit (ICU).

METABOLISM: CRITICAL ILLNESS VERSUS STARVATION

Starvation is characterized by initial use of glycogen, fat mobilization, and ketosis and preservation of skeletal and visceral protein until fat stores have been exhausted. Physicians are most likely to encounter this scenario in patients with advanced cancer, cachexia, psychiatric eating disorders or substance abuse problems. Starvation differs from malnutrition, in which calorie intake may be sufficient but where intake of some required dietary component is inadequate. Macronutrient deficiency usually involves inadequate protein intake (sometimes called kwashiorkor) and, perhaps, essential fatty acids, while micronutrient deficiency involves vitamins or minerals. The critically ill starved or malnourished patient[3,4] is particularly vulnerable to both the intense hypercatabolic effects of critical illness[5] and the concomitant risk of refeeding syndrome (Table 68.1).[6]

Injury, infection, or surgery activate adaptive homeostatic mechanisms. The initial response assures adequate substrate delivery to organs essential for survival, notably the heart and brain. This phase is followed by activation of inflammation

and tissue repair and, ultimately, recovery.[5] In most forms of acute critical illness, adaptive mechanisms are inadequate and intervention is required. Inadequate perfusion, i.e., shock, requires intervention with fluids and perhaps vasopressors, prolonging the initial phase of the normal response. Abnormalities in the inflammatory phase may be excessive, inadequate or simply inappropriate; in some cases (e.g., sepsis), all three forms may occur concurrently. This inflammatory process is modulated by immune (including cytokine-mediated), neural and endocrine mechanisms.[5,7] All three are energy-requiring activities with an initial dependence on glucose and glutamine metabolism, which are required by white blood cells and preferred by neurons. In addition, tissue repair requires substrate in the form of amino acids for protein synthesis. Once glycogen is depleted, emphasis shifts to hepatic gluconeogenesis, primarily from alanine and glutamine, and recycling of lactate (the Cori cycle). The need for protein for repair and energy leads to breakdown of skeletal muscle by a process recently termed "autophagy"[5,8–10] Prolonged starvation overwhelms autophagy and may contribute to chronic critical illness syndrome.[10,11]

The cumulative impact of the catabolic response to critical illness is a devastating loss of lean body mass (LBM)—up to 20% of skeletal muscle is lost (~1 kg/day) within 10 days of admission to the ICU.

ASSESSMENT OF NUTRITIONAL STATUS

While tools such as anthropometrics and visceral protein status have been used to assess nutritional status, they have not been appropriately validated in critically ill patients. At the onset of critical illness, patients may be obese/overweight, well nourished, malnourished or undernourished (Fig. 68.1). Importantly, malnutrition may exist despite normal or elevated BMI and patients may be malnourished for micronutrients or macronutrients (see Fig. 68.1). Undernourished and malnourished patients have very poor critical care outcomes.[2,12] Conversely, recent data suggest that obesity may be

TABLE 68.1	Signs of Refeeding Syndrome.
System	Impact
Metabolic	Hypophosphatemia
	Hypocalcemia
	Hypomagnesemia
	Vitamin deficiency (thiamine)
	Hyponatremia
Neurological	Confusion
	Delirium
	Convulsions
	Coma
	Cranial nerve palsy
	Korsakoff's psychosis
	Wernicke's encephalopathy
	Motor and sensory neuropathy
Neuromuscular	Tetany/spasm
	Tremors/muscle weakness
	Paresthesia
Respiratory	Hypercarbia (increased CO_2 production)
	Respiratory failure
Cardiovascular	Cardiac arrhythmias
	Acute heart failure
Renal	Rhabdomyolysis
	Metabolic acidosis
	Acute kidney injury
	Water overload - peripheral edema
Hematopoietic	Bone marrow failure
	Pancytopenia

ventilators found poor correlation with indirect calorimetry.[18,19] While many practitioners recommend starting critically ill patients on a regimen of 25 kcal/kg/day, including 1.2–2 g/kg of protein, this approach has not been subjected to rigorous evaluation[14].

Patients with pre-existing malnutrition are at risk for refeeding syndrome, which occurs when uncontrolled nutrition is restored to undernourished patients who have adapted to very low energy intake.[6] It is associated with rapid transfer of electrolytes—principally phosphate (which falls by >30% from baseline), magnesium and calcium into cells along with depletion in cofactors, such as thiamine. The syndrome is characterized by dramatic fluid shifts that may precipitate pulmonary edema and cardiac dysfunction secondary to magnesium and phosphate depletion. The dramatic increase in substrate utilization can increase CO_2 production, further compromising ventilation. Clinical manifestations of refeeding syndrome are summarized in Table 68.1. While it has been recommended that feeding at-risk patients be initiated at 10 kcal/kg/day and gradually increased, this approach is not evidence based (Fig. 68.2).

ENTERAL NUTRITION OR PARENTERAL NUTRITION

Early enteral nutrition in acute critical illness has been administered in the hope of attenuating loss of LBM, preserving gut integrity and preventing secondary complications. In postsurgical patients, the preponderance of evidence indicates that early enteral nutrition is associated with shorter hospital stays.[20] These findings may not, however, translate to the critically ill. In these patients, technical difficulties, positioning and gastrointestinal (GI)/intra-abdominal pathobiology may limit the initiation and acceleration of GI feeding. Despite a lack of evidence, some clinicians avoid administration of enteral nutrition to patients on vasopressor therapy due to concerns about mesenteric ischemia.[14] It would seem that use of parenteral nutrition would facilitate meeting nutritional goals in a timely manner. Early studies on small numbers of patients favored the use of enteral nutrition, noting a lower incidence of infectious complications, principally catheter-related bloodstream infections (CLABSI), and shorter ICU length of stay.[21] Recent emphasis on prevention of CLABSI

protective in sepsis.[13] Actual determination of nutritional status may, however, be difficult. Two malnutrition scoring systems, NUTRIC and NRS 2002, have been recommended for use in the critically ill in the United States,[14] but not in Europe.[15] Importantly, neither has been thoroughly validated. Similarly, calculation of nutritional requirements in the critically ill is problematic. Use of formulae derived and validated in patients who are not critically ill underestimates requirements.[16,17] Determination of resting energy expenditure from measurements of oxygen consumption (VO_2) and carbon dioxide production (VCO_2) involves specialized equipment and does not assess protein requirements. A study comparing measurements of VO_2 and VCO_2 by modern

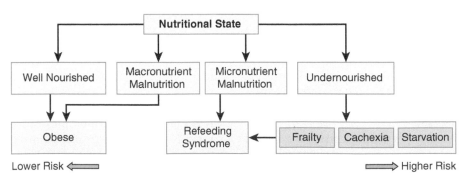

Fig. 68.1 Assessment of Nutritional Status.

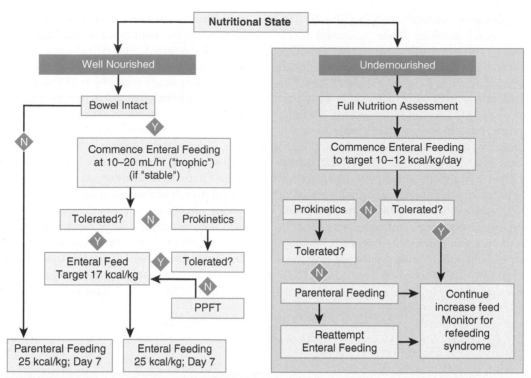

Fig. 68.2 A Suggested Approach to Feeding Critically Ill Patients. *Y,* yes; *N,* No; *PPFT,* postpyloric feeding tube. "Tolerated" indicates that the patient is not vomiting, regurgitating or does not have gastric residual volumes >500 mL. "Stable" is a clinical decision—patients should not be enterally fed if receiving rapidly escalating doses of vasopressors, are undergoing massive resuscitation, or in the early stage of mechanical support of the cardiovascular system.

and other infectious complications reduced the frequency of these problems.[22,23] However, there remained a need for direct evidence.

CALORIES was a large publicly funded study of 2400 patients with unplanned (i.e., not following elective surgery) admission to 33 ICUs in England.[24] Patients were randomized to either early enteral nutrition or early parenteral nutrition; the median time for commencement of support was <24 hours in both groups. The feeding strategy was continued for 5 days following admission or until the patient transitioned to oral feeding. Energy targets were set at 25 kcal per kilogram of actual body weight per day. Mortality at 30 days (33.1% early parenteral nutrition group vs. 34.2% in the early enteral nutrition group; $P = .57$) or 90 days (37.3% early parenteral nutrition vs. 39.1% early enteral nutrition, $P = .4$) was similar, as was the incidence of infectious complications (0.22% early parenteral nutrition vs. 0.21% early enteral nutrition; $P = .72$). Importantly, most patients in both groups failed to meet their nutritional targets.

NUTRIREA-2, the largest clinical trial of critically ill patients that compared early enteral nutrition and early parenteral nutrition, was conducted in 44 French ICUs and included 2410 patients.[25] Patients were randomized within 24 hours of requiring mechanical ventilation or ICU admission. Vasopressor or inotrope therapy was a recruitment requirement and most of the patients received norepinephrine; only 2% received dobutamine alone. Parenteral nutrition was continued for 7 days or until vasopressor therapy was discontinued. The

trial was stopped early because no differences were detected at the first interim analysis, making it inappropriate to draw conclusions.

In summary, there is no evidence supporting the hypothesis that use of either early enteral or early parenteral nutrition confers an outcome benefit in critical illness

EARLY OR LATE PARENTERAL NUTRITION (IN PATIENTS UNSUITABLE FOR /INTOLERANT OF ENTERAL NUTRITION)

The majority of patients can tolerate a short period of fasting but experts suggest that nutritional therapy be initiated after 48 hours in intensive care.[15] In general, oral or enteral nutrition is preferred because it is simpler and less expensive. In patients who are mechanically ventilated or unwilling/unable to eat, feeding via nasoenteral tube can be considered despite an absence of supporting evidence. However, clinicians may encounter patients who cannot receive or tolerate EF. This situation requires choice from among several less-than-ideal approaches.

Despite viewing the same data, international guideline committees in Europe and North America delivered different recommendations for initiation of parenteral nutrition in patients in whom enteral nutrition is not an option. The European Society of Parenteral Nutrition (ESPEN) guidelines recommended parenteral nutrition within 2 days of ICU admission.[26] Conversely, the North American groups recommended hypocaloric enteral nutrition, if tolerated, and delaying parenteral nutrition ("late parenteral nutrition") for 7 days.[27,28] To resolve this controversy, EPaNIC, a government-funded, multicentre randomized controlled trial (RCT) was conducted in Belgium (Table 68.2).[29] The investigators randomized 4640 patients to either early parenteral nutrition ($n = 2312$), within 48 hours of ICU admission, or late parenteral nutrition ($n = 2328$), initiated on day 8 or later. A protocol for enteral nutrition was also applied to all patients. Thus, EPaNIC compared hypocaloric enteral nutrition + early parenteral nutrition to hypocaloric enteral nutrition + late parenteral nutrition. The primary endpoint of EPaNic was the number of days spent in the ICU before being judged suitable for discharge. Outcomes were better in the late parenteral nutrition cohort: there was a 3.5% absolute increase in the likelihood of being discharged alive from the ICU after 8 days ($P = .04$). This group also had fewer ICU infections (22.8 vs. 26.2%, $P = .008$), a lower incidence of

cholestasis, spent fewer days on mechanical ventilation and on renal replacement therapy. No difference in 90-day mortality was detected. Interestingly, the subgroup of patients who could not be given enteral nutrients because of anatomical contraindications ($n = 517$)—that is, the group that would have been predicted to benefit maximally from parenteral nutrition—had worse than average outcomes.

These data are consistent with the Veteran's Administration of parenteral nutrition in high-risk patients undergoing major surgery.[30] In that study, patients were randomized to receive parenteral nutrition started preoperatively and continued postop or parenteral nutrition first started 3 days following surgery. Outcomes were indistinguishable in patients who were initially mildly or moderately malnourished; benefit was reported only in a tiny subgroup of patients who were severely malnourished prior to surgery.[31]

In summary, data suggest that parenteral nutrition can be withheld for up to 7 days in previously well-nourished

TABLE 68.2 Major Clinical Trials of Critical Care Nutrition (2010–2018).

Study	Number	Year	Question	Outcome	Inx Group	Control Group	P value
EPaNIC[29]	4640	2011	Early (full calorie) feeding with PN within 48 h vs. with HEN & LPN (day 8)	Discharge alive from ICU	71.7% (EEN + EPN)	75.2%[a] (HEN + LPN)	.04
CALORIES[24]	2400	2014	EPN vs. EEN for the first 5 days	30-day mortality	33% (EPN)	34.2% (EEN)	.57
NUTRIREA-2[25]	2410	2018	EPN vs. EEN	28-day mortality	35% (EPN)	37% (EEN)	.33
EARLY PN[32]	1372	2013	EPN (within 24 h) vs. HEN or no feeding for 7 days	60-day mortality	21.5% (EPN)	22.8% (EN or no feed)	.6
NIH EN trial[42]	200	2011	TF vs. IEN in ARDS (2003–2009)	Ventilator-free days by day 28	23 days (TF)	23 days (IEN)	.9
EDEN[43]	1000	2012	TF vs. IEN in ARDS (2008–2011)	Ventilator-free days by day 28	14.9 days (TF)	15 days (IEN)	.89
PermiT[44]	894	2015	HEN vs. IEN	90-day mortality	27.2% (HEN)	28.9% (IEN)	.29
TARGET[45]	3967	2018	1.5 kcal/mL (ED-EF) vs. 1.9 kcal/mL (S-EF)	90-day mortality	26.8% (early, dense EF)	25.7% (S-EF)	.41
EAT-ICU[46]	203	2017	Early IEN – EN ± PN vs. standard nutrition (target 25 kcal/kg)	Physical component summary score of SF-36 at 6 months	22.9 EGDN	23 SEN	.99
PYTHON[50]	208	2014	EEN (within 24 h) vs. delayed (after 72 h) EN in acute pancreatitis	6-month mortality	11% EEN	7% DEN	.033

[a]Better outcome.
ARDS, acute respiratory distress syndrome; *DEN*, delayed enteral nutrition (EN delayed until ≥72 h after admission); *ED-EF*, energy dense enteral feed/formula (1.5 kcal/mL enteral feed); *EEN*, early enteral nutrition (commenced within 24 h of ICU admission); *EF*, enteral feeding; *EGDN*, early goal-directed nutrition (PN delivered in addition to EN to achieve nutritional goal); *EN*, enteral nutrition; *EPN*, early parenteral nutrition (delivered within 24 h of ICU admission); *HEN*, hypocaloric enteral nutrition (deliberately administering <70% of patient's nutritional goals); *IEN*, isocaloric enteral nutrition (administering 100% of patient's nutritional goals); *LPN*, late parenteral nutrition (delivered 7 days or more after ICU admission); *PN*, parenteral (intravenous) nutrition; *S-EF*, standard enteral feed/formula (1.0 kcal/mL enteral feed); *TF*, trophic feeds (delivering ≤20 mL/h of enteral feed).

patients admitted to the ICU following surgery. The benefits of early parenteral nutrition in malnourished or undernourished patients in critical care, or of hypocaloric parenteral nutrition, are unknown.

PARENTERAL NUTRITION VERSUS LIMITED OR NO NUTRITION

The long-held assumption that withholding nutrition would be associated with worse outcomes in critical illness was not finally tested until the 2010s. Doig and colleagues performed a multicenter RCT of 1372 patients in 31 hospitals in Australia and New Zealand over 5 years (2006–2011: the Early-PN Trial).[32] Patients enrolled had relative contraindications to early enteral nutrition and were expected to remain in the ICU longer than 2 days. Most of the participants were surgical patients; almost 50% of the operations were elective. Patients were randomized to standard care (29.2% received enteral nutrition, 27.3% received parenteral nutrition, and 40.8% were not fed), usually started on postop day 2, or to early enteral nutrition, started within 1 hour of enrolment. Patients in the latter group received significantly more calories and protein during the first 7 days. No differences in 60-day mortality (22.8% for standard care vs. 21.5% for early parenteral nutrition; $P = .60$) or infection rates were detected. Early parenteral nutrition patients spent marginally less time on mechanical ventilation and may have retained more fat and lean tissue.

In summary, this study was unable to demonstrate the utility of early parenteral nutrition to caloric goal compared with delayed nutrition.

ENTERAL FEEDING—STOMACH OR POSTPYLORIC

Placement of a gastric feeding tube (usually nasogastric [NG]) is significantly easier and more reliable than achieving postpyloric feeding access. This results in earlier initiation of enteral feeds. NG feeding is tolerated by the majority of patients. However, it has been speculated that gastroparesis or large gastric residual volumes may limit nutritional intake in some patients. Moreover, a variety of systematic reviews have suggested that postpyloric feeding may achieve the patients nutritional needs more rapidly than gastric feeding, while also limiting the risk of aspiration and pneumonia.[14,15,33] and that patients with greater severity of illness are more likely to achieve their nutritional goals when fed directly into the small bowel.[34]

The largest multicenter RCT of critically ill patients with large gastric residuals was published by Davies et al in 2012.[35] Patients were randomized to postpyloric vs. continued gastric feeding. Despite rapid placement of the postpyloric feeding tube, no difference in targeted energy intake (roughly 71% for both groups), vomiting, aspiration, ventilator-associated pneumonia, diarrhea or mortality could be identified. There was a slight increase in the incidence of minor GI bleeding in the postpyloric feeding tube group (13 vs. 3%; $P = .02$).[35]

Thus such data as exist do not favor use of either route over the other.

ENTERAL FEEDING—GASTRIC RESIDUAL VOLUME

Previous guidelines have recommended monitoring the absorption of enteral feeds by intermittently checking gastric residual volumes,[36] with some arbitrary level—150 mL, 250 mL, 500 mL, etc.—designated as excessive.[37] NUTRIREA-1, a French multicentre RCT randomized 452 patients who were mechanically ventilated to either an approach that checked gastric residual volumes (control) or one that did not (intervention).[38] A residual volume of >250 mL or overt vomiting was considered to indicate intolerance in the control group. Vomiting alone indicated intolerance in the intervention group. The study was unable to demonstrate a difference in the incidence of ventilator-associated pneumonia diagnosed within 90 days, the duration of ICU stay, or of mechanical ventilation, infection rate, or mortality.

In summary, it is probably unnecessary and unhelpful to routinely check gastric residual volumes.

ENTERAL FEEDING—BOLUS OR CONTINUOUS

Enteral nutrition may be delivered by intermittent infusion, bolus, cyclically or continuously. Generally, postpyloric or jejunal feeding is administered continuously, but the stomach may be "bloused." Studies comparing the different approaches tend to be small with weak endpoints, and the data are insufficient to recommend any specific approach.

DELIBERATE UNDERFEEDING (HYPOCALERIC) AND TROPHIC FEEDING

Acute illness is associated with anorexia.[11] Although the need for nutrition is widely acknowledged, the timing is unclear and deliberately feeding patients to meet all of their presumed energy requirements may undermine adaptive responses such as autophagy.[11] INTACT, a trial that randomized patients to receive either aggressively targeted energy requirements or standard care, was stopped early due to increased mortality in the investigation group.[39] A posthoc analysis suggested that the negative impact was due to high early (<7 days) energy intake.[40] These findings suggest that early isocaloric feeding is neither necessary nor desirable.

Deliberately administering only 60–70% of calculated energy requirements, either with or without a full protein load, is referred to as hypocaloric nutrition. "Trophic" feeding involves low-volume enteral nutrition that is targeted at feeding only the bowel mucosa—continued for 4 or 5 days—and then gradually increased (Fig. 68.3). A recent review indicates that outcomes are similar with either approach.[41] While patients fed using low-level nutrition received less calories,[42–46] the studies could not demonstrate an effect on mortality,[42–46] duration of mechanical ventilation,[42] ICU or hospital length of stay,[42,44–46] or ventilator free day.[43] Some

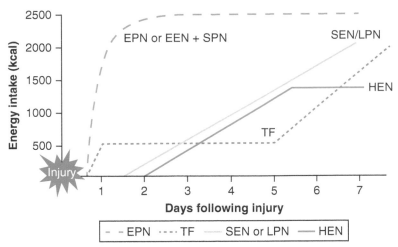

Fig. 68.3 Nutritional intake over the first 7 days of critical illness, illustrating the various strategies used in clinical trials.

studies reported feeding intolerance in patients receiving feedings to meet full calculated energy requirements.[43] Studies comparing hypocaloric or trophic feeding to no feeding need to be performed. Studies examining the need for meeting calculated protein requirements are also required.[1,47]

Thus while it might seem that hypocaloric feeding is a reasonable approach in early critical illness, available data do not justify this conclusion. The role of protein during this phase also remains unclear. Indeed, a large international observational trial suggested that greater protein intake over the duration of ICU stay was associated with improved outcomes.[1]

NUTRITION IN ACUTE PANCREATITIS

Acute pancreatitis is a common diagnosis for critical care admission. The optimal feeding strategy (oral, NG, nasoenteral feeding, parenteral) has long been controversial. A 2010 meta-analysis of 8 trials, including 348 patients, of parenteral vs. enteral nutrition in pancreatitis suggested that the former was associated with increased risk of death, multiorgan failure, sepsis, the need for surgery, and prolonged hospital stay.[48] Enteral nutrition is believed to promote GI motility, prevent bacterial overgrowth, and preserve barrier integrity. Many centers use early enteral nutrition in the belief that it will "rouse the bowel."[49] Conversely, enteral nutrition is uncomfortable for patients and often complicated by delivery issues that include tube placement and obstruction requiring manipulation or even replacement. The PYTHON (Pancreatitis, Very Early Compared with Selective Delayed Start of Enteral Feeding) trial was designed to look at early enteral nutrition vs. delayed or "on demand" feeding in 208 severely ill (APACHE II score of ≥ 8, mean of 11) patients with acute pancreatitis at 19 Dutch hospitals.[50] The study, which compared early NG feeding with nutrition delayed 72 hours, did not demonstrate differences in major infection (pneumonia, pancreatic necrosis or pseudocyst, bloodstream infections, etc., 25% EG vs. 26% OD; *P* = .87) or mortality at 6 months

(11% ED vs. 7% OD; *P* = .33).[50] Importantly, 69% of the patients randomized to a delayed oral diet tolerated the approach without the need for an EF tube. Criticisms of this study have centered around the use of nasojejunal feeding, the fact that patient outcomes were better than expected, and that the study was probably underpowered.

In summary, enteral nutrition is well-tolerated in patients with acute pancreatitis, but the preferred site of delivery or time of initiation is unknown.

> **AUTHORS' RECOMMENDATIONS**
> - The principal purpose of critical care nutrition is to arrest the loss of lean body mass and to maintain and restore energy-dependent homeostatic functions.
> - There is no well-validated tool to evaluate the nutritional status of the critically ill patient. Therefore most recommendations reflect expert opinion based on clinical evaluation of nutritional status.
> - Evidence does not demonstrate a benefit to meeting nutritional goals early in the course of critical illness. Evidence does, however, indicate that parenteral nutrition can be withheld for 7 days in previously well-nourished patients admitted to the ICU following surgery or with critical illness.
> - There appears to be no benefit in using either enteral or parenteral nutrition early in critical illness.
> - Outcome differences associated with either early or late initiation of nutritional support have not been identified.
> - Parenteral nutrition is not associated with increased infection risk. Enteral nutrition is associated with GI complications, principally vomiting, that are likely to be clinically insignificant.
> - Enteral nutrition is safe to administer to patients receiving vasoactive drugs after the initial shock period.
> - The addition of supplemental parenteral nutrition to enteral nutrition to increase caloric intake has not been shown to improve outcomes in early critical illness. There may be a benefit to supplemental parenteral nutrition in later-stage

critical illness in patients who cannot achieve caloric goals with enteral nutrition alone.

- Evidence does not support a need for postpyloric enteral access in most patients. It also does not support routine determination of gastric residual volumes.
- Evidence demonstrates that enteral nutrition is superior to parenteral nutrition in patients with acute pancreatitis. Appropriate timing of initiation is unclear, but it is unnecessary to feed within 24 hours of diagnosis.

REFERENCES

1. Compher C, Chittams J, Sammarco T, Nicolo M, Heyland DK. Greater protein and energy intake may be associated with improved mortality in higher risk critically ill patients: a multicenter, multinational observational study. *Crit Care Med.* 2017;45(2):156-163.

2. Compher C, Chittams J, Sammarco T, Higashibeppu N, Higashiguchi T, Heyland DK. Greater nutrient intake is associated with lower mortality in Western and Eastern critically ill patients with low BMI: a multicenter, multinational observational study. *JPEN J Parenter Enteral Nutr.* 2019;43(1):63-69.

3. Mullen JT, Moorman DW, Davenport DL. The obesity paradox: body mass index and outcomes in patients undergoing nonbariatric general surgery. *Ann Surg.* 2009;250(1):166-172.

4. Lew CCH, Yandell R, Fraser RJL, Chua AP, Chong MFF, Miller M. Association between malnutrition and clinical outcomes in the intensive care unit: a systematic review. *JPEN J Parenter Enteral Nutr.* 2017;41(5):744-758.

5. Preiser JC, Ichai C, Orban JC, Groeneveld AB. Metabolic response to the stress of critical illness. *Br J Anaesth.* 2014;113(6):945-954.

6. van Zanten AR. Nutritional support and refeeding syndrome in critical illness. *Lancet Respir Med.* 2015;3(12):904-905.

7. Ingels C, Gunst J, Van den Berghe G. Endocrine and metabolic alterations in sepsis and implications for treatment. *Crit Care Clin.* 2018;34(1):81-96.

8. Plank LD, Hill GL. Similarity of changes in body composition in intensive care patients following severe sepsis or major blunt injury. *Ann N Y Acad.Sci.* 2000;904:592-602.

9. Crouser ED. Autophagy, the first step towards recovery from critical illness. *Crit Care Med.* 2013;41(1):358-359.

10. Gunst J. Recovery from critical illness-induced organ failure: the role of autophagy. *Crit Care.* 2017;21(1):209.

11. Rosenthal MD, Carrott P, Moore FA. Autophagy: should it play a role in ICU management? *Curr Opin Crit Care.* 2018;24(2):112-117.

12. Mogensen KM, Robinson MK, Casey JD, et al. Nutritional status and mortality in the critically ill. *Crit Care Med.* 2015;43(12):2605-2615.

13. Pepper DJ, Demirkale CY, Sun J, et al. Does obesity protect against death in sepsis? A retrospective cohort study of 55,038 adult patients. *Crit Care Med.* 2019;47(5):643-650.

14. McClave SA, Taylor BE, Martindale RG, et al. Guidelines for the provision and assessment of nutrition support therapy in the adult critically ill patient: Society of Critical Care Medicine (SCCM) and American Society for Parenteral and Enteral Nutrition (A.S.P.E.N.). *JPEN J Parenter Enteral Nutr.* 2016; 40(2):159-211.

15. Singer P, Blaser AR, Berger MM, et al. ESPEN guideline on clinical nutrition in the intensive care unit. *Clin Nutr.* 2019; 38(1):48-79.

16. Subramaniam A, McPhee M, Nagappan R. Predicting energy expenditure in sepsis: Harris-Benedict and Schofield equations versus the Weir derivation. *Crit Care Resusc.* 2012;14(3):202-210.

17. Reid CL. Poor agreement between continuous measurements of energy expenditure and routinely used prediction equations in intensive care unit patients. *Clin Nutr.* 2007;26(5):649-657.

18. Kagan I, Zusman O, Bendavid I, Theilla M, Cohen J, Singer P. Validation of carbon dioxide production (VCO_2) as a tool to calculate resting energy expenditure (REE) in mechanically ventilated critically ill patients: a retrospective observational study. *Crit Care.* 2018;22(1):186.

19. Singer P, Anbar R, Cohen J, et al. The tight calorie control study (TICACOS): a prospective, randomized, controlled pilot study of nutritional support in critically ill patients. *Intensive Care Med.* 2011;37(4):601-609.

20. Herbert G, Perry R, Andersen HK, et al. Early enteral nutrition within 24 hours of lower gastrointestinal surgery versus later commencement for length of hospital stay and postoperative complications. *Cochrane Database Syst Rev.* 2018;10:CD004080.

21. Elke G, van Zanten AR, Lemieux M, et al. Enteral versus parenteral nutrition in critically ill patients: an updated systematic review and meta-analysis of randomized controlled trials. *Crit Care.* 2016;20(1):117.

22. Palomar M, Álvarez-Lerma F, Riera A, et al. Impact of a national multimodal intervention to prevent catheter-related bloodstream infection in the ICU: the Spanish experience. *Crit Care Med.* 2013;41(10):2364-2372.

23. Pronovost P, Needham D, Berenholtz S, et al. An intervention to decrease catheter-related bloodstream infections in the ICU. *N Engl J Med.* 2006;355(26):2725-2732.

24. Harvey SE, Parrott F, Harrison DA, et al. Trial of the route of early nutritional support in critically ill adults. *N Engl J Med.* 2014;371(18):1673-1684.

25. Reignier J, Boisramé-Helms J, Brisard L, et al. Enteral versus parenteral early nutrition in ventilated adults with shock: a randomised, controlled, multicentre, open-label, parallel-group study (NUTRIREA-2). *Lancet.* 2018;391(10116):133-143.

26. Singer P, Berger MM, Van den Berghe G, et al. ESPEN guidelines on parenteral nutrition: intensive care. *Clin Nutr.* 2009; 28(4):387-400.

27. Heyland DK, Dhaliwal R, Drover JW, Gramlich L, Dodek P; Canadian Critical Care Clinical Practice Guidelines Committee. Canadian clinical practice guidelines for nutrition support in mechanically ventilated, critically ill adult patients. *JPEN J Parenter Enteral Nutr.* 2003;27(5):355-373.

28. Martindale RG, McClave SA, Vanek VW, et al. Guidelines for the provision and assessment of nutrition support therapy in the adult critically ill patient: Society of Critical Care Medicine and American Society for Parenteral and Enteral Nutrition: Executive Summary. *Crit Care Med.* 2009;37(5):1757-1761.

29. Casaer MP, Mesotten D, Hermans G, et al. Early versus late parenteral nutrition in critically ill adults. *N Engl J Med.* 2011;365(6):506-517.

30. Veterans Affairs Total Parenteral Nutrition Cooperative Study Group. Perioperative total parenteral nutrition in surgical patients. *N Engl J Med.* 1991;325(8):525-532.

31. Assmann SF, Pocock SJ, Enos LE, Kasten LE. Subgroup analysis and other (mis)uses of baseline data in clinical trials. *Lancet.* 2000;355(9209):1064-1069.

32. Doig GS, Simpson F, Sweetman EA, et al. Early parenteral nutrition in critically ill patients with short-term relative contraindications to early enteral nutrition: a randomized controlled trial. *JAMA*. 2013;309(20):2130-2138.

33. Alkhawaja S, Martin C, Butler RJ, Gwadry-Sridhar F. Post-pyloric versus gastric tube feeding for preventing pneumonia and improving nutritional outcomes in critically ill adults. *Cochrane Database Syst Rev*. 2015;(8):CD008875.

34. Huang HH, Chang SJ, Hsu CW, Chang TM, Kang SP, Liu MY. Severity of illness influences the efficacy of enteral feeding route on clinical outcomes in patients with critical illness. *J Acad Nutr Diet*. 2012;112(8):1138-1146.

35. Davies AR, Morrison SS, Bailey MJ, et al. A multicenter, randomized controlled trial comparing early nasojejunal with nasogastric nutrition in critical illness. *Crit Care Med*. 2012; 40(8):2342-2348.

36. McClave SA, Martindale RG, Vanek VW, et al. Guidelines for the provision and assessment of nutrition support therapy in the adult critically ill patient: Society of Critical Care Medicine (SCCM) and American Society for Parenteral and Enteral Nutrition (A.S.P.E.N.). *JPEN J Parenter Enteral Nutr*. 2009;33(3):277-316.

37. Wang Z, Ding W, Fang Q, Zhang L, Liu X, Tang Z. Effects of not monitoring gastric residual volume in intensive care patients: A meta-analysis. *Int J Nurs Stud*. 2019;91:86-93.

38. Reignier J, Mercier E, Le Gouge A, et al. Effect of not monitoring residual gastric volume on risk of ventilator-associated pneumonia in adults receiving mechanical ventilation and early enteral feeding: a randomized controlled trial. *JAMA*. 2013;309(3):249-256.

39. Braunschweig CA, Sheean PM, Peterson SJ, et al. Intensive nutrition in acute lung injury: a clinical trial (INTACT). *JPEN J Parenter Enteral Nutr*. 2015;39(1):13-20.

40. Braunschweig CL, Freels S, Sheean PM, et al. Role of timing and dose of energy received in patients with acute lung injury on mortality in the Intensive Nutrition in Acute Lung Injury Trial (INTACT): a post hoc analysis. *Am J Clin Nutr*. 2017; 105(2):411-416.

41. Silva CFA, de Vasconcelos SG, da Silva TA, Silva FM. Permissive or trophic enteral nutrition and full enteral nutrition had similar effects on clinical outcomes in intensive care: a systematic review of randomized clinical trials. *Nutr Clin Pract*. 2018;33(3):388-396.

42. Rice TW, Mogan S, Hays MA, Bernard GR, Jensen GL, Wheeler AP. Randomized trial of initial trophic versus full-energy enteral nutrition in mechanically ventilated patients with acute respiratory failure. *Crit Care Med*. 2011;39(5):967-974.

43. National Heart, Lung, and Blood Institute Acute Respiratory Distress Syndrome (ARDS) Clinical Trials Network, Rice TW, Wheeler AP, et al. Initial trophic vs. full enteral feeding in patients with acute lung injury: the EDEN randomized trial. *JAMA*. 2012;307(8):795-803.

44. Arabi YM, Aldawood AS, Haddad SH, et al. Permissive underfeeding or standard enteral feeding in critically ill adults. *N Engl J Med*. 2015;372(25):2398-2408.

45. TARGET Investigators, for the ANZICS Clinical Trials Group, Chapman M, Peake SL, et al. Energy-dense versus routine enteral nutrition in the critically ill. *N Engl J Med*. 2018; 379(19):1823-1834.

46. Allingstrup MJ, Kondrup J, Wiis J, et al. Early goal-directed nutrition versus standard of care in adult intensive care patients: the single-centre, randomised, outcome assessor-blinded EAT-ICU trial. *Intensive Care Med*. 2017;43(11):1637-1647.

47. Arabi YM, Aldawood AS, Al-Dorzi HM, et al. Permissive underfeeding or standard enteral feeding in high- and low-nutritional-risk critically ill adults. post hoc analysis of the PermiT trial. *Am J Respir Crit Care Med*. 2017;195(5):652-662.

48. Al-Omran M, Albalawi ZH, Tashkandi MF, Al-Ansary LA. Enteral versus parenteral nutrition for acute pancreatitis. *Cochrane Database Syst Rev*. 2010;(1):CD002837.

49. Petrov MS, Windsor JA. Nutritional management of acute pancreatitis: the concept of 'gut rousing'. *Curr Opin Clin Nutr Metab Care*. 2013;16(5):557-563.

50. Bakker OJ, van Brunschot S, van Santvoort HC, et al. Early versus on-demand nasoenteric tube feeding in acute pancreatitis. *N Engl J Med*. 2014;371(21):1983-1993.

69

What Does Critical Illness Do to the Liver?

Michael Bauer and Andreas Kortgen

Liver alterations are common in critical illness. These changes can be attributed to diverse factors, including systemic inflammation and poor perfusion but also to drugs and parenteral nutrition.[1-4] Damage ranges from self-limited abnormalities in liver chemistry to fulminant organ failure. In addition, critical illness elicits profound changes in the concentrations of acute-phase proteins, plasma peptides synthesized by the liver as part of the response to a "danger" signal. Although some of these proteins help to control damage, the functions of others are obscure. Critical illness also induces a reprogramming of metabolic function. Finally, there is a severity-dependent disruption of phase I and II biotransformation and bile transport (i.e., excretory failure with important implications for pharmacotherapy in the intensive care unit [ICU]). The hepatobiliary excretory machinery appears exceptionally sensitive to inflammation.[5,6] As a result, impaired excretion occurs in the absence of traditional markers of (ischemic) liver cell death, such as serum transaminases.[3] Importantly, these changes—acute-phase protein elaboration, altered metabolism, and disrupted biotransformation—occur in parallel. With increasing severity of liver impairment, other functions, most notably synthesis of coagulation proteins and glucose homeostasis, fail, and impaired clearance of toxic compounds affects other organs, as occurs in hepatic encephalopathy. Although fulminant liver failure in previously healthy patients is rare, deterioration of preexisting liver disease is more common. The extent of dysfunction is often underestimated, especially in surgical patients, and is associated with substantial morbidity and mortality. Episodes of decompensated cirrhosis are manifested as variceal bleeding, renal insufficiency, and encephalopathy.

MECHANISMS AND MANIFESTATION OF LIVER DYSFUNCTION

The liver is a highly perfused organ, and complex mechanisms regulate liver microcirculatory blood flow. Under pathophysiologic conditions, these regulatory mechanisms can become ineffective and impaired. An altered microcirculation may lead to profound changes in critically ill patients and may even reduce effective sinusoidal blood flow. Globally reduced (e.g., in hemorrhagic shock, right heart failure, mechanical ventilation) or redistributed (i.e., sepsis, anaphylaxis, endocrinopathies)

blood flow with shunting are mechanisms for ischemic damage. Shunts can be intrahepatic or extrahepatic. In patients with chronic liver disease and portal hypertension, an especially large amount of portal blood can be redirected via extrahepatic shunts. Conversely, increased liver blood flow in acute hepatitis has also been described.

Ischemic damage to the liver may accompany low flow states (i.e., shock) or reflect congestion as a consequence of right heart failure. When severe, ischemia characteristically leads to pericentral cell death that is reflected in an increase in serum levels of glutamate dehydrogenase. Hypoxic hepatitis leading to centrolobular hepatocellular necrosis is associated with a rapid increase in serum aminotransferases (aspartate and alanine aminotransferase) with levels up to 20 times the upper limit of normal.[1]

Impaired excretory function is a frequent manifestation of critical illness. Development of jaundice as a complication of severe trauma or life-threatening disease was only observed with the widespread establishment of ICUs in the 1960s. This finding may well be related to prototypical therapeutic ICU interventions such as multiple transfusions, parenteral nutrition, and potentially hepatotoxic medications.[7] In a large Austrian multicentric cohort, an early increase in plasma bilirubin (>2 mg/dL), noted in approximately 10% of critically ill intensive care patients, was a strong independent risk factor for mortality.[8]

Hepatocellular excretory dysfunction in the critically ill might result from altered blood flow or transmembrane transport; however, it is more frequently associated with systemic inflammation than with ischemic damage. Sepsis accounts for approximately 20% of jaundice cases. This number is surpassed as a cause only by malignant compression of the bile duct.[9] Many basolateral and canalicular transport proteins are downregulated in critically ill patients. This response most likely reflects sensitivity to inflammatory stimuli.[3,10] Alterations in hepatocellular enzyme expression and activity, including those modulating phase I and II metabolism, may lead to profound changes in endobiotic and xenobiotic detoxification.[4] Ductal cholestasis is another characteristic of hepatic dysfunction in the critically ill. This abnormality is most often seen in association with prolonged shock, in which impaired arterial perfusion may result in ischemic injury to the biliary system. Although hepatocellular impairment is most often fully reversible, ductular damage can lead to persistent alterations that may progress to secondary sclerosing cholangitis, an underappreciated long-term sequel of critical illness that carries a very poor prognosis.[11]

The incidence of excretory impairment is underestimated by traditional "static" measures, such as serum transaminases or bilirubin. In contrast, "dynamic" tests, such as solute clearance, are much more sensitive. Hepatobiliary transport systems are essential for the uptake and excretion of various compounds, including bile acids and xenobiotics, and this partial function is best monitored by a functional test such as dye excretion.

IMPACT OF LIVER DYSFUNCTION ON CRITICAL CARE PHARMACOLOGY

Liver disease induces complex changes in the handling of drugs. These alterations are often unpredictable and may affect pharmacokinetics and pharmacodynamics. Therefore administration of medications to these patients must be carefully evaluated and strictly controlled, a mandate that is especially important when dosing drugs with a narrow therapeutic index. The additional risk of (hepatotoxic) side effects must be taken into account, and extreme caution is recommended when such drugs are used. Whenever possible, therapeutic monitoring should be performed, and dosage should be adjusted based on measured pharmacokinetic and pharmacodynamic properties. For some drugs, such as sedatives or analgesics, titrating dosage according to clinical effect may be sufficient; however, in the critically ill, it is essential that initial underdosing be avoided. This issue is especially germane with respect to antibiotic therapy in septic patients, where early and effective drug levels are essential for patient survival. In general, the following recommendations for dosing of drugs eliminated by hepatic metabolism and excretion should be observed in critically ill patients:

1. In drugs with a high extraction ratio (>0.6), oral/enteral application leads to high first-pass metabolism and therefore low bioavailability. A reduction in hepatic blood flow due to shunting (intrahepatic, extrahepatic, or artificial following transjugular intrahepatic portosystemic shunt) or cirrhosis may substantially increase the bioavailability of such drugs. Thus, reducing initial doses and titrating maintenance doses should be considered for drugs with a high hepatic extraction ratio.

2. Intravenous administration of drugs is usually more reliable and predictable. If liver blood flow is reduced, then maintenance doses should be reduced. Conversely, administration of prodrugs that have to be metabolized to their active form in the liver can result in reduced availability of the active form (e.g., clopidogrel, enalapril).[12]

3. For drugs with a low hepatic extraction ratio (<0.3), clearance is dependent on the intrinsic capacity of the elimination pathway and on the fraction of drug that is not protein bound. Impairment of specific elimination mechanisms must be taken into account. For drugs with protein binding less than 90%, maintenance, but not

initial, doses should be reduced. The amount of reduction can be estimated based on the severity of liver dysfunction. For example, in patients with liver dysfunction consistent with Child-Turcotte-Pugh (CTP) Class A, doses should be dropped to 50% of normal. A decrease to 25% of the normal dose is recommended in Class B dysfunction, whereas the more severe impairment associated with Class C requires the use of drug monitoring.[12] These recommendations have limitations because the CTP score represents a rough approximation of impairment and each individual elimination mechanism may be differentially affected. Because phase II metabolism may be less severely impaired, drugs solely metabolized via this pathway should be preferentially used.

4. For drugs with a low hepatic extraction ratio and high protein binding, changes in pharmacokinetics are unpredictable. Therefore drug monitoring is recommended wherever possible, and the unbound fraction should be measured.

5. For hydrophilic substances, such as β-lactam antibiotics, an increased initial dosage should be considered in patients with ascites and edema because the volume of distribution may be substantially increased;[12] however, for maintenance dosage of these drugs, the potential for renal dysfunction must be considered.

Recent reports suggest that liver function tests can be used to predict the required drug dosages. For example, the disappearance rate of indocyanine green from the plasma may be used to determine the appropriate argatroban maintenance dose in critically ill patients with heparin-induced thrombocytopenia type II, whereas the methacetin breath test can predict the increase in tacrolimus trough levels after liver transplantation.[13–15] In the future, such testing might be used to govern therapy in which monitoring drug levels is not possible or where correct determination of the initial dose is crucial with respect to toxicity/side effects or therapeutic effect.

HEPATIC ADAPTATION TO CRITICAL ILLNESS: THE ACUTE-PHASE RESPONSE

Critical illness elicits profound changes in the plasma proteome. Many of the affected peptides are predominantly synthesized in the liver and are referred to as "acute-phase proteins." Proteins may be upregulated (as in the case of C-reactive protein) or downregulated (as in the case of albumin). The response is presumed to be adaptive, and, indeed, some acute-phase proteins have been shown to control damage and to participate in tissue repair; however, the role of many acute-phase reactants is unknown. In the clinical setting, measurements of acute-phase proteins have diagnostic or prognostic value. Reprogramming of metabolic function occurs in parallel with a severity-dependent disruption of phase I and II biotransformation and canalicular transport. Thus activation of the acute-phase response may not be entirely adaptive but may be associated with excretory impairment.

Overall, a deterioration of hepatobiliary excretion reflects an early and poor prognostic event in the critically ill.

This change has important implications for monitoring and pharmacotherapy in the ICU. Early recognition, supportive care, and effective treatment of the underlying disease process as well as avoidance of hepatotoxic drugs are the cornerstones of management of liver dysfunction in the critical care setting.

AUTHORS' RECOMMENDATIONS

- Liver dysfunction in critical illness can be attributed to diverse factors, including systemic inflammation and poor perfusion but also to drugs and parenteral nutrition.
- The hepatobiliary excretory machinery appears exceptionally sensitive to inflammation; changes in acute phase protein elaboration, altered metabolism, and disrupted biotransformation may occur without changes in traditional liver function tests (e.g., transaminases).
- Hyperbilirubinemia or frank jaundice is a common complication of critical illness—and strongly predicts mortality. It results from downregulation of many basolateral and canalicular transport proteins.
- Liver disease induces complex changes in the handling of drugs. It is essential that initial underdosing be avoided—particularly with antibiotics. Drug dosing should be adjusted for hepatic extraction ratio, protein binding, and the type of metabolism (phase I vs. phase II).
- Plasma protein levels may change in critical illness, specifically reprioritization of visceral proteins for acute phase compounds (such as CRP). It is unclear whether this is adaptive or pathologic.

REFERENCES

1. Fuhrmann V, Jäger B, Zubkova A, Drolz A. Hypoxic hepatitis – epidemiology, pathophysiology and clinical management. *Wien Klin Wochenschr*. 2010;122:129-139.
2. Vanwijngaerden YM, Wauters J, Langouche L, et al. Critical illness evokes elevated circulating bile acids related to altered hepatic transporter and nuclear receptor expression. *Hepatology*. 2011; 54:1741-1752.
3. Kortgen A, Paxian M, Werth M, et al. Prospective assessment of hepatic function and mechanisms of dysfunction in the critically ill. *Shock*. 2009;32:358-365.
4. Recknagel P, Gonnert FA, Westermann M, et al. Liver dysfunction and phosphatidylinositol-3-kinase signalling in early sepsis: experimental studies in rodent models of peritonitis. *PLoS Med*. 2012;9:e1001338.
5. Geier AP, Fickert M, Trauner M. Mechanisms of disease: mechanisms and clinical implications of cholestasis in sepsis. *Nat Clin Pract Gastroenterol Hepatol*. 2006;3:574-585.
6. Gonnert FA, Recknagel P, Hilger I, Claus RA, Bauer M, Kortgen A. Hepatic excretory function in sepsis: implications from biophotonic analysis of transcellular xenobiotic transport in a rodent model. *Crit Care*. 2013;17:R67.
7. Marshall JC. New translational research provides insights into liver dysfunction in sepsis. *PLoS Med*. 2012;9:e1001341.
8. Kramer L, Jordan B, Druml W, Bauer P, Metnitz PG. Incidence and prognosis of early hepatic dysfunction in critically ill patients-a prospective multicenter study. *Crit Care Med*. 2007;35:1099-1104.
9. Whitehead MW, Hainsworth I, Kingham JG. The causes of obvious jaundice in South West Wales: perceptions versus reality. *Gut*. 2001;48:409-413.
10. Andrejko KM, Raj NR, Kim PK, Cereda M, Deutschman CS. IL-6 modulates sepsis-induced decreases in transcription of hepatic organic anion and bile acid transporters. *Shock*. 2008; 29:490-496.
11. Ruemmele P, Hofstaedter F, Gelbmann CM. Secondary sclerosing cholangitis. *Nat Rev Gastroenterol Hepatol*. 2009; 6:287-295.
12. Delcò F, Tchambaz L, Schlienger R, Drewe J, Krähenbühl S. Dose adjustments in patients with liver disease. *Drug Saf*. 2005;28:529-545.
13. Link A, Girndt M, Selejan S, Mathes A, Böhm M, Rensing H. Argatroban for anticoagulation in continuous renal replacement therapy. *Crit Care Med*. 2009;37:105-110.
14. Parker BM, Cywinski JB, Alster JM, et al. Predicting immunosuppressant dosing in the early postoperative period with noninvasive indocyanine green elimination following orthotopic liver transplantation. *Liver Transpl*. 2008;14:46-52.
15. Lock JF, Malinowski M, Schwabauer E, et al. Initial graft function is a reliable predictor of tacrolimus trough levels during the first post-transplant week. *Clin Transplant*. 2011;25:436-443.

70

How Do I Manage a Patient With Acute Liver Failure?

Mark T. Keegan

Acute liver failure (ALF) is a catastrophic condition that can result in multiple organ failure. The severity of the illness and rapidity of clinical deterioration in a previously healthy individual is alarming to patients, their families, and the health-care team. Care of the patient with ALF requires full armamentarium of therapies available in a modern intensive care unit (ICU) and may require orthotopic liver transplantation (OLT).[1] Survival rates have increased significantly in recent years, and advances in ICU management have driven improved outcomes.[2–7]

ALF (the preferred term) is defined as the onset of hepatic encephalopathy (HE) and coagulopathy within 26 weeks of jaundice in a patient without preexisting liver disease. Terms that base classification on the duration of illness are popular but less useful because they do not have prognostic significance distinct from the etiology.[8–10]

In 2011 the American Association for the Study of Liver Diseases (AASLD) updated its position paper detailing the management of ALF.[11] Recommendations of the U.S. Acute Liver Failure Study Group for the ICU management of such patients were published in 2007.[12] The European Association for the Study of the Liver (EASL) and the American Gastroenterological Association Institute both published guidelines on ALF in 2017.[6,13] The rarity, heterogeneity, severity, and speed of progression of ALF mean that there is a paucity of randomized controlled trials (RCTs) evaluating therapies, and many interventions are empiric or based on expert opinion.

EPIDEMIOLOGY

ALF is rare. In developed countries, the reported incidence is between 1 and 6 cases/million persons per year, with approximately 2000 cases/year in the United States.[14–16] Rates are probably higher in locations with high rates of infective hepatitis and/or lack of resources for treatment, but data are sparse. The etiology of ALF differs depending on the geographic location. In the United States and Europe, medications are responsible for most cases.[1,6] Acetaminophen accounted for 46% of the 1696 cases of adult ALF in the U.S. Acute Liver Failure Registry, many from unintentional overdose and many in women.[3,17,18] In other parts of the world, a viral etiology (especially hepatitis A, B, D, and E) predominates. Other causes of ALF are detailed in Box 70.1.[19] Despite the presence of a

preexisting liver disease, patients with an acute presentation of chronic autoimmune hepatitis, Wilson disease, and Budd–Chiari syndrome are considered as having ALF if they develop encephalopathy in the context of appropriate abnormalities in liver blood tests and coagulation profile.[6]

CLINICAL PRESENTATION

Although ALF originates with a liver insult, it becomes a multisystem disease by inducing a three-phase (initiation, propagation, and resolution) systemic inflammatory response syndrome (SIRS). Hepatocyte death initiates a massive proinflammatory response, likely caused by activation of Kupffer cells (macrophages). This SIRS activates a compensatory antiinflammatory response.[20] Systemic organ dysfunction occurs involving vasodilation, encephalopathy and cerebral edema, coagulopathy, acute kidney injury (AKI), immunosuppression, and metabolic acidosis. The stigmata of chronic liver disease are absent. HE and coagulopathy are characteristic features of ALF and may progress rapidly over days or even hours. Diagnosis of ALF is made on clinical grounds, aided by laboratory analysis. Imaging studies (e.g., hepatic ultrasound to assess the patency of the liver's vascular supply) are usually performed. Routine liver biopsy is not advisable; although it may change the diagnosis in a minority of cases, it will usually not change therapy.[13]

INITIAL ASSESSMENT AND MANAGEMENT

When ALF is diagnosed, a referral center with a liver transplant program should be contacted for management advice and consideration for transfer.[1,3,6,11] When encephalopathy develops in a patient with ALF, ICU care is usually warranted because of the potential for further deterioration and the potential need for urgent interventions, such as intubation, mechanical ventilation, and hemodynamic support. Several institutions have developed formal protocols for management of patients with ALF.[21]

PROGNOSIS

With supportive therapy, some patients with ALF will spontaneously recover hepatic function. In many other cases,

BOX 70.1   Etiologies of Acute Liver Failure.

Viral
Hepatitis A virus, Hepatitis B virus ± Hepatitis D virus, Hepatitis E virus, Herpes simplex virus, Cytomegalovirus, Epstein Barr virus, Varicella zoster virus, adenovirus, hemorrhagic fever viruses

Drugs and Toxins
Dose-dependent: Acetaminophen, carbon tetrachloride, yellow phosphorus, *Amanita phalloides*, *Bacillus cereus* toxin, sulfonamides, tetracycline, methyldioxymethamphetamine (ecstasy), herbal remedies
Idiosyncratic: Volatile anesthetics (especially halothane), isoniazid, rifampicin, valproic acid, nonsteroidal antiinflammatory drugs, disulfiram

Vascular
Right heart failure, Budd–Chiari syndrome, veno-occlusive disease, shock liver (ischemic hepatitis), heat stroke

Metabolic
Acute fatty liver of pregnancy, Wilson disease, Reye syndrome, galactosemia, hereditary fructose intolerance, tyrosinemia

Miscellaneous
Malignant infiltration (liver metastases, lymphoma), autoimmune hepatitis, sepsis

Indeterminate
Includes primary graft nonfunction in liver transplant recipients

Modified from Saas DA, Shakil AO. Fulminant hepatic failure. *Liver Transpl.* 2005;11(6):594-605.

however, the patient will die without OLT. Of 1696 patients with ALF in the U.S. Acute Liver Failure Study Group dataset, overall patient survival was 71%.[3] Outcomes have improved over time. The 21-day survival rates in patient cohorts treated in 1998–2005 and 2006–2013 were 67.1 and 75.3%, respectively. Transplant-free survival improved from 45.1% during 1998–2005 to 56.2% during 2006–2013, and posttransplantation survival increased from 88.3 to 96.3%.[7]

Nonetheless, ALF remains a life-threatening disease entity. The main causes of death are cerebral edema with subsequent herniation and multiple organ failure. In data reported by Lee,[3] 660 (39%) of 1696 patients were listed for transplantation, 409 were transplanted, with 371 survivors and 38 deaths. Without transplantation, 826 survived and 461 died.[3] In a 2-year follow-up, long-term survival was significantly higher in transplant recipients than in patients who survived without the need for transplantation, perhaps because of underlying comorbidities.[22]

The timing of transplantation is crucial. Delay in listing for transplantation may result in the patient's demise before a donor organ is found or may result in perioperative mortality. Premature listing may result in OLT procedure in patients who might have otherwise spontaneously recovered liver function. Multiple prognostic scoring systems have been

developed to identify patients at high risk of mortality.[11,23] The most commonly used, the King's College Criteria (KCC), were developed in a cohort of 588 patients with ALF who were managed medically between 1973 and 1985.[24] The KCC differentiate between acetaminophen-induced ALF and ALF caused by other causes and use pH, international normalized ratio (INR), creatinine, encephalopathy grade, age, duration of jaundice, and bilirubin level for prognostication. These characteristics have clinically acceptable specificity but more limited sensitivity.[25] Other prognostic systems include the Clichy criteria (which use encephalopathy grade, factor V concentration, and age), the Japanese criteria (age, encephalopathy grade, bilirubin level, and coagulopathy), and the ALF early dynamic model (international normalized ratio [INR], serum bilirubin, arterial ammonia, and HE).[9,10,26] There are insufficient data to recommend a particular scheme.[12,27] Box 70.2 identifies potentially helpful indicators of poor prognosis in patients with ALF.[28] The etiology of ALF appears to be the most important factor, albeit with imperfect sensitivity and specificity.

The United Network for Organ Sharing (UNOS), the donor organ allocation body in the United States, has criteria that must be satisfied before a patient may be listed as a Status IA candidate for liver transplantation (the highest priority for organ allocation). These include "ALF with a life expectancy of less than 7 days without a liver transplant" or "primary graft nonfunction, hepatic artery thrombosis, and acute Wilson disease."

SPECIFIC CAUSES AND RELATED THERAPIES

The cause of ALF has implications for both therapy and prognosis.[6,11] *N*-acetylcysteine (NAC) is effective in the treatment of acetaminophen toxicity and an acetaminophen level should be drawn in every patient with ALF.[6,11,18,29,30] Acetaminophen toxicity may be indicated by the presence of very high serum transaminases and low bilirubin levels and assays for toxicity-related serum acetaminophen-containing protein adducts. Intravenous (IV) NAC should be administered even if there is doubt regarding the timing or dose of ingestion or of the plasma acetaminophen concentration. The duration of administration is determined by clinical condition rather than by time or serum acetaminophen concentration.[11,12] In addition to NAC administration, patients with known or suspected acetaminophen overdose within 4 hours of presentation should be administered activated charcoal prior to starting NAC.[11]

Nonacetaminophen, drug-induced hepatotoxicity is usually idiosyncratic. In acute drug toxicity, the serum aminotransaminase concentration is characteristically extremely elevated (>10,000 IU/L) and bilirubin levels may be normal. Lower transaminase levels may be seen in accidental staggered toxicity. Antibiotics (especially antituberculous medications), nonsteroidal antiinflammatory drugs, and anticonvulsants are most commonly implicated.[3,31,32] There are no specific antidotes. In unexplained ALF, potential drug or toxin exposure should be investigated. In the U.S. Acute Liver Failure Study Group data, 11% patients had (nonacetaminophen)

BOX 70.2 Potentially Helpful Indicators of Poor Prognosis[a] in Patients With Acute Liver Failure.

Etiology
- Idiosyncratic drug reaction
- Acute hepatitis B (and other non-hepatitis A viral infections)
- Autoimmune hepatitis
- Mushroom poisoning
- Wilson disease
- Budd–Chiari syndrome
- Indeterminate cause

Coma grade on admission
- III or IV

King's College criteria
- Acetaminophen-induced ALF
  - Strongly consider OLT listing if arterial lactate >3.5 mmol/L after early fluid resuscitation
  - List for OLT if pH <7.3 or arterial lactate >3.0 mmol/L after adequate fluid resuscitation
  - List for OLT if all three of the following occur within a 24-h period: grade III or IV HE, INR >6.5, creatinine >3.4 mg/dL
- Nonacetaminophen-induced ALF
  - List for OLT if INR >6.5 and encephalopathy present (irrespective of grade)
  - List for OLT if encephalopathy present (irrespective of grade) and any three of the following are present:
    - Age <10 or >40 years[b]
    - Jaundice for >7 days before development of encephalopathy†
    - INR ≥3.5
    - Serum bilirubin ≥17 mg/dL
    - Unfavorable cause such as Wilson disease, idiosyncratic drug reaction, seronegative hepatitis

[a] Note that none of these factors, with the exception of Wilson disease and possibly mushroom poisoning, are either necessary or sufficient to indicate the need for immediate liver transplantation.
[b] These criteria, in particular, have not been found to be predictive of outcome in recent analyses.
ALF, acute liver failure; HE, hepatic encephalopathy; INR, international normalized ratio; OLT, orthotopic liver transplantation.
From Lee WM, Stravitz RT, Larson AM. Introduction to the revised American Association for the Study of Liver Diseases Position Paper on acute liver failure 2011. *Hepatology.* 2012;55(3):965-967.

drug-induced ALF, and the entity was especially common in women and minorities.[32] Transplant-free (3-week) survival was poor (27.1%), but with highly successful transplantation occurring in 42.1%; overall survival was 66.2%.

Hepatitis A and B accounted for 4 and 8%, respectively, of ALF cases in the U.S. multicenter cohort.[3,17] Viral hepatitis is more common elsewhere. Acute hepatitis D may cause acute liver dysfunction in a patient with preexisting hepatitis B, and hepatitis E may cause ALF in endemic areas, especially during pregnancy. Care of a patient with acute viral hepatitis is mainly supportive. Lamivudine may be of use in hepatitis B-associated ALF, although a clinical trial has not been performed.[11] Acyclovir and consideration for transplantation are recommended for cases of the (rarely seen) herpes simplex or varicella-zoster-induced ALF.

ALF may develop as an acute presentation of autoimmune hepatitis and should be suspected in patients presenting with other autoimmune disorders, elevated globulin fraction, and autoantibodies.[6] Corticosteroids (prednisolone starting at 40–60 mg/day) are often administered in this scenario, but steroid administration is not supported by the large retrospective analysis of Karkhanis et al.[33] Transplantation may be required.

Acute fatty liver of pregnancy is a rare disease that may occur in the third trimester. It resolves with delivery of the fetus. OLT has been performed for this condition but should not be necessary with early diagnosis and prompt delivery.[34] HELLP syndrome (hemolysis, elevated liver enzymes, and low platelets) is also a disease of pregnancy, usually in association with preeclampsia. Prompt delivery is indicated and is usually associated with a good outcome.

Wilson disease is an uncommon cause of ALF (2–3% of cases in the U.S. Acute Liver Failure Group cohort) but carries a grim prognosis without transplantation. Features include low serum ceruloplasmin, high serum and urinary copper, hemolysis, Kayser–Fleischer rings (seen on slit-lamp examination), very low serum alkaline phosphatase and uric acid, and a bilirubin (mg/dL) to alkaline phosphatase (IU/L) ratio of >2.[35] Although penicillamine treatment may be used in Wilson disease, it is not recommended in the setting of ALF.[36] Rather, other measures to reduce serum copper and prevent further hemolysis (e.g., plasmapheresis) should be initiated while the patient is waiting to undergo an emergent liver transplant.

Patients with mushroom poisoning (the most hepatotoxic of which is *Amanita phalloides*) typically present with gastrointestinal symptoms. Mushroom poisoning has been treated with penicillin G, NAC, and silibinin although controlled trials have not been performed, and the latter is not available as a licensed drug in the United States.[37]

When ALF is caused by an acute ischemic injury or severe congestive heart failure, treatment of the underlying cause is required, and prognosis is related to the response to therapy of the inciting insult.

Abdominal pain, prominent hepatomegaly, and ascites may indicate acute hepatic vein thrombosis (Budd–Chiari syndrome), which may present as ALF.[38] Liver transplantation is indicated based on high survival rates in case series, provided underlying malignancy is excluded. Malignant infiltration of the liver sufficient to cause ALF is a contraindication to liver transplantation and indicates a very poor prognosis. Other conditions that may cause ALF but are not an indication for OLT include hemophagocytic lymphohistiocytosis and infections such as malaria, dengue fever, and rickettsiosis.

ALF may be caused by extensive liver resection (e.g., hemihepatectomy) or vascular complications after liver surgery. Most patients recover if the resection is performed in the absence of advanced liver disease.

HEPATIC ENCEPHALOPATHY

Ammonia produced in the gut is usually converted to urea in the liver's urea cycle. In hepatic failure, ammonia accumulates and is shunted to the systemic circulation. Hyperammonemia causes neuronal dysfunction, leading to HE, one of the hallmarks of ALF.[39] In contrast to patients with chronic liver disease, the development of encephalopathy in a patient with ALF is often associated with the development of cerebral edema and elevations in intracranial pressure (ICP), with potential herniation. The correlation between arterial ammonia concentration and cerebral edema, although imperfect, is stronger in patients with ALF than in those with cirrhosis; an arterial ammonia >200 μmol/L within 24 hours of the development of grade III or IV HE is predictive of herniation.[40]

Encephalopathy may develop rapidly in patients with ALF. In the West Haven grading system, there are four grades of encephalopathy (Table 70.1). The grade of encephalopathy correlates with the development of cerebral edema and with outcome. For patients who become comatose, the Full Outline of Unresponsiveness or FOUR score is more discriminating because it includes brain stem and respiration assessment, which are not further differentiated in the West Haven system.[41] Cerebral edema is uncommon in grade I or II, but it occurs in 25–35% and 65–75% in patients with grades III and IV encephalopathy, respectively.

Treatment of Hepatic Encephalopathy and Elevated Intracranial Pressure

Grades I and II Hepatic Encephalopathy

Patients with grade I HE may be managed in a general ward with skilled nursing; however, in most institutions, patients with ALF should be managed in an ICU. If and when grade II HE develops, ICU care is indicated. A computed tomography (CT) scan of the head should be performed to exclude other causes of mental status change (e.g., intracranial hemorrhage, space-occupying lesion). Although CT scans may demonstrate cerebral edema in patients with HE, intracranial hypertension may not be detected.[39]

Administration of sedatives to patients with grade I or II HE should be avoided if possible because they will confound progression detection. Nonetheless, small doses of short-acting agents (e.g., haloperidol, benzodiazepines, or dexmedetomidine) may be required to control agitation. Lactulose administration has been associated with a small increase in survival time but no difference in the severity of encephalopathy or overall outcome.[42] Nonabsorbable antibiotics (rifaximin, neomycin) have also not proven to be beneficial in ALF, and neomycin carries a risk of nephrotoxicity.

Grades III and IV Hepatic Encephalopathy

A patient who progresses to grade III HE requires endotracheal intubation for airway protection. There are no studies to demonstrate the advantage of one sedative or anesthetic agent over another in this circumstance. It is intuitive that a drug regimen that minimizes the risk of increasing ICP should be used, and propofol is a reasonable choice. If needed, a nondepolarizing neuromuscular blocker (e.g., cisatracurium) offers some advantages over succinylcholine in terms of its effect on ICP.

Intracranial Pressure Monitoring

The use of ICP monitoring devices in ALF is controversial.[11,43,44] The traditionally used device, an epidural catheter, has relatively lower associated risks for intracranial hemorrhage but may be less accurate than other devices. Subdural or intraparenchymal monitors provide improved reliability but are associated with an increased risk of bleeding, and ICP monitor-associated hemorrhage may be catastrophic. Definitive recommendations for international normalized ratio (INR) or platelet count prior to ICP monitor insertion are not available.

In the recent U.S. data, ICP monitoring was used in 140 (22%) of 169 patients with ALF.[45,46] Hemorrhagic complications were rare. Overall 21-day mortality was similar in patients with ICP monitors (33%) and controls (38%; $P = .24$). In acetaminophen-induced ALF, no difference in 21-day mortality could be detected when comparing patients with ICP monitoring with unmonitored individuals; however, in ALF from other causes, use of ICP monitoring was associated with an increased 21-day mortality. A randomized clinical trial to determine the effectiveness of ICP monitoring in ALF would be logistically difficult and has not been performed. The AASLD position paper states that "ICP monitoring is

TABLE 70.1	Grades of Hepatic Encephalopathy.		
Grade	Mental Status	Tremor	EEG
I	Euphoria; occasional depression; fluctuant mild confusion; slowness of mentation and affect; untidy, slurred speech; disorder in sleep rhythm	Slight	Usually normal
II	Accentuation of grade I; drowsiness; inappropriate behavior; able to maintain sphincter control	Present (easily elicited)	Abnormal; generalized slowing
III	Sleeps most of the time but arousable; incoherent speech; marked confusion	Usually present if patient can cooperate	Always abnormal
IV	Not arousable; may or may not respond to painful stimuli	Usually absent	Always abnormal

EEG, electroencephalogram.
Modified from Sass DA, Shakil AO. Fulminant hepatic failure. *Gastroenterol Clin North Am.* 2003;32(4):1195-1211.

recommended in ALF patients with high-grade HE, in centers with expertise in ICP monitoring, and in patients awaiting and undergoing liver transplantation."[11] The European Guidelines advise consideration of ICP monitoring "in a highly selected subgroup of patients who have progressed to grade III or IV coma, are intubated and ventilated, and deemed to be at high risk of intracranial hemorrhage based on the presence of more than one of the following variables: a) young patients with hyperacute or acute presentations, b) ammonia level more than 150–200 μmol/L that does not drop with initial treatment intervention, c) renal impairment, and d) vasopressor support."

Maintenance of Cerebral Perfusion Pressure

The management goal for patients with cerebral edema is to limit ICP while maintaining cerebral persursion pressure (CPP). Targets for CPP are subjects of debate, but a goal ICP <25 mm Hg and a CPP >60 mm Hg seem reasonable.[11] A CPP >70 mm Hg may be of further advantage if that level can be achieved.[11] An ICP >40 mm Hg and a prolonged period of time with a CPP <50 mm Hg are strongly associated with poor neurological recovery, although the data are not sufficient to contraindicate OLT.[47] It may be necessary to pharmacologically elevate mean arterial pressure (MAP) to attain and maintain a satisfactory CPP.

Control of Elevations of Intracranial Pressure in Patients With Grade III or IV Hepatic Encephalopathy

General Measures: Patients with elevated ICP (defined as an ICP >20–25 mm Hg for >1 minute or a CPP <50 mm Hg) should be managed in a quiet environment with head elevated to 20–30 degrees. Obstruction to venous return (e.g., head rotation, tight endotracheal tube ties) should be avoided, endotracheal tube suctioning should be kept to a minimum, and consideration should be given to administration of a bolus of a sedative agent such as propofol or lidocaine before suctioning. Hypoxemia and hypercapnia will increase ICP, and every effort should be made to avoid these.

Sedation and Analgesia: Sedation to control ICP has been recommended in patients with grade III or IV HE. Propofol is a reasonable choice.[48] The induction of "barbiturate coma" with pentobarbital or sodium thiopental has been used to treat refractory intracranial hypertension in ALF, but the value of this approach is based on uncontrolled studies.[49] Side effects are numerous and include hemodynamic compromise and apnea. Patients receiving infusions of propofol or barbiturates may require pressor support to maintain optimum hemodynamics.

Opiate infusions are often used to treat discomfort and as adjunctive sedatives. Fentanyl is a better choice than morphine or meperidine because these two are longer acting and have active metabolites that may accumulate in hepatic or renal dysfunction.

Mannitol: Mannitol is the only therapy proven in a controlled trial to reduce intracranial hypertension and improve survival in patients with ALF. Canalese et al.[50] randomized 44 patients with ALF to receive mannitol (1 g/kg as required), dexamethasone (32 mg IV, then 8 mg IV every 6 hours), both drugs, or neither drug for the treatment of elevated ICP.[50] The EASL guidelines recommend a bolus of 50 mL of 20% mannitol to be administered over 20 minutes. Limitations to the use of mannitol include the development of acute renal failure or hyperosmolality (serum osmolality >320 mOsm/L). The prophylactic administration of mannitol in ALF has not been studied.

Hypertonic Saline: Hypertonic saline, administered to maintain serum sodium concentrations between 145 and 155 mEq/L in patients with ALF and encephalopathy, reduced the incidence and severity of intracranial hypertension but not survival.[51] The role of prophylactic hypertonic saline remains unproven, but its use is recommended by the AASLD "in patients at highest risk of developing cerebral edema."[11] The EASL guidelines recommend that mannitol or hypertonic saline be administered for surges in ICP. Hypotonic solutions and hyponatremia should be avoided because of the risk of worsening cerebral edema.

Treatment of Fever: Fever exacerbates intracranial hypertension, and measures to maintain normothermia, including cooling blankets and fans, should be used in the febrile patient. Nonsteroidal antiinflammatory drugs and acetaminophen are relatively contraindicated because of the potential for nephrotoxicity and further hepatotoxicity.[1,52]

Hyperventilation: Hyperventilation to a partial pressure of carbon dioxide in arterial blood ($PaCO_2$) of <30 mm Hg causes cerebral vasoconstriction and rapidly reduces ICP in patients with cerebral edema. Prophylactic hyperventilation, however, did not reduce the incidence of cerebral edema in an RCT of 20 patients with ALF.[53] Furthermore, marked hypocapnia (to a $PaCO_2$ ≤25 mm Hg) or sustained hypocapnia may cause cerebral ischemia. Accordingly, the use of therapeutic hyperventilation is reserved for situations in which life-threatening cerebral edema is present and has proven refractory to other measures. Use of hyperventilation in this circumstance should be temporary for at most a few hours.[11] Maintenance of $PaCO_2$ between 30 and 40 mm Hg is a reasonable goal.[12]

Seizure Prophylaxis: The development of seizures will markedly increase cerebral oxygen requirements, increase ICP, and may cause or worsen cerebral edema. Subclinical seizure activity was noted in 30% of patients with ALF.[54] Phenytoin administration is recommended for control of seizures when they occur, although supporting data are scarce.[11] Benzodiazepines may also be administered for both their antiseizure and sedative properties, but their metabolism and clearance are greatly decreased in liver failure. Prophylactic IV phenytoin was shown to reduce the incidence of seizures in a group of 42 patients; however, the beneficial effects of phenytoin could not be documented in a confirmatory study.[55] The use of prophylactic phenytoin is not supported by current evidence. Electroencephalography should be performed in grade III or IV HE if myoclonus is present, if a sudden unexplained deterioration in neurologic status occurs, or when barbiturate coma is being used for management of cerebral edema.[12,55]

Indomethacin: Tofteng and Larsen[56] administered bolus doses of indomethacin to a series of 12 patients with

ALF and cerebral edema and demonstrated a reduction in ICP and an increase in CPP, but further studies have not been forthcoming.

Other agents: Nonabsorbable disaccharides, benzodiazepine receptor antagonists, or dopaminergic agonists have not been proven to be beneficial for the treatment of HE, nor has L-ornithine L-aspartate (LOLA), a drug that is supposed to facilitate the detoxification and excretion of ammonia.

COAGULOPATHY

The development of coagulopathy is a hallmark of ALF. Coagulopathy may be due to platelet dysfunction (quantitative and qualitative), hypofibrinogenemia, and inadequate coagulation factor synthesis. Overall hemostasis, however, may be preserved by compensatory mechanisms despite marked elevation of INR and a rebalancing of coagulation may actually be slightly biased toward thrombosis.[57] The thromboelastogram to aid in the management of coagulopathy (especially in patients undergoing OLT) has been shown to decrease transfusions.[58,59] In the absence of bleeding, administration of fresh frozen plasma (FFP) is not required and may confound assessment of disease progression.[11] Indeed, almost 40 years ago, Gazzard et al.[60] showed that FFP administration did not reduce morbidity or mortality in ALF. Spontaneous and postprocedure bleeding complications are actually uncommon in patients with ALF. Nonetheless, such complications, especially in the setting of ICP monitor placement, may be catastrophic. When invasive procedures are planned or when the patient is bleeding, it may be appropriate to treat coagulopathy, although a more conservative approach to transfusion is now encouraged.[11,12,58] Many clinicians advocate treatment of extreme coagulopathy (e.g., INR >7), even if invasive procedures are not planned.[11] Vitamin K is typically given to patients with ALF because some have subclinical vitamin K deficiency at the time of presentation. In the absence of bleeding or plans for invasive procedures, a platelet count of greater than 10–20 × 10⁹/L seems acceptable. If invasive procedures are planned, a platelet count of at least 50 × 10⁹/L has been recommended. Cryoprecipitate administration has been recommended when the fibrinogen level is <100 mg/dL. Recombinant factor VIIa (40 μg/kg) transiently corrected the coagulopathy of ALF and allowed performance of invasive procedures in two nonrandomized studies in a total of 26 patients who met KCC for liver transplantation.[61] Thrombosis is a potential side effect. The use of prothrombin complex concentrates has yet to be sufficiently investigated in patients with ALF.

INFECTION

Individuals with ALF are at risk for bacterial and fungal infection. Gram-positive cocci, enteric gram-negative bacilli, and *Candida* species are the most commonly isolated organisms. Disseminated infection may be a contraindication to transplantation. Prophylactic antimicrobial therapy may reduce the incidence of infection in ALF but does not impact survival, nor does antimicrobial therapy alter the relationship between SIRS and encephalopathy.[62] Surveillance for infection is empirically recommended in patients with ALF.[11] Antibiotics have been empirically recommended when surveillance cultures reveal significant isolates, in grade III or IV HE, in the presence of refractory hypotension, and if SIRS is present.[12] Broad-spectrum antibacterial agents are typically used and vancomycin added if intravascular catheter-related bloodstream infection or methicillin-resistant *Staphylococcus aureus* infection is suspected.

ACUTE KIDNEY INJURY

In one cohort of 1604 patients with ALF, 70% developed acute kidney injury and 30% underwent renal replacement therapy (RRT).[63] AKI affected short- and long-term outcomes, but it rarely resulted in chronic kidney disease (only 4% of survivors were dialysis-dependent). Early initiation of RRT should be considered in patients with ALF, especially in those with markedly elevated ammonia, significant acidosis, and progressive HE.[6] Continuous RRT (CRRT) is associated with less hemodynamic compromise and is less likely to provoke an elevation in ICP or pulmonary pressures than is intermittent dialysis, and it is the dialysis method of choice in patients with ALF.[6,64] CRRT may be continued in the operating room during liver transplantation.[65]

HEMODYNAMIC SUPPORT

Patients with ALF often develop distributive shock. Hypovolemia usually reflects transudation of fluid into the extravascular space and decreased oral intake. Despite adequate fluid resuscitation, a low systemic vascular resistance in ALF often results in persistent hypotension, and vasopressors may be required. The recommended goal MAP is 75 mm Hg, but this is not supported by data, and there are no data evaluating the need for higher pressures to augment CPP or lower pressures to reduce ICP.[11,66] Similarly, there are no definitive trials to identify the best vasoactive agent to augment blood pressure. Most centers use norepinephrine, which can minimize tachycardia while preserving splanchnic (thereby hepatic) blood flow.[11,66] Vasopressin use is controversial, and a small study of terlipressin in ALF (six patients with ALF and HE) at a dose that did not alter systemic hemodynamics demonstrated worsening of cerebral hyperemia and intracranial hypertension.[67]

Adrenal insufficiency may be present in patients with liver failure. Some data support the use of corticosteroids (e.g., hydrocortisone 200 mg/day) for refractory hypotension in patients with chronic liver failure; however, significant controversy exists regarding steroid supplementation in patients with ALF and, indeed, in all critically ill patients.[68]

MECHANICAL VENTILATION

Intubation is indicated when ALF with grade III hepatic encephalopathy placed patients at risk for aspiration. Mechanical ventilation may be used to correct respiratory failure or severe metabolic acidosis. Acute respiratory distress syndrome has been reported in association with ALF. The use of lung-protective ventilation may be at odds with the need for relative respiratory alkalosis to manage elevated ICP. Therefore the use of permissive hypercapnia should be avoided. Obstruction of hepatic venous outflow by positive end-expiratory pressure (PEEP) is of theoretical concern and should not prevent the use of PEEP to aid in oxygenation and recruitment.[69]

GASTROINTESTINAL BLEEDING

There is a significant risk of gastrointestinal bleeding in individuals with ALF, although this risk is presumably less than that in patients with cirrhosis, portal hypertension, and esophageal or gastric varices. In two controlled trials involving 75 patients, H2 blockers, but not antacids, were associated with a decreased incidence of bleeding in patients with ALF. Accordingly, H2 blockers or, by extension, proton pump inhibitors may be administered to patients with ALF.[11,70]

METABOLIC CONCERNS

Severe metabolic acidosis is common in patients with ALF, especially when accompanied by acute renal failure. Infusions of sodium bicarbonate or a nonsodium buffer such as tris(hydroxymethyl) aminomethane or initiation of CRRT with a bicarbonate-rich infusate have been used, but evidence supporting this practice is limited. Lactic acidosis may result from a combination of hypoperfusion and decreased lactate clearance. Profound hypoglycemia secondary to impaired hepatic gluconeogenesis can occur. Boluses of 50% dextrose solutions and continuous 10% dextrose infusions have been administered to maintain normoglycemia; however, bolus administration carries a risk of osmotic shifts that may contribute to cerebral edema and intracranial hypertension. Phosphate and magnesium levels may be low. Hypophosphatemia is a favorable prognostic sign and appears to be associated with liver regeneration.[71] Fluid resuscitation and, if necessary, hypertonic saline solutions should be targeted to maintain serum sodium at 140–145 mEq/L, although rapid changes in sodium should be avoided.[6]

NUTRITION

Patients with ALF are catabolic with increased energy requirements;[72] however, studies on the value of nutritional support are limited. The enteral route has been recommended although studies comparing enteral and parenteral nutrition are inconclusive. A European study of nutritional support in patients with ALF demonstrated that 25 of 33 responding units used parenteral nutrition.[73] The AASLD position paper recommends 60 g of protein per day, but this does not account for patient body habitus or age; requirements determined on a g/kg basis seem more appropriate.[11] Studies on the beneficial effect of branched-chain amino acids in ALF are equivocal.[74] Lipid emulsions appear to be safe in patients with ALF; however, there is a moderate risk of pancreatitis.

TRANSPLANTATION

Although ALF may resolve with only supportive interventions, especially in patients with acetaminophen-induced ALF, OLT is the only definitive therapy for the condition. The therapy has not been evaluated in a prospective clinical trial for patients with ALF, but there is little doubt as to its effectiveness. Overall survival for patients with ALF has increased from 15% in the pretransplant era to ≥60% in the posttransplant era.[17] Some of the improved survival rates reflect improvements in ICU management that have also enhanced spontaneous survival rates. ALF is the only condition designated as UNOS Status I (highest priority for donor liver allocation). OLT is not universally available, and only 8–10% of liver transplantations are performed in patients with ALF.[6,75,76] In the U.S. Acute Liver Failure Study Group series, 29% of patients underwent OLT and 25% of patients listed for transplantation died on the waiting list.[17] A "look-back" study of adult patients admitted to the King's College liver center in London between 1973 and 2008 demonstrated that 387 (18%) of 2095 patients with ALF underwent OLT.[2] In the Nordic countries' experience, 73% of 315 patients listed received a transplant, and 16% died without transplant.[15] Mortality after OLT in the first year is higher for patients with ALF than for patients transplanted for other reasons (1-year survival rate was 79% for OLT in setting of ALF vs. approximately 90% for other causes), and most deaths occur from infection within the first 3 months.[76] Outcome is worse for older recipients, those who receive older or partial grafts, and those receiving non-ABO identical grafts.[76,77] Longer-term survival, however, is better than in those transplanted for chronic liver disease. Perioperative management of liver transplant patients is beyond the scope of this chapter.

AREAS OF CONTROVERSY

Therapeutic Hypothermia

Hypothermia (cooling to core temperature of 33°C–34°C) to decrease brain edema has been used as a "bridge to transplant" or to control ICP during transplant surgery in small series.[78,79] A multicenter retrospective cohort study evaluating the impact of mild-moderate hypothermia on the prevention of elevations in ICP and the occurrence of transplant-free survival in high-risk patients with ALF and grade III-IV HE was unable to demonstrate an effect on 21-day survival or transplant-free interval.[80] A multicenter RCT of prophylactic hypothermia (34°C for 72 hours) in 43 patients with ALF at high risk of cerebral edema was terminated early owing to futility.[81] Adverse effects of therapeutic hypothermia appear to relate closely to the minimum temperatures achieved and include sepsis and arrhythmias. Theoretical concerns with worsening of coagulopathy and reduction in hepatic regeneration have not been seen in the ALF hypothermia trials. Hypothermia cannot be recommended as a routine management strategy for patients with ALF, though the EASL guidelines state that "mild hypothermia.... may be considered in uncontrolled intracranial hypertension."

N-acetylcysteine for Nonacetaminophen-Induced ALF

NAC may have a role in nonacetaminophen-induced ALF; however, the supporting evidence is weak at this time. In a randomized, double-blind, multicenter, placebo-controlled trial, IV NAC improved transplant-free survival in patients with early-stage nonacetaminophen-induced ALF, although patients with advanced coma grades did not benefit.[82] Other evidence is observational;[83] however, the most recent guidelines from the American Gastroenterological Institute, presumably on the basis of sparse or inconclusive data, provided "No recommendation" for the use of NAC in nonacetaminophen ALF.

Hepatectomy and Auxiliary Transplantation

The use of hepatectomy to decrease liver-derived proinflammatory cytokines has been advocated in patients with ALF, refractory circulatory dysfunction, and intracranial hypertension, assuming that OLT will be performed thereafter.[84] Data to support such a practice, however, are sparse and consist of case reports and uncontrolled case series. Hepatectomy cannot be recommended at this time.

Auxiliary liver transplantation is a technique in which a partial liver graft is placed either heterotopically or orthotopically while leaving part of the native liver in situ in the hope that the native liver will regenerate. If the native liver does regenerate, immunosuppression can be withdrawn, allowing the transplanted liver to atrophy. A European multicenter study demonstrated the feasibility and potential utility of this technique, but there are considerable technical difficulties.[85] Subtotal hepatectomy and auxiliary liver transplantation have been performed for acetaminophen-induced ALF with encouraging early results in nonrandomized case series.[86] At this time, no clear indications for auxiliary liver transplantation exist, and a randomized clinical trial has not been performed.[6]

Liver Support Systems

The "holy grail" for the treatment of ALF is a liver support device to replace the detoxification, metabolic, and synthetic functions of the liver.[87] Such a system could be used as a bridge to liver transplantation or preferably to complete recovery of the patient's native liver. Trials for the assessment of liver support devices are complicated by the fact that many patients are diverted to liver transplantation before the response to therapy with the device can be established. "Bioartificial livers" have been developed using hepatocytes harvested from pigs or derived from human hepatocellular cancer cells. A randomized, clinical trial evaluating a porcine bioartificial liver in 171 patients with ALF failed to demonstrate a survival benefit.[88] Metaanalyses (based on few subjects) evaluating the utility of artificial liver support systems in ALF have provided conflicting results.[89,90] A new generation of biological devices will begin clinical trials soon.

"Non-biologic" systems combine hemodialysis with adsorption to albumin or charcoal. Use of commercially available artificial systems based on albumin dialysis (Molecular Adsorbent Recirculating System or MARS) and fractionated plasma separation and adsorption (Prometheus) has not been associated with improved survival, although most studies have been in patients with acute or chronic liver failure.[91] A single study examining treatment with high-volume plasma exchange identified an association with increased transplant-free survival.[92] Further investigations are awaited.

SUMMARY

ALF is a complex, multisystem illness that develops after a catastrophic hepatic insult. It is characterized by coagulopathy and HE accompanied by cerebral edema and elevated ICP. The etiology is dependent on geographic location, with drugs and toxins causing more than half of the cases in developed countries. Care of the patient requires a multidisciplinary approach and full armamentarium of ICU support (Tables 70.2 and 70.3). The rarity of the condition and the rapidity of its development mean that there is a paucity of randomized clinical trials evaluating therapies. The U.S. Acute Liver Failure Study Group has published a consensus document with recommendations for specific aspects of ICU care of these patients, and the EASL has also published clinical practical guidelines. Although some patients recover spontaneously, for patients with poor prognosis, liver transplantation is the only definitive treatment. Survival rates after liver transplantation are approximately 75–90%. The efficacy of artificial liver support devices in ALF remains unproven.

TABLE 70.2 Important Summary Documents and Guidelines for the Management of Acute Liver Failure.

Authors	Year	Organization	Type of Document
Lee et al.	2012	American Association for the Study of Liver Diseases	Position paper on the management of acute liver failure: Update
Stravitz et al.	2007	United States Acute Liver Failure Study Group	Recommendations for intensive care of patients with acute liver failure
Wendon et al.	2017	European Association for the Study of the Liver	Clinical practice guidelines on the management of acute (fulminant) liver failure
Flamm et al	2017	American Gastroenterological Association Institute	Guidelines for the diagnosis and management of acute liver failure

TABLE 70.3   Selected Randomized Studies in the Management of Acute Liver Failure.

Study, Year	Number of Subjects (Intervention, No Intervention)	Study Design	Intervention	Control	Outcomes
Canalese et al. 1982	44 patients with ALF (4 groups)	Prospective, randomized, controlled trial	Dexamethasone alone, mannitol alone, both dexamethasone and mannitol	Neither	Dexamethasone did not affect survival among patients who developed cerebral edema, survival was better in mannitol group
Bhatia et al. 2004	42 patients with ALF (22 patients given prophylactic phenytoin, 22 controls)	Prospective, randomized, controlled trial	Prophylactic phenytoin administration	Usual therapy	Similar rates of cerebral edema, need for mechanical ventilation, incidence of seizures, mortality
Gazzard et al. 1975	20 patients with acetaminophen-induced ALF (10 intervention, 10 controls)	Prospective, randomized, controlled trial	FFP 300 mL every 6 h	Usual therapy	No difference in morbidity or mortality between intervention and control groups
Davenport et al. 1993	32 patients (12 intermittent RRT, 20 continuous RRT)	Prospective, randomized, controlled trial of patients with ALF and acute renal failure	Continuous RRT	Intermittent RRT	Patients in intermittent RRT had significantly lower cardiac indices and MAP
Demetriou et al. 2004	171 patients (85 bioartificial liver, 86 control)	Prospective, randomized, controlled, multicenter trial in patients with severe ALF	HepatAssist bioartificial liver (patients were allowed to undergo liver transplantation)	Usual therapy (including potential liver transplantation)	30-day survival 71% for bioartificial liver vs. 62% for control ($P = .26$).
Acharya et al. 2009	201 patients	Prospective, randomized, placebo-controlled, trial in patients with ALF	LOLA infusions (30 g daily over 3 days) HepatAssist bioartificial liver (patients were allowed to undergo liver transplantation)	Placebo	No improvement in encephalopathy grade or survival with LOLA administration
Bernal et al. 2016	43 patients with ALF (17 in the hypothermia group, 26 in the control group)	Prospective, randomized, controlled, multicenter trial in patients with ALF, HE and ICP monitoring	Targeted temperature management to 34°C for 72 h	Targeted temperature management to 36°C for 72 h	No significant difference between the groups in the prevention of intracranial hemorrhage or in overall survival
Lee et al. 2009	173 patients with ALF (81 received N-acetyl cysteine, 92 received placebo)	Randomized, double-blind, multicenter placebo controlled trial in patients with non-acetaminophen-related ALF	Intravenous N-acetyl cysteine infusion for 72 h	Placebo	Improved transplant-free survival at 3 weeks in patients with early-stage ALF but not in those with advanced HE.

ALF, acute liver failure; *FFP,* fresh frozen plasma; *HE,* hepatic encephalopathy; *LOLA,* L-ornithine L-aspartate; *MAP,* mean arterial pressure; *RRT,* renal replacement therapy.

AUTHOR'S RECOMMENDATIONS

- The diagnosis of ALF should prompt discussion with a referral center for consideration of transfer and potential liver transplantation.
- The U.S. Acute Liver Failure Study Group and the European Association for the Study of the Liver have both published recommendations for the management of patients with ALF.
- The cause of ALF should be determined because specific therapies exist for certain conditions. Acetaminophen overdose is a common cause of ALF and should be treated with NAC. The utility of NAC in non-acetaminophen ALF remains controversial
- Use of ICP monitoring has not been demonstrated to improve mortality in patients with ALF; however, some centers empirically target an ICP <25 mm Hg and a CPP >60 mm Hg.
- Coagulopathy should be treated only if invasive procedures are planned, if the patient is actively bleeding, or if the coagulopathy is extreme.
- Transplantation is the only definitive treatment for ALF, and, provided there are no contraindications, the patient should receive a highest priority listing for liver transplantation.

REFERENCES

1. Bernal W, Wendon J. Acute liver failure. *N Engl J Med.* 2013; 369(26):2525-2534.
2. Bernal W, Hyyrylainen A, Gera A, et al. Lessons from look-back in acute liver failure? A single centre experience of 3300 patients. *J Hepatol.* 2013;59(1):74-80.
3. Lee WM. Acute liver failure. *Semin Respir Crit Care Med.* 2012;33(1):36-45.
4. Bernal W, Lee WM, Wendon J, Larsen FS, Williams R. Acute liver failure: a curable disease by 2024? *J Hepatol.* 2015;62(suppl 1):S112-120.
5. Khan R, Koppe S. Modern management of acute liver failure. *Gastroenterol Clin North Am.* 2018;47(2):313-326.
6. European Association for the Study of the Liver, Wendon J, Cordoba J, et al. EASL Clinical practical guidelines on the management of acute (fulminant) liver failure. *J Hepatol.* 2017;66(5):1047-1081.
7. Reuben A, Tillman H, Fontana RJ, et al. Outcomes in adults with acute liver failure between 1998 and 2013: an observational cohort study. *Ann Intern Med.* 2016;164(11):724-732.
8. O'Grady JG, Schalm SW, Williams R. Acute liver failure: redefining the syndromes. *Lancet.* 1993;342(8866):273-275.
9. Bernuau J, Rueff B, Benhamou JP. Fulminant and subfulminant liver failure: definitions and causes. *Semin Liver Dis.* 1986;6(2): 97-106.
10. Mochida S, Nakayama N, Matsui A, Nagoshi S, Fujiwara K. Re-evaluation of the guideline published by the Acute Liver Failure Study Group of Japan in 1996 to determine the indications of liver transplantation in patients with fulminant hepatitis. *Hepatol Res.* 2008;38(10):970-979.
11. Lee WM, Stravitz RT, Larson AM. Introduction to the revised American Association for the Study of Liver Diseases Position Paper on acute liver failure 2011. *Hepatology.* 2012;55:965-967.
12. Stravitz RT, Kramer AH, Davern T, et al. Intensive care of patients with acute liver failure: recommendations of the U.S. Acute Liver Failure Study Group. *Crit Care Med.* 2007;35(11):2498-2508.

13. Flamm SL, Yang YX, Singh S, Falck-Ytter YT. American Gastro-enterological Association Institute guidelines for the diagnosis and management of acute liver Failure. *Gastroenterology.* 2017; 152(3):644-647.
14. Bower WA, Johns M, Margolis HS, Williams IT, Bell BP. Population-based surveillance for acute liver failure. *Am J Gastroenterol.* 2007;102(11):2459-2463.
15. Brandsaeter B, Höckerstedt K, Friman S, et al. Fulminant hepatic failure: outcome after listing for highly urgent liver transplantation-12 years experience in the nordic countries. *Liver Transpl.* 2002;8(11):1055-1062.
16. Escorsell A, Mas A, de la Mata M. Acute liver failure in Spain: analysis of 267 cases. *Liver Transpl.* 2007;13(10):1389-1395.
17. Ostapowicz G, Fontana RJ, Schiødt FV, et al. Results of a prospective study of acute liver failure at 17 tertiary care centers in the United States. *Ann Intern Med.* 2002;137(12):947-954.
18. Larson AM, Polson J, Fontana RJ, et al. Acetaminophen-induced acute liver failure: results of a United States multicenter, prospective study. *Hepatology.* 2005;42(6):1364-1372.
19. Sass DA, Shakil AO. Fulminant hepatic failure. *Liver Transpl.* 2005;11(6):594-605.
20. Bernsmeier C, Antoniades CG, Wendon J. What's new in acute liver failure? *Intensive Care Med.* 2014;40(10):1545-1548.
21. Patton H, Misel M, Gish RG. Acute liver failure in adults: an evidence-based management protocol for clinicians. *Gastroenterol Hepatol (N Y).* 2012;8(3):161-212.
22. Fontana RJ, Ellerbe C, Durkalski VE, et al. Two-year outcomes in initial survivors with acute liver failure: results from a prospective, multicentre study. *Liver Int.* 2015;35(2):370-380.
23. Shakil AO, Kramer D, Mazariegos GV, Fung JJ, Rakela J. Acute liver failure: clinical features, outcome analysis, and applicability of prognostic criteria. *Liver Transpl.* 2000;6(2):163-169.
24. O'Grady JG, Alexander GJ, Hayllar KM, Williams R. Early indicators of prognosis in fulminant hepatic failure. *Gastroenterology.* 1989;97:439-445.
25. McPhail MJ, Wendon JA, Bernal W. Meta-analysis of performance of Kings's College Hospital Criteria in prediction of outcome in non-paracetamol-induced acute liver failure. *J Hepatol.* 2010; 53(3):492-499.
26. Kumar R, Sharma H, Goyal R, et al. Prospective derivation and validation of early dynamic model for predicting outcome in patients with acute liver failure. *Gut.* 2012;61(7):1068-1075.
27. Wlodzimirow KA, Eslami S, Chamuleau RA, Nieuwoudt M, Abu-Hanna A. Prediction of poor outcome in patients with acute liver failure-systematic review of prediction models. *PLoS One.* 2012;7(12):e50952.
28. Bernal W, Auzinger G, Dhawan A, Wendon J. Acute liver failure. *Lancet.* 2010;376(9736):190-201.
29. Smilkstein MJ, Knapp GL, Kulig KW, Rumack BH. Efficacy of oral N-acetylcysteine in the treatment of acetaminophen overdose. Analysis of the national multicenter study (1976 to 1985). *N Engl J Med.* 1988;319(24):1557-1562.
30. Keays R, Harrison PM, Wendon JA, et al. Intravenous acetylcysteine in paracetamol induced fulminant hepatic failure: a prospective controlled trial. *BMJ.* 1991;303(6809):1026-1029.
31. Leise MD, Poterucha JJ, Talwalkar JA. Drug-induced liver injury. *Mayo Clin Proc.* 2014;89(1):95-106.
32. Reuben A, Koch DG, Lee WM. Drug-induced acute liver failure: results of a U.S. multicenter, prospective study. *Hepatology.* 2010; 52(6):2065-2076.
33. Karkhanis J, Verna EC, Chang MS, et al. Steroid use in acute liver failure. *Hepatology.* 2014;59(2):612-621.

34. Hay JE. Liver disease in pregnancy. *Hepatology.* 2008;47(3): 1067-1076.

35. Korman JD, Volenberg I, Balko J, et al. Screening for Wilson disease in acute liver failure: a comparison of currently available diagnostic tests. *Hepatology.* 2008;48(4):1167-1174.

36. Roberts EA, Schilsky ML. A practice guideline on Wilson disease. *Hepatology.* 2003;37(6):1475-1492.

37. Broussard CN, Aggarwal A, Lacey SR, et al. Mushroom poisoning—from diarrhea to liver transplantation. *Am J Gastroenterol.* 2001;96(11):3195-3198.

38. Menon KV, Shah V, Kamath PS. The Budd-Chiari syndrome. *N Engl J Med.* 2004;350(6):578-585.

39. Wijdicks EF. Hepatic encephalopathy. *N Engl J Med.* 2016; 375(17):1660-1670.

40. Clemmesen JO, Larsen FS, Kondrup J, Hansen BA, Ott P. Cerebral herniation in patients with acute liver failure is correlated with arterial ammonia concentration. *Hepatology.* 1999;29(3): 648-653.

41. Mouri S, Tripon S, Rudler M, et al. FOUR score, a reliable score for assessing overt hepatic encephalopathy in cirrhotic patients. *Neurocrit Care.* 2015;22(2):251-257.

42. Alba L, Hay JE, Angulo P, LEE WM. Lactulose therapy in acute liver failure. *J Hepatol.* 2002;36:33.

43. Wendon JA, Larsen FS. Intracranial pressure monitoring in acute liver failure. A procedure with clear indications. *Hepatology.* 2006;44(2):504-506.

44. Bernuau J, Durand F. Intracranial pressure monitoring in patients with acute liver failure: a questionable invasive surveillance. *Hepatology.* 2006;44(2):502-504.

45. Vaquero J, Fontana RJ, Larson AM, et al. Complications and use of intracranial pressure monitoring in patients with acute liver failure and severe encephalopathy. *Liver Transpl.* 2005; 11(12):1581-1589.

46. Karvellas CJ, Fix OK, Battenhouse H, Durkalski V, Sanders C, Lee WM. Outcomes and complications of intracranial pressure monitoring in acute liver failure: a retrospective cohort study. *Crit Care Med.* 2014;42(5):1157-1167.

47. McCashland TM, Shaw Jr BW, Tape E. The American experience with transplantation for acute liver failure. *Semin Liver Dis.* 1996; 16(4):427-433.

48. Wijdicks EF, Nyberg SL. Propofol to control intracranial pressure in fulminant hepatic failure. *Transplant Proc.* 2002;34(4): 1220-1222.

49. Forbes A, Alexander GJ, O'Grady JG, et al. Thiopental infusion in the treatment of intracranial hypertension complicating fulminant hepatic failure. *Hepatology.* 1989;10(3):306-310.

50. Canalese J, Gimson AE, Davis C, Mellon PJ, Davis M, Williams R. Controlled trial of dexamethasone and mannitol for the cerebral oedema of fulminant hepatic failure. *Gut.* 1982;23(7): 625-629.

51. Murphy N, Auzinger G, Bernel W, Wendon J. The effect of hypertonic sodium chloride on intracranial pressure in patients with acute liver failure. *Hepatology.* 2004;39(2):464-470.

52. Wendon J, Lee W. Encephalopathy and cerebral edema in the setting of acute liver failure: pathogenesis and management. *Neurocrit Care.* 2008;9(1):97-102.

53. Ede RJ, Gimson AE, Bihari D, Williams R. Controlled hyperventilation in the prevention of cerebral oedema in fulminant hepatic failure. *J Hepatol.* 1986;2(1):43-51.

54. Ellis AJ, Wendon JA, Williams R. Subclinical seizure activity and prophylactic phenytoin infusion in acute liver failure: a controlled clinical trial. *Hepatology.* 2000;32(3):536-541.

55. Bhatia V, Batra Y, Acharya SK. Prophylactic phenytoin does not improve cerebral edema or survival in acute liver failure—a controlled clinical trial. *J Hepatol.* 2004;41(1):89-96.

56. Tofteng F, Larsen FS. The effect of indomethacin on intracranial pressure, cerebral perfusion and extracellular lactate and glutamate concentrations in patients with fulminant hepatic failure. *J Cereb Blood Flow Metab.* 2004;24(7):798-804.

57. Stravitz RT, Lisman T, Luketic VA, et al. Minimal effects of acute liver injury/acute liver failure on hemostasis as assessed by thromboelastography. *J Hepatol.* 2012;56(1):129-136.

58. De Pietri L, Bianchini M, Montalti R, et al. Thrombelastography-guided blood product use before invasive procedures in cirrhosis with severe coagulopathy: a randomized, controlled trial. *Hepatology.* 2016;63(2):566-573.

59. Wang SC, Shieh JF, Chang KY, et al. Thromboelastography-guided transfusion decreases intraoperative blood transfusion during orthotopic liver transplantation: randomized clinical trial. *Transplant Proc.* 2010;42(7):2590-2593.

60. Gazzard BG, Henderson JM, Williams R. Early changes in coagulation following a paracetamol overdose and a controlled trial of fresh frozen plasma therapy. *Gut.* 1975;16(8): 617-620.

61. Shami VM, Caldwell SH, Hespenheide EE, Arseneau KO, Bickston SJ, Macik BG. Recombinant activated factor VII for coagulopathy in fulminant hepatic failure compared with conventional therapy. *Liver Transpl.* 2003;9(2):138-143.

62. Rolando N, Wade J, Davalos M, Wendon J, Philpott-Howard J, Williams R. The systemic inflammatory response syndrome in acute liver failure. *Hepatology.* 2000;32(4 Pt 1):734-739.

63. Tujios SR, Hynan LS, Vazquez MA, et al. Risk factors and outcomes of acute kidney injury in patients with acute liver failure. *Clin Gastroenterol Hepatol.* 2015;13(2):352-359.

64. Davenport A. Renal replacement therapy in the patient with acute brain injury. *Am J Kidney Dis.* 2001;37(3):457-466.

65. Nadim MK, Annanthapanyasut W, Matsuoka L, et al. Intraoperative hemodialysis during liver transplantation: a decade of experience. *Liver Transpl.* 2014;20(7):756-764.

66. Stravitz RT, Kramer DJ. Management of acute liver failure. *Nat Rev Gastroenterol Hepatol.* 2009;6(9):542-553.

67. Shawcross DL, Davies NA, Mookerjee RP, et al. Worsening of cerebral hyperemia by the administration of terlipressin in acute liver failure with severe encephalopathy. *Hepatology.* 2004; 39(2):471-475.

68. Marik PE. Adrenal-exhaustion syndrome in patients with liver disease. *Intensive Care Med.* 2006;32(2):275-280.

69. Saner FH, Olde Damink SW, Pavlakovifá G, et al. Positive end-expiratory pressure induces liver congestion in living donor liver transplant patients: myth or fact. *Transplantation.* 2008; 85(12):1863-1866.

70. Macdougall BR, Bailey RJ, Williams R. H2-receptor antagonists and antacids in the prevention of acute gastrointestinal haemorrhage in fulminant hepatic failure. Two controlled trials. *Lancet.* 1977;1(8012):617-619.

71. Schmidt LE, Dalhoff K. Serum phosphate is an early predictor of outcome in severe acetaminophen-induced hepatotoxicity. *Hepatology.* 2002;36(3):659-665.

72. Walsh TS, Wigmore SJ, Hopton P, Richardson R, Lee A. Energy expenditure in acetaminophen-induced fulminant hepatic failure. *Crit Care Med.* 2000;28(3):649-654.

73. Schütz T, Bechstein WO, Neuhaus P, Lochs H, Plauth M. Clinical practice of nutrition in acute liver failure—a European survey. *Clin Nutr.* 2004;23(5):975-982.

74. Als-Nielsen B, Koretz RL, Kjaergard LL, Gluud C. Branched-chain amino acids for hepatic encephalopathy. *Cochrane Database Syst Rev.* 2003(2):CD001939.

75. Simpson KJ, Bates CM, Henderson NC, et al. The utilization of liver transplantation in the management of acute liver failure: comparison between acetaminophen and non-acctaminophen etiologies. *Liver Transpl.* 2009;15(6):600-609.

76. Germani G, Theocharidou E, Adam R, et al. Liver transplantation for acute liver failure in Europe: outcomes over 20 years from the ELTR database. *J Hepatol.* 2012;57(2):288-296.

77. Bernal W, Cross TJ, Auzinger G, et al. Outcome after wait-listing for emergency liver transplantation in acute liver failure: a single centre experience. *J Hepatol.* 2009;50(2):306-313.

78. Vaquero J. Therapeutic hypothermia in the management of acute liver failure. *Neurochem Int.* 2012;60(7):723-735.

79. Jalan R, Damink SW, Deutz NE, Lee A, Hayes PC. Moderate hypothermia for uncontrolled intracranial hypertension in acute liver failure. *Lancet.* 1999;354(9185):1164-1168.

80. Karvellas CJ, Todd Stravitz R, Battenhouse H, Lee WM, Schilsky ML, US Acute Liver Failure Study Group. Therapeutic hypothermia in acute liver failure: a multicenter retrospective cohort analysis. *Liver Transpl.* 2015;21(1):4-12.

81. Bernal W, Murphy N, Brown S, et al. A multicentre randomized controlled trial of moderate hypothermia to prevent intracranial hypertension in acute liver failure. *J Hepatol.* 2016;65(2):273-279.

82. Lee WM, Hynan LS, Rossaro L, et al. Intravenous N-Acetylcysteine improves transplant-free survival in early stage non-acetaminophen acute liver failure. *Gastroenterology.* 2009;137(3):856-864.

83. Darweesh SK, Ibrahim MF, El-Tahawy MA. Effect of N-Acetylcysteine on mortality and liver transplantation rate in non-acetaminophen-induced acute liver failure: A multicenter study. *Clin Drug Investig.* 2017;37(5):473-482.

84. Jalan R, Pollok A, Shah SH, Madhavan K, Simpson KJ. Liver derived pro-inflammatory cytokines may be important in producing intracranial hypertension in acute liver failure. *J Hepatol.* 2002;37(4):536-538.

85. Chenard-Neu MP, Boudjema K, Bernuau J, et al. Auxiliary liver transplantation: regeneration of the native liver and outcome in 30 patients with fulminant hepatic failure—a multicenter European study. *Hepatology.* 1996;23(5):1119-1127.

86. Rajput I, Prasad KR, Bellamy MC, Davies M, Attia MS, Lodge JP. Subtotal hepatectomy and whole graft auxiliary transplantation for acetaminophen-associated acute liver failure. *HPB (Oxford).* 2014;16(3):220-228.

87. Williams R. The elusive goal of liver support—quest for the Holy Grail. *Clin Med (Lond).* 2006;6(5):482-487.

88. Demetriou AA, Brown Jr RS, Busuttil RW, et al. Prospective, randomized, multicenter, controlled trial of a bioartificial liver in treating acute liver failure. *Ann Surg.* 2004;239(5):660-667, discussion 667-670.

89. Stutchfield BM, Simpson K, Wigmore SJ. Systematic review and meta-analysis of survival following extracorporeal liver support. *Br J Surg.* 2011;98(5):623-631.

90. Zheng Z, Li X, Li Z, Ma X. Artificial and bioartificial liver support systems for acute and acute-on-chronic hepatic failure: a meta-analysis and meta-regression. *Exp Ther Med.* 2013;6(4):929-936.

91. Saliba F, Camus C, Durand F, et al. Albumin dialysis with a noncell artificial liver support device in patients with acute liver failure: a randomized, controlled trial. *Ann Intern Med.* 2013;159(8):522-531.

92. Larsen FS, Schmidt LE, Bernsmeier C, et al. High-volume plasma exchange in patients with acute liver failure: an open randomised controlled trial. *J Hepatol.* 2016;64(1):69-78.

93. Davenport A, Will EJ, Davidson AM. Improved cardiovascular stability during continuous modes of renal replacement therapy in critically ill patients with acute hepatic and renal failure. *Crit Care Med.* 1993;21(3):328-38.

94. Acharya SK, Bhatia V, Sreenivas V, Khanal S, Panda SK. Efficacy of L-ornithine L-aspartate in acute liver failure: a double-blind, randomized, placebo-controlled study. *Gastroenterology.* 2009;136(7):2159-68.

71

Is There a Place for Anabolic Hormones in Critical Care?

Nicholas Heming, Virginie Maxime, Hong Tuan Ha Vivien, and Djillali Annane

Anabolism is the enzymatic process by which nutrients and energy are used to synthesize molecules in living cells. In contrast, catabolism involves chemical reactions that lead to the degradation of molecules. During growth, anabolic processes dominate, either through increased biosynthesis or decreased molecular degradation. In healthy subjects, energy is produced through the catabolism of carbohydrates and fat, whereas proteins and amino acids are used to generate new structures (i.e., for anabolism). When patients become acutely ill, amino acids from muscle are used to synthesize acute-phase proteins and for gluconeogenesis; however this process is limited and adaptive. In critical illness, two distinct metabolic phases have been described.[1] The first is similar to what is seen in acute illness and is characterized by the diversion of energy and anabolism toward vital organs and the immune system. This response is mediated in part by the endocrine system. Protracted critical illness constitutes the second phase. It is often maladaptive, with uncompensated catabolism leading to major nitrogen loss and muscle wasting, and is characterized by a globally decreased endocrine response.[2] Increased catabolism may be responsible for insufficient wound healing, prolonged mechanical ventilation, and extended lengths of hospital stay. Aggressive nutritional support during this second phase does not prevent muscle wasting.[3,4] It has been hypothesized that hormone supplementation during the protracted phase of critical illness may favor anabolism. Four hormones having anabolic properties may be of interest in the critical care setting: androgens, insulin, growth hormone, and thyroid hormone. The following chapter reviews the evidence regarding the safety and efficacy of anabolic hormone supplementation in critically ill adults.

ANDROGENS

Androgens, or male sex hormones, are synthesized from cholesterol by a series of enzymatic reactions. This synthetic pathway is detailed in Fig. 71.1. Of note, 17-OH-pregnenolone and 17-OH-progesterone are also precursors of cortisol. Di-hydro-epi-androsterone (DHEA, as well as DHEA-S, the sulfated form of DHEA that predominates in the circulation) and androstenedione, although adrenal androgens, are considered to be largely inactive.[5,6] Serum DHEA levels are increased during septic shock, whereas those of DHEA-S are decreased. The increase in DHEA concentration may follow the increase in cortisol levels seen during septic shock.[7] Testosterone can also be converted to estradiol by the aromatase enzyme.

Testosterone is the most abundantly produced and most clinically relevant androgen. It is secreted by the interstitial cells of Leydig in the testes and by the adrenal glands in both males and females.[5,8] Testosterone secretion is regulated by luteinizing hormone (LH) produced in the anterior pituitary. LH secretion is stimulated by gonadotropin-releasing hormone (GnRH), which is produced by the hypothalamus. Circulating testosterone is bound to albumin or to the sex hormone-binding globulin.[9] Serum concentrations of testosterone are 12–31 nmol/L in healthy males and 0.52–2.6 nmol/L in healthy females. Testosterone remains in the circulation for no more than a few hours, after which it is either transported to its target tissues or degraded. At a cellular level, testosterone or its intracellular metabolite, dihydrotestosterone, binds to a nuclear receptor protein complex. This complex migrates to the cell nucleus and induces DNA transcription. Testosterone has well-documented anabolic properties.[10] It induces hypertrophy of type I and II muscle fibers and increases the number of skeletal muscle satellite cells.[11,12] Testosterone also promotes the differentiation of multipotent mesenchymal cells into myocytes and inhibits their differentiation into adipocytes.[13,14] Finally, androgens may alter other physiologic parameters via nongenomic signaling pathways that involve lipid and protein metabolism.[15]

Studies in animal models of trauma, hemorrhage, and sepsis have demonstrated that females have stronger immune responses and better survival rates than males[16,17]; however, in the critically ill, clinical evidence of an association between female gender and improved outcome is weak and relies on inconclusive or contradictory literature.[18,19]

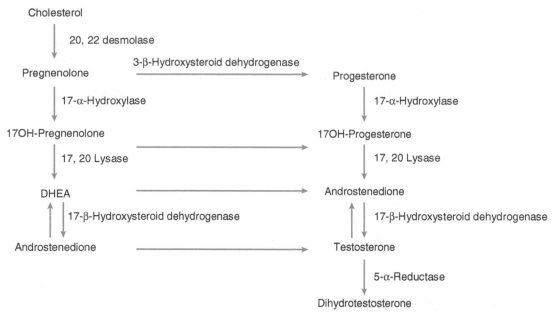

Fig. 71.1 Biosynthesis of Androgens. *DHEA,* dehydroepiandrosterone. (Modified from Miller WL, Auchus RJ. The molecular biology, biochemistry, and physiology of human steroidogenesis and its disorders. *Endocr Rev.* 2011;32[1]:81–151.)

During acute illness, testosterone concentrations are low, whereas LH levels are increased.[20] In patients with prolonged critical illness, serum testosterone, LH, and GnRH concentrations are low.[21,22] For example, in some patients with chronic obstructive pulmonary disease or human immunodeficiency virus-associated wasting syndromes, administration of synthetic androgens induced a gain in muscle mass and strength and improved respiratory function.[23,24] In men with severe burn injuries, testosterone reduced protein catabolism.[25] The synthetic androgen oxandrolone, which has been approved by the US Food and Drug Administration as an adjunctive therapy after surgery or trauma, may reduce weight loss, improve functional status, and increase wound healing[26,27]; however, a large trial involving oxandrolone administration to trauma patients failed to demonstrate any significant benefit.[28] Another trial, performed in ventilator-dependent surgical patients, found that oxandrolone prolonged the duration of mechanical ventilation.[29] Data from trials assessing the effect of testosterone supplementation in critically ill patients on patient-centered outcomes are scarce, with ongoing clinical trials (ClinicalTrials.gov: NCT03038919). Although data are limited, the safety profile of androgens may be favorable. Likewise, data on use of testosterone precursors such as DHEA in the critically ill are also lacking.

Overall, in the critically ill, androgen supplementation may have some benefits on nutritional endpoints in select subgroups of patients. Additional trials are still needed before the routine use of such a therapeutic approach could be suggested for caring for the critically ill.

INSULIN

Insulin is formed by two peptide chains—a 21-amino acid A chain and a 30-amino acid B chain—that are linked by disulfide bonds.[30] The hormone regulates carbohydrate metabolism by promoting glucose entry into some types of cells. Insulin is produced by the beta cells of the islets of Langerhans of the pancreas.[5] The gene encoding insulin is highly conserved and yields a single chain precursor. Various factors, including glucose, glucagon, cholecystokinin, and gastric inhibitory polypeptide, induce insulin secretion. Insulin secretion is inhibited by catecholamines and somatostatin. Monomers of insulin, the active form of the hormone, are mostly unbound in the circulation. The half-life of circulating insulin is extremely short, approximately 6 minutes, ensuring that carbohydrate homeostasis occurs almost instantaneously. The fasting serum concentration of insulin ranges from 28 to 108 pmol/L in healthy individuals.

The insulin receptor has strong analogies with the insulin-like growth factor-1 (IGF-1) receptor. Both belong to the receptor tyrosine kinase family.[31] On ligand binding, intracellular portions of the receptor are activated by phosphorylation. Activation is followed by the recruitment and phosphorylation of adaptor proteins and downstream signaling proteins.[32] One of the downstream signals involves the mitogen-activated protein (MAP) kinase cascade, which plays a role in modulating cellular proliferation, differentiation, and survival. Insulin receptors can also recruit the insulin receptor substrate adaptor, inducing the activation of phosphoinositide 3-kinase. This enzyme indirectly increases the amount of glucose that is captured by the organism.[33] In addition to its effect on carbohydrate metabolism, insulin also plays a role in protein metabolism and storage, but the mechanics leading to the modification of protein metabolism are poorly understood.

Insulin increases the translation of mRNA as well as the rate of transcription of select DNA sequences. Insulin inhibits the catabolism of proteins, decreases the rate of amino acid release by muscle cells, and stimulates the transport of amino acids into the cells. Insulin inhibits the activity of enzymes promoting gluconeogenesis. Because gluconeogenesis relies on amino acids, insulin indirectly conserves protein and amino acid stores.[34] Insulin promotes protein synthesis in cultured cells, in isolated muscles, and in vivo in animal models.[35,36] A trial conducted in healthy human volunteers, using isotopic tracers, showed that insulin promotes muscle anabolism by stimulating protein synthesis.[37] Trials conducted in severely burned patients indicate that insulin improves protein synthesis.[38,39]

Numerous trials of glycemic control by insulin administration in critically ill patients have been conducted since 2000. The aim of these trials was to assess the effect of glucose control on mortality; thus they did not focus on the anabolic effect of insulin. A large monocentric trial found that surgical intensive care unit (ICU) patients treated with intensive insulin therapy (target blood glucose levels between 80 and 110 mg/dL) had lower ICU mortality than patients managed with conventional treatment (blood glucose between 180 and 200 mg/dL).[40] A second monocentric trial did not find significant differences in survival rates in medical ICU patients with or without intensive insulin therapy.[41] Subgroup analyses revealed that intensive insulin therapy reduced the mortality rate in patients hospitalized in the ICU for more than 3 days.[41] The GLUCONTROL multicenter trial compared intensive insulin therapy (target blood glucose between 80 and 110 mg/dL) with conventional treatment (target blood glucose between 140 and 180 mg/dL) in the critically ill.[42] In this trial, which was prematurely stopped because of a high number of protocol violations, ICU mortality was similar in both groups. Intensive insulin therapy was associated with an increased incidence of hypoglycemia.[42] The NICE-SUGAR trial, including more than 6000 patients, compared intensive insulin therapy (target blood glucose range of 81 to 108 mg/dL), to conventional treatment (target of ≤180 mg/dL).[43] Mortality at day 90 and the incidence of hypoglycemia were significantly higher in the intensive insulin therapy group.[43] The VISEP (Efficacy of Volume Substitution and Insulin Therapy in Severe Sepsis) trial included ICU patients with severe sepsis. In this trial, the mean score for organ failure and the number of deaths at 28 days were not significantly different between the intensive insulin therapy group (target blood glucose levels 80–110 mg/dL) and the conventional treatment group (target blood glucose levels 180–200 mg/dL). This trial was stopped prematurely because of a significant increase in the incidence of hypoglycemia with the experimental intervention.[44] Lastly, glucose variability might be an independent prognostic factor in critically ill patients.[45,46]

Current guidelines for the management of sepsis recommend administering insulin to control hyperglycemia.[47] As a general rule, physicians should target a blood glucose level of less than 180 mg/dL during ICU stay. There is no specific recommendation for the administration of insulin as an anabolic hormone.

GROWTH HORMONE

Growth hormone (GH) is structurally similar to prolactin and placental lactogen. Production of GH is positively controlled by the GH releasing hormone (GHRH) and ghrelin. Both are subjected to pulsatile release from the hypothalamus and act on the anterior pituitary to induce pulsatile release of GH. Ghrelin is also produced by the stomach and pancreas.[48,49] Stress, physical exercise, hypoglycemia, and elevated insulin concentrations induce GHRH production. By contrast, somatostatin, hyperglycemia, obesity, and hypercortisolism inhibit GHRH production.[50,51] The serum half-life of GH ranges between 20 and 30 minutes. The fasting serum concentration of GH in healthy adults is less than 5 ng/mL. GH plays an anabolic role in protein and glucose metabolism, and stimulates bone growth.[52] The hormone acts either directly through the GH receptors or via the effect of other growth hormones that have a structure similar to proinsulin and stimulate the uptake of amino acids and inhibit the degradation of muscle proteins.[53,54] The most important of these hormones is IGF-1, produced by hepatocytes under the influence of GH.[55] IGF-1 is a negative feedback regulator of GH and GHRH. IGF-1 stimulates protein synthesis and decreases the degradation of skeletal muscle proteins.[54] More than 90% of circulating IGF-1 is bound to IGF binding proteins (IGFBPs).[50]

Critically ill patients suffer from major nitrogen loss associated with muscle wasting. This state has some similarities to that of patients suffering from chronic GH deficiency.[56] The acute phase of critical illness is characterized by increased production of pituitary hormones, especially GH, and peripheral resistance to their effects. Overall production of GH is raised through an upsurge in the number and the intensity of GHRH ghrelin pulses and is associated with heightened GH concentrations between pulses and attenuated oscillatory activity.[57] Underlying mechanisms may include increased levels of GHRH and decreased levels of somatostatin. In the ICU, elevated GH concentrations seem to be associated with an increased risk of death.[58] In addition, IGF-1 levels are decreased because of the downregulated expression of liver GH receptors[59] or decreased levels of the main carrier protein IGFBP-3, which is also regulated by GH. These changes are considered adaptive because they could direct the use of glucose, fatty acids, and amino acids toward the production of energy rather than anabolism.[60] During the chronic phase of critical illness, GH and IGF-1 levels decrease even further because of the dramatically reduced pulse amplitude only partially offset by the increased frequency of these same pulses. This neuroendocrine dysfunction seems to be secondary to decreased ghrelin levels. Indeed, high concentrations of ghrelin are associated with a favorable outcome.[61]

IGF-I promotes proliferation and differentiation in muscle cell lines.[62] The administration of GH or of IGF-1 to healthy animals induces muscle hypertrophy.[63] Both GH and IGF-1 administration to animals suffering from burns or major surgery are associated with improved nitrogen balance and immune responses.[64,65]

Exploratory trials in humans showed that GH supplementation is associated with a positive nitrogen balance both in patients with and without sepsis.[66,67] One trial reported that GH supplementation after major surgery was associated with a positive nitrogen balance and improved peripheral muscular testing[68]; however, two separate multicenter trials in general ICU populations showed that the administration of recombinant human GH was associated with increased in-hospital mortality rates.[69] Current guidelines do not recommend the use of GH in the critically ill.[70] The administration of GH releasing peptide-2 (GHRP-2), which is an agonist of ghrelin, is more effective than GHRH for increasing circulating levels of GH, IGF-1, and IGFBP.[71] Additional studies are needed to confirm the efficacy and safety of this treatment. The administration of insulin to the critically ill increases circulating levels of GH and peripheral resistance to GH.[72] Peripheral resistance to GH during protracted illness could be protective.[50]

Opotherapy for GH deficiency is harmful during the acute phase of critical illness. Further studies are needed to examine the effects of GHRH on anabolism during protracted critical illness.

THYROID HORMONES

Thyroid hormones (THs) are synthesized in the thyroid gland. TH synthesis requires the prohormone thyroglobulin and iodine, obtained through normal dietary intake. Tyrosine residues on thyroglobulin can bind iodine once, forming monoiodotyrosine (MIT), or twice, forming diiodotyrosine (DIT). The combination of two DIT residues results in the formation of thyroxine (T_4). The combination of one MIT with one DIT residue results in the formation of triiodothyronine (T_3) or of the biologically inactive 3,3',5'-triiodothyronine (reverse T_3 or rT_3).[73] These hormones have the same thyronine structure but differ by the number and position of iodine atoms. T_4 is converted by type 1 deiodinase into the more active T_3. Type 2 deiodinase converts T_4 into T_3 and also converts rT_3 into T_2 (diiodothyronine). Type 3 deiodinase degrades THs, converting T_4 into rT_3 and T_3 into T_2. The hypothalamic thyroid-releasing hormone (TRH) controls the release of thyroid-stimulating hormone (TSH), which originates in the pituitary gland. In turn, TSH stimulates the production of T_3 and T_4. TSH has a basal level of constant secretion over which pulses are released. TSH is inhibited by somatostatin and dopamine as well as feedback from T_3 and T_4.[74] Approximately 80% of THs are transported bound to T_4-binding globulin, whereas 20% are bound to transthyretin or albumin. Serum concentration of free T_3 ranges between 4 and 9 pmol/L, while the concentration of free T_4 is between 9 and 25 pmol/L and that of TSH between 0.1 and 4.5 μIU/mL. The half-life of T_4 is 6 to 7 days, whereas that of T_3 is 24 hours. THs enter the cell and bind to nuclear receptors, which mediate the activity of THs via modification of transcriptional activity. THs upregulate all cellular metabolic activities by increasing the number and the activity of mitochondria and accelerating the active transport of ions (potassium, sodium) and glucose across cell membranes. THs also upregulate metabolic activities via nongenomic pathways (i.e., through other means than TH nuclear receptor binding).[75] Physiologic amounts of THs have an anabolic effect and enhance protein synthesis.

In animal models, THs are necessary for anabolism,[76] while supraphysiologicl levels of THs are catabolic. In the ICU, up to 70% of patients have a "nonthyroidal illness syndrome" in which levels of T_3 are diminished and T_4 levels are normal or lowered in the absence of thyroidal disease. TSH is not increased.[77] These anomalies are caused by peripheral mechanisms. Type 1 deiodinase activity is decreased; thus less T_4 is deiodinated into T_3, whereas the activity of type 3 deiodinase is increased, inactivating THs.[78] The activity of type 2 deiodinase remains almost unchanged during the acute phase of critical illness. Patients also exhibit reduced levels of TH-binding protein, causing lower levels of circulating T_4. Decreased levels of intracellular transport and of intranuclear receptor expression could be an adaptive mechanism, aimed at increasing tissue levels of the hormones, especially in the liver and the skeletal muscle.[79,80]

During protracted illness, hormonal disturbances are the consequence of hypothalamic-pituitary axis insufficiency: TRH and TSH levels are low.[81] Decreased TRH secretion could be induced by raised levels of T_3 at the hypothalamic level, either via upregulation of type 2 deiodinase or a downregulation of type 3 deiodinase activity.[82] Consequently, secretion of TSH is also modified. TSH pulsatility is lost, and the amplitude of each pulse is decreased. The pathophysiologic mechanisms explaining these modifications are incompletely understood but may involve imbalance in proinflammatory and antiinflammatory cytokines.

Clinical trials of TH supplementation were undertaken in several small cohorts. T_4 supplementation increased mortality in patients with acute renal failure.[83] T_3 supplementation increased heart rate and vascular resistances without affecting mortality after major cardiac surgery.[84] The administration of TRH, associated with GHRH or GHRP-2, restored normal TSH and T_3 levels without increasing rT_3 levels.[85] None of these trials showed any clinically relevant beneficial effect of TH supplementation in adults previously devoid of thyroidal disease.

Overall, there is no evidence suggesting any significant benefit from the administration of THs or GHs to the critically ill. Anabolic steroid androgens might improve surrogate outcomes such as weight gain after major surgery or burns. Finally, insulin, which is now broadly given to ICU patients to control blood glucose, may also provide some anabolic effects.

AUTHORS' RECOMMENDATIONS
- Administration of TH or GH to the critically ill is not recommended.
- The synthetic androgen oxandrolone may be used as an adjunctive therapy to promote weight gain after surgery or trauma.
- Insulin, used as part of a blood glucose control strategy, may have some anabolic effects.

REFERENCES

1. Van den Berghe G, de Zegher F, Bouillon R. Clinical review 95: acute and prolonged critical illness as different neuroendocrine paradigms. *J Clin Endocrinol Metab.* 1998;83:1827-1834.
2. Puthucheary ZA, Rawal J, McPhail M, et al. Acute skeletal muscle wasting in critical illness. *JAMA.* 2013;310:1591-1600.
3. Streat SJ, Beddoe AH, Hill GL. Aggressive nutritional support does not prevent protein loss despite fat gain in septic intensive care patients. *J Trauma.* 1987;27:262-266.
4. Hart DW, Wolf SE, Herndon DN, et al. Energy expenditure and caloric balance after burn: increased feeding leads to fat rather than lean mass accretion. *Ann Surg.* 2002;235:152-161.
5. Guyton AC. *Textbook of Medical Physiology.* 11th ed. Philadelphia, PA: Saunders; 2005.
6. Shea JL, Wong PY, Chen Y. Free testosterone: clinical utility and important analytical aspects of measurement. *Adv Clin Chem.* 2014;63:59-84.
7. Arlt W, Hammer F, Sanning P, et al. Dissociation of serum dehydroepiandrosterone and dehydroepiandrosterone sulfate in septic shock. *J Clin Endocrinol Metab.* 2006;91:2548-2554.
8. Federman DD. The biology of human sex differences. *N Engl J Med.* 2006;354:1507-1514.
9. Fortunati N. Sex hormone-binding globulin: not only a transport protein. What news is around the corner? *J Endocrinol Invest.* 1999;22:223-234.
10. Bhasin S, Storer TW, Berman N, et al. The effects of supraphysiologic doses of testosterone on muscle size and strength in normal men. *N Engl J Med.* 1996;335:1-7.
11. Sinha-Hikim I, Artaza J, Woodhouse L, et al. Testosterone-induced increase in muscle size in healthy young men is associated with muscle fiber hypertrophy. *Am J Physiol Endocrinol Metab.* 2002;283:E154-E164.
12. Sinha-Hikim I, Roth SM, Lee MI, Bhasin S. Testosterone-induced muscle hypertrophy is associated with an increase in satellite cell number in healthy, young men. *Am J Physiol Endocrinol Metab.* 2003;285:E197-E205.
13. Singh R, Artaza JN, Taylor WE, Gonzalez-Cadavid NF, Bhasin S. Androgens stimulate myogenic differentiation and inhibit adipogenesis in C3H 10T1/2 pluripotent cells through an androgen receptor-mediated pathway. *Endocrinology.* 2003;144:5081-5088.
14. Bhasin S, Taylor WE, Singh R, et al. The mechanisms of androgen effects on body composition: mesenchymal pluripotent cell as the target of androgen action. *J Gerontol A Biol Sci Med Sci.* 2003;58:M1103-M1110.
15. Mauras N, Hayes V, Welch S, et al. Testosterone deficiency in young men: marked alterations in whole body protein kinetics, strength, and adiposity. *J Clin Endocrinol Metab.* 1998;83:1886-1892.
16. Wichmann MW, Ayala A, Chaudry IH. Male sex steroids are responsible for depressing macrophage immune function after trauma-hemorrhage. *Am J Physiol.* 1997;273:C1335-C1340.
17. Zellweger R, Wichmann MW, Ayala A, Stein S, DeMaso CM, Chaudry IH. Females in proestrus state maintain splenic immune functions and tolerate sepsis better than males. *Crit Care Med.* 1997;25:106-110.
18. Croce MA, Fabian TC, Malhotra AK, Bee TK, Miller PR. Does gender difference influence outcome? *J Trauma.* 2002;53:889-894.
19. Valentin A, Jordan B, Lang T, Hiesmayr M, Metnitz PG. Gender-related differences in intensive care: a multiple-center cohort study of therapeutic interventions and outcome in critically ill patients. *Crit Care Med.* 2003;31:1901-1907.
20. Lephart ED, Baxter CR, Parker Jr CR. Effect of burn trauma on adrenal and testicular steroid hormone production. *J Clin Endocrinol Metab.* 1987;64:842-848.
21. Sharshar T, Bastuji-Garin S, De Jonghe B, et al. Hormonal status and ICU-acquired paresis in critically ill patients. *Intensive Care Med.* 2010;36:1318-1326.
22. Van den Berghe G, Weekers F, Baxter RC, et al. Five-day pulsatile gonadotropin-releasing hormone administration unveils combined hypothalamic-pituitary-gonadal defects underlying profound hypoandrogenism in men with prolonged critical illness. *J Clin Endocrinol Metab.* 2001;86:3217-3226.
23. Schols AM, Soeters PB, Mostert R, Pluymers RJ, Wouters EF. Physiologic effects of nutritional support and anabolic steroids in patients with chronic obstructive pulmonary disease. A placebo-controlled randomized trial. *Am J Respir Crit Care Med.* 1995;152:1268-1274.
24. Strawford A, Barbieri T, Van Loan M, et al. Resistance exercise and supraphysiologic androgen therapy in eugonadal men with HIV-related weight loss: a randomized controlled trial. *JAMA.* 1999;281:1282-1290.
25. Ferrando AA, Sheffield-Moore M, Wolf SE, Herndon DN, Wolfe RR. Testosterone administration in severe burns ameliorates muscle catabolism. *Crit Care Med.* 2001;29:1936-1942.
26. Demling RH, Orgill DP. The anticatabolic and wound healing effects of the testosterone analog oxandrolone after severe burn injury. *J Crit Care.* 2000;15:12-17.
27. Jeschke MG, Finnerty CC, Suman OE, Kulp G, Mlcak RP, Herndon DN. The effect of oxandrolone on the endocrinologic, inflammatory, and hypermetabolic responses during the acute phase postburn. *Ann Surg.* 2007;246:351-360.
28. Gervasio JM, Dickerson RN, Swearingen J, et al. Oxandrolone in trauma patients. *Pharmacotherapy.* 2000;20:1328-1334.
29. Bulger EM, Jurkovich GJ, Farver CL, Klotz P, Maier RV. Oxandrolone does not improve outcome of ventilator dependent surgical patients. *Ann Surg.* 2004;240:472-478.
30. Adams MJ, Blundell TL, Dodson EJ, et al. Structure of rhombohedral 2 zinc insulin crystals. *Nature.* 1969;224:491-495.
31. Hubbard SR, Till JH. Protein tyrosine kinase structure and function. *Annu Rev Biochem.* 2000;69:373-398.
32. De Meyts P, Whittaker J. Structural biology of insulin and IGF1 receptors: implications for drug design. *Nat Rev Drug Discov.* 2002;1:769-783.
33. Pessin JE, Saltiel AR. Signaling pathways in insulin action: molecular targets of insulin resistance. *J Clin Invest.* 2000;106:165-169.
34. Barthel A, Schmoll D. Novel concepts in insulin regulation of hepatic gluconeogenesis. *Am J Physiol Endocrinol Metab.* 2003;285:E685-E692.
35. Manchester KL, Young FG. The effect of insulin on incorporation of amino acids into protein of normal rat diaphragm in vitro. *Biochem J.* 1958;70:353-358.
36. Airhart J, Arnold JA, Stirewalt WS, Low RB. Insulin stimulation of protein synthesis in cultured skeletal and cardiac muscle cells. *Am J Physiol.* 1982;243:C81-C86.
37. Biolo G, Declan Fleming RY, Wolfe RR. Physiologic hyperinsulinemia stimulates protein synthesis and enhances transport of selected amino acids in human skeletal muscle. *J Clin Invest.* 1995;95:811-819.
38. Sakurai Y, Aarsland A, Herndon DN, et al. Stimulation of muscle protein synthesis by long-term insulin infusion in severely burned patients. *Ann Surg.* 1995;222:283-294, 294-297.
39. Ferrando AA, Chinkes DL, Wolf SE, Matin S, Herndon DN, Wolfe RR. A submaximal dose of insulin promotes net skeletal

muscle protein synthesis in patients with severe burns. *Ann Surg.* 1999;229:11-18.

40. Van den Berghe G, Wouters P, Weekers F, et al. Intensive insulin therapy in critically ill patients. *N Engl J Med.* 2001;345:1359-1367.

41. Van den Berghe G, Wilmer A, Hermans G, et al. Intensive insulin therapy in the medical ICU. *N Engl J Med.* 2006;354:449-461.

42. Preiser JC, Devos P, Ruiz-Santana S, et al. A prospective randomised multi-centre controlled trial on tight glucose control by intensive insulin therapy in adult intensive care units: the Glucontrol study. *Intensive Care Med.* 2009;35:1738-1748.

43. NICE-SUGAR Study Investigators, Finfer S, Chittock DR, et al. Intensive versus conventional glucose control in critically ill patients. *N Engl J Med.* 2009;360:1283-1297.

44. Brunkhorst FM, Engel C, Bloos F, et al. Intensive insulin therapy and pentastarch resuscitation in severe sepsis. *N Engl J Med.* 2008;358:125-139.

45. Hermanides J, Vriesendorp TM, Bosman RJ, Zandstra DF, Hoekstra JB, Devries JH. Glucose variability is associated with intensive care unit mortality. *Crit Care Med.* 2010;38:838-842.

46. Meyfroidt G, Keenan DM, Wang X, Wouters PJ, Veldhuis JD, Van den Berghe G. Dynamic characteristics of blood glucose time series during the course of critical illness: effects of intensive insulin therapy and relative association with mortality. *Crit Care Med.* 2010;38:1021-1029.

47. Rhodes A, Evans LE, Alhazzani W, et al. Surviving sepsis campaign: international guidelines for management of severe sepsis and septic shock: 2016. *Crit Care Med.* 2017;45:486-552.

48. Kojima M, Hosoda H, Date Y, Nakazato M, Matsuo H, Kangawa K. Ghrelin is a growth-hormone-releasing acylated peptide from stomach. *Nature.* 1999;402:656-660.

49. Nass R, Gaylinn BD, Thorner MO. The ghrelin axis in disease: potential therapeutic indications. *Mol Cell Endocrinol.* 2011;340:106-110.

50. Mesotten D, Van den Berghe G. Changes within the GH/IGF-I/IGFBP axis in critical illness. *Crit Care Clin.* 2006;22:17-28.

51. Giustina A, Veldhuis JD. Pathophysiology of the neuroregulation of growth hormone secretion in experimental animals and the human. *Endocr Rev.* 1998;19:717-797.

52. Berneis K, Keller U. Metabolic actions of growth hormone: direct and indirect. *Baillieres Clin Endocrinol Metab.* 1996;10:337-352.

53. Humbel RE. Insulin-like growth factors I and II. *Eur J Biochem.* 1990;190:445-462.

54. Froesch ER, Schmid C, Schwander J, Zapf J. Actions of insulin-like growth factors. *Annu Rev Physiol.* 1985;47:443-467.

55. Brown GM, Kirpalani SH. A critical review of the clinical relevance of growth hormone and its measurement in the nuclear medicine laboratory. *Semin Nucl Med.* 1975;5:273-285.

56. Ruokonen E, Takala J. Dangers of growth hormone therapy in critically ill patients. *Curr Opin Clin Nutr Metab Care.* 2002;5:199-209.

57. Ross R, Miell J, Freeman E, et al. Critically ill patients have high basal growth hormone levels with attenuated oscillatory activity associated with low levels of insulin-like growth factor-I. *Clin Endocrinol (Oxf).* 1991;35:47-54.

58. Schuetz P, Müller B, Nusbaumer C, Wieland M, Christ-Crain M. Circulating levels of GH predict mortality and complement prognostic scores in critically ill medical patients. *Eur J Endocrinol.* 2009;160:157-163.

59. Dahn MS, Lange MP, Jacobs LA. Insulinlike growth factor 1 production is inhibited in human sepsis. *Arch Surg.* 1988;123:1409-1414.

60. Van den Berghe G. Dynamic neuroendocrine responses to critical illness. *Front Neuroendocrinol.* 2002;23:370-391.

61. Koch A, Sanson E, Helm A, Voigt S, Trautwein C, Tacke F. Regulation and prognostic relevance of serum ghrelin concentrations in critical illness and sepsis. *Crit Care.* 2010;14:R94.

62. Florini JR, Ewton DZ, Coolican SA. Growth hormone and the insulin-like growth factor system in myogenesis. *Endocr Rev.* 1996;17:481-517.

63. Adams GR, McCue SA. Localized infusion of IGF-I results in skeletal muscle hypertrophy in rats. *J Appl Physiol.* 1998;84:1716-1722.

64. Inaba T, Saito H, Fukushima R, et al. Effects of growth hormone and insulin-like growth factor 1 (IGF-1) treatments on the nitrogen metabolism and hepatic IGF-1-messenger RNA expression in postoperative parenterally fed rats. *JPEN J Parenter Enteral Nutr.* 1996;20:325-331.

65. Shimoda N, Tashiro T, Yamamori H, Takagi K, Nakajima N, Ito I. Effects of growth hormone and insulin-like growth factor-1 on protein metabolism, gut morphology, and cell-mediated immunity in burned rats. *Nutrition.* 1997;13:540-546.

66. Voerman BJ, Strack van Schijndel RJ, Groeneveld AB, de Boer H, Nauta JP, Thijs LG. Effects of human growth hormone in critically ill nonseptic patients: results from a prospective, randomized, placebo-controlled trial. *Crit Care Med.* 1995;23:665-673.

67. Voerman HJ, van Schijndel RJ, Groeneveld AB, et al. Effects of recombinant human growth hormone in patients with severe sepsis. *Ann Surg.* 1992;216:648-655.

68. Jiang ZM, He GZ, Zhang SY, et al. Low-dose growth hormone and hypocaloric nutrition attenuate the protein-catabolic response after major operation. *Ann Surg.* 1989;210:513-524.

69. Takala J, Ruokonen E, Webster NR, et al. Increased mortality associated with growth hormone treatment in critically ill adults. *N Engl J Med.* 1999;341:785-792.

70. Critical evaluation of the safety of recombinant human growth hormone administration: statement from the Growth Hormone Research Society. *J Clin Endocrinol Metab.* 2001;86:1868-1870.

71. Van den Berghe G, Wouters P, Weekers F, et al. Reactivation of pituitary hormone release and metabolic improvement by infusion of growth hormone-releasing peptide and thyrotropin-releasing hormone in patients with protracted critical illness. *J Clin Endocrinol Metab.* 1999;84:1311-1323.

72. Mesotten D, Wouters PJ, Peeters RP, et al. Regulation of the somatotropic axis by intensive insulin therapy during protracted critical illness. *J Clin Endocrinol Metab.* 2004;89:3105-3113.

73. Bianco AC, Salvatore D, Gereben B, Berry MJ, Larsen PR. Biochemistry, cellular and molecular biology, and physiological roles of the iodothyronine selenodeiodinases. *Endocr Rev.* 2002;23:38-89.

74. Yen PM. Physiological and molecular basis of thyroid hormone action. *Physiol Rev.* 2001;81:1097-1142.

75. Davis PJ, Davis FB. Nongenomic actions of thyroid hormone. *Thyroid.* 1996;6:497-504.

76. Flaim KE, Li JB, Jefferson LS. Effects of thyroxine on protein turnover in rat skeletal muscle. *Am J Physiol.* 1978;235:E231-E236.

77. Farwell AP. Nonthyroidal illness syndrome. *Curr Opin Endocrinol Diabetes Obes.* 2013;20:478-484.

78. Peeters RP, Wouters PJ, Kaptein E, van Toor H, Visser TJ, Van den Berghe G. Reduced activation and increased inactivation of thyroid hormone in tissues of critically ill patients. *J Clin Endocrinol Metab.* 2003;88:3202-3211.

79. Thijssen-Timmer DC, Peeters RP, Wouters P, et al. Thyroid hormone receptor isoform expression in livers of critically ill patients. *Thyroid.* 2007;17:105-112.

80. Chopra IJ, Huang TS, Beredo A, Solomon DH, Chua Teco GN, Mead JF. Evidence for an inhibitor of extrathyroidal conversion of thyroxine to 3,5,3'-triiodothyronine in sera of patients with nonthyroidal illnesses. *J Clin Endocrinol Metab*. 1985;60:666-672.

81. Fliers E, Noppen NW, Wiersinga WM, Visser TJ, Swaab DF. Distribution of thyrotropin-releasing hormone (TRH)-containing cells and fibers in the human hypothalamus. *J Comp Neurol*. 1994;350:311-323.

82. Arem R, Wiener GJ, Kaplan SG, Kim HS, Reichlin S, Kaplan MM. Reduced tissue thyroid hormone levels in fatal illness. *Metabolism*. 1993;42:1102-1108.

83. Acker CG, Singh AR, Flick RP, Bernardini J, Greenberg A, Johnson JP. A trial of thyroxine in acute renal failure. *Kidney Int*. 2000;57:293-298.

84. Klemperer JD, Klein I, Gomez M, et al. Thyroid hormone treatment after coronary-artery bypass surgery. *N Engl J Med*. 1995;333:1522-1527.

85. Van den Berghe G, Wouters P, Carlsson L, Baxter RC, Bouillon R, Bowers CY. Leptin levels in protracted critical illness: effects of growth hormone-secretagogues and thyrotropin-releasing hormone. *J Clin Endocrinol Metab*. 1998;83:3062-3070.

72

How Do I Diagnose and Manage Acute Endocrine Emergencies in the ICU?

Joseph Fernandez-Moure, Anna E. Garcia Whitlock, and Carrie A. Sims

Endocrine emergencies are frequently encountered in the intensive care unit (ICU). This chapter will focus on several common disorders including diabetic ketoacidosis (DKA), hyperosmolar hyperglycemia, thyroid storm, myxedema coma, and vasopressin deficiency. Adrenal insufficiency is addressed elsewhere in this volume. Understanding the pathophysiology of these different states will enable the intensivist to make a rapid diagnosis, initiate appropriate therapy, and avoid major pitfalls.

DIABETIC KETOACIDOSIS

DKA is a life-threatening hyperglycemic condition that accounts for more than 168,000 annual hospital admissions.[1,2] The mortality associated with DKA has significantly decreased to <1% in the last 10 years; however, the cost of care for patients with DKA has dramatically increased with aggregate health-care charges reaching $5.1 billion in the United States in 2014.[3] While DKA was once considered a pathognomonic complication of insulin-dependent diabetes (type 1), up to 35% of DKA occurs in people with type 2 diabetes.[4]

Pathophysiology

DKA is a dysregulated catabolic state that occurs in the setting of insulin deficiency coupled with high levels of counterregulatory hormones such as glucagon, cortisol, catecholamines, and growth hormone.[5] This hormonal imbalance leads to impaired glucose uptake, increased gluconeogenesis, and increased glycogenolysis, culminating in a marked increase in the serum glucose level.[6,7] An elevated glucose level leads to increased serum osmolarity and water is shifted from the intracellular to the extracellular compartment. Because the kidney cannot effectively reabsorb water in the presence of marked hyperglycemia, an osmotic diuresis ensues, precipitating with hypovolemia and profound electrolyte depletion.

The increased production of glucose in the setting of relative insulin deficiency is followed by a preferential shift toward fat metabolism. As the liver oxidizes free fatty acids, ketones (acetone, beta-hydroxybutyrate, and acetoacetate) are generated. Ketones are the hallmark of DKA. As relatively strong acids, ketones deplete the body's buffering capacity and directly contribute to acidosis.[1]

Precipitating Factors

DKA may be the initial presentation of newly diagnosed diabetes. Of particular relevance in the ICU, DKA is frequently associated with infection.[1] Other diagnoses of consequence to the intensivist are myocardial ischemia, stroke, or trauma. Various medications frequently encountered in the ICU are associated with DKA, including glucocorticoids, thiazides, pentamidine, second-generation antipsychotics, vasopressors, and sympathomimetic agents including cocaine.[8] Interestingly, oral diabetes medications that act to inhibit the sodium-glucose cotransporter-2 inhibitors, such as canagliflozin (Invokana) and dapagliflozin (Farxiga), are associated with a euglycemic form of DKA.[9] In these cases, there is often no overt precipitating cause; thus clinicians must have a low threshold to consider these medications in patients presenting with clinical signs of DKA with a glucose level <200 mg/dL.

Clinical Presentation

The symptoms of DKA are directly related to hyperglycemia and acidosis. Hyperglycemia leads to polyuria, polydipsia, and dehydration. The generation of ketoacids results in nausea, vomiting, and abdominal pain. Metabolic acidosis also triggers compensatory hyperventilation with acetone excretion leading to a classic fruity odor on the patient's breath and the pathognomonic, labored Kussmaul breathing.

Defining laboratory features of DKA include metabolic acidosis (arterial pH <7.35 with bicarbonate <16 mEq/L), hyperglycemia (>250 mg/dL), and ketonemia. The severity of DKA can be graded as mild, moderate, or severe according to the degree of metabolic acidosis and the presence of an altered mental status (Table 72.1).[6,10] An increased white blood cell count is common even in the absence of an infection; however, fever is rare and should prompt an aggressive search for infection. Likewise, an altered mental status cannot solely be attributed to DKA and warrants further investigation. Patients also exhibit a hypercoagulable state, potentially caused by elevated circulating levels of proinflammatory cytokines (e.g., tumor necrosis factor [TNF]-α, interleukins [ILs], and C-reactive proteins) or elevated plasminogen activator inhibitor-1.[11,12]

Therapy

In 2006 the American Diabetes Association published a consensus statement regarding the management of DKA in terms

TABLE 72.1   Laboratory Findings in Diabetic Ketoacidosis and Hyperosmolar Hyperglycemic State.

	Diabetic Ketoacidosis	Hyperosmolar Hyperglycemic State
Anion gap acidosis	pH <7.3 Bicarbonate <18 Anion gap >10	pH >7.3 Bicarbonate >18 Anion gap variable
Osmolality	<320	>320
Hyperglycemia	>250	>600
Ketonemia/ ketonuria	Present	Rare

From Maletkovic J, Drexler A. Diabetic ketoacidosis and hyperglycemic hyperosmolar state. *Endocr Metab Clin North Am.* 2013;42(4): 677-695.

of fluids, electrolytes, and insulin therapy, which continues to remain clinically relevant.[5] An overview of the guidelines including additional recent recommendations is provided further.

Initial Evaluation

The presence of a blood glucose level >250 mg/dl is diagnostic and mandate initiation of therapy. If the level is between 200 mg/dl and 250 mg/dl, measurement should be re-checked hourly. Blood and urine electrolyte profiles should be obtained, including ketones, in order to document hyperglycemia, ketonemia, and ketonuria. DKA is further confirmed by the presence of arterial pH <7.35 or bicarbonate <16 mEq/L. Given the potential for profound electrolyte shifts, an electrocardiogram should be obtained with consideration of continuous cardiac telemetry. An infectious workup should be initiated including urinalysis, chest X-ray, and blood cultures.

Fluid and Electrolyte Replacement

Rapid volume replacement is the recommended initial therapy, and isotonic saline (0.9% NaCl) should be infused rapidly (1 L/hour) even if the serum sodium level is elevated. It is necessary to correct for the osmolarity of hyperglycemia when evaluating serum sodium levels, adding 1.6 mEq/L to sodium for every 200 mg/dL of glucose. Isotonic saline (0.9%) should be used at 250–500 mL/hour if the corrected serum sodium level is <135 mEq/L, whereas half normal saline (0.45%) should be used if the corrected sodium is normal or >145 mEq/L.[1,5,13] After 2–3 hours of resuscitation, the corrected sodium and urine output are used to determine the type and rate of fluids to be infused.

Almost all patients with DKA have a potassium deficiency secondary to urinary losses. Serum potassium, however, is often initially elevated because potassium is shifted out of cells in response to the insulin deficiency,

hyperosmolality, and acidosis.[6] With insulin therapy, potassium returns to the intracellular space, resulting in profound, potentially life-threatening hypokalemia. Therefore, potassium levels <3.3 mEq/L should be corrected prior to insulin initiation. Otherwise, potassium replacement should be initiated when the serum potassium concentration falls below 5.2 mEq/L.[13]

Phosphate levels in DKA may be deceptively elevated despite total body depletion. Although phosphate replacement has not been associated with improved clinical outcomes, supplementation is prudent when the serum phosphate concentration is <1.0 mg/dL to avoid cardiopulmonary muscle weakness.[14]

Finally, supplemental bicarbonate is rarely needed and may contribute to worsening intracellular acidosis, an increased risk of hypokalemia, and cerebral edema. A recent review suggests that the decision to administer bicarbonate even for an arterial pH <6.9 should be individualized, particularly in hemodynamically unstable patients or those with concomitant hyperchloremic metabolic acidosis.[15]

Insulin Therapy

Insulin therapy should only be initiated after adequate volume replacement and if the serum potassium level is ≥3.3 mEq/L. A continuous infusion of regular insulin is recommended. Glucose levels should decrease by 50–70 mg/dL per hour; if reduction in the first hour is inadequate, a bolus should be considered. The insulin infusion rate should be doubled until there is a steady rate of decline in the serum glucose concentration and should be continued until serum glucose reaches 200 mg/dL. Glucose should be monitored hourly by finger stick and confirmed by frequent serum glucose measurements.[13]

It is important to note that the serum glucose will normalize before ketoacid production stops. An abrupt discontinuation of insulin can lead to a recurrence of hyperglycemia and worsening of ketoacidosis. Therefore, both insulin therapy and supplemental glucose should be continued until the anion gap normalizes.[13]

Complications

Both cerebral and pulmonary edemas are DKA-specific complications. Cerebral edema is uncommon and primarily occurs in children.[16] Clinical symptoms include headache and behavioral/mental status changes that may rapidly progress to seizures, coma, and death. If neurologic findings progress beyond lethargy and behavioral changes, the mortality rate exceeds 70% and only 7–14% of survivors recover without permanent disability. Treatment is primarily supportive. Use of mannitol, hypertonic saline, and dexamethasone has not been rigorously validated.[6] Pulmonary edema occurs more frequently in older adults in the setting of overzealous fluid replacement, poor cardiac function, or reduced osmotic pressure.

HYPEROSMOLAR HYPERGLYCEMIC STATE

Hyperglycemia-induced volume depletion without acidosis—"hyperosmolar hyperglycemic state" (HHS)—is an insidiously developing life-threatening medical emergency.[17] HHS commonly occurs in the elderly with type 2 diabetes and is characterized by markedly elevated blood glucose levels (600–1000 mg/dL) and hyperosmolality (>320 mOsm/kg) with minimal to no ketosis or acidosis.[18] Mortality in HHS is higher than that in DKA, ranging from 10 to 20%.[18,19] Patients do not usually die owing to severe hypertonicity, rather they succumb to dehydration and the comorbidities that precipitate HHS or develop during its treatment.

Pathophysiology

HHS is actually associated with a state of relative insulin deficiency that is complicated by ongoing hepatic gluconeogenesis and lipolysis[20] and impaired glucose utilization that reflect an unopposed response to glucagon, catecholamines, and other regulatory hormones. Glucosuria leads to a significant diuresis.[18] If adequate fluid intake and renal perfusion are maintained, glucose clearance will be preserved and major hyperglycemia will not develop; however, if renal function deteriorates owing to underlying kidney disease or intravascular volume depletion, severe hyperglycemia and hyperosmolality will lead to an exuberant osmotic diuresis and severe dehydration.[17]

Precipitating Factors

Infection is the most common inciting event in HHS accounting for approximately 57% cases; however, any severe illness or proinflammatory state can provoke HHS.[17] In fact, up to 20% of patients will have no previous history of insulin resistance with HHS; thus a diagnosis of diabetes may first be recognized during critical illness.[11] Interestingly, elevated levels of proinflammatory cytokines, such as IL-6, IL-8, IL-β, and TNF-α, observed in HHS often resolve with initiation of appropriate insulin therapy.[11,13]

HHS is also common among patients with type 2 diabetes and poor medication compliance. Elderly diabetics are particularly at risk owing to underlying comorbidities, decreased thirst response, poor water intake, and use of medications such as glucocorticoids, thiazide diuretics, phenytoin, and beta blockers that affect carbohydrate metabolism. An association with alcohol and cocaine use has also been observed.[2]

Clinical Presentation

HHS is characterized by severe hyperglycemia (glucose level >600 mg/dL) and plasma hyperosmolality (>320 mOsm/kg) in the absence of significant ketoacidosis. A mild ketonemia, however, does not preclude the diagnosis (see Table 72.1).[21] HHS patients are profoundly volume depleted with an average total body water deficit of 8–10 L.[2,22]

Altered mental status and neurologic symptoms are the most common presenting symptoms and typically manifest when the osmolality reaches 230–330 mOsm/kg.[23,24] Other symptoms include polydipsia, polyuria, fatigue, visual disturbances, weakness, anorexia, weight loss, dizziness, confusion, and lethargy.[18] Hallmarks of DKA including Kussmaul breathing, fruity odor, and positive urine ketones are not expected.

Therapy

Although the treatments of DKA and HHS are very similar, insulin and fluid requirements are notably different.

Insulin Therapy

As with DKA, intravascular volume and electrolyte resuscitation should precede instituting insulin therapy. The profound volume depletion leads to lower insulin requirements; volume expansion addresses hyperglycemia, hyperosmolarity, and volume depletion. Serum glucose levels should be maintained at 250–300 mg/dL until the plasma osmolality is ≤315 mOsm/kg and the patient is mentally alert. To meet these goals, an initial bolus of insulin should be followed by an infusion until the serum glucose is 250–300 mg/dL.[6,18] If the glucose level does not appropriately fall, the rate can be doubled. Once the blood glucose level is <300 mg/dL, insulin can be titrated via sliding scale.[5]

Fluid and Electrolyte Replacement

Volume resuscitation is the mainstay of therapy and can lower serum glucose level by as much as 75–100 mg/hour. Electrolyte deficits are often profound but may not be appreciated prior to resuscitation. Initial management includes infusion of isotonic saline at 15–20 mL/kg during the first 1–2 hours and then individualized based on patient's clinical degree of hypovolemia (i.e., symptoms of malperfusion or shock), corrected serum sodium, and clinical comorbidities.

Accurate identification of volume status, osmolarity, and potential risk for cerebral edema may require calculation of a corrected serum sodium level using the following equation[16]

$$\text{Corrected Na}^+ = 1.6(\text{glucose} - 100)/100.$$

Free water deficit can be estimated as:

$$\text{Free water deficit} = \text{TBW} \times \left(\left([\text{Na}^+]_{calc} / [\text{Na}^+]_{normal}\right) - 1\right)$$

where total body water (TBW) = body weight (kg) $\times$ 0.6 for males or 0.5 for females.

Patients with elevated corrected serum sodium (>145 mEq/L) should be treated with 0.45% NaCl, while 0.9% NaCl is recommended for those with lower corrected serum sodium (<135 mEq/L). In general, one half of the fluid deficit should be replaced within the initial 18–24 hours[18]; however, more gradual administration may be needed to avoid cerebral edema, especially in patients aged <20 years.[18,25]

Patients with HHS are often significantly potassium deficit despite having initial levels that are normal or even elevated. This deficit is exacerbated once insulin is initiated and potassium is shifted intracellular. Therefore, once urine output is sufficient, replacement should be initiated when serum potassium values are 3.3–5.3 mEq/L. Phosphate, calcium, and magnesium replacement are only needed when levels are extremely low.[18,26]

Complications

Prothrombotic states and subclinical rhabdomyolysis can occur in HHS and may contribute to acute renal failure. Also, it is important to be mindful of treatment-associated complications such as cerebral and pulmonary edema.[18]

AUTHORS' RECOMMENDATIONS

- HHS is characterized by glucose level >600 mg/dL and dehydration in the absence of ketoacidosis.
- Elderly and diabetics are at the highest risk; infection is the most common inciting event.
- Dehydration is often more profound in HHS than in DKA and should be addressed within the first 24 hours unless precluded by the patient's cardiac function, age, or corrected sodium level.
- Supplemental potassium chloride should be given when the serum potassium concentration is ≤5.3 mEq/L. Replacement should be initiated before insulin therapy if the serum concentration is <3.3 mEq/L.
- Low dose IV insulin therapy includes a bolus followed by an infusion to maintain glucose levels at 250–300 mg/dL until the osmolality is ≤315 mOsm/kg and the patient is mentally alert.

THYROTOXIC CRISIS

Thyrotoxic crisis or thyroid storm is an acute, potentially life-threatening state that occurs in patients with untreated or incompletely treated, hyperthyroidism. Although the prevalence of hyperthyroidism is roughly 1.3% in the United States, only 1–5% of hyperthyroid patients develop thyroid storm.[27] If left untreated, thyrotoxicosis is almost universally lethal; however, even with early management, the mortality

from thyroid storm is surprisingly high (10–20%).[28] Therefore early recognition and prompt treatment are paramount.

Pathophysiology

Thyroid hormone secretion is tightly regulated by the hypothalamic–pituitary–thyroid axis. Thyrotropin-releasing hormone (TRH) is released from the hypothalamus and stimulates the synthesis and secretion of thyroid-stimulating hormone (TSH). In turn, TSH controls the synthesis and secretion of thyroxine (T_4) and triiodothyronine (T_3). T_4 has limited activity and must be converted to T_3 by tissue deiodinases that are primarily found in the kidney and liver. T_3 directly binds to cytoplasmic thyroid hormone receptor complexes and in conjunction with additional regulatory elements, migrates to the nucleus to directly modulate the expression of genes controlling cellular metabolism, adrenergic responsiveness, and thermoregulation.[28] Free T_4 and T_3 decrease further secretion of TSH and TRH—a classic negative feedback loop. More than 99.5% of serum T_4 and T_3 are protein bound and metabolically inactive.[29]

Hyperthyroidism typically results from an overactive thyroid nodule or gland. Less commonly, excessive TSH secretion or thyroid hormone ingestion can lead to hyperthyroidism.[27] The pathologic transition from hyperthyroidism to thyroid storm is not fully understood but usually occurs in the setting of surgery, sepsis, injury, or other acute medical illness. Elevated catecholamines in acute illness or trauma may further stimulate the synthesis and release of thyroid hormone. Although total thyroid hormone levels may not be significantly higher than those observed in uncomplicated thyrotoxicosis, higher levels of free thyroid hormone and lower levels of binding proteins have been demonstrated.[30]

Precipitating Factors

An infection, acute medical illness, or sympathomimetic agents may precipitate the development of thyroid storm by increasing circulating catecholamines.[31] Amiodarone and other iodinated medications may also precipitate thyrotoxicosis and subsequent thyroid crisis in those with underlying thyroid disease.[32] Finally, withdrawal or noncompliance with antithyroid medications may contribute to the development of thyrotoxicosis.

Clinical Presentation

Thyroid storm most frequently occurs as a complication of Graves disease.[33] Patients classically present with fever ($>38.5°C$) and a range of multisystem complaints.[31,34] Cardiac findings include profound tachycardia, atrial fibrillation, congestive heart failure, hypotension, and shock. Gastrointestinal symptoms include nausea, vomiting, diarrhea, abdominal pain, and occasionally liver failure. In fact, gastrointestinal fluid losses may be so profound that dehydration contributes to the development of multiorgan failure. Central nervous system symptoms are also common and range from confusion to psychosis to coma.[34]

Serum T_4 or T_3 values cannot be used to differentiate thyrotoxicosis from thyroid storm; the diagnosis must be made on clinical grounds. In 1993 Burch and Wartofsky[29] developed

TABLE 72.2 Diagnostic Scoring System for Thyroid Storm.

Physiologic Parameters	Points
Thermoregulatory Dysfunction Temperature (°F)	
99–99.9	5
100–100.9	10
101–101.9	15
102–102.9	20
103–103.9	25
≥104.0	30
Central Nervous System Dysfunction	
Absent	0
Mild (agitation)	10
Moderate (delirium, psychosis, extreme lethargy)	20
Severe (seizures, coma)	30
Gastrointestinal-Hepatic Dysfunction	
Absent	0
Moderate (nausea, vomiting, diarrhea, abdominal pain)	10
Severe (unexplained jaundice)	20
Cardiovascular Dysfunction Tachycardia (beats/minute)	
90–109	5
110–119	10
120–129	15
≥140	25
Congestive Heart Failure	
Absent	0
Mild (pedal edema)	5
Moderate (bibasilar rales)	10
Severe (pulmonary edema)	15
Atrial Fibrillation	
Absent	0
Present	10
Precipitating Event	
Absent	0
Present	10

Modified from Burch HB, Wartofsky L. Life-threatening thyrotoxicosis: thyroid storm. *Endocrinol Metab Clin North Am.* 1993;22(2):263-277.

a clinical scoring system to standardize the diagnosis based on the severity of organ dysfunction (Table 72.2). A score of ≥45 is highly suggestive of thyroid storm, whereas a score of <25 makes thyroid storm unlikely.

In addition to altered thyroid parameters, abnormal clinical labs include elevated blood urea nitrogen and creatinine, elevated liver function tests, hypercalcemia, anemia, thrombocytopenia, leukocytosis or leukopenia, and hyperglycemia.[30] Concomitant adrenal insufficiency, especially in the setting of Graves disease, should be ruled out by measuring a random cortisol.[35]

Treatment

The therapeutic goals of treating thyroid storm are to (1) decrease hormone production and secretion, (2) block the conversion of T_4 to T_3, and (3) antagonize the catecholaminergic effects of thyroid hormone (Table 72.3).

Decreasing Hormone Production and Secretion

Thionamides, such as propylthiouracil and methimazole, effectively block new thyroid hormone synthesis, but they do not prevent the release of stored hormone. Thionamides have immunosuppressive properties that decrease the expression of antithyroptropin-receptor antibodies. Propylthiouracil inhibits the peripheral conversion of T_4 to T_3 but must be given two to three times per day and has been associated with severe liver toxicity. Methimazole can be given once daily.[27,36]

High-dose iodine, such as saturated potassium iodide solutions or potassium iodide-iodine (Lugol's solution), can acutely block the release of T_4 and T_3.[37] Iodine products, however, should only be given after thyroid synthesis has been blocked for several hours. If synthetic function is not adequately inhibited, the iodine will enhance thyroid hormone synthesis and can exacerbate the thyrotoxicosis.[33]

Iopanoic acid and other iodinated oral radiographic contrast agents have extremely high iodine concentrations and have been used off-label in lieu of iodine solutions. In addition to decreasing thyroid hormone release, these agents attenuate the effects of thyroid hormone by decreasing hepatic uptake of T_4, inhibiting peripheral conversion of T_4 to T_3, and blocking cellular binding of T_4 and T_3.[38,39] Thyroid synthesis should be blocked before use to prevent enriched thyroid hormone production.

Lithium carbonate can also block the formation and release of thyroid hormone[33]; however, lithium is not considered a first-line therapy because of a narrow therapeutic window and is reserved for patients with an iodine allergy. L-carnitine blocks nuclear uptake of thyroid hormone and has been suggested as a treatment of thyrotoxicosis in combination with methimazole.[40]

Decreasing Peripheral Conversion of T_4 to T_3

Glucocorticoids effectively reduce the peripheral deiodination of T_4 to T_3 and may be helpful in modulating autoimmune disorders such as Graves disease. Glucocorticoids are traditionally used even in patients with "normal" cortisol levels because of their presumed overall benefit and concern for concomitant adrenal insufficiency.[36] As mentioned, propylthiouracil and iopanoic acid also decrease the peripheral deiodination of T_4 to T_3.

Oral cholestyramine reduces circulating thyroid hormone by inhibiting enterohepatic recirculation.[41] There are case reports describing the use of plasmaphoresis, hemoperfusion, and plasma exchange to reduce autoimmune antibodies, immune complexes, and thyroid levels in critically ill patients refractory to conventional therapies.[42]

TABLE 72.3	Pharmacologic Management of Thyroid Storm.	
Medication	**Mechanism of Action**	**Dosage**
Propylthiouracil	Inhibits new hormone synthesis; decreases T_4 to T_3 conversion	200–400 mg po q 6–8 h
Methimazole	Inhibits new hormone synthesis	20–25 mg po q 6 h
Lugol solution	Blocks release of hormone from gland	4–8 drops po q 6–8 h
Saturated solution of potassium iodide	Blocks release of hormone from gland	5 drops po q 6 h
Iopanoic acid	Blocks release of hormone from gland; inhibits T_4 to T_3 conversion	1 g po q 8 hour for 24 h then 500 mg po q 12 h
Lithium carbonate	Blocks release of hormone from gland; inhibits new hormone synthesis	300 mg po q 8 h
Cholestyramine	Decreases enterohepatic resorption of thyroid hormone	4 g po qid
Propranolol	β-Adrenergic blockade; decreases T_4 to T_3 conversion	1–2 mg IV q 10–15 min 20–120 mg po q 4–6 h
Esmolol	β-Adrenergic blockade	50–100 µg/kg/min
Diltiazem	Decreases adrenergic symptoms	5–10 mg/hour IV 60–120 mg po q 6–8 h
Reserpine	Decreases secretion of catecholamines	2.5–5 mg IM q 4–6 h
Guanethidine	Decreases secretion of catecholamines	30–40 mg po q 6 h
Hydrocortisone	Decreases T_4 to T_3 conversion; vasomotor stability	100 g IV q 8 h

IM, intramuscular; *IV,* intravenous; T_3, triiodothyronine; T_4, thyroxine.

Antagonizing the Adrenergic Effects of Thyroid Hormone

Beta blockade counteracts adrenergic-mediated effects of thyroid hormones. In addition, beta blockers inhibit the peripheral conversion of T_4 to T_3. These agents reduce tachycardia, markedly improve agitation, confusion, psychosis, diaphoresis, diarrhea, and fever.[33] Beta blockers should be used cautiously in patients with congestive heart failure. Diltiazem, a calcium channel antagonist, may provide an alternative method of controlling adrenergic symptoms.[43]

Supportive Care

Supportive care is essential and should be provided in an ICU environment. Atrial fibrillation is observed in up to 40% of patients with thyroid storm. Many patients require vigorous fluid resuscitation. If hypotension persists despite adequate volume resuscitation, vasopressors should be added and hydrocortisone should be considered.

Hyperpyrexia should be treated with external cooling methods and acetaminophen. Salicylates, such as aspirin, should be avoided because they can inhibit hormone-protein binding and increase free hormone levels.[33]

Definitive Treatment

Patients with a history of thyroid storm should undergo definitive treatment with either radioactive iodine ablation or surgical thyroidectomy. Use of iodine in the initial management eliminated radioactive ablation as an acute approach; this form of therapy should be postponed for several months until the iodine stores are depleted. Surgical resection can be performed after treatment with iodine, although there is an increased risk of perioperative thyroid storm.

AUTHORS' RECOMMENDATIONS
- Thyroid storm is a rare condition that presents with exaggerated features of hyperthyroidism.
- Thyroid function tests cannot be used that differentiate thyrotoxicosis from thyroid storm.
- Pharmacologic treatment of thyroid storm includes thionamides to decrease hormone synthesis, a beta blocker to antagonize the adrenergic effects, a steroid to decrease peripheral hormone conversion, and occasionally iodine to prevent hormone release.
- Hydrocortisone is given for the increased risk of concomitant adrenal insufficiency and to inhibit the peripheral conversion of T4 to T3.
- After resolution of the crisis, patients should be evaluated for definitive management with radioiodine ablation or surgical thyroidectomy.

MYXEDEMA COMA

Myxedema coma is the result of severe, decompensated hypothyroidism. The condition is characterized by a depressed mental status, hypotension, and hypothermia. It is a serious, but rare, medical emergency that carries a high mortality rate (20–50%) even with early diagnosis and appropriate therapy.[44]

Pathophysiology

Primary hypothyroidism occurs when there is permanent loss or atrophy of thyroid tissue. This condition accounts for 90–95% of cases of myxedema coma. Serum TSH is elevated, whereas free T_4 values are low. Less than 5% of cases of myxedema coma result from hypothalamic or pituitary dysfunction (central hypothyroidism). These patients will have a normal or low TSH and a low free T_4 concentration.[44] Decreased thyroid function results in systemically depressed metabolic function and impaired energy production.

Precipitating Factors

The presence of a precipitating infection or concurrent acute illness should be investigated. Typical signs of infection (e.g., fever, tachycardia) may not be present in the patient with myxedema coma, and patients who die frequently have unrecognized infection and sepsis.

Clinical Presentation

Patients with hypothyroidism are frequently elderly women. Physical findings include dry skin, thin hair, a hoarse voice, and delayed deep tendon reflexes. Classically, mucin deposition (myxedema) may cause nonpitting edema of the hands and feet, periorbital swelling, and macroglossia.[45]

Progression to myxedema coma is characterized by mental status changes and hypothermia. In a retrospective review of 24 patients, 88% presented with a temperature less than 94°F (34°C).[46] Mortality from myxedema correlates directly with the degree of hypothermia.[44]

Although hypothyroidism has broad systemic effects, the cardiovascular system is particularly affected. Decreased β-adrenergic responses (bradycardia, decreased cardiac output, low blood pressure, diminished cerebral blood flow) and diminished thermogenesis lead to increased vascular resistance, diastolic hypertension, decreased blood volume, QT interval prolongation, and heart block. Without the administration of thyroid hormone, hypotension may become refractory to vasopressor support.[44,47]

Central respiratory depression and respiratory muscle weakness may cause hypoventilation, respiratory acidosis, and hypoxemia that often require mechanical ventilation.[45] Finally, decreased gastrointestinal motility limits the use of oral medications and enteral nutrition. Thyroid hormone should be given intravenously.[44]

Laboratory values are notable for hyponatremia and hypoglycemia.[48] Although infection is frequently a precipitating cause of myxedema coma, an elevated white blood cell count is frequently absent.

Therapy

Given the lethality of untreated myxedema coma, therapy should be instituted without waiting for laboratory confirmation. Appropriate hormonal supplementation will normalize the basal metabolic rate and reverse most symptoms and signs of hypothyroidism[48]; some neuromuscular and psychiatric symptoms may take months to disappear.[49]

Hormonal Replacement Therapy

There are no randomized clinical trials comparing treatment regimens. Thyroid hormone therapy is critical but may precipitate cardiac arrhythmias or ischemia. In addition, thyroid replacement may unmask coexisting adrenal insufficiency and precipitate an adrenal crisis. Hydrocortisone should be given in conjunction with thyroid replacement.[44]

Because the conversion of T_4 to T_3 is impaired in severe hypothyroidism, IV T_3 may be preferable and may positively affect survival.[50] T_3 crosses the blood-brain barrier more readily than T_4 and may hasten the improvement of neurologic symptoms. Treatment with IV T_4 can also be used but the need to peripherally convert T_4 to T_3 may lengthen the time to effective therapy.[51]

A theoretical argument can be made for administration of both a subtherapeutic dose of T_3 and a loading dose of T_4; however, there are no clinical studies validating this approach.[44] IV T4 (200–400 mcg) followed by a daily dose of 50–100 mcg can be administered until the patient is tolerating an oral diet. IV T3 (5–20 mcg) is given concurrently, followed by 2.5–10 mcg every 8 hours until clinically stable. Lower doses of both T4 and T3 should be given in older patients and those at risk for cardiac complications including arrhythmias.

Monitoring Therapy

Patients should be carefully monitored for the development of tachyarrhythmias or myocardial ischemia during IV thyroid administration. Initially, TSH and free T_4 levels should be closely followed to prevent overtreatment. In patients with central hypothyroidism, TSH levels will not reflect the adequacy of treatment. Free T_4 levels should be monitored and maintained in the upper normal range.

AUTHORS' RECOMMENDATIONS
- Treatment of myxedema coma should be initiated without waiting for the results of thyroid function tests.
- The optimal strategy for thyroid hormone replacement remains controversial. Regimens include IV T3, T4, or a combination of both hormones.
- IV hydrocortisone should be given in conjunction with thyroid hormone replacement.
- Empiric antibiotics should be initiated until cultures are proven negative.

VASOPRESSIN DEFICIENCY IN SHOCK

Shock, defined as inadequate tissue perfusion and oxygenation leading to cellular ischemia, is associated with mortality rates as high as 40–60%.[52,53] Patients with either septic or hemorrhagic shock demonstrate a high incidence of arginine vasopressin (AVP) deficiency, and exogenous replacement during resuscitation is effective in augmenting blood pressure.

Pathophysiology

AVP, which causes vasoconstriction and renal water retention, is synthesized in the hypothalamus and released into circulation by the posterior pituitary in response to hypotension and hyperosmolarity. In early shock, AVP release can increase up to 200-fold; however, shock is also associated with impaired AVP synthesis and decreased peripheral vasopressin receptor density. With prolonged or severe shock, serum AVP levels can decline precipitously, leaving patients refractory to catecholamine supplementation and volume resuscitation.[54,55] Patients in shock who have AVP levels <10 pg/mL are considered to have absolute deficiency and those with 10–130 pg/mL have relative deficiency.[56]

Clinical Presentation

Clinically, patients with either absolute or relative AVP deficiency have an increased need for vasopressor support, fluid resuscitation, and blood product transfusion as well as an increase in ICU length of stay.[54] AVP administration to patients with septic or hemorrhagic can have pronounced hemodynamic effects.[56] AVP doses higher than 0.04 U/minute, however, decrease portosystemic blood flow and increase the potential for end organ ischemia.[57]

Therapy

Although the therapeutic approaches to patients in septic and hemorrhagic shock are significantly different, resuscitation strategies in both states may benefit from AVP supplementation.

The addition of AVP to norepinephrine does not change overall mortality in septic shock[58]; however, a relative reduction in 28-day mortality was observed in a subset of patients in the VASST trial who required <15 µg/mL of norepinephrine.[58] A metaanalysis of nine randomized controlled trials concluded that AVP in combination with norepinephrine was associated with a reduction in mortality and in vasopressor dependence.[59,60]

The treatment of hemorrhagic shock focuses on hemorrhage control, volume resuscitation, and the correction of coagulopathy.[61] In general, vasopressor use is avoided in trauma; however, AVP supplementation in experimental hemorrhagic shock improved survival and was associated with reduced blood product administration and crystalloid use in clinical trials.[62,63]

An AVP infusion at 0.03–0.04 U/minute[55,64] will restore the serum concentration to 100 pmol/L. Increasing the dose above 0.04 U/minute increases the risk of ischemic complications but may be renal protective. In a recent study of septic patients, Gordon et al.[65] compared AVP (up to 0.06 U/minute) with norepinephrine (max 12 mcg/minute).[65] While the use of AVP did not improve kidney failure-free days, less renal replacement therapy was required, suggesting the need for a larger trial.

Similarly, the use of AVP has been investigated in both animal models and clinical trials. In uncontrolled hemorrhage models, the use of AVP significantly improved survival when compared with either fluid resuscitation or norepinephrine.[66,67] In clinical trials, AVP supplementation appears to decrease the overall volume needed for resuscitation. Larger trials, however, are needed to determine if AVP significantly reduces mortality or serious complications.[63]

AUTHORS' RECOMMENDATIONS
- In septic shock, AVP should be initiated early in combination with norepinephrine.
- AVP supplementation is associated with decreased volume requirements and should be initiated early as an adjunct to resuscitation.

- While the optimal dose of AVP remains unclear, a dose of 0.03–0.04 U/minute is known to restore physiologic levels of AVP and is considered the standard dose.

REFERENCES

1. Umpierrez G, Korytkowski M. Diabetic emergencies - ketoacidosis, hyperglycaemic hyperosmolar state and hypoglycaemia. *Nat Rev Endocrinol.* 2016;12(4):222-232.
2. Umpierrez GE, Smiley D, Kitabchi AE. Narrative review: ketosis-prone type 2 diabetes mellitus. *Ann Intern Med.* 2006;144(5):350-357.
3. Centers for Disease Control and Prevention. *National Diabetes Statistics Report, 2017.* Atlanta, GA: Centers for Disease Control and Prevention, US Dept of Health and Human Services; 2017.
4. Desai D, Mehta D, Mathias P, Menon G, Schubart UK. Health care utilization and burden of diabetic ketoacidosis in the U.S. over the past decade: a nationwide analysis. *Diabetes Care.* 2018;41(8):1631-1638.
5. Kitabchi AE, Umpierrez GE, Murphy MB, Kreisberg RA. Hyperglycemic crises in adult patients with diabetes: a consensus statement from the American Diabetes Association. *Diabetes Care.* 2006;29(12):2739-2748.
6. Nyenwe EA, Kitabchi AE. The evolution of diabetic ketoacidosis: An update of its etiology, pathogenesis and management. *Metabolism.* 2016;65(4):507-521.
7. Wolfsdorf J, Glaser N, Sperling MA, American Diabetes Association. Diabetic ketoacidosis in infants, children, and adolescents: A consensus statement from the American Diabetes Association. *Diabetes Care.* 2006;29(5):1150-1159.
8. Delaney MF, Zisman A, Kettyle WM. Diabetic ketoacidosis and hyperglycemic hyperosmolar nonketotic syndrome. *Endocrinol Metab Clin North Am.* 2000;29(4):683-705, V.
9. Rosenstock J, Ferrannini E. Euglycemic diabetic ketoacidosis: a predictable, detectable, and preventable safety concern with SGLT2 inhibitors. *Diabetes Care.* 2015;38(9):1638-1642.
10. Westerberg DP. Diabetic ketoacidosis: evaluation and treatment. *Am Fam Physician.* 2013;87(5):337-346.
11. Stentz FB, Umpierrez GE, Cuervo R, Kitabchi AE. Proinflammatory cytokines, markers of cardiovascular risks, oxidative stress, and lipid peroxidation in patients with hyperglycemic crises. *Diabetes.* 2004;53(8):2079-2086.
12. Dalton RR, Hoffman WH, Passmore GG, Martin SL. Plasma C-reactive protein levels in severe diabetic ketoacidosis. *Ann Clin Lab Sci.* 2003;33(4):435-442.
13. Kitabchi AE, Umpierrez GE, Miles JM, Fisher JN. Hyperglycemic crises in adult patients with diabetes. *Diabetes Care.* 2009;32(7):1335-1343.
14. Miller DW, Slovis CM. Hypophosphatemia in the emergency department therapeutics. *Am J Emerg Med.* 2000;18(4):457-461.
15. Kamel KS, Halperin ML. Acid-base problems in diabetic ketoacidosis. *N Engl J Med.* 2015;372(6):546-554.
16. Fayfman M, Pasquel FJ, Umpierrez GE. Management of hyperglycemic crises: diabetic ketoacidosis and hyperglycemic hyperosmolar state. *Med Clin North Am.* 2017;101(3):587-606.
17. Pasquel FJ, Umpierrez GE. Hyperosmolar hyperglycemic state: a historic review of the clinical presentation, diagnosis, and treatment. *Diabetes Care.* 2014;37(11):3124-3131.

18. Stoner GD. Hyperosmolar hyperglycemic state. *Am Fam Physician*. 2005;71(9):1723-1730.

19. Fadini GP, de Kreutzenberg SV, Rigato M, et al. Characteristics and outcomes of the hyperglycemic hyperosmolar non-ketotic syndrome in a cohort of 51 consecutive cases at a single center. *Diabetes Res Clin Pract*. 2011;94(2):172-179.

20. Schade DS, Eaton RP. Dose response to insulin in man: differential effects on glucose and ketone body regulation. *J Clin Endocrinol Metab*. 1977;44(6):1038-1053.

21. Arieff AI, Carroll HJ. Hyperosmolar nonketotic coma with hyperglycemia: abnormalities of lipid and carbohydrate metabolism. *Metabolism*. 1971;20(6):529-538.

22. Umpierrez GE, Kelly JP, Navarrete JE, Casals MM, Kitabchi AE. Hyperglycemic crises in urban blacks. *Arch Intern Med*. 1997;157(6):669-675.

23. Misra UK, Kalita J, Bhoi SK, Dubey D. Spectrum of hyperosmolar hyperglycaemic state in neurology practice. *Indian J Med Res*. 2017;146(suppl):S1-S7.

24. Daugirdas JT, Kronfol NO, Tzamaloukas AH, Ing TS. Hyperosmolar coma: cellular dehydration and the serum sodium concentration. *Ann Intern Med*. 1989;110(11):855-857.

25. Siperstein MD. Diabetic ketoacidosis and hyperosmolar coma. *Endocrinol Metab Clin North Am*. 1992;21(2):415-432.

26. Kitabchi AE, Umpierrez GE, Murphy MB, et al. Hyperglycemic crises in diabetes. *Diabetes Care*. 2004;27(Suppl. 1):S94-S102.

27. De Leo S, Lee SY, Braverman LE. Hyperthyroidism. *Lancet*. 2016;388(10047):906-918.

28. Nayak B, Burman K. Thyrotoxicosis and thyroid storm. *Endocrinol Metab Clin North Am*. 2006;35(4):663-686, vii.

29. Burch HB, Wartofsky L. Life-threatening thyrotoxicosis: thyroid storm. *Endocrinol Metab Clin North Am*. 1993;22(2):263-277.

30. Dabon-Almirante CL, Surks MI. Clinical and laboratory diagnosis of thyrotoxicosis. *Endocrinol Metab Clin North Am*. 1998;27(1):25-35.

31. Papi G, Corsello SM, Pontecorvi A. Clinical concepts on thyroid emergencies. *Front Endocrinol (Lausanne)*. 2014;5:102.

32. Danzi S, Klein I. Amiodarone-induced thyroid dysfunction. *J Intensive Care Med*. 2015;30(4):179-185.

33. Klubo-Gwiezdzinska J, Wartofsky L. Thyroid emergencies. *Med Clin North Am*. 2012;96(2):385-403.

34. Wartofsky L. Clinical criteria for the diagnosis of thyroid storm. *Thyroid*. 2012;22(7):659-660.

35. Bornstein SR. Predisposing factors for adrenal insufficiency. *N Engl J Med*. 2009;360(22):2328-2339.

36. Carroll R, Matfin G. Endocrine and metabolic emergencies: thyroid storm. *Ther Adv Endocrinol Metab*. 2010;1(3):139-145.

37. Emerson CH, Anderson AJ, Howard WJ, Utiger RD. Serum thyroxine and triiodothyronine concentrations during iodide treatment of hyperthyroidism. *J Clin Endocrinol Metab*. 1975;40(1):33-36.

38. Pandey CK, Raza M, Dhiraaj S, Agarwal A, Singh PK. Rapid preparation of severe uncontrolled thyrotoxicosis due to Graves' disease with Iopanoic acid—a case report. *Can J Anaesth*. 2004;51(1):38-40.

39. Tyer NM, Kim TY, Martinez DS. Review of oral cholecystographic agents for the management of hyperthyroidism. *Endocr Pract*. 2014;20(10):1084-1092.

40. Benvenga S, Ruggeri RM, Russo A, Lapa D, Campenni A, Trimarchi F. Usefulness of L-carnitine, a naturally occurring peripheral antagonist of thyroid hormone action, in iatrogenic hyperthyroidism: a randomized, double-blind, placebo-controlled clinical trial. *J Clin Endocrinol Metab*. 2001;86(8):3579-3594.

41. Solomon BL, Wartofsky L, Burman KD. Adjunctive cholestyramine therapy for thyrotoxicosis. *Clin Endocrinol (Oxf)*. 1993;38(1):39-43.

42. Carhill A, Gutierrez A, Lakhia R, Nalini R. Surviving the storm: two cases of thyroid storm successfully treated with plasmapheresis. *BMJ Case Rep*. 2012;2012:bcr2012006696.

43. Keleştimur F, Aksu A. The effect of diltiazem on the manifestations of hyperthyroidism and thyroid function tests. *Exp Clin Endocrinol Diabetes*. 1996;104(1):38-42.

44. Wartofsky L. Myxedema coma. *Endocrinol Metab Clin North Am*. 2006;35(4):687-698, vii-viii.

45. Mathew V, Misgar RA, Ghosh S, et al. Myxedema coma: a new look into an old crisis. *J Thyroid Res*. 2011;2011:493462.

46. Reinhardt W, Mann K. [Incidence, clinical picture and treatment of hypothyroid coma. Results of a survey]. *Med Klin (Munich)*. 1997;92(9):521-524.

47. Kwaku MP, Burman KD. Myxedema coma. *J Intensive Care Med*. 2007;22(4):224-231.

48. Fliers E, Wiersinga WM. Myxedema coma. *Rev Endocr Metab Disord*. 2003;4(2):137-141.

49. Zulewski H, Müller B, Exer P, Miserez AR, Staub JJ. Estimation of tissue hypothyroidism by a new clinical score: evaluation of patients with various grades of hypothyroidism and controls. *J Clin Endocrinol Metab*. 1997;82(3):771-776.

50. Bigos ST, Ridgway EC, Kourides IA, Maloof F. Spectrum of pituitary alterations with mild and severe thyroid impairment. *J Clin Endocrinol Metab*. 1978;46(2):317-325.

51. Hylander B, Rosenqvist U. Treatment of myxoedema coma—factors associated with fatal outcome. *Acta Endocrinol (Copenh)*. 1985;108(1):65-71.

52. Curry N, Hopewell S, Dorée C, Hyde C, Brohi K, Stanworth S. The acute management of trauma hemorrhage: a systematic review of randomized controlled trials. *Crit Care*. 2011;15(2):R92.

53. Nasa P, Juneja D, Singh O. Severe sepsis and septic shock in the elderly: An overview. *World J Crit Care Med*. 2012;1(1):23-30.

54. Sims CA, Guan Y, Bergey M, et al. Arginine vasopressin, copeptin, and the development of relative AVP deficiency in hemorrhagic shock. *Am J Surg*. 2017;214(4):589-595.

55. Anand T, Skinner R. Arginine vasopressin: the future of pressure-support resuscitation in hemorrhagic shock. *J Surg Res*. 2012;178(1):321-329.

56. Landry DW, Oliver JA. The pathogenesis of vasodilatory shock. *N Engl J Med*. 2001;345(8):588-595.

57. Krejci V, Hiltebrand LB, Jakob SM, Takala J, Sigurdsson GH. Vasopressin in septic shock: effects on pancreatic, renal, and hepatic blood flow. *Crit Care*. 2007;11(6):R129.

58. Russell JA, Walley KR, Singer J, et al. Vasopressin versus norepinephrine infusion in patients with septic shock. *N Engl J Med*. 2008;358(9):877-887.

59. Thompson BT. Greater treatment effect with lower disease severity: VASST insights. *Crit Care Med*. 2017;45(6):1094-1095.

60. Serpa Neto A, Nassar AP, Cardoso SO, et al. Vasopressin and terlipressin in adult vasodilatory shock: a systematic review and meta-analysis of nine randomized controlled trials. *Crit Care*. 2012;16(4):R154.

61. Cannon JW. Hemorrhagic shock. *N Engl J Med*. 2018;378(19):1852-1853.

62. Cohn SM. Potential benefit of vasopressin in resuscitation of hemorrhagic shock. *J Trauma*. 2007;62(suppl 6):S56-S57.

63. Cohn SM, McCarthy J, Stewart RM, Jonas RB, Dent DL, Michalek JE. Impact of low-dose vasopressin on trauma outcome: prospective randomized study. *World J Surg*. 2011;35(2):430-439.

64. Mutlu GM, Factor P. Role of vasopressin in the management of septic shock. *Intensive Care Med.* 2004;30(7): 1276-1291.

65. Gordon AC, Mason AJ, Thirunavukkarasu N, et al. Effect of early vasopressin vs. norepinephrine on kidney failure in patients with septic shock: the VANISH randomized clinical trial. *JAMA.* 2016;316(5):509-518.

66. Voelckel WG, Raedler C, Wenzel V, et al. Arginine vasopressin, but not epinephrine, improves survival in uncontrolled hemorrhagic shock after liver trauma in pigs. *Crit Care Med.* 2003;31(4):1160-1165.

67. Morales D, Madigan J, Cullinane S, et al. Reversal by vasopressin of intractable hypotension in the late phase of hemorrhagic shock. *Circulation.* 1999;100(3):226-229.

73

What is the Current Role for Corticosteroids in Critical Care?

Craig Lyons and Leo G. Kevin

INTRODUCTION

Corticosteroids are commonly used in critical care. The merits of these drugs are fully established in some disease states, such as an adrenal crisis, anaphylaxis and vasculitic crises; however, there are several conditions that are regularly seen in the critical care unit where corticosteroid treatment is the subject of debate, controversy and ongoing clinical trials. In this chapter, we examine the evidence-base in those critical illnesses for which corticosteroid use is particularly contested, namely septic shock, acute respiratory distress syndrome, community acquired pneumonia, acute exacerbation of chronic obstructive pulmonary disease, acute severe asthma, and traumatic spinal cord injury (TSCI).

SEPTIC SHOCK

In 1976, William Schumer published the first trial comparing use of methylprednisolone (30 mg/kg) or dexamethasone (3 mg/kg) with placebo.[1] Both regimens were associated with a substantial reduction in mortality (methylprednisolone—1.6%; dexamethasone—9.3%; placebo—38.4%). In the 1980s however, four randomized controlled trials of varying design failed to validate a mortality benefit and instead suggested potential for harm. All used high-dose regimens, typically methylprednisolone 30 mg/kg.[2–5]

In the 1990s, with growing interest in the phenomenon of relative adrenocortical insufficiency during critical illness, and in use of "low-dose" corticosteroids to mitigate this, four small randomized controlled trials totaling 165 patients, demonstrated faster shock reversal with use of low-dose hydrocortisone.[6–9] These findings reignited the debate regarding the merits of corticosteroids in septic shock and prompted a number of large-scale trials for the new millennium.

The first of these, from Annane et al., randomized 300 patients with septic shock to receive either placebo or 50mg hydrocortisone every 6 hours, plus fludrocortisone 50 µg daily for 7 days.[10] Twenty-eight day mortality was reduced in those patients who received corticosteroids (55 vs. 61%). A subgroup analysis isolated the mortality benefit to those patients with inadequate adrenal reserve on the basis of their response to an ACTH stimulation test. This prompted the Corticosteroid Therapy of Septic Shock (CORTICUS) trial.[11]

CORTICUS randomized 499 patients with septic shock to receive 50 mg hydrocortisone or placebo every 6 hours for 5 days, after which the dose was tapered. Corticosteroid administration did not reduce 28-day mortality, irrespective of the response to ACTH stimulation.

2018 saw the publication of two large randomized controlled trials, the "Hydrocortisone plus Fludrocortisone for Adults with Septic Shock" (APROCCHSS) trial,[12] and the "Adjunctive Glucocorticoid Therapy in Patients with Septic Shock" (ADRENAL) trial.[13] These offer the most informative evidence to date of corticosteroid use in septic shock, but their divergent results fail to offer a definitive direction for clinical practice.

In APROCCHSS, a combination of hydrocortisone 50 mg every 6 hours and 50 mcg enteral fludrocortisone were administered for 7 days without tapering. The intervention arm had a reduction in 90-day mortality compared to placebo (43 vs. 49.1%). Secondary outcomes were also in favor of corticosteroid use, with patients weaned more quickly from mechanical ventilation and vasopressor therapies. Hyperglycemia was more commonly observed in the steroid arm but other side effects occurred at a similar rate in both groups.

ADRENAL randomized 3800 patients with septic shock who required mechanical ventilation to receive 200 mg hydrocortisone per day by continuous infusion, or placebo, for 7 days. Ninety-day mortality was 27.9% in the hydrocortisone group and 28.8% in the placebo group (OR 0.9; 95% confidence interval 0.82–1.10, $P = .50$). No mortality difference was observed in six prespecified groups: admission type (medical vs. surgical), gender, APACHE II score (<25 vs. ≥25), duration of shock at time of randomization, and dose of catecholamine infusions (norepinephrine or epinephrine at doses of <15 µg/min or >15 µg/min). Interestingly, however, there were advantages of hydrocortisone in some secondary outcomes: resolution of shock occurred more rapidly (median 3 days vs. 4 days), there was a lower incidence of blood transfusion (37.0 vs. 41.7%) and there was a shorter time to discharge from the intensive care unit (10 days vs. 12 days), although time to hospital discharge was not different between groups.

Based on current evidence, chiefly the ADRENAL trial by magnitude of patient enrolment, and a 2018 metaanalysis,[14] it can be concluded that corticosteroids do not reduce mortality in patients with septic shock. There are some caveats, however. Patients in APROCCHSS were sicker, requiring much higher doses of vasopressors at enrolment, perhaps pointing to a specific subgroup that does benefit. The role for fludrocortisone remains unclear and it is not widely used. Where these two trials agree is in the finding that corticosteroid treatment favorably alters the course of disease and does not appear to increase the risk of myopathy, infections or wound dehiscence. Some clinicians may reasonably seek to justify corticosteroid administration for the reported secondary benefits, all of which may improve resource utilization.

A separate question is whether corticosteroids have the potential to prevent the *development* of shock in septic patients. This was examined in the HYPRESS trial, where 200mg hydrocortisone was given for 5 days and then tapered.[15] No difference was found in rates of progression to septic shock (21.2 vs. 22.9%) or 28-day mortality (8.8 vs. 8.2%).

ACUTE RESPIRATORY DISTRESS SYNDROME

The first report of acute respiratory distress syndrome (ARDS) in 1967 proposed a role for corticosteroids,[16] but more than 50 years later, their role in this condition remains unresolved. Several trials have been performed, some focusing on preventing the development of ARDS in at-risk patients, others on improving outcomes in the early phase of the disease, and still others at preventing lung fibrosis later on. Interpretation of this literature is complicated by differences in selected corticosteroid, in the duration and dose of corticosteroid treatment, and in the variable inclusion of patients with septic shock. Moreover, since the publication of many of these trials, there have been major changes in the definition of ARDS and in many aspects of critical care management, particularly mechanical ventilation strategies.

Prevention of ARDS

Four randomized controlled trials have tested methylprednisolone in the prevention of ARDS in at-risk patients. When subjected to metaanalysis they pointed to an increased, rather than a decreased, risk of ARDS, and a higher risk of mortality in those who subsequently developed ARDS.[17]

Treatment of Established ARDS

In 1987 Bernard et al. randomized 99 patients with ARDS to a short course of high-dose methylprednisolone (30 mg/kg every 6 hours for 4 doses) or placebo.[18] The mean interval between the clinical onset of ARDS and entry to the trial was 31 hours. At 45 days, there were no differences between the groups in measures of gas exchange, lung mechanics or mortality. Importantly, there was also no evidence of increased infection in the corticosteroid group. Interest in use of high dose corticosteroids to treat ARDS waned, although the question of longer treatments and lower doses remained to be tested.

In 2006, a retrospective analysis of patients with ARDS in a sepsis trial, where patients were treated with hydrocortisone, pointed to improved survival and an increase in ventilator-free days[10,19]; however, these benefits occurred only in those patients who had failed a corticotropin stimulation test. Furthermore, patients in the treatment group were given fludrocortisone in addition to hydrocortisone. Meduri et al. then reported a randomized controlled trial in which a long course of low-dose methylprednisolone was given to patients within 72 hours of disease onset.[20] Intensive care mortality was 20.6% in the treatment group vs. 42.9% in the placebo group (*P* = .03); however, the trial comprised only 91 patients, and there were striking between-group differences at baseline, most notably in the rate of catecholamine-dependent shock which was much higher in the placebo group.

Late Treatment in Persistent ARDS

Meduri et al. administered methylprednisolone 2 mg/kg per day (tapered from day 14) or placebo to patients with ARDS who had been ventilated for at least 7 days without evidence of improvement.[21] The trial was stopped early after only 24 patients, when none of 16 patients in the methylprednisolone group had died compared to 5 out of 8 patients in the placebo group. There were also improvements in oxygenation and lung mechanics, and less organ dysfunction. The NIH NHLBI ARDS Network then trialed the same protocol in 180 patients.[22] Once again, compared to patients in the placebo group, those in the methylprednisolone group showed improvements in oxygenation and lung mechanics. Moreover, they liberated from mechanical ventilation sooner (14 days vs. 23 days), although they were later more likely to need a return to assisted ventilation (28 vs. 9%). Most importantly however, on this occasion methylprednisolone gave survival benefit. Also of note, in the subset of patients randomized 14 or more days after the onset of ARDS, those in the methylprednisolone group had a higher mortality, suggesting that corticosteroid treatment might be harmful if started late in the course of the disease.

COMMUNITY ACQUIRED PNEUMONIA

Corticosteroids are widely used in the treatment of community acquired pneumonia (CAP) albeit without a strong evidence base. Blum et al. published the largest RCT on steroid use in CAP in 2015, randomizing 785 patients to receive either 50mg prednisolone daily or placebo for 7 days.[23] The primary endpoint, time to attainment of stable vital signs, was achieved more quickly in the corticosteroid group (3 days vs. 4.4 days). Median time to discharge from hospital was 1 day shorter but there was no reduction in mortality. Patients with severe disease were inadequately represented, limiting generalizability of results to critically ill patients with CAP. Indeed, there is little data pertaining specifically to severe CAP. Torres et al. assessed benefit of a 5-day course of methylprednisolone in patients with CAP, 73% of whom were classified with Pneumonia Severity Index class IV or V, a larger representation of such patients than in most studies.[24] A composite primary outcome of treatment failure, which was typically diagnosed by radiographic progression of pneumonia, occurred less commonly in those patients receiving methylprednisolone (13 vs. 31%).

A metaanalysis of relevant trials of CAP of all grades did not demonstrate a mortality benefit, although there were reductions in time to clinical stability and in lengths of critical care and hospital stay.[25] A further metaanalysis isolated a survival benefit to the subgroup of patients with severe pneumonia.[26]

Corticosteroid benefits, if they exist, may be partly dependent on the infecting pathogen. Although the evidence is of low-grade, corticosteroid therapy is standard at treatment initiation for Pneumocystis jiroveci pneumonia,[27,28] whereas potential harm is reported in viral pneumonia.[29,30]

In summary, corticosteroid therapy does not have an established place in treatment of pneumonia although there is some evidence of benefits in those with severe disease. The Extended Steroids in CAPe (ESCAPEe) trial (NCT01283009), currently in progress, aims to provide more clarity to this question.

ACUTE EXACERBATION OF CHRONIC OBSTRUCTIVE PULMONARY DISEASE

Corticosteroid administration during acute exacerbations of chronic obstructive pulmonary disease (COPD) improves indices of pulmonary function in the first 72 hours of therapy and shortens hospital stay, but there is little evidence that it reduces mortality.[31] Of note, the majority of patients in trials of corticosteroid therapy for COPD exacerbation do not have an illness severity sufficient to warrant critical care admission. Indeed, some trials regard it as an exclusion criterion. There is conflicting evidence from the few trials that focused specifically on critically ill patients. Some have found less progression to invasive mechanical ventilation and shorter duration of invasive ventilation in corticosteroid treated patients,[32] whereas others have not.[33]

Guidelines issued by the Global Initiative for Chronic Obstructive Lung Disease (GOLD) advise the use of 40 mg prednisolone daily or equivalent for 5 days.[34] The American Thoracic Society recommends therapy up to 14 days in duration.[35] Evidence for a short course comes from the Reduction in the Use of Corticosteroids in Exacerbated COPD (REDUCE) trial, which compared 40 mg prednisolone daily for 5 vs. 14 days.[36] No difference was observed in measures of lung function or in the likelihood of further exacerbation within 6 months. Patients with a higher eosinophil count may represent a subpopulation more likely to derive benefit from steroid therapy.[37]

ACUTE SEVERE ASTHMA

Systemic corticosteroid administration accelerates improvements in airflow limitation in patients with acute asthma who are failing to respond to standard bronchodilator therapy, although published studies are underpowered to detect a mortality benefit.[38,39] Administration within 1 hour of emergency department admission is recommended. Patients who have not been receiving steroids preadmission seem to derive greater benefit.[40]

High doses provide no advantage over lower doses,[41] whilst oral and intravenous routes of administration are equally effective.[42,43] Likelihood of relapse appears similar for 5 and 10 day courses.[44] In practice, patients with severe or life-threatening exacerbations typically receive corticosteroids intravenously and for a longer duration. This is at least partly related to concerns that these groups have been underrepresented in controlled trials. Various recommendations exist, including hydrocortisone 100 mg 6-hourly and prednisolone 40–50 mg daily for 5 days.[45]

TRAUMATIC SPINAL CORD INJURY

Evidence for corticosteroids in TSCI comes largely from the National Acute Spinal Cord Injury Studies (NASCIS) II and III, published in 1990 and 1997, respectively.[46,47] NASCIS II randomized 487 acute TSCI patients to receive methylprednisolone or placebo. Methylprednisolone was administered as a 30 mg/kg bolus followed by maintenance infusion of 5.4 mg/kg per hour for 23 hours. There was no significant difference in neurological outcomes between the groups[46]; however, a posthoc analysis showed improved motor function in those patients who had received methylprednisolone within 8 hours of injury.[48] In response to this, NASCIS III randomized 499 patients to receive methylprednisolone within 8 hours of injury and then for either 24 or 48 hours. For patients that received their steroid bolus within 3 hours of injury, there was no difference in outcomes at 1 year between groups. For patients treated between 3 and 8 hours after injury, those who received 48 hours of methylprednisolone attained greater motor but not functional recovery. They also had a higher incidence of severe pneumonia, whilst mortality was unchanged.[47]

There was some, but not universal adoption of corticosteroids for spinal cord injuries. Much skepticism remains. Major problems concerning the statistical analysis of the NASCIS data have been identified,[49] and there is the obvious lack of a placebo group in NASCIS III. Recent metaanalyses provide no support for routine use of corticosteroids and indeed raise concerns about serious adverse effects.[50] Current US guidelines expressly discourage use of corticosteroids in TSCI.[51]

CONCERNS REGARDING CORTICOSTEROID USE

Accepted adverse effects of corticosteroids in critically ill patients include hyperglycemia and electrolyte disorders. Less certain, but more concerning, adverse effects include gastrointestinal bleeding, muscle weakness and increased secondary infections. An early report of severe muscle weakness in asthmatic patients treated with corticosteroids and muscle relaxants[52] had a profound impact on the use of both these drug classes in critically ill patients, particularly in combination. Animal studies confirm an effect of corticosteroids on skeletal muscle.[53] The recent, large trials of corticosteroids in critically ill patients offer inconclusive and sometimes conflicting results on the question of these adverse events.

For example, in both CORTICUS[11] and ADRENAL,[13] there were insufficient cases of neuromuscular weakness reported to allow a firm conclusion while there were increased rates of secondary infections in CORTICUS but not in ADRENAL. Accepted practice is to limit duration of corticosteroid administration to as short a time as possible, particularly when muscle relaxants are coadministered.

AUTHORS' RECOMMENDATIONS

- Corticosteroids can be considered in septic shock, to aid reversal of shock.
- Corticosteroids should not be given late in the course of ARDS (from 14 days).
- Corticosteroids are recommended in acute severe asthma and acute exacerbations of COPD. Evidence does not indicate a mortality benefit but does support more rapid resolution of bronchospasm and there may be benefits in other outcomes.
- Although widely used, there is no clear evidence of benefit from corticosteroids in community acquired pneumonia.
- After much controversy, corticosteroids are not recommended in traumatic acute spinal cord injury.
- Due to concerns about secondary infections and ICU-acquired weakness, corticosteroid treatment duration should be limited, especially in patients also receiving muscle relaxants.

REFERENCES

1. Schumer W. Steroids in the treatment of clinical septic shock. *Ann Surg.* 1976;184(3):333-341.
2. Lucas CE, Ledgerwood AM. The cardiopulmonary response to massive doses of steroids in patients with septic shock. *Arch Surg.* 1984;119(5):537-541.
3. Sprung CL, Caralis PV, Marcial EH, et al. The effects of high-dose corticosteroids in patients with septic shock. A prospective, controlled study. *N Engl J Med.* 1984;311(18):1137-1143.
4. Bone RC, Fisher Jr CJ, Clemmer TP, Slotman GJ, Metz CA, Balk RA. A controlled clinical trial of high-dose methylprednisolone in the treatment of severe sepsis and septic shock. *N Engl J Med.* 1987;317(11):653-658.
5. Veterans Administration Systemic Sepsis Cooperative Study Group. Effect of high-dose glucocorticoid therapy on mortality in patients with clinical signs of systemic sepsis. *N Engl J Med.* 1987;317(11):659-665.
6. Bollaert PE, Charpentier C, Levy B, Debouverie M, Audibert G, Larcan A. Reversal of late septic shock with supraphysiologic doses of hydrocortisone. *Crit Care Med.* 1998;26(4):645-650.
7. Briegel J, Forst H, Haller M, et al. Stress doses of hydrocortisone reverse hyperdynamic septic shock: a prospective, randomized, double-blind, single-center study. *Crit Care Med.* 1999;27(4):723-732.
8. Chawla K, Kupfer Y, Goldman I, Tessler S. Hydrocortisone reverses refractory septic shock. *Crit Care Med.* 1999;27(1):33A.
9. Yildiz O, Doganay M, Aygen B, Güven M, Keleştimur F, Tutuû A. Physiological-dose steroid therapy in sepsis. *Crit Care.* 2002;6(3):251-259.
10. Annane D, Sébille V, Charpentier C, et al. Effect of treatment with low doses of hydrocortisone and fludrocortisone on mortality in patients with septic shock. *JAMA.* 2002;288(7):862-871.
11. Sprung CL, Annane D, Keh D, et al. Hydrocortisone therapy for patients with septic shock. *N Engl J Med.* 2008;358(2):111-124.
12. Annane D, Renault A, Brun-Buisson C, et al. Hydrocortisone therapy for patients with septic shock. *N Engl J Med.* 2008;358(2):111-124.
13. Venkatesh B, Finfer S, Cohen J, et al. Adjunctive glucocorticoid therapy in patients with septic shock. *N Engl J Med.* 2018;378(9):797-808.
14. Rygård SL, Butler E, Granholm A, et al. Low-dose corticosteroids for adult patients with septic shock: a systematic review with meta-analysis and trial sequential analysis. *Intensive Care Med.* 2018;44(7):1003-1016.
15. Keh D, Trips E, Marx G. Effect of hydrocortisone on development of shock among patients with severe sepsis: the HYPRESS randomized clinical trial. *JAMA.* 2016;316(17):1775-1785.
16. Ashbaugh DG, Bigelow DB, Petty TL, Levine BE. Acute respiratory distress in adults. *Lancet.* 1967;2(7511):319-323.
17. Peter JV, John P, Graham PL, Moran JL, George IA, Bersten A. Corticosteroids in the prevention and treatment of acute respiratory distress syndrome (ARDS) in adults: meta-analysis. *BMJ.* 2008;336(7651):1006-1009.
18. Bernard GR, Luce JM, Sprung CL, et al. High-dose corticosteroids in patients with the adult respiratory distress syndrome. *N Engl J Med.* 1987;317(25):1565-1570.
19. Annane D, Sébille V, Bellissant E, Ger-Inf-05 Study Group. Effect of low doses of corticosteroids in septic shock patients with or without early acute respiratory distress syndrome. *Crit Care Med.* 2006;34(1):22-30.
20. Meduri GU, Golden E, Freire AX, et al. Methylprednisolone infusion in early severe ARDS: results of a randomized controlled trial. *Chest.* 2007;131(4):954-963.
21. Meduri GU, Headley AS, Golden E, et al. Effect of prolonged methylprednisolone therapy in unresolving acute respiratory distress syndrome: a randomized controlled trial. *JAMA.* 1998;280(2):159-165.
22. Steinberg KP, Hudson LD, Goodman RB, et al. Efficacy and safety of corticosteroids for persistent acute respiratory distress syndrome. *N Engl J Med.* 2006;354(16):1671-1684.
23. Blum CA, Nigro N, Briel M, et al. Adjunct prednisone therapy for patients with community-acquired pneumonia: a multicentre, double-blind, randomised, placebo-controlled trial. *Lancet.* 2015;385(9977):1511-1518.
24. Torres A, Sibila O, Ferrer M, et al. Effect of corticosteroids on treatment failure among hospitalized patients with severe community-acquired pneumonia and high inflammatory response: a randomized clinical trial. *JAMA.* 2015;313(7):677-686.
25. Wan YD, Sun TW, Liu ZQ, Zhang SG, Wang LX, Kan QC. Efficacy and safety of corticosteroids for community-acquired pneumonia: a systematic review and meta-analysis. *Chest.* 2016;149(1):209-219.
26. Nie W, Zhang Y, Cheng J, Xiu Q. Corticosteroids in the treatment of community-acquired pneumonia in adults: a meta-analysis. *PLoS One.* 2012;7(10):e47926.
27. Montaner JS, Lawson LM, Levitt N, Belzberg A, Schechter MT, Ruedy J. Corticosteroids prevent early deterioration in patients with moderately severe Pneumocystis carinii pneumonia and the acquired immunodeficiency syndrome (AIDS). *Ann Intern Med.* 1990;113(1):14-20.

28. Gagnon S, Boota AM, Fischl MA, Baier H, Kirksey OW, La Voie L. Corticosteroids as adjunctive therapy for severe Pneumocystis carinii pneumonia in the acquired immunodeficiency syndrome. A double-blind, placebo-controlled trial. *N Engl J Med.* 1990; 323(21):1444-1450.

29. Rodrigo C, Leonardi-Bee J, Nguyen-Van-Tam J, Lim WS. Corticosteroids as adjunctive therapy in the treatment of influenza. *Cochrane Database Syst Rev.* 2016;3:CD010406.

30. Moreno G, Rodríguez A, Reyes LF, et al. Corticosteroid treatment in critically ill patients with severe influenza pneumonia: a propensity score matching study. *Intensive Care Med.* 2018; 44(9):1470-1482.

31. Walters JA, Tan DJ, White CJ, Gibson PG, Wood-Baker R, Walters EH. Systemic corticosteroids for acute exacerbations of chronic obstructive pulmonary disease. *Cochrane Database Syst Rev.* 2014;(9):CD001288.

32. Alía I, de la Cal MA, Esteban A, et al. Efficacy of corticosteroid therapy in patients with an acute exacerbation of chronic obstructive pulmonary disease receiving ventilatory support. *Arch Intern Med.* 2011;171(21):1939-1946.

33. Abroug F, Ouanes-Besbes L, Fkih-Hassen M, et al. Prednisone in COPD exacerbation requiring ventilatory support: an open-label randomised evaluation. *Eur Respir J.* 2014;43(3): 717-724.

34. Gold: UpToDate: Global Initiative for Chronic Obstructive Lung Disease (GOLD). *Global Strategy for the Diagnosis, Management and Prevention of Chronic Obstructive Pulmonary Disease.* 2018. Available at: http://www.goldcopd.org. Accessed September 24, 2018.

35. Wedzicha JA Ers Co-Chair, Miravitlles M, Hurst JR. Management of COPD exacerbations: a European Respiratory Society/ American Thoracic Society guideline. *Eur Respir J.* 2017;49(3): pii: 1600791.

36. Leuppi JD, Schuetz P, Bingisser R, et al. Short-term vs. conventional glucocorticoid therapy in acute exacerbations of chronic obstructive pulmonary disease: the REDUCE randomized clinical trial. *JAMA.* 2013;309(21):2223-2231.

37. Bafadhel M, Davies L, Calverley PM, Aaron SD, Brightling CE, Pavord ID. Blood eosinophil guided prednisolone therapy for exacerbations of COPD: a further analysis. *Eur Respir J.* 2014;44(3):789-791.

38. Lin RY, Pesola GR, Bakalchuk L, et al. Rapid improvement of peak flow in asthmatic patients treated with parenteral methylprednisolone in the emergency department: a randomized controlled study. *Ann Emerg Med.* 1999;33(5):487-494.

39. Fanta CH, Rossing TH, McFadden Jr ER. Glucocorticoids in acute asthma. A critical controlled trial. *Am J Med.* 1983; 74(5):845-851.

40. Rowe BH, Spooner C, Ducharme FM, Bretzlaff JA, Bota GW. Early emergency department treatment of acute asthma with systemic corticosteroids. *Cochrane Database Syst Rev.* 2001; (1):CD002178.

41. Manser R, Reid D, Abramson M. Corticosteroids for acute severe asthma in hospitalised patients. *Cochrane Database Syst Rev.* 2001;(1):CD001740.

42. Harrison BD, Stokes TC, Hart GJ, Vaughan DA, Ali NJ, Robinson AA. Need for intravenous hydrocortisone in addition to oral prednisolone in patients admitted to hospital with severe asthma without ventilatory failure. *Lancet.* 1986;1(8474):181-184.

43. Ratto D, Alfaro C, Sipsey J, Glovsky MM, Sharma OP. Are intravenous corticosteroids required in status asthmaticus? *JAMA.* 1988;260(4):527-529.

44. Jones AM, Munavvar M, Vail A, et al. Prospective, placebo-controlled trial of 5 vs. 10 days of oral prednisolone in acute adult asthma. *Respir Med.* 2002;96(11):950-954.

45. Scottish Intercollegiate Guidelines Network. *British Guideline on the Management of Asthma.* 2016. Available at: https://www.sign.ac.uk/assets/sign153.pdf. Accessed September 24, 2018.

46. Bracken MB, Shepard MJ, Collins WF, et al. A randomized, controlled trial of methylprednisolone or naloxone in the treatment of acute spinal-cord injury. Results of the Second National Acute Spinal Cord Injury Study. *N Engl J Med.* 1990; 322(20):1405-1411.

47. Bracken MB, Shepard MJ, Holford TR, et al. Administration of methylprednisolone for 24 or 48 hours or tirilazad mesylate for 48 hours in the treatment of acute spinal cord injury. Results of the Third National Acute Spinal Cord Injury Randomized Controlled Trial. National Acute Spinal Cord Injury Study. *JAMA.* 1997;277(20):1597-1604.

48. Bracken MB, Shepard MJ, Collins Jr WF, et al. Methylprednisolone or naloxone treatment after acute spinal cord injury: 1-year follow-up data. Results of the second National Acute Spinal Cord Injury Study. *J Neurosurg.* 1992;76(1):23-31.

49. Coleman WP, Benzel D, Cahill DW, et al. A critical appraisal of the reporting of the National Acute Spinal Cord Injury Studies (II and III) of methylprednisolone in acute spinal cord injury. *J Spinal Disord.* 2000;13(3):185-199.

50. Evaniew N, Belley-Côté EP, Fallah N, Noonan VK, Rivers CS, Dvorak MF. Methylprednisolone for the treatment of patients with acute spinal cord injuries: a systematic review and meta-analysis. *J Neurotrauma.* 2016;33(5):468-481.

51. Hurlbert RJ, Hadley MN, Walters BC, et al. Pharmacological therapy for acute spinal cord injury. *Neurosurgery.* 2013;72 (Suppl. 2):93-105.

52. MacFarlane IA, Rosenthal FD. Severe myopathy after status asthmaticus. *Lancet.* 1977;2(8038):615.

53. Massa R, Carpenter S, Holland P, Karpati G. Loss and renewal of thick myofilaments in glucocorticoid-treated rat soleus after denervation and reinnervation. *Muscle Nerve.* 1992;15(11): 1290-1298.

74

How Should Trauma Patients Be Managed in the Intensive Care Unit?

Brian P. Smith and Patrick M. Reilly

Each year, in the United States, more than 2.5 million people are killed or hospitalized as a result of traumatic injuries.[1] Over one quarter of these patients are treated in an intensive care unit (ICU) at some point during their hospital stay.[2] With mortality rates exceeding 20% for the most severely injured patients (injury severity score [ISS] >25),[3] it stands to reason that the delivery of high-quality health care to trauma patients in an ICU setting plays a paramount role in their resuscitation and recovery.

INFRASTRUCTURE

Trauma patients should be cared for at hospitals with specialty trauma services. Population-based estimates have demonstrated a relative risk (RR) for mortality of 0.80 (95% confidence interval [CI], 0.66 to 0.98) for trauma patients treated at trauma centers compared with case mix-matched patients treated at facilities without designated trauma center status.[4] Multiple studies have confirmed that this model of care is successful and cost effective.[4-6] There remains debate regarding the source of this outcome advantage. Specifically, it is unclear whether the advantage derives from the absolute volume of the trauma center or the level of trauma center designation (and the resources associated with that designation).[7-10]

There is much less uncertainty about the role of intensivists in caring for these patients. In a large multicenter prospective cohort study in 2006, Nathens and colleagues demonstrated that, when compared with "open" ICUs, the intensivist model was associated with an RR of death of 0.78.[11] This effect was more pronounced among elderly patients (RR of death, 0.55), in ICUs in trauma centers (RR of death, 0.64), and in units directed by surgically trained intensivists (RR of death, 0.67). Similar data have shown not only improved mortality but also lower ICU mortality, lower ventilator-associated pneumonia rates, and increased ventilator-free days in ICUs that actively engage intensivists in the care of trauma patients.[12-14] This model has been expanded to trauma care in the combat zone, with favorable effects on morbidity and mortality among combat-injured patients cared for by intensivists.[15] The role played by an inhouse trauma attending physician should also be considered. These doctors do seem to expedite the transfer of patients from the emergency area into the ICU, and there is some evidence suggesting that the presence of an inhouse trauma physician attendings is associated with decreased ICU length of stay.[16,17] However, the exact nature of the influence of inhouse trauma attendings on ICU efficiency metrics remains unclear.

Perhaps the most important factor contributing to the better care afforded by trauma centers and staffed with specifically trained personnel is the availability of ICU beds themselves. Emergency department lengths of stay continue to increase, and much of the early part of resuscitation occurs within the confines of the emergency department or the trauma bay.[18,19] Providing ICU-level care within the trauma bay can be a challenging task. Evidence suggests that emergency department length of stay is directly linked to increased rates of pneumonia and death.[20,21] One response to this problem is implementation of an "open trauma bed" protocol to improve throughput from the trauma bay. In this study sample, institution of the protocol decreased the emergency department length of stay by nearly 1 hour.[22] Other investigators have demonstrated similar results, supported by cost-effectiveness data, by staffing an open ICU bed with an otherwise unassigned charge nurse.[23] However, it remains unclear how these protocols affect patients who are displaced from the ICU to generate bed availability.

RESUSCITATION

The primary goal of the intensivist caring for a trauma patient should be the recognition of shock and the implementation of resuscitation strategies to capture and reverse the associated abnormal physiology. The diagnosis of shock must be made with a high clinical index of suspicion because ongoing occult hypoperfusion (which occurs in up to 85% of severely injured trauma patients) has been associated with increased morbidity and mortality.[24–26] Several modalities of quantifying resuscitative efforts beyond standard vital signs have been proposed. They can be classified broadly into invasive monitors (such as pulmonary artery [PA] catheters, peripheral arterial catheters, and gastric tonometers), noninvasive monitors (such as bedside ultrasonography and bioreactance monitoring), and biomarkers (such as arterial or venous lactate, base deficit, and arterial or mixed venous oxygen saturation).

Invasive Hemodynamic Monitoring

Optimal oxygen (O_2) delivery relies on adequate cardiac performance. Therefore, optimization of cardiac output (CO) is a key feature of any resuscitative effort. Historically, PA catheterization was the mainstay of invasive hemodynamic monitoring. However, routine use of these devices has become less common,[27] and they seem most efficacious among older trauma patients and those who arrive in severe shock.[28]

Several commercially available products are available to estimate CO with less intrusion than PA catheterization. For instance, the lithium indicator dilution technique utilizes central venous catheterization and cannulation of the femoral or axillary artery to measure heart function. Similarly, there exist proprietary algorithms capable of estimating CO via transpulmonary thermodilution methods. Finally, volume responsiveness based on stroke volume variation transduced by a peripherally inserted arterial catheter can be calculated by several devices. Although all of these systems show promise in regards to their low complication rates, their efficacy in guiding fluid resuscitation of trauma patients remains unknown. Animal hemorrhagic shock models suggest that these devices might be unreliable, most commonly underestimating CO.[29–31] It is conceivable that as these technologies evolve, they will be capable of estimating cardiac function similar to pulmonary arterial cannulation without the need to traverse the right side of the heart and dwell within the pulmonary arterial system.

Noninvasive Hemodynamic Monitoring

Impedance cardiography and bioreactance are two methods of quantifying cardiac function without invasive monitoring. Both methods use electrophysiology to measure how changes in aortic blood volume and flow influence transmission of a known electrical current across the thorax. These technologies have been studied in multiple ICU settings and show modest correlation with traditional PA catheter thermodilution.[32,33] To date, there is one prospective observational study of this technology in trauma patients, demonstrating an association of bioreactance monitoring and shortened hospital length of stay.[34] However, it should be noted that the comparison groups were historic controls, and changes in hospital admission and discharge practices might have confounded the analysis.

Ultrasonography has been used as a triage tool in the trauma bay for many years and has recently become an important tool for the intensivist who cares for trauma patients.

Several investigators have shown that bedside ultrasonography of the cava and heart can demonstrate hypovolemic shock and the response to plasma expansion.[35–38] Most of these studies are limited by their retrospective nature; however, a recent randomized trial indicated that use of limited transthoracic echocardiograms during trauma resuscitation was associated with decreased intravenous fluid administration and improved survival.[39] Confirmatory studies are required. However, the repeatability, relatively low cost, and noninvasiveness of this diagnostic tool seem promising.

Biomarkers

The mainstay of trauma resuscitation has been biochemical endpoints of resuscitation. Although many have been investigated, the two that have been most useful in caring for trauma patients are serum lactate and base deficit. Both of these tests are sensitive measures of hypoperfusion[40,41]; however, the interpretation of these tests can be clouded by hepatic and/or renal dysfunction. Abnormal lactate and base deficit have been associated with morbidity and mortality.[42,43] Measurement of lactate and base deficit might be useful guides for resuscitative progress because mortality has been associated with increased time to normalization of serum lactate.[44] Likewise, in one study of trauma patients with increasing base deficit despite resuscitation, 65% were found to have ongoing hemorrhage, suggesting the potential utility of this test as an adjunct to the resuscitative efforts.[45] The most recent recommendation on the topic was developed by the Eastern Association for the Surgery of Trauma and suggests using at least one of these measures to quantify the need for ongoing resuscitation.[24]

There is mounting evidence that these studies, performed as point-of-care (POC) tests, decrease the time to diagnosis and intervention, reduce the total volume of blood draws, and shorten ICU lengths of stay.[46–48] POC thromboelastography can also be considered to help guide blood product administration during resuscitation in the trauma bay as well as in the ICU.[49,50] Mounting evidence demonstrates that resuscitations guided by thromboelastography not only reduce overall utilization of blood products, but also improve survival among severely injured patients.[51,52]

Special Considerations of Shock
Hypovolemic Shock

Hypovolemic shock from uncontrolled hemorrhage is the quintessential form of shock among trauma patients. Much work has been done to advance the care of trauma patients, both in the control of hemorrhage (permissive hypotension, fluid restrictive resuscitation, damage control surgery, applications of tourniquets, topical hemostatic agents, endovascular occlusion, etc.) as well as in the replacement of intravascular volume (colloid, isotonic and hypertonic crystalloid, balanced salt solutions, blood products, massive transfusion protocols, etc.). Details of these techniques can be found elsewhere in this volume. Suffice it to say that mastery of hemorrhage control and fluid resuscitation is critical to the cessation and reversal of hemorrhagic shock.

Septic Shock

Trauma patients with septic shock should be cared for according to the Surviving Sepsis Guidelines.[53] Although no studies, to date, have demonstrated any outcome advantage in particular to trauma patients, this body of work remains the most comprehensive summary of sepsis management in most patients. Particular mention should be made of two details. First, source control can be particularly challenging in trauma patients with multiple injured systems. Practitioners must rely heavily on physical examination, coupled with various methods of diagnostic imaging to guide interventions. This is particularly true in hostile abdomens and thoraces, in which some patients will undoubtedly benefit from percutaneous drainage rather than more traditional surgical exposures. Second, antibiotic stewardship is fundamental to trauma ICUs. The data supporting deescalation of antibacterial therapy as a means of quelling antibiotic resistance are lacking. However, the recent emergence of increasingly resistant organisms coincident with the common practice of empiric broad-spectrum antibiotic therapy lends strong credence to a linkage between these phenomena. Consequentially, strong consideration should be given to narrowing antibacterial coverage when culture data are available in appropriate patient groups.[54–56] There is no evidence that trauma patients (even those with much "spillage" or "contamination") benefit from extended empiric coverage. Likewise, the "open abdomen" strategy of patient care does not necessarily mandate the use of antibiotics in the absence of other indicators of infection.[57]

In addition, those practitioners who care for trauma patients must remain vigilant for signs of sepsis or septic shock throughout the duration of each patient's encounter. Either might very well be the inciting event leading to a patient's trauma and admission, or might bring a trauma patient back to the hospital from inpatient physical therapy, skilled nursing, or even home. Further, patients remain susceptible to the diagnosis at every point in between.

Neurogenic Shock

The incidence of neurogenic shock in patients with cervical spinal cord injuries is 20%.[58] The optimal treatment of the bradycardia and hypotension that define this pathophysiology remains unknown, but treatment with intravascular volume expansion as well as pharmacologic management with vasoactive, chronotropic, and inotropic medications might be indicated.[58–60] On occasion, the use of electrical cardiac stimulation, by way of percutaneous or intravascular pacers, might be valuable.[61] Therefore, the ICU should be capable of managing these various modes of hemodynamic support for patients with this injury complex.

Cardiogenic Shock

The combination of increasing age among trauma patients and higher numbers of high-speed motor vehicle accidents has contributed to increasing numbers of clinically significant cardiac injuries. It is estimated that up to 20% of road traffic deaths are associated with blunt injuries to the heart.[62]

Recognition of cardiac compromise can be challenging because many of these patients suffer concomitant injuries resulting in mixed shock physiology.[63,64] Signs of systemic hypotension in the face of elevated central venous pressure should raise concern for cardiogenic shock. Otherwise, clinicians must maintain a high index of suspicion based on the mechanism of injury despite potentially silent clinical signs. Patients with suspected blunt cardiac injury should be screened with electrocardiogram and troponin I. The negative predictive value of these combined tests approaches 100%.[64] The care of patients with cardiogenic shock is detailed elsewhere in this text. The care of trauma patients, in particular, must be guided by experienced traumatologists, in consultation with cardiologists, weighing the risks and benefits of interventions in the setting of potentially competing priorities.

Special Considerations of Trauma Patients
The Open Cavity

The use of damage control surgery and resuscitation has resulted in many critically ill trauma patients presenting to the ICU with open body cavities.[65,66] It is not unusual for patients to spend days recovering from the initial physiologic insult before these cavities can be closed. In this regard, it is paramount that ICUs specializing in the care of trauma patients be familiar with management of severe biomechanical and physiologic derangements that occur as chest and abdominal wall geometry are altered. Advanced modes of mechanical ventilation may be necessary for patients with packed thoraces. Likewise, the open abdomen requires skilled nursing wound care with negative pressure dressings and supplemented nutritional strategies for gastrointestinal drainage and discontinuity.

Traction/Immobility

Damage control orthopedic surgery (early external fixation followed by definitive treatment) has become increasingly common among polytrauma patients.[67–70] Therefore, the number of patients with large external fixation devices in the ICU has increased. Likewise, ICU patients might be cared for with pelvic stabilization devices (sheets and commercially available pelvic binders) and/or spinal column stabilizing devices (cervical spine bracing devices such as cervical collars or Halo systems, thoracolumbosacral orthosis braces). Although these techniques are helpful to the recovery of various injuries, they oftentimes limit mobility and access to soft tissue care. Therefore, particular attention must be paid to these trauma patients to ensure adequate wound care and prevention of the secondary complications of immobility.

Venous Thromboembolism Prophylaxis

Venous thromboembolism (VTE) is a common complication in patients with major trauma.[71] The risk is compounded by various factors, such as the systemic inflammatory response to major trauma, immobility, and the hypercoagulable state associated with major surgery, bone fractures, and the use of invasive vascular devices. It is important for the ICU to practice aggressive evaluation for VTE with protocolized care to help prevent the (potentially fatal) sequelae of VTE.[72,73] Implementation of VTE prevention strategies in the form of "smart order sets" or risk assessment models has been associated with decreased rates of radiographically documented VTE (2.5% vs. 0.7%) and a 39% RR reduction of hospital-acquired VTE in some patient groups.[74,75] Clinicians must also be familiar with evidence-based best practice guidelines to help reduce VTE risk, particularly for trauma patients.[76,77]

INTENSIVE CARE UNIT PROTOCOLS

Guideline-based care (in the form of agreed-upon practice patterns, guidelines, or protocols) plays an important role in the delivery of high-quality intensive care therapies to patients with traumatic injuries. Studies have demonstrated that implementation of trauma systems, including things such as early management guidelines and consensus-developed clinical practice guidelines and protocols, are associated with decreasing odds of death (odds ratio [OR] 0.45; 95% CI, 0.27 to 0.76), standardized care, and improved resource utilization.[78,79] They are natural extensions of the algorithmic approach to the triage of life-threatening injuries suggested by the Advanced Trauma Life Support (ATLS) curriculum.[80] It is impossible to list every ICU trauma guideline but consideration should be given to several management strategies. Indeed, this approach has been advocated for management of, among others, elevated intracranial pressure, spinal cord injury and rehabilitation, sedation and delirium, pain control, mechanical ventilation and weaning, use of enteral and parenteral nutrition, glucose control, utilization of bladder catheters, blood transfusions, antibiotic stewardship, prophylaxis of stress ulcers and venous thromboembolic disease, early mobilization and physical therapy, and use of various ICU devices (such as central and peripherally inserted catheters, arterial lines, and ICU specialty beds). Importantly, virtually none of these interventions is based on high-level evidence. However, the central theme of the guidelines (i.e., improved outcomes for injured patients) can be obtained through better organization, and planning of trauma care should be maintained.[81] Some researchers have found that major deviations from clinical management guidelines are associated with a 3-fold increase in mortality among trauma patients (adjusted OR 3.28; 95% CI, 1.53 to 7.03).[82] Similarly, an intervention as simple as strict adherence to a daily rounding checklist has been linked to improved outcomes, such as decreased ventilator-associated pneumonia rates, relative to partial compliance with the same checklist (3.5% vs. 13.4%, $P = .04$).[83]

TERTIARY EXAMINATION

A common pitfall of caring for trauma patients (particularly those who are critically ill) is failure to recognize missed injuries.[84] This results from many variables, including severe physiologic derangements, inability of the patient to participate in the history and physical examination, handoffs of care, and multiple service lines assuming care of different injury complexes. So-called "missed injuries" can result in significant morbidity and even death.[85,86] Several mechanisms have been proposed to help decrease the rate of missed injuries. Most are extensions of the tertiary survey proposed by Enderson in 1990.[87] Technological advances should also help to reduce missed injury rates as faster and more detailed medical imaging becomes increasingly affordable and mobile. Access to electronic medical records and the use of handheld communication devices and electronic checklists should also help expedite recognition and communication of previously undocumented injuries.

THE EXTENDED INTENSIVE CARE UNIT TEAM

Nursing

There are differences in the needs of family and friends of trauma ICU patients compared with those of families of general ICU patients. These differences primarily surround the sensation of shock and personal distress experienced by the families in the trauma ICU, but they also extend to the reported needs of the families and the ways in which those families perceive patient care, which has significant implications for the ways in which bedside care (in all forms) is delievered.[88] This is particularly germane to nursing staff who undertake a significant portion of family counseling, and might explain why nurses in trauma ICU environments have higher than average scores in subjective reporting of moral distress situations.[89]

Physical Therapy

More than 25% of patients with multiple injuries and extended ICU lengths of stay develop long-term limitations of range of motion unrelated to their injuries, 30% are unable to return to work, and nearly 50% suffer permanent sensory deficits.[90,91] Early mobilization plays a fundamental role in the battle against ICU-acquired weakness. Therefore, integration of an aggressive physical and occupational therapy service into the daily care of these patients is paramount in their recovery.[92-95] This seems particularly true among patients requiring blood transfusions during the ICU stay.[96]

Pharmacy

There is increasing evidence that the presence of a clinical pharmacist at ICU rounds improves outcomes of ICU patients.[97-100] Clinical pharmacists serve as a direct link to the main hospital pharmacies. They are often well versed in hospital antibiograms, they have critical training in drug–drug interactions, and they provide continuity of care among the prehospital setting, the ICU stay, and the transition to other levels of care. There is good evidence demonstrating an association between engaged clinical pharmacists and decreased adverse drug events, as well as cost savings in trauma centers.[101]

SUMMARY

Traumatic injuries account for many ICU admissions each year. These patients are best served at dedicated trauma centers with access to multimodality diagnostic and treatment options. Care teams should be led by intensive trained physicians with knowledge and experience in various resuscitative techniques, and team members should represent various disciplines including nursing, pharmacy, and physical therapy. The ICU should be capable of and familiar with POC testing, invasive and noninvasive monitoring, and appropriate triage of critically ill patients. Most importantly, the care of the trauma patient in the ICU should integrate algorithmic approaches to diagnosis and treatment, incorporating resources from evidence-based guidelines and expert-level opinions.

AUTHORS' RECOMMENDATIONS

- Critically ill trauma patients should be cared for by a team of trained intensive care practitioners in a designated trauma center ICU.
- Intensive care team members should be well trained in the recognition and treatment of shock, and they should maintain a high index of suspicion for various shock states based on history, physical examination, and mechanism of injury.
- Trauma ICUs should be familiar with and capable of monitoring patients with invasive, noninvasive, and POC testing based on patient needs and severity of illness.
- ICU protocols should be used to guide trauma care, with particular attention paid to VTE prophylaxis. ICU care should also account for the management of open body cavities and trauma variables such as skeletal traction.

REFERENCES

1. Centers for Disease Control and Prevention. *Web-Based Injury Statistics Query and Reporting System (WISQARS)*. Available at: http://www.cdc.gov/injury/WISQARS/. Accessed November 14, 2018.
2. Nathens AB, Maier RV, Jurkovich GJ, Monary D, Rivara FP, Mackenzie EJ. The delivery of critical care services in US trauma centers: is the standard being met? *J Trauma*. 2006;60:773-784.
3. Dutton RP, Stansbury LG, Leone S, Kramer E, Hess JR, Scalea TM. Trauma mortality in mature trauma systems: are we doing better? An analysis of trauma mortality patterns, 1997-2008. *J Trauma*. 2010;69:620-626.
4. MakKenzie EJ, Rivara FP, Jurkavich GJ, et al. A national evaluation of the effect of trauma-center care on mortality. *N Engl J Med*. 2006;354:366-378.
5. Sampalis JS, Denis R, Lavoie A, et al. Trauma care regionalization: a process-outcome evaluation. *J Trauma*. 1999;46:565-579.
6. MacKenzie EJ, Weir S, Rivara FP, et al. The value of trauma center care. *J Trauma*. 2010;69:1-10.
7. Nathens AB, Jurkovich GJ, Maier RV, et al. Relationship between trauma center volume and outcomes. *JAMA*. 2001;285:1164-1171.
8. Demetriades D, Martin M, Salim A, Rhee P, Brown C, Chan L. The effect of trauma center designation and trauma volume on outcome in specific severe injuries. *J Trauma*. 2005;242:512-517.
9. Bennett KM, Vaslef S, Pappas TN, Scarborough JE. The volume-outcomes relationship for United States level I trauma centers. *J Surg Res*. 2011;167:19-23.
10. Minei JP, Fabian TC, Guffey DM, et al. Increased trauma center volume is associated with improved survival after severe injury: results of a Resuscitation Outcomes Consortium study. *Ann Surg*. 2014;260:456-465.
11. Nathens AB, Rivara FP, MacKenzie EJ, et al. The impact of an intensivist-model ICU on trauma-related mortality. *Ann Surg*. 2006;244:545-552.
12. Multz AS, Chalfin DB, Samson IM, et al. A "closed" medical intensive care unit (MICU) improves resource utilization when compared with an "open" MICU. *Am J Respir Crit Care Med*. 1998;157:1468-1473.
13. Ghorra S, Reinert SE, Cioffi W, Buczko G, Simms HH. Analysis of the effect of conversion from open to closed surgical intensive care unit. *Ann Surg*. 1999;229:163-171.
14. Pronovost PJ, Jenckes MW, Dorman T, et al. Organizational characteristics of intensive care units related to outcomes of abdominal aortic surgery. *JAMA*. 1999;281:1310-1317.
15. Lettieri CJ, Shah AA, Greenburg DL. An intensivist-directed intensive care unit improves clinical outcomes in a combat zone. *Crit Care Med*. 2009;37:1256-1260.
16. van der Vliet QMJ, van Maarseveen OEC, Smeeing DPJ, et al. Severely injured patients benefit from in-house attending trauma surgeons. *Injury*. 2019;50(1):20-26. doi:10.1016/j.injury.2018.08.006.
17. Cox JA, Bernard AC, Bottiggi AJ, et al. Influence of in-house attending presence on trauma outcomes and hospital efficiency. *J Am Coll Surg*. 2014;218:734-738.
18. Fromm Jr RE, Gibbs LR, McCallum WG, et al. Critical care in the emergency department: a time-based study. *Crit Care Med*. 1993;21:970-976.
19. Derlet RW, Richards JR. Overcrowding in the nation's emergency departments: complex causes and disturbing effects. *Ann Emerg Med*. 2000;35:63-68.
20. Carr BG, Kaye AJ, Wiebe DJ, Gracias VH, Schwab CW, Reilly PM. Emergency department length of stay: a major risk factor for pneumonia in intubated blunt trauma patients. *J Trauma*. 2007;63:9-12.
21. Mowery NT, Dougherty SD, Hildreth AN, et al. Emergency department length of stay is an independent predictor of hospital mortality in trauma activation patients. *J Trauma*. 2011;70:1317-1325.
22. Bhakta A, Bloom M, Warren H, et al. The impact of implementing a 24/7 open trauma bed protocol in the surgical intensive care unit on throughput and outcomes. *J Trauma Acute Care Surg*. 2013;75:97-101.
23. Fryman L, Talley C, Kearney P, Bernard A, Davenport D. Maintaining an open trauma intensive care unit bed for rapid admission can be cost-effective. *J Trauma Acute Care Surg*. 2015;79:98-103.
24. Tisherman SA, Barie P, Bokhari F, et al. Clinical practice guideline: endpoints of resuscitation. *J Trauma*. 2004;57:898-912.
25. Scalea TM, Maltz S, Yelon J, Trooskin SZ, Duncan AO, Sclafani SJ. Resuscitation of multiple trauma and head injury: role of crystalloid fluids and inotropes. *Crit Care Med*. 1994;20:1610-1615.
26. Abou-Khalil B, Scalea TM, Trooskin SZ, Henry SM, Hitchcock R. Hemodynamic responses to shock in young trauma patients: need for invasive monitoring. *Crit Care Med*. 1994;22:633-639.
27. Rajaram SS, Desai NK, Kalra A, et al. Pulmonary artery catheters for adult patients in intensive care. *Cochrane Database Syst Rev*. 2013;(2):CD003408.
28. Friese RS, Shafi S, Gentilello LM. Pulmonary artery catheter use is associated with reduced mortality in severely injured

patients: a National Trauma Data Bank analysis of 53,312 patients. *Crit Care Med*. 2006;34:1597-1601.

29. Lee CH, Wang JY, Huang KL, et al. Unreliability of pulse contour-derived cardiac output in piglets simulating acute hemorrhagic shock and rapid volume expansion. *J Trauma*. 2010;68:1357-1361.

30. Piehl MD, Manning JE, McCurdy SL, et al. Pulse contour cardiac output analysis in a piglet model of severe hemorrhagic shock. *Crit Care Med*. 2008;36:1189-1195.

31. Cooper ES, Muir WW. Continuous cardiac output monitoring via arterial pressure waveform analysis following severe hemorrhagic shock in dogs. *Crit Care Med*. 2007;37:1724-1729.

32. Kamath SA, Dranzer MH, Tassisa G, Rogers JG, Stevenson LW, Yancy CW. Correlation of impedance cardiography with invasive hemodynamic measurements in patients with advanced heart failure: the BioImpedance CardioGraphy (BIG) substudy of the Evaluation Study of Congestive Heart Failure and Pulmonary Artery Catheterization Effectiveness (ESCAPE) Trial. *Am Heart J*. 2009;158:217-223.

33. Kieback AG, Borges AC, Schink T, Baumann G, Laule M. Impedance cardiography versus invasive measurements of stroke volume index in patients with chronic heart failure. *Int J Cardiol*. 2010;143:211-213.

34. Dunham CM, Chirichella TJ, Gruber BS, et al. Emergency department noninvasive (NICOM) cardiac outputs are associated with trauma activation, patient injury severity and host conditions and mortality. *J Trauma Acute Care Surg*. 2012;73:479-485.

35. Ferrada P, Vanguri P, Anand RJ, et al. A, B, C, D, echo: limited transthoracic echocardiogram is a useful tool to guide therapy for hypotension in the trauma bay—a pilot study. *J Trauma Acute Care Surg*. 2013;74:220-223.

36. Yanagawa Y, Sakamoto T, Okada Y. Hypovolemic shock evaluated by sonographic measurement of the inferior vena cava during resuscitation in trauma patients. *J Trauma*. 2007;63:1245-1248.

37. Carr BG, Dean AJ, Everett WW, et al. Intensivist bedside ultrasound (INBU) for volume assessment in the intensive care unit: a pilot study. *J Trauma*. 2007;63:495-500.

38. Nguyen A, Plurad DS, Bricker S, et al. Flat or fat? Inferior vena cava ratio is a marker for occult shock in trauma patients. *J Surg Res*. 2014;192:263-267.

39. Ferrada P, Evans D, Wolfe L, et al. Findings of a randomized controlled trial using limited transthoracic echocardiogram (LTTE) as a hemodynamic monitoring tool in the trauma bay. *J Trauma Acute Care Surg*. 2014;76:31-37.

40. Rutherford EJ, Morris JA Jr, Reed GW, Hall KS. Base deficit stratifies mortality and determines therapy. *J Trauma*. 1992;33:417-423.

41. Manikis P, Jankowski S, Zhang H, Kahn RJ, Vincent JL. Correlation of serial blood lactate levels to organ failure and mortality after trauma. *Am J Emerg Med*. 1995;13:619-622.

42. McNelis J, Marini CP, Jurkiewicz A, et al. Prolonged lactate clearance is associated with increased mortality in the surgical intensive care unit. *Am J Surg*. 2001;182:481-485.

43. Davis JW, Kaups KL. Base deficit in the elderly: a marker of severe injury and death. *J Trauma*. 1998;45:873-877.

44. Abramson D, Salea TM, Hitchcock R, Trooskin SZ, Henry SM, Greenspan J. Lactate clearance and survival following injury. *J Trauma*. 1993;35:584-588.

45. Davis JW, Shackford SR, Mackersie SC, Hoyt DB. Base deficit as a guide to volume resuscitation. *J Trauma*. 1988;28:1464-1467.

46. Weber CF, Görlinger K, Meininger G, et al. Point-of-care testing: a prospective, randomized clinical trial of efficacy in coagulopathic cardiac surgery patients. *Anesthesiology*. 2012;117:531-547.

47. Rossi AF, Khan DM, Hannan R, Bolivar J, Zaidenweber M, Burke R. Goal-directed medical therapy and point-of-care testing improve outcomes after congenital heart surgery. *Intensive Care Med*. 2005;31:98-104.

48. Meybohm P, Zacharowski K, Weber C. Point-of-care coagulation management in intensive care medicine. *Crit Care*. 2013;17:218-227.

49. Feinman M, Cotton BA, Haut ER. Optimal fluid resuscitation in trauma: type, timing, and total. *Curr Opin Crit Care*. 2014;20:366-372.

50. Tapia NM, Chang A, Norman M. TEG-guided resuscitation is superior to standardized MTP resuscitation in massively transfused penetrating trauma patients. *J Trauma Acute Care Surg*. 2013;74:378-385.

51. Wikkelsø A, Wetterslev J, Møller AM, Afshari A. Thromboelastography (TEG) or thromboelastometry (ROTEM) to monitor haemostatic treatment versus usual care in adults or children with bleeding. *Cochrane Database Syst Rev*. 2016;(8):CD007871.

52. Gonzalez E, Moore EE, Moore HB, et al. Goal-directed hemostatic resuscitation of trauma-induced coagulopathy: a pragmatic randomized clinical trial comparing a viscoelastic assay to conventional coagulation assays. *Ann Surg*. 2016;263:1051-1059.

53. Dellinger RP, Levy MM, Rhodes A, et al. Surviving sepsis campaign: international guidelines for management of severe sepsis and septic shock: 2012. *Crit Care Med*. 2013;41:580-637.

54. Eachempati SR, Hydo LJ, Shou J, Barie PS. Does de-escalation of antibiotic therapy for ventilator-associated pneumonia affect the likelihood of recurrent pneumonia or mortality in critically ill surgical patients? *J Trauma*. 2009;66:1343-1348.

55. Rello J, Vidaur L, Sandiumenge A, et al. De-escalation therapy in ventilator-associated pneumonia. *Crit Care Med*. 2004;32:2183-2190.

56. Masterton R. Antibiotic de-escalation. *Crit Care Clin*. 2011;27:149-162.

57. Dutton WD, Diaz JJ Jr, Miller RS. Critical care issues in managing complex open abdominal wound. *J Intensive Care Med*. 2012;27:167-171.

58. Guly HR, Bouamra O, Lecky FE, Trauma Audit and Research Network. The incidence of neurogenic shock in patients with isolated spinal cord injury in the emergency department. *Resuscitation*. 2008;76:57-62.

59. Zipnick RI, Scalea TM, Trooskin SZ, et al. Hemodynamic responses to penetrating spinal cord injuries. *J Trauma*. 1993;35:578-582.

60. Dumont RJ, Verma S, Okonkwo DO, et al. Acute spinal cord injury, part II: contemporary pharmacotherapy. *Clin Neuropharmacol*. 2001;24:265-279.

61. Bilello JF, Davis JW, Cunningham MA, Groom TF, Lemaster D, Sue LP. Cervical spinal cord injury and the need for cardiovascular intervention. *Arch Surg*. 2003;138:1127-1129.

62. Parmly LF, Manion WC, Mattingly TW. Nonpenetrating traumatic injury of the heart. *Circulation*. 1958;18:371-396.

63. Prêtre R, Chilcott M. Blunt trauma to the heart and great vessels. *N Engl J Med*. 1997;336:626-632.

64. Clancy K, Velopulos C, Bilaniuk JW, et al. Screening for blunt cardiac injury: an Eastern Association for the Surgery of Trauma practice management guideline. *J Trauma Acute Care Surg*. 2012;73:s301-s306.

65. Rotondo MF, Schwab CW, McGonigal MD, et al. 'Damage control': an approach for improved survival in exsanguinating penetrating abdominal injury. *J Trauma*. 1993;35:375-382.

66. Burch JM, Ortiz VB, Richardson RJ, Martin RR, Mattox KL, Jordan Jr GL. Abbreviated laparotomy and planned reoperation for critically injured patients. *Ann Surg.* 1992;215:476-484.

67. Hoey BA, Schwab CW. Damage control surgery. *Scand J Surg.* 2009;91:92-103.

68. Nowotarski PJ, Turen CH, Brumback RJ, Scarboro JM. Conversion of external fixation to intramedullary nailing for fractures of the shaft of the femur in multiply injured patients. *J Bone Joint Surg Am.* 2000;82:781-788.

69. Pape HC, Hildebrand F, Pertschy S, et al. Changes in the management of femoral shaft fractures in polytrauma patients: from early total care to damage control orthopedic surgery. *J Trauma.* 2002;53:452-461.

70. Taeger G, Ruchholtz S, Waydhas C, Lewan U, Schmidt B, Nast-Kolb D. Damage control orthopedics in patients with multiple injuries is effective, time saving, and safe. *J Trauma.* 2005;59:409-416.

71. Geerts WH, Code KI, Jay RM, Chen E, Szalai JP. A prospective study of venous thromboembolism after major trauma. *N Engl J Med.* 1994;331:1601-1606.

72. Tooher R, Middleton P, Pham C, et al. A systematic review of strategies to improve prophylaxis for venous thromboembolism in hospitals. *Ann Surg.* 2005;241:397-415.

73. Maynard G, Stein J. Designing and implementing effective venous thromboembolism prevention protocols: lessons from collaborative efforts. *J Thromb Thrombolysis.* 2010;29:159-166.

74. Zeidan AM, Streiff MB, Lau BD, et al. Impact of a venous thromboembolism prophylaxis "smart order set": improved compliance, fewer events. *Am J Hematol.* 2013;88:545-549.

75. Maynard GA, Morris TA, Jenkins IH, et al. Optimizing prevention of hospital-acquired venous thromboembolism (VTE): prospective validation of a VTE risk assessment model. *J Hosp Med.* 2010;5:10-18.

76. Rogers FB, Cipolle MD, Velmahos G, Rozycki G, Luchette FA. Practice management guidelines for the prevention of venous thromboembolism in trauma patients: the EAST practice management guidelines work group. *J Trauma.* 2002; 53:142-164.

77. Guyatt GH, Akl EA, Crowther M, et al. Executive summary: antithrombotic therapy and prevention of thrombosis, 9th ed: American College of Chest Physicians Evidence-Based Clinical Practice Guidelines. *Chest.* 2012;141:7s-47s.

78. Brennan PW, Everest ER, Griggs WM, et al. Risk of death among cases attending South Australian Major Trauma Services after severe trauma: the first 4 years of operation of a state trauma system. *J Trauma.* 2002;53:333-339.

79. Simons R, Eliopoulos V, Laflamme D, Brown DR. Impact on process of trauma care delivery 1 year after the introduction of a trauma program in a provincial trauma center. *J Trauma.* 1999;46:811-816.

80. American College of Surgeons Committee on Trauma. *Advanced Trauma Life Support Program for Doctors.* 9th ed. Chicago, IL: American College of Surgeons; 2013.

81. Mock C, Lormond JD, Goosen J, et al. *Guidelines for Essential Trauma Care.* Geneva, Switzerland: World Health Organization; 2004.

82. Rice TW, Morris S, Tortella BJ, Wheeler AP, Christensen MC. Deviations from evidence-based clinical management guidelines increase mortality in critically injured trauma patients. *Crit Care Med.* 2012;40:778-786.

83. Dubose J, Teixeira PGR, Inaba K, et al. Measurable outcomes of quality improvement using a daily quality rounds checklist: one-year analysis in a trauma intensive care unit with sustained ventilator-associated pneumonia reduction. *J Trauma.* 2010;69: 855-860.

84. Angle N, Coimbra R, Hoyt DB. Pitfalls in the management of the trauma patient in the intensive care unit. *Trauma.* 1999;1:301-305.

85. Janjua KJ, Sugrue M, Deane SA. Prospective evaluation of early missed injuries and the role of tertiary trauma survey. *J Trauma.* 1998;44:1000-1006.

86. Buduhan G, McRitchie DI. Missed injuries in patients with multiple trauma. *J Trauma.* 2000;49:600-605.

87. Enderson BL, Reath DB, Meadors J, Dallas W, DeBoo JM, Maull KI. The tertiary trauma survey: a prospective study of missed injury. *J Trauma.* 1990;30:666-669.

88. Mitchell M, Dwan T, Takashima M, et al. The needs of familes of trauma intensive care patients: A mixed methods study. *Intensive Crit Care Nurs.* 2019;50:11-20.

89. Mason VM, Leslie G, Clark K, et al. Compassion fatigue, moral distress, and work engagement in surgical intensive care unit trauma nurses: a pilot study. *Dimens Crit Care Nurs.* 2014; 33:215-225.

90. Grotz M, Hohensee A, Remmers D, Wagner TO, Regel G. Rehabilitation results of patients with multiple injuries and multiple organ failure and long-term intensive care. *J Trauma.* 1997;42:919-926.

91. Baldry Currens JA. Evaluation of disability and handicap following injury. *Injury.* 2000;31:99-106.

92. De Jonghe B, Lacherade J-C, Sharshar T, et al. Intensive care unit-acquired weakness: risk factors and prevention. *Crit Care Med.* 2009;37:s309-s315.

93. Griffiths RD, Hall JB. Intensive care unit-acquired weakness. *Crit Care Med.* 2010;38:779-787.

94. Nordon-Craft A, Moss M, Quan D, Schenkman M. Intensive care unit-acquired weakness: implications for physical therapist management. *Phys Ther.* 2012;92(12):1494-1506.

95. Yosef-Brauner O, Adi N, Ben Shahar T, Yehezkel E, Carmeli E. Effect of physical therapy on muscle strength, respiratory muscles and functional parameters in patients with intensive care unit-acquired weakness. *Clin Respir J.* 2015;9:1-6.

96. Parsons EC, Kross EK, Ali NA, et al. Red blood cell transfusion is associated with decreased in-hospital muscle strength among critically ill patients requiring mechanical ventilation. *J Crit Care.* 2013;28:1079-1085.

97. Papadopoulos J, Rebuck JA, Lober C, et al. The critical care pharmacist: an essential intensive care practitioner. *Pharmacotherapy.* 2002;22:1484-1488.

98. Kane SL, Weber RJ, Dasta JF. The impact of critical care pharmacists on enhancing patient outcomes. *Intensive Care Med.* 2003;29:691-698.

99. MacLaren R, Bond CA, Martin SJ, Fike D. Clinical and economic outcomes of involving pharmacists in the direct care of critically ill patients with infections. *Crit Care Med.* 2008;36:3184-3189.

100. Preslaski CR, Lat I, MacLaren R, Poston J. Pharmacist contributions as members of the multidisciplinary ICU team. *Chest.* 2013;144:1687-1695.

101. Hamblin S, Rumbaugh K, Miller R. Prevention of adverse drug events and cost savings associated with PharmD interventions in an academic Level I trauma center: an evidence-based approach. *J Trauma Acute Care Surg.* 2012;73:1484-1490.

75

What Is Abdominal Compartment Syndrome and How Should It Be Managed?

Michael A. Vella and Lewis J. Kaplan

Intraabdominal hypertension (IAH) and abdominal compartment syndrome (ACS) fall on a spectrum of pathophysiologic abnormalities resulting from elevations in intraabdominal pressure (IAP). Diagnostic criteria have been articulated by the World Society of the Abdominal Compartment Syndrome (WSACS; www.wsacs.org).[1,2] IAH is defined as the sustained or repetitive elevation of IAP to ≥12 mm Hg (normal 5–11 mm Hg) and is graded according to a four-tiered continuum (Table 75.1).[1,3] ACS occurs when an elevated IAP >20 mm Hg results in end-organ dysfunction.[1] In an era of restrictive fluid practices, the incidence of ACS has decreased, and diagnosis can be challenging.[4,5,6] The clinician with little experience managing ACS must maintain a high index of suspicion in at-risk patients and be prepared to quickly institute corrective measures, ideally through a protocolized approach. This chapter describes the pathophysiology, monitoring, categorization, and management of IAH and ACS.

PATHOPHYSIOLOGY AND MECHANISM OF ACTION

The pathophysiology of ACS is complex. A disequilibrium in the abdominal compartment's normal pressure-volume (PV) relationship maintained by arterial inflow, venous outflow, and the space occupied by viscera and intraabdominal fluid (i.e., blood, ascites) leads to rising IAP. This process is similar to the PV dynamics observed when a space occupying lesion within the skull leads to elevated intracranial pressure, although the abdomen is obviously a more compliant structure. The initial response to rising IAP includes reshaping of the abdominal cavity, stretching of the abdominal wall musculature and cephalad displacement of the diaphragm. Once these mechanisms are exhausted, IAP begins to increase exponentially, and ACS is likely to result.[7] Typical adult IAP ranges from 0 to 5 mm Hg, however, obesity, pregnancy, and advanced age may elevate baseline abdominal pressures. One study showed an increase of between 0.14 and 0.23 mm Hg for each body mass index (BMI) unit and 0.20 mm Hg for each year increase in age.[8] Open abdominal operations may also elevate the measured IAP.[1]

ACS is traditionally classified as primary, secondary, or recurrent. *Primary* ACS develops as the direct result of an abdominal injury or other abdominal surgical emergency (e.g., intestinal perforation or ischemia). *Secondary* ACS results from a condition that is not of primary abdominal origin. This is often the sequela of visceral edema and/or the acute accumulation of ascites as seen in massive volume resuscitation following thermal injury, acute pancreatitis, or extra-abdominal septic shock. Lastly, *recurrent* or *tertiary* ACS develops after successful medical or surgical therapy for primary or secondary ACS. Recurrent ACS may occur in an open abdomen following initial successful surgical decompression even if a temporary closure device has been applied. Blood, ascites, or visceral edema (or any combination of the three) may increase the IAP and recreate the ACS. Similarly, external compression from an excessively tight binder can also elevate IAP.

More recently, *quaternary* ACS has been used to describe the compartment syndrome that can develop in patients undergoing elective complex abdominal wall reconstruction/hernia repair. This type of ACS is thought to be physiologically distinct from recurrent ACS in that it is not caused by the inflammation and endovascular dysfunction of a secondary insult.[7] Regardless of cause, ACS affects every organ system in a deleterious fashion.[1,3,9]

Risk factors for the development of ACS are detailed in Box 75.1. Importantly, IAH/ACS can occur in both medical and surgical patient populations.

DIAGNOSIS

Physical examination performs poorly as a diagnostic aid in IAH, with a sensitivity of 60%.[10]

Pressure-Volume Metrics

Pressure Volume metrics that aid in monitoring IAP include the following:
1. Bladder pressures: IAP can be estimated using an indwelling bladder catheter and the use of a protocolized transbladder technique such as that which has been approved by the WSACS. Problematic measurements may result when the patient is agitated, not supine, when the transducer is not zeroed at the mid-axillary line, or when measurements are not obtained at end-expiration. It is recommended that ICU patients are screened for IAH/ACS risk factors upon

TABLE 75.1 Intraabdominal Hypertension Grading Classification.

Grade	Intraabdominal Pressure (mm Hg)
I	12–15
II	16–20
III	21–25
IV	>25

From Harman PK, Kron IL, McLaachlan HD, et al. Elevated intraabdominal pressure and renal function. *Ann Surg.* 1982;196: 594-597.

BOX 75.1 Risk Factors for the Development of Abdominal Compartment Syndrome.

Acidosis (pH <7.2)
Hypothermia (core temperature <33°C)
Massive transfusion (>10 U of packed red blood cells) or resuscitation (>5L of colloid or crystalloid per 24 hour)
Coagulopathy (platelets <55,000 or activated partial thromboplastin greater than 2 times normal or international normalized ratio >1.5
Severe sepsis/septic shock (AECC definitions) regardless of source
Bacteremia
Intraabdominal infection and/or abscess
Hepatic dysfunction or cirrhosis with ascites
Mechanical ventilation
Elevated PEEP or the presence of auto-PEEP
Abdominal surgery (especially with tight fascial closures or massive incisional hernia repair)
Cardiac surgery
Disordered intestinal motility
Intestinal volvulus or intestinal obstruction (mechanical or functional)
Peritoneal or retroperitoneal space occupying lesions
Major burn injury
Major traumatic injury
Body mass index >30
Prone patient positioning
Acute pancreatitis
Damage control laparotomy
Laparoscopy with excessive inflation pressures
Peritoneal dialysis
Emergent aortic aneurysm repair
Obstetrical complications (e.g., preeclampsia, HELLP syndrome)

AECC, American-European Consensus Conference; *HELLP,* Hemolysis Elevated Liver enzymes, and Low Platelet count; *PEEP,* positive end-expiratory pressure. Data from The Abdominal Compartment Society (website). 2013. Available at www.wsacs.org. Accessed September 12, 2018; Malbrain MNG, Cheatham ML, Kirkpatrick A, et al. Results from the international conference of experts on intra-abdominal hypertension and abdominal compartment syndrome. *Intensive Care Med.* 2006; 32:1722-1732; Rogers WK, Garcia L. Intraabdominal hypertension, abdominal compartment syndrome, and the open abdomen. *Chest.* 2018; 153(1):238-250.

admission or with new or progressive organ failure. If two or more risk factors are present, a baseline IAP measurement should be obtained. If elevated, serial measurements should continue.[1, 2, 3]

2. Abdominal perfusion pressure (APP) is defined as mean arterial pressure (MAP) minus intraabdominal pressure (IAP) and has a normal value >50 mm Hg:

$$APP = MAP - IAP$$

Trending the APP may be a useful parameter to follow progression of IAH. However, the absolute number does not define ACS. At this time, the World Society of ACS recommends maintaining an APP above 50–60 mm Hg in patients with IAH/ACS.[1]

Adjunctive Measurements

1. Urine output may identify incipient acute kidney injury (AKI) secondary to rising IAP. Oliguria in this condition generally reflects renal vein hypertension rather than decreased arterial inflow. Nonetheless, this measure is problematic when there is AKI, chronic kidney disease (stage III or greater), and is without merit in those with anuria and dialysis dependence.[11]

2. Pulmonary pressures can be helpful in identifying dynamic changes in abdominal PV relationships. The pressure to be measured depends on the mode of mechanical ventilation. When on volume-cycled ventilation, increased abdominal pressure can manifest as an increase in peak airway (Paw_{peak}) and plateau ($Paw_{plateau}$) pressures from baseline. It is unclear what amount of change is significant, as the increase does not necessarily reflect worsening lung compliance. In contrast, when using pressure control ventilation, the tidal volume ($VT_{resultant}$) will be adversely affected. Escalating abdominal pressures will decrease the release volume ($VT_{release}$) on Airway Pressure Release Ventilation (APRV).[12]

SYSTEMIC IMPACT OF ACS

Increased IAP may lead to dysfunction of the respiratory, cardiovascular, renal, and gastrointestinal systems.[13] Elevated ICP and depressed cerebral perfusion pressure (CPP) also may result from increased IAP.[14]

Cardiovascular System

Increases in IAP elevate intravascular and intrapleural pressures. Flow per unit time and the stroke volume per cardiac cycle are typically reduced by elevated IAP, despite elevated intrathoracic pressures.[13–15]

Cardiac output (CO) decreases progressively as the IAP increases, principally as a result of decreased venous return, diminished pulmonary flow and subsequent impairment of left ventricular filling.[13] The magnitude of the decline in CO may depend on the patient's intravascular volume, as hypovolemia exacerbates the cardiovascular effects of IAH and ACS. One study demonstrated a 53% decrease in CO in hypovolemic animals subjected to increased IAP up to 30 mm Hg but only a 17% decrease when euvolemic.[16] Although intravenous volume expansion may enhance cardiac performance, it will not salvage kidneys already impacted by AKI.[17,18]

Respiratory System

Progressive increases in IAP displace the hemi-diaphragms cephalad, limiting alveolar gas filling and creating basilar and posterior alveolar collapse, leading to ventilation-perfusion mismatch. The decrease in pulmonary artery cross-sectional area may create a relative increase in pulmonary artery pressure against which the right ventricle must eject, leading to a decreased RV ejection fraction. This sequence can decrease net pulmonary flow, further exacerbating impaired oxygen loading and carbon dioxide offloading. Complicating these untoward effects is the decrease in venous return (VR) that is caused by progressive inferior vena cava (IVC) compression as IAP continues to rise.[19]

Common interim steps to offset this sequence include increasing positive end-expiratory pressure (PEEP), a maneuver that may further impede VR.[20–22] Plasma volume expansion may improve VR but may increase extravascular lung water due to the capillary leak that is associated with ACS and the underlying etiology for IAH. Increased extra-vascular lung water may further compromise gas exchange and reduces pulmonary compliance and elastance. It is clear that the management priority is to relieve the excessive IAH in order to restore homeostasis.

Renal System

In patients with normal renal function and IAH, oliguria (urine output <0.5 mL/kg per hour for 6 hours) is the most commonly identified initial abnormality.[23] While hypovolemic oliguria should respond to stressed volume expansion, in the presence of euvolemia the oliguria of IAH and ACS often does not, or does so only transiently. A number of factors may contribute to this abnormality. Decreased perfusion secondary to altered cardiac output may compromise renal blood flow and glomerular filtration rate.[24] At the same time, IVC and renal vein compression impair outflow. These derangements may both decrease glomerular filtration pressure and increase proximal tubular pressure (PTP). PTP elevation may be directly affected by IAP. The combination of abnormalities can compromise the renal filtration gradient and renal perfusion pressure.[25] While IAP and renal vein compression recreate the findings of ACS in a laboratory model, extrinsic renal parenchymal compression does not.

The second component of routine renal assessment is laboratory profiling, principally focused on blood urea nitrogen (BUN) and serum creatinine (SCr). Recent refinements in the clinical criteria characterize renal injury by stage.[26–28] Within the framework identified by RIFLE (Risk, Injury, Failure, Loss and End stage disease) criteria, these stages directly correlate with mortality.[29] Importantly, plasma volume expansion may not reverse AKI (as measured by elevations in SCr) even when titrated using invasive measures of cardiac performance. Models of abdominal decompression also fail to restore normal biochemistry once ACS has occurred

despite clearly restoring a normal IAP.[24,30] Therefore, timely management of IAH to mitigate progression to ACS and limit the extent of AKI is paramount.

Non-Renal Viscera

Clinically, progressive increases in IAP that lead to IAH/ACS are paralleled by changes in abdominal girth, abdominal distention, and splanchnic blood flow. Animal models indicate that, in addition to impairing organ perfusion, increases in IAP specifically decrease ileal and gastric mucosal blood flow.[31] Hepatic arterial, portal venous, and hepatic microcirculatory blood flow decrease as IAH progresses, effecting hepatic energy production and small bowel tissue oxygen delivery and utilization. This compromised gastrointestinal blood flow has been associated with immune activation and the initiation of a proinflammatory cascade.[32–37] Unrelieved IAH creates physiology similar to nonocclusive mesenteric ischemia and may lead to intestinal infarction and the need for intestinal resection.

Central Nervous System

Central nervous system dysfunction may occur relatively late in the course of IAH evolving into ACS. Animal studies indicate that elevated IAP leads to increased ICP and decreased CPP.[38–40] Two processes likely contribute to this observation. Decreased venous return and stroke volume/cardiac output reduce cerebral blood flow (CBF) and may provoke cerebral ischemia (<20 mL O_2/min per 100 gm tissue). In addition, IAP-induced elevation in central venous pressure impairs cerebral venous drainage, which may further elevate ICP. Indeed, abdominal decompression has been shown to reverse elevated ICP and augment CPP.[40] Given the frequent association of abdominal injury with traumatic brain injury (TBI), this relationship is clinically relevant as TBI perturbs normal CBF autoregulation. Accordingly, limited clinical experience suggests that abdominal decompression in the setting of intractable intracranial hypertension and IAH is advisable.[41,42]

Ocular System

The ACS has been associated with the rupture of retinal capillaries, resulting in the sudden onset of decreased central vision (Valsalva retinopathy). The mechanism behind this clinical entity is likely related to venous hypertension. Retinal hemorrhage usually resolves within days to months, and no specific treatment is necessary.[43] This diagnosis should be considered in any patient with ACS who develops visual changes.

MANAGEMENT APPROACHES

The primary therapy for IAH and ACS is reduction in IAP through both nonoperative and operative techniques, and early surgical consultation should be obtained. Although the strict definition of ACS requires an IAP >20 mm Hg, deleterious effects on end-organ perfusion have been reported at lower abdominal pressures. In a recent study that included 53 patients managed with an open abdomen approach for ACS, the median peak IAP was 25 mm Hg but with a range of 12–40 mm Hg.[44] In one medical ICU population over a 3 month period, 87 (58%) patients had ≥2 risk factors for IAH/ACS, and 59 (68%) developed IAH. Although none met strict ACS criteria, the presence of IAH was associated with longer ICU and hospital length of stays.[45] These findings are likely the result of abnormal and reduced APP in the context of non-ACS qualifying elevations in IAP. The fashion with which IAP reduction is achieved, therefore, depends on where a patient falls on the IAH-ACS spectrum, the presence of end-organ dysfunction, and the etiology of the increased IAP.

Interventions to alleviate IAH include positional changes (avoiding head of bed elevation >30 degrees), gastric and/or colonic decompression to evacuate intraluminal contents, and sedation/analgesia and temporary neuromuscular blockade to improve abdominal and/or thoracic wall compliance. Constricting abdominal dressings or binders should be loosened, burn eschar should be divided, and enteral nutrition should be provided with caution. Limiting excessive crystalloid resuscitation is recommended in order to avoid salt and water excess and promotion of ascites and visceral edema.[46] A neutral fluid balance should be maintained when feasible, although the role of albumin, hypertonic fluids, diuretics, and renal support techniques in managing extraluminal and intraperitoneal salt and water volume remain unclear.[1] Importantly, when the above measures fail to reverse clinically important IAH and/or the ACS has occurred, other approaches are warranted.

Secondary compartment syndrome from ascites may respond to ultrasound guided percutaneous drainage to alleviate IAH and prevent recurrence.[47–50] A recent nonrandomized study compared 31 cases of IAH/ACS managed with a 14FR pigtail catheter with 31 case controls: 81% (25 of 31) of the patients undergoing catheter drainage avoided laparotomy, and 58% survived to discharge. The authors noted that evacuation of 1000 mL of volume or a decrease in abdominal pressure by 9 mm Hg was a predictor of successful percutaneous management of IAH without need for laparotomy. Importantly, the control cohort was surgically decompressed when ACS developed, whereas the treatment group was often decompressed before the development of ACS. Six of 31 patients managed with percutaneous drainage developed a subsequent compartment syndrome and required laparotomy.[49] Catheter based management is not recommended for management of visceral edema, retroperitoneal hematoma or intraperitoneal hemorrhage.[1]

The gold standard for the management of IAH that progresses to ACS is decompressive laparotomy. In fact, increasing mortality has been associated with longer interval times to decompression.[44] While traditionally performed in the OR, a decompressive laparotomy may be safely undertaken in the ICU with minimal OR resources aside from equipment. Management with advanced ventilation appears to drive the need to operate in the ICU just as strongly as does hemodynamic instability that precludes safe and/or timely transport.[51] Repeat laparotomy, lavage, and temporary closure may also be safely achieved in the ICU setting.[52]

The initial unpacking of a patient who has undergone a damage control procedure is best undertaken in the OR, but immediate relief of ACS due to a temporary closure that has become too tight should be performed in the ICU without delay. Because APP may be reduced prior to development of true ACS, there may be a role for laparotomy outside of the traditional criteria, especially when there is concomitant evidence of incipient or progressive organ dysfunction.[53] Such decisions are ideally made during early consultation with a surgeon for at-risk patients.

Abdominal decompression can be associated with precipitous hemodynamic changes. Heart rate often falls, MAP rises, pulse pressure widens, and peak/mean/plateau pressures fall with a rise in SaO_2. Alveolar recruitment occurs more readily, as the diaphragms are no longer displaced cephalad. The use of APRV and pressure-based ventilation may result in substantial pulmonary distension, as larger volumes of gas are delivered into increasingly compliant lungs prior to reaching the pressure threshold for flow termination.

On occasion, abdominal decompression may trigger unanticipated abrupt or worsened hypotension. Two possible etiologies have been proposed for this phenomenon, including: (1) an acute dilatation of the precapillary arteriolar sphincters[54] and (2) reperfusion injury mediated by vasoactive byproducts including a large metabolic acid load.[55]

Vacuum-based devices are currently recommended for the management of the open abdomen due to their ease of placement, capacity for fluid management, and ability to thoroughly separate viscera from the posterior aspect of the anterior abdominal wall; accordingly, many temporary closure systems are available.[56,57] A systematic review regarding closure of the open abdomen surmised that negative pressure wound vacuum therapy may result in improved facial closure rates and may be associated with improved outcomes over alternative abdominal closure techniques. However, the study acknowledged a lack of prospective data, with only two randomized controlled studies largely forming the basis of this conclusion.[57]

Regardless of the technique selected, management priorities remain the same. The ability to easily gain access to the abdominal cavity for planned or unplanned reoperations is crucial. The abdominal viscera must be protected from the exterior environment and from evaporative losses. Aspirated fluid across the open abdomen contains roughly 2 grams of protein per liter removed, and this should be anticipated and addressed in the nutritional prescription.[58]

Finally, timing of definitive abdominal closure after abdominal decompression remains controversial. The open abdomen is associated with significant morbidity. Loss of abdominal domain and lateralization of the abdominal fascia may lead to large soft tissue deficits. Indeed, management with an open abdomen approach that leads to a giant ventral hernia is strongly associated with a reduced quality of life for up to 5 years after the index laparotomy.[59] Enterocutaneous or enteroatmospheric fistula are estimated to occur in 20% of patients managed with an open abdomen and are associated with large bowel resections, large volume fluid resuscitations, and increasing number of abdominal reexplorations.[60–62]

Evidence suggests that complication risk, principally entero-atmospheric fistulization, increases if primary closure is delayed beyond 8 days following the initial decompression. Direct peritoneal resuscitation, a technique whereby a glucose-rich peritoneal dialysis solution is continuously instilled into the open abdomen, has been shown to decrease time to and success of primary closure as well as intraabdominal (i.e., abscess) complications.[63]

The World Society of the Abdominal Compartment Syndrome has endorsed protocolized efforts to obtain an early or at least same-hospital-stay abdominal fascial closure through reductions in variations in care.[1] However, the best method of definitive closure remains controversial. Primary fascial closure is associated with a 30% rate of hernia formation and is not always possible, whereas the use of biologic mesh closure is associated with hernia rates of 80%.[64–66] When necessary, hernia repair is delayed at least 6–12 months after the index operation.[65,67,68]

For the intensivist managing patients with an open abdomen, there is some evidence to suggest that brief use of neuromuscular blockade and 3% hypertonic saline fluid administration may facilitate early primary fascial closure, although these approaches are not standard of care, nor standard practice.[69,70] Interestingly, and in contradistinction to prior conventional wisdom, recent evidence supports that some patients with an open abdomen do not require mechanical ventilation and can be safely extubated postoperatively if hemodynamics and respiratory status permit.[71] In this situation it is imperative to maintain excellent negative pressure spanning the fascial gap to provide some abdominal wall support during negative pressure ventilation.

AUTHORS' RECOMMENDATIONS

- Early recognition and treatment are of prime importance when managing patients with IAH and ACS.
- Plasma volume expansion and relief of IAH or ACS may not reverse the untoward impact on end-organ function, especially within the renal system.
- ACS deleteriously impacts both blood flow and oxygen delivery in every organ system.
- Early intervention to manage IAH may retard progression to ACS and should be undertaken in a tiered fashion.
- It is important to measure bladder pressure in the correct fashion. Instilling too much irrigant may cause falsely elevated IAP readings and lead to overly aggressive treatment.
- ACS may occur even after decompressive laparotomy has been performed, requiring loosening of the temporary abdominal dressings or unplanned laparotomy for management.

REFERENCES

1. Kirkpatrick AW, Roberts DJ, De Waele J, et al. Intra-abdominal hypertension and the abdominal compartment syndrome: updated consensus definitions and clinical practice guidelines from the World Society of Abdominal Compartment Syndrome. *Intensive Care Med.* 2013;39:1190-1206.
2. WSACS. The Abdominal Compartment Society. 2013. Available at: https://www.wsacs.org. Accessed September 12, 2018.
3. Malbrain ML, Cheatham ML, Kirkpatrick A, et al. Results from the international conference of experts on intra-abdominal hypertension and abdominal compartment syndrome. *Intensive Care Med.* 2006;32:1722-1732.
4. Rogers WK, Garcia L. Intraabdominal hypertension, abdominal compartment syndrome, and the open abdomen. *Chest.* 2018;153(1):238-250.
5. Strang SG, Van Lieshout EMM, Verhoeven RA, et al. Recognition and management of intra-abdominal hypertension and abdominal compartment syndrome; a survey amount Dutch surgeons. *Eur J Trauma Emerg Surg.* 2017;43(1):85-98.
6. Hunt L, Frost SA, Newton PJ, Salamonson Y, Davidson PM. A survey of critical care nurses' knowledge of intra-abdominal hypertension and abdominal compartment syndrome. *Aust Crit Care.* 2017;30(1):21-27.
7. Kirkpatrick AW, Nickerson D, Roberts DJ, et al. Intra-abdominal hypertension and abdominal compartment syndrome after abdominal wall reconstruction: quaternary syndromes? *Scan J Surg.* 2017;106(2):97-106.
8. Wilson A, Longhi J, Goldman C, Mcnatt S. Intra-abdominal pressure and the morbidly obese patient: the effect of body mass index. *J Trauma.* 2010;69(1):78-83.
9. Gracias VH, Braslow B, Johnson J, et al. Abdominal compartment syndrome in the open abdomen. *Arch Surg.* 2002;137:1298-1300.
10. Sugrue M, Bauman A, Jones F, et al. Clinical examination is an inaccurate predictor of intraabdominal pressure. *World J Surg.* 2002;26:1428-1431.
11. Mohmand H, Goldfarb S. Renal dysfunction associated with intra-abdominal hypertension and the abdominal compartment syndrome. *J Am Soc Nephrol.* 2011;22(4):615-621.
12. Pelosi P, Quintel M, Malbrain ML. Effect of intra-abdominal pressure on respiratory mechanics. *Acta Clin Belg.* 2007;62(Suppl 1):78-88.
13. Schein M, Wittmann DH, Aprahamian CC, Condon RE. The abdominal compartment syndrome: The physiological and clinical consequences of elevated intra-abdominal pressure. *J Am Coll Surg.* 1995;180:745-753.
14. Cheatham ML. Abdominal compartment syndrome: pathophysiology and definitions. *Scand J Trauma Resusc Emerg Med.* 2009;17:10.
15. Cheatham M, Malbrain M. Abdominal perfusion pressure. In: Ivatury R, Cheatham M, Malbrain M, Sugrue M, eds. *Abdominal Compartment Syndrome.* Georgetown, TX: Landes Bioscience; 2006:69-81.
16. Wauters J, Claus P, Brosens N, et al. Relationship between abdominal pressure, pulmonary compliance, and cardiac preload in a porcine model. *Crit Care Res Pract.* 2012;2012:1-6.
17. Ridings PC, Bloomfield GL, Blocher CR, Sugerman HJ. Cardiopulmonary effects of raised intra-abdominal pressure before and after intravascular volume expansion. *J Trauma.* 1995;39:1071-1075.
18. Kashtan J, Green JF, Parsons EQ, Holcroft JW. Hemodynamic effects of increased abdominal pressure. *J Surg Res.* 1981;30:249-255.
19. Wittmann D. The compartment syndrome of the abdominal cavity. *J Intensive Care Med.* 2000;15:201-220.
20. Burchard KW, Ciombor DM, McLeod MK, Slothman GJ, Gann DS. Positive end expiratory pressure with increased intra-abdominal pressure. *Surg Gynecol Obstet.* 1985;161:313-318.

21. Regli A, Mahendran R, Fysh ET, et al. Matching positive end-expiratory pressure to intra-abdominal pressure improves oxygenation in a porcine sick lung model of intra-abdominal hypertension. *Crit Care*. 2012;16(5):R208.

22. Krebs J, Pelosi P, Tsagogiorgas C, Alb M, Luecke T. Effects of positive end-expiratory pressure on respiratory function and hemodynamics in patients with acute respiratory failure with and without intra-abdominal hypertension: a pilot study. *Crit Care*. 2009;13(5):R160.

23. Dennen P, Douglas IS, Anderson R. Acute kidney injury in the intensive care unit: an update and primer for the intensivist. *Crit Care Med*. 2010;38(1):261-275.

24. Doty JM, Saggi BH, Blocher CR, et al. Effects of increased renal parenchymal pressure on renal function. *J Trauma*. 2000;48(5):874-877.

25. De Waele JJ, De Laet I. Intra-abdominal hypertension and the effect on renal function. *Acta Clin Belg*. 2007;62(Suppl 2):371-374.

26. Bellomo R, Ronco C, Kellum JA, Mehta RL, Palevsky P. Acute renal failure - definition, outcome measures, animal models, fluid therapy and information technology needs: the Second International Consensus Conference of the Acute Dialysis Quality Initiative (ADQI) Group. *Crit Care*. 2004;8(4):R204.

27. Mehta RL, Kellum JA, Shah SV, et al. Acute Kidney Injury Network: Report of an initiative to improve outcomes in acute kidney injury. *Crit Care*. 2007;11(2):R31.

28. Kidney Disease: Improving Global Outcomes (KDIGO) Acute Kidney Injury Work Group. KDIGO clinical practice guideline for acute kidney injury. *Kidney Int Suppl*. 2009;(113):S1-S130.

29. Uchino S, Bellomo R, Goldsmith D, Bates S, Ronco C. An assessment of the RIFLE criteria for acute renal failure in hospitalized patients. *Crit Care Med*. 2006;34:1913-1917.

30. Mohmand H, Goldfarb S. Renal dysfunction associated with intra-abdominal hypertension and the abdominal compartment syndrome. *J Am Soc Nephrol*. 2011;22(4):615-621.

31. Diebel LN, Dulchavsky SA, Wilson RF. Effect of increased intra-abdominal pressure on mesenteric arterial and intestinal mucosal blood flow. *J Trauma*. 1992;33:45-49.

32. Caldwell CB, Ricotta JJ. Changes in visceral blood flow with elevated intraabdominal pressure. *J Surg Res*. 1987;43:14-20.

33. Diebel LN, Dulchavsky SA, Brown WJ. Splanchnic ischemia and bacterial translocation in the abdominal compartment syndrome. *J Trauma*. 1996;40:78.

34. Nakatani T, Sakamoto Y, Kaneko I, Ando H, Kobayashi K. Effects of intraabdominal hypertension on hepatic energy metabolism in a rabbit model. *J Trauma*. 1998;44(3):446-453.

35. Pusajó JF, Bumaschny E, Agurrola A, et al. Postoperative intra-abdominal pressure: Its relation to splanchnic perfusion, sepsis, multiple organ failure and surgical reintervention. *Intensive Crit Care Dig*. 1994;13:2-4.

36. Bongard F, Pianim N, Dubecz S, et al. Adverse consequences of increased intraabdominal pressure on bowel tissue oxygen. *J Trauma*. 1995;39:519-525.

37. Eleftheriadis E, Kotzampassi K, Papanotas K, Heliadis N, Sarris K. Gut ischemia, oxidative stress, and bacterial translocation in elevated abdominal pressure in rats. *World J Surg*. 1996;20:11-16.

38. Bloomfield GL, Ridings PC, Blocher CR, et al. Increased pleural pressure mediates the effects of elevated intra-abdominal pressure upon the central nervous and cardiovascular systems. *Surg Forum*. 1995;46:572-574.

39. Bloomfield GL, Ridings PC, Blocher CR, Marmarou A, Sugerman HJ. Effects of increased intra-abdominal pressure upon intracranial and cerebral perfusion pressure before and after volume expansion. *J Trauma*. 1996;40:936-943.

40. Bloomfield GL, Ridings PC, Blocher CR, Marmarou A, Sugerman HJ. A proposed relationship between increased intra-abdominal, intrathoracic, and intracranial pressure. *Crit Care Med*. 1997; 25:496-503.

41. Joseph DK, Dutton RP, Arabi B, Scalea TM. Decompressive laparotomy to treat intractable intracranial hypertension after traumatic brain injury. *J Trauma*. 2004;57(4):687-693.

42. Dorfman JD, Burns JD, Green DM, DeFusco C, Agarwal S. Decompressive laparotomy for refractory intracranial hypertension after traumatic brain injury. *Neurocrit Care*. 2011;15(3):516-518.

43. Priluck IA, Blodgett DW. The effects of increased intra-abdominal pressure on the eyes. *Nebr Med J*. 1996;81:8-9.

44. Seternes A, Rekstad LC, Mo S, et al. Open abdomen treated with negative pressure wound therapy: indications, management, and survival. *World J Surg*. 2017;41(1):152-161.

45. Santa-Teresa P, Muñoz J, Montero I, et al. Incidence and prognosis of intra-abdominal hypertension in critically ill medical patients: a prospective epidemiological study. *Ann Intensive Care*. 2012;2(Suppl 1):S3.

46. Joseph B, Zangbar B, Pandit V, et al. The conjoint effect of reduced crystalloid administration and decreased damage control laparotomy use in the development of abdominal compartment syndrome. *J Trauma*. 2014;76(2):457-461.

47. Reed SF, Britt RC, Collins J, Weireter L, Cole F, Britt LD. Aggressive surveillance and early catheter-directed therapy in the management of intra-abdominal hypertension. *J Trauma*. 2006;61:1359-1365.

48. Radenkovic DV, Bajec D, Ivancevic N, et al. Decompressive laparotomy with temporary abdominal closure versus percutaneous puncture with placement of abdominal catheter in patients with abdominal compartment syndrome during acute pancreatitis: background and design of multicenter, randomized, controlled study. *BMC Surg*. 2010;10:22.

49. Cheatham ML, Safcsak K. Percutaneous catheter decompression in the treatment of elevated intraabdominal pressure. *Chest*. 2011;140:1428-1435.

50. Latenser BA, Kowal-Vern A, Kimball D, Chakrin A, Dujovny N. A pilot study comparing percutaneous decompression with decompressive laparotomy for acute abdominal compartment syndrome in thermal injury. *J Burn Care Rehabil*. 2002;23:190-195.

51. Piper G, Maerz LL, Schuster KM, et al. When the ICU is the operating room. *J Trauma Acute Care Surg*. 2013;74(3):871-875.

52. Diaz JJ, Mejia V, Subhawong AP, et al. Protocol for bedside laparotomy in trauma and emergency general surgery: a low return to the operating room. *Am Surg*. 2005;71(11):986-991.

53. Sugrue M. Abdominal compartment syndrome and the open abdomen: any unresolved issues? *Curr Opin Crit Care*. 2017; 23(1):73-78.

54. Shelly MP, Robinson AA, Hesford JW, Park GR. Haemodynamic effects following surgical release of increased intra-abdominal pressure. *Br J Anaesth*. 1987;59:800-805.

55. Morris Jr JA, Eddy VA, Blinman TA, Rutherford EJ, Sharp KW. The staged celiotomy for trauma: Issues in unpacking and reconstruction. *Ann Surg*. 1993;217:576-586.

56. Perez D, Wildi S, Demartines N, Bramkamp M, Koehler C, Clavien PA. Prospective evaluation of vacuum-assisted closure in abdominal compartment syndrome and severe abdominal sepsis. *J Am Coll Surg*. 2007;205:586-592.

57. Roberts DJ, Zygun DA, Grendar J, et al. Negative-pressure wound therapy for critically ill adults with open abdominal

wounds: a systematic review. *J Trauma Acute Care Surg.* 2012; 73(3):629-639.

58. Cheatham ML, Safcsak K, Brzezinski SJ, Lube MW. Nitrogen balance, protein loss, and the open abdomen. *Crit Care Med.* 2007;35:127.

59. Zarzaur BL, DiCocco JM, Fabian TC. Quality of life after abdominal reconstruction following open abdomen. *J Trauma.* 2011;285-291.

60. Miller RS, Morris Jr JA, Diaz Jr JJ, Herring MB, May AK. Complications after 344 damage-control open celiotomies. *J Trauma.* 2005;59(6):1365.

61. Rao M, Burke D, Finan P J, Sagar PM. The use of vacuum-assisted closure of abdominal wounds: a word of caution. *Colorectal Dis.* 2007;9(3):266-268.

62. Bradley MJ, DuBose JJ, Scalea TM, et al. Independent predictors of enteric fistula and abdominal sepsis after damage control surgery. *JAMA Surg.* 2013;148(10):947-954.

63. Smith JW, Matheson PJ, Franklin GA, Harbrecht BG, Richardson JD, Garrison RN. Randomized controlled trial evaluating the efficacy of peritoneal resuscitation in the management of trauma patients undergoing damage control surgery. *J Am Coll Surg.* 224(4):396-404.

64. DiCocco JM, Magnotti LJ, Emmett KP, et al. Long-term follow-up of abdominal wall reconstruction after planned ventral hernia: a 15-year experience. *J Am Coll Surg.* 2010;210(5):686-695, 695-698.

65. Diaz Jr JJ, Guy J, Berkes MB, Guillamondegui O, Miller RS. Acellular dermal allograft for ventral hernia repair in the compromised surgical field. *Am Surg.* 2006;72(12):1181-1187; discussion 1187-1188.

66. Jin J, Rosen MJ, Blatnik J, et al. Use of acellular dermal matrix for complicated ventral hernia repair: does technique affect outcomes? *J Am Coll Surg.* 2007;205(5):654-660.

67. Jernigan TW, Fabian TC, Croce MA, et al. Staged management of giant abdominal wall defects: acute and long-term results. *Ann Surg.* 2003;238(3):349-355; discussion 355-357.

68. Diaz Jr JJ, Dutton WD, Ott MM, et al. Eastern Association for the Surgery of Trauma: a review of the management of the open abdomen—part 2 "Management of the open abdomen". *J Trauma.* 2011;71(2):502-512.

69. Abouassaly CT, Dutton WD, Zaydfudim V, et al. Postoperative neuromuscular blocker use is associated with higher primary fascial closure rates after damage control laparotomy. *J Trauma.* 2010;69(3):557-561.

70. Harvin JA, Mims MM, Duchesne JC, et al. Chasing 100%: the use of hypertonic saline to improve early primary fascial closure after damage control laparotomy. *J Trauma Acute Care Surg.* 2013;74(2):426-432.

71. Sujka JA, Safcsak K, Cheatham ML, Ibrahim JA. Trauma patients with an open abdomen following damage control laparotomy can be extubated prior to abdominal closure. *World J Surg.* 2018; 42(10):3210-3214.

76

How Should Patients With Burns Be Managed in the Intensive Care Unit?

Marc G. Jeschke

More than 500,000 burn injuries occur annually in the United States.[1] Although most are minor, approximately 40,000–60,000 burn patients require admission to a hospital or major burn center for appropriate treatment.[2] The devastating consequences of burns have resulted in the allocation of significant clinical and research resources. Indeed, preventive strategies and improved care have resulted in a 50% decline in burn-related deaths and hospital admissions in the United States during the past 20 years.[3,4] Advances in therapy strategies, based on implementation of critical care bundles, improved understanding of resuscitation, enhanced wound coverage, better support of the hypermetabolic response to injury, more appropriate infection control, and better treatment of inhalation injury have improved the clinical outcome of this unique patient population. It is important to recognize that successful management of burn patients requires a diversified and multidisciplinary approach. This chapter gives an overview of the evidence-based management of severely burned patients in the intensive care unit (ICU).

INITIAL ASSESSMENT AND EMERGENCY TREATMENT

All burned patients should initially be managed as trauma patients, following the guidelines of the American College of Surgeons Committee on Trauma and the Advanced Trauma Live Support Center.[5] The algorithms for trauma evaluation should be diligently applied to the burn patient. In particular, any wheezing, stridor, hoarseness, or tachypnea may be a sign of airway compromise. Tracheal tugging, carbonaceous sputum, soot around the patient's airway passages, and singed facial or nasal hair may suggest an airway burn or smoke inhalation. As in any trauma patient, progression to the next step in the primary survey is delayed until a proper airway is established and maintained.

Cardiac performance may be difficult to evaluate in the burn victim. In particular, burned extremities may impede the ability to obtain a blood pressure reading. In these situations, arterial lines, particularly femoral lines, are useful to monitor continuous blood pressure readings. Use of a pulmonary artery catheter (PAC) may be beneficial in the assessment of cardiovascular performance in certain situations

(e.g., inadequate noninvasive monitoring, difficult-to-define end points of resuscitation),[6] but the general practicability, risk-to-benefit ratio, and lack of mortality reduction when the PAC is used have been widely criticized. Currently, there are no studies in burn patients that provide evidence-based recommendations. Because of the disadvantages of PAC use, less-invasive techniques have been developed.[7] None of these, however, is of specific value in burn patients. Several descriptive studies using PiCCO technology, in which cardiac performance is approximated with an arterial thermodilution catheter, have been conducted in burn patients.[8,9] Prospective trials are underway.

FLUID RESUSCITATION

Severe burns cause significant hemodynamic changes. These must be managed carefully to optimize intravascular volume, maintain end-organ tissue perfusion, and maximize oxygen delivery to the tissues.[10] Massive fluid shifts after severe burn injury result in the sequestration of fluid in burned and unburned tissue.[11] The result of this generalized edema may be burn shock, a leading cause of mortality in severely burned patients.[12–14] Therefore, early and accurate fluid resuscitation of patients with major burns is critical.[15] Calculations of fluid requirements are based on the amount of body surface involved in second- or third-degree (but not first-degree) burns. The "rule of nines" (Fig. 76.1A) has been used to estimate the area of burned body surface, but this rule has limitations, particularly in children, in whom the head accounts for a disproportionate fraction of body mass. In these cases, a more accurate assessment can be made by using the Lund and Browder chart, which takes into account changes associated with growth (Fig. 76.1B). Various resuscitation formulas have been used. These differ in the amount of crystalloid and colloid to be given and in fluid tonicity (Table 76.1).[10,16] The modified Brooke and Parkland (Baxter) formulas are most commonly used for early resuscitation,[17] but no formula will accurately predict the volume requirements of an individual patient. Recently, the American Burn Association recommended that the initial volume of resuscitative fluid be decreased from 4 to 2 cc/kg/% burn. It is currently not known whether decreased fluids are associated with improved outcomes. A recent study showed that resuscitation

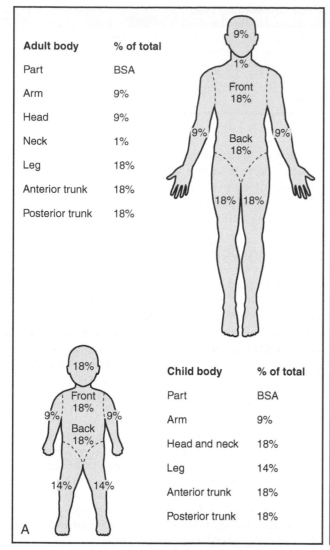

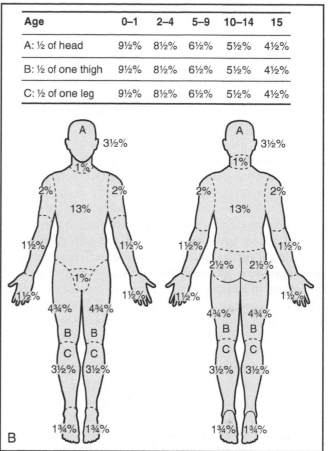

Fig. 76.1 (A) Estimation of burn size with the "rule of nines." (B) Estimation of burn size with the Lund and Browder method. *BSA,* body surface area.

Age	0–1	2–4	5–9	10–14	15
A: ½ of head	9½%	8½%	6½%	5½%	4½%
B: ½ of one thigh	9½%	8½%	6½%	5½%	4½%
C: ½ of one leg	9½%	8½%	6½%	5½%	4½%

Adult body — **% of total**

Part	BSA
Arm	9%
Head	9%
Neck	1%
Leg	18%
Anterior trunk	18%
Posterior trunk	18%

Child body — **% of total**

Part	BSA
Arm	9%
Head and neck	18%
Leg	14%
Anterior trunk	18%
Posterior trunk	18%

TABLE 76.1 Formulas for Estimating Adult Burn Patient Resuscitation Fluid Needs.

Colloid Formula	Electrolyte	Colloid
Evans	Normal saline, 1.0 mL/kg/% burn	1.0 cc/kg/% burn
Brooke	Lactated Ringer solution, 1.5 mL/kg/% burn	0.5 mL/kg
Slater	Lactated Ringer solution, 2 L/24 h	Fresh-frozen plasma, 75 mL/kg/24 h
Crystalloid formulas		
Parkland	Lactated Ringer solution	4 mL/kg/% burn
Modified	Lactated Ringer solution	2 mL/kg/% burn
Hypertonic saline solutions		
Monafo	Volume to maintain urine output at 30 mL/h; fluid contains 250 mEq Na/L.	
Warden	Lactated Ringer solution +50 mEq $NaHCO_3$ (180 mEq Na/L) for 8 hours to maintain urine output at 30-50 mL/h. Lactated Ringer solution to maintain urine output at 30-50 mL/h beginning 8 hours postburn.	
Dextran formula (Demling)	Dextran 40 in saline, 2 mL/kg for 8 hours. Lactated Ringer solution, volume to maintain urine output at 30 mL/h. Fresh-frozen plasma, 0.5 mL/kg/h for 18 hours beginning 8 hours postburn.	

Na, sodium; *$NaHCO_3$,* sodium bicarbonate.
From Warden GD. Burn shock resuscitation. *World J Surg.* 1992;16(1):16-23.

TABLE 76.2   Formulas for Estimating Pediatric Resuscitation Needs.

Cincinnati Shriners Burns Hospital	$4\ mL \times kg \times \%$ total BSA burn + 1500 mL $\times\ m^2$ BSA	1st 8 hours 2nd 8 hours 3rd 8 hours	Lactated Ringer's solution + 50 mg $NaHCO_3$ Lactated Ringer's solution Lactated Ringer's solution + 12.5 g albumin
Galveston Shriners Burns Hospital	$5000\ mL/m^2$ BSA burn + $2000\ mL/m^2$ BSA	Lactated Ringer's solution + 12.5 g albumin	

BSA, body surface area; *NaHCO₃,* sodium bicarbonate.

under 4 cc/kg per %burn was associated with a significantly greater incidence of renal failure and did not improve outcome.[18]

In children, maintenance requirements must be added to the resuscitation formula. The Galveston and Cincinnati Shriners Burns Hospitals have devised useful formulas (Table 76.2). Intravascular volume status must be reevaluated frequently during the acute phase. Fluid balance during burn shock resuscitation is typically measured by hourly urine output through an indwelling urethral catheter. It has been recommended that urine output be maintained at approximately 0.5 mL/kg per hour in adults[19] and 0.5–1.0 mL/kg per hour in patients weighing less than 30 kg.[20] However, no clinical studies have identified the hourly urine output that is truly required to maintain vital organ perfusion during burn shock resuscitation. Because large volumes of fluid and electrolytes are administered initially and throughout the course of resuscitation, it is important to obtain baseline laboratory measurements.[21] Crystalloid, in particular lactated Ringer's solution, is the most popular resuscitation fluid currently in use for burn patients.[22] Other crystalloid solutions and colloids have been used. Despite extensive study no outcome differences between the two have been identified.[23–26] Proponents of crystalloid solutions alone report that colloids offer no added value and are more expensive.[27] Nonetheless, most burn surgeons agree that patients with low serum albumin during burn shock may benefit from albumin supplementation to maintain oncotic pressure.[28]

INHALATION INJURY

Inhalation injury is one of the most critical problems accompanying thermal insult, with mortality paralleling that for acute respiratory distress syndrome in patients requiring ventilator support for more than 1 week.[29,30] Early diagnosis of bronchopulmonary injury is initiated by a history of closed-space exposure; facial burns; or carbonaceous debris in the mouth, pharynx, or sputum.[31] There are few evidence-based data regarding inhalation injury. Therefore the standard diagnostic method is bronchoscopy. Endorf and Gamelli established a grading system for inhalation injury (0, 1, 2, 3, and 4) derived from findings at initial bronchoscopy and based on Abbreviated Injury Score criteria.[32] Bronchoscopic criteria that are consistent with inhalation injury included airway edema, inflammation, mucosal necrosis, presence of soot and charring in the airway, tissue sloughing, or carbonaceous material in the airway. At this time, however, there are neither uniform diagnosis criteria nor standardized treatment

guidelines. Management of inhalation injury consists of ventilatory support, aggressive pulmonary toilet, bronchoscopic removal of casts, and nebulization therapy.[10] The American Burn Association guidelines do not recommend the use of prophylactic antibiotics.

INFECTION/SEPSIS

Severely burned patients are susceptible to various infectious complications.[33] Because burns induce a systemic inflammatory response,[34] specific guidelines for the diagnosis and treatment of wound infection and sepsis in burns have been formulated (Box 76.1). That said, the burn community realized that sepsis is very complex, and while an ideal definition of sepsis does not currently exist, studies are ongoing to develop a burn-specific definition of sepsis.

BOX 76.1   Definition of Burn Sepsis.

American Burn Association Consensus Definition on Burn Sepsis

- At least 3 of the following parameters:
- T $>38.5°$ C or $<36.5°$ C
- Progressive tachycardia >90 beats/min in adults or >2 SD above age-specific norms in children
- Progressive tachypnea >30 breaths/min in adults or >2 SD above age-specific norms in children
- WBC $>12,000$ or <4000 in adults or >2 SD above age-specific norms in children
- Refractory hypotension: SBP <90 mm Hg, MAP <70, or an SBP decrease >40 mm Hg in adults or <2 SD below normal for age in children
- Thrombocytopenia: Platelet count $<100,000/\mu L$ in adults, <2 SD below norms in children
- Hyperglycemia: Plasma glucose >110 mg/dL or 7.7 mM/L in the absence of diabetes
- Enteral feeding intolerance (residual >150 mL/h in children or 2 times feeding rate in adults; diarrhea >2500 mL/day for adults or >400 mL/day in children)
  and
  Pathologic tissue source identified: >105 bacteria on quantitative wound tissue biopsy or microbial invasion on biopsy
  Bacteremia or fungemia
  Documented infection as defined by Centers for Disease Control.

MAP, mean arterial pressure; *SBP,* systolic blood pressure; *SD,* standard deviation; *T,* temperature; *WBC,* white blood cell count. From Greenhalgh DG, Saffle JR, Holmes JH, et al. American Burn Association consensus conference to define sepsis and infection in burns. *J Burn Care Res.* 2007; 28:776-790.

BURN WOUND EXCISION

Methods for handling burn wounds have changed in recent decades. Increasingly, aggressive early tangential excision of the burn tissue and early wound closure primarily by skin grafts have led to significant improvement in survival and have substantially lowered costs in this patient population.[10,35–38] Early wound closure also has been associated with decreased severity of hypertrophic scarring, joint contractures and stiffness, and with quicker rehabilitation.[10,35] Techniques of burn wound excision have evolved substantially over the past decade. Published estimates of bleeding associated with these operations range between 3.5% and 5% of the blood volume for every 1% of the body surface excised.[39,40] Burn wound excision should occur in the operating room soon after the patient is admitted; however, sometimes excision in the ICU may be necessary.

METABOLIC RESPONSE AND NUTRITIONAL SUPPORT

The metabolic consequences of severe burn injury are profound, and their modulation constitutes an ongoing challenge. Metabolic rates of burn victims exceed those of most other critically ill patients and cause marked wasting of lean body mass within days of injury.[41] Failure to meet the subsequent energy and protein requirements may result in impaired wound healing, organ dysfunction, increased susceptibility to infection, and death.[42] Thus, adequate nutrition is imperative. Because of the significant increase in postburn energy expenditure, high-calorie nutritional support was thought to decrease muscle metabolism,[43] but a randomized, double-blind, prospective study found that aggressive high-calorie feeding with a combination of enteral and parenteral nutrition was associated with increased mortality.[44] Therefore most investigators recommend adequate calorie intake through early enteral feeding and avoidance of overfeeding.[10,41] Different formulas have been developed to address the specific energy requirements of burned adult and pediatric patients[45–47] (Tables 76.3 and 76.4). The caloric requirements in adult burn patients most often are calculated using the Curreri formula. This calls for 25 kcal/kg per day plus 40 kcal/%BSAB (percentage of total body surface area burned) per day.[48] Recommendations suggest administration

of 1 to 2 g/kg per day of protein.[42] Because of glucose intolerance and futile cycling in critical illness, most ICUs provide a significant amount of caloric requirements as fat.[42,49] However, burn patients exhibit lipid intolerance that may result in hyperlipidemia and fatty liver infiltration. These complications are associated with a higher incidence of infection and higher postoperative mortality rates.[50–53] Thus the extent to

TABLE 76.4 Formulas for Estimating Caloric Requirements in Pediatric Burn Patients.

Formula	Sex/Age	Equation (Daily Requirement in kcal)
WHO[89]	Males	
	0–3 years	$(60.9 \times W) - 54$
	3–10 years	$(22.7 \times W) + 495$
	10–18 years	$(17.5 \times W) + 651$
	Females	
	0–3 years	$(61.0 \times W) - 51$
	3–10 years	$(22.5 \times W) + 499$
	10–18 years	$(12.2 \times W) + 746$
RDA[90]	0–6 months	$108 \times W$
	6 months to 1 year	$98 \times W$
	1–3 years	$102 \times W$
	4–10 years	$90 \times W$
	11–14 years	$55 \times W$
Curreri junior[91]	<1 year	RDA + (15 × %BSAB)
	1–3 years	RDA + (25 × %BSAB)
	4–15 years	RDA + (40 × %BSAB)
Galveston infant[92]	0–1 years	2100 kcal/m² BSA + 1000 kcal/m² BSAB
Galveston revised[47]	1–11 years	1800 kcal/m² BSA + 1300 kcal/m² BSAB
Galveston adolescent[93]	12+	1500 kcal/m² BSA + 1500 kcal/m² BSAB

BSA, body surface area; BSAB, body surface area burned; %BSAB, percentage of total body surface area burned; RDA, Recommended Dietary Allowance (US); W, weight (kg); WHO, World Health Organization.

TABLE 76.3 Formulas for Estimating Caloric Requirements in Adult Burn Patients.

Formula	Age/Sex	Equation
Harris-Benedict[88]	Men	BEE (kcal/day) = 66.5 + (13.75 × W) + (5.03 × H) − (6.76 × A)
	Women	BEE (kcal/day) = 655 + (9.56 × W) + (1.85 × H) − (4.68 × A)
Comment: Multiply BEE by stress factor of 1.2–2.0 (1.2–1.5 sufficient for most burns) to estimate caloric requirement.		
Curreri[45]	Age: 16–59 years	Calories (kcal/day) = (25 × W) + (40 × %BSAB)
	Age: >60 years	Calories = (20 × W) + (65 × %BSAB)
Comment: Specific for burns, may significantly overestimate energy requirements, maximum 50% BSAB.		

A, age (year); BEE, basal energy expenditure; %BSAB, percentage of total body surface area burned; H, height (cm); W, weight (kg).

which exogenous lipid can be used as an energy source is limited.[49,54,55] Studies in a large cohort of severely burned children demonstrated that patients receiving a low-fat, high-carbohydrate diet had a significantly lower incidence of fatty liver on autopsy. Relative to historic controls, these patients had a significantly lower incidence of sepsis, prolonged survival, and significantly shorter stays in the ICU (grade C data). On the basis of these findings, nutritional regimens for treatment of burn patients which include a significantly reduced proportion of fat as the source of total caloric intake are recommended.

Diminished gastrointestinal absorption, increased urinary losses, altered distribution, and altered carrier protein concentrations after severe burns may lead to micronutrient (trace elements and vitamins [such as Cu, Fe, Se, Zn, vitamins C and E]) deficiency in major burns.[56-58] Such deficiencies may, in turn, lead to infectious complications, delayed wound healing, and stunting in children.[59] Thus supplementation would seem appropriate, but evidence-based practice guidelines are not currently available. Enhancing trace element status and antioxidant defenses by supplementing selenium, zinc, and copper was shown to decrease the incidence of nosocomial pneumonia in critically ill, severely burned patients in two consecutive, randomized double-blind trials.[60] Caution should be used to avoid toxic side effects.

MODULATION OF THE HORMONAL AND ENDOCRINE RESPONSE

Modification of adverse components of the hypermetabolic response to burn injury, particularly protein catabolism, would seem to be desirable. β-adrenergic blockade, β-adrenergic supplementation, anabolic steroids, recombinant growth hormone, and insulin-like growth factor (IGF) are under active investigation. Various studies have demonstrated the potential beneficial effect of β blockers in burn patients. In a single-center study, administration of propranolol in doses that decrease the heart rate by approximately 15% to 20% from baseline reduced the release of free fatty acids from adipose tissue, decreased hepatic triacylglycerol storage and fat accumulation, and reversed muscle protein catabolism.[61-63] In a retrospective study of adult burn patients, use of β blockers was associated with decreased mortality, wound infection rate, and wound healing time.[64] Therefore β blockers appear to have high potential as an anticatabolic treatment in severely burned patients.

Treatment with anabolic agents, such as oxandrolone, a testosterone analog, improved muscle protein catabolism through enhanced protein synthesis efficiency,[65] reduced weight loss, and increased donor site wound healing.[66] In a prospective randomized study, Wolf and colleagues demonstrated that administration of 10 mg of oxandrolone every 12 hours decreased hospital length of stay.[67] In a large prospective, double-blind, randomized single-center study, oxandrolone given at a dose of 0.1 mg/kg every 12 hours shortened acute hospital length of stay, maintained lean body mass, and improved body composition and hepatic protein synthesis.[68]

The use of recombinant human growth hormone in daily subcutaneous doses has been reported to accelerate donor site healing and restore earlier positive nitrogen balance.[69-71] Indeed, administration of 0.05 mg/kg of recombinant human growth hormone given over a 12-month period after burn injury significantly improved height, weight, lean body mass, bone mineral content, cardiac function, and muscle strength.[72] These findings are in contrast to those of Takala and colleagues in adults with critical illness from multiple etiologies[73] and with studies showing that growth hormone treatment induced hyperglycemia and insulin resistance.[71,74] It is likely that the prolonged catabolic nature of burn injury and perhaps the dose account for these discrepant results. IGF-1 has been shown to decrease the metabolic rate after burn injury and to increase whole-body anabolic activity without hyperglycemia or insulin resistance.[75] Studies by Van den Berghe and colleagues indicate that the use of IGF-1 alone is not effective in critically ill patients without burns.[76] Again, the prolonged catabolic nature of burn injury may explain the difference.

GLUCOSE CONTROL

A prominent component of the hypermetabolic response after burn injury is hyperglycemia and insulin resistance.[77] These result from both an increase in hepatic gluconeogenesis and impaired insulin-mediated glucose transport into skeletal muscle, cardiac muscle and adipose tissue.[78-81] Hyperglycemia and elevations in circulating insulin concentration are of serious clinical concern. Hyperglycemia has been linked to impaired wound healing, increased infectious complications, and increased mortality.[82-85] A randomized controlled trial in severely burned pediatric patients indicated superiority for glucose control using insulin.[86] Care providers need to be vigilant of an increased incidence of hypoglycemia that is associated with a 4- to 9-fold increase in morbidity and mortality. A recent Phase I/II prospective trial in burn patients showed safety, significantly less hypoglycemia when compared to insulin, and efficacy of metformin in burn patients and currently, larger trials are being designed to test metformin as a glucose modulating agent in the setting of burn patients.[87]

AUTHOR'S RECOMMENDATIONS
- Burn patients should be managed initially as trauma patients. Algorithms for trauma evaluation should be diligently applied to the burn patient.
- Early and accurate fluid resuscitation of patients with major burns is critical for survival, but overaggressive resuscitation should be avoided, particularly in small children younger than 4 years.
- Early diagnosis of bronchopulmonary injury is critical. Management of inhalation injury consists of ventilatory support, aggressive pulmonary toilet, bronchoscopic removal of casts, and nebulization therapy.

- Adequate nutritional intake through enteral tube feeding will aid in the control of stress ulceration, preserve intestinal mucosal integrity, and provide fuel for the resulting hypermetabolic state. Nutritional regimes for the treatment of burn patients include a significantly reduced proportion of fat as the source of total caloric intake.
- Modulation of the hypermetabolic response improves outcomes.
- Hyperglycemia in burn patients is associated with increased complications and needs to be controlled to a target level of 130 mg/dL. Hypoglycemia needs to be avoided because it leads to increased mortality after burn.
- Hyperlipidemia should be treated to avoid fatty infiltration of organs.

REFERENCES

1. American Burn Association/American College of Surgeons. Guidelines for the operation of burn centers. *J Burn Care Res.* 2007;28:134-141.
2. Nguyen TT, Gilpin DA, Meyer NA, Herndon DN. Current treatment of severely burned patients. *Ann Surg.* 1996;223:14-25.
3. Brigham PA, McLoughlin E. Burn incidence and medical care use in the United States: estimates, trends, and data sources. *J Burn Care Rehabil.* 1996;17:95-107.
4. Wolf SE. Critical care in the severely burned: organ support and management of complications. In: Herndon DN, ed. *Total Burn Care* 3rd ed. London: Saunders; 2007.
5. American College of Surgeons Committee on Trauma. *Resources of Optimal Care of the Injured Patient.* Chicago: American College of Surgeons; 1993.
6. Pulmonary Artery Catheter Consensus conference: consensus statement. *Crit Care Med.* 1997;25:910-925.
7. Della Rocca G, Costas MG. Intrathoracic blood volume: clinical applications. In: Jean-Louis V, ed. *Yearbook of Intensive Care and Emergency Medicine.* Berlin: Springer; 2006:142-151.
8. Branski LK, Herndon DN, Byrd JF, et al. Transpulmonary thermodilution for hemodynamic measurements in severely burned children. *Crit Care.* 2011;15(2):R118.
9. Kraft R, Herndon DN, Branski LK, Finnerty CC, Leonard KR, Jeschke MG. Optimized fluid management improves outcomes of pediatric burn patients. *J Surg Res.* 2013;181(1):121-128.
10. Ramzy PI, Barret JP, Herndon DN. Thermal injury. *Crit Care Clin.* 1999;15:333-352. ix.
11. Fodor L, Fodor A, Ramon Y, Shoshani O, Rissin Y, Ullmann Y. Controversies in fluid resuscitation for burn management: literature review and our experience. *Injury.* 2006;37:374-379.
12. Carvajal HF. Fluid resuscitation of pediatric burn victims: a critical appraisal. *Pediatr Nephrol.* 1994;8:357-366.
13. Youn YK, LaLonde C, Demling R. The role of mediators in the response to thermal injury. *World J Surg.* 1992;16:30-36.
14. Warden GD. Burn shock resuscitation. *World J Surg.* 1992; 16:16-23.
15. Wolf SE, Rose JK, Desai MH, Mileski JP, Barrow RE, Herndon DN. Mortality determinants in massive pediatric burns: an analysis of 103 children with > or = 80% TBSA burns (> or = 70% full-thickness). *Ann Surg.* 1997;225:554-565; discussion 565-569.
16. Pham TN, Cancio LC, Gibran NS. American Burn Association practice guidelines burn shock resuscitation. *J Burn Care Res.* 2008;29:257-266.
17. Holm C. Resuscitation in shock associated with burns: tradition or evidence-based medicine. *Resuscitation.* 2000;44:157-164.
18. Mason SA, Nathens AB, Jeschke MG. Hold the pendulum: rates of acute kidney injury are increased in patients who receive resuscitation volumes less than predicted by the Parkland Equation. *Ann Surg.* 2017;266(6):e108.
19. Baxter CR, Shires T. Physiological response to crystalloid resuscitation of severe burns. *Ann N Y Acad Sci.* 1968;150:874-894.
20. Schwartz SI. Supportive therapy in burn care: consensus summary on fluid resuscitation. *J Trauma.* 1979;19(suppl 11):876-877.
21. Fabri PJ. Monitoring of the burn patient. *Clin Plast Surg.* 1986; 13:21-27.
22. Greenhalgh DG. Burn resuscitation: the results of the ISBI/ABA survey. *Burns.* 2010;36(2):176-182.
23. Perel P, Roberts I. Colloids versus crystalloids for fluid resuscitation in critically ill patients. *Cochrane Database Syst Rev.* 2007;4:CD000567.
24. Alderson P, Bunn F, Lefebvre C, et al. Human albumin solution for resuscitation and volume expansion in critically ill patients. *Cochrane Database Syst Rev.* 2004;4:CD001208.
25. Vincent JL, Sakr Y, Reinhart K, et al. Is albumin administration in the acutely ill associated with increased mortality? Results of the SOAP study. *Crit Care.* 2005;9:R745-R754.
26. Cartotto R, Callum J. A review of the use of human albumin in burn patients. *J Burn Care Res.* 2012;33(6):702-717.
27. Pruitt Jr BA, Mason Jr AD, Moncrief JA. Hemodynamic changes in the early postburn patient: the influence of fluid administration and of a vasodilator (hydralazine). *J Trauma.* 1971;11:36-46.
28. Warden GD. Fluid resuscitation and early management. In: Herndon DN, ed. *Total Burn Care.* 3rd ed. London: Saunders; 2007:107-118.
29. Finnerty CC, Herndon DN, Jeschke MG. Inhalation injury in severely burned children does not augment the systemic inflammatory response. *Crit Care.* 2007;11:R22.
30. Thompson PB, Herndon DN, Traber DL, Abston S. Effect on mortality of inhalation injury. *J Trauma.* 1986;26:163-165.
31. Sheridan RL. Burns. *Crit Care Med.* 2002;30(suppl 11);S500-S514.
32. Endorf FW, Gamelli RL. Inhalation injury, pulmonary perturbations, and fluid resuscitation. *J Burn Care Res.* 2007;28:80-83.
33. Pruitt Jr BA. Infection and the burn patient. *Br J Surg.* 1990; 77:1081-1082.
34. Greenhalgh DG, Saffle JR, Holmes JH, et al. American Burn Association consensus conference to define sepsis and infection in burns. *J Burn Care Res.* 2007;28:776-790.
35. Atiyeh BS, Dham R, Kadry M, et al. Benefit-cost analysis of moist exposed burn ointment. *Burns.* 2002;28:659-663.
36. Lofts JA. Cost analysis of a major burn. *N Z Med J.* 1991;104:488-490.
37. Munster AM, Smith-Meek M, Sharkey P. The effect of early surgical intervention on mortality and cost-effectiveness in burn care, 1978–91. *Burns.* 1994;20:61-64.
38. Chan BP, Kochevar IE, Redmond RW. Enhancement of porcine skin graft adherence using a light-activated process. *J Surg Res.* 2002;108:77-84.
39. Budny PG, Regan PJ, Roberts AH. The estimation of blood loss during burns surgery. *Burns.* 1993;19:134-137.
40. Housinger TA, Lang D, Warden GD. A prospective study of blood loss with excisional therapy in pediatric burn patients. *J Trauma.* 1993;34:262-263.
41. Herndon DN, Tompkins RG. Support of the metabolic response to burn injury. *Lancet.* 2004;363:1895-1902.

42. Abdullahi A, Jeschke MG. Nutrition and anabolic pharmaco-therapies in the care of burn patients. *Nutr Clin Pract.* 2014;29(5):621-630.

43. Hart DW, Wolf SE, Chinkes DL, et al. Effects of early excision and aggressive enteral feeding on hypermetabolism, catabolism, and sepsis after severe burn. *J Trauma.* 2003;54:755-761; discussion 761-764.

44. Herndon DN, Barrow RE, Stein M, et al. Increased mortality with intravenous supplemental feeding in severely burned patients. *J Burn Care Rehabil.* 1989;10:309-313.

45. Curreri PW, Richmond D, Marvin J, Baxter CR. Dietary requirements of patients with major burns. *J Am Diet Assoc.* 1974;65:415-417.

46. Allard JP, Pichard C, Hoshino E, et al. Validation of a new formula for calculating the energy requirements of burn patients. *JPEN J Parenter Enteral Nutr.* 1990;14:115-118.

47. Hildreth MA, Herndon DN, Desai MH, Broemeling LD. Current treatment reduces calories required to maintain weight in pediatric patients with burns. *J Burn Care Rehabil.* 1990;11:405-409.

48. Herndon DN, Curreri PW. Metabolic response to thermal injury and its nutritional support. *Cutis.* 1978;22:501-506. 514.

49. Demling RH, Seigne P. Metabolic management of patients with severe burns. *World J Surg.* 2000;24:673-680.

50. Garrel DR, Razi M, Larivière F, et al. Improved clinical status and length of care with low-fat nutrition support in burn patients. *JPEN J Parenter Enteral Nutr.* 1995;19:482-491.

51. Mochizuki H, Trocki O, Dominioni L, Ray MB, Alexander JW. Optimal lipid content for enteral diets following thermal injury. *JPEN J Parenter Enteral Nutr.* 1984;8:638-646.

52. Barret JP, Jeschke MG, Herndon DN. Fatty infiltration of the liver in severely burned pediatric patients: autopsy findings and clinical implications. *J Trauma.* 2001;51:736-739.

53. Aarsland A, Chinkes D, Wolfe RR. Contributions of de novo synthesis of fatty acids to total VLDL-triglyceride secretion during prolonged hyperglycemia/hyperinsulinemia in normal man. *J Clin Invest.* 1996;98:2008-2017.

54. Jeschke MG, Herndon DN. Burns in children: standard and new treatments. *Lancet.* 2014;383(9923):1168-1178.

55. Herndon DN, Nguyen TT, Wolfe RR, et al. Lipolysis in burned patients is stimulated by the beta 2-receptor for catecholamines. *Arch Surg.* 1994;129:1301-1304; discussion 1304-1305.

56. Cuthbertson DP, Fell GS, Smith CM, Tilstone WJ. Metabolism after injury. I. Effects of severity, nutrition, and environmental temperature on protein potassium, zinc, and creatine. *Br J Surg.* 1972;59:926-931.

57. Shakespeare PG. Studies on the serum levels of iron, copper and zinc and the urinary excretion of zinc after burn injury. *Burns Incl Therm Inj.* 1982;8:358-364.

58. Berger MM, Cavadini C, Bart A, et al. Cutaneous copper and zinc losses in burns. *Burns.* 1992;18:373-380.

59. Berger MM, Raffoul W, Shenkin A. Practical guidelines for nutritional management of burn injury and recovery: a guideline based on expert opinion but not including RCTs. *Burns.* 2008;34:141-143.

60. Berger MM, Eggimann P, Heyland DK, et al. Reduction of nosocomial pneumonia after major burns by trace element supplementation: aggregation of two randomised trials. *Crit Care.* 2006;10:R153.

61. Herndon DN, Hart DW, Wolf SE, Chinkes DL, Wolfe RR. Reversal of catabolism by beta-blockade after severe burns. *N Engl J Med.* 2001;345:1223-1229.

62. Aarsland A, Chinkes D, Wolfe RR, et al. Beta-blockade lowers peripheral lipolysis in burn patients receiving growth hormone. Rate of hepatic very low density lipoprotein triglyceride secretion remains unchanged. *Ann Surg.* 1996;223:777-787; discussion 787-789.

63. Morio B, Irtun O, Herndon DN, Wolfe RR. Propranolol decreases splanchnic triacylglycerol storage in burn patients receiving a high-carbohydrate diet. *Ann Surg.* 2002;236:218-225.

64. Arbabi S, Ahrns KS, Wahl WL, et al. Beta-blocker use is associated with improved outcomes in adult burn patients. *J Trauma.* 2004;56:265-269; discussion 269-271.

65. Hart DW, Wolf SE, Ramzy PI, et al. Anabolic effects of oxandrolone after severe burn. *Ann Surg.* 2001;233:556-564.

66. Demling RH, Orgill DP. The anticatabolic and wound healing effects of the testosterone analog oxandrolone after severe burn injury. *J Crit Care.* 2000;15:12-17.

67. Wolf SE, Edelman LS, Kemalyan N, et al. Effects of oxandrolone on outcome measures in the severely burned: a multicenter prospective randomized double-blind trial. *J Burn Care Res.* 2006;27:131-139; discussion 140-141.

68. Jeschke MG, Finnerty CC, Suman OE, Kulp G, Mlcak RP, Herndon DN. The effect of oxandrolone on the endocrinologic, inflammatory, and hypermetabolic responses during the acute phase postburn. *Ann Surg.* 2007;246:351-360; discussion 360-362.

69. Gilpin DA, Barrow RE, Rutan RL, Broemeling L, Herndon DN. Recombinant human growth hormone accelerates wound healing in children with large cutaneous burns. *Ann Surg.* 1994;220:19-24.

70. Meyer NA, Muller MJ, Herndon DN. Nutrient support of the healing wound. *New Horiz.* 1994;2:202-214.

71. Demling RH. Comparison of the anabolic effects and complications of human growth hormone and the testosterone analog, oxandrolone, after severe burn injury. *Burns.* 1999;25:215-221.

72. Przkora R, Herndon DN, Suman OE, et al. Beneficial effects of extended growth hormone treatment after hospital discharge in pediatric burn patients. *Ann Surg.* 2006;243:796-801; discussion 801-803.

73. Takala J, Ruokonen E, Webster NR, et al. Increased mortality associated with growth hormone treatment in critically ill adults. *N Engl J Med.* 1999;341:785-792.

74. Gore DC, Honeycutt D, Jahoor F, Rutan T, Wolfe RR, Herndon DN. Effect of exogenous growth hormone on glucose utilization in burn patients. *J Surg Res.* 1991;51:518-523.

75. Kupfer SR, Underwood LE, Baxter RC, Clemmons DR. Enhancement of the anabolic effects of growth hormone and insulin-like growth factor I by use of both agents simultaneously. *J Clin Invest.* 1993;91:391-396.

76. Mesotten D, Van den Berghe G. Changes within the growth hormone/insulin-like growth factor I/IGF binding protein axis during critical illness. *Endrocrinol Metab Clin North Am.* 2006;35:793-805.

77. Jeschke MG. Clinical review: Glucose control in severely burned patients - current best practice. *Crit Care.* 2013;17(4):232.

78. Jahoor F, Herndon DN, Wolfe RR. Role of insulin and glucagon in the response of glucose and alanine kinetics in burn-injured patients. *J Clin Invest.* 1986;78:807-814.

79. Gearhart MM, Parbhoo SK. Hyperglycemia in the critically ill patient. *AACN Clin Issues.* 2006;17:50-55.

80. Xin-Long C, Zhao-Fan X, Dao-Feng B, Jian-Guang T, Duo W. Insulin resistance following thermal injury: An animal study. *Burns.* 2007;33:480-483.

81. Zauner A, Nimmerrichter P, Anderwald C, et al. Severity of insulin resistance in critically ill medical patients. *Metabolism.* 2007;56:1-5.
82. Guvener M, Pasaoglu I, Demircin M, Oc M. Perioperative hyperglycemia is a strong correlate of postoperative infection in type II diabetic patients after coronary artery bypass grafting. *Endocr J.* 2002;49:531-537.
83. McCowen KC, Malhotra A, Bistrian BR. Stress-induced hyperglycemia. *Crit Care Clin.* 2001;17:107-124.
84. Christiansen C, Toft P, Jørgensen HS, Andersen SK, Tønnesen E. Hyperglycaemia and mortality in critically ill patients: a prospective study. *Intensive Care Med.* 2004;30:1685-1688.
85. Jeschke MG, Pinto R, Herndon DN, Finnerty CC, Kraft R. Hypoglycemia is associated with increased postburn morbidity and mortality in pediatric patients. *Crit Care Med.* 2014; 42(5):1221-1231.
86. Jeschke MG, Kulp GA, Kraft R, et al. Intensive insulin therapy in severely burned pediatric patients: a prospective randomized trial. *Am J Respir Crit Care Med.* 2010;182:351-359.
87. Jeschke MG, Abdullahi A, Burnett M, Rehou S, Stanojcic M. Glucose control in severely burned patients using metformin: an interim safety and efficacy analysis of a phase II randomized controlled trial. *Ann Surg.* 2016;264(3):518-527.
88. Harris JA, Benedict FG. A biometric study of human basal metabolism. *Proc Natl Acad Sci USA.* 1918;4:370-373.
89. Kleinman RE, Barness LA, Finberg L. History of pediatric nutrition and fluid therapy. *Pediatr Res.* 2003;54:762-772.
90. Food and Nutrition Board, Institute of Medicine. *Dietary Reference Intakes.* Washington, DC: National Academy Press; 2002.
91. Day T, Dean P, Adams M, et al. Nutritional requirements of the burned child: The Curreri Junior formula. *Proc Am Burn Assoc.* 1986;18(86).
92. Hildreth MA, Herndon DN, Desai MH, Broemeling LD. Caloric requirements of patients with burns under one year of age. *J Burn Care Rehabil.* 1993;14:108-112.
93. Hildreth MA, Herndon DN, Desai MH, Duke MA. Caloric needs of adolescent patients with burns. *J Burn Care Rehabil.* 1989;10:523-526.

77

What Is the Best Approach to Resuscitation In Trauma?

Samuel A. Tisherman, Megan T. Quintana, and Jason S. Radowsky

INTRODUCTION/BACKGROUND

Exsanguinating hemorrhage is a major cause of death from trauma. Rapid fluid resuscitation accompanied by aggressive efforts at hemostasis is required to save lives. Many questions regarding fluid resuscitation remain. These include the choice of fluid, indications for blood products, managing the coagulopathy of trauma, and monitoring the adequacy of fluid resuscitation, both before and after hemostasis is achieved.

In the early 1960s, Shires and colleagues documented the value of crystalloid administration to correct the fluid shifts that characterized the response to hemorrhage.[1] Adoption of crystalloid resuscitation during the Vietnam conflict decreased renal failure but likely contributed to "Da Nang lung" or "shock lung"—either acute respiratory distress syndrome (ARDS) or hydrostatic pulmonary edema. Administration of lactated Ringer's (LR) quickly became a standard of care in prehospital and emergency department (ED) resuscitation of civilian trauma victims. Possible immunologic effects of LR[2] and findings of detrimental effects of excessive crystalloid administration[3] have led to questions related to this practice and interest in finding better alternatives.

Blood administration, another mainstay of resuscitation from hemorrhagic shock (HS), has evolved from use of whole blood to components—packed red blood cells (PRBC), fresh frozen plasma (FFP) and platelets. Recent studies have suggested that rapid resuscitation with blood components that essentially reconstitute whole blood may prevent and/or treat the coagulopathy of trauma.[4] Transfusions, however, have potentially deleterious effects that merit discussion.[5]

Finally, the endpoints for fluid resuscitation have been reconsidered. In ongoing hemorrhage (uncontrolled HS) normalization of blood pressure may increase bleeding and worsen outcome. Limited, or hypotensive, fluid resuscitation may be appropriate. Once hemostasis has been achieved, determining the adequacy of resuscitation is critical. Standard parameters may leave patients underresuscitated, in "compensated hemorrhagic shock". Adjuvant tests are necessary to recognize this condition and assure restoration of homeostasis.[6]

PATHOPHYSIOLOGY OF HEMORRHAGIC SHOCK

Blood pressure and heart rate are the typical clinical parameters used to determine the severity of HS, but they lack sensitivity. In general, patients need to lose at least 30–40% of their blood volume to become hypotensive.[7] An individual's response to hemorrhage may be affected by age, comorbid conditions, medications, and ingestion of drugs and alcohol. Recognition and reversal of "compensated shock" is critical to achieve optimal outcomes.

Approximately 6–9% of trauma patients are in shock on admission. Of these, one third have exsanguinating hemorrhage, which can present as a lack of response to fluid resuscitation.[7] These patients invariably require operative intervention and aggressive fluid resuscitation, including blood products, or they will die within minutes to hours. Another third of patients, classified as transient responders, are hypotensive initially and will show hemodynamic improvement during fluid resuscitation, only to deteriorate again. They have less active bleeding than the first group, but their transient response can lull clinicians into a sense of complacency. Without ongoing resuscitation, operative intervention as necessary, and vigilance, they, too, have a high risk of dying or developing multiple organ dysfunction. The final third of patients respond appropriately to fluid resuscitation and spontaneously achieve hemostasis. These patients are still at risk of hypoperfusion and organ dysfunction. In all trauma patients, early recognition of hypoperfusion, rapid restoration of homeostasis, and continued resuscitation to appropriate endpoints can reduce the risk of early cardiovascular collapse, development of organ system dysfunction, and death.

The inflammatory response to trauma may affect the coagulation system and may increase the risk of organ dysfunction and late death from trauma.[8] Although laboratory studies have suggested therapies that could mitigate these deleterious cascades, none of these agents have been used in the clinical setting. Nonetheless, it seems that late deaths from multiple organ dysfunction and sepsis are actually rare.[9]

PRESENTATION OF AVAILABLE DATA BASED ON SYSTEMATIC REVIEW

Choice of Fluid

Although the use of crystalloids for resuscitation from traumatic HS has long been the standard of care, it seems that these solutions are not as innocuous as originally believed. Administration of crystalloids may have specific, detrimental effects.

Laboratory studies have demonstrated that crystalloids may exacerbate cellular injury. Lactated Ringer's solution can increase oxidative burst and expression of adhesion molecules on neutrophils in human blood and during HS in pigs.[10–12] Saline is the most commonly administered crystalloid, but its safety has been questioned in retrospective observational studies and experimental models because the high chloride load may decrease renal cortical blood flow, increase the need for renal replacement therapy, and increase the risk of death.[13]

Until recently, no trial had directly compared the different crystalloids (Table 77.1). Small studies, such as the Saline vs. Plasma-Lyte for ICU fluid Therapy (SPLIT) trial, compared Plasma-Lyte to normal saline in critically ill patients who required crystalloids, and did not demonstrate a difference in the primary outcome of acute kidney injury or requirement

TABLE 77.1   Summary of Clinical Trials.

Study, Year	Number of Subjects (Intervention/ No Intervention)	Study Design (DB, Double-Blind; P, Placebo-Controlled)	Intervention	Control	Outcomes
Balanced Crystalloids Compared to Saline					
2018[13]	7942 balanced crystalloid 7860 NS	Cluster randomized, crossover by ICU	LR or Plasma-Lyte A	NS	Lower rate of the composite outcome of death from any cause, new renal-replacement therapy, or persistent renal dysfunction.
2015[14]	1152 buffered crystalloid 1110 NS	DB, prospective, randomized	Plasma-Lyte 148	NS	No difference in acute kidney injury.
Hypertonic Saline for Hemorrhagic Shock					
2011[29]	376 NS 256 HTS 220 HSD	DB, prospective, randomized	HTS/HSD	NS	No difference in 28-day survival.
2007[2]	36 HSD 26 LR	DB, prospective, randomized	HSD	LR	Inhibit CD11b. Trend toward increased IL-1β, IL-10.
2007[28]	110 HSD 99 LR	DB, prospective, randomized	HSD	LR	No difference in ARDS-free survival. Improved ARDS-free survival if >10u blood given.
2006[27]	13 HSD 14 NS	DB, prospective, randomized	HSD	NS	Promotes a more balanced inflammatory response.
2003[26]	120 HSD 110 NS	DB, prospective, randomized	HSD	NS	Survival 83% vs. 76% overall (NS), 85% vs. 67% for patients requiring surgery ($P = .01$).
1993[23]	85 HTS 89 HS 84 NS	DB, prospective, randomized	HS or HSD	LR	HS improved survival compared to TRISS.
1992[22]	35 HS 35 HSD 35 NS	DB, prospective, randomized	HS or HSD	NS	No difference in survival. Better blood pressure and volume expansion. Less fluid needed.
1991[21]	83 HSD 83 LR	DB, prospective, randomized	HSD	LR	Improved BP. No change in survival.
1991[20]	211 HSD 211 Crystalloid	DB, prospective, randomized	HSD	Crystalloid	No difference in survival, except patient who required operation. Improved blood pressure, fewer complications.
1990[19]	32 HS 23 HSD 51 LR	DB, prospective, randomized	HSD HS	LR	No safety issues, except mild hyperchloremic acidosis.

Continued

TABLE 77.1   Summary of Clinical Trials.—cont'd

Study, Year	Number of Subjects (Intervention/ No Intervention)	Study Design (DB, Double-Blind; P, Placebo-Controlled)	Intervention	Control	Outcomes
Transfusion					
2017[82]	PRBC storage 2457 Short-term 2462 Long-term	DB, prospective, randomized	Short-term storage	Standard issue	No difference in mortality.
2016[81]	PRBC storage 6936 Short-term 13,922 Long-term	Prospective, randomized	Short-term storage	Long-term storage	No difference in mortality.
2015[80]	1211 Fresh PRBCs 1219 Standard issue PRBCs	DB, prospective, randomized	Fresh PRBCs	Standard issue PRBCs	No difference in mortality or complications.
2007[84]	240 depleted 439 standard	Retrospective	Leukocyte depleted PRBC	Standard PRBC	No difference in LOS or mortality.
2006[83]	132 leukoreduced 136 standard	Prospective, randomized	Leukocyte depleted PRBC	Standard PRBC	No difference in infections, organ failures, mortality.
2006[78]	93 transfused 117 Not transfused	Prospective Operation Iraqi Freedom	Transfused	Not transfused	Higher ISS, HR, lower Hct, increased infection rate, ICU, LOS.
2005[79]	102	Prospective, observational			The amount of transfused blood is independently associated with both the development of ARDS and hospital mortality.
Clotting Factor and Platelet Replacement					
2018[59]	230 Plasma 271 Standard care	Prospective, randomized	Plasma during air transport	Standard care	Prehospital administration of thawed plasma decreased mortality and decreased prothrombin-time ratio.
2015[4]	Plasma:platelets: PRBC ratio 338 1:1:1 342 1:1:2	Prospective, randomized	Transfuse 1:1:1 FFP:platelets: PRBCs	Transfuse 1: 1:2 FFP: platelets: PRBCs	No difference in mortality. More patients in the 1:1:1 group achieved hemostasis and fewer died from exsanguination in the first 24 hours.
2013[50]	905 patients who received ≥3 units of blood products within 24 hours	Prospective, cohort			Early administration of higher plasma and platelet ratios were associated with decreased mortality.
2013[49]	Units PRBC transfused 353 1–3 237 4–9 152 ≥10	Retrospective			Time-dependent analysis found no association between low FFP: PRBC ratio and mortality. Conventional analysis demonstrated a protective effect of high FFP: PRBC ratio.
2011[48]	Platelet:RBC ratio 211 >1:20 216 1:2 216 1:1	Retrospective			Higher ratios were associated with improved early and late survival, decreased death from hemorrhage, and an increase in death from multiple organ failure.
2011[57]	61 DCR 57 Standard	Prospective and retrospective	Permissive hypotension, less crystalloid	Standard care, historical controls	DCR resulted in less crystalloid, more FFP, improved survival, OR 0.4 (CI: 0.18–0.9).

TABLE 77.1   Summary of Clinical Trials.—cont'd

Study, Year	Number of Subjects (Intervention/ No Intervention)	Study Design (DB, Double-Blind; P, Placebo-Controlled)	Intervention	Control	Outcomes
2011[56]	108 Hypotension 82 Standard	Prospective and retrospective	Permissive hypotension, less crystalloid	Standard care, historical controls	DCR was associated with increased survival, OR 2.5 (CI: 1.1–5.6).
2011[45]	438	Retrospective			Plasma deficit (#units PRBC − FFP) per hour may be more sensitive than overall PRBC:FFP ratios. Early plasma repletion was associated with less blood product use.
2010[43]	214	Prospective and retrospective	Massive transfusion protocol	Standard care, historical controls	Factors that influenced survival were FFP:PRBC, platelets:PRBC, ISS, age and total PRBC.
2010[44]	Platelet:PRBC ratio 171 <1:18 77 ≥1:18 and <1:12 249 ≥1:12 and <1:6 160 ≥1:6	Retrospective			Increased platelet:PRBC ratio was associated with increased survival.
2009[41]	FFP:PRBC ratio 62 ≤1:8 95 >1:8 and ≤1:3 111 >1:3 and ≤1:2 115 >1:2	Retrospective			Higher FFP:PRBC ratio up to 1:3 was an independent predictor of survival. Higher ratio was not associated with a further increased survival.
2009[40]	466 patients receiving massive transfusion	Retrospective			Early administration of high ratios of FFP and platelets to PRBC associated with improved survival and decreased need for PRBC.
2009[58]	442 preemptive 390 historical controls	Prospective and retrospective	Preemptive FFP and platelets	Standard care, historical controls	Mortality decreased from 31% to 20% long term. Thromboelastography was used to titrate products.
2009[42]	37 1:1.5 40 Standard	Prospective and retrospective	1:1.5 FFP:PRBC, more rapid product availability	Standard care, historical controls	No difference in ratios, but more rapid administration was associated with improved mortality.
2008[38]	484 PRBC:FFP >1:1 114 PRBC:FFP 0.9–1.1:1 115 PRBC:FFP <0.9	Retrospective			Lower PRBC:FFP ratio was associated with lower mortality.
2008[39]	467	Retrospective			High plasma:RBC ratio (≥1:2) relative to those with low plasma:RBC ratio and high platelet:RBC ratio (≥1:2) relative to those with low platelet:RBC ratio were associated with improved survival.
2008[52]	806	Prospective, nonrandomized			There was no association between PRBC:FFP ratio and intensive care unit days, hospital days, or mortality, including patients who received massive transfusion (≥10 U).

Continued

TABLE 77.1 Summary of Clinical Trials.—cont'd					
Study, Year	Number of Subjects (Intervention/ No Intervention)	Study Design (DB, Double-Blind; P, Placebo-Controlled)	Intervention	Control	Outcomes
Limited Fluid Resuscitation for Uncontrolled Hemorrhage					
2015[95]	97 Controlled 95 Standard	Prospective, randomized	Controlled crystalloid resuscitation	Standard crystalloid resuscitation	The volume of crystalloid administered was different between groups. Overall mortality was not different, except that 24-hour mortality in patients with blunt trauma was less with controlled resuscitation.
2011[93]	44 MAP >50 46 MAP >65	Prospective, randomized, intraoperative	MAP >50	MAP >65	Lower MAP group required fewer blood products, had less coagulopathy and decreased early death.
2002[90]	55 SBP >70 55 SBP >100	Randomized	SBP >70	SBP >100	Survival 93% with no difference between groups.
1996[91]	526 RIS 451 matched controls	Retrospective	Rapid Infusion System used	Historical controls	Increase risk of dying 4.8×.
1994[88]	309 delayed 289 immediate	Randomized day of month	Delayed resuscitation	Immediate resuscitation	Improved survival: 70% vs. 62%. Decreased LOS.
1990[87]	6855	Retrospective			No difference in mortality if fluids were administered prehospital.

ARDS, acute respiratory distress syndrome; *DCR*, damage control resuscitation; *Hb*, hemoglobin; *Hct*, hematocrit; *HR*, hazard ratio; *HS*, hemorrhagic shock; *HSD*, hypertonic saline dextran; *HTS*, hypertonic saline; *IL*, interlukin; *ISS*, injury severity score; *LOS*, length of stay; *LR*, lactated Ringer's; *MAP*, mean arterial pressure; *NS*, normal saline; *OR*, odds ratio; *PRBC*, packed red blood cells; *SBP*, systolic blood pressure; *TRISS*, trauma and injury severity score.

for renal replacement therapy.[14] There was also no difference in hospital mortality. The larger Isotonic Solutions and Major Adverse Renal Events Trial (SMART) assigned ICU patients to receive balanced crystalloid or normal saline according to randomization of the ICU in which they were admitted.[13] This study, with an adequate power, suggested that patients who received balanced crystalloids had lower rates of death from any cause, need for new renal replacement therapy, or persistent renal dysfunction than those who received normal saline. These results have been questioned because the study was at a single center, not blinded, and because subjects did not receive significant amounts of either fluid. Multicenter, blinded trials are ongoing.

As balanced crystalloid solutions have gained favor over normal saline in the resuscitation of critically ill patients, research has also concentrated on ways to improve these solutions. Modifications of LR, e.g., substituting the L-isomer of lactate or substitution of pyruvate or ketone bodies (β-hydroxybutyrate) for racemic lactate can decrease the neutrophil activation and apoptosis.[15,16] Hypertonic saline (HTS) and fresh whole blood, in contrast, do not cause neutrophil activation. HTS can attenuate immune-mediated cellular injury after trauma.[2]

Several small clinical trials have suggested the benefits of hypertonic solutions (HTS alone or HTS + colloid such as

dextran [HSD]) for trauma resuscitation (see Table 77.1). Multiple studies demonstrated that HTS or HSD increased blood pressure and volume expansion better than crystalloids.[17–28] Given the potential physiologic benefit of HTS and the tactical advantage of small volume resuscitation for the military, the Resuscitation Outcomes Consortium (ROC) conducted a multicenter, prehospital, prospective, double-blind, randomized trial comparing normal saline, HTS, and HSD as the first resuscitation fluid in hypotensive trauma patients.[29] Survival to 28 days was not significantly different between groups. If anything, patients who received hypertonic solutions and were not transfused in the first 24 hs had poorer outcomes than those who received normal saline. The authors postulated that the hypertonic saline may have led to early mortality before blood transfusion or a change in physician behavior regarding recognition of shock because of the short-term hemodynamic effect of the hypertonic fluid.

Beyond the choice of crystalloid, the administration of too much crystalloid can have adverse clinical outcomes in critically ill patients. Kasotakis, et al., found that the amount of crystalloid administered to blunt trauma victims correlated with ventilator days; length of stay; development of multiple organ failure, infections, and compartment syndromes (abdominal and extremity), but not mortality.[3]

Colloid was thought to be a reasonable alternative to crystalloids for volume expansion. However, the most recent Cochrane review of albumin administration found no benefit for patients with hypovolemia, burns, or hypoalbuminemia.[30] Increasing evidence suggests that starch solutions do not improve survival in the general intensive care unit (ICU) population and may increase the need for renal replacement therapy[31] or death.[32] These fluids currently have no role in trauma resuscitation.

Because the plasma substitutes discussed so far do not carry oxygen, there has long been interest in developing hemoglobin-based carriers (HBOCs) utilizing hemoglobin from red blood cells. Unconjugated hemoglobin has severe renal and tissue toxicity. Researchers have sought to identify techniques to decrease the nephrotoxicity and increase plasma half-life. A study using Diaspirin cross-linked hemoglobin (HemAssist, Baxter Healthcare, Round Lake, Illinois), the first product to undergo a randomized clinical trial in trauma patients, but was discontinued early because of increased mortality in the subjects exposed to the product.[33] More recently, polymerized hemoglobin derived from human blood (PolyHeme, Northfield Laboratories, Evanston, Illinois) was compared to PRBCs in a small, randomized trial for trauma patients who required operations.[34] A pivotal, randomized trial of Polyheme compared to prehospital LR administration and early in-hospital blood transfusion demonstrated decreased allogeneic blood transfusion requirements, but no mortality benefit.[35] Consequently, no HBOCs are currently available.

TRANSFUSION

The mechanisms underlying the coagulopathy of trauma are complex.[36] They include dilution or consumption of clotting factors, intravascular coagulation, fibrinolysis, hypothermia, acidosis, inflammation, and other factors. Although prothrombin time, activated partial thromboplastin time, and platelet counts are typically used to monitor coagulation status, thromboelastography (TEG) or rotational thromboelastometry may better represent overall clotting function and allow for more targeted therapy. Traditionally, management of the coagulopathy has been reactionary, i.e., administering FFP, cryoprecipitate, platelets and calcium once the patient is coagulopathic. Military and civilian data suggests that a more proactive approach may be beneficial.[37–51] The unavailability of fresh whole blood has resulted in the use of a "hemostatic resuscitation" or "damage control resuscitation" approach that involves the administration of FFP, platelets, and PRBC in a 1:1:1 ratio (see Table 77.1). In addition, higher early infusion rates for FFP and platelets may be associated with improved survival.[49,51] These retrospective studies have been criticized for potential survival bias and other studies have not demonstrated a positive effect.[46] For patients who do not require massive transfusion, in particular, the administration of FFP is associated with an increased risk of complications, including acute respiratory distress syndrome, multiple organ failure, pneumonia, and sepsis.[52–55]

Several studies of specific massive transfusion protocols have suggested benefit compared to historic controls.[56–58] In a prospective, randomized trial, a 1:1:1 ratio of FFP:platelets:PRBCs was shown to be superior to a 1:1:2 ratio in terms of 24-hour mortality from bleeding, but no difference in 24-hour or 30-day all-cause mortality.[4] The Prehospital Air Medical Plasma trial demonstrated that early plasma administration (during air medical transport) improved survival and decreased prothrombin-time ratio in patients at risk for hemorrhagic shock.[59]

This hemostatic resuscitation strategy is most likely to benefit patients who are at a high risk of requiring a massive transfusion. The ABC score, which utilizes easily-obtained clinical parameters in the ED (penetrating mechanism, systolic blood pressure of ≤ 90 mm Hg, heart rate of ≥ 120 bpm, or positive focused assessment by sonography for trauma) is a tool that may predict the need for massive transfusions (area under the receiver operating characteristic curve of 0.84).[60] Because vital signs are constantly changing in critically injured patients, integration of continuous vital sign data, even over as short a time as 5 min, can be predictive of the need for massive transfusions.[61]

Tranexamic acid (TxA), an inhibitor of fibrinolysis, can decrease transfusion requirements during a variety of elective surgical procedures. The doubled-blind Clinical Randomization of an Antifibrinolytic in Significant Hemorrhage 2 (CRASH-2) study compared TxA with placebo in 20,211 patients in 274 hospitals in 40 countries.[62] The study demonstrated that TxA significantly decreased mortality without increasing the risk of vascular occlusive events. Subset analysis of this study revealed that the benefit was limited to patients who received TxA in the first 3 hs following trauma; waiting longer resulted in worse outcomes.

The role for other agents to reverse the complex coagulopathy of trauma, including activated Factor VIIa, fibrinogen concentrate, and prothrombin complex concentrates, remains unclear. Recombinant activated Factor VII is seldom used in trauma patients because of cost and lack of clear benefit.[63] Hypofibrinogenemia, typically managed with cryoprecipitate, is common in trauma patients. Fibrinogen products are available in some countries and may have benefits.[64–67] Prothrombin complex concentrates are available, although data on efficacy in the absence of warfarin-induced coagulopathy are variable.[68–70] Lyophilized plasma is another product that shows promise.[71] Perhaps titration of these agents using readily-available, point-of-care tests, such as thromboelastometry, could, by identifying patients with a hyperfibrinolytic phenotype, prove useful.[72] These patients may be harmed by TxA, whereas patients with a hypofibrinolytic phenotype may benefit from TxA.[73] The most recent guidelines from the Eastern Association for the Surgery of Trauma suggested that a massive transfusion/damage control resuscitation protocol should be instituted and that high ratios of FFP and platelets to PRBCs should be administered.[74] Early use of TxA was conditionally recommended. The guideline did not recommend for or against the use of activated Factor VII.

After the initial resuscitation and achievement of euvolemia, the indication for blood transfusion is based primarily upon hemoglobin level. In the general ICU population, a restrictive transfusion threshold (Hb <7 g/dL) was as good, and possibly better, than a more liberal threshold (<10 g/dL).[75] A subset analysis of trauma patients found no differences in outcomes between the two transfusion thresholds, suggesting that the more restrictive strategy was safe.[76] Several studies have demonstrated strong associations between the amount of blood transfused in trauma patients and injury severity score (ISS), organ failure, length of stay and mortality.[5,77–79] Administration of blood stored for more prolonged periods of time may increase risk of infection. However, large prospective investigations, such as the ABLE, INFORM, and TRANSFUSE trials, suggest that age of transfused blood has no negative effect on mortality in heterogeneous patient populations.[80–82] Though some have postulated that complications of transfusions are related to leukocytes, leukocyte-depleted PRBCs seem to provide no benefit.[83,84] Additionally, a more restrictive fluid resuscitation approach, along with a lung-protective strategy, may decrease the risk of ARDS following trauma.[85]

UNCONTROLLED HEMORRHAGIC SHOCK

Minimizing hypoperfusion and tissue ischemia would seem to dictate rapid volume resuscitation in the actively bleeding patient, but this strategy could worsen bleeding and increase mortality. This has been demonstrated in a variety of animal models.[86] The optimal blood pressure goal during uncontrolled HS depends upon the injury pattern, as well as the type and rate of fluid resuscitation. The safe duration of this limited, hypotensive fluid resuscitation is similarly unclear.

In a retrospective study, Kaweski, et al. found that prehospital administration of fluids had no impact on mortality compared to no fluid administration[87] (see Table 77.1). A randomized clinical trial by Bickell, et al. demonstrated slightly improved survival (70% vs. 62%) in delayed resuscitation from HS.[88] In contrast, Turner, et al., found no difference in outcome comparing standard prehospital fluid resuscitation and no fluid resuscitation strategies.[89]

Dutton, et al., explored hypotensive resuscitation in hospital patients who had sustained either blunt or penetrating trauma and were unable to demonstrate any difference in outcome, although survival was high in both groups.[90] In a separate study, these investigators found that initial aggressive fluid resuscitation in severely injured trauma victims using the Rapid Infusion System increased the risk of dying almost 5-fold.[91]

Duke, et al., retrospectively examined the effect of "restrictive" fluid resuscitation in conjunction with a damage control resuscitation and damage control surgery strategy and found that the restrictive approach was associated with improved survival.[92] Morrison, et al., demonstrated that hypotensive resuscitation of trauma patients in the operating room was associated with less coagulopathy and

blood transfusion requirements, as well as decreased early deaths from hemorrhage.[93]

In a metaanalysis, Wang, et al., reviewed four randomized clinical trials and seven observational studies comparing a restrictive fluid resuscitation strategy and a more liberal strategy in trauma patients.[94] They found an increased risk of mortality with a liberal strategy in both randomized controlled trials and observational studies.

Schreiber, et al., prospectively evaluated a controlled, restrictive crystalloid resuscitation strategy (goal systolic blood pressure of 70 mm Hg vs. 110 mm Hg) until hemostasis was achieved in hypotensive trauma patients.[95] The restrictive strategy was associated with decreased early mortality in blunt trauma patients but did not affect ventilator or ICU free days, acute kidney injury, or hospital mortality. No differences were found with victims of penetrating trauma. They suggested that larger studies are needed to more clearly define the blood pressure goals for restrictive, hypotensive resuscitation.

ENDPOINTS OF RESUSCITATION

Once hemostasis is achieved, the first goal of fluid resuscitation in hypotensive trauma patients is to restore end organ perfusion. While normalization of blood pressure, heart rate and urine output is initially sought, vital signs alone may not identify "compensated shock", leaving some vascular beds inadequately perfused. Other clinical data are needed to identify this state and monitor further resuscitation.

Initially, small randomized trials attempting to replicate the high cardiac output, oxygen delivery, and oxygen consumption that characterized survivors of traumatic HS [96,97] suggested that these supranormal oxygen delivery values could improve survival.[98,99] Others have not been able to replicate these results.[100] In more recent studies, decreasing the oxygen delivery goals produced similar outcomes with less fluid and blood product administration.[101]

Systemic evidence of inadequate tissue perfusion, i.e., compensated shock, can be identified by evidence of anaerobic metabolism. Lactate levels, base deficit, and serum bicarbonate correlate with survival.[102–106] Lactate levels can be measured at the point-of-care, even during air medical transport[107] and may assist with triage. Failure to rapidly normalize these parameters is associated with increased mortality,[108,109] though not all studies have demonstrated good correlation between lactate levels and mortality.[110]

The compensatory reserve index (CRI) applies an advanced machine learning algorithm to arterial waveform characteristics and generates a noninvasive measure of the body's capacity to compensate for hypoperfusion. In trauma patients at risk for hemorrhage, Johnson, et al., demonstrated that the CRI correlates relatively well with lactate in terms of identifying hypoperfusion and, perhaps, improved perfusion with resuscitation.[111]

Near-infrared spectroscopy[112] and heart rate variability[113] hold promise as continuous, noninvasive parameters to optimize resuscitation. Arterial pressure waveform analysis can help predict volume responsiveness in critically ill patients.[114] The use of ultrasonographic/echocardiographic estimation of volume status, expected volume responsiveness, and cardiac performance has become standard in the ICU.[115,116] Recent studies show that the Focused Rapid Echocardiographic Evaluation (FREE) does, in fact, alter care among ICU patients by providing clinical data that may not otherwise be easily obtained at the bedside.[117] To date, none of these strategies have been shown to outperform standard clinical and acid-base parameters. A recent Eastern Association for the Surgery of Trauma guideline suggested that focused ultrasound and arterial pressure waveform analysis could be useful for predicting volume responsiveness and may predict complications and organ failures, but not mortality.[6]

SUMMARY

Optimal early management of trauma victims with HS requires simultaneous efforts at hemostasis and fluid resuscitation. Balanced crystalloids are the initial plasma substitutes of choice. Early transfusions of PRBC, FFP and platelets in a 1:1:1 manner are life-saving, but should be limited to the quantity that is absolutely necessary. While the patient is actively bleeding, fluid resuscitation should be limited to not aggravate bleeding, but still maintain a pulse and adequate organ perfusion. Once hemostasis has been achieved, fluid resuscitation should be aggressive to normalize hemodynamics and mitigate anaerobic metabolism as evidenced by improving lactate or base deficit.

AUTHORS' RECOMMENDATIONS

- HS causes tissue ischemia followed by reperfusion injury and a systemic inflammatory response that can lead to multiple organ system dysfunction and death.
- Crystalloids remain the initial fluid of choice for resuscitation of patients with mild HS. Blood products should be administered early in patients with severe shock.
- During active hemorrhage, fluid resuscitation should be limited to avoid exacerbating hemorrhage. Once hemostasis has been achieved, fluid resuscitation should be aggressive to reverse tissue ischemia.
- Following hemostasis, transfusions should be limited to maintain hemoglobin >7 gm/dL. FFP and platelets should be administered to correct the coagulopathy of trauma.

REFERENCES

1. McClelland RN, Shires GT, Baxter CR, Coln CD, Carrico J. Balanced salt solution in the treatment of hemorrhagic shock. Studies in dogs. *JAMA*. 1967;199(11):830-834.
2. Bulger EM, Cuschieri J, Warner K, Maier RV. Hypertonic resuscitation modulates the inflammatory response in patients with traumatic hemorrhagic shock. *Ann Surg*. 2007;245(4):635-641.
3. Kasotakis G, Sideris A, Yang Y, et al. Aggressive early crystalloid resuscitation adversely affects outcomes in adult blunt trauma patients: an analysis of the Glue Grant database. *J Trauma Acute Care Surg*. 2013;74:1215-1222.
4. Holcomb JB, Tilley BC, Baraniuk S, et al. Transfusion of plasma, platelets, and red blood cells in a 1:1:1 vs. a 1:1:2 ratio and mortality in patients with severe trauma: the PROPPR randomized clinical trial. *JAMA*. 2015;313(5):471-482.
5. Malone DL, Dunne J, Tracy JK, Putnam AT, Scalea TM, Napolitano LM. Blood transfusion, independent of shock severity, is associated with worse outcome in trauma. *J Trauma*. 2003;54(5):898-905.
6. Plurad DS, Chiu W, Raja AS, et al. Monitoring modalities and assessment of fluid status: a practice management guideline from the Eastern Association for the Surgery of Trauma. *J Trauma Acute Care Surg*. 2017;84:37-49.
7. American College of Surgeons Committee on Trauma. Shock. In: *Advanced Trauma Life Support® Student Course Manual*. 10th ed. Chicago, IL: American College of Surgeons; 2018:42-61.
8. Tompkins RG. Genomics of injury: the Glue Grant experience. *J Trauma Acute Care Surg*. 2015;78:671-686.
9. Tisherman SA, Schmicker RH, Brasel KJ, et al. Detailed description of all deaths in both the shock and traumatic brain injury hypertonic saline trials of the Resuscitation Outcomes Consortium. *Ann Surg*. 2015;261(3):586-590.
10. Stanton K, Alam HB, Rhee P, et al. Human polymorphonuclear cell death after exposure to resuscitation fluids in vitro: apoptosis versus necrosis. *J Trauma*. 2003;54(6):1065-1074.
11. Alam HB, Stanton K, Koustova E, et al. Effect of different resuscitation strategies on neutrophil activation in a swine model of hemorrhagic shock. *Resuscitation*. 2004;60(1):91-99.
12. Koustova E, Stanton K, Gushchin V, Alam HB, Stegalkina S, Rhee PM. Effects of lactated Ringer's solutions on human leukocytes. *J Trauma*. 2002;52(5):872-878.
13. Self WH, Semler MW, Wanderer JP, et al. Balanced crystalloids versus saline in noncritically ill adults. *N Engl J Med*. 2018;378(9):819-828.
14. Young P, Bailey M, Beasley R, et al. Effect of a buffered crystalloid solution vs. saline on acute kidney injury among patients in the intensive care unit: the SPLIT randomized clinical trial. *JAMA*. 2015;314:1701-1710.
15. Koustova E, Rhee P, Hancock T, et al. Ketone and pyruvate Ringer's solutions decrease pulmonary apoptosis in a rat model of severe hemorrhagic shock and resuscitation. *Surgery*. 2003;134(2):267-274.
16. Ayuste EC, Chen H, Koustova E, et al. Hepatic and pulmonary apoptosis after hemorrhagic shock in swine can be reduced through modifications of conventional Ringer's solution. *J Trauma*. 2006;60(1):52-63.
17. Holcroft JW, Vassar MJ, Perry CA, Gannaway WL, Kramer GC. Use of a 7.5% NaCl/6% Dextran 70 solution in the resuscitation of injured patients in the emergency room. *Prog Clin Biol Res*. 1989;299:331-338.
18. Maningas PA, Mattox KL, Pepe PE, Jones RL, Feliciano DV, Burch JM. Hypertonic saline-dextran solutions for the prehospital management of traumatic hypotension. *Am J Surg*. 1989;157(5):528-533.
19. Vassar MJ, Perry CA, Holcroft JW. Analysis of potential risks associated with 7.5% sodium chloride resuscitation of traumatic shock. *Arch Surg*. 1990;125(10):1309-1315.
20. Mattox KL, Maningas PA, Moore EE, et al. Prehospital hypertonic saline/dextran infusion for post-traumatic hypotension. The U.S.A. Multicenter Trial. *Ann Surg*. 1991;213(5):482-491.

21. Vassar MJ, Perry CA, Gannaway WL, Holcroft JW. 7.5% sodium chloride/dextran for resuscitation of trauma patients undergoing helicopter transport. *Arch Surg.* 1991;126(9):1065-1072.

22. Younes RN, Aun F, Accioly CQ, Casale LP, Szajnbok I, Birolini D. Hypertonic solutions in the treatment of hypovolemic shock: a prospective, randomized study in patients admitted to the emergency room. *Surgery.* 1992;111(4):380-385.

23. Vassar MJ, Perry CA, Holcroft JW. Prehospital resuscitation of hypotensive trauma patients with 7.5% NaCl versus 7.5% NaCl with added dextran: a controlled trial. *J Trauma.* 1993;34(5):622-632.

24. Wade CE, Kramer GC, Grady JJ, Fabian TC, Younes RN. Efficacy of hypertonic 7.5% saline and 6% dextran-70 in treating trauma: a meta-analysis of controlled clinical studies. *Surgery.* 1997;122(3):609-616.

25. Mauritz W, Schimetta W, Oberreither S, Pölz W. Are hypertonic hyperoncotic solutions safe for prehospital small-volume resuscitation? Results of a prospective observational study. *Eur J Emerg Med.* 2002;9(4):315-319.

26. Wade CE, Grady JJ, Kramer GC. Efficacy of hypertonic saline dextran fluid resuscitation for patients with hypotension from penetrating trauma. *J Trauma.* 2003;54(5 suppl):S144-S148.

27. Rizoli SB, Rhind SG, Shek PN, et al. The immunomodulatory effects of hypertonic saline resuscitation in patients sustaining traumatic hemorrhagic shock: a randomized, controlled, double-blinded trial. *Ann Surg.* 2006;243(1):47-57.

28. Bulger EM, Jurkovich GJ, Nathens AB, et al. Hypertonic resuscitation of hypovolemic shock after blunt trauma: a randomized controlled trial. *Arch Surg.* 2007;143(2):139-148.

29. Bulger EM, May S, Kerby JD, et al. Out-of-hospital hypertonic resuscitation after traumatic hypovolemic shock: a randomized, placebo controlled trial. *Ann Surg.* 2011;253(3):431-441.

30. Albumin Reviewers. Human albumin solution for resuscitation and volume expansion in critically ill patients. *Cochrane Database Syst Rev.* 2011(10):CD001208.

31. Myburgh JA, Finfer S, Bellomo R, et al. Hydroxyethyl starch or saline for fluid resuscitation in intensive care. *N Engl J Med.* 2012;367(20):1901-1911.

32. Zarychanski R, Abou-Setta AM, Turgeon AF, et al. Association of hydroxyethyl starch administration with mortality and acute kidney injury in critically ill patients requiring volume resuscitation: a systematic review and meta-analysis. *JAMA.* 2013;309(7):678-688.

33. Sloan EP, Koenigsberg M, Gens D, et al. Diaspirin cross-linked hemoglobin (DCLHb) in the treatment of severe traumatic hemorrhagic shock: a randomized controlled efficacy trial. *JAMA.* 1999;282(19):1857-1864.

34. Gould SA, Moore EE, Hoyt DB, et al. The first randomized trial of human polymerized hemoglobin as a blood substitute in acute trauma and emergent surgery. *J Am Coll Surg.* 1998;187(2):113-120.

35. Moore EE, Moore FA, Fabian TC, et al. Human polymerized hemoglobin for the treatment of hemorrhagic shock when blood is unavailable: the USA multicenter trial. *J Am Coll Surg.* 2009;208(1):1-13.

36. Hess JR, Brohi K, Dutton RP, et al. The coagulopathy of trauma: a review of mechanisms. *J Trauma.* 2008;65(4):748-754.

37. Borgman MA, Spinella PC, Perkins JG, et al. The ratio of blood products transfused affects mortality in patients receiving massive transfusions at a combat support hospital. *J Trauma.* 2007;63(4):805-813.

38. Maegele M, Lefering R, Paffrath T, et al. Red-blood-cell to plasma ratios transfused during massive transfusion are associated with mortality in severe multiple injury: a retrospective analysis from the Trauma Registry of the Deutsche Gesellschaft für Unfallchirurgie. *Vox sang.* 2008;95(2):112-119.

39. Holcomb JB, Wade CE, Michalek JE, et al. Increased plasma and platelet to red blood cell ratios improves outcome in 466 massively transfused civilian trauma patients. *Ann Surg.* 2008;248(3):447-458.

40. Zink KA, Sambasivan CN, Holcomb JB, Chisholm G, Schreiber MA. A high ratio of plasma and platelets to packed red blood cells in the first 6 hours of massive transfusion improves outcomes in a large multicenter study. *Am J Surg.* 2009;197(5):565-570.

41. Teixeira PG, Inaba K, Shulman I, et al. Impact of plasma transfusion in massively transfused trauma patients. *J Trauma.* 2009;66(3):693-697.

42. Riskin DJ, Tsai TC, Riskin L, et al. Massive transfusion protocols: the role of aggressive resuscitation versus product ratio in mortality reduction. *J Am Coll Surg.* 2009;209(2):198-205.

43. Shaz BH, Dente CJ, Nicholas J, et al. Increased number of coagulation products in relationship to red blood cell products transfused improves mortality in trauma patients. *Transfusion.* 2010;50(2):493-500.

44. Inaba K, Lustenberger T, Rhee P, et al. The impact of platelet transfusion in massively transfused trauma patients. *J Am Coll Surg.* 2010;211(5):573-579.

45. de Biasi AR, Stansbury LG, Dutton RP, Stein DM, Scalea TM, Hess JR. Blood product use in trauma resuscitation: plasma deficit versus plasma ratio as predictors of mortality in trauma (CME). *Transfusion.* 2011;51(9):1925-1932.

46. Wafaisade A, Maegele M, Lefering R, et al. High plasma to red blood cell ratios are associated with lower mortality rates in patients receiving multiple transfusion (4≤red blood cell units<10) during acute trauma resuscitation. *J Trauma.* 2011;70:81-89.

47. Rajasekhar A, Gowing R, Zarychanski R, et al. Survival of trauma patients after massive red blood cell transfusion using a high or low red blood cell to plasma transfusion ratio. *Crit Care Med.* 2011;39(6):1507-1513.

48. Holcomb JB, Zarzabal LA, Michalek JE, et al. Increased platelet:RBC ratios are associated with improved survival after massive transfusion. *J Trauma.* 2011;71(2 suppl 3):S318-S328.

49. Halmin M, Boström F, Brattström O, et al. Effect of plasma-to-RBC ratios in trauma patients: a cohort study with time-dependent data. *Crit Care Med.* 2013;41:1905-1914.

50. Holcomb JB, del Junco DJ, Fox EE, et al. The Prospective, Observational, Multicenter, Major Trauma Transfusion (PROMMTT) study: comparative effectiveness of a time-varying treatment with competing risks. *JAMA Surg.* 2013;148:127-136.

51. Simms ER, Hennings DL, Hauch A, et al. Impact of infusion rates of fresh frozen plasma and platelets during the first 180 minutes of resuscitation. *J Am Coll Surg.* 2014;219(2):181-188.

52. Scalea TM, Bochicchio KM, Lumpkins K, et al. Early aggressive use of fresh frozen plasma does not improve outcome in critically injured trauma patients. *Ann Surg.* 2008;248(4):578-584.

53. Sarani B, Dunkman WJ, Dean L, Sonnad S, Rohrbach JI, Gracias VH. Transfusion of fresh frozen plasma in critically ill surgical patients is associated with an increased risk of infection. *Crit Care Med.* 2008;36:1114-1118.

54. Watson GA, Sperry JL, Rosengart MR, et al. Fresh frozen plasma is independently associated with a higher risk of multiple organ

failure and acute respiratory distress syndrome. *J Trauma*. 2009; 67:221-230.

55. Inaba K, Branco BC, Rhee P, et al. Impact of plasma transfusion in trauma patients who do not require massive transfusion. *J Am Coll Surg*. 2010;210:957-965.

56. Cotton BA, Reddy N, Hatch QM, et al. Damage control resuscitation is associated with a reduction in resuscitation volumes and improvement in survival in 390 damage control laparotomy patients. *Ann Surg*. 2011;254(4):598-605.

57. Duchesne JC, Barbeau JM, Islam TM, Wahl G, Greiffenstein P, McSwain Jr NE. Damage control resuscitation: from emergency department to the operating room. *Am Surg*. 2011; 77(2):201-206.

58. Johansson PI, Stensballe J. Effect of haemostatic control resuscitation on mortality in massively bleeding patients: a before and after study. *Vox Sang*. 2009;96(2):111-118.

59. Sperry JL, Guyette FX, Brown JB, et al. Prehospital plasma during air medical transport in trauma patients at risk for hemorrhagic shock. *N Engl J Med*. 2018;379:315-326.

60. Nunez TC, Voskresensky IV, Dossett LA, Shinall R, Dutton WD, Cotton BA. Early prediction of massive transfusion in trauma: simple as ABC (assessment of blood consumption)? *J Trauma*. 2009;66(2):346-352.

61. Parimi N, Hu PF, Mackenzie CF, et al. Automated continuous vital signs predict use of uncrossed matched blood and massive transfusion following trauma. *J Trauma Acute Care Surg*. 2016;80:897-906.

62. CRASH-2 trial collaborators. Effects of tranexamic acid on death, vascular occlusive events, and blood transfusion in trauma patients with significant haemorrhage (CRASH-2): a randomised, placebo-controlled trial. *Lancet*. 2010;376(9734): 23-32.

63. Hauser CJ, Boffard K, Dutton R, et al. Results of the CONTROL trial: efficacy and safety of recombinant activated Factor VII in the management of refractory traumatic hemorrhage. *J Trauma*. 2010;69(3):489-500.

64. Meyer MA, Ostrowski SR, Windeløv NA, Johansson PI. Fibrinogen concentrates for bleeding trauma patients: what is the evidence? *Vox Sang*. 2011;101(3):185-190.

65. Ponschab M, Voelckel W, Pavelka M, Schlimp CJ, Schöchl H. Effect of coagulation factor concentrate administration on ROTEM® parameters in major trauma. *Scand J Trauma Resusc Emerg Med*. 2015;23:84.

66. Yamamoto K, Yamaguchi A, Sawano M, et al. Pre-emptive administration of fibrinogen concentrate contributes to improved prognosis in patients with severe trauma. *Trauma Surg Acute Care Open*. 2016;1(1):e000037.

67. McQuilten ZK, Bailey M, Cameron PA, et al. Fibrinogen concentration and use of fibrinogen supplementation with cryoprecipitate in patients with critical bleeding receiving massive transfusion: a bi-national cohort study. *Br J Haematol*. 2017; 179(1):131-141.

68. Joseph B, Aziz H, Pandit V, et al. Prothrombin complex concentrate versus fresh-frozen plasma for reversal of coagulopathy of trauma: is there a difference? *World J Surg*. 2014;38(8): 1875-1881.

69. Matsushima K, Benjamin E, Demetriades D. Prothrombin complex concentrate in trauma patients. *Am J Surg*. 2015;209: 413-417.

70. Jehan F, Aziz H, O'Keeffe T, et al. The role of 4-factor prothrombin complex concentrate in coagulopathy of trauma: a propensity matched analysis. *J Trauma Acute Care Surg*. 2018;85(1):18-24.

71. Garrigue D, Godier A, Glacet A. et al. French lyophilized plasma versus fresh frozen plasma for the initial management of trauma-induced coagulopathy: a randomized open-label trial. *J Thromb Haemost*. 2018;16(3):481-489.

72. Schöchl H, Nienaber U, Hofer G, et al. Goal-directed coagulation management of major trauma patients using thromboelastometry (ROTEM)-guided administration of fibrinogen concentrate and prothrombin complex concentrate. *Crit Care*. 2010;14(2):R55.

73. Moore HB, Moore EE, Huebner BR, et al. Tranexamic acid is associated with increased mortality in patients with physiological fibrinolysis. *J Surg Res*. 2017;220:438-443.

74. Cannon JW, Khan MA, Raja AS, et al. Damage control resuscitation in patients with severe traumatic hemorrhage: a practice management guideline from the Eastern Association for the Surgery of Trauma. *J Trauma Acute Care Surg*. 2017;82(3):605-617.

75. Hébert PC, Wells G, Blajchman MA, et al. A multicenter, randomized, controlled clinical trial of transfusion requirements in critical care. Transfusion Requirements in Critical Care Investigators, Canadian Critical Care Trials Group. *N Engl J Med*. 1999;340(6):409-417.

76. McIntyre L, Hebert PC, Wells G, et al. Is a restrictive transfusion strategy safe for resuscitated and critically ill trauma patients? *J Trauma*. 2004;57(3):563-568.

77. Dunne JR, Malone DL, Tracy JK, Napolitano LM. Allogenic blood transfusion in the first 24 hours after trauma is associated with increased systemic inflammatory response syndrome (SIRS) and death. *Surg Infect (Larchmt)*. 2004;5(4):395-404.

78. Dunne JR, Riddle MS, Danko J, Hayden R, Petersen K. Blood transfusion is associated with infection and increased resource utilization in combat casualties. *Am Surg*. 2006;72(7):619-625.

79. Silverboard H, Aisiku I, Martin GS, Adams M, Rozycki G, Moss M. The role of acute blood transfusion in the development of acute respiratory distress syndrome in patients with severe trauma. *J Trauma*. 2005;59(3):717-723.

80. Lacroix J, Hébert PC, Fergusson DA, et al. Age of transfused blood in critically ill adults. *N Engl J Med*. 2015;372(15):1410-1418.

81. Heddle NM, Cook RJ, Arnold DM, et al. Effect of short-term vs. long-term blood storage on mortality after transfusion. *N Engl J Med*. 2016;375(20):1937-1945.

82. Cooper DJ, McQuilten ZK, Nichol A, et al. Age of red cells for transfusion and outcomes in critically ill adults. *N Engl J Med*. 2017;377(19):1858-1867.

83. Nathens AB, Nester TA, Rubenfeld GD, Nirula R, Gernsheimer TB. The effects of leukoreduced blood transfusion on infection risk following injury: a randomized controlled trial. *Shock*. 2006;26(4):342-347.

84. Phelan HA, Sperry JL, Friese RS. Leukoreduction before red blood cell transfusion has no impact on mortality in trauma patients. *J Surg Res*. 2007;138(1):32-36.

85. Plurad D, Martin M, Green D, et al. The decreasing incidence of late posttraumatic acute respiratory distress syndrome: the potential role of lung protective ventilation and conservative transfusion practice. *J Trauma*. 2007;63(1):1-7.

86. Mapstone J, Roberts I, Evans P. Fluid resuscitation strategies: a systematic review of animal trials. *J Trauma*. 2003;55(3): 571-589.

87. Kaweski SM, Sise MJ, Virgilio RW. The effect of prehospital fluids on survival in trauma patients. *J Trauma*. 1990; 30(10):1215-1218.

88. Bickell WH, Wall Jr MJ, Pepe PE, et al. Immediate versus delayed fluid resuscitation for hypotensive patients with

penetrating torso injuries. *N Engl J Med.* 1994;331(17): 1105-1109.

89. Turner J, Nicholl J, Webber L, Cox H, Dixon S, Yates D. A randomised controlled trial of prehospital intravenous fluid replacement therapy in serious trauma. *Health Technol Assess.* 2000;4:1-57.

90. Dutton RP, Mackenzie CF, Scalea TM. Hypotensive resuscitation during active hemorrhage: impact on in-hospital mortality. *J Trauma.* 2002;52(6):1141-1146.

91. Hambly PR, Dutton RP. Excess mortality associated with the use of a rapid infusion system at a level 1 trauma center. *Resuscitation.* 1996;31(2):127-133.

92. Duke MD, Guidry C, Guice J, et al. Restrictive fluid resuscitation in combination with damage control resuscitation: time for adaptation. *J Trauma Acute Care Surg.* 2012;73(3):674-678.

93. Morrison CA, Carrick MM, Norman MA, et al. Hypotensive resuscitation strategy reduces transfusion requirements and severe postoperative coagulopathy in trauma patients with hemorrhagic shock: preliminary results of a randomized controlled trial. *J Trauma.* 2011;70(3):652-663.

94. Wang CH, Hsieh WH, Chou HC, et al. Liberal versus restricted fluid resuscitation strategies in trauma patients: a systematic review and meta-analysis of randomized controlled trials and observational studies. *Crit Care Med.* 2014;42(4):954-961.

95. Schreiber MA, Meier EN, Tisherman SA, et al. A controlled resuscitation strategy is feasible and safe in hypotensive trauma patients: results of a prospective randomized pilot trial. *J Trauma Acute Care Surg.* 2015;78(4):687-695.

96. Shoemaker WC, Montgomery ES, Kaplan E, Elwyn DH. Physiologic patterns in surviving and nonsurviving shock patients. Use of sequential cardiorespiratory variables in defining criteria for therapeutic goals and early warning of death. *Arch Surg.* 1973;106(5):630-636.

97. Bishop MH, Shoemaker WC, Appel PL, et al. Relationship between supranormal circulatory values, time delays, and outcome in severely traumatized patients. *Crit Care Med.* 1993;21(1):56-63.

98. Bishop MH, Shoemaker WC, Appel PL, et al. Prospective, randomized trial of survivor values of cardiac index, oxygen delivery, and oxygen consumption as resuscitation endpoints in severe trauma. *J Trauma.* 1995;38(5):780-787.

99. Fleming A, Bishop M, Shoemaker W, et al. Prospective trial of supranormal values as goals of resuscitation in severe trauma. *Arch Surg.* 1992;127(10):1175-1179.

100. Velmahos GC, Demetriades D, Shoemaker WC, et al. Endpoints of resuscitation of critically injured patients: normal or supranormal? A prospective randomized trial. *Ann Surg.* 2000;232(3):409-418.

101. McKinley BA, Kozar RA, Cocanour CS, et al. Normal versus supranormal oxygen delivery goals in shock resuscitation: the response is the same. *J Trauma.* 2002;53(5):825-832.

102. Rutherford EJ, Morris Jr JA, Reed GW, Hall KS. Base deficit stratifies mortality and determines therapy. *J Trauma.* 1992; 33(3):417-423.

103. Davis JW, Shackford SR, Mackersie RC, Hoyt DB. Base deficit as a guide to volume resuscitation. *J Trauma.* 1988;28(10): 1464-1467.

104. Davis JW, Kaups KL, Parks SN. Base deficit is superior to pH in evaluating clearance of acidosis after traumatic shock. *J Trauma.* 1998;44(1):114-118.

105. Kincaid EH, Miller PR, Meredith JW, Rahman N, Chang MC. Elevated arterial base deficit in trauma patients: a marker of impaired oxygen utilization. *J Am Coll Surg.* 1998;187(4): 384-392.

106. Cerović O, Golubović V, Spec-Marn A, Kremzar B, Vidmar G. Relationship between injury severity and lactate levels in severely injured patients. *Intensive Care Med.* 2003;29(8): 1300-1305.

107. Brown JB, Lerner EB, Sperry JL, Billiar TR, Peitzman AB, Guyette FX. Prehospital lactate improves accuracy of prehospital criteria for designating trauma activation level. *J Trauma Acute Care Surg.* 2016;81:445-452.

108. Odom SR, Howell MD, Silva GS, et al. Lactate clearance as a predictor of mortality in trauma patients. *J Trauma Acute Care Surg.* 2013;74:999-1004.

109. Dezman ZD, Comer AC, Smith GS, Narayan M, Scalea TM, Hirshon JM. Failure to clear elevated lactate predicts 24-hour mortality in trauma patients. *J Trauma Acute Care Surg.* 2015; 79:580-585.

110. Pal JD, Victorino GP, Twomey P, Liu TH, Bullard MK, Harken AH. Admission serum lactate levels do not predict mortality in the acutely injured patient. *J Trauma.* 2006;60(3):583-587.

111. Johnson MC, Alarhayem A, Convertino V, et al. Comparison of compensatory reserve and arterial lactate as markers of shock and resuscitation. *J Trauma Acute Care Surg.* 2017;83:603-608.

112. Cohn SM. Near-infrared spectroscopy: potential clinical benefits in surgery. *J Am Coll Surg.* 2007;205(2):322-332.

113. Ryan ML, Ogilvie MP, Pereira BM, et al. Heart rate variability is an independent predictor of morbidity and mortality in hemodynamically stable trauma patients. *J Trauma.* 2011; 70(6):1371-1380.

114. Cecconi M, Monti G, Hamilton MA, et al. Efficacy of functional hemodynamic parameters in predicting fluid responsiveness with pulse power analysis in surgical patients. *Minerva Anestesiol.* 2012;78(5):527-533.

115. Ferrada P, Murthi S, Anand RJ, Bochicchio GV, Scalea T. Transthoracic focused rapid echocardiographic examination: real-time evaluation of fluid status in critically ill trauma patients. *J Trauma.* 2011;70(1):56-62.

116. Murthi SB, Hess JR, Hess A, Stansbury LG, Scalea TM. Focused rapid echocardiographic evaluation versus vascular cather-based assessment of cardiac output and function in critically ill trauma patients. *J Trauma Acute Care Surg.* 2012;72(5):1158-1164.

117. Murthi SB, Markandaya M, Fang R, et al. Focused comprehensive, quantitative, functionally based echocardiographic evaluation in the critical care unit is feasible and impacts care. *Mil Med.* 2015;180(3 suppl):74-79.

78

How Do I Diagnose and Treat Major Gastrointestinal Bleeding?

Charles R. Vasquez and Niels D. Martin

INTRODUCTION

The incidence of hospitalizations for acute upper gastrointestinal (GI) bleeding has declined in the United States over the past several decades, from approximately 100 per 100,000 population in the 1990s to 60 per 100,000 population by 2012. This change has largely been driven by decreased rates of bleeding from gastritis and peptic ulcer disease (PUD).[1] Hospitalization for acute lower GI bleeding has also declined from 41 to 35 per 100,000 population. In this case, the decline is primarily related to decreased rates of diverticular bleeding.[1,2] Overall, mortality from acute GI bleeding is approximately 2–4%. Lower GI bleeding is slightly less common than upper GI bleeding, and increases slightly with age.[1,2] The clinical presentation of upper GI bleeding is extremely varied, from asymptomatic to overt shock with decreased tissue perfusion. Both upper and lower GI bleeding may present with hematochezia, although upper GI bleeds are more likely to present as hematemesis or melena or with weakness, dyspnea, and anemia.

ETIOLOGIES

The most common etiologies of acute bleeding vary by location. PUD, including duodenal ulcers, gastric ulcers and gastritis, account for approximately 50% of cases.[3,4] Other common causes include esophageal and gastric varices (seen in patients with portal hypertension). These are responsible for about 15% of cases. Other rare causes include arteriovenous malformations, Mallory-Weiss tears, tumors, and Dieulafoy lesions. Diverticular disease is the most common cause of lower GI bleeding (30%) and is particularly common in older patients (>65 years). Angiodysplasia (8%) is another condition seen more commonly in older patients. In contrast, hemorrhoids (5%) are seen in a younger population. Other common causes of lower GI bleeding include polyps (18%), malignancies (18%), and colitis (18%). However, roughly 15% of cases are idiopathic (Table 78.1).[4]

Acute GI bleeding can be classified based upon point of origin, with the ligament of Treitz as the major geographic landmark distinguishing the upper GI tract from lower GI tract. Predisposing factors for upper GI bleeds include pharmacologic agents such as aspirin and other antiplatelet medications, nonsteroidal antiinflammatory drugs (NSAIDs), corticosteroids, and anticoagulants, as well as cigarettes and alcohol.[3] Vascular malformations along the GI tract may predispose to acute bleeding, as can coagulopathies, malignancies, and any disease process that alters the GI mucosa (e.g., diverticulosis, inflammatory bowel disease, or esophagitis).[3,4]

EVIDENCE

Management of Nonvariceal Upper Gastrointetsinal Bleeding

Nonvariceal upper GI bleeding is the most common cause of GI bleeding.[3] As with any critically ill patient, immediate hemodynamic resuscitation should occur as needed. A large randomized controlled trial (RCT) of 921 patients with acute upper GI bleeding demonstrated the safety of a restrictive (hemoglobin maintained at >7 g/dL) transfusion strategy relative to a liberal transfusion strategy (Hb maintained at >9 g/dL); indeed, the restrictive approach was associated with 1) improved survival at 6 weeks (95% vs. 91%, hazard ratio 0.55, 95% confidence interval [CI] 0.33–0.92, P =.02), 2) lower rebleeding rates (10% vs. 16%, P = .01) and 3) lower adverse events (40% vs. 48%, P = .02).[5] In retrospective studies on patients taking antiplatelet medications, no benefit was derived from prophylactic platelet transfusion in patients without thrombocytopenia; indeed, prophylactic platelet transfusion may worsen mortality.[6]

The European Society of Gastrointestinal Endoscopy currently recommends initial medical therapy with high-dose intravenous proton pump inhibitors (PPI) while awaiting endoscopy.[7] A systematic review and metaanalysis by Sachar et al. in 2014 did not find a significant benefit of continuous PPI over intermittent PPI therapy.[8]

Administration of a single dose of erythromycin has been associated with improved gastric mucosa visualization, decreased need for repeat endoscopy, decreased red blood cell (RBC) transfusions and a reduced hospital length of stay.[7] The European Society no long recommends routine use of nasogastric aspiration/lavage, as it has low ability to identify severe upper GI bleeding (sensitivity 77% [95% CI 57–90%], specificity 76% [95% CI 32–95%]), which is similar to other clinical and laboratory signs.[7,9] Along the same lines, endotracheal intubation is not recommended prior to

TABLE 78.1 Common Causes of Gastrointestinal Bleeding.

Source	Presentation	Common Causes
Upper gastrointestinal	Hematemesis, melena, hematochezia (uncommon)	Peptic ulcer (duodenal or gastric), varices (esophageal or gastric), Mallory-Weiss tear, acute hemorrhagic gastritis
Lower gastrointestinal	Hematochezia, melena	Diverticular disease, arteriovenous malformation, colitis, neoplasm, benign anorectal disease

endoscopy unless the patient requires intubation for another reason.

Early upper GI endoscopy should be performed within 24 hours after hemodynamic resuscitation. A large retrospective analysis of 400,000 patients demonstrated increased mortality in patients for whom endoscopy was delayed for more than 1 day (OR 1.3, 95% CI 1.26–1.38).[7,10] Very early (<12 hours) endoscopy should be considered in patients with hemodynamic instability despite ongoing resuscitation, bloody emesis/NGT aspirate or with strong contraindications to cessation/interruption of anticoagulation.[7] One retrospective analysis of patients with upper GI bleeding demonstrated that, in a subset of patients with a high Glasgow-Blatchford Score (>12), the time between presentation to endoscopy was the only independent risk factor for mortality and that a cutoff time of 13 hours was best able to discriminate survivors from nonsurvivors.[11]

Endoscopic management begins by identifying potential lesions and classifying them using the Forrest classification system (Table 78.2).

Patients with FIa and FIb lesions should have combination therapy with epinephrine injection and a second mechanical hemostasis modality (e.g., thermal energy device, clip, or sclerotherapy). In a metaanalysis of 19 RCTs (N = 2033 patients), this combination therapy was found to reduce rebleeding (OR 0.53, 95% CI 0.35–0.81) and the need for

TABLE 78.2 Forrest Classification of Upper Gastrointestinal Bleeding.

Class	Lesion
Ia	Spurting hemorrhage
Ib	Oozing hemorrhage
IIa	Nonbleeding visible vessel
IIb	Adherent clot
IIc	Flat pigmented spot
III	Clean base ulcer

emergent surgery (OR 0.68, 95% CI 0.50–0.93) when compared to monotherapy with epinephrine.[7,12]

Following endoscopic therapy, intravenous PPI therapy should be continued for at least 72 hours.[7] In patients at high risk of rebleeding, the long-term use of high-dose esomeprazole (40 mg twice daily) may reduce rebleeding risk when compared to standard dose (40 mg daily).[13] Routine second-look endoscopy does not appear to have a clinical benefit in patients without evidence of recurrent bleeding.[7] However, repeat endoscopy should be performed in patients with evidence of rebleeding. If rebleeding occurs after a second endoscopy, adjunctive diagnostic and therapeutic modalities should be pursued. If an upper GI site of bleeding is confirmed, transcatheter arterial embolization (TAE) should be attempted prior to consideration of surgery. If the bleeding vessel is not identified, it is prudent to perform embolization of the most likely arterial feeder vessel. For esophageal and gastric fundal bleeding, the left gastric artery is the most common arterial supply, whereas suspected duodenal bleeding is best treated by gastro-duodenal artery embolization.[14] A retrospective study of 48 patients who underwent TAE identified anticoagulant or corticosteroid use before admission, vasopressor use at time of TAE, and use of coils only for embolization (vs. coils plus additional embolic material) as significant risk factors for TAE failure.[15]

Surgical therapy remains a treatment of last resort for upper GI bleeding but should be considered in patients who have failed repeated endoscopic treatment and TAE or who develop hemodynamic instability and/or shock despite aggressive resuscitation.[16]

If peptic ulcers are identified on endoscopy, *Helicobacter pylori* testing should be performed in the acute setting.[7] If positive, treatment should be initiated promptly, with the choice of regimen guided by local factors, such as medication availability. Due to an increased false-negative rate of testing in the setting of acute bleeding episodes, patients with a negative test should be retested after four weeks.[7]

Management of Acute Variceal Bleeding

Both endoscopic and pharmacologic therapies are recommended for treatment of acutely bleeding varices.[17,18] General supportive therapy should be initiated in all patients. In addition, pharmacologic therapy aimed at increased splanchnic vasoconstriction is indicated. Currently available medications include vasopressin (often used in combination with nitroglycerin to prevent excessive peripheral vasoconstriction), terlipressin, and somatostatin analogues such as octreotide. A 2003 Cochrane review and clinical guidelines from the American College of Gastroenterology in 2007 did not find sufficient evidence to recommend one agent over the other.[19,20] Antibiotic prophylaxis should be administered, typically with a quinolone (oral or IV), in patients with Child's A cirrhosis and with IV ceftriaxone in patients with Child's B or C cirrhosis or at institutions where there is a high rate of quinolone resistance. This approach has been shown to reduce the risk of spontaneous bacterial peritonitis and other infections and is associated with a reduction in mortality compared to not giving prophylactic antibiotics.[17]

Endoscopic therapy should be performed within 12 hours in patients with suspected variceal hemorrhage. A metaanalysis of 14 studies (N = 1236) comparing endoscopic variceal ligation to sclerotherapy demonstrated that the former was associated with a lower rebleeding rate (relative risk [RR] 0.68, 95% CI 0.57–0.81) and lower complication rate (RR 0.28, 95% CI 0.13–0.58), but no significant difference in mortality (RR 0.95, 95% CI 0.77–1.17).[21] Combined pharmacologic and endoscopic therapy is associated with improved control of bleeding and lower rebleeding rates over the subsequent 5 days relative to either therapy alone. Combination therapy was not, however, associated with a difference in mortality relative to monotherapy.

Approximately 10–20% of patients presenting with acute variceal bleeding will fail standard pharmacologic and endoscopic therapy and should be considered for transjugular intrahepatic portosystemic shunt (TIPS).[17] The use of TIPS preemptively (within 24–72 hours) after initial endoscopic therapy, irrespective of treatment failure, has been studied by several groups in both RCTs and in large observational studies. In Child class C disease, this approach appears to be associated with a reduction in mortality (22% vs. 47%, $P = .002$, number needed to treat of 4.2 (CI 2.6–24.4)).[22]

Small Intestine Bleeding

Isolated small intestine bleeding accounts for 5–10% of all patients presenting with acute GI bleeding.[23] Small intestine bleeding, distal to the ampulla of Vater and proximal to the ileocecal valve, should be considered in patients with GI bleeding who have had normal upper and lower GI endoscopy. In cases of suspected small intestine bleeding, second look endoscopy should be performed. Consideration should be given to performing a push enteroscopy at second-look, in order to evaluate the proximal small intestine beyond the ligament of Treitz, although this typically only allows visualization of an additional 45–90 cm.[23] Video-capsule endoscopy (VCE) should be performed if bleeding is not detected on second look; this approach may also be used as a first-line test for small intestine bleeding. VCE has been shown to have high positive (97%) and high negative (83%) predictive value for GI bleeding.[24] In a metaanalysis, VCE has been shown to increase diagnostic yield (56% vs. 26%) compared to push enteroscopy for small bowel bleeding.[25] VCE should not be performed in patients with suspected intestinal obstruction or strictures. In these patients, CT enterography (CTE) may be considered, with a large metaanalysis demonstrating similar diagnostic yield to VCE (40% vs. 53%).[26]

Balloon-assisted enteroscopy, requiring specialized equipment, may be performed from the mouth or rectum and is an additional technique to facilitate visualization of a longer length of bowel than can be achieved with standard or push enteroscopy, but complete visualization rates are highly variable operator-dependent.[23] Both push enteroscopy and balloon-assisted enteroscopy allow for treatment of identified lesions. The same principles described above for nonvariceal

GI bleeding apply to small bowel lesions. As is the case at other anatomic locations, angiographic embolization or surgical therapy should be considered in cases of refractory bleeding.

Lower Gastrointestinal Bleeding

Classically, lower GI bleeding is classified as confined to the colon and rectum. Initial assessment and management of suspected lower GI bleeding proceeds along the same clinical pathway as upper GI bleeding. If diagnostic uncertainty exists, upper GI bleeding should be ruled out via nasogastric aspiration and lavage.[27] Conversely, the presence of red blood and clots makes lower GI bleeding much more likely.[9] Underlying patient factors associated with poor outcomes include age >60 years, anemia, elevated creatinine, history of diverticulosis or angioectasia and comorbid illnesses.[28] Additionally, patients presenting with hemodynamic instability and ongoing bleeding have more frequent adverse outcomes.

Every effort should be made to perform an adequate bowel preparation prior to colonoscopy to improve diagnostic and therapeutic yield. Without bowel preparation, the technical success rate, as measured by ability to achieve cecal intubation, is low (55–70%).[27]

Urgent colonoscopy should be performed within 24 hours in patients with ongoing bleeding, significant comorbid conditions or high-risk clinical features. One small prospective trial demonstrated an increased rate of definitive diagnosis with urgent colonoscopy.[29] This trial and an additional prospective study did not demonstrate a difference in rebleeding, need for surgery, mortality or cost.[29,30] However, multiple retrospective studies have shown an association between urgent colonoscopy and increased diagnostic and therapeutic yield as well as decreased hospital length of stay. Repeat colonoscopy may be performed in cases of recurrent bleeding. Once bleeding is localized, multiple therapeutic modalities may be utilized. Approaches include injection of dilute epinephrine, thermal devices (e.g., bipolar electrocoagulation, argon plasma coagulation, etc.) or mechanical devices (e.g., endoscopic clips and bands). The authors are not aware of any prospective studies demonstrating superiority of any of the above methods in achieving definitive hemostasis. As such, choice of therapeutic intervention should be guided by the location and etiology of bleeding, local resources and operator experience.[27]

Patients taking NSAIDs, antiplatelet agents and anticoagulants are at increased risk for rebleeding. If possible, NSAIDs should be avoided immediately after a GI bleed. Studies evaluating specific timing in specific clinical situations for resumption of antiplatelet therapy are lacking.

In patients who have failed endoscopic management, adjunctive diagnostic studies such as tagged RBC scintigraphy and CT angiography may aid in the localization of active bleeding. RBC scintigraphy is able to detect bleeding at rates of 0.05–0.1 mL/min, whereas CT angiography can detect bleeding at rates >0.25 mL/min.[31] The data comparing these two modalities is sparse. In general, tagged RBC scintigraphy is thought to be more sensitive, but CT angiography may be a reasonable first-line screening test in recurrent lower GI bleeding after failed colonoscopy due to its widespread availability and greater specificity in anatomic localization.[27] Reported sensitivity and specificity of CT angiography vary, but in general, range from sensitivity of 78% to >90% and specificity >90%. False negative CT angiogaphic studies may be due to the short acquisition time.[31] The CT angiogram is performed in three phases (noncontrast, arterial, and venous) and can also detect extraluminal sources of GI bleeding, such as hemobilia. Continued advances in imaging technology have improved the ability of interventional radiologists to assist in the management of acute GI bleeding. Other advanced modalities include cone-beam CT, which allows for improved anatomic discrimination compared to traditional two-dimensional angiography.[32] In addition, three-dimensional reconstruction and vessel tracking software improve the ability to localize the target vessel, improving subsequent success of an IR intervention.[32] Once localized, a variety of embolization materials (e.g., gelatin sponges, particles, coils, and glue) may be used and currently, there are no evidence-based recommendations for which material is preferable.

In situations where repeated episodes of occult bleeding have occurred, provocative intraarterial administration of vasodilators (e.g., Verapamil or nitroglycerin), anticoagulants (e.g., Heparin) or thrombolytics (e.g., tissue plasminogen activator) may be considered.[33] However, at this time, these techniques have not been validated.

Surgical therapy should be considered as a last resort in patients who have failed less invasive therapies and continue to have ongoing bleeding. Considerable debate exists regarding the threshold to proceed with surgical management. It is the opinion of the authors, in line with expert opinion, that emergency surgery should be considered in patients with active bleeding and hemodynamic instability, persistent recurrent bleeding with appropriate localization, and a significant acute transfusion requirement.[27] Retrospective data suggest that patients who received >10 units of PRBC within 24 hours had significantly higher mortality compared to those who received <10 units of PRBC in 24 hours (45% vs. 7%).[34]

Management of Patients Receiving Anticoagulation

Frequently, patients presenting with GI bleeding are taking anticoagulant and/or antiplatelet medications. Recommendations for management of these agents reflect the results of small observational studies or expert consensus. Per the American College of Gastroenterology and the European Society of Gastrointestinal Endoscopy, patients with an INR >2.5 should be given reversal agents prior to endoscopic therapy.[7,27] The choice of reversal agent should be individualized to the patient's underlying comorbidities and the reason for anticoagulation. Patients with thrombocytopenia (platelet count <50 × 10⁹/L) and severe bleeding should receive platelet transfusion.[7,27] In patients requiring massive transfusion, typically defined as >10 units of packed RBCs in 24 hours, the appropriate blood product transfusion ratio is unclear. As such, consensus recommendations are extrapolated from the trauma literature, and currently favor a balanced transfusion strategy adhering to a 1:1:1 ratio of RBCs, plasma and platelets.[35] Two recently published retrospective studies of nontrauma patients that required massive transfusion did not demonstrate a mortality benefit in patients who received a FFP:PRBC higher than 1:1.[36,37]

In patients requiring long-term anticoagulation, the timing of resuming anticoagulation should be decided on a case by case basis. Retrospective, observational studies have demonstrated a roughly two-fold increased bleeding risk if warfarin is restarted with seven days.[7] Conversely, restarting warfarin beyond 30 days was associated with increased thromboembolism and mortality risk.[7,38] Early resumption of anticoagulation using bridging therapy should be considered in patients at high risk of thromboembolism (e.g., chronic atrial fibrillation with previous embolic event, CHADS$_2$ >3, mechanical heart valve, recent deep vein thrombosis or pulmonary embolism [within three months] or known hypercoagulable disorder).[39] There is currently no consensus guidelines or evidence to provide specific recommendations for patients taking direct oral anticoagulants.

Prophylactic aspirin should be discontinued and the risks and benefits of continuing therapy should be discussed with cardiology input.[7,27] Aspirin may be restarted as early as day 3 in patients taking it for secondary prophylaxis. In patients prescribed dual antiplatelet therapy, cardiology consultation should be obtained in order to discuss timing and need for anticoagulation.[7,27] These patients should be discharged on PPI therapy, which significantly decreased rates of GI bleeding (OR 0.24, 95% CI 0.09–0.62; $P =$.003) compared to no PPI therapy following an acute GI bleed.[40]

CONTROVERSIES

- The precise dose, delivery and duration of PPI therapy in upper GI bleeding is unclear.
- In acute variceal hemorrhage, early TIPS appears to be beneficial, at least in patients with Child C disease or Child B disease with high risk bleeding stigmata, but larger trials are needed to define where TIPS should most appropriately be situated within the treatment algorithm.
- In patients with acute massive hemorrhage from GI bleeding, the appropriate blood product ratio is not well defined. Current practice is extrapolated from the trauma literature.

AUTHORS' RECOMMENDATIONS
- Active, goal-directed resuscitation in an ICU setting is appropriate for all major GI bleeding.
- Early endoscopic evaluation (within 24 hours) is recommended for major upper and lower GI bleeding.
- Adjunctive pharmacologic intervention (PPIs, etc.) should be initiated early for all patients with acute GI bleeding.
- Adjunctive diagnostic and therapeutic options should be understood by the intensivist so that timely, informed communication can be initiated with consultative services.

• Anticoagulation and antiplatelet agents should be reversed in acute bleeding. Timing of restarting these agents should occur after multidisciplinary risk stratification.

REFERENCES

1. Laine L, Yang H, Chang SC, Datto C. Trends for incidence of hospitalization and death due to GI complications in the United States from 2001-2009. *Am J Gastroenterol*. 2012;107: 1190-1195.
2. Wuerth BA, Rockey DC. Changing epidemiology of upper gastrointestinal hemorrhage in the last decade: a nationwide analysis. *Dig Dis Sci*. 2018;63:1286-1293.
3. Laine L. Upper gastrointestinal bleeding due to a peptic ulcer. *N Engl J Med*. 2016;374:2367-2376.
4. Lanas A, García-Rodriguez LA, Polo-Thomás M, et al. Time trends and impact of upper and lower gastrointestinal bleeding and perforation in clinical practice. *Am J Gastroenterol*. 2009;104:1633-1641.
5. Viallanueva C, Colomo A, Bosch A. Transfusion strategies for acute upper gastrointestinal bleeding. *N Engl J Med*. 2013; 368:11-21.
6. Zakko L, Rustagi T, Douglas M, Laine L. No benefit from platelet transfusion for gastrointestinal bleeding in patients taking antiplatelet agents. *Clin Gastroenterol Hepatol*. 2017;15:46-52.
7. Gralnek IM, Dumonceau JM, Kuipers EJ, et al. Diagnosis and management of nonvariceal upper gastrointestinal hemorrhage: European Society of Gastrointestinal Endoscopy (ESGE) Guideline. *Endoscopy*. 2015;47:1-46.
8. Sachar H, Vaidya K, Laine L. Intermittent vs. continuous proton pump inhibitor therapy for high-risk bleeding ulcers: a systematic review and meta-analysis. *JAMA Intern Med*. 2014; 174(11):1755-1762.
9. Srygley FD, Gerardo CJ, Tran T, Fisher DA. Does this patient have a severe upper gastrointestinal bleed? *JAMA*. 2012;307: 1072-1079.
10. Wysocki JD, Srivastav S, Winstead NS. A nationwide analysis of risk factors for mortality and time to endoscopy in upper gastrointestinal haemorrhage. *Aliment Pharmacol Ther*. 2012;36:30-36.
11. Lim LG, Ho KY, Chan YH, et al. Urgent endoscopy is associated with lower mortality in high-risk but not low-risk nonvariceal upper gastrointestinal bleeding. *Endoscopy*. 2011;43:300-306.
12. Vergara M, Bennett C, Calvet X, Gisbert JP. Epinephrine injection versus epinephrine injection and a second endoscopic method in high risk bleeding ulcers. *Cochrane Database Syst Rev*. 2014;(10):CD005584.
13. Cheng HC, Wu CT, Chang WL, Cheng WC, Chen WY, Sheu BS. Double oral esomeprazole after a 3-day intravenous esomeprazole infusion reduces recurrent peptic ulcer bleeding in high-risk patients: a randomized controlled study. *Gut*. 2014;63:1864-1872.
14. Abdel-Aal AK, Bag AK, Saddekni S, Hamed MF, Ahmed FY. Endovascular management of nonvariceal upper gastrointestinal hemorrhage. *Eur J Gastroenterol Hepatol*. 2013;25:755-763.
15. Lundgren JA, Matsushima K, Lynch FC, Frankel H, Cooney RN. Angiographic embolization of nonvariceal upper gastrointestinal bleeding: predictors of clinical failure. *J Trauma*. 2011;70:1208-1212.
16. Ali A, Ahmed BH, Nussbaum MS. Surgery for peptic ulcer disease. In: Yeo C, ed. *Shackelford's Surgery of the Alimentary Tract*. 8th ed. Philadelphia: Elsevier; 2019:673-701.
17. Garcia-Tsao G, Bosch J. Management of varices and variceal hemorrhage in cirrhosis. *N Engl J Med*. 2010;362:823-832.
18. Satapathy SK, Sanyal AJ. Nonendoscopic management strategies for acute esophagogastric variceal bleeding. *Gastroenterol Clin North Am*. 2014;43:819-833.
19. Ioannou GN, Doust J, Rockey DC. Terlipressin for acute esophageal variceal hemorrhage. *Cochrane Database Syst Rev*. 2003;1:CD002147.
20. Garcia-Tsao G, Sanyal AJ, Grace ND, et al. Prevention and management of gastroesophageal varices and variceal hemorrhage in cirrhosis. *Am J Gastroenterol*. 2007;102:2086-2102.
21. Dai C, Liu WX, Jiang M, Sun MJ. Endoscopic variceal ligation compared with injection sclerotherapy for treatment of esophageal variceal hemorrhage: a meta-analysis. *World J Gastroenterol*. 2015;21(8):2534-2541.
22. Hernández-Gea V, Procopet B, Giráldez Á, et al. Preemptive-TIPS improves outcome in high-risk variceal bleeding: an observational study. *Hepatology*. 2018.
23. Gerson LB, Fidler JL, Cave DR, Leighton JA. ACG clinical guideline: diagnosis and management of small bowel bleeding. *Am J Gastroenterol*. 2015;110:1265-1287.
24. Pennazio M, Santucci R, Rondonotti E, et al. Outcome of patients with obscure gastrointestinal bleeding after capsule endoscopy: report of 100 consecutive cases. *Gastroenterology*. 2004;126:643-653.
25. Triester SL, Leighton JA, Leontiadis GI, et al. A meta-analysis of the yield of capsule endoscopy compared to other diagnostic modalities in patients with obscure gastrointestinal bleeding. *Am J Gastroenterol*. 2005;100:2407-2418.
26. Wang Z, Chen JQ, Liu JL, Qin XG, Huang Y. CT enterography in obscure gastrointestinal bleeding: a systematic review and meta-analysis. *J Med Imaging Radiat Oncol*. 2013;57:263-273.
27. Strate LL, Gralnek IM. ACG clinical guideline: management of patients with acute lower gastrointestinal bleeding. *Am J Gastroenterol*. 2016;111:459-474.
28. Strate LL, Saltzman JR, Ookubo R, Mutinga ML, Syngal S. Validation of a clinical prediction rule for severe acute lower intestinal bleeding. *Am J Gastroenterol*. 2005;100:1821-1827.
29. Green BT, Rockey DC, Portwood G, et al. Urgent colonoscopy for evaluation and management of acute lower gastrointestinal hemorrhage: a randomized controlled trial. *Am J Gastroenterol*. 2005;100:2395-2402.
30. Laine L, Shah A. A randomized trial of urgent vs. elective colonoscopy in patients hospitalized with lower GI bleeding. *Am J Gastroenterol*. 2010;105:2636-2641.
31. Wortman JR, Landman W, Fulwadhva UP, Viscomi SG, Sodickson AD. CT angiography for acute gastrointestinal bleeding: what the radiologist needs to know. *Br J Radiol*. 2017;90:20170076.
32. Ierardi AM, Urbano J, De Marchi G. New advances in lower gastrointestinal bleeding management with embolotherapy. *Br J Radiol*. 2016;89:20150934.
33. Zurkiya O, Walker TG. Angiographic evaluation and management of nonvariceal gastrointestinal hemorrhage. *AJR Am J Roentgenol*. 2015;205:753-763.
34. Bender JS, Wiencek RG, Bouvman DL. Morbidity and mortality following total abdominal colectomy for massive lower gastrointestinal bleeding. *Am Surg*. 1991;57:536-541.
35. Holcomb JB, Tilley BC, Baraniuk S, et al. Transfusion of plasma, platelets, and red blood cells in a 1:1:1 vs. a 1:1:2 ratio

and mortality in patients with severe trauma The PROPPR randomized clinical trial. JAMA. 2015;313(5):471-482.

36. Mesar T, Larentzakis A, Dzik W, Chang Y, Velmahos G, Yeh DD. Association between ratio of fresh frozen plasma to red blood cells during massive transfusion and survival among patients without traumatic injury. JAMA Surg. 2017;152(6): 574-580.

37. Etchill EW, Myers SP, McDaniel L, et al. Should all massively transfused patients be treated equally? An analysis of massive transfusion ratios in the nontrauma setting. *Crit Care Med.* 2017;45(8):1311-1316.

38. Witt DM, Delate T, Garcia DA, et al. Risk of thromboembolism, recurrent hemorrhage, and death after warfarin therapy interruption for gastrointestinal tract bleeding. *Arch Intern Med.* 2012;172:1484-1491.

39. Qureshi W, Mittal C, Patsias I, et al. Restarting anticoagulation and outcomes after major gastrointestinal bleeding in atrial fibrillation. *Am J Cardiol.* 2014;113:662-668.

40. Cardoso RN, Benjo AM, DiNicolantonio JJ, et al. Incidence of cardiovascular events and gastrointestinal bleeding in patients receiving clopidogrel with and without proton pump inhibitors: an updated meta-analysis. *Open Heart.* 2015;2:e000248.

79

How Should the Critically Ill Pregnant Patient Be Managed?

Ariel Tamara Slavin and Lauren A. Plante

INTRODUCTION

A critically ill pregnant woman presents many challenges to the intensivist who must consider the needs of both mother and fetus in clinical decision-making.

Fortunately, the need for critical care services in the obstetric population is uncommon. Estimates on the incidence of obstetric admissions later requiring care in the intensive care unit (ICU) ranged from 2.4 to 8 per 1000.[1–3] Furthermore, another 1–2% of critically ill women are treated in a labor and delivery unit or a specialized obstetric care unit.[4,5] These numbers may understate the severity of the problem because a large national population-based study of severe maternal morbidity conducted from 2008 to 2009 found that nearly 1.6% of delivery and postpartum hospitalizations in the United States, excluding antepartum admissions, were associated with severe maternal complications.[6] The decision to admit or transfer an obstetric patient to the ICU varies with the range of services available at the institution, a fact that is illustrated by the large discrepancy between state-level reports of ICU utilization.[7] A state-level analysis from 1998 to 2008 in Maryland calculated the ICU utilization rate as 419 per 100,000 deliveries.[8] Extrapolating to the nearly 4 million births in the United States every year,[9] nearly 17,000 pregnant or postpartum women in the United States should require ICU admission annually, at least 64,000 should sustain a major complication, and somewhere between 40,000 and 80,000 with a critical illness or potentially life-threatening complication should be treated within obstetric units, with or without the input of critical care specialists. Most obstetric patients admitted to ICU are postpartum rather than undelivered, so the fetus is no longer a concern, although pregnancy physiology persists.[1,10,11]

The trend toward establishing a lowered threshold for ICU admission among obstetric patients, combined with improved access and increasing number of ICU beds,[12] means that the intensivist should be involved in the care of a greater number of pregnant or postpartum women. Special considerations in obstetrics include the "two-patient problem" (i.e., the balance of needs between mother and fetus) and the need for the clinician to factor in the effects of the physiology of pregnancy. Further complicating clinical decision-making is the paucity of research specifically focused on the critically ill pregnant patients. What follows is information, such as it exists, to assist the clinician caring for a pregnant or postpartum patient who has sepsis or acute respiratory distress syndrome (ARDS) and requires ventilator support. In most cases it is necessary to extrapolate from research performed on nonpregnant adults.

SEPSIS IN PREGNANCY

Most treatment trials explicitly exclude pregnant patients. Because sepsis and septic shock (aside from unsafe abortion) are not common in pregnancy, the epidemiology of sepsis in this population is not as well described as in a general medical-surgical population. The World Health Organization in 2014 noted sepsis to the be third most common cause of maternal death, with an estimated 11% of sepsis cases in developing countries thought to be due to pregnancy-related infection.[13] Criteria for sepsis have been met in 3–9 cases per 10,000 deliveries in Europe.[14,15] A population-based cohort study using data from the Nationwide Inpatient Sample reported the incidence of sepsis among delivering and postpartum patients to be 29.4 per 100,000 births; antepartum hospitalizations not resulting in delivery were not included in this estimation.[16] Varying definitions for "sepsis" complicate any discussion of the medical literature. Virtually nothing has been published applying the Sepsis-3 criteria to pregnant and postpartum patients.

The case-fatality rate for sepsis in the obstetric population is not known with any degree of certainty; however, the case-fatality rate for puerperal sepsis has been reported as 15% globally.[17] Calculations based on birth statistics and the National Inpatient Sample,[6] although not provided in the original paper, would put the overall case-fatality rate for sepsis at delivery or postpartum at approximately 9%.

Sepsis may be obstetric or nonobstetric. Causes of obstetric sepsis include uterine infection (chorioamnionitis if undelivered, endomyometritis if postpartum), septic abortion, and wound infection (cesarean or episiotomy wound). In addition, sepsis may follow invasive procedures such as amniocentesis, chorionic villus sampling, cervical cerclage, or percutaneous umbilical blood sampling. One of the few case series in the US literature on septic shock in pregnancy[18] reported that half of the cases had an obstetric cause; sepsis from nonobstetric causes in most of the other half of the patients originated in the urinary tract. However, more recent data from the Case Mix Programme, a high quality database of patient outcomes in the United Kingdom, showed that 40% of maternal sepsis cases were due to pneumonia and 9% were due to a urinary source.[19,20]

IDENTIFYING AND DIAGNOSING SEPSIS IN PREGNANT OR POSTPARTUM PATIENT

The Sepsis-1/Sepsis-2 criteria for sepsis may not be applicable in pregnancy, labor, or the immediate puerperium because of overlap between the normal physiologic parameters of pregnancy and criteria used to identify the systemic inflammatory response syndrome (SIRS). This problem contributed to both high false-negative and false-positive rates. Sepsis-3, published in 2016, redefined sepsis as "life-threatening organ dysfunction caused by dysregulated host response to infection" and provided evidence-based clinical criteria (a Sequential Organ Failure Assessment [SOFA] score ≥ 2) to identify patients with the disorder.[21] This formulation eliminated "severe sepsis" and the reliance on SIRS criteria.[21] Septic shock was defined as "sepsis where underlying circulatory and/or metabolic abnormality are sufficient to increase the risk of mortality" and could be clinically identified by persistent hypotension requiring vasopressors and a serum lactate level >2 after adequate volume resuscitation. Sepsis-3 also recommended using the quick SOFA (qSOFA, quick Sequential Organ Failure Assessment) score comprising three elements: respiratory rate ≥ 22 breaths/minute, altered mentation, and systolic blood pressure ≤ 100 mm Hg. The presence of two or three of these should prompt the clinician to consider sepsis, look further for organ dysfunction, and escalate therapy or monitoring.[21]

Prior definitions of maternal sepsis were vague and inconsistent, and the need for a clear and widely applicable update was apparent. In 2017, following the changes reflected in Sepsis-3, the WHO released a new maternal sepsis definition that similarly emphasizes organ dysfunction rather than a physiologic or inflammatory response specifically: "Maternal sepsis is a life-threatening condition defined as organ dysfunction resulting from infection during pregnancy, childbirth, postabortion, or postpartum period".[22] The WHO expert panel did not, however, settle on a set of clinical criteria analogous to SOFA or qSOFA because of the persistent concern about the effect of normal pregnancy physiology on the parameters that comprise these scores. A large international cross-sectional study was conducted late in 2017, which was designed, among other things, to assess both prevalence of maternal sepsis and criteria for identification[23]; however, results have not been published yet.

Sepsis scoring systems other than SOFA have been developed to improve diagnostic sensitivity, to stratify illness severity, and to expedite and direct treatment. Use of these alternatives in the obstetric population is limited because the normal physiologic changes of pregnancy act as a significant confounder. For example, the normal mild changes in respiratory rate, heart rate, and white blood cell count observed in pregnancy may be sufficient to meet previously recognized SIRS criteria, leading to overdiagnosis.[24] Several pregnancy-specific modifications of scoring systems have been suggested in hopes of improving diagnostic accuracy.

A large, retrospective, case-control study[25] examined the predictive validity for mortality of the Sepsis in Obstetrics Score (SOS). However, the SOS was not superior to four other systems that had been previously validated in the general population. Of these, the Multiple Organ Dysfunction Score (MODS) was the most accurate in predicting mortality regardless of pregnancy status. Overall, organ dysfunction-based scores (MODS and SOFA) tend to be superior to other scoring systems (Acute Physiology and Chronic Health Evaluation II or APACHE II score and Simplified Acute Physiology Score II or SAPS II) that are based on physiologic criteria, even after these systems (SOS) are adjusted to control for normal changes in pregnancy.

The Society of Obstetric Medicine of Australia and New Zealand, cognizant of the need for different criteria for organ dysfunction in pregnancy, has proposed both an obstetrically modified SOFA score and an obstetrically modified qSOFA score.[26] They suggest that the obstetrically modified qSOFA score assigns 1 point for systolic blood pressure ≤ 90 mm Hg, respiratory rate ≥ 25 breaths/minute, and mental status as not alert; a score of 2 or 3 would be abnormal. This modified score accounts for the normal vasodilation and lower blood pressure as well as the augmented minute ventilation expected in pregnancy. It has not yet been extensively tested or validated.

MANAGEMENT OF SEPSIS

The Surviving Sepsis Campaign (SSC)[27] is a multiorganizational effort to improve outcomes in sepsis and septic shock based on the best available evidence via the use of care "bundles". Subsequent research showed a decrease in hospital mortality after the implementation of these bundles in totality with a specific time frame (6 hours initial, modified to 3 hours in 2016).[28] In 2018 SSC recommendations focus on initiation of broad-spectrum antibiotics and fluid resuscitation along with cultures and lactate measurement within 1 hour.[29] The Royal College of Obstetricians and Gynecologists had recommended application based on the need for more specific, evidence-based management guidelines[22] of the SSC 6-hour bundle in pregnancy despite the absence of pregnancy-specific data.[30] Because pregnant patients are excluded from most studies, large-scale randomized control trials on the management of sepsis in the obstetric population are lacking.[22] It seems prudent to recommend that pregnant and postpartum patients with sepsis not be exempted from the SSC 1-hour bundle. However, overly aggressive fluid resuscitation may precipitate pulmonary edema in pregnant women, in whom the gradient between colloid osmotic pressure and left ventricular end-diastolic pressure is lower than that in other healthy adults.[31]

In the absence of pregnancy-specific recommendations, the authors suggest that the following elements of the SSC guidelines be applied to the pregnant patient.

1. Lactate levels do not change in pregnancy and may therefore be used to guide treatment.

2. Blood cultures should be obtained before starting antibiotic therapy unless this approach significantly delays starting antimicrobial therapy. One study in Finland reported on this specific policy for obstetric patients; 2% (of >40,000) were cultured for fever and had broad-spectrum antibiotics immediately administered. Bacteremia was confirmed in 5% of cases; only 1 of the 798 patients cultured had septic shock, for an incidence of 0.1%.[32]

3. Broad-spectrum antibiotic therapy should be initiated within 1 hour of diagnosis. Most but not all antibiotics can be used in pregnancy; however, dose adjustments may be required because of changes in pharmacokinetics (e.g., expanded plasma volume, increased glomerular filtration rate, increased protein binding).[33] Broad-spectrum coverage is reasonable in obstetrics patients; in a recent Finnish study of peripartum sepsis, more than 40 organisms were cultured, including aerobic gram-positive and gram-negative as well as anaerobic bacteria.[32] The presence of beta-lactamase–producing microbes should be considered in patients who do not respond to initial therapy.

   Begin resuscitation with crystalloid fluids.

   Importantly, the hemodynamic state that characterizes pregnancy is similar to that observed in sepsis. Specifically, normal pregnancy includes increased cardiac output, increased heart rate, decreased systemic vascular resistance, and a somewhat lower basal blood pressure.[34]

4. There is no evidence suggesting any advantage to the use of colloid in pregnant patients with sepsis. Trials comparing crystalloid with colloid prior to conduction of axis (spinal or epidural) anesthesia for elective cesarean delivery have been performed, but extrapolation to sepsis would be inappropriate. Because the gradient between colloid oncotic pressure and pulmonary artery occlusion pressure is lower in pregnancy,[34] there may be more risk of pulmonary edema with aggressive fluid loading than in the nonobstetric patient.

   Vasopressors, preferably norepinephrine, should be started for a mean arterial pressure (MAP) <65 mm Hg.

   This MAP goal does not, however, account for the fact that pregnancy is a volume-loaded, vasodilated state. Indeed, a MAP as low as 60 mm Hg may be normal in pregnancy.[35] There is no data to recommend a lower MAP limit in pregnancy. While norepinephrine has been used in obstetric crises, such as shock, data on the use of any vasopressor in human pregnancy are limited. Norepinephrine infusion during spinal anesthesia for cesarean section maintains MAP as effectively as phenylephrine and more effectively improved cardiac output[36] without any adverse neonatal events.[37] There are no data in obstetric sepsis.

It is important to note that the uteroplacental circulation does not autoregulate and compromised placental perfusion may be apparent by examination of the electronic fetal heart rate tracing. Therefore, using the tracing as a resource for evaluating tissue perfusion may allow for individualization of the target MAP for the mother.

ACUTE RESPIRATORY DISTRESS SYNDROME IN PREGNANCY

ARDS is uncommon in pregnancy, with an incidence estimated at 0.014–0.06% of deliveries, which appears to be increasing over time.[38–40] The incidence of acute lung injury (including ARDS) is estimated at roughly 80 per 100,000 patient-years in the general US population.[41] The incidence of ARDS in pregnancy is calculated as 21–46 per 100,000 person-years[2] in the obstetric population, which is lower than the rate in the general population (although not, obviously, age-adjusted). The mortality rate for ARDS among obstetric patients was estimated as 24–44% among older case series.[38,39,41,42] In a more recent US series from 2006 to 2012, the mortality rate was lower at 9–15% compared with the general population case-fatality rate of 38%.[40,41] A national review of Canadian hospital admissions between 1991 and 2002 found that the case-fatality rate among obstetric patients with ARDS in the absence of any major preexisting condition (e.g., diabetes, heart disease) was only 6%.[43]

WHAT IS THE OPTIMUM STRATEGY FOR MECHANICAL VENTILATION IN A PREGNANT PATIENT?

There are no randomized controlled trials of ventilator strategies in the obstetric population. Many authorities recommend maintaining maternal oxygen saturation by pulse oximetry (SpO_2) greater than 95% or partial pressure of oxygen in arterial blood (PaO_2) greater than 60 mm Hg "to preserve fetal wellbeing," but it is unclear what evidence supports this recommendation, at least in humans. Uteroplacental blood flow rather than maternal oxygenation *per se* is the major determinant of fetal oxygen delivery. The model for gas transport across the human placenta is thought to be that of a concurrent exchanger. The gradient between maternal and fetal oxygen content drives transfer. Because the oxygen content of fetal blood is low, the gradient is easily preserved: normal fetal umbilical venous partial pressure of oxygen (the most highly oxygenated blood in the fetal circulation) is only 31–42 mm Hg.[44] The nature of a concurrent exchanger is such that oxygen saturation at the most highly oxygenated end of the fetal side is still lower than the least oxygenated end of the maternal circulation, represented by the uterine vein, or approximately the mixed venous saturation of oxygen. Only in the extreme case of a venous equilibrator could the two be equal, and under no circumstances can the fetal side be higher than the maternal venous side. Oxygen delivery to the fetus and fetal organs, as to the adult, is represented by the product of blood flow and oxygen content. Adaptive strategies in the fetus include higher affinity of fetal hemoglobin for oxygen and high cardiac output relative to size.

There is one experimental trial of deliberate hypoxia in human pregnancy.[45] Ten women with normal pregnancies near term were exposed to a hypoxic gas mixture with a fraction of inspired oxygen of approximately 0.1 (50% room air, 50% nitrogen) for 10 minutes, during which time SpO_2 decreased by 15%. Fetal parameters that are thought to represent fetal oxygenation (i.e., heart rate baseline and variability, fetal umbilical artery Doppler indices, and fetal middle cerebral artery Doppler indices) did not change during experimental maternal hypoxia. Direct sampling of fetal blood was not performed in this study.

In case series from the era preceding low-tidal-volume ventilation for ARDS, barotrauma rates were high in obstetric patients who underwent mechanical ventilation (i.e., 36–44%).[39,40] This compares unfavorably with the background rate of barotrauma of 11% among nonobstetric patients ventilated with "traditional" tidal volumes in ARDS.[46]

In contemporary practice, pregnant patients with ARDS are usually treated with the usual low-tidal-volume ventilator strategy. The limited available data suggests that it is safe for mother and fetus.[47]

When undertaking a standard low-tidal-volume ventilation strategy for pregnant women with ARDS, the maternal partial pressure of carbon dioxide in arterial blood ($PaCO_2$) is probably at least as important as the PaO_2. CO_2 transfer across the placenta also requires a gradient; in this case the higher $PaCO_2$ of fetal blood diffuses across placental interface to the lower $PaCO_2$ of maternal blood. High maternal $PaCO_2$, as in permissive hypercapnia, would be expected to impede fetomaternal CO_2 transfer and promote fetal acidemia. In a small trial of CO_2 rebreathing in 35 healthy pregnant women, an increase in the maternal end-tidal CO_2 as high as 60 torr was associated with a loss of fetal heart rate variability in 57% of fetuses monitored, this being a proxy for fetal acidemia; 90% of fetuses thus affected normalized the tracing after test.[48]

Thus it would seem that a pregnant woman ventilated with the standard low-tidal-volume strategy could have the fetal heart rate tracing continuously monitored as a way of assessing fetal oxygenation and acid-base status. This would be irrelevant at very early gestational ages (e.g., before 24 weeks). If the tracing shows signs of fetal compromise, then interventions might include decreasing positive end-expiratory pressure (to improve uterine blood flow by improving cardiac output) or increasing tidal volume so as to increase maternal pH and decrease maternal $PaCO_2$.

Additional therapies that have been used for ARDS in the general population may be applied in the case of pregnancy, including inhaled nitric oxide and prone positioning, although creative use of buttresses or mattress cutouts may be required for proning depending on the size of the gravid uterus. Fetal concerns should not be allowed to interfere with appropriate sedation of the mother. Neuromuscular blocking agents, if used, do not cross the placenta.

Delivery in itself does not seem to improve maternal survival in ARDS.[40,49,50] Fetal survival, however, is tightly linked to gestational age at delivery: this would imply a fetal benefit to continuing rather than interrupting pregnancy, assuming maternal and fetal condition permits.

WHAT IS THE ROLE OF EXTRACORPOREAL MEMBRANE OXYGENATION IN REFRACTORY ACUTE RESPIRATORY DISTRESS SYNDROME IN OBSTETRIC PATIENTS?

Extracorporeal membrane oxygenation (ECMO) has become increasingly common and more generally available in adult patients with respiratory failure. The Conventional Versus ECMO for Severe Adult Respiratory Failure (CESAR) trial[51] showed a survival benefit of transfer to ECMO specialty centers for consideration of this intervention. Survival rates were 63% among patients who received ECMO compared with 47% of those not considered for ECMO. Although there were no obstetric patients enrolled in the CESAR trial, the year of the trial's publication also saw the worldwide pandemic of a novel influenza A virus, H1N1, which was significantly more severe among pregnant women than most other groups. A pragmatic approach to H1N1 respiratory failure, pioneered in Australia and New Zealand, meant that an unprecedented number of pregnant (and postpartum) patients were treated with ECMO.[52–54] This recent experience has led to an increasing willingness to consider ECMO in obstetric patients, in most cases for refractory respiratory failure. A compilation of data from case reports and case series suggests that maternal survival on ECMO is approximately 75–80% and fetal survival is approximately 65%.[55,56] Experience is more extensive with venovenous cannulation. Both antepartum and postpartum bleeding are of concern and may be catastrophic. Attention should also be paid to adequate venous drainage because the gravid uterus may compress the inferior vena cava when the patient is prone; thus, alterations in patient positioning or the addition of another venous outflow cannula may be required. ECMO in pregnancy is a high-stakes situation, which should only be undertaken in centers with appropriate experience and a full spectrum of resources.

CONCLUSION

Care of the critically ill obstetric patient requires interpretation and adaptation of studies performed in the nonobstetric population. In most situations of critical illness in pregnancy, there are no randomized trials to guide the practitioner, and none are likely to be performed. Pregnancy physiology, uteroplacental perfusion, and fetal issues may require modifications in ICU management. A multidisciplinary approach, with careful assessment of treatment options, is expected to serve these patients best.

AUTHORS' RECOMMENDATIONS

- Most obstetric patients in the ICU have been admitted after delivery, most commonly as a result of hypertensive disease of pregnancy or postpartum hemorrhage.
- Pregnant patients have been specifically excluded from all major critical care trials.
- In general, what is good for the mother is good for the fetus. A multidisciplinary approach involving intensivists, obstetricians, and midwives/nurses with careful assessment of treatment options is expected to serve these patients best.
- Sepsis in pregnancy may be due to obstetric or nonobstetric causes, but should not be treated differently.
- Maternal sepsis has recently been redefined as a life-threatening condition defined as organ dysfunction resulting from infection during pregnancy, childbirth, postabortion, or postpartum period. The specific criteria qualifying as organ dysfunction have not been fully worked out since modification for the physiologic changes of pregnancy is needed.
- Fluid resuscitation in septic shock: pregnant women may be more susceptible to pulmonary edema with aggressive fluid resuscitation.
- Norepinephrine is the vasopressor of choice.
- ARDS in pregnancy should be treated with a standard lung-protective strategy. The fetal heart rate tracing may be a guide as to the lower limit for maternal PaO_2 or upper limit of $PaCO_2$. Delivery does not improve outcome.
- ECMO has been used successfully in pregnancy but should be limited to centers with experience.

REFERENCES

1. Zwart JJ, Dupuis JR, Richters A, Ory F, van Roosmalen J. Obstetric intensive care unit admission: a 2-year nationwide population-based cohort study. *Intensive Care Med.* 2010;36:256-263.
2. Keizer JL, Zwart JJ, Meerman RH, Harinck BI, Feuth HD, van Roosmalen J. Obstetric intensive care admissions: a 12-year review in a tertiary care centre. *Eur J Obstet Gynecol Reprod Biol.* 2006;128:152-156.
3. Munnur U, Karnad DR, Bandi VD, et al. Critically ill obstetric patients in an American and an Indian public hospital: comparison of case-mix, organ dysfunction, intensive care requirements, and outcomes. *Intensive Care Med.* 2005;31:1087-1094.
4. Ryan M, Hamilton V, Bowen M, McKenna P. The role of a high-dependency unit in a regional obstetric hospital. *Anaesthesia.* 2000;55:1155-1158.
5. Zeeman GG, Wendel Jr GD, Cunningham FG. A blueprint for obstetric critical care. *Am J Obstet Gynecol.* 2003;188:532-536.
6. Callaghan WM, Creanga AA, Kuklina EV. Severe maternal morbidity among delivery and postpartum hospitalizations in the United States. *Obstet Gynecol.* 2012;120:1029-1036.
7. Oud L. Epidemiology of pregnancy-associated ICU utilization in Texas: 2001-2010. *J Clin Med Res.* 2017;9:143-153.
8. Wanderer JP, Leffert LR, Mhyre JM, Kuklina EV, Callaghan WM, Bateman BT. Epidemiology of obstetric-related intensive care unit admissions in Maryland: 1999-2008. *Crit Care Med.* 2013;41:1844-1852.
9. Hamilton BE, Martin JA, Osterman MJK, Curtin SC. Births: preliminary data for 2013. *Natl Vital Stat Rep.* 2014;63(2). Available at: https://www.cdc.gov/nchs/data/nvsr/nvsr63/nvsr63_02.pdf. Accessed November 28, 2018.
10. Intensive Care National Audit and Research Centre. Female admissions (aged 16-50 years) to adult, general critical care units in England, Wales and Northern Ireland reported as 'currently pregnant' or 'recently pregnant'. 2013. Available at: https://www.oaa-anaes.ac.uk/assets/_managed/cms/files/Obstetric%20admissions%20to%20critical%20care%202009-2012%20-%20FINAL.pdf. Accessed November 28, 2018.
11. Paxton JL, Presneill J, Aitken L. Characteristics of obstetric patients referred to intensive care in an Australian tertiary hospital. *Aust N Z J Obstet Gynaecol.* 2014;54:445-449.
12. Gooch RA, Kahn JM. ICU bed supply, utilization, and health care spending: an example of demand elasticity. *JAMA.* 2014;311:567-568.
13. Say L, Chou D, Gemmill A, et al. Global causes of maternal death: a WHO systematic analysis. *Lancet Glob Health.* 2014;2:e323-e333.
14. Waterstone M, Bewley S, Wolfe C. Incidence and predictors of severe obstetric morbidity: case-control study. *BMJ.* 2001;322:1089-1094.
15. Zhang WH, Alexander S, Bouvier-Colle MH, Macfarlane A. Incidence of severe pre-eclampsia, postpartum haemorrhage and sepsis as a surrogate marker for severe maternal morbidity in a European population-based study: the MOMS-B survey. *BJOG.* 2005;112:89-96.
16. Al-Ostad G, Kezouh A, Abenhaim HA. Incidence of and risk factors for sepsis mortality in labor, delivery, and postpartum. *Am J Obstet Gynecol.* 2015;212:S241-S242.
17. Dolea C, Stein C. *Global Burden of Maternal Sepsis in the Year 2000: Evidence and Information for Policy (EIP).* Geneva, Switzerland: World Health Organization; 2003. Available at: https://www.who.int/healthinfo/statistics/bod_maternalsepsis.pdf. Accessed November 28, 2018.
18. Mabie WC, Barton JR, Sibai B. Septic shock in pregnancy. *Obstet Gynecol.* 1997;90:553-561.
19. Acosta CD, Kurinczuk JJ, Lucas DN, et al. Severe maternal sepsis in the UK, 2011-2012: A national case-control study. *PLoS Med.* 2014;11(7):e1001672.
20. Acosta CD, Harrison DA, Rowan K, Lucas DN, Kurinczuk JJ, Knight M. Maternal morbidity and mortality from severe sepsis: a national cohort study. *BMJ Open.* 2016;6:e012323.
21. Singer M, Deutschman CS, Seymour CW, et al. The third international consensus definitions for sepsis and septic shock (Sepsis-3). *JAMA.* 2016;315:801-810.
22. World Health Organization. *Statement on Maternal Sepsis.* Geneva, Switzerland: WHO; 2017. Available at: http://apps.who.int/iris/bitstream/handle/10665/254608/WHO-RHR-17.02-eng.pdf;jsessionid=A4B12115B0D094925A5DB5E04E4F6615?sequence=1. Accessed November 28, 2018.
23. Bonet M, Souza JP, Abalos E, et al. The global maternal sepsis study and awareness campaign (GLOSS): study protocol. *Reprod Health.* 2018;15:16.
24. Bauer ME, Bauer ST, Rajala B, et al. Maternal physiologic parameters in relationship to systemic inflammatory response syndrome criteria: a systematic review and meta-analysis. *Obstet Gynecol.* 2014;124:535-541.
25. Aarvold AB, Ryan HM, Magee LA, von Dadelszen P, Fjell C, Walley KR. Multiple organ dysfunction score is superior to the obstetric-specific sepsis in obstetrics score in predicting mortality in septic obstetric patients. *Crit Care Med.* 2017;45:e49-e57.
26. Bowyer L, Robinson HL, Barrett H, et al. SOMANZ guidelines for the investigation and management sepsis in pregnancy. *Aust N Z J Obstet Gynaecol.* 2017;57:540-551.

27. Dellinger RP, Levy MM, Rhodes A, et al. Surviving Sepsis Campaign: international guidelines for management of severe sepsis and septic shock: 2012. *Crit Care Med.* 2013;41:580-637.

28. Levy MM, Dellinger RP, Townsend SR, et al. The Surviving Sepsis Campaign: results of an international guideline-based performance improvement program targeting severe sepsis. *Intensive Care Med.* 2010;36:222-231.

29. Levy MM, Evans LE, Rhodes A. The Surviving Sepsis Campaign bundle: 2018 update. *Intensive Care Med.* 2018;44:925-928.

30. Morgan M, Hughes RG, Kinsella SM. Bacterial sepsis following pregnancy. *Royal College of Obstetricians & Gynaecologists.* Green-top guideline No. 64b. 2012.

31. Dennis AT, Solnordal CB. Acute pulmonary oedema in pregnant women. *Anaesthesia.* 2012;67:646-659.

32. Kankuri E, Kurki T, Carlson P, Hiilesmaa V. Incidence, treatment and outcome of peripartum sepsis. *Acta Obstet Gynecol Scand.* 2003;82:730-735.

33. Nahum GG, Uhl K, Kennedy DL. Antibiotic use in pregnancy and lactation: what is known and not know about teratogenic and toxic risks. *Obstet Gynecol.* 2006;107:1120-1138.

34. Clark SL, Cotton DB, Lee W, et al. Central hemodynamic assessment of normal term pregnancy. *Am J Obstet Gynecol.* 1989;161:1439-1442.

35. Macedo ML, Luminoso D, Savvidou MD, McEniery CM, Nicolaides KH. Maternal wave reflections and arterial stiffness in normal pregnancy as assessed by applanation tonometry. *Hypertension.* 2008;51:1047-1051.

36. Ngan Kee WD, Lee SW, Ng FF, Tan PE, Khaw KS. Randomized double-blinded comparison of norepinephrine and phenylephrine for maintenance of blood pressure during spinal anesthesia for cesarean delivery. *Anesthesiology.* 2015;122:736-745.

37. Ngan Kee WD, Lee SWY, Ng FF, Khaw KS. Prophylactic norepinephrine infusion for preventing hypotension during spinal anesthesia for cesarean delivery. *Anesth Analg.* 2018;126:1989-1994.

38. Mabie WC, Barton JR, Sibai BM. Adult respiratory distress syndrome in pregnancy. *Am J Obstet Gynecol.* 1992;167:950-957.

39. Catanzarite V, Willms D, Wong D, Landers C, Cousins L, Schrimmer D. Acute respiratory distress syndrome in pregnancy and the puerperium: causes, courses, and outcomes. *Obstet Gynecol.* 2001;97:760-764.

40. Rush B, Martinka P, Kilb B, McDermid RC, Boyd JH, Celi LA. Acute respiratory distress syndrome in pregnant women. *Obstet Gynecol.* 2017;129:530-535.

41. Rubenfeld GD, Caldwell E, Peabody E, et al. Incidence and outcomes of acute lung injury. *N Engl J Med.* 2005;353:1685-1693.

42. Perry Jr KG, Martin RW, Blake PG, Roberts WE, Martin Jr JN. Maternal mortality associated with adult respiratory distress syndrome. *South Med J.* 1998;91:441-444.

43. Wen SW, Huang L, Liston R, et al. Severe maternal morbidity in Canada, 1991-2001. *CMAJ.* 2005;173:759-764.

44. Nicolaides KH, Economides DL, Soothill PW. Blood gases, pH, and lactate in appropriate- and small-for-gestational-age fetuses. *Am J Obstet Gynecol.* 1989;161:996-1001.

45. Erkkola R, Pirhonen J, Polvi H. The fetal cardiovascular function in chronic placental insufficiency is different from experimental hypoxia. *Ann Chir Gynaecol Suppl.* 1994;208:76-79.

46. Acute Respiratory Distress Syndrome Network, Brower RG, Matthay MA, et al. Ventilation with lower tidal volumes as compared with traditional tidal volumes for acute lung injury and the acute respiratory distress syndrome. *N Engl J Med.* 2000;342:1301-1308.

47. Lapinsky SE, Rojas-Suarez JA, Crozier TM, et al. Mechanical ventilation in critically-ill pregnant women: a case series. *Int J Obstet Anesth.* 2015;24:323-328.

48. Fraser D, Jensen D, Wolfe LA, Hahn PM, Davies GAL. Fetal heart rate response to maternal hypocapnia and hypercapnia in late gestation. *J Obstet Gynaecol Can.* 2008;30(4):312-316.

49. Grisaru-Granovsky S, Ioscovich A, Hersch M, Schimmel M, Elstein D, Samueloff A. Temporizing treatment for the respiratory-compromised gravida: an observational study of maternal and neonatal outcome. *Int J Obstet Anesth.* 2007;16:261-264.

50. Tomlinson MW, Caruthers TJ, Whitty JE, Gonik B. Does delivery improve maternal condition in the respiratory-compromised gravida? *Obstet Gynecol.* 1998;91:108-111.

51. Peek GJ, Mugford M, Tiruvoipati R, et al. Efficacy and economic assessment of conventional ventilatory support versus extracorporeal membrane oxygenation for severe adult respiratory failure (CESAR): a multicentre randomised controlled trial. *Lancet.* 2009;374:1351-1363.

52. ANZIC Influenza Investigators and Australasian Maternity Outcomes Surveillance System. Critical illness due to 2009 A/H1N1 influenza in pregnant and postpartum women: population based cohort study. *BMJ.* 2010;340:c1279.

53. Oluyomi-Obi T, Avery L, Schneider C, et al. Perinatal and maternal outcomes in critically ill obstetrics patients with pandemic H1N1 influenza A. *J Obstet Gynaecol Can.* 2010;32:443-447.

54. Dubar G, Azria E, Tesnière A, et al. French experience of 2009 A/H1N1v influenza in pregnant women. *PLoS One.* 2010;5(10):e13112.

55. Sharma NS, Wille KM, Bellot SC, Diaz-Guzman E. Modern use of extracorporeal life support in pregnancy and postpartum. *ASAIO J.* 2015;61(1):110-114.

56. Moore SA, Dietl CA, Coleman DM. Extracorporeal life support during pregnancy. *J Thorac Cardiovasc Surg.* 2016;151(4):1154-1160.

80

How Do I Diagnose and Manage Patients Admitted to the Intensive Care Unit After Common Poisonings?

Jakub Furmaga and Kurt Kleinschmidt

Critically ill poisoned patients pose significant diagnostic and therapeutic challenges to intensive care staff. Unfortunately, there is no universally accepted management algorithm to aid in evaluation, despite the presence of so many harmful agents. The clinical history is often unavailable, and physicians must rely on physical exam, knowledge of toxidromes, and laboratory data to guide diagnosis and management.

In this chapter we review diagnostic strategies using toxidromes and laboratory testing, describe acetaminophen and salicylate toxicity, clarify the appropriate use of N-acetyl cysteine (NAC) as an antidote for acetaminophen (paracetamol) overdose, review the evidence behind urine alkalinization for salicylate overdose, and discuss the evidence behind various decontamination strategies.

DIAGNOSIS

Toxidromes

Toxidromes are constellations of signs and symptoms consistent with a specific group of xenobiotics and their unique effects on neuroreceptors (Table 80.1). The diagnostic benefit of using toxidromes diagnostically is that they enable management to be started without identifying the specific causative agent. For example, drugs that block acetylcholine at the muscarinic receptors can cause anticholinergic toxidrome which presents with tachycardia, dry skin, hypoactive bowel sounds, urinary retention, mydriasis, and delirium. Regardless if it was caused by an antihistamine such as diphenhydramine, an antipsychotic such as clozapine, or a plant such as Jimsonweed, anticholinergic symptoms should improve with the administration of physostigmine, a cholinesterase inhibitor. The sympathomimetic toxidrome is caused by norepinephrine and dopamine receptor agonists, such as cocaine or amphetamine, and this toxidrome is characterized by tachycardia, diaphoresis, mydriasis, and delirium. Regardless of the ingested agent, treatment with benzodiazepines will improve symptoms. The anticholinergic and sympathomimetic toxidromes may initially appear similar; however, anticholinergic patients are "dry as a bone", whereas sympathomimetic patients are usually diaphoretic. The cholinergic toxidrome is the opposite of anticholinergic and results from overstimulation of muscarinic and nicotinic receptors. It manifests with diaphoresis, salivation, lacrimation, urination, defecation, miosis, muscle twitching, and the life-threatening symptoms of bradycardia, bronchospasm, and bronchorrhea. The prototypical agents that cause a cholinergic toxidrome are organophosphate and carbamate pesticides and are treated with atropine, an anticholinergic agent. The opioid toxidrome results from overstimulation of the mu, kappa, and delta opiate receptors and manifests as pinpoint pupils, respiratory depression, and decreased mental status. Antagonists of the opioid receptors, such as naloxone, reverse these symptoms. The sedative/hypnotics toxidrome is similar to that of opioids, except that it has no pupillary changes and usually much less respiratory depression. There is no antidote for most sedative/hypnotic agents, except for flumazenil which reverses benzodiazepine-induced toxicity.

Toxidromes can guide antidote selection without having to know the exact agent involved. However, identification of a toxidrome is difficult in patients that present after polydrug ingestions which, based on their mechanisms of action, can both stimulate and block each other's receptors. In addition, most ingested agents either do not have a unique toxidrome or have a long quiescent/asymptomatic period, like in acetaminophen (paracetamol) overdoses. Therefore, in addition to physical exam, the use of laboratory testing can help diagnose poisoned patients.

Laboratory

Urine drug screens (UDS) are available in most hospitals. However, their routine use does not alter patient management or outcomes.[1] Interpretation of results can be difficult because different urine assays vary as to which agents, within a class, will be detected. Thus, the list of known false-positive and false-negative results will vary from institution to institution. However, some summary points exist. A "positive" UDS does not automatically equate to current intoxication as clinical symptoms are generally gone long before the test itself becomes "negative." For example, the cannabinoid UDS can remain positive for 3 days after a single marijuana exposure and for positive over a month after cessation of heavy chronic use.[2] Benzodiazepine assays often yield false-negative results as not all of the benzodiazepines are metabolized to the same metabolites, nordiazepam and oxazepam, that are targeted by the assay. Amphetamines are often associated with false-positive results because of their structural similarity to many medications such as pseudoephedrine or bupropion.[2]

TABLE 80.1 **Toxidromes—The Clinical Presentations.**

Toxidrome	Vital Signs	Signs
Anticholinergic	HR ↑	Bowel sounds ↓
		Delirium[a]
		Dry mouth
		Mydriasis or normal
		Skin - dry, flushed
Sympathomimetic	HR ↑	Agitated
	BP ↑	Delirium[a]
		Mydriasis
		Skin—diaphoretic
Opioid	RR ↓ and/or shallow	Bowel sounds ↓
		Mental status ↓
		Miosis
Sedative-hypnotic	RR normal or ↓[b]	Mental status ↓
Cholinergic	HR ↓	Bronchoconstriction
		Bronchorrhea
		Diaphoresis
		Lacrimation
		Miosis
		Salivation
		Urination

[a]If severe
[b]If combined with other sedatives
BP, blood pressure; *HR,* heart rate; *RR,* respiratory rate; ↑, increased; ↓, decreased.

Serum concentrations of acetaminophen (paracetamol), salicylate, lithium, digoxin, methanol, and ethylene glycol are measured, following ingestion, as the concentration of these agents impacts on treatment and the level of care required. Phenytoin, valproic acid, and carbamazepine levels in serum are measured to guide therapeutic dose. However, in an overdose, an elevated serum concentration is most useful in confirming the drug's presence rather than affecting management. Treatment is focused on observation until clinical improvement, rather than improvement in lab results. Serum concentrations can modify patient evaluation. For example, if a patient has altered mental status in the setting of medication overdose with elevated drug concentrations, then additional testing for other etiologies of delirium may be obviated.

DANGEROUS POISONINGS: TWO IMPORTANT AGENTS

Most toxic exposures in the United States are nonfatal. According to the 2016 report from the American Association of Poison Control Centers' National Poison Data System, only 0.1% of the reported toxic exposures resulted in death.[3] However, acetaminophen (paracetamol) and acetaminophen-containing products accounted for 16.9% of deaths (313 of the 1852 exposure-related fatalities) and salicylates for 3.5% (65 of the 1852).[3] Errors occur in the evaluation and treatment of both of these common exposures. For example, a 2008

Maryland Poison Center study suggested that intravenous NAC administration errors for acetaminophen poisoning occurred in approximately one-third of cases and these included incorrect doses, incorrect rate, interruption of therapy, and unnecessary administration of NAC.[4] In addition, acetaminophen and salicylates are often confused for each other because they are both commonly used over-the-counter analgesics, despite each having completely different toxicities and treatments. Thus, the following section details the treatment of acetaminophen and salicylate overdoses.

Acetaminophen (Paracetamol)

The chemical name for acetaminophen is acetyl-para-aminophenol (APAP). At therapeutic doses, 90–95% of the ingested APAP is glucuronidated or sulfated inactive metabolites that are renally eliminated. The remaining 5–10% is oxidized by the Cytochrome P450 system into the hepatotoxic *N*-acetyl-*p*-benzoquinoneimine (NAPQI).[5] NAPQI is detoxified via conjugation with glutathione, which produces a nontoxic species that is renally eliminated[6] (Fig. 80.1). In APAP overdose, however, glucuronidation and sulfation pathways become saturated and the excess APAP is metabolized to NAPQI. As the glutathione is rapidly depleted in conjugation with NAPQI, undetoxified free NAPQI causes hepatotoxicity. Hepatitis (as defined by aspartate aminotransferase [AST] >1000 IU/L),[7] often occurs after an ingestion of 150 mg/kg.[8] Higher doses can lead to acute liver failure (ALF).[9]

As APAP toxicity has no early symptoms, a serum acetaminophen concentration is obtained in all cases of suspected overdose. The Rumack–Matthew nomogram (Fig. 80.2) guides the use of NAC in acute single exposure overdoses when time of ingestion is known.[10] The treatment line is based on a 4-hour half-life starting with a toxic 4-hour serum concentration of 150 mcg/mL. This screening tool has a sensitivity of almost 100% when strictly applied in a single acute overdose (not chronic, and not involving multiple doses) and a known time of exposure.[11] Serum drug concentration from time 0 to 4 hours post ingestion do not necessarily guide therapy but they do indicate the level of exposure. Except in the setting of massive overdose (more than 80–100 tablets) or co-ingestants that slow down gastrointestinal motility, serial APAP concentrations are unnecessary due to acetaminophen's

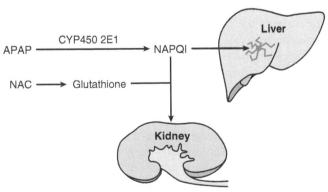

Fig. 80.1 Acetaminophen Metabolism.

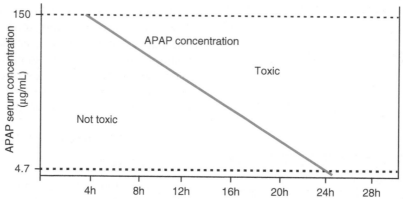

Fig. 80.2 Rumack–Matthew Nomogram. (Redrawn with permission of DallasTox.com.)

predictable pharmacokinetics. In cases of massive APAP ingestion, absorption is delayed and the elimination half-life can be prolonged up to 20.3 hours.[12]

Previously, in the US, a toxic concentration was treated with oral NAC for 72 hours (140 mg/kg followed by 70 mg/kg every 4 hours for 17 doses). However, in 2004, the Food and Drug Administration approved Acetadote, a pyrogen-free intravenous form of NAC. Similar products are available in 200mg/ml preparations in other countries (e.g. Parvolex). Intravenous NAC is recommended for patients who present within 10 hours of acute ingestion and is administered using a 21-hour protocol: 150 mg/kg of NAC in 200 mL of 5% dextrose solution (D5) over 1 hour, then 50 mg/kg in 500 mL of D5 over 4 hours, and then 100 mg/kg in 1000 mL of D5 over 16 hours. A 2009 cost analysis indicated that this intravenous NAC regimen may be less expensive than the generic oral NAC due to shortened hospital stay.[13] Both regimens are equally effective when started early[14]; however, one meta-analysis showed that for treatment started more than 18 hours post ingestion (late presenters), the 72-hour oral NAC formulation was more effective at preventing hepatotoxicity than the intravenous formulation. This difference was attributed to oral NAC protocol's larger cumulative dose (1330 mg/kg vs. 300 mg/kg) and longer duration of treatment (72 hours vs. 21 hours).[15] Importantly, late presenters who have already developed ALF may still benefit from NAC administration: they have lower mortality and less progression to grade III/IV encephalopathy when compared with untreated patients.[16] Toxicologists advocate giving additional NAC (i.e., Acetadote bag #2: 50 mg/kg in 500 mL of D5W over 4 hours, or Acetadote bag #3: 100 mg/kg in 1000 mL of D5W over 16 hours) following the 21-hour infusion protocol to patients with continuously rising AST and for those with ongoing hepatitis. Administration of Acetadote bag #2 results in a dose of 12.5 mg/kg per hour of NAC, whereas administration of Acetadote bag #3 results in a dose of only 6.25 mg/kg per hour of NAC and is preferentially given to the sicker patients. NAC treatment is appropriate even if APAP concentrations become undetectable as it is the unmeasured metabolite NAPQI that is causing the liver injury.

Salicylates

Aspirin, or acetylsalicylic acid (ASA) poisoning is very common due to its availability in many over the counter pharmaceutical products.[17] The acute salicylate toxidrome includes vomiting, hyperpnea, diaphoresis, dizziness, and hearing changes such as muffled hearing and/or tinnitus. In severe poisoning, patients may develop cerebral and/or pulmonary edema. Arterial blood gas analysis may demonstrate mixed respiratory alkalosis and a widened anion-gap metabolic acidosis. In chronic ingestion, patients may present with altered mental status, mimicking infection.[18]

Serum salicylate concentrations are most commonly reported in milligrams/deciliter (mg/dL), although some laboratories report them in mg/L, which may result in a misinterpretation of the concentration by a factor of 10. Therapeutic concentrations range from 10 to 30 mg/dL. Toxicity results from tissue distribution and not from the salicylate in the blood. Consequently serum concentrations and toxicity do not always correlate. For example, a serum salicylate concentration may be decreasing due to salicylate redistribution into tissues (the patient is deteriorating) or the salicylate is being eliminated by the kidneys (and the patient is recovering). Toxicity is considered to be resolving if (1) serial salicylate concentrations are no longer toxic (<30 mg/dL) and decreasing, and (2) the patient is clinically improving. It must be emphasized that salicylate evaluation is very different from that of APAP (where treatment is primarily dictated by laboratory results) because management of ASA toxicity depends on serial serum concentrations in conjunction with symptomatology.

Treatment of salicylate toxicity is focused on increased excretion. Urine alkalinization enhances salicylate elimination by "trapping" the salicylate ion in the renal tubules and improving its removal (Fig. 80.3). In a 1982 study by Prescott and colleagues, urine alkalinization was achieved by adding three 8.4% (50mls, 1mEq/ml) ampules of sodium bicarbonate into 1 L of D5W with 40 mEq of potassium chloride and infusing this mixture at 375 ml/hour (1.5 L total) for 4 hours.[19] The mean urine pH in these patients was 8.1 ± (SD) 0.5. This significantly increased the amount of salicylate found in the urine. In that same study, forced diuresis was shown to be less effective at improving elimination, suggesting that these patients should only receive fluids required to reach euvolemia.[19] It is important to note that the positive data presented refers to only 6 patients in a study

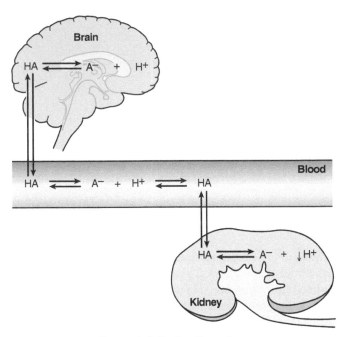

Fig. 80.3 Salicylate Excretion.

of 44 patients in total, and represents the only data available to support alkalinzation of urine. Hypokalemia must be avoided in order to optimally eliminate the salicylate. Serum hypokalemia will trigger intercalated cells in the distal tubules to secrete hydrogen ions in exchange for potassium, thus preventing urine alkalinization.

In the more severe cases, hemodialysis should be considered. The following are indications for emergent hemodialysis for salicylate toxicity[20]:

- any patient with altered mental status
- any patient with acute respiratory distress requiring supplemental O_2
- concentration of 100 mg/dL or more in acute ingestion
- concentration of 90 mg/dL or more in those with impaired renal function
- severe acidosis with pH $\leq$ 7.20.

MANAGEMENT PRINCIPLES

Prior to the 1960s, the standard treatment of poisoned patients was with medications that would have the opposite effect on neuroreceptors than the ingested substance (i.e., sedative ingestions would be treated with stimulants, stimulant exposures with sedatives). However, this approach caused many iatrogenic complications. In 1961, the "Scandinavian method" for treating patients after barbiturate poisoning was described.[21] It used observation and respiratory support instead of the previously employed gastric lavage and central analeptics. This new method decreased the mortality from barbiturate overdose from 20% to 1–2%.[21] This study shifted the treatment of poisoned patients to primarily supportive care (i.e. respiratory and circulatory support).

If there is suspicion of opiate overdose in a respiratory depressed patient, naloxone administration is appropriate. The competitive benzodiazepine antagonist flumazenil may improve respiratory status and prevent intubation in benzodiazepine overdose. The drug should be initially administerd in low doses due to the risk of precipitating intractable seizures in benzodiazepine dependent patients.[22]

DECONTAMINATION AND ENHANCED ELIMINATION

Decontamination refers to interventions that attempt to minimize the patient's further exposure to the toxin. In theory, gastrointenstinal (GI) decontamination decreases ongoing absorption of the remaining drug in the intestines. These strategies include gastric emptying (GE) through induction of emesis with ipecac or using gastric lavage, binding of unabsorbed toxins via single dose activated charcoal (AC), and improved excretion with whole bowel irrigation. The effectiveness of these decontamination techniques is debatable; a few of the more influential clinical trials are discussed below.

GE eliminates substances still within the stomach through induction of emesis with ipecac or lavage with a large bore oral gastric tube. In a prospective study performed by Merigian et al.,[23] 808 poisoned patients were given AC with or without GE. GE yielded no clinical benefit. In fact, those treated with GE were admitted to the intensive care unit twice as often, were intubated nearly four times more often, and experienced more aspiration pneumonia (GE had 8 vs. 0 for no-GE).[23]

Whole bowel irrigation (WBI) uses polyethylene glycol to mechanically flush out the contents of the gastrointestinal tract. While volunteer studies reflect that WBI decreases absorption of ingested drugs, no clinical improvement has been demonstrated. WBI is contraindicated in patients with bowel obstruction, perforation, ileus, hemodynamic instability, or compromised airways. WBI should be considered for sustained-release drugs, enteric-coated medications, iron, and packets of illicit drugs.[24]

Multidose activated charcoal (MDAC) enhances elimination of already absorbed medications. MDAC involves repeated oral dosing of AC (first dose 50 g of AC with sorbitol and then 25 g of AC without sorbitol every 4 hours) to maintain the drug concentration gradient between the gut and the blood. This encourages migration of the drug from blood into the intestinal lumen ("gut dialysis"), where it binds to AC and is excreted. In addition, the persistent presence of AC disrupts the enterohepatic circulation of agents that undergo biliary elimination, thus enhancing their elimination. Certain toxins such as ASA are known to form bezoars, which MDAC may neutralize. Although MDAC significantly increases drug elimination in animal and volunteer studies, it has not been shown to affect clinical outcomes.[25]

To summarize, the various decontamination techniques do not appear to improve clinical outcomes. However, the studies of clinical outcomes are likely too small and have beta-error. As such, there are some patients who may benefit from decontamination. Many toxicologists recommend gastric lavage and AC for patients who present within 1 hour of ingestions of very toxic substances. Examples of such substances include salicylates, beta-blockers, and calcium channel blockers.

AUTHORS' RECOMMENDATIONS

- The diagnosis of critically ill poisoned patients is facilitated by correct identification of toxidromes.
- A prolonged course of NAC should be administered to those with ongoing liver toxicity after acetaminophen overdose.
- Urine alkalinization enhances salicylate elimination.
- Good supportive care is the primary management for most poisoned patients.
- GE techniques with ipecac or gastric lavage have not been shown to benefit patients and may actually cause harm.
- AC may be considered in an awake and alert patient with a potentially fatal ingestion in whom aspiration is unlikely.
- WBI is useful in eliminating substances that are not affected by AC (such as iron or lithium).
- MDAC should be considered for patients poisoned with lethal amounts of salicylate, carbamazepine, dapsone, phenobarbital, quinine, or theophylline.

REFERENCES

1. Kellermann AL, Fihn SD, LoGerfo JP, Copass MK. Impact of drug screening in suspected overdose. *Ann Emerg Med*. 1987;16(11):1206-1216.
2. Moeller KE, Lee KC, Kissack JC. Urine drug screening: practical guide for clinicians. *Mayo Clin Proc*. 2007;83(1):66-76.
3. Gummin DD, Mowry JB, Spyker DA, et al. 2016 annual report of the American Association of Poison Control Centers' National Poison Data System (NPDS): 34th annual report. *Clin Toxicol (Phila)*. 2017;55(10):1072-1252.
4. Hayes BD, Klein-Schwartz W, Doyon S. Frequency of medication errors with intravenous acetylcysteine for acetaminophen overdose. *Ann Pharmacother*. 2008;42(4):766-770.
5. Corcoran GB, Mitchell JR, Vaishnav YN, Horning EC. Evidence that acetaminophen and *N*-hydroxyacetaminophen form a common arylating intermediate, *N*-acetyl-*p*-benzoquinoneimine. *Mol Pharmacol*. 1980;18(3):536-542.
6. Miller RP, Roberts RJ, Fischer LJ. Acetaminophen elimination kinetics in neonates, children, and adults. *Clin Pharmacol Ther*. 1976;19(3):284-294.
7. Smilkstein MJ, Knapp GL, Kulig KW, Rumack BH. Efficacy of oral *N*-acetylcysteine in the treatment of acetaminophen overdose. Analysis of the national multicenter study (1976 to 1985). *N Engl J Med*. 1988;319(24):1557-1562.
8. Prescott LF. Paracetamol overdosage. Pharmacological considerations and clinical management. *Drugs*. 1983;25(3):290-314.
9. Makin A, Williams R. The current management of paracetamol overdosage. *Br J Clin Pract*. 1994;48(3):144-148.
10. Rumack BH, Matthew H. Acetaminophen poisoning and toxicity. *Pediatrics*. 1975;55(6):871-876.
11. Smilkstein MJ, Douglas DR, Daya MR. Acetaminophen poisoning and liver function. *N Engl J Med*. 1994;331(19):1310-1312.
12. Gosselin S, Juurlink DN, Kielstein JT, et al. Extracorporeal treatment for acetaminophen poisoning: Recommendations from the EXTRIP workgroup. *Clin Toxicol (Phila)*. 2014;52(8):856-867.
13. Marchetti A, Rossiter R. Managing acute acetaminophen poisoning with oral versus intravenous N-acetylcysteine: a provider-perspective cost analysis. *J Med Econ*. 2009;12(4):384-391.
14. Green JL, Heard KJ, Reynolds KM, Albert D. Oral and intravenous acetylcysteine for treatment of acetaminophen toxicity: a systematic review and meta-analysis. *West J Emerg Med*. 2013;14(3):218-226.
15. Yarema MC, Johnson DW, Berlin RJ, et al. Comparison of the 20-hour intravenous and 72-hour oral acetylcysteine protocols for the treatment of acute acetaminophen poisoning. *Ann Emerg Med*. 2009;54(4):606-614.
16. Harrison PM, Keays R, Bray GP, Alexander GJ, Williams R. Improved outcome of paracetamol-induced fulminant hepatic failure by late administration of acetylcysteine. *Lancet*. 1990;335(8705):1572-1573.
17. Karsh J. Adverse reactions and interactions with aspirin. Considerations in the treatment of the elderly patient. *Drug Saf*. 1990;5(5):317-327.
18. Leatherman JW, Schmitz PG. Fever, hyperdynamic shock, and multiple-system organ failure. A pseudo-sepsis syndrome associated with chronic salicylate intoxication. *Chest*. 1991;100(5):1391-1396.
19. Prescott LF, Balali-Mood M, Critchley JA, Johnstone AF, Proudfoot AT. Diuresis or urinary alkalinisation for salicylate poisoning? *Br Med J (Clin Res Ed)*. 1982;285(6352):1383-1386.
20. Juurlink DN, Gosselin S, Kielstein JT, et al. Extracorporeal treatment for salicylate poisoning: systematic review and recommendations from the EXTRIP workgroup. *Ann Emerg Med*. 2015;66(2):165-181.
21. Clemmesen C, Nilsson E. Therapeutic trends in the treatment of barbiturate poisoning. The Scandinavian method. *Clin Pharmacol Ther*. 1961;2:220-229.
22. Höjer J, Baehrendtz S. The effect of flumazenil (Ro 15-1788) in the management of self-induced benzodiazepine poisoning. A double-blind controlled study. *Acta Med Scand*. 1988;224(4):357-365.
23. Merigian KS, Woodard M, Hedges JR, et al. Prospective evaluation of gastric emptying in the self-poisoned patient. *Am J Emerg Med*. 1990;8(6):479-483.
24. Position paper: whole bowel irrigation. *J Toxicol Clin Toxicol*. 2004;42(6):843-854.
25. Position statement and practice guidelines on the use of multi-dose activated charcoal in the treatment of acute poisoning. American Academy of Clinical Toxicology; European Association of Poisons Centres and Clinical Toxicologists. *J Toxicol Clin Toxicol*. 1999;37(6):731-751.

81

When Is Transfusion Therapy Indicated in Critical Illness and When Is It Not?

Babak Sarani and Cheralyn J. Hendrix

INTRODUCTION

Transfusion of blood products is one of the most common therapies ordered in the intensive care unit (ICU). It is estimated that 4 million patients are transfused 8–12 million units of packed red blood cells (PRBC) annually in the United States alone and that the majority of transfusions occur in either surgical or critically ill patients. Several studies in various countries have documented that the incidence of PRBC transfusion in the ICU varies between 20 and 50%.[1–5] In addition to anemia approximately 40% of critically ill patients have a low platelet count or elevation in their coagulation parameters at some point during their ICU stay. Most of these hematological derangements, however, are asymptomatic, and numerous studies have shown that outcomes are either not changed or worsened following transfusion to normalize these values. While there are some well-designed trials that may be used to formulate guidelines regarding transfusion of PRBC in critically ill patients, there are no good studies that can be used to determine which patients will likely benefit from platelet or plasma transfusion in the ICU. This chapter reviews the available evidence on best transfusion practices in the ICU, including a review of the use of recombinant factor VIIa and four-factor prothrombin complex concentrate (PCC).

BASIS FOR TRANSFUSION OF BLOOD PRODUCTS—BENEFITS AND RISKS

Outcomes related to transfusion practices are only now being studied in well-designed prospective trials. Although there are many trials related to transfusion of PRBC, there is a dearth of information related to practice patterns and outcomes from the use of non-RBC products in patients who are not actively hemorrhaging.

Packed Red Blood Cell Transfusion

The normal blood volume is 7–8% of ideal body weight. This corresponds to a hemoglobin (Hb) level of 14–16 g/dL

and hematocrit level of 40–45%. Transfusion of RBCs can restore both circulating blood volume and oxygen-carrying capacity.

The body has many adaptive responses to increase oxygen delivery in the face of anemia (Box 81.1). Clinically, the easiest initial maneuver to increase oxygen delivery is to increase the oxygen saturation or Hb concentration because increasing cardiac output can increase myocardial oxygen demand and may precipitate ischemia in patients with coronary artery disease.[6]

Historically, the ideal Hb / hematocrit values in hospitalized patients were considered to be 10 g/dL or 30%. The basis for this claim lies partially on rheological principles, which suggest that there is an optimal balance between oxygen-carrying capacity (where high is better) and viscosity (where low is better). Such a balance would minimize cardiac work and maintain peripheral oxygen delivery. As recently as the 1990s, this recommendation was supported by two large retrospective studies in Jehovah's Witness populations that showed a significant increase in perioperative mortality if the preoperative Hb was 6 g/dL as opposed to 12 g/dL (odds ratio of 2.5 for each gram that the postoperative Hb was <8 g/dL; Table 81.1).[7,8] The risk of death was highest in patients with known cardiovascular disease.

Trials in postoperative patients have called into question the validity of these retrospective studies and suggest that transfusion thresholds should be individualized based on the documentation of end-organ hypoxia. Two randomized studies of post-cardiac surgery patients found no difference in morbidity in those randomized to a liberal vs. restrictive transfusion strategy.[9,10] However, the study by Hajjar et al.[9] found a dose-dependent increase in morbidity following transfusion, whereas the study by Murphy et al.[10] found an increase in mortality but no change in morbidity in those randomized to the restrictive transfusion arm of the study. Reasons for these findings are uncertain considering that the mean difference in the Hb level between the two arms was only 1 g/dL. Thus although a restrictive strategy for blood transfusion following cardiac surgery may be desirable, the

BOX 81.1   Physiologic Mechanisms to Increase Oxygen Delivery in Anemia.

Mechanisms that increase arterial oxygen content
- Increased production of erythropoietin leading to increased hemoglobin synthesis and concentration
- Rightward shift of hemoglobin saturation curve due to increased 2,3-diphosphoglycerate permitting increased oxygen "off-loading" at capillary P_{O_2}

Mechanisms that increase cardiac output
- Increased heart rate
- Increased myocardial contractility
- Decreased blood viscosity leading to decreased peripheral vascular resistance (afterload)

TABLE 81.1   Postoperative Outcomes of Anemic Jehovah's Witnesses.

Preoperative Hemoglobin Level (g/dL)	Mortality (%)
<6	61.5
6.1–8	33
8.1–10	0
>10	7.1

From Carson JL, Poses RM, Spence RK, Bonavita G. Severity of anaemia and operative mortality and morbidity. *Lancet.* 1988;1(8588): 727–729.

actual Hb trigger has yet to be determined. Similarly, another randomized study of elderly patients undergoing total hip arthroplasty found no difference in morbidity or mortality in those randomized to Hb transfusion threshold of 10 g/dL vs. 8 g/dL,[11] whereas a retrospective study in a similar patient population found a significant increase in perioperative morbidity and no change in mortality.[12]

In a single prospective, randomized, blinded study, blood transfusion used as part of a sepsis bundle was found to improve survival in patients with septic shock whose hemodynamic parameters did not correct with intravenous fluids.[13] However, because the interventions in this study were delivered as a bundle, it was not possible to determine the relative impact of transfusion on outcomes. Subsequently, an adequately-powered, randomized, prospective study of critically ill patients with septic shock found no difference in mortality or need for ongoing critical care interventions, such as mechanical ventilation, vasopressor use, or renal replacement therapy, between patients assigned to transfusion at Hb trigger of 7 g/dL vs. 9 g/dL.[14] Moreover, there was no change in the results in the subgroups of patients aged >70 years nor in those with known cardiovascular disease, though patients with acute coronary syndrome were excluded from this study. "Three small RCTs failed to demonstrate a benefit from PRBC transfusion, in terms of oxygen delivery or uptake, in septic critically ill patients."[15–17]

Many studies have addressed the role of PRBC transfusion in asymptomatic, hemodynamically stable, nonbleeding, anemic, critically ill patients. A single, randomized, blinded, prospective study in 1999, along with several subsequent observational studies, found that patients who are transfused above the Hb value of 7 g/dL have either the same or better outcomes than those who are transfused the Hb value of 10 g/dL.[3–5] These findings are consistent with other studies and one metaanalysis that also documented an increased risk of infection following PRBC transfusion.[3,5,18–25] Other studies have documented an increased risk of death following RBC transfusion.[3,5] Based on these data, current guidelines regarding PRBC transfusion in critically ill but asymptomatic and resuscitated patients call for the Hb transfusion trigger of 7 g/dL (Boxes 81.2 and 81.3).[26]

There are no randomized studies evaluating a threshold for PRBC transfusion in patients with unstable angina or acute coronary syndrome (ACS). However, a large, *post hoc* analysis from the combined patient pool of three studies that were originally designed to evaluate the efficacy of antiplatelet agents in those with myocardial ischemia found a significant increase in the hazard ratio in patients who were transfused to a hematocrit >25%.[27] This finding has been corroborated in multiple other retrospective studies.[28–30] Conversely, a recent, retrospective analysis of a highly selected cohort of patients with ACS suggested a decrease in mortality for those transfused for a Hb trigger of 9 g/dL.[31] However, the authors caution that the cohort enrolled in the study was not representative of typical patients with ACS; therefore, the results of the trial may not be generalizable to the overall population of patients with ACS. Thus, although there are insufficient data upon which to strongly recommend a transfusion threshold below the Hb level of 10 g/dL in this cohort, transfusion to the Hb level of 8–10 g/dL may

BOX 81.2   Thresholds for Transfusion in Stable Anemic Patients Without Risk for Potential Acute Blood Loss or Acute Surgical Stress.

Hemoglobin <8–10 g/dL
Acute myocardial infarction or acute coronary syndrome
Hemoglobin ≤7 g/dL
All other patients

BOX 81.3   Thresholds for Transfusion in Stable Patients at High Risk for Acute Blood Loss.

Hemoglobin ≤10 g/dL
Known disorders of hemostasis or red blood cell dyscrasia (e.g., sickle cell anemia)
All with anticipated estimated blood loss ≥1000 mL
Hemoglobin ≤7 g/dL
All other patients

be reasonable in most patients. Furthermore, the need for transfusion to a higher Hb level may be more appropriately reserved for patients with the evidence of ongoing end-organ ischemia.

Transfusion of blood products carries many risks. These include transmission of blood-borne pathogens, transfusion-associated circulatory overload (TACO), transfusion-related acute lung injury (TRALI), and transfusion-related immunomodulation (TRIM). Clinically significant transfusion reaction is rare under current guidelines and is most commonly due to clerical error. Interestingly, this adverse event is rarely observed in exsanguinating patients. This is likely due to alterations in the immune system resulting from severe injury necessitating massive transfusion.[32] TRALI and TRIM are most likely variants of the same disorder—an exaggerated inflammatory response and altered or deranged immune system due to transfusion of foreign protein—and may explain the increased risk for infection.[33] TRALI may result from local (pulmonary) inflammation, whereas TRIM may represent systemic immune derangement. Both entities are likely underreported due to a lack of unique diagnostic criteria and adequately-designed studies aimed at addressing their incidence.

TRALI is defined as noncardiogenic pulmonary edema that occurs within 4–6 hours of transfusion. It has a reported incidence of 1:5000 to 1:10,000 transfusions[34] and is most common following plasma transfusion. TRIM is best exemplified by reports showing the association between PRBC transfusion and infection[19,20,22,23,35,36] and reports documenting a chimeric state where donor epitopes can be expressed by cells of transfused trauma patients years after the transfusion itself.[37–39] Mechanisms underlying TRIM are only now being elucidated. Cotransfusion of soluble proteins, such as human leukocyte antigen or fibrinogen/fibrin degradation products, or cotransfusion of disrupted white blood cell products have been proposed as possible explanations.[33]

Plasma Transfusion

The plasma portion of donated whole blood contains most of the necessary clotting factors of the coagulation cascade. Although there are decreased concentrations of factors V, VII, and VIII, as a result of degradation and fibrinogen (factor I) due to dilution, spontaneous hemorrhage rarely occurs with factor concentrations >25%.[40,41] Plasma is dosed as 10–15 mL/kg (ideal body weight) and generally, 4 units will result in 40–60% factor recovery.[41] It is important to note that transfusion of 5 units of random donor platelets or 1 unit of single donor platelets also results in the transfusion of 1 unit-equivalent of plasma since platelets are suspended in plasma.[40] Plasma is commonly used in the ICU to rapidly treat coagulopathy with concomitant hemorrhage or in anticipation of an invasive procedure in a patient with coagulopathy.

Warfarin is a commonly used oral anticoagulant to prevent thromboembolic disease from various causes. A retrospective study found that each 30-minute delay in the administration of the first unit of plasma decreases the odds of correction of warfarin-induced coagulopathy by 20% in patients with intracerebral bleeding, underscoring the need for rapid and accurate reversal of the drug in hemorrhaging patients.[42] Because the speed with which plasma can be administered is limited by its supply and the time required to thaw and prepare the product, the use of PCCs to quickly restore clotting ability is becoming increasingly common. PCCs provide a concentrated source of three or four vitamin K-dependent coagulation factors. PCCs are stored in a lyophilized state and only require reconstitution. A type/screen is not needed, the product does not need to be thawed, and the total volume of drug to be administered is <100 mL, thus making administration significantly faster and eliminating the risk of TACO. Multiple international organizations, including the American College of Chest Physicians, recommend a combination of PCC and vitamin K for emergency anticoagulation reversal.[43] A 2013 study by Sarode et al.[44] evaluated the efficacy and safety of PCC compared with plasma in patients on vitamin K antagonists presenting with major bleeding. Rapid international normalized ratio (INR) reduction was achieved in 62% of patients receiving PCC vs. 10% of patients receiving. The safety profile was similar between groups.[44]

There is wide variability in the manner in which physicians utilize fresh frozen plasma (FFP) in nonbleeding patients with coagulopathy.[45] Many physicians use FFP prophylactically to reverse coagulopathy in nonbleeding patients despite published guidelines recommending against this, along with an unknown risk-benefit ratio.[46,47] Others cite mild coagulopathy as a reason to use FFP as a volume expander in nonbleeding, volume-depleted patients.[48] To date, there are no guidelines universally agreed upon for the use of FFP in nonbleeding patients. Suggested indications and dosing are shown in Box 81.4.

Historically, plasma transfusion was associated with a high incidence of TRALI. However, this risk has diminished to the point where TRALI is now rarely associated with plasma transfusion because most transfused plasma is collected from men and women who are either nulliparous or have had very few babies. The proposed mechanism to account for this phenomenon is a decrease in the variability of plasma proteins found in these individuals compared with multiparous women. This hypothesis is supported by a randomized, blinded, crossover study that found that the

---

BOX 81.4   Indications for Transfusion of Plasma.

Emergency reversal of warfarin-induced coagulopathy[a]
Replacement of isolated coagulation protein deficiency
Massive transfusion
Disseminated intravascular coagulation with serious active bleeding
Liver disease with clinical bleeding and evidence of coagulation defect
Thrombotic thrombocytopenic purpura
Replacement of clotting factors after apheresis therapy

[a]Consider prothrombin complex concentrate in lieu of plasma.

risk of TRALI is higher following plasma transfusion obtained from multiparous women.[49] Transfusion of plasma may be associated with TRIM. A retrospective study identified a three-fold higher relative risk of infection in critically ill surgical patients who received FFP, a finding that is consistent with the risk of infection following PRBC transfusion.[50] This study has not been repeated because the donor pool for procurement of plasma was altered to try to exclude multiparous women. Finally, hemolytic transfusion reactions also are possible following plasma transfusion as plasma contains variable titers of anti-A and anti-B antibody.

Single-center studies have suggested that the use of PCC may be effective in treating non-vitamin K antagonist-related coagulopathy, reducing the need for plasma transfusion. One study involving severely injured patients found that use of PCC plus plasma (compared with plasma alone) was associated with a significant reduction in the time required to lower the INR below 1.5 as well as the need for both RBC and plasma transfusion.[51] There was no difference in thromboembolic event risk. Another study found that the INR could be lowered significantly in patients who were coagulopathic due to either sepsis or liver failure.[52] However, both of these studies require validation in larger, appropriately-designed studies.

Cryoprecipitate Transfusion

Cryoprecipitate is the precipitated fraction obtained from thawing FFP at 4°C. This method of isolation means that cryoprecipitate is pooled from the FFP obtained from multiple donors. Cryoprecipitate is rich is factor VIII, von Willebrand factor, factor XIII, and fibronectin. Most importantly, it contains concentrated fibrinogen and thus the main indication for its use is the treatment of coagulopathy due to hypofibrinogenemia.[47] It may therefore be useful in the management of disseminated intravascular coagulation (DIC) with hemorrhage and in the reversal of thrombolytic agents (Box 81.5). While an adequate dose of plasma can replete fibrinogen, hypofibrinogenemia can be reversed more quickly using cryoprecipitate or, better, fibrinogen concentrate. Cryoprecipitate is dosed as a 10-pack transfusion; each 10-pack raises the fibrinogen level 75%.[41] Bleeding patients with known von Willebrand deficiency also should receive cryoprecipitate to optimize platelet function, while nonbleeding patients with this disorder can be treated with desmopressin.

BOX 81.5 Indications for Transfusion of Cryoprecipitate.

Hemophilia A (factor VIII deficiency)
von Willebrand's disease
Fibrinogen deficiency
Dysfibrinogenemia
Factor XIII deficiency
Uremic platelet dysfunction

Risks associated with transfusion of cryoprecipitate are the same as those reported for the other blood components. However, the incidence of TRALI and TRIM is probably lower than that associated with plasma transfusion because the total volume of cryoprecipitate transfused is much less than that of plasma, thereby minimizing the recipient's exposure to foreign protein antigen. The risk of transmission of blood-borne pathogens, however, may be higher due to the pooled nature of this product. There are no well-designed studies assessing outcomes or adverse events related to transfusion of cryoprecipitate.

Platelet Transfusion

Platelet transfusion is less common than RBC or plasma transfusion. The most common indication for platelet transfusion is decreased production followed by the increased destruction of cells.[40] In the critically ill population, where DIC is more prevalent, increased consumption of platelets can also lead to thrombocytopenia. Although the absolute platelet count may not correlate with function and ability to form a stable clot, it is generally accepted that spontaneous bleeding can occur with platelet counts <10,000 cells/μL.[53] Although not validated in studies, many clinicians recommend that a minimum platelet count of 50,000 cells/μL should be maintained, if possible, for patients at significant risk of bleeding (e.g., trauma postoperative patients, or those about to undergo an invasive procedure associated with a significant risk of hemorrhage), and a target of 80,000–100,000 cells/μL is recommended for patients who are actively bleeding or at risk for intracranial hemorrhage.[40,54] However, the authors stress that there is no evidence-based basis for this practice, and it is very likely that platelet number and physiologic impact on clot formation/stability do not have a linear relationship.

Despite the fact that the platelet count can be determined easily and quickly, there is no simple method for testing platelet function. A possible exception is thromboelastography (TEG), a method of assessing clot formation and lysis. Limited evidence from observational and retrospective data suggests that TEG is able to detect platelet dysfunction following trauma.[55–57] However, these studies also demonstrate a high rate of inhibition of both the arachidonic acid and adenosine diphosphate pathways in the platelet following even minor injury or relatively mild critical illness. Thus, in contrast to serum coagulation parameters, there are no studies that can be used to direct platelet transfusion in critically ill patients. The critical care practitioner should be aware of the high incidence of platelet dysfunction in the critically ill patient and base the decision to transfuse platelets on the clinical scenario at hand.

There are no studies that can be used to recommend timing and volume of platelet transfusion in nonbleeding, critically ill patients. Further, although there are no studies to determine the impact that use of aspirin or nonsteroidal antiinflammatory agents have on hemorrhage following injury, a review of the literature suggests that use of aspirin may worsen intracranial hemorrhage following traumatic brain injury.[58–60] An open-label, ex-vivo study in volunteers showed that platelet transfusion can reverse the platelet dysfunction caused by clopidrogel.[61] Two studies demonstrate that platelet transfusion is effective in reversing the degree of platelet inhibition caused by aspirin or clopidogrel, although the studies were not appropriately designed to describe a dose-response curve.[57,62] The authors recommended utilizing serial TEG measurements to determine the efficacy after each platelet transfusion.

MASSIVE EXSANGUINATION AND TRANSFUSION

Patients requiring massive transfusion are a unique cohort in whom aggressive transfusion is needed for hemodynamic support and reversal of coagulopathy (Table 81.2). The most commonly utilized definition of massive transfusion is the administration of 10 units of PRBC within 24 hours. This does not address the coagulopathy that also exists in these patients and fuels the process underlying the hemorrhage.[63] Non-controlled and retrospective studies suggest that aggressive transfusion using plasma:RBC ratios that approach 1:1 within a pre-defined massive transfusion protocol may result in earlier arrest of hemorrhage, as well as a mortality benefit.[64–66] The PROMMTT trial prospectively evaluated 1245 trauma patients who received at least one unit of RBCs within 6 hours of admission. Increased ratios of plasma:RBCs and platelets:RBCs were independently associated with a decrease in 6-hour mortality. Patients with ratios less than 1:2 were 3–4 times more likely to die than patients with ratios of 1:1 or higher.[67] The PROPPR trial found no difference in mortality, but a decrease in hemorrhage and transfusion need in trauma patients who received a 1:1 vs. 1:2 transfusion strategy.[68] Until similar studies are carried out in the non-trauma population, it may be prudent to treat exsanguinating, critically ill patients with

BOX 81.6	Causes of Abnormal Bleeding in Surgery and Trauma.
Release of tissue thromboplastin
Massive transfusion
Autotransfusion
Disseminated intravascular coagulation
Platelet dysfunction
Hypothermia

aggressive transfusion of plasma and platelets in addition to RBCs while also preventing hypothermia, acidosis, and other causes of on-going coagulopathy.[69] Common causes of abnormal bleeding in critically ill patients are noted in Box 81.6.

RECOMBINANT FACTOR VIIA

Mechanism of Action and Clinical Use

Recombinant factor VIIa is approved for use in hemophiliacs with antibodies to factor VIII or IX. However, many case reports and small series found that it may also have a role in arresting hemorrhage from other causes. Recombinant factor VIIa works by binding to exposed tissue factor in an area of endothelial injury, thereby activating platelets and platelet plug formation. Factor VIIa then stimulates the coagulation cascade by activating thrombin on the platelet plug. Fibrinolysis is inhibited through factor VIIa-mediated activation of thrombin activatable fibrinolysis inhibitor.

Factor VIIa has been shown to reduce hemorrhage following injury. Two parallel, randomized, blinded, placebo-controlled studies found that the drug was associated with a 50% relative reduction in severity of hemorrhage in bluntly injured patients but did not have a transfusion-sparing effect in victims of penetrating trauma.[70] However, the potential transfusion-sparing effect was only seen at very high doses, a difference that has substantial cost implications. The only large, randomized, blinded, placebo-controlled study on the use of factor VIIa in injured patients (CONTROL trial) was stopped early for futility when the control arm was noted to have a substantially lower mortality than anticipated.[71] Given the drug's cost, lack of mortality benefit, its association with thrombotic events (see later), and the availability of PCC, factor VIIa is no longer routinely used in trauma or critically ill patients.

Adverse Events Associated with Recombinant Factor VIIa

Factor VIIa has been associated with thromboembolic complications, particularly when used off-label. Reports from the Food and Drug Administration suggest that the incidence of thromboembolic disease is 0.02% in hemophiliacs, but the incidence of myocardial infarction, stroke, or pulmonary embolism may be as high as 8% when the agent is used in other populations.[72] Moreover, there is an almost equal incidence of

TABLE 81.2	Transfusion Guidelines for Patients who are Acutely Bleeding.
Clinical Situation	**Recommended Response**
Rapid acute hemorrhage without immediate control, estimated blood loss >30–40%, or presence of symptoms of severe blood loss	Transfuse PRBC. Initiate massive transfusion protocol with 1:1 RBC:FFP transfusion.[a]
Estimated blood loss <25–30% without uncontrolled hemorrhage	Crystalloid resuscitation, proceed to blood transfusion if hemorrhage is not quickly arrested
Presence of comorbid factors	Consider transfusion with lesser degrees of blood loss

[a]May require uncrossmatched or type-specific blood.
FFP, fresh frozen plasma; *PRBC*, packed red blood cells.

arterial and venous thrombi following administration of the drug. However, the CONTROL trial did not find any difference in complications between trauma patients who did and did not receive factor VIIa.[71]

TRANEXAMIC ACID

Mechanism of Action and Clinical Use

Tranexamic acid (TXA) is a synthetic lysine derivative that inhibits fibrinolysis by binding to and inhibiting plasminogen. A review of 53 studies incorporating 3836 persons undergoing elective surgery found that administration of this agent resulted in a 39% reduction in blood transfusion. CRASH-2, a multinational, randomized, blinded, placebo-controlled study, that included 270 hospitals and enrolled over 20,000 injured patients, found that administration of TXA within 8 hours of injury resulted in a statistically significant 1.5% decrease in the risk of death from any cause.[73] Further analysis suggested that the biggest reduction was in hemorrhage-related death. Subgroup analysis found that this benefit was confined to patients who received tranexamic acid within 3 hours of injury.[74] Persons who were treated with the medication 3–8 hours following injury actually had a higher mortality than the placebo group. The study has been criticized for enrolling patients who were actually hemorrhaging as well as those perceived to be at risk of hemorrhage based on the judgment of the bedside clinician. Furthermore, although the study found a significant decrease in the probability of hemorrhage-related death, there was no difference in the amount of blood transfused in surviving patients.

The MaTTERS and MaTTERS II trials are retrospective studies of the same patient cohort and evaluated the benefits of TXA in soldiers wounded in battle.[75,76] Similar to the CRASH-2 trial, these studies also found a significant decrease in hemorrhage-related mortality, but the study cohort consisted solely of patients requiring a massive transfusion. Maximal benefit from administration of TXA was found in patients who received both a 1:1:1 ratio of PRBC:FFP as well as cryoprecipitate. The risk of venous thromboembolic disease was 2–3%. The number needed to treat to prevent one hemorrhage-related death in the MaTTERS study was 7.

Reports have been published suggesting an increase in mortality associated with TXA administration in patients who do not have fibrinolysis evident on TEG, a condition referred to as "fibrinolysis shut down."[77-79] These studies suggest that TXA administration to persons with an LY30 value <0.8% is associated with an increase in mortality, whereas TXA administration to persons with an LY30 value >3% is associated with a reduction in death risk. As such, until randomized trials validating these findings are published, it may be prudent to check the degree of thrombolysis present prior to administrating this agent, if possible. Lastly, these findings have not been validated in noninjured patients, and the risk/benefit analysis of TXA as a treatment for sepsis or other related causes of thrombolysis remains uncertain.

CONCLUSION

There remains a paucity of high-level evidence to guide transfusion practice in the ICU. Studies to date argue for a restrictive policy of PRBC transfusion in critically ill patients who are not hemorrhaging and are not manifesting signs of end-organ ischemia. Similarly, patients who have other asymptomatic derangements in coagulation should not be transfused unless an invasive procedure, with propensity for hemorrhage, is planned. The use of PCC may be superior to the use of FFP in this setting. Patients who require ongoing transfusion support should be aggressively treated with transfusion of PRBC, plasma, and platelets. Further studies are needed to better evaluate pharmacologic adjuncts and laboratory-guided transfusion therapy, particularly viscoelastogram-guided therapy, in hemorrhaging patients.

AUTHORS' RECOMMENDATIONS

Red blood cell transfusion
- Used to augment the oxygen-carrying capacity of blood
- Evidence-based transfusion trigger in critically ill, resuscitated patients is Hb 7 g/dL
- Transfusion trigger in patients with end-organ dysfunction or shock remains uncertain. Common practice uses Hb 9–10 g/dL as a trigger for transfusion if the patient fails crystalloid resuscitation
- Complication of transfusion can be grouped into: transfusion reaction (clerical), volume overload (TACO), and immune dysfunction (TRALI and TRIM)

Plasma transfusion
- Used to reverse diffuse coagulopathy
- Dosed as 10–15 mL/kg
- Has the highest association with TRALI
- Consider treating vitamin K-dependent coagulopathy with PCC.

Cryoprecipitate transfusion
- Contains factor VIII, von Willebrand factor, factor XIII, and fibronectin
- Used to treat DIC or to reverse thrombolytic-induced hemorrhage (i.e., hypofibrinogenemia)

Platelet transfusion
- May be used to reverse clopidogrel (and possibly aspirin)-induced thrombocytopathy
- Platelet count of 50,000–100,000 cells/dL are needed for operation, depending on the nature of the procedure planned
- Other than TEG, there is no readily available test to clinically evaluate platelet function
- Platelet dysfunction is common in critically ill or injured patients. Platelet transfusion should be carried out in the appropriate clinical setting and not solely to reverse this dysfunction

Massive transfusion
- Retrospective studies suggest that a ratio approaching 1:1:1 of RBC:FFP:platelet may decrease net transfusion needs
- TXA acid may be associated with a survival benefit in hemorrhaging patients who have demonstrable thrombolysis but may also be associated with a rise in mortality in persons who do not

REFERENCES

1. French CJ, Bellomo R, Finfer SR, Lipman J, Chapman M, Boyce NW. Appropriateness of red blood cell transfusion in Australasian intensive care practice. *Med J Aust.* 2002;177:548-551.
2. Walsh TS, Garrioch M, Maciver C, et al. Red cell requirements for intensive care units adhering to evidence-based transfusion guidelines. *Transfusion.* 2004;44:1405-1411.
3. Corwin HL, Gettinger A, Pearl RG, et al. The CRIT Study: Anemia and blood transfusion in the critically ill—current clinical practice in the United States. *Crit Care Med.* 2004;32:39-52.
4. Hébert PC, Wells G, Blajchman MA, et al. A multicenter, randomized, controlled clinical trial of transfusion requirements in critical care. Transfusion Requirements in Critical Care Investigators, Canadian Critical Care Trials Group. *N Engl J Med.* 1999;340:409-417.
5. Vincent JL, Baron JF, Reinhart K, et al. Anemia and blood transfusion in critically ill patients. *JAMA.* 2002;288:1499-1507.
6. Hayes MA, Timmins AC, Yau EH, Palazzo M, Hinds CJ, Watson D. Elevation of systemic oxygen delivery in the treatment of critically ill patients. *N Engl J Med.* 1994;330:1717-1722.
7. Carson JL, Duff A, Poses RM, et al. Effect of anaemia and cardiovascular disease on surgical mortality and morbidity. *Lancet.* 1996;348:1055-1060.
8. Carson JL, Noveck H, Berlin JA, Gould SA. Mortality and morbidity in patients with very low postoperative Hb levels who decline blood transfusion. *Transfusion.* 2002;42:812-818.
9. Hajjar LA, Vincent JL, Galas FR, et al. Transfusion requirements after cardiac surgery: the TRACS randomized controlled trial. *JAMA.* 2010;304:1559-1567.
10. Murphy GJ, Pike K, Rogers CA, et al. Liberal or restrictive transfusion after cardiac surgery. *N Engl J Med.* 2015;372:997-1008.
11. Carson JL, Terrin ML, Noveck H, et al. Liberal or restrictive transfusion in high-risk patients after hip surgery. *N Engl J Med.* 2011;365:2453-2462.
12. Frisch NB, Wessell NM, Charters MA, Yu S, Jeffries JJ, Silverton CD. Predictors and complications of blood transfusion in total hip and knee arthroplasty. *J Arthroplasty.* 2014;29:189-192.
13. Rivers E, Nguyen B, Havstad S, et al. Early goal-directed therapy in the treatment of severe sepsis and septic shock. *N Engl J Med.* 2001;345:1368-1377.
14. Holst LB, Haase N, Wetterslev J, et al. Lower versus higher hemoglobin threshold for transfusion in septic shock. *N Engl J Med.* 2014;371:1381-1391.
15. Dietrich KA, Conrad SA, Hebert CA, Levy GL, Romero MD. Cardiovascular and metabolic response to red blood cell transfusion in critically ill volume-resuscitated nonsurgical patients. *Crit Care Med.* 1990;18:940-944.
16. Fernandes CJ Jr, Akamine N, De Marco FV, et al. Red blood cell transfusion does not increase oxygen consumption in critically ill septic patients. *Crit Care.* 2001;5:362-367.
17. Lorente JA, Landin L, De Pablo R, Renes E, Rodríguez-Díaz R, Liste D. Effects of blood transfusion on oxygen transport variables in severe sepsis. *Crit Care Med.* 1993;21:1312-1318.
18. Chang H, Hall GA, Geerts WH, Greenwood C, McLeod RS, Sher GD. Allogeneic red blood cell transfusion is an independent risk factor for the development of postoperative bacterial infection. *Vox Sang.* 2000;78:13-18.
19. Claridge JA, Sawyer RG, Schulman AM, McLemore EC, Young JS. Blood transfusions correlate with infections in trauma patients in a dose-dependent manner. *Am Surg.* 2002;68:566-572.
20. Hill GE, Frawley WH, Griffith KE, Forestner JE, Minei JP. Allogeneic blood transfusion increases the risk of postoperative bacterial infection: a meta-analysis. *J Trauma.* 2003;54:908-914.
21. Malone D, Dunne J, Tracy K, Putnam AT, Scalea TM, Napolitano LM. Blood transfusion, Independent of shock severity, is associated with worse outcome in trauma. *J Trauma.* 2003;54:898-907.
22. Shorr AF, Duh MS, Kelly KM, Kollef MH. Red blood cell transfusion and ventilator-associated pneumonia: a potential link? *Crit Care Med.* 2004;32:666-674.
23. Taylor RW, Manganaro L, O'Brien J, Trottier SJ, Parkar N, Veremakis C. Impact of allogenic packed red blood cell transfusion on nosocomial infection rates in the critically ill patient. *Crit Care Med.* 2002;30:2249-2254.
24. Vamvakas EC. Perioperative blood transfusion and cancer recurrence: meta-analysis for explanation. *Transfusion.* 1995;35:760-768.
25. Taylor RW, O'Brien J, Trottier SJ, et al. Red blood cell transfusions and nosocomial infections in critically ill patients. *Crit Care Med.* 2006;34:2302-2308; quiz 2309.
26. Napolitano LM, Kurek S, Luchette FA, et al. Clinical practice guideline: red blood cell transfusion in adult trauma and critical care. *Crit Care Med.* 2009;37:3124-3157.
27. Rao SV, Jollis JG, Harrington RA, et al. Relationship of blood transfusion and clinical outcomes in patients with acute coronary syndromes. *JAMA.* 2004;292:1555-1562.
28. Alexander KP, Chen AY, Wang TY, et al. Transfusion practice and outcomes in non-ST-segment elevation acute coronary syndromes. *Am Heart J.* 2008;155:1047-1053.
29. Aronson D, Dann EJ, Bonstein L, et al. Impact of red blood cell transfusion on clinical outcomes in patients with acute myocardial infarction. *Am J Cardiol.* 2008;102:115-119.
30. Singla I, Zahid M, Good CB, Macioce A, Sonel AF. Impact of blood transfusions in patients presenting with anemia and suspected acute coronary syndrome. *Am J Cardiol.* 2007;99:1119-1121.
31. Salisbury AC, Reid KJ, Marso SP, et al. Blood transfusion during acute myocardial infarction: association with mortality and variability across hospitals. *J Am Coll Cardiol.* 2014;64:811-819.
32. Dutton RP, Shih D, Edelman BB, Hess J, Scalea TM. Safety of uncrossmatched type-O red cells for resuscitation from hemorrhagic shock. *J Trauma.* 2005;59:1445-1449.
33. Vamvakas EC. Possible mechanisms of allogeneic blood transfusion-associated postoperative infection. *Transfus Med Rev.* 2002;16:144-160.
34. Stainsby D, Cohen H, Jones H, et al. Serious Hazards of Transfusion (SHOT) Annual Report 2003; 2004.
35. Carson JL, Altman DG, Duff A, et al. Risk of bacterial infection associated with allogeneic blood transfusion among patients undergoing hip fracture repair. *Transfusion.* 1999;39:694-700.
36. Dutton RP, Lefering R, Lynn M. Database predictors of transfusion and mortality. *J Trauma.* 2006;60:S70-S77.
37. Reed W, Lee TH, Norris PJ, Utter GH, Busch MP. Transfusion-associated microchimerism: a new complication of blood transfusions in severely injured patients. *Semin Hematol.* 2007;44:24-31.
38. Utter GH, Nathens AB, Lee TH, et al. Leukoreduction of blood transfusions does not diminish transfusion-associated microchimerism in trauma patients. *Transfusion.* 2006;46:1863-1869.
39. Utter GH, Owings JT, Lee TH, et al. Blood transfusion is associated with donor leukocyte microchimerism in trauma patients. *J Trauma.* 2004;57:702-707; discussion: 707-708.

40. American College of Pathologists. Practice parameter for the use of fresh-frozen plasma, cryoprecipitate, and platelets. *JAMA*. 1994;271:777-781.

41. Puget Sound Blood Center. *Blood Component Therapy*. 2012. Available at: http://www.psbc.org/therapy/ffp.htm. Accessed March 15, 2015.

42. Goldstein JN, Thomas SH, Frontiero V, et al. Timing of fresh frozen plasma administration and rapid correction of coagulopathy in warfarin-related intracerebral hemorrhage. *Stroke*. 2006;37:151-155.

43. Holbrook A, Schulman S, Witt DM, et al. Evidence-based management of anticoagulant therapy: Antithrombotic Therapy and Prevention of Thrombosis, 9th ed: American College of Chest Physicians Evidence-Based Clinical Practice Guidelines. *Chest*. 2012;141:e152S-e184S.

44. Sarode R, Milling Jr TJ, Refaai MA, et al. Efficacy and safety of a 4-factor prothrombin complex concentrate in patients on vitamin K antagonists presenting with major bleeding: a randomized, plasma-controlled, phase IIIb study. *Circulation*. 2013;128:1234-1243.

45. Dara SI, Rana R, Afessa B, Moore SB, Gajic O. Fresh frozen plasma transfusion in critically ill medical patients with coagulopathy. *Crit Care Med*. 2005;33:2667-2671.

46. Contreras M, Ala FA, Greaves M, et al. Guidelines for the use of fresh frozen plasma. British Committee for Standards in Haematology, Working Party of the Blood Transfusion Task Force. *Transfus Med*. 1992;2:57-63.

47. O'Shaughnessy DF, Atterbury C, Bolton Maggs P, et al. Guidelines for the use of fresh-frozen plasma, cryoprecipitate and cryosupernatant. *Br J Haematol*. 2004;126:11-28.

48. Lauzier F, Cook D, Griffith L, Upton J, Crowther M. Fresh frozen plasma transfusion in critically ill patients. *Crit Care Med*. 2007;35:1655-1659.

49. Palfi M, Berg S, Ernerudh J, Berlin G. A randomized controlled trial of transfusion-related acute lung injury: is plasma from multiparous blood donors dangerous? *Transfusion*. 2001;41:317-322.

50. Sarani B, Dunkman WJ, Dean L, Sonnad S, Rohrbach JI, Gracias VH. Transfusion of fresh frozen plasma in critically ill surgical patients is associated with an increased risk of infection. *Crit Care Med*. 2008;36:1114-1118.

51. Jehan F, Aziz H, O'Keeffe T, et al. The role of four-factor prothrombin complex concentrate in coagulopathy of trauma: a propensity matched analysis. *J Trauma Acute Care Surg*. 2018;85:18-24.

52. Young H, Holzmacher JL, Amdur R, Gondek S, Sarani B, Schroeder ME. Use of four-factor prothrombin complex concentrate in the reversal of warfarin-induced and nonvitamin K antagonist-related coagulopathy. *Blood Coagul Fibrinolysis*. 2017;28:564-569.

53. NIH Consensus Conference. Platelet transfusion therapy. *JAMA*. 1987;257:1777-1780.

54. British Committee for Standards in Haematology and Blood Transfusion Task Force. Guidelines for the use of platelet transfusions. *Br J Haematol*. 2003;122:10-23.

55. Wohlauer MV, Moore EE, Thomas S, et al. Early platelet dysfunction: an unrecognized role in the acute coagulopathy of trauma. *J Am Coll Surg*. 2012;214:739-746.

56. Hase T, Sirajuddin S, Maluso P, Bangalore R, DePalma L, Sarani B. Platelet dysfunction in critically ill patients. *Blood Coagul Fibrinolysis*. 2017;28:475-478.

57. Sirajuddin S, Valdez C, DePalma L, et al. Inhibition of platelet function is common following even minor injury. *J Trauma Acute Care Surg*. 2016;81:328-332.

58. Joseph B, Pandit V, Sadoun M, et al. A prospective evaluation of platelet function in patients on antiplatelet therapy with traumatic intracranial hemorrhage. *J Trauma Acute Care Surg*. 2013;75:990-994.

59. Naidech AM, Rosenberg NF, Bernstein RA, Batjer HH. Aspirin use or reduced platelet activity predicts craniotomy after intracerebral hemorrhage. *Neurocrit Care*. 2011;15:442-446.

60. Sakr M, Wilson L. Best evidence topic report. Aspirin and the risk of intracranial complications following head injury. *Emerg Med J*. 2005;22:891-892.

61. Vilahur G, Choi BG, Zafar MU, et al. Normalization of platelet reactivity in clopidogrel-treated subjects. *J Thromb Haemost*. 2007;5:82-90.

62. Holzmacher JL, Reynolds C, Patel M, et al. Platelet transfusion does not improve outcomes in patients with brain injury on antiplatelet therapy. *Brain Inj*. 2018;32:325-330.

63. Holcomb JB, Jenkins D, Rhee P, et al. Damage control resuscitation: directly addressing the early coagulopathy of trauma. *J Trauma*. 2007;62:307-310.

64. Cotton BA, Reddy N, Hatch QM, et al. Damage control resuscitation is associated with a reduction in resuscitation volumes and improvement in survival in 390 damage control laparotomy patients. *Ann Surg*. 2011;254:598-605.

65. Young PP, Cotton BA, Goodnough LT. Massive transfusion protocols for patients with substantial hemorrhage. *Transfus Med Rev*. 2011;25:293-303.

66. Borgman MA, Spinella PC, Perkins JG, et al. The ratio of blood products transfused affects mortality in patients receiving massive transfusions at a combat support hospital. *J Trauma*. 2007;63:805-813.

67. Holcomb JB, del Junco DJ, Fox EE, et al. The prospective, observational, multicenter, major trauma transfusion (PROMMTT) study: comparative effectiveness of a time-varying treatment with competing risks. *JAMA Surg*. 2013;148:127-136.

68. Holcomb JB, Tilley BC, Baraniuk S, et al. Transfusion of plasma, platelets, and red blood cells in a 1:1:1 vs. a 1:1:2 ratio and mortality in patients with severe trauma: the PROPPR randomized clinical trial. *JAMA*. 2015;313:471-482.

69. McDaniel LM, Neal MD, Sperry JL, et al. Use of a massive transfusion protocol in nontrauma patients: activate away. *J Am Coll Surg*. 2013;216:1103-1109.

70. Boffard KD, Riou B, Warren B, et al. Recombinant factor VIIa as adjunctive therapy for bleeding control in severely injured trauma patients: two parallel randomized, placebo-controlled, double-blind clinical trials. *J Trauma*. 2005;59:8-15; discussion: 15-18.

71. Hauser CJ, Boffard K, Dutton R, et al. Results of the CONTROL trial: efficacy and safety of recombinant activated Factor VII in the management of refractory traumatic hemorrhage. *J Trauma*. 2010;69:489-500.

72. O'Connell KA, Wood JJ, Wise RP, Lozier JN, Braun MM. Thromboembolic adverse events after use of recombinant human coagulation factor VIIa. *JAMA*. 2006;295:293-298.

73. Shakur H, Roberts I, Bautista R, et al. Effects of tranexamic acid on death, vascular occlusive events, and blood transfusion in trauma patients with significant haemorrhage (CRASH-2): a randomised, placebo-controlled trial. *Lancet*. 2010;376:23-32.

74. Roberts I, Shakur H, Afolabi A, et al. The importance of early treatment with tranexamic acid in bleeding trauma patients: an exploratory analysis of the CRASH-2 randomised controlled trial. *Lancet.* 2011;377:1096-1101, 1101. e1-2.

75. Morrison JJ, Dubose JJ, Rasmussen TE, Midwinter MJ. Military Application of Tranexamic Acid in Trauma Emergency Resuscitation (MATTERs) Study. *Arch Surg.* 2012;147: 113-119.

76. Morrison JJ, Ross JD, Dubose JJ, Jansen JO, Midwinter MJ, Rasmussen TE. Association of cryoprecipitate and tranexamic acid with improved survival following wartime injury: findings from the MATTERs II Study. *JAMA Surg.* 2013;148:218-225.

77. Moore HB, Moore EE, Gonzalez E, et al. Hyperfibrinolysis, physiologic fibrinolysis, and fibrinolysis shutdown: the spectrum of postinjury fibrinolysis and relevance to antifibrinolytic therapy. *J Trauma Acute Care Surg.* 2014;77:811-817; discussion: 817.

78. Moore HB, Moore EE, Huebner BR, et al. Fibrinolysis shutdown is associated with a fivefold increase in mortality in trauma patients lacking hypersensitivity to tissue plasminogen activator. *J Trauma Acute Care Surg.* 2017;83:1014-1022.

79. Moore HB, Moore EE, Liras IN, et al. Acute fibrinolysis shutdown after injury occurs frequently and increases mortality: a multicenter evaluation of 2,540 severely injured patients. *J Am Coll Surg.* 2016;222:347-355.

82

Is There a Role for Granulocyte-Macrophage Colony-Stimulating Factor and/or Erythropoietin in Critical Illness?

McKenzie K. Hollen, Philip A. Efron, and Alicia M. Mohr

CHRONIC CRITICAL ILLNESS

Chronic critical illness (CCI) is defined by some as continued organ dysfunction while in an intensive care unit (ICU) for >14 days. Patients with CCI are typically immunosuppressed with an increased susceptibility to hospital-acquired complications and secondary infections as well as prolonged anemia. Several factors contribute to these abnormalities, including T-cell apoptosis, expansion of T regulatory cells, expansion and persistence of myeloid-derived suppressor cells, deterioration of lymphocyte number and function, and inadequacy of erythropoiesis to improve anemia.[1] Much of the pathology can be linked to altered bone marrow/stem cell function. In addition, the neuroendocrine stress response, patient's age, and patient's comorbidities collectively play a role in dysregulated myelopoiesis and hematopoietic function.[2] This chapter will explore potential targeted therapies in these patients.

ROLE OF GRANULOCYTE-MACROPHAGE COLONY-STIMULATING FACTOR

Despite improvements in the management of nosocomial infections in critically ill patients, financial burdens and the rise of bacterial resistance pose new challenges that require novel approaches.[3] Both a severe insult and treatment for critical illness contribute to long-term changes to patients' innate and adaptive immune systems that may leave the patient highly vulnerable to subsequent infections. Granulocyte-macrophage colony-stimulating factor (GM-CSF) is a heterodimeric myelopoietic growth factor, and is naturally occurring. GM-CSF was initially identified as a factor capable of mobilizing bone marrow precursor cells and promoting dendritic cell maturation; however, it is currently recognized for its role in governing mature myeloid populations during the host inflammatory response.[4] In vitro GM-CSF promotes cell survival, proliferation, differentiation, and activation of neutrophils, basophils, eosinophils, and monocytes (Fig. 82.1).[3] These properties have obvious clinical potential.[3] Exogenous GM-CSF has been administered to chemotherapy patients with acquired secondary myelosuppression and chemotherapy-induced neutropenia.[5] The analogy in critically ill patients with immunosuppressive clinical phenotypes comparable to those seen during chemotherapy is clear. Thus, GM-CSF has been investigated as an immune-stimulant capable of restoring the antigen-presenting cell (APC) function of myeloid cells as well as the potential to boost host adaptive immunity in other ways.[3,6] In certain illnesses, GM-CSF administration has shortened the duration of granulocytopenia and promoted immune cell proliferation and function by increasing bone marrow production and decreasing neutrophil migration from tissues at the site of inflammation.[6–8]

GM-CSF exerts extensive effects that may be both proinflammatory and antiinflammatory.[9] Studies in knock-out mice have demonstrated that GM-CSF is associated with type I natural killer T cells and lung macrophage differentiation, although macrophage activation requires an additional stimulus, for example, a proinflammatory cytokine (PIC; e.g., interleukin-1 [IL-1] and tumor-necrosis factor [TNF]).[3] GM-CSF improves host adaptive immunity, increases macrophage cytotoxicity, and exerts a significant proinflammatory role in mature myeloid populations by increasing monocyte expression of human leukocyte antigen DR (mHLA-DR), thus promoting APC function.[6,10] Without TNFα, IL-1, lipopolysaccharide, or other stimulus, activation of GM-CSF in vitro is limited.[11–13] GM-CSF is produced in T lymphocytes, keratinocytes, smooth muscle cells, endothelial and epithelial cells, and neurons.[12,14]

CLINICAL STUDIES

Although GM-CSF has been extensively studied, its potential therapeutic benefits in septic and critically ill patients remain unclear. One conundrum plaguing the management of the critically ill is the need to concurrently manage persistent inflammation and adaptive immunosuppression.[3] GM-CSF has been examined as an agent that might resolve this issue. Research has demonstrated that GM-CSF therapy can result in an improved recovery time after infection, a decrease in the length of hospital stay, and a decrease in patient days on mechanical ventilation.

Pinder et al.[15] evaluated the administration of subcutaneous GM-CSF injections as an immunomodulatory strategy to

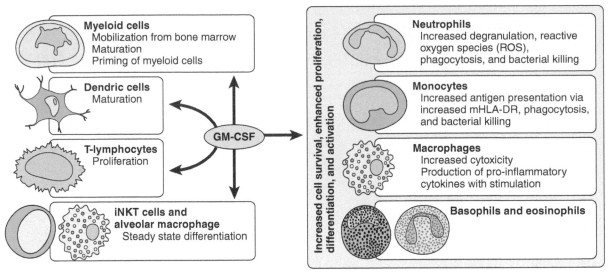

Fig. 82.1 The proinflammatory and steady-state function of granulocyte-macrophage colony-stimulating factor (GM-CSF). In vitro GM-CSF mobilizes myeloid populations from the bone marrow and their precursors in the blood. It primes myeloid cells for activation while promoting cell survival, maturation, and proliferation of granulocytes and monocytes. GM-CSF stimulates dendritic cell maturation, T cell proliferation, and is involved in the homeostatic differentiation of invariant natural killer T cells and macrophages. When administered or released systemically in response to infection, GM-CSF mirrors in vitro effects. (Redrawn from Mathias B, Szpila BE, Moore FA, Efron PA, Moldawer LL. A review of GM-CSF therapy in sepsis. *Medicine* [Baltimore]. 2015;94(50):e2044.)

combat neutropenia in critically ill patients. In a targeted cohort of critically ill patients with impaired neutrophil function, Pinder et al.[15] conducted a double-blinded study that compared subcutaneous GM-CSF (3 mg/kg per day) to placebo for 4 days. Neutrophil capacity at day 2, neutrophil phagocytic capacity at day 9, and increased circulating mHLA-DR expression on CD14+ monocytes (consistent with improved cell function[10]) were improved in the GM-CSF cohort.[15] GM-CSF-induced increases in mHLA-DR expression have been demonstrated in ex vivo studies. In addition, GM-CSF was associated with upregulation of cell adhesion molecules found on the surface of neutrophils and monocytes and on the endothelial cells of injured tissues, thus aiding in migration.[3] A randomized, double-blinded, placebo-controlled, multiinstitutional prospective study demonstrated that administration of GM-CSF for 8 days to patients in a severe state of sepsis or in septic shock with low levels of mHLA-DR was associated with increased numbers of neutrophils, monocytes, and T lymphocytes, elevated mHLA-DR expression, and increased serum levels of IL-6, TNFα, and IL-10. Changes in function were not reported.[3,10,16] GM-CSF administration was also associated with trends towards decreased hospital days, length of mechanical ventilation, and disease severity scores. Importantly, no adverse effects were reported, though no significant difference in 28-day mortality was determined.[16] A similar randomized, placebo-controlled trial revealed upregulation of functional inflammatory markers, increases in total leukocyte counts, improved disease clearance, and better overall clinical outcomes in septic, neutropenic patients receiving GM-CSF therapy.[17] No significant differences in mortality or clinical

organ failure scores were observed. The heterogeneous population of septic patients may have confounded these results.[3] An additional randomized, double-blinded, placebo-controlled clinical trial attempted to control for these factors by excluding perioperative patients with nontraumatic abdominal sepsis patients. GM-CSF therapy was associated with decreases in hospital stay, median antibiotic treatment duration, quantity of infectious complications, and direct financial burdens.[18] This study suggests that GM-CSF therapies may be beneficial for specific subsets of patients. Further human studies are needed to explicate functional qualitative differences in immune cells.

HETEROGENEITY OF TRIALS

The use for GM-CSF in sepsis is still considered to be "off-label", partially reflecting the heterogeneity of published clinical trials. Time of administration is an important inadequately examined variable; it is unclear if GM-CSF should be administered prophylactically, based on immunosuppressive/clinical biomarkers, or at some specific time following the onset of illness. In addition, some trials have used continuous infusion while others incorporated protocols with doses that differed day-to-day. The optimal route of administration, local versus systemically, is also unclear; studies suggest that systemic administration is associated with migration of cells from the bone marrow, while local administration induces the proinflammatory effects observed in vitro. Other factors that must be addressed include the manufacturing process, individual patient characteristics, comorbidities, age, and genetic variance.[19,20]

PATHOPHYSIOLOGY OF ANEMIA IN INTENSIVE CARE UNIT PATIENTS

Anemia is extremely common in ICU patients who frequently receive red blood cell (RBC) transfusions. Studies have demonstrated that 95% of patients receiving treatment in the ICU for at least 3 days become anemic[21] and 55% of all critically ill trauma patients receive a transfusion, half of which occur >5 days following ICU admission.[2] However, administration of allogenic blood has been associated with immune or infectious risks, for example, transfusion-related lung-injury.[22–24] Thus, strategies to limit the use of transfusions might improve outcomes in the critically ill. While the pathophysiology (Fig. 82.2) of persistent injury-associated anemia is not fully understood,[2] it has been

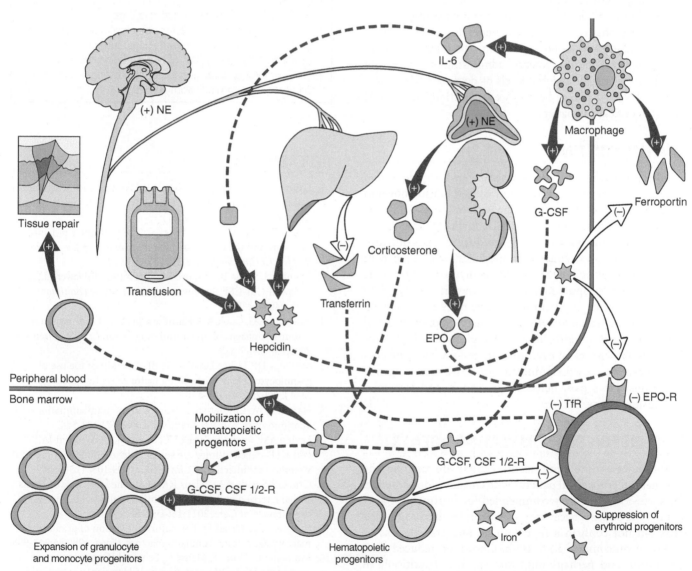

Fig. 82.2 Hypothesis for the pathophysiology of persistent injury-associated anemia in intensive care unit patients. Neuroendocrine activation, hyperinflammation, and allogenic red blood cell transfusions suppress adequate erythroid progenitor growth, iron regulation, and mobilization of hematopoietic stem cells to injured tissues. *CSF1/2-R*, colony-stimulating factor 1 receptor and colony-stimulating factor 2 receptor; *EPO*, erythropoietin; *EPO-R*, erythropoietin receptor; *G-CSF*, granulocyte colony–stimulating factor; *NE*, norepinephrine; *TfR*, transferrin receptor. (Redrawn from Loftus TJ, Mira JC, Miller ES, et al. The postinjury inflammatory state and the bone marrow response to anemia. *Am J Respir Crit Care Med.* 2018;198(5):629-638.)

hypothesized that contributing factors include neuroendocrine-mediated suppression of erythroid progenitor growth.[2,25,26] These findings have led to the examination of erythropoietin (EPO) in critically ill patients.

Animal studies have demonstrated complex and multifactorial links between EPO, erythropoietin receptor expression, hepcidin, and iron in persistent injury-associated anemia.[27] High levels of EPO did not improve anemia. Elevated serum EPO levels were associated with decreased EPO receptor expression in the bone marrow and a reduction in available iron stores, which is consistent with persistent injury-associated anemia. Factors influencing erythropoiesis include β-adrenergic receptor blockade, iron availability, IL-6,[28,29] and hepcidin.[2] The hyperadrenergic state that follows severe trauma is associated with bone marrow dysfunction and prolonged hematopoietic progenitor cell mobilization with decreased growth of erythroid progenitors.[30] This complex pathophysiology clearly demonstrates that ICU-associated anemia is too multifaceted to be treated solely by blood transfusion. Iron supplementation and exogenous erythropoietin administration have not reliably increased hemoglobin levels or decreased RBC transfusions.[2,31–33] Better strategies are needed to stimulate erythropoiesis in critically ill patients.[2]

ERYTHROPOIETIN

In addition to the role EPO plays in erythropoiesis and maturation of erythroid progenitor cells, it is also known to serve as a multifunctional cytokine with immuno-modulating characteristics.[34] Erythropoiesis normally occurs at a steady-state in the bone marrow, but during times of stress, erythropoiesis can occur in extramedullary sites, namely in the liver and spleen.[27] During anemia, hypoxia triggers the release of erythropoietin. During ischemic injury, EPO plays both cardiac and neuroprotective roles and is known to promote neovascularization, mobilization of endothelial progenitors, and an upregulation of angiogenesis.[34] In addition to EPO's effects on erythroid progenitor cells, the hormone has also shown significant protective effects against conditions like sepsis, hemorrhagic shock, and ischemia/reperfusion injury.[35,36]

ERYTHROPOIESIS-STIMULATING AGENTS

Erythropoiesis-stimulating agents (ESAs) are used in the treatment of critically ill patients with chronic kidney disease. ESAs are not currently recommended for treatment of anemia in ICU patients because multiple randomized controlled trials did not confirm a reduction in RBC transfusions or improved outcomes.[22] ESA use has, however, reduced RBC transfusion and perhaps improved survival in critically ill patients also administered EPO.[37,38]

IRON SUPPLEMENTATION

A recent metaanalysis of five randomized controlled trials of iron supplementation (four intravenous [IV] iron, one oral iron) in adult critical care with 665 patients found no difference in RBC transfusions, hemoglobin level, mortality, in-hospital infection, or length of stay. However, there is considerable heterogeneity between trials.[39] Smaller studies demonstrated conflicting results.[40,41] Most recently, the IRONMAN trial compared IV iron to placebo in 140 critically ill patients. This study was unable to demonstrate statistically significant effects other than on hemoglobin level at discharge.[40] Additional well-designed trials are needed to investigate the optimal iron-dosing regimens in ICU patients and strategies to identify which patients are most likely to benefit from iron, together with patient-focused outcomes.

AUTHORS' RECOMMENDATIONS
- Use of EPO, ESAs, or iron supplementation in the critically ill cannot be recommended at this time.
- Current treatment options for iron-restricted anemia seen in the ICU include RBC transfusions and direct treatment of the underlying disorder to reduce inflammation.
- New emerging treatments are evaluating the hepcidin pathway and vitamin D administration.

REFERENCES

1. Loftus TJ, Mohr AM, Moldawer LL. Dysregulated myelopoiesis and hematopoietic function following acute physiologic insult. *Curr Opin Hematol.* 2018;25(1):37-43.
2. Loftus TJ, Mira JC, Miller ES, et al. The postinjury inflammatory state and the bone marrow response to anemia. *Am J Respir Crit Care Med.* 2018;198(5):629-638.
3. Mathias B, Szpila BE, Moore FA, Efron PA, Moldawer LL. A review of GM-CSF therapy in sepsis. *Medicine (Baltimore).* 2015;94(50):e2044.
4. Fleetwood AJ, Cook AD, Hamilton JA. Functions of granulocyte-macrophage colony-stimulating factor. *Crit Rev Immunol.* 2005;25(5):405-428.
5. Stephens DP, Fisher DA, Currie BJ. An audit of the use of granulocyte colony-stimulating factor in septic shock. *Intern Med J.* 2002;32(4):143-148.
6. Hamilton JA. Colony-stimulating factors in inflammation and autoimmunity. *Nat Rev Immunol.* 2008;8(7):533-544.
7. Levine AM, Reed JA, Kurak KE, Cianciolo E, Whitsett JA. GM-CSF–deficient mice are susceptible to pulmonary group B streptococcal infection. *J Clin Invest.* 1999;103(4):563-569.
8. Otto GP, Sossdorf M, Claus RA, et al. The late phase of sepsis is characterized by an increased microbiological burden and death rate. *Crit Care.* 2011;15(4):R183.
9. Burgess AW, Metcalf D. The nature and action of granulocyte-macrophage colony stimulating factors. *Blood.* 1980;56:947-958.
10. Monneret G, Venet F, Meisel C, Schefold JC. Assessment of monocytic HLA-DR expression in ICU patients: analytical issues for multicentric flow cytometry studies. *Crit Care.* 2010;14(4):432.
11. Zucali JR, Dinarello CA, Oblon DJ, Gross MA, Anderson L, Weiner RS. Interleukin 1 stimulates fibroblasts to produce granulocyte-macrophage colony-stimulating activity and prostaglandin E2. *J Clin Invest.* 1986;77:1857-1863.

12. Bagby Jr GC, Dinarello CA, Wallace P, Wagner C, Hefeneider S, McCall E. Interleukin 1 stimulates granulocyte macrophage colony-stimulating activity release by vascular endothelial cells. *J Clin Invest.* 1986;78:1316-1323.

13. Filonzi EL, Zoellner H, Stanton H, Hamilton JA. Cytokine regulation of granulocyte macrophage colony stimulating factor and macrophage colony-stimulating factor production in human arterial smooth muscle cells. *Atherosclerosis.* 1993;99:241-252.

14. Hotchkiss RS, Moldawer LL. Parallels between cancer and infectious disease. *N Engl J Med.* 2014; 371:380-383.

15. Pinder EM, Rostron AJ, Hellyer TP, et al. Randomised controlled trial of granulocyte macrophage colony stimulating factor in critically ill patients with impaired neutrophil function. *Am Thorac Soc.* 2016;A2727-A2727.

16. Meisel C, Schefold JC, Pschowski R, et al. Granulocyte–macrophage colony-stimulating factor to reverse sepsis-associated immunosuppression. *Am J Respir Crit Care Med.* 2009;180(7):640-648.

17. Rosenbloom AJ, Linden PK, Dorrance A, Penkosky N, Cohen-Melamed MH, Pinsky MR. Effect of granulocyte-monocyte colony-stimulating factor therapy on leukocyte function and clearance of serious infection in nonneutropenic patients. *Chest.* 2005;127:2139-2150.

18. Orozco H, Arch J, Medina-Franco H, et al. Molgramostim (GM-CSF) associated with antibiotic treatment in nontraumatic abdominal sepsis: a randomized, double-blind, placebo-controlled clinical trial. *Arch Surg.* 2006;141:150-153, discussion 154.

19. Nacionales DC, Gentile LF, Vanzant E, et al. Aged mice are unable to mount an effective myeloid response to sepsis. *J Immunol.* 2014;192(2):612-622.

20. Nacionales DC, Szpila B, Ungaro R, et al. A detailed characterization of the dysfunctional immunity and abnormal myelopoiesis induced by severe shock and trauma in the aged. *J Immunol.* 2015;195(5):2396-2407.

21. Corwin HL, Gettinger A, Pearl RG, et al. The CRIT Study: anemia and blood transfusion in the critically ill—Current clinical practice in the United States. *Crit Care Med.* 2004; 32(1):39-52.

22. Jelkmann I, Jelkmann W. Impact of erythropoietin on intensive care unit patients. *Transfus Med Hemother.* 2013;40(5): 310-318.

23. Marik PE, Corwin HL. Efficacy of red blood cell transfusion in the critically ill: a systematic review of the literature. *Crit Care Med.* 2008;36:2667-2674.

24. Napolitano LM, Kurek S, Luchette FA, et al. Clinical practice guideline: red blood cell transfusion in adult trauma and critical care. *Crit Care Med.* 2009;37:3124-3157.

25. Fonseca RB, Mohr AM, Wang L, Sifri ZC, Rameshwar P, Livingston DH. The impact of a hypercatecholamine state on erythropoiesis following severe injury and the role of IL-6. *J Trauma.* 2005;59:884-889, discussion 889-890.

26. Fonseca RB, Mohr AM, Wang L, et al. Adrenergic modulation of erythropoiesis following severe injury is mediated through bone marrow stroma. *Surg Infect (Larchmt).* 2004;5: 385-393.

27. Alamo IG, Kannan KB, Smith MA, Efron PA, Mohr AM. Characterization of erythropoietin and hepcidin in the regulation of persistent injury-associated anemia. *J Trauma Acute Care Surg.* 2016;81(4):705-712

28. Abel J, Spannbrucker N, Fandrey J, Jelkmann W. Serum erythropoietin levels in patients with sepsis and septic shock. *Eur J Haematol.* 1996;57(5):359-363.

29. Finberg KE. Regulation of systemic iron homeostasis. *Curr Opin Hematol.* 2013;20:208-214.

30. Alamo IG, Kannan KB, Bible LE, et al. Daily propranolol administration reduces persistent injury-associated anemia after severe trauma and chronic stress. *J Trauma Acute Care Surg.* 2017;82(4):714-721.

31. Lin DM, Lin ES, Tran MH. Efficacy and safety of erythropoietin and intravenous iron in perioperative blood management: a systematic review. *Transfus Med Rev.* 2013;27:221-234.

32. Corwin HL, Gettinger A, Fabian TC, et al. Efficacy and safety of epoetin alfa in critically ill patients. *N Engl J Med.* 2007;357:965-976.

33. Pieracci FM, Stovall RT, Jaouen B, et al. A multicenter, randomized clinical trial of IV iron supplementation for anemia of traumatic critical illness. *Crit Care Med.* 2014;42:2048-2057.

34. Sherbini SAE, Ali AA, Kamal S, Marzouk H, Rashed L. Promising roles of erythropoietin and lymphotoxin alpha in critical illness: A pilot study in critically ill children. *Egypt Pediatr Assoc Gaz.* 2018;66(1):28-34.

35. Abdelrahman M, Sharples EJ, McDonald MC, et al. Erythropoietin attenuates the tissue injury associated with hemorrhagic shock and myocardial ischemia. *Shock.* 2004;22(1):63-69.

36. Calvillo L, Latini R, Kajstura J, et al. Recombinant human erythropoietin protects the myocardium from ischemia-reperfusion injury and promotes beneficial remodeling. *Proc Natl Acad Sci U S A.* 2003;100(8):4802-4806.

37. Patel NS, Collino M, Yaqoob MM, Thiemermann C. Erythropoietin in the intensive care unit: beyond treatment of anemia. *Ann Intensive Care.* 2011;1(1):40.

38. Corwin HL, Gettinger A, Pearl RG, Fink MP, Levy MM, Shapiro MJ, Corwin MJ, Colton T; EPO Critical Care Trials Group. Efficacy of recombinant human erythropoietin in critically ill patients: a randomized controlled trial. *JAMA.* 2002 Dec 11;288(22):2827-35.

39. Shah A, Roy NB, McKechnie S, Doree C, Fisher SA, Stanworth SJ. Iron supplementation to treat anemia in adult critical care patients: a systematic review and meta-analysis. *Crit Care.* 2016; 20(1):306.

40. Napolitano LM. Anemia and red blood cell transfusion: advances in critical care. *Crit Care Clin.* 2017;33(2):345-364.

41. Pieracci FM, Henderson P, Rodney JR, et al. Randomized, double-blind, placebo-controlled trial of effects of enteral iron supplementation on anemia and risk of infection during surgical critical illness. *Surg Infect (Larchmt).* 2009;10(1): 9-19.

83

What Anticoagulants Should Be Used in the Critically Ill Patient? How Do I Choose?

Cheralyn J. Hendrix, Lisbi Rivas, and Babak Sarani

The critically ill patient in the intensive care unit (ICU) is at risk for arterial and venous thromboembolic events, including pulmonary embolism (PE), deep venous thrombosis (DVT), stroke (cerebrovascular accident [CVA]), and acute coronary syndrome (ACS). Appropriate use of anticoagulant prophylaxis and therapy is essential. This discussion is limited to inhibitors of the coagulation cascade.

WARFARIN

Warfarin is a classic vitamin K antagonist (VKA) that is frequently used for the prevention of thromboembolic events. However, its efficacy is limited by factors noted in Box 83.1.[1] Patient compliance with warfarin can also be problematic due to the complex dosing regimen needed to maintain appropriate blood levels and the need for frequent outpatient monitoring of blood levels.

Warfarin is primarily metabolized by the CYP2C9 hepatic microsomal enzyme system. This system is inducible by many other medications and carries genetic variability that can alter activity.[2] Warfarin is strongly protein bound, and it is the non-protein-bound fraction that is biologically active. The drug is water soluble and is readily absorbed in the small bowel following oral administration.[3,4] The biological half-life is 36–42 hours.

Warfarin interferes with the biosynthesis of the vitamin-K-dependent coagulation factors II, VII, IX, and X and the natural anticoagulant proteins C and S.[3,5] Because the half-life of proteins C and S is shorter than the coagulation factors, warfarin produces a transient prothrombotic state. Fortunately, this is not clinically relevant in most instances, However, it is important to note that the desired anticoagulant effects of warfarin are delayed by approximately 48–72 hours. The length of this delay depends on the clearance of normal clotting factors, particularly prothrombin, from the circulation.[3,6] This characteristic as well as the long half-life make warfarin a less-desirable agent for initiation of anticoagulation in the ICU.

Despite these characteristics, warfarin remains a well-established therapy for patients with PE, DVT, atrial fibrillation, and mechanical heart valves. It may be most useful in the presence of severely impaired renal function, which limits the feasibility of other long-acting agents. It is, however, problematic to reinstitute if discontinued. The BRIDGE trial demonstrated a significantly increased risk of bleeding in patients who were chronically anticoagulated with warfarin for nonvalvular atrial fibrillation and who had the drug stopped for elective surgery.[7] Specifically, use of low-molecular-weight heparin (LMWH) as a bridge to the resumption of anticoagulation with warfarin was associated with a significantly higher incidence of bleeding than the group that did not receive LMWH. Moreover, the latter group did not have a higher thromboembolic risk. Of note, the study cohort consisted mainly of persons with a CHADS$_2$ score 1–3.

Monitoring warfarin levels is accomplished by measurement of the international normalized rate (INR), defined as the ratio of the patient's prothrombin time (PT) to a normal sample (control). A therapeutic INR is defined according to the indication for anticoagulation: goal INR for a DVT is usually in the range of 2.0–2.5 and goal INR for mechanical heart valves is usually 2.5–3.5, depending on the location of the valve.[3]

Because of the many interactions between warfarin and food/medications, the INR can vary greatly from week to week. This, in turn, results in a varying propensity for hemorrhage, which is probably the reason that warfarin is associated with a higher rate of spontaneous hemorrhage (especially intracerebral hemorrhage) when compared with other anticoagulants.[8] It is therefore not surprising that the United States Food and Drug Administration (FDA) favors the use of direct oral anticoagulants (DOACs; see below), which have a lower incidence of cerebral hemorrhage, for anticoagulation in patients with venous thromboembolism (VTE) and nonvalvular atrial fibrillation.

Traditionally, the antidote to warfarin has been fresh frozen plasma (FFP) and vitamin K. The dose of FFP required to re-establish a normal coagulation profile varies based on the INR and there is no general consensus on a specific regimen. In 2013, the FDA approved use of a four-factor prothrombin complex concentrate, KCentra, for immediate reversal of warfarin in hemorrhaging patients and those who require urgent operation.[9] KCentra has notable advantages over plasma and vitamin K; namely, more rapid INR reduction and smaller volume of infusion with reduction in risk of transfusion-associated circulatory overload (TACO).[10,11] Although KCentra is significantly more expensive (approximately US$3000–5000 per dose vs. approximately US$80—100/unit of FFP), after factoring in the added cost of mechanical ventilation per day in the ICU, the cost of KCentra is quickly offset by the decreased risk of TACO.[12,13]

UNFRACTIONATED HEPARIN

Heparin is a naturally occurring polysaccharide consisting of molecular chains of varying lengths or molecular weights.[14,15] Unfractionated heparin (UFH) potentiates the action of antithrombin III, inactivating thrombin and activated coagulation factors IX, X, XI, XII, and plasmin, thereby preventing the conversion of fibrinogen to fibrin.[16] Heparin is primarily metabolized by the liver, but it may be partially metabolized in the reticuloendothelial system. The elimination half-life of heparin is approximately 1–2 hours. Because anticoagulation with UFH can be challenging in the individual patient, administration is commonly guided by dosing protocols designed to reach a goal of therapeutic activated partial thromboplastin time (aPTT) and maintain the aPTT afterwards.[17]

UFH has been, traditionally, the parenteral agent of choice for anticoagulation. A rare group of patients who are deficient in antithrombin III will be resistant to UFH activity. When dosed in small subcutaneous aliquots, its use for prevention of DVT is ubiquitous in the ICU.[18] Intravenous UFH is the preferred agent for systemic anticoagulation in severe renal failure (creatinine clearance <30 mL/min) because all other medications are renally metabolized or excreted. The short half-life of UFH permits quick reversal, and UFH has a specific reversal agent, protamine sulfate. While anaphylaxis to protamine sulfate was once problematic, the drug is now made via recombinant DNA technology and therefore no longer carries this risk.

A rare but serious complication of heparin exposure is heparin-induced thrombocytopenia (HIT), a syndrome in which antibodies to the complex of heparin and platelet factor IV trigger platelet activation, causing major arterial and/or venous thrombosis.[19] Paradoxically, the risk of HIT is maximum while the patient is thrombocytopenic. Treatment of this life-threatening complication is to immediately terminate all heparin exposure and initiate anticoagulation with a non-heparin alternative such as a direct thrombin inhibitor (DTI). Once a patient has developed HIT, reexposure to heparin should be avoided because of the risk of accelerated thrombocytopenia and venous/arterial thrombus formation.

LOW-MOLECULAR-WEIGHT HEPARIN

LMWHs are short polysaccharide chains fractionated from heparin. These drugs have increased bioavailability and are thus more clinically reliable.[14,15] As with UFHs, LMWHs work via activation of antithrombin III. Other advantages of LMWH relative to UFH are longer duration of anticoagulant action, fixed dosing (obviating the need for routine laboratory monitoring), and a lower risk of HIT.[20] Multiple meta-analyses indicate that subcutaneous LMWH is more effective than UFH for the treatment of VTE, exhibiting higher rates of thrombus regression and lower rates of recurrent thrombosis, major bleeding, and mortality.[21–24] Despite these presumed clinical advantages, randomized trials of LMWH vs. UFH for thromboprophylaxis in the ICU have yielded inconsistent results.[25,26] A multicenter randomized trial of 3754 ICU patients compared dalteparin with twice-daily UFH for thromboprophylaxis. There was no difference (hazard ratio 0.92; 95% confidence interval [CI] 0.68–1.23; $P = .57$) between groups in the primary outcome variable—the incidence of proximal leg DVT.[27] However, dalteparin significantly lowered the incidence of PE (hazard ratio 0.51; 95% CI 0.30–0.88; $P = .01$) and HIT (hazard ratio 0.27; 95% CI 0.08–0.98; $P = .05$).

Systematic reviews have demonstrated a lower incidence of HIT in postoperative patients undergoing thromboprophylaxis with LMWH when compared with UFH (risk ratio 0.25; 95% CI 0.07–0.82; $P = .02$).[28,29] In the analysis for HIT complicated by VTE,[29] LMWH was associated with an 80% risk reduction for this complication compared with UFH (risk ratio 0.20; 95% CI 0.04–0.90; $P = .04$).

The lack of a routine test to measure the effects of LMWH can be problematic in patients for whom bleeding is particularly dangerous and in morbidly obese patients where standard dosing may be insufficient to achieve the desired clinical effect.

There is no specific reversal agent for LMWH. While protamine sulfate has been used, it has reported anticoagulant reversal rates of only 60–80%.[30,31] The FDA has (approved) a novel, nonselective antidote, andexanet alfa, for all medications that inhibit factor X (see below). Although the FDA approval for this agent is restricted to the factor Xa antagonists apixaban and rivaroxaban, the ANNEXA-4 study included patients who were on LMWH and demonstrated that andexanet alfa restored a normal coagulation profile in some patients.[32] However, use of this drug for reversal of LMWH remains off-label.

INTRAVENOUS DIRECT THROMBIN INHIBITORS

In contrast to the heparins, DTIs provide anticoagulation regardless of antithrombin III levels and have the ability to inhibit fibrin-bound thrombin, allowing more complete anticoagulant activity.[19,33,34] DTIs also are more predictable because they do not bind to other plasma proteins. Currently, available intravenous DTIs include lepirudin, desirudin, bivalirudin, and argatroban. The last two are the most common because they have a broader range of approved indications.

Bivalirudin is an analog of hirudin, an anticoagulant found in the saliva of leeches. Bivalirudin binds to thrombin directly and causes anticoagulation within 5 minutes.[19] This DTI is primarily used to anticoagulate critically ill patients with HIT. Binding is reversible because the molecule is cleaved by thrombin, which leads to a short half-life (25 minutes) in patients with normal or mildly reduced renal function. Metabolism of the drug is primarily renal and proteolytic.[33,35] The anticoagulant effect can be monitored using the activated clotting time (ACT), but there are no set standards for the degree of anticoagulation required for a particular indication (e.g., VTE vs. arterial clot). Although no rapid reversal agent exists, the drug is cleared by hemodialysis.[35] Because acute kidney injury is common in the ICU, this drug is not frequently used.

Argatroban is an alternative to bivalirudin. This drug also reversibly binds to an active site on thrombin, causing direct inhibition. Argatroban is used primarily for is anticoagulation in patients with HIT.[36,37] Because of its rapid onset and short half-life, argatroban is typically given by infusion. Some references suggest administering a bolus of the drug prior to starting the infusion, but significant bleeding may result. In contrast to bivalirudin, argatroban is primarily metabolized by the liver and can be used in patients with renal insufficiency.[38,39] Monitoring can be performed with either an ACT or aPTT. Because argatroban affects thrombin-dependent coagulation tests, PT and INR may be altered—an important consideration when transitioning to warfarin. There is no reversal agent for this drug.

PARENTERAL INDIRECT FACTOR XA INHIBITORS

Fondaparinux is an indirect factor Xa inhibitor that is a synthetic analog of a natural pentasaccharide contained in heparin and LMWH. Fondaparinux interrupts the coagulation cascade upstream of thrombin. The lack of thrombin inhibition prevents rebound thrombin generation. The drug has a half-life of 17–21 hours and is administered as a daily subcutaneous injection. Peak plasma concentrations are achieved within 2 hours of injection.[40] A 2011 trial demonstrated that the bioavailability of fondaparinux after subcutaneous injection was not significantly affected by vasopressor therapy in critically ill patients.[41] Clearance is significantly decreased in

the setting of renal failure. The effects of fondaparinux can be followed with serial measurement of factor Xa activity, but routine monitoring is not standard. The PT, INR, and aPTT are typically not affected. There is no specific reversal agent for fondaparinux,[42] although andexanet alfa should be effective in antagonizing this agent as well.

In a randomized controlled trial ($N = 849$ acute medical patients >60 years, 35 centers from 8 countries), fondaparinux as compared with placebo significantly reduced the risk of VTE by 46.7% from 10.5% to 5.6% ($P < .05$) with no increase in bleeding risk.[38,43] A meta-analysis (cumulative $N > 13,000$ medical and surgical patients, 8 randomized trials) confirmed a 20% reduction in mortality from VTE with fondaparinux as compared with the control groups of placebo or LMWH.[44] Beyond thromboprophylaxis for VTE, a series of randomized controlled trials have established a role for fondaparinux in the management of ACS (managed with and without coronary angiography),[45–47] although the use of this agent for this indication is still not common.

Fondaparinux has been successfully used in the treatment of HIT, and, although there are few reported cases of HIT caused by fondaparinux, its value as a pharmacologic alternative in patients with HIT is well reported.[48] Fondaparinux is considered a nonheparin anticoagulant, despite being a synthetic version of a natural pentasaccharide contained in heparin. This natural pentasaccharide does not interact with platelet factor 4 (PF4), thereby giving this agent a potential role in the treatment of HIT.[49]

DIRECT ORAL ANTICOAGULANTS

Dabigatran etexilate is an oral DTI.[50] DTIs inhibit free and fibrin-bound direct thrombin inhibition, which is an advantage over heparin. Dabigatran has a rapid onset, reaching peak plasma concentrations within 1.5 hours, and has a half-life of 12–14 hours.[1,51] Adjustment for renal dysfunction is required because 80% of the drug undergoes renal elimination. Current indications include prophylaxis and treatment of VTE and thromboembolic prophylaxis in nonvalvular atrial fibrillation. The drug is not approved for use as prophylaxis against thrombus formation in patients with mechanical heart valves.

A large randomized trial compared twice-daily dabigatran with warfarin in atrial fibrillation patients who were at increased risk for stroke.[52] In patients receiving a high dose (150 mg given twice daily), the incidence of stroke during the median 2-year follow-up was lower than warfarin, without an increased risk of major bleeding. Subsequent studies have confirmed that although the use of dabigatran is associated with a risk of ischemic stroke and spontaneous intracerebral hemorrhage, it is also associated with a higher risk of gastrointestinal bleeding.[53,54] Guidelines now endorse dabigatran as an alternative to warfarin in selected patients with atrial fibrillation (Class I recommendation; level of evidence B).[55]

There is no clinically useful test to monitor the level of dabigatran, which poses a significant challenge in patients who present with hemorrhage. As such, the clinician must decide on the need for active reversal of the agent. The thrombin time is overly sensitive to dabigatran's effect.[1] The ecarin clotting time, another option, is not routinely available, and the absolute aPTT value does not correlate to actual concentrations of dabigatran.[56,57]

There is a specific reversal agent, idarucizumab (Praxbind), for dabigatran:[58,59] A monoclonal antibody to the drug. The cost of idarucizumab is US$3000–5000 per dose. In the authors' institution, clinical judgment is used when ordering the reversal agent, weighing factors such as the location and severity of hemorrhage (e.g., intracranial vs. extremity), time that the patient last took the parent drug, and the presence of renal insufficiency. Of note, plasma is not effective in reversing dabigatran and the use of prothrombin concentrate to do so is off-label and unproven.[60]

ORAL DIRECT FACTOR XA INHIBITORS

The oral direct factor Xa inhibitors are also a new class of anticoagulants that includes rivaroxaban and apixaban.[61] Both agents inhibit factor Xa, independent of antithrombin III. They do not cause rebound thrombin generation. Both available drugs possess high bioavailability and half-lives in the range of 8–12 hours.

Rivaroxaban is primarily eliminated via the kidneys, and should not be used in patients with severe renal dysfunction.[61] As with dabigatran, current indications for rivaroxaban include the prevention and treatment of VTE and prevention of arterial emboli in patients with nonvalvular atrial fibrillation. Furthermore, as in the comparison of dabigatran with warfarin, use of rivaroxaban (15 mg twice daily followed by 20 mg once daily) for the treatment of symptomatic VTE or PE is associated with a lower rate of cerebral hemorrhage than warfarin.[54]

Apixaban is also approved for prevention and treatment of VTE and prevention of arterial emboli in patients with nonvalvular atrial fibrillation. Although apixaban is also eliminated via the kidneys, it is extensively metabolized in the liver and can be given to patients with renal insufficiency in a dose-adjusted fashion.

As with dabigatran, there is no reliable and readily available clinical test to measure the presence of either rivaroxaban or apixaban in the serum. The PT may be elevated in the presence of these drugs, but lack of an elevated PT does not correlate with absence of drug in the serum.[56] A more promising test, the chromogenic antifactor Xa assay, is not widely available.[62,63]

In May 2018, the FDA approved the first reversal agent for both apixaban and rivaroxaban: andexanet-α.[32,64] This is a synthetic molecule that resembles the Xa receptor and therefore acts as a decoy receptor for the parent drug. It has higher affinity for either DOAC than the actual Xa receptor. Given its mechanism of action, theoretically, it is effective for

reversal of all factor Xa inhibiting drugs, although there are few data to support this assumption aside from the ANNEXA-4 trial.[32] As it works via competitive inhibition, administration of the agent involves a bolus followed by a 2-hour infusion. Parent drug levels rebound quickly upon cessation of andexenet-alpha,[65] and it is possible that repeat dosing may be needed in hemorrhaging patients. Due to its mechanism of action, andexenet-alpha does not reverse the effects of dabigatran.

HOW DO I CHOOSE IN THE ICU: WHICH ANTICOAGULANT FOR WHICH PATIENT?

Choosing the optimal anticoagulant for the ICU patient depends on multiple factors. Consideration of whether the need is for prophylaxis or treatment of VTE is of paramount importance. A key consideration in the ICU is the potential for hemorrhage and/or need for an urgent invasive procedure. Choosing an agent that has a short half-life and/or reversal agent may be appropriate based on these concerns. It may also be important to consider the patient's post-ICU anticoagulation goals. Short-term anticoagulation may be addressed with an intravenous or subcutaneous medication. However, if the patient requires extended treatment, a longer-acting oral agent may be preferable. Other factors related to the specific drug should be considered, including half-life and primary metabolic and elimination pathways. Patient factors such as hepatic and renal function must also be considered, and dose adjustment in the critically ill may be necessary. Concerns regarding the risk for HIT may eliminate the use of heparins. The ability to monitor the degree of anticoagulation is an important consideration in choosing an anticoagulant and the lack of routine monitoring may be problematic in the critically ill patient who may have impaired absorption of the drug.

Evidence-based clinical practice guidelines offer recommendations on the various available drugs.[20,55,66–68] However, most of these recommendations do not consider the complex critically ill patient. As the indications for the direct oral anticoagulant agents continue to expand, these agents may play an increased role in the critical care setting. Table 83.1 summarizes the various commonly used anticoagulants, mechanisms of action, and reversal agents.

AUTHORS' RECOMMENDATIONS
- Anticoagulation in critically ill patients is necessary given the multiple factors that increase their risk for the development of thromboembolism.
- The choice of a particular anticoagulant in the ICU patient should be determined by the indication for therapy, patient factors, and drug factors, including reversibility.
- Intensivists should be aware of the spectrum of available anticoagulant agents and their specific reversal agents.

TABLE 83.1	Commonly Used Anticoagulant Agents and Their Key Characteristics.			
Drug	**Mechanism of Action**	**Metabolism Site**	**Half-Life**	**Reversal Agent**
Warfarin	Inhibits vitamin-K-mediated synthesis of factors II, VII, IX, and X	Liver	36–42 hours	Prothrombin complex concentrate or plasma *and* vitamin K
Unfractionated heparin	Activates antithrombin III	Liver	1–2 hours	Protamine sulfate
Low-molecular-weight heparin	Activates antithrombin III and inhibits factor X	Liver	6 hours	Protamine sulfate or andexanet alfa or pro-thrombin complex concentrate[a]
Bivalirudin	Inhibits thrombin	Liver and kidney	25 minutes	None
Argatroban	Inhibits thrombin	Liver	45 minutes	None
Fondaparinux	Activates antithrombin III and inhibits factor Xa	Liver	20 hours	Andexanet alfa or prothrombin complex concentrate[a]
Dabigatran	Inhibits thrombin	Kidney	12 hours	Idarucizumab
Rivaroxaban	Inhibits factor Xa	Liver and kidney	8 hours	Andexanet alfa
Apixaban	Inhibits factor Xa	Liver	12 hours	Andexanet alfa

[a]There are no FDA-approved reversal agents for this drug. There are no good studies to date suggesting that the above strategies are efficacious in most persons.

REFERENCES

1. Augoustides JG. Advances in anticoagulation: focus on dabigatran, an oral direct thrombin inhibitor. *J Cardiothorac Vasc Anesth.* 2011;25:1208-1212.
2. Johnson JA, Cavallari LH. Warfarin pharmacogenetics. *Trends Cardiovasc Med.* 2015;25:33-41.
3. Freedman MD. Oral anticoagulants: pharmacodynamics, clinical indications and adverse effects. *J Clin Pharmacol.* 1992;32:196-209.
4. Lee MT, Klein TE. Pharmacogenetics of warfarin: challenges and opportunities. *J Hum Genet.* 2013;58:334-338.
5. Thornsberry LA, LoSicco KI, English JC, 3rd. The skin and hypercoagulable states. *J Am Acad Dermatol.* 2013;69:450-462.
6. Warkentin TE. Anticoagulant failure in coagulopathic patients: PTT confounding and other pitfalls. *Expert Opin Drug Saf.* 2014;13:25-43.
7. Douketis JD, Spyropoulos AC, Kaatz S, et al. Perioperative bridging anticoagulation in patients with atrial fibrillation. *N Engl J Med.* 2015;373:823-833.
8. U.S. Food and Drug Administration (2015). Atrial fibrillation and new oral anticoagulant drugs. Available at: https://www.fda.gov/drugs/newsevents/ucm405148.htm. Accessed May 22, 2018.
9. U.S. Food and Drug Administration (2018). KCentra (Prothrombin complex concentrate, Human). Available at: https://www.fda.gov/BiologicsBloodVaccines/BloodBloodProducts/ApprovedProducts/LicensedProductsBLAs/FractionatedPlasmaProducts/ucm350130.htm. Accessed May 25, 2018.
10. Sarode R, Milling Jr TJ, Refaai MA, et al. Efficacy and safety of a 4-factor prothrombin complex concentrate in patients on vitamin K antagonists presenting with major bleeding: a randomized, plasma-controlled, phase IIIb study. *Circulation.* 2013;128:1234-1243.
11. Thigpen JL, Limdi NA. Reversal of oral anticoagulation. *Pharmacotherapy.* 2013;33:1199-1213.
12. Dasta JF, McLaughlin TP, Mody SH, Piech CT. Daily cost of an intensive care unit day: the contribution of mechanical ventilation. *Crit Care Med.* 2005;33:1266-1271.
13. Frumkin K. Rapid reversal of warfarin-associated hemorrhage in the emergency department by prothrombin complex concentrates. *Ann Emerg Med.* 2013;62:616-626. e8.
14. Casu B, Naggi A, Torri G. Re-visiting the structure of heparin. *Carbohydr Res.* 2015;403:60-68.
15. Weitz JI. Low-molecular-weight heparins. *N Engl J Med.* 1997;337:688-698.
16. Hirsh J, Bauer KA, Donati MB, Gould M, Samama MM, Weitz JI. Parenteral anticoagulants: American College of Chest Physicians Evidence-Based Clinical Practice Guidelines (8th Edition). *Chest.* 2008;133:141S-159S.
17. Hylek EM, Regan S, Henault LE, et al. Challenges to the effective use of unfractionated heparin in the hospitalized management of acute thrombosis. *Arch Intern Med.* 2003;163:621-627.
18. Alhazzani W, Lim W, Jaeschke RZ, Murad MH, Cade J, Cook DJ. Heparin thromboprophylaxis in medical-surgical critically ill patients: a systematic review and meta-analysis of randomized trials. *Crit Care Med.* 2013;41:2088-2098.
19. Augoustides JG. Update in hematology: heparin-induced thrombocytopenia and bivalirudin. *J Cardiothorac Vasc Anesth.* 2011;25:371-375.
20. Linkins LA, Dans AL, Moores LK, et al. Treatment and prevention of heparin-induced thrombocytopenia: Antithrombotic Therapy and Prevention of Thrombosis, 9th ed: American College of Chest Physicians Evidence-Based Clinical Practice Guidelines. *Chest.* 2012;141:e495S-e530S.
21. Castellucci LA, Cameron C, Le Gal G, et al. Clinical and safety outcomes associated with treatment of acute venous thromboembolism: a systematic review and meta-analysis. *JAMA.* 2014;312:1122-1135.
22. Erkens PM, Prins MH. Fixed dose subcutaneous low molecular weight heparins versus adjusted dose unfractionated heparin for venous thromboembolism. *Cochrane Database Syst Rev.* 2010;(9):CD001100.
23. Gould MK, Dembitzer AD, Doyle RL, Hastie TJ, Garber AM. Low-molecular-weight heparins compared with unfractionated heparin for treatment of acute deep venous thrombosis. A

meta-analysis of randomized, controlled trials. *Ann Intern Med*. 1999;130:800-809.

24. Segal JB, Streiff MB, Hofmann LV, Thornton K, Bass EB. Management of venous thromboembolism: a systematic review for a practice guideline. *Ann Intern Med*. 2007;146:211-222.

25. Cade JF. High risk of the critically ill for venous thromboembolism. *Crit Care Med*. 1982;10:448-450.

26. De A, Roy P, Garg VK, Pandey NK. Low-molecular-weight heparin and unfractionated heparin in prophylaxis against deep vein thrombosis in critically ill patients undergoing major surgery. *Blood Coagul Fibrinolysis*. 2010;21:57-61.

27. Cook D, Meade M, Guyatt G, et al. Dalteparin versus unfractionated heparin in critically ill patients. *N Engl J Med*. 2011; 364:1305-1314.

28. Junqueira DR, Perini E, Penholati RR, Carvalho MG. Unfractionated heparin versus low molecular weight heparin for avoiding heparin-induced thrombocytopenia in postoperative patients. *Cochrane Database Syst Rev*. 2012;(9):CD007557.

29. Warkentin TE, Sheppard JI, Heels-Ansdell D, et al. Heparin-induced thrombocytopenia in medical surgical critical illness. *Chest*. 2013;144:848-858.

30. van Veen JJ, Maclean RM, Hampton KK, et al. Protamine reversal of low molecular weight heparin: clinically effective? *Blood Coagul Fibrinolysis*. 2011;22:565-570.

31. Smythe MA, Priziola J, Dobesh PP, Wirth D, Cuker A, Wittkowsky AK. Guidance for the practical management of the heparin anticoagulants in the treatment of venous thromboembolism. *J Thromb Thrombolysis*. 2016;41:165-186.

32. Connolly SJ, Milling TJ, Jr., Eikelboom JW, et al. Andexanet alfa for acute major bleeding associated with factor Xa inhibitors. *N Engl J Med*. 2016;375:1131-1141.

33. Lee CJ, Ansell JE. Direct thrombin inhibitors. *Br J Clin Pharmacol*. 2011;72:581-592.

34. Untereiner O, Seince PF, Chterev V, et al. Management of direct oral anticoagulants in the perioperative setting. *J Cardiothorac Vasc Anesth*. 2015;29:741-748.

35. Reed MD, Bell D. Clinical pharmacology of bivalirudin. *Pharmacotherapy*. 2002;22:105S-111S.

36. Alatri A, Armstrong AE, Greinacher A, et al. Results of a consensus meeting on the use of argatroban in patients with heparin-induced thrombocytopenia requiring antithrombotic therapy—a European Perspective. *Thromb Res*. 2012;129:426-433.

37. Smythe MA, Koerber JM, Forsyth LL, Priziola JL, Balasubramaniam M, Mattson JC. Argatroban dosage requirements and outcomes in intensive care versus non-intensive care patients. *Pharmacotherapy*. 2009;29:1073-1081.

38. Nutescu EA, Shapiro NL, Chevalier A. New anticoagulant agents: direct thrombin inhibitors. *Cardiol Clin*. 2008;26:169-187, v-vi.

39. Retter A, Barrett NA. The management of abnormal haemostasis in the ICU. *Anaesthesia*. 2015;70(Suppl 1):121-7, e40-e41.

40. Flato UA, Buhatem T, Merluzzi T, Bianco AC. New anticoagulants in critical care settings. *Rev Bras Ter Intensiva*. 2011;23: 68-77.

41. Cumbo-Nacheli G, Samavati L, Guzman JA. Bioavailability of fondaparinux to critically ill patients. *J Crit Care*. 2011;26: 342-346.

42. Bijsterveld NR, Moons AH, Boekholdt SM, et al. Ability of recombinant factor VIIa to reverse the anticoagulant effect of the pentasaccharide fondaparinux in healthy volunteers. *Circulation*. 2002;106:2550-2554.

43. Cohen AT, Davidson BL, Gallus AS, et al. Efficacy and safety of fondaparinux for the prevention of venous thromboembolism in older acute medical patients: randomised placebo controlled trial. *BMJ*. 2006;332:325-329.

44. Eikelboom JW, Quinlan DJ, O'Donnell M. Major bleeding, mortality, and efficacy of fondaparinux in venous thromboembolism prevention trials. *Circulation*. 2009;120:2006-2011.

45. Karthikeyan G, Mehta SR, Eikelboom JW. Fondaparinux in the treatment of acute coronary syndromes: evidence from OASIS 5 and 6. *Expert Rev Cardiovasc Ther*. 2009;7:241-249.

46. Steg PG, Jolly SS, Mehta SR, et al. Low-dose vs. standard-dose unfractionated heparin for percutaneous coronary intervention in acute coronary syndromes treated with fondaparinux: the FUTURA/OASIS-8 randomized trial. *JAMA*. 2010;304:1339-1349.

47. van Rees Vellinga TE, Peters RJ, Yusuf S, et al. Efficacy and safety of fondaparinux in patients with ST-segment elevation myocardial infarction across the age spectrum. Results from the Organization for the Assessment of Strategies for Ischemic Syndromes 6 (OASIS-6) trial. *Am Heart J*. 2010;160:1049-1055.

48. Warkentin TE, Pai M, Sheppard JI, Schulman S, Spyropoulos AC, Eikelboom JW. Fondaparinux treatment of acute heparin-induced thrombocytopenia confirmed by the serotonin-release assay: a 30-month, 16-patient case series. *J Thromb Haemost*. 2011;9:2389-2396.

49. Warkentin TE, Cook RJ, Marder VJ, et al. Anti-platelet factor 4/heparin antibodies in orthopedic surgery patients receiving antithrombotic prophylaxis with fondaparinux or enoxaparin. *Blood*. 2005;106:3791-3796.

50. Hankey GJ, Eikelboom JW. Dabigatran etexilate: a new oral thrombin inhibitor. *Circulation*. 2011;123:1436-1450.

51. Levy JH, Faraoni D, Spring JL, Douketis JD, Samama CM. Managing new oral anticoagulants in the perioperative and intensive care unit setting. *Anesthesiology*. 2013;118:1466-1474.

52. Connolly SJ, Ezekowitz MD, Yusuf S, et al. Dabigatran versus warfarin in patients with atrial fibrillation. *N Engl J Med*. 2009;361:1139-1151.

53. Ezekowitz MD, Nagarakanti R, Noack H, et al. Comparison of dabigatran and warfarin in patients with atrial fibrillation and valvular heart disease: the RE-LY trial (Randomized Evaluation of Long-Term Anticoagulant Therapy). *Circulation*. 2016;134:589-598.

54. Miller CS, Grandi SM, Shimony A, Filion KB, Eisenberg MJ. Meta-analysis of efficacy and safety of new oral anticoagulants (dabigatran, rivaroxaban, apixaban) versus warfarin in patients with atrial fibrillation. *Am J Cardiol*. 2012;110:453-460.

55. Wann LS, Curtis AB, Ellenbogen KA, et al. 2011 ACCF/AHA/HRS focused update on the management of patients with atrial fibrillation (update on dabigatran): a report of the American College of Cardiology Foundation/American Heart Association Task Force on practice guidelines. *J Am Coll Cardiol*. 2011;57:1330-1337.

56. Miyares MA, Davis K. Newer oral anticoagulants: a review of laboratory monitoring options and reversal agents in the hemorrhagic patient. *Am J Health Syst Pharm*. 2012;69:1473-1484.

57. Vanden Daelen S, Peetermans M, Vanassche T, Verhamme P, Vandermeulen E. Monitoring and reversal strategies for new oral anticoagulants. *Expert Rev Cardiovasc Ther*. 2015;13:95-103.

58. Pollack CV, Jr., Reilly PA, Eikelboom J, et al. Idarucizumab for dabigatran reversal. *N Engl J Med*. 2015;373:511-520.

59. Reardon DP, Owusu K. Idarucizumab for dabigatran reversal guideline. *Crit Pathw Cardiol*. 2016;15:33-35.

60. Babilonia K, Trujillo T. The role of prothrombin complex concentrates in reversal of target specific anticoagulants. *Thromb J*. 2014;12:8.

61. Augoustides JG. Breakthroughs in anticoagulation: advent of the oral direct factor Xa inhibitors. *J Cardiothorac Vasc Anesth.* 2012;26:740-745.

62. Hillarp A, Gustafsson KM, Faxälv L, et al. Effects of the oral, direct factor Xa inhibitor apixaban on routine coagulation assays and anti-FXa assays. *J Thromb Haemost.* 2014;12: 1545-1553.

63. Samama MM. Which test to use to measure the anticoagulant effect of rivaroxaban: the anti-factor Xa assay. *J Thromb Haemost.* 2013;11:579-580.

64. U.S Food and Drug Administration. (2018). Summary basis for regulatory action. Available at: https://www.fda.gov/downloads/biologicsbloodvaccines/cellulargenetherapy-products/approvedproducts/ucm610006.pdf. Accessed June 1, 2018.

65. Siegal DM, Curnutte JT, Connolly SJ, et al. Andexanet alfa for the reversal of factor Xa inhibitor activity. *N Engl J Med.* 2015;373:2413-2424.

66. Ansell J, Hirsh J, Hylek E, Jacobson A, Crowther M, Palareti G. Pharmacology and management of the vitamin K antagonists: American College of Chest Physicians Evidence-Based Clinical Practice Guidelines (8th Edition). *Chest.* 2008;133:160S-198S.

67. Holbrook A, Schulman S, Witt DM, et al. Evidence-based management of anticoagulant therapy: Antithrombotic Therapy and Prevention of Thrombosis, 9th ed: American College of Chest Physicians Evidence-Based Clinical Practice Guidelines. *Chest.* 2012;141:e152S-e184S.

68. Wadhera RK, Russell CE, Piazza G. Cardiology patient page. Warfarin versus novel oral anticoagulants: how to choose? *Circulation.* 2014;130:e191-e193.

84

Is There a Better Way to Deliver Optimal Critical Care Services?

Ian J. Barbash and Jeremy M. Kahn

INTRODUCTION

Critical illness is defined by life-threatening organ dysfunction leading to excess morbidity and mortality. While overall mortality in hospitalized patients is less than 5%, more than 10% of patients die after admission to the intensive care unit (ICU).[1,2] In the most severe forms of critical illness such as septic shock and acute respiratory distress syndrome, mortality approaches 50%.[3,4] In addition to this human toll, critical illness imposes substantial financial costs: annual ICU spending in the United States exceeds US$100 billion and accounts for nearly 15% of hospital costs and almost 1% of the gross domestic product.[5]

Given our tremendous social and financial investment in critical care, it is imperative that we optimize the organization and management of critical care delivery. For most of their history, ICUs were physically separate from other areas of the hospital but were managed without specific attention to physician staffing patterns or team-based care models. In the 21st century, a growing body of evidence supports specific approaches to optimal ICU organization and management. Simultaneously, in the era of value-based care, there is increasing interest from payers, government agencies, and regulators in implementing strategies that improve the outcomes of critically ill patients while minimizing costs.[6–8] These maturing forces—an increasingly robust evidence base and the drive to implement strategies that improve the value of health care—have created an environment in which the tools of evidence-based medicine are essential to optimizing the delivery of ICU services.

An evidence-based approach is particularly important because the effectiveness of a given approach to critical care delivery often depends on the local context in which it is implemented—that is, ICU organization and management are not "one size fits all." This observation parallels the precision medicine movement for patient-level treatments, in which there is increasing recognition that a particular intervention may be more effective for some critically ill patients

than for others.[9] For many organizational strategies, there is a mix of studies with "positive" and "negative" results; rather than this representing evidence of ineffectiveness, it is likely that contextual factors render a given organizational strategy more effective in some ICUs than in others.

THE INTERPROFESSIONAL TEAM

There is a growing consensus that the key to a high-quality ICU is a collaborative team of individuals from multiple health professions.[10] In their most expansive forms, these teams comprise intensive care physicians and advanced practice providers, nurses, respiratory therapists, clinical pharmacists, physical and occupational therapists, speech and language pathologists, dieticians, social workers, case managers, and spiritual support. It is impractical to expect representatives from all of these disciplines to participate directly in daily ICU rounding, and many of these individuals have competing responsibilities beyond the ICU that necessitate communication outside a formal rounding structure. However, compared with isolated physician rounding, some form of interprofessional rounding is associated with reductions in ICU length of stay, medication errors, and mortality.[11,12] The best evidence supports, at a minimum, the inclusion of the ICU physician, bedside nurse, and clinical pharmacist in a synchronous discussion on rounds.[11] Clearly, engaging respiratory therapists is essential for patients with respiratory failure, for whom protocolized daily spontaneous breathing trials speed liberation from mechanical ventilation.[13,14] Depending on local ICU case mix, integrating additional professions into daily bedside rounds may prove beneficial.

It seems intuitive that ICU quality depends not only on the physical presence of multiple health professionals but also on how they function together as a team. Well-functioning teams are characterized by role clarity, shared goals, effective information exchange, and collaborative processes for decision making and conflict resolution.[15,16] A recent systematic review of interventions to improve team functioning in the

ICU found that simulation-based team training can improve team climate.[17] Other hospital- and ICU-based interventions addressing teamwork and collective efforts to identify and mitigate errors can improve the climate of safety.[18,19] In general, even studies showing a robust effect of interventions on team function did not show a significant impact on patient-centered outcomes. In part, this probably reflects the difficulty in defining and measuring team performance, which is an important area of future research in ICU teamwork, and its impact on patient outcomes.

INTENSIVIST STAFFING MODELS

Under the current gold-standard model of the interprofessional ICU team, an intensivist physician provides leadership and directs the overall plan of care.[20] This intensivist is typically board-certified with specific subspecialty training in critical care medicine. There are two traditional models under which an ICU can operate: a "closed" unit, in which the intensivist takes direct responsibility for all patients admitted to the ICU; or an "open" unit, in which a nonintensivist primary physician retains responsibility for patients admitted to the ICU and consults an intensivist for co-management for some patients. Early versions of ICU organization guidelines endorsed the closed models as the preferred approach.[21] However, a large study in 69 US centers failed to show a difference in outcomes between closed and open ICUs, and current guidelines no longer emphasize that a closed model is paramount.[2,20]

While there is general agreement that some form of intensivist involvement benefits critically ill patients, several systematic reviews point to a lack of consensus as to the optimal intensity of physician staffing patterns during daylight hours.[22-24] Most studies compared "high-intensity" with "low-intensity" physician staffing models: a high-intensity model is a closed ICU or one with mandatory intensivist consultation; a low-intensity model is an open ICU without

intensivists or with elective intensivist consultation. Whereas earlier systematic reviews, including studies from the 1980s and 1990s, indicated a potential mortality benefit to high-intensity staffing, data from the most recent decade are less convincing.[24,25] Table 84.1 summarizes existing multicenter studies that compared mortality in critically ill patients under high-intensity vs. low-intensity staffing models,[25-32] and Table 84.2 provides an overview of the four major staffing models. The fact that high-intensity daytime intensivist physician staffing is not strongly and independently associated with mortality in the modern era may reflect the fact that other aspects of critical care delivery, including interprofessional, team-based care, are more widely available and improve components of quality previously addressed primarily by individual physicians.

In addition to the debate regarding high-intensity vs. low-intensity daytime staffing, a recent systematic review suggests that "around-the-clock," 24-hour in-house intensivist coverage does not improve mortality in most ICUs.[33] This review evaluated one randomized controlled trial (RCT) and 17 observational studies; the pooled odds ratio for mortality associated with 24-hour intensivist coverage was 0.99, with a 95% confidence interval (CI) of 0.75–1.29. The single RCT compared in-house intensivist coverage by critical care attendings and fellows to intensivist consultation by phone to in-house residents and nurses.[34] In-house nocturnal intensivist coverage did not reduce ICU length of stay (rate ratio for the time to ICU discharge 0.98; 95% CI 0.88–1.09; $P = .72$) or ICU mortality (relative risk 1.07; 95% CI 0.90–1.28). The primary limitation of this study was that it was conducted in a single academic center, and even the control intervention included on-demand consultation with intensivists by phone, constraining its generalizability to other environments.

We should not take from these intensivist staffing data a message that intensivists "don't matter," but rather that their impact is probably context-dependent. The optimal physician staffing of a small, 8-bed ICU in a rural hospital with few

TABLE 84.1 Summary of Multicenter Cohort Studies on Intensivist Physician Staffing for Critically Ill Adults.

Study	Population	Centers (N)	Patients (N)	Outcome Measure	Risk Estimate[a]
Pronovost et al., 1999[26]	Abdominal aortic surgery	46	2987	In-hospital mortality	0.33 (0.20–0.52)
Diringer and Edwards, 2001[27]	Intracerebral hemorrhage	42	1038	In-hospital mortality	0.39 (0.22–0.67)
Dimick et al., 2001[28]	Esophageal resection	35	366	In-hospital mortality	0.66 (0.16–2.5)
Nathens et al., 2006[29]	Trauma	68	2599	In-hospital mortality	0.78 (0.58–1.04)
Treggiari et al., 2007[30]	Acute lung injury	23	1,075	In-hospital mortality	0.68 (0.53–0.89)
Levy et al., 2008[31]	All ICU patients	100	101,832	In-hospital mortality	1.40 (NP)
Kim et al., 2012[32]	Severe sepsis	25	251	In-hospital mortality	0.46 (0.22–0.93)
Costa et al., 2015[25]	All ICU patients	49	65,752	In-hospital mortality	0.86 (0.65–1.14)

[a]Adjusted odds ratio or risk ratio comparing patients managed under a high-intensity staffing model to patients managed under a low-intensity staffing model. Definitions of high- and low-intensity staffing models differed among studies; high-intensity staffing typically refers to complete transfer of care to an intensivist or a mandatory consult model.

ICU, intensive care unit; *NP*, not provided.

TABLE 84.2 Overview of Daytime Intensivist Staffing Models.

High-Intensity Models	Low-Intensity Models
Closed	**Open, Optional Consult**
• All patients are seen by an intensivist on daily rounds • Intensivist takes primary responsibility for all aspects of patient care • Other physicians may be involved as consultants	• Nonintensivist physician takes primary responsibility for patient care • Intensivist sees some patients as a consultant at the discretion of the primary physician
Open, Mandatory Consult	**Open, no Intensivist**
• All patients are seen by an intensivist on daily rounds • Intensivist shares responsibility for patient care with primary physician • Additional physicians may be involved as consultants	• Nonintensivist physician takes primary responsibility for patient care • There is not an intensivist available for in-person consultation

mechanically ventilated patients is unlikely to mirror that of a 24-bed ICU in a large tertiary referral hospital. In addition, many of the mechanisms by which intensivists improved outcomes in the past may be less important in the modern age of highly functional, interprofessional ICU teams using standardized protocols to deliver evidence-based critical care. Indeed, even ICUs with dedicated intensivists can fail to comply with evidence-based practices.[4] The shortage of intensivists and physicians in general[35] along with the relatively high costs of physician salaries present barriers to universal adoption of high-intensity care models; given the existing evidence, some hospitals and ICUs might reasonably apply models of care other than one involving high-intensity daytime intensivist coverage with an in-house nocturnal intensivist.

ADVANCED PRACTICE PROVIDERS

In light of the debate surrounding the effectiveness and practicality of universal intensivist physician staffing, there is increasing interest in the role of advanced practice providers such as nurse practitioners (NPs) and physician assistants (PAs) in critical care.[36] The most recent systematic review on this topic is over a decade old; the included studies generally showed that inclusion of advanced practice providers in critical care teams was well-received by team members and associated with equivalent or somewhat improved processes of care and outcomes.[37] In recent years, as more hospitals and ICUs have adopted advanced practice providers, several studies have confirmed that, in critical care environments, they achieve outcomes that are at least equivalent to those under alternative care models.[38,39] In addition, a number of studies suggest that including advanced practice providers in ICU teams can improve the experience of resident and fellow

critical care trainees, perhaps by mitigating physician trainee workload.[40,41] With increasing numbers of advanced practice providers entering the ICU workforce, the question is not whether to incorporate them into ICU care models, but how to do so in ways that optimize team function as well as patient and financial outcomes.

PROTOCOLIZATION AND DECISION SUPPORT

Many decisions in medicine depend upon the judgment of clinicians, which is tailored to individual patients, but an increasing number of evidence-based practices lend themselves to standardization and protocolization for near-universal application. Several archetypal best practices relevant to the ICU are daily spontaneous breathing trials paired with daily interruption of sedation to facilitate liberation from mechanical ventilation in ICU patients.[13,42] Importantly, the studies establishing the efficacy of these practices have employed standardized protocols driven by respiratory therapists and bedside nurses. In the years since these initial studies, systematic reviews of numerous other studies have confirmed that standardized, protocol-based approaches to sedation management and ventilator weaning improve patient outcomes by improving adherence to best practices.[43,44] A 2008 survey of ICU directors in 90 academic medical centers confirmed that these protocols are common, with 86% of ICUs using respiratory therapist-driven ventilator weaning protocols and 73% using nurse-driven sedation protocols. Other protocols addressed lung-protective ventilation,[45] early sepsis resuscitation, and postoperative glucose control.[46–47]

Rounding checklists can theoretically synergize with these protocols by helping ICU teams set shared goals, identify opportunities to improve adherence with evidence-based practices, and improve efficiency.[48,49] ICU teams prefer checklists that are shorter, clinically relevant, and integrate seamlessly into rounding workflow.[49] The evidence supporting the impact of checklists on care processes and outcomes is generally weak.[50] A recent landmark cluster-randomized clinical trial evaluated the effect of a multicomponent intervention that included rounding checklists, goal setting, and clinician prompts in more than 100 Brazilian ICUs.[51] This study showed that the intervention did improve several relevant care processes, including sedation practices, central venous catheter utilization, and lung-protective ventilation, although the magnitude of the changes was relatively small. There were no significant differences in any patient-centered clinical outcomes between the intervention and control arms. Future work will need to better define the contexts in which ICU checklists are most likely to be beneficial.

As more hospitals adopt electronic health records (EHRs), automated clinical decision support systems (CDSS) operating within the EHR are an increasingly feasible approach to preventing errors and standardizing the delivery of accepted evidence-based practices. Existing CDSS based on relatively straightforward decision rules may reduce medication errors, improve compliance with blood transfusion guidelines, and increase rates of prophylaxis for venous thromboembolism.[52–55] The future of CDSS in the ICU will include machine learning techniques employing more complex algorithms to identify deteriorating patients and gaps in evidence-based care, facilitating earlier interventions. However, clinical applications of machine learning in the ICU are currently limited by compartmentalization of data across platforms, issues with data precision and accuracy, and challenges in applying statistical models to the complex and dynamic conditions of critical illness.[56] Ultimately, in order to add value to the clinical environment, CDSS must provide timely, actionable, and novel information to ICU teams without an excessive false-negative rate that contributes to alarm fatigue.

QUALITY MEASUREMENT AND IMPROVEMENT

As more hospitals adopt and refine their EHRs, ICUs directors have increasing access to timely, granular data on patient treatment processes and outcomes; these data can facilitate quality measurement and process improvement activities. Multiple critical care professional societies endorse the importance of developing and using both process- and outcome-based measures at multiple levels within the heath system, including in the ICU.[20,57] Measurement alone, however, does not drive improvement—the measures must be tied to specific strategies to implement changes that improve processes and outcomes. Traditional approaches generally link evidence-based protocols with educational initiatives, performance measurement, and feedback of these results to spur behavior change in low performers. These resource-intensive strategies can be difficult to implement and sustain, and the effects are often modest.[58] A complementary approach, known as pay for performance, links quality measurement to physician payment, although existing data suggest that pay for performance is associated with marginal improvements in treatment or outcomes for patients in the hospital and ICU.[59,60] Thus, while the increasing availability of electronic data may facilitate quality measurement, the process of changing behavior in ways that improves patient care and outcomes remains a challenge.

REGIONALIZATION

Regionalization is a system-wide approach to critical care organization and management by which selected patients are systematically transferred to regional referral centers.[61,62] Regionalization leverages the observation that hospitals caring for higher case volumes have better patient outcomes in a variety of conditions, including sepsis,[63,64] acute respiratory failure requiring mechanical ventilation,[65,66] and acute myocardial infarction.[67] However, the benefits of widespread regionalization of critical care services are largely theoretical,[66,68] and need to be balanced against the potential harms, including delays in the early management of time-sensitive conditions[69] and overwhelming the capacity available at tertiary facilities. New evidence also suggests that a regionalized

approach may help some critically ill patients but not others,[70,71] again highlighting the fact that the benefits of a particular ICU organizational strategy are probably contextual, and varying, based on local and regional case mix and other patient and hospital factors.

ICU TELEMEDICINE

In areas without local access to intensivist physicians, telemedicine is an approach that may bring the benefits of intensivist involvement in patient care without physically transferring patients to regional referral centers.[68] Multiple models of ICU telemedicine exist, ranging from continuous multibed monitoring of an entire ICU to more selective monitoring and/or on-demand consultation.[72] Studies of the impact of ICU telemedicine are largely limited by a before-and-after design, and systematic reviews indicate inconsistent effects on patient-centered outcomes despite substantial up-front financial investments.[73–77] The largest national study of telemedicine adoption compared 132 hospitals that adopted ICU telemedicine programs to 389 similar control hospitals that did not adopt ICU telemedicine programs.[75] In the overall comparison, ICU telemedicine adoption was associated with a small reduction in mortality among ICU admissions (relative risk 0.96; 95% CI 0.95–0.98), although there was dramatic heterogeneity, and only 16 individual hospitals experienced a statistically significant drop in mortality following ICU telemedicine adoption. This heterogeneity in effectiveness is probably due to a number of barriers and facilitators to telemedicine adoption, which are variably present across institutions and telemedicine programs.[78]

FUTURE DIRECTIONS

We have come a long way from a system that simply centralized critically ill patients in a single location within a hospital to one that emphasizes team-based, interprofessional care. ICU directors must consider a number of variables that may affect patient outcomes, including the nature of intensivist staffing, the use of advanced practice providers, protocolization and decision support, quality measurement, regionalization, and ICU telemedicine. We are increasingly understanding that the impact of any one of these organizational strategies depends not on *whether* but *how* we use them, and the context in which we do so. Future research should seek to refine existing organizational strategies and better understand the contextual factors that mediate their success or failure in reference to important patient-centered outcomes.

AUTHORS' RECOMMENDATIONS
- Interprofessional, team-based care is consistently associated with improved patient outcomes and is the gold-standard model of ICU medicine.
- Intensivist physician staffing may benefit many critically ill patients, although there are probably contexts in which intensivist involvement does not improve mortality.

- Complementary care models may bring some of the benefits of intensivist staffing and can help overcome barriers related to physician shortages and the direct financial costs of full-time intensivist staffing. These complementary care models include:
  - using advanced practice providers to increase the efficiency of intensivist leadership
  - protocolization and decision support systems to increase the consistent application of evidence-based practices
  - quality measurement to identify opportunities for improvement and monitor progress of improvement efforts
  - regionalization of critical care services to match patient severity of illness to the level of care needed
  - ICU telemedicine to expand the reach of intensivist expertise to locations where intensivists are not physically present.
- The impact of these complementary care models probably depends on local context; patient, provider, and financial implications should be evaluated prior to and following the process of implementing a new organizational strategy in an ICU.

REFERENCES

1. Liu V, Escobar GJ, Greene JD, et al. Hospital deaths in patients with sepsis from 2 independent cohorts. *JAMA*. 2014;312: 90-92.
2. Checkley W, Martin GS, Brown SM, et al. Structure, process, and annual ICU mortality across 69 centers: United States Critical Illness and Injury Trials Group Critical Illness Outcomes Study. *Crit Care Med*. 2014;42:344-356.
3. Seymour CW, Liu VX, Iwashyna TJ, et al. Assessment of clinical criteria for sepsis. *JAMA*. 2016;315:762.
4. Bellani G, Laffey JG, Pham T, et al. Epidemiology, patterns of care, and mortality for patients with acute respiratory distress syndrome in intensive care units in 50 countries. *JAMA*. 2016;315:788-800.
5. Halpern NA, Goldman DA, Tan KS, Pastores SM. Trends in critical care beds and use among population groups and Medicare and Medicaid beneficiaries in the United States: 2000-2010. *Crit Care Med*. 2016;44:1490-1499.
6. Costa DK, Kahn JM. Organizing critical care for the 21st century. *JAMA*. 2016;315:751.
7. Angus DC, Shorr AF, White A, Dremsizov TT, Schmitz RJ, Kelley MA. Critical care delivery in the United States: distribution of services and compliance with Leapfrog recommendations. *Crit Care Med*. 2006;34:1016-1024
8. Hershey TB, Kahn JM. State sepsis mandates—a new era for regulation of hospital quality. *N Engl J Med*. 2017;376(24): 2311-2313.
9. Iwashyna TJ, Burke JF, Sussman JB, Prescott HC, Hayward RA, Angus DC. Implications of heterogeneity of treatment effect for reporting & analysis of randomized trials in critical care. *Am J Respir Crit Care Med*. 2015;192(9):1045-1051.
10. Donovan AL, Aldrich JM, Gross AK, et al. Interprofessional care and teamwork in the ICU. *Crit Care Med*. 2018;46:980-990.
11. Lane D, Ferri M, Lemaire J, McLaughlin K, Stelfox HT. A systematic review of evidence-informed practices for patient care rounds in the ICU. *Crit Care Med*. 2013;41:2015-2029.
12. Kim MM, Barnato AE, Angus DC, Fleisher LA, Kahn JM. The effect of multidisciplinary care teams on intensive care unit mortality. *Arch Intern Med*. 2010;170:369-376.
13. Esteban A, Frutos F, Tobin MJ, et al. A comparison of four methods of weaning patients from mechanical ventilation. *N Engl J Med*. 1995;332:345-350.
14. Robertson TE, Sona C, Schallom L, et al. Improved extubation rates and earlier liberation from mechanical ventilation with implementation of a daily spontaneous-breathing trial protocol. *J Am Coll Surg*. 2008;206:489-495.
15. Reader TW, Flin R, Mearns K, Cuthbertson BH. Developing a team performance framework for the intensive care unit. *Crit Care Med*. 2009;37:1787-1793.
16. Ervin JN, Kahn JM, Cohen TR, Weingart LR. Teamwork in the intensive care unit. *Am Psychol*. 2018;73:468-477.
17. Dietz AS, Pronovost PJ, Mendez-Tellez PA, et al. A systematic review of teamwork in the intensive care unit: What do we know about teamwork, team tasks, and improvement strategies? *J Crit Care*. 2014;29:908-914.
18. Sexton JB, Berenholtz SM, Goeschel CA, et al. Assessing and improving safety climate in a large cohort of intensive care units. *Crit Care Med*. 2011;39:934-939.
19. Weaver SJ, Lubomksi LH, Wilson RF, Pfoh ER, Martinez KA, Dy SM. Promoting a culture of safety as a patient safety strategy. *Ann Intern Med*. 2013;158:369.
20. Weled BJ, Adzhigirey LA, Hodgman TM, et al. Critical care delivery: the importance of process of care and ICU structure to improved outcomes: an update from the American College of Critical Care Medicine Task Force on Models of Critical Care. *Crit Care Med*. 2015;43:1520-1525.
21. Brilli RJ, Spevetz A, Branson RD, et al. Critical care delivery in the intensive care unit: defining clinical roles and the best practice model. *Crit Care Med*. 2001;29:2007-2019.
22. Young MP, Birkmeyer JD. Potential reduction in mortality rates using an intensivist model to manage intensive care units. *Eff Clin Pract*. 2000;3:284-289.
23. Pronovost PJ, Angus DC, Dorman T, Robinson KA, Dremsizov TT, Young TL. Physician staffing patterns and clinical outcomes in critically ill patients: a systematic review. *JAMA*. 2002;288: 2151-2162.
24. Wilcox ME, Chong CA, Niven DJ, et al. Do intensivist staffing patterns influence hospital mortality following ICU admission? A systematic review and meta-analyses. *Crit Care Med*. 2013;41:2253-2274.
25. Costa DK, Wallace DJ, Kahn JM. The association between daytime intensivist physician staffing and mortality in the context of other ICU organizational practices. *Crit Care Med*. 2015;43: 2275-2282.
26. Pronovost PJ, Jenckes MW, Dorman T, et al. Organizational characteristics of intensive care units related to outcomes of abdominal aortic surgery. *JAMA*. 1999;281:1310-1317.
27. Diringer MN, Edwards DF. Admission to a neurologic/neurosurgical intensive care unit is associated with reduced mortality rate after intracerebral hemorrhage. *Crit Care Med*. 2001; 29:635-640.
28. Dimick JB, Pronovost PJ, Heitmiller RF, Lipsett PA. Intensive care unit physician staffing is associated with decreased length of stay, hospital cost, and complications after esophageal resection. *Crit Care Med*. 2001;29:753-758.
29. Nathens AB, Rivara FP, MacKenzie EJ, et al. The impact of an intensivist-model ICU on trauma-related mortality. *Ann Surg*. 2006;244:545-554.

30. Treggiari MM, Martin DP, Yanez ND, Caldwell E, Hudson LD, Rubenfeld GD. Effect of intensive care unit organizational model and structure on outcomes in patients with acute lung injury. *Am J Respir Crit Care Med.* 2007;176:685-690.

31. Levy MM, Rapoport J, Lemeshow S, Chalfin DB, Phillips G, Danis M. Association between critical care physician management and patient mortality in the intensive care unit. *Ann Intern Med.* 2008;148:801-809.

32. Kim JH, Hong SK, Kim KC, et al. Influence of full-time intensivist and the nurse-to-patient ratio on the implementation of severe sepsis bundles in Korean intensive care units. *J Crit Care.* 2012;27:414.e11-414.e21.

33. Kerlin MP, Adhikari NKJ, Rose L, et al. An official American Thoracic Society Systematic Review: the effect of nighttime intensivist staffing on mortality and length of stay among intensive care unit patients. *Am J Respir Crit Care Med.* 2017;195: 383-393.

34. Kerlin MP, Small DS, Cooney E, et al. A randomized trial of nighttime physician staffing in an intensive care unit. *N Engl J Med.* 2013;368:2201-2209.

35. Halpern NA, Pastores SM, Oropello JM, Kvetan V. Critical care medicine in the United States: addressing the intensivist shortage and image of the specialty. *Crit Care Med.* 2013;41: 2754-2761.

36. Hoffman LA, Guttendorf J. Preparation and evolving role of the acute care nurse practitioner. *Chest.* 2017;152:1339-1345.

37. Kleinpell RM, Ely EW, Grabenkort R. Nurse practitioners and physician assistants in the intensive care unit: an evidence-based review. *Crit Care Med.* 2008;36:2888-2897.

38. Landsperger JS, Semler MW, Wang L, Byrne DW, Wheeler AP. Outcomes of nurse practitioner-delivered critical care. *Chest.* 2016;149:1146-1154.

39. Scherzer R, Dennis MP, Swan BA, Kavuru MS, Oxman DA. A comparison of usage and outcomes between nurse practitioner and resident-staffed medical ICUs. *Crit Care Med.* 2017;45:e132-e137.

40. Joffe AM, Pastores SM, Maerz LL, Mathur P, Lisco SJ. Utilization and impact on fellowship training of non-physician advanced practice providers in intensive care units of academic medical centers: a survey of critical care program directors. *J Crit Care.* 2014;29:112-115.

41. Kahn SA, Davis SA, Banes CT, Dennis BM, May AK, Gunter OD. Impact of advanced practice providers (nurse practitioners and physician assistants) on surgical residents' critical care experience. *J Surg Res.* 2015;199:7-12.

42. Girard TD, Kress JP, Fuchs BD, et al. Efficacy and safety of a paired sedation and ventilator weaning protocol for mechanically ventilated patients in intensive care (Awakening and Breathing Controlled trial): a randomised controlled trial. *Lancet.* 2008;371:126-134.

43. Jackson DL, Proudfoot CW, Cann KF, Walsh T. A systematic review of the impact of sedation practice in the ICU on resource use, costs and patient safety. *Crit Care.* 2010; 14:R59.

44. Blackwood B, Burns KEA, Cardwell CR, O'Halloran P. Protocolized versus non-protocolized weaning for reducing the duration of mechanical ventilation in critically ill adult patients. *Cochrane Database Syst Rev.* 2014;(11):CD006904.

45. Prasad M, Christie JD, Bellamy SL, Rubenfeld GD, Kahn JM. The availability of clinical protocols in US teaching intensive care units. *J Crit Care.* 2010;25(4):610–619.

46. Rivers E, Nguyen B, Havstad S, et al. Early goal-directed therapy in the treatment of severe sepsis and septic shock. *N Engl J Med.* 2001;345:1368-1377.

47. Van den Berghe G, Wouters P, Weekers F, et al. Intensive insulin therapy in critically ill patients. *N Engl J Med.* 2001;345: 1359-1367.

48. Centofanti JE, Duan EH, Hoad NC, et al. Use of a daily goals checklist for morning ICU rounds. *Crit Care Med.* 2014;42: 1797-1803.

49. Hallam BD, Kuza CC, Rak K, et al. Perceptions of rounding checklists in the intensive care unit: a qualitative study. *BMJ Qual Saf.* 2018;27(10):836-843 .

50. Ko HCH, Turner TJ, Finnigan MA. Systematic review of safety checklists for use by medical care teams in acute hospital settings—limited evidence of effectiveness. *BMC Health Serv Res.* 2011;11:211.

51. Cavalcanti AB, Bozza FA, Machado FR, et al. Effect of a quality improvement intervention with daily round checklists, goal setting, and clinician prompting on mortality of critically ill patients. *JAMA.* 2016;315:1480.

52. Kaushal R, Shojania KG, Bates DW. Effects of computerized physician order entry and clinical decision support systems on medication safety. *Arch Intern Med.* 2003;163:1409.

53. Prgomet M, Li L, Niazkhani Z, Georgiou A, Westbrook JI. Impact of commercial computerized provider order entry (CPOE) and clinical decision support systems (CDSSs) on medication errors, length of stay, and mortality in intensive care units: a systematic review and meta-analysis. *J Am Med Informatics Assoc.* 2017;24(2):413-422.

54. Hibbs SP, Nielsen ND, Brunskill S, et al. The impact of electronic decision support on transfusion practice: a systematic review. *Transfus Med Rev.* 2015;29:14-23.

55. Borab ZM, Lanni MA, Tecce MG, Pannucci CJ, Fischer JP. Use of computerized clinical decision support systems to prevent venous thromboembolism in surgical patients: a systematic review and meta-analysis. *JAMA Surg.* 2017;152:638-645.

56. Johnson AEW, Ghassemi MM, Nemati S, Niehaus KE, Clifton DA, Clifford GD. Machine learning and decision support in critical care. *Proc IEEE Inst Electr Electron Eng.* 2016;104: 444-466.

57. Kahn JM, Gould MK, Krishnan JA, et al. An official American Thoracic Society workshop report: developing performance measures from clinical practice guidelines. *Ann Am Thorac Soc.* 2014;11:S186-S195.

58. Sinuff T, Muscedere J, Adhikari NKJ, et al. Knowledge translation interventions for critically ill patients: a systematic review. *Crit Care Med.* 2013;41:2627-2640.

59. Mendelson A, Kondo K, Damberg C, et al. The effects of pay-for-performance programs on health, health care use, and processes of care: a systematic review. *Ann Intern Med.* 2017;166: 341-353.

60. Barbash IJ, Pike F, Gunn SR, Seymour CW, Kahn JM. Effects of physician-targeted pay for performance on use of spontaneous breathing trials in mechanically ventilated patients. *Am J Respir Crit Care Med.* 2017;196:56-63.

61. Thompson DR, Clemmer TP, Applefeld JJ, et al. Regionalization of critical care medicine: task force report of the American College of Critical Care Medicine. *Crit Care Med.* 1994;22: 1306-1313.

62. Kahn JM, Branas CC, Schwab CW, Asch DA. Regionalization of medical critical care: What can we learn from the trauma experience? *Crit Care Med.* 2008;36:3085-3088.

63. Walkey AJ, Wiener RS. Hospital case volume and outcomes among patients hospitalized with severe sepsis. *Am J Respir Crit Care Med*. 2014;189:548-555.

64. Gaieski DF, Edwards JM, Kallan MJ, Mikkelsen ME, Goyal M, Carr BG. The relationship between hospital volume and mortality in severe sepsis. *Am J Respir Crit Care Med*. 2014;190:665-674.

65. Kahn JM, Goss CH, Heagerty PJ, Kramer AA, O'Brien CR, Rubenfeld GD. Hospital volume and the outcomes of mechanical ventilation. *N Engl J Med*. 2006;355:41-50.

66. Kahn JM, Linde-Zwirble WT, Wunsch H, et al. Potential value of regionalized intensive care for mechanically ventilated medical patients. *Am J Respir Crit Care Med*. 2008;177:285-291.

67. Ross JS, Normand SLT, Wang Y, et al. Hospital volume and 30-day mortality for three common medical conditions. *N Engl J Med*. 2010;362:1110-1118.

68. Nguyen YL, Kahn JM, Angus DC. Reorganizing adult critical care delivery. *Am J Respir Crit Care Med*. 2010;181:1164-1169.

69. Faine BA, Noack JM, Wong T, et al. Interhospital transfer delays appropriate treatment for patients with severe sepsis and septic shock: a retrospective cohort study. *Crit Care Med*. 2015;43:2589-2596.

70. Ofoma UR, Dahdah J, Kethireddy S, Maeng D, Walkey AJ. Case volume–outcomes associations among patients with severe sepsis who underwent interhospital transfer. *Crit Care Med*. 2017;45:615-622.

71. Greenberg JA, Hohmann SF, James BD, et al. Hospital volume of immunosuppressed sepsis patients and sepsis mortality. *Ann Am Thorac Soc*. 2018;15(8):962-969.

72. Kahn JM, Hill NS, Lilly CM, et al. The research agenda in ICU telemedicine: a statement from the Critical Care Societies Collaborative. *Chest*. 2011;140:230-238.

73. Morrison JL, Cai Q, Davis N, et al. Clinical and economic outcomes of the electronic intensive care unit: results from two community hospitals. *Crit Care Med*. 2010;38:2-8.

74. Young LB, Chan PS, Lu X, Nallamothu BK, Sasson C, Cram PM. Impact of telemedicine intensive care unit coverage on patient outcomes: a systematic review and meta-analysis. *Arch Intern Med*. 2011;171:498-506.

75. Kahn JM, Le TQ, Barnato AE, et al. ICU telemedicine and critical care mortality. *Med Care*. 2016;54:319-325.

76. Kumar G, Falk DM, Bonello RS, Kahn JM, Perencevich E, Cram P. The costs of critical care telemedicine programs. *Chest*. 2013;143:19-29.

77. Chen J, Sun D, Yang W, et al. Clinical and economic outcomes of telemedicine programs in the intensive care unit: a systematic review and meta-analysis. *J Intensive Care Med*. 2018;33:383-393.

78. Ray KN, Felmet KA, Hamilton MF, et al. Clinician attitudes toward adoption of pediatric emergency telemedicine in rural hospitals. *Pediatr Emerg Care*. 2017;33:250-257.

85

How Do Critical Care Pharmacists Contribute to Team-Based Care?

Judith Jacobi

INTRODUCTION

Clinical pharmacists are licensed practitioners with advanced education and training who practice in all types of patient care settings with a focus on comprehensive medication management (CMM). CMM is defined as the standard of care in ensuring that each patient's medications (prescription, nonprescription, supplements, or herbals) are individually assessed to determine whether they are appropriate for the patient, effective for the condition, safe for use with concurrent comorbidities and therapies, and that the patient is able to take them.[1] An individualized care plan defines the goals, monitoring, and intended outcome. These specialized pharmacists are focused on achieving optimal use of medications, emphasizing dosing, monitoring, identification of adverse effects, and economic efficiency for optimal patient outcomes. They are a primary source of scientifically valid information on the safe, appropriate, and cost-effective use of medications. Critical care pharmacists apply this activity to the complex and rapidly changing patients in that setting. They work as essential members of the critical care team and need to have time dedicated to those direct patient care roles. The history of critical care pharmacists has been described in detail.[2] Their participation began in the 1970's with a small group of pharmacists who individually developed practices in intensive care unit (ICU) settings and progressively grew the discipline through the development of clinical training programs and, ultimately, through formal training programs in critical care pharmacy.

DEFINITION OF CLINICAL PHARMACY

The American College of Clinical Pharmacy is the parent organization of clinical pharmacists with a primary focus on development, advancement, and positioning of clinical pharmacists among other providers, public, and professional societies. There are over 17,000 members, but many other pharmacists practice direct patient care. Clinical pharmacy is defined as a health science discipline where pharmacists provide care that optimizes medication therapy and promotes health, wellness, and disease prevention.[3]

Many critical care pharmacists consider the Society of Critical Care Medicine (SCCM) to be their primary specialty organization. The SCCM was founded as a multiprofessional organization where all critical care practitioners share full membership rights. Critical care pharmacists have been a part of the governing council since the late 1990's and have served in the executive committee and as president. Committees are multiprofessional, and pharmacists have led and contributed toward much of the organization's work product, including programming and publications.

The American Society of Parenteral and Enteral Nutrition and the Neurocritical Care Society are similarly multiprofessional, and pharmacists have had leadership roles and been contributing members since their inception.

CLINICAL TEAMS DEFINED

The American College of Physicians has described the clinical care team in the United States as the health professionals—physicians, advanced practice registered nurses, other registered nurses, physician assistants, clinical pharmacists, and other health care professionals—with the training and skills needed to provide high-quality, coordinated care specific to the patient's clinical needs and circumstances).[4] While the composition of teams may vary, the responsibility and authority for specific aspects of care are optimally assigned to the person most appropriate for the task. Optimal team effectiveness relies on a culture of trust, shared goals, effective communication, and mutual respect. The best interests of the patient should be the driving force for team activities. Teamwork is the standard for critical care patient management. High functioning multiprofessional teams facilitate optimal patient outcomes.[5] Pharmacists contribute to these teams through CMM, educating members on critical therapies, and supporting the medication use process. Pharmacists also evaluate medication use for performance improvement opportunities, identify and manage errors and adverse medication events, and participate in clinical research. Other activities include defining best practice for drug therapy and organization of treatment ordering pathways that ensure consistency.

TRAINING AND CERTIFICATION

A pharmacist in the United States is eligible for licensure after 6 years of college education and attainment of a Doctor of Pharmacy degree. While not required, many of these graduates already have a Bachelor of Science in another field. Pharmacists who are interested in direct patient care roles are encouraged to seek additional training in postgraduate year-one residency programs in acute care or ambulatory care settings. These are broad-based accredited experiences in clinical care, drug information, administration, teaching methods, and project/research over 12 months.[6] For hospital specialty practice, such as critical care, cardiology, or emergency medicine, a second year of training in the focused area is essential.[7] There are approximately 140 critical care pharmacy residency programs. Additional research fellowship training may follow, especially for those interested in an academic or research role.

Following didactic and experiential training, many clinical pharmacists seek Board of Pharmacy Specialties (BPS) certification.[8] There are more than 38,000 pharmacists worldwide who are BPS board certified in 12 pharmacy specialties, currently including cardiology and critical care, with emergency medicine in the future. Board certification is a validation that the pharmacist has advanced knowledge and experiences to optimize patient outcomes. There are approximately 2000 Board Certified Critical Care Pharmacists. Board certified pharmacists must pass a rigorous examination and then maintain accreditation through continuing education or additional testing every 7 years. Board certification is a typical requirement to achieve privileges for independent or collaborative practice. It is also a requirement to serve as a critical care pharmacy residency program director and will be a minimum credential for Fellowship eligibility in the American College of Critical Care Medicine of SCCM.

Clinical pharmacists may practice under a formal collaborative practice agreement with physicians in their practice area or as granted by the hospital.[9] For example, pharmacists may modify the dose, frequency, or route of administration of medications covered by a collaborative practice agreement or other hospital protocol. They may also initiate serum concentration monitoring or order other applicable laboratory tests to monitor the effects of the therapy. Quality assessment has demonstrated the value of these programs.[10] In a growing number of hospitals, clinical pharmacists are granted practice-specific privileges through mechanisms similar to other providers. The laws for pharmacist activities are governed by individual states and local hospital regulation.

The size of the current or potential critical care pharmacist workforce is not known. There are almost 2500 pharmacists in the Clinical Pharmacy and Pharmacology Section of SCCM and over 3000 in the American College of Clinical Pharmacy critical care practice and research network. There are likely many other pharmacists who practice in the critical care environment who are not members of a professional society.

While the critical care specialist will be most visible, there is a network of pharmacists and technicians working together to ensure timely and accurate medication availability and safe administration and documentation. Parenteral medications are a mainstay of critical care patient therapy, and pharmacists and technicians have specialized in the preparation of these products in an aseptic environment that meets United States Pharmacopeia 797 standards for sterile product compounding.[11] Standardized procedures for cleanroom design, cleaning, inspection, and product handling are applied to minimize the risk of contamination and patient harm. Pharmacists assess and verify the appropriateness of medication orders, with the assistance of computerized decision support systems within the electronic medical record. Technicians manage the preparation and delivery of nonparenteral medications on a per-patient basis or through automated dispensing cabinets. Hospital pharmacy technicians are certified upon the successful completion of a national examination.

PRACTICE FRAMEWORK

A framework for critical care pharmacy services was published in 2000 to define activities as fundamental, desirable, or optimal.[12] Activities such as prospective evaluation of drug therapy, management of adverse drug events (ADEs), pharmacokinetic consultation, communication and optimization of critical care formularies, and quality assurance activities were considered to be fundamental. Where resources permitted and hospital volume/acuity required, activities such as rounding, resuscitation participation, education of students and residents, medication history documentation, and scholarly activities were considered desirable. Optimal activities included provision of continuing education, management of pharmacy residencies, conducting independent research, and development of new pharmacy programs. A recent review of these same services by a group of critical care pharmacists has reclassified many of these activities as standard work, and will be defined as fundamental aspects of practice in a future paper on pharmacist roles. Some activities remain resource and expertise dependent or pertain to settings where specialized patient populations are managed. Clinicians will have a new reference to measure the depth of their involvement and a tool to direct role expansion when this updated document is published.

In the United Kingdom, pharmacy practice has a defined framework for pharmacist training and advancement. Specialist critical care pharmacists (SCCP) have developed a competency framework and process for credentialing that includes a career advancement pathway.[13,14] Once demonstrate their ability to work at the advanced or mastery level, they have additional privileges, including prescribing, when at the level of mastery/consultant.

A survey in 2005 described similar critical care clinical pharmacist roles in 24 countries outside North America.[15]

ROLE OF CRITICAL CARE PHARMACISTS

Critical care pharmacists work in all types of ICUs and provide a spectrum of services. There is no such thing as a typical day, but like their medical colleagues, the pharmacists evaluate new patients for medication history and allergies and document in the medical record, provide CMM, individualize drug doses through serum concentration monitoring, round with the clinical care team, educate nurses formally and informally, provide drug information, educate patients and families, respond to medical emergencies, and document their activities. The pharmacist will also perform medication order review and verification, evaluate potential drug interactions, monitor for and document adverse events, and assure adherence to hospital protocols. Education and mentoring of pharmacy students and residents, committee activities, performance improvement assessments, and formal research activities may also be done. Management of problems, such as drug shortages, and development of new treatment guidelines are other common challenges.[16]

IMPACT OF CRITICAL CARE PHARMACISTS

Pharmacists targeting practice changes have demonstrated their value as members of the multiprofessional team as well as in direct patient care roles through consistent implementation of best practices worldwide. Pharmacists in Australia have described medication therapy interventions for hospitalized inpatients and demonstrated their ability to reduce length of stay (LOS) and to account for over $4 million in annualized hospital cost savings in eight hospitals.[17] While a majority were targeted to reduce drug expenditure, 6.9% were independently judged to reduce LOS, and 11.1% had reduced readmission. Over 25% of the interventions were rated as major or life-saving.

Most studies evaluating the role of the pharmacist are before and after cohorts and thus study design demonstrates an association. Pharmacists work within a team of practitioners on complex and unstable patients; thus it is challenging to show an impact from a single provider.

Critical care pharmacists in the Netherlands have significantly reduced prescribing errors and potential patient harm by their presence in the ICU compared with the baseline central pharmacy services.[18]

One of the most significant reports is from French critical care pharmacists. This study demonstrated a reduction in ICU (1.4 days [2.3–0.5]; $P < .01$) and hospital LOS (3.7 days [5.2–2.3]; $P < .001$) by leading in the application of a quality bundle.[19] The bundle included antimicrobial de-escalation, optimal sedation titration, and nonmedication elements of protective ventilation, head of bed elevation, and removal of central lines and urinary catheters. The effectiveness of the bundle is a testament to their integration in the critical care team and illustrates that all team members can influence outcomes. While the before and after study design may have been influenced by other practice changes, the individual bundle elements have previously been shown to improve outcome. Further, the pragmatic design did not allow for matching based on severity of illness. The pharmacists did not abandon the traditional role of medication optimization, error prevention, and detection. The economic benefit of the interventions (13.8% reduction of hospital cost per stay or a mean of □ 2560 [3728–1392]; $P < .001$ savings per patient) exceeded the salaries of the pharmacists, indicating that practicing to a full extent sometimes referred to "at the top of their license" is a fiscally beneficial role. Much of the cost saving was related to reduced consumption of sedatives and antimicrobial agents. These pharmacists provide an excellent return on investment. In contrast, a prospective, randomized trial that compared drug costs in patients after the involvement of a critical care pharmacist with matched controls was not able to demonstrate a significant benefit on mean daily drug costs in a single ICU without excluding high-cost drugs, considered to be outliers.[20] Data analysis was confounded by differences in drug costs and LOS despite matching for clinical variables likely to influence outcome in this underpowered study. Interestingly, the pharmacist time per patient was 24.1 ± 8.2 minutes, similar to the UK report of 22.5 ± 9.5 minutes per patient.[21]

Pharmacists have addressed components of the French bundle individually. Sedation of critically ill patients is a fine balance to achieve appropriate levels of patient comfort and nursing workload, while avoiding prolonged periods of mechanical ventilation that can increase the risk of infections while waiting for the patient to awaken. Pharmacists have developed sedation protocols and supervised medication titration to reduce the duration of mechanical ventilation in single-center studies of various sizes. A before and after study of a pharmacist managed the sedation protocol in two medical ICUs. Daily assessment of sedation by a pharmacist reduced ICU LOS from 380 ± 325 hours to 238 ± 206 hours ($P = .001$) during a 3-month intervention in 156 patients.[22] Pharmacist-directed down-titration of medications in oversedated patients reduced the daily dose of midazolam from 87 mg/vent day to 12 mg/vent day ($P = .0012$). A team of hospital pharmacists collaborated with the intensivists and nurses to develop a sedation weaning protocol based on the SCCM pain, agitation, and delirium guidelines as a part of the quality improvement bundle.[23] Pharmacists evaluated hemodynamic stability, ventilator settings, and sedative infusion dose and weaned eligible patients from continuous to intermittent therapy given as needed. Neuroleptic agents were added for treatment of delirium in conjunction with measures to prevent delirium. A cohort of 436 patients in medical ICU was compared with historical controls from 6 months prior to the study. The initiative was associated with a reduction in ventilator duration from 5.6 to 4 days ($P = .03$), increased patient mobility, and has sustained the benefits over 1.5 years. Overall cost of care for these patients declined, and the reduction in spending for sedative agents was substantial.

Pharmacists have demonstrated a role in infection control, as previously discussed regarding the French quality improvement bundle, and as related to need for a central line. Pharmacists in a pediatric ICU reviewed their interventions over 11 years, and 79.8% were accepted by the clinical team.[24] Changes in the drug dose regimen and drug selection were most frequent. A focused effort to reduce the use of intravenous antibiotics by converting to oral agents contributed to a reduced utilization of central lines and risk of central line infections. Central line entries per patient decreased from 25.2 in 2007 to 12.4 per 1000 central line days in 2013 ($P = .006$).

Critical care pharmacists regularly implement antimicrobial stewardship plans that are promulgated by the antimicrobial stewardship pharmacists. Antimicrobial stewardship programs have been endorsed by numerous professional organizations as a method to reduce inappropriate utilization and stem the development of resistance. The Center for Disease Control Core Elements suggests the appointment of a pharmacist as the drug expert member within antimicrobial stewardship programs.[25] However, consistent compliance with guidelines by a critical care team member such as the critical care pharmacist is likely needed.

Early administration of antimicrobials is a cornerstone of sepsis therapy and is now recommended during the first hour of sepsis care.[26] Once the order is generated, the pharmacy department must respond promptly to make the medication available. Pharmacists in the emergency department employ strategies such as stocking in an automated dispensing cabinet for rapid availability and administration of the first dose as an intravenous push rather than a slower infusion. An inpatient "code sepsis" program with pharmacist involvement reduced time from sepsis identification to antimicrobial administration from 427 minutes at baseline to 31 minutes for patients in the ICU, and with similar magnitude outside the ICU.[27] The pharmacist role on the sepsis team included antibiotic ordering in 18% of cases, but for most, the pharmacy team facilitated the order verification and medication delivery process. Implementation of this sepsis initiative was associated with a 16% reduction in the adjusted mortality index for sepsis.

MacLaren et al.[28] demonstrated an association between critical care clinical pharmacists and improved clinical and economic outcomes of medicare patients with infections. Within this large billing database, mortality from nosocomial infection in units without a critical care pharmacist was 23.6% higher ($P < .001$, 386 extra deaths) than that with a pharmacist. Mortality was similarly 16.2% and 4.8% higher for community-acquired infection and sepsis, respectively. LOS was longer and medicare billing was approximately 12% higher in units without a critical care pharmacist. This type of big-data analysis does not demonstrate other differences between hospitals, but the magnitude of benefit was consistent between infection types. Specific activities contributing to the benefit are not identified in this type of study; however, as the prior report suggested, the timeliness of antimicrobial delivery and administration in conjunction with optimal antimicrobial stewardship are likely important contributing factors.

Prevention of medication errors is at the core of critical care pharmacist focus. The majority of earlier studies attempting to examine the effectiveness of critical care pharmacists in preventing medication errors did not demonstrate a benefit when those trials were examined in a metaanalysis.[29] However, the metaanalysis did indicate that pharmacists may significantly reduce preventable ADEs and prescribing errors. More recently, a large prospective, multicenter, observational study in 21 ICUs in the United Kingdom reported 3294 critical care pharmacist interventions over 14 days.[30] The clinical impact of the interventions was scored by an investigator in a blinded fashion. Medication error prevention occurred in 42% of the interventions and 19% were designated as high impact and 48.3% moderate impact potential errors. Interventions made by a pharmacy specialist were of a higher impact and more frequent than those made by less experienced pharmacists.[21] More interventions occurred on Monday, indicating a potential benefit of 7-day staffing by a critical care pharmacist.

In a pediatric ICU study, many interventions were identified by the critical care pharmacist for this high-risk population. Participation by the pharmacist during the ordering phase may help to proactively prevent ordering errors. The pediatric ICU pharmacists reported potential prevention of 1056 ADEs.[24] Pharmacists who know the medication treatment plan can more easily detect ordering errors and prevent ADEs. In another report, a critical care pharmacist more effectively identified and prevented ADEs more often than pharmacists involved in order entry and verification, and avoided the potential expenditure of over $210,000 in 4.5 months.[31]

Many other studies that show improvements in the management of infections, anticoagulation therapy, sedation, and analgesia for patients receiving mechanical ventilation and in emergency response help to justify the need for clinical pharmacy services for critically ill patients and are summarized in published reviews.[32–34]

RESEARCH ROLE

Critical care pharmacists have an active role in quality improvement activities and formal research. A pharmacist-managed clinical trials group has recently been incorporated into the SCCM Discovery network, with the hope of larger projects and greater inclusion. On a smaller scale, pharmacists are working with their critical care teams to develop treatment protocols and ensure standardization of care when appropriate. Measurement of the effectiveness of the treatments and appropriate utilization of medications is a standard activity.

AUTHOR'S RECOMMENDATIONS

- Critical care pharmacists are an integral part of the team in a multiprofessional model of ICU practice
- Critical care pharmacists contribute to care via:
  - evaluation of new patients
  - individualization of drug doses through serum concentration monitoring
  - provision of education to other members of the critical care team
  - participation in medical emergencies
  - review of medication ordering and verification
  - evaluation of potential drug interactions
  - adverse event monitoring and evaluation
  - hospital protocol review
  - management of drug shortages
  - development guidelines
- There are limited examples in the literature of the impact and contributions of critical care pharmacists to optimal patient outcomes.

REFERENCES

1. American College of Clinical Pharmacy. Comprehensive Medication Management in Team-Based Care. Available at: www.accp.com/docs/positions/misc/CMM%20Brief.pdf. Accessed November 5, 2018.
2. Benedict N, Hess MM. History and future of critical care pharmacy practice. *Am J Health Syst Pharm.* 2015;72(23):2101-2105.
3. American College of Clinical Pharmacy. The definition of clinical pharmacy. *Pharmacotherapy.* 2008;28(6):816-817.
4. Doherty RB, Crowley RA, Health and Public Policy Committee of the American College of Physicians. Principles supporting dynamic clinical care teams: an American College of Physicians position paper. *Ann Intern Med.* 2013;159(9):620-626.
5. Dietz AS, Pronovost PJ, Mendez-Tellez PA, et al. A systematic review of teamwork in the intensive care unit: what do we know about teamwork, team tasks, and improvement strategies? *J Crit Care.* 2014;29(6):908-914.
6. American Society of Health-System Pharmacists. ASHP Accreditation Standard for Postgraduate Year One (PGY1) Pharmacy Residency Programs. 2016. Available at: www.ashp.org/-/media/assets/professional-development/residencies/docs/pgy1-residency-accreditation-standard-2016.ashx?la=en&hash=9FF7C76962C10562D567F73184FAA45BA7E186CB. Accessed November 5, 2018.
7. American Society of Health-System Pharmacists. Required Competency Areas, Goals, and Objectives for Postgraduate Year Two (PGY2) Critical Care Pharmacy Residencies. 2016. Available at: www.ashp.org/-/media/assets/professional-development/residencies/docs/pgy2-newly-approved-critical-care-pharmacy-2016.ashx?la=en&hash=8861F9DD0BD06308FAA06FABA45E575567738C07A. Accessed November 5, 2018.
8. Board of Pharmacy Specialties. Available at: www.bpsweb.org/. Accessed November 5, 2018.
9. American College of Clinical Pharmacy, McBane SE, Dopp AL, et al. Collaborative drug therapy management and comprehensive medication management—2015. *Pharmacotherapy.* 2015;35(4):e39-e50.
10. Isetts BJ, Brown LM, Schondelmeyer SW, Lenarz LA. Quality assessment of a collaborative approach for decreasing drug-related morbidity and achieving therapeutic goals. *Arch Intern Med.* 2003;163(15):1813-1820.
11. United States Pharmacopeia. General Chapter <797> Pharmaceutical Compounding—Sterile Preparations. 2008. Available at: www.usp.org/compounding/general-chapter-797. Accessed November 5, 2018.
12. Rudis MI, Brandl KM. Position paper on critical care pharmacy services. Society of Critical Care Medicine and American College of Clinical Pharmacy Task Force on Critical Care Pharmacy Services. *Crit Care Med.* 2000;28(11):3746-3750.
13. Competency Development & Evaluation Group. Advanced Level Practice. Available at: http://www.codeg.org/advanced-level-practice/. Accessed November 5, 2018.
14. McKenzie C, Borthwick M, Thacker M, et al. Developing a process for credentialing advanced level practice in the pharmacy profession using a multi-source evaluation tool. *Pharm J.* 2011;286:1-5.
15. LeBlanc JM, Seoane-Vazquez EC, Arbo TC, Dasta JF. International critical care hospital pharmacist activities. *Intensive Care Med.* 2008;34(3):538-542.
16. Jurado LV, Steelman JD. The role of the pharmacist in the intensive care unit. *Crit Care Nurs Q.* 2013;36(4):407-414.
17. Dooley MJ, Allen KM, Doecke CJ, et al. A prospective multicentre study of pharmacist initiated changes to drug therapy and patient management in acute care government funded hospitals. *Br J Clin Pharmacol.* 2004;57(4):513-521.
18. Klopotowska JE, Kuiper R, van Kan HJ, et al. On-ward participation of a hospital pharmacist in a Dutch intensive care unit reduces prescribing errors and related patient harm: an intervention study. *Crit Care.* 2010;14(5):R174.
19. Leguelinel-Blache G, Nguyen TL, Louart B, et al. Impact of quality bundle enforcement by a critical care pharmacist on patient outcome and costs. *Crit Care Med.* 2018;46(2):199-207.
20. Claus BO, Robays H, Decruyenaere J, Annemans L. Expected net benefit of clinical pharmacy in intensive care medicine: a randomized interventional comparative trial with matched before-and-after groups. *J Eval Clin Pract.* 2014;20(6):1172-1179.
21. Rudall N, McKenzie C, Landa J, Bourne RS, Bates I, Shulman R. PROTECTED-UK - Clinical pharmacist interventions in the UK critical care unit: exploration of relationship between intervention, service characteristics and experience level. *Int J Pharm Pract.* 2017;25(4):311-319.
22. Marshall J, Finn CA, Theodore AC. Impact of a clinical pharmacist-enforced intensive care unit sedation protocol on duration of mechanical ventilation and hospital stay. *Crit Care Med.* 2008;36(2):427-433.
23. Louzon P, Jennings H, Ali M, Kraisinger M. Impact of pharmacist management of pain, agitation, and delirium in the intensive care unit through participation in multidisciplinary bundle rounds. *Am J Health Syst Pharm.* 2017;74(4):253-262.
24. Tripathi S, Crabtree HM, Fryer KR, Graner KK, Arteaga GM. Impact of clinical pharmacist on the pediatric intensive care practice: an 11-year tertiary center experience. *J Pediatr Pharmacol Ther.* 2015;20(4):290-298.

25. Centers for Disease Control and Prevention. Antibiotic Prescribing and Use in Hospitals and Long-Term Care. Core Elements of Hospital Antibiotic Stewardship Programs. 2017. Available at: www.cdc.gov/antibiotic-use/healthcare/implementation/core-elements.html. Accessed November 5, 2018.

26. Levy MM, Evans LE, Rhodes A. The Surviving Sepsis Campaign Bundle: 2018 update. *Crit Care Med*. 2018;46(6):997-1000.

27. Beardsley JR, Jones CM, Williamson J, Chou J, Currie-Coyoy M, Jackson T. Pharmacist involvement in a multidisciplinary initiative to reduce sepsis-related mortality. *Am J Health Syst Pharm*. 2016;73(3):143-149.

28. MacLaren R, Bond CA, Martin SJ, Fike D. Clinical and economic outcomes of involving pharmacists in the direct care of critically ill patients with infections. *Crit Care Med*. 2008; 36(12):3184-3189.

29. Wang T, Benedict N, Olsen KM, et al. Effect of critical care pharmacist's intervention on medication errors: a systematic review and meta-analysis of observational studies. *J Crit Care*. 2015;30(5):1101-1106.

30. Shulman R, McKenzie CA, Landa J, et al. Pharmacist's review and outcomes: treatment-enhancing contributions tallied, evaluated, and documented (PROTECTED-UK). *J Crit Care*. 2015;30(4):808-813.

31. Kopp BJ, Mrsan M, Erstad BL, Duby JJ. Cost implications of and potential adverse events prevented by interventions of a critical care pharmacist. *Am J Health Syst Pharm*. 2007;64(23):2483-2487.

32. Preslaski CR, Lat I, MacLaren R, Poston J. Pharmacist contributions as members of the multidisciplinary ICU team. *Chest*. 2013;144(5):1687-1695.

33. Bauer SR, Kane-Gill SL. Outcome assessment of critical care pharmacist services. *Hosp Pharm*. 2016;51(7):507-513.

34. Chant C, Dewhurst NF, Friedrich JO. Do we need a pharmacist in the ICU? *Intensive Care Med*. 2015;41(7):1314-1320.

86

What Is the Role of Advanced Practice Nurses and Physician Assistants in the ICU?

Ruth Kleinpell and W. Robert Grabenkort

It is estimated that more than 5.7 million patients are admitted annually to intensive care units (ICUs) in the United States for intensive or life-sustaining treatments for acute and critical care conditions. Additionally, approximately 20% of acute care admissions are to an ICU and up to 58% of emergency department admissions result in an ICU admission.[1] Research indicates that the demand will create a 35% shortfall of intensivist hours by 2020.[1,2]

One strategy for meeting ICU workforce needs is the addition of advanced practice professionals to ICU teams.[3,4] Advanced practice providers (APPs), including nurse practitioners (NPs) and physician assistants (PAs), are an increasingly important component of the nation's health-care workforce. More than 370,000 (>250,000 NPs and >120,000 PAs) practice in the US health-care system.[5,6] Consistent with the Institute of Medicine's report,[7] NPs and PAs play a vital role in delivering patient care, promoting multiprofessional collaboration, and advancing team approaches to care. These clinicians provide primary, acute, and specialty care services to patients in countless acute and nonacute care settings.

NURSE PRACTITIONER AND PHYSICIAN ASSISTANT ROLES

NPs are registered nurses who are prepared at either the master's or doctoral level, have an independent license, and are required to pass a national certification examination in most states to practice. NPs practice autonomously in most states with a scope of practice that is dependent on education, licensure, certification, and program accreditation. To be in compliance with the National Council of State Boards of Nursing's recommendations for the Advanced Practice Registered Nurse Consensus Model for practice in the ICU setting, NPs should be certified in either acute care or adult gerontology acute care.[8] Similarly, PAs are health-care professionals who are certified by a national examination process. Most PAs are prepared at the graduate level, but some have bachelor's degrees.[6] PAs are state-licensed health-care professionals who practice under the supervision of a sponsoring physician who must be available for consultation by phone or in person.[6]

NPs and PAs often have similar roles in the ICU, but in some settings differences exist. PAs focus on direct medical management or surgical assistance, whereas NP care encompasses direct patient care in addition to continuity of care components such as discharge planning; nursing, patient, and family education; and quality improvement/research, among with other additional duties (Table 86.1).[9-11]

USE OF NURSE PRACTITIONERS AND PHYSICIAN ASSISTANTS IN THE ICU

Data from national surveys on the use of NPs and PAs indicate that utilization in hospital settings has increased because of the higher acuity of hospitalized patients, restrictions placed on medical resident work hours, the need for continuity of care, and workforce shortages.[12] In university-based hospital settings where the new Accreditation Council for Graduate Medical Education duty-hour regulations for physicians in training have been implemented, the integration of NPs and PAs into multidisciplinary provider models represents a solution to the gap in coverage.[12] A study of 25 academic medical centers indicated that an additional role for NP and PA care has resulted from the need for improved access, improved continuity of care, patient throughput, and medical resident training restrictions, among others (Fig. 86.1).[12] Role components of NPs and PAs in the ICU are detailed in Box 86.1.[13]

Several studies have linked improved quality and reduced costs to the participation of NPs and PAs in care (Table 86.2). Because ICU care is often team based, assessing the impact of NPs and PAs in the ICU can be difficult. However, several studies have demonstrated that NP- and PA-provided care resulted in improved outcomes (Box 86.2).[14-26]

On the basis of reports of established and developing models of care with NPs and PAs and research demonstrating their effectiveness, the use of NPs and PAs in the ICU is now a recognized solution to workforce challenges in managing critically ill patients.[27] Integrating NPs and PAs in the ICU can help to facilitate the delivery of high-quality medical care and can provide continuity of care. NPs and PAs can become important elements of multiprovider ICU teams.[28]

TABLE 86.1   NP and PA Role Comparisons.

Category	PA	NP
Definition	Health-care professionals licensed to practice medical care with physician supervision. Currently, the American Academy of Physician Assistants (AAPA) is exploring the Optimal Team Practice model, which does not require the establishment of a specific, sponsoring physician	Registered nurses with advanced education and training who have an independent license
Philosophy/model	Medical/physician model, disease centered, with emphasis on the biological/pathologic aspects of health, assessment, diagnosis, treatment. Practice model is a team approach relationship with physicians	Medical/nursing model, biopsychosocial centered, with emphasis on disease adaptation, health promotion, wellness, and prevention. Practice model is a collaborative relationship with physicians
Education	Affiliated with *medical schools*. Previous health-care experience required; most require entry-level bachelor's degree. The program curriculum is advanced science based. Approximately 2000 clinical hours. All PAs are trained as generalists. Education is procedure and skill oriented with emphasis on diagnosis, treatment, surgical skills, and patient education. Currently, most programs award master's degrees and the remaining programs are currently transitioning to the master's level. Some graduate PAs elect to receive optional, advanced postgraduate specialty training in areas such as critical care medicine	Affiliated with *nursing schools*. BSN is prerequisite and education is at master's or doctoral level; curriculum is biopsychosocial based, based on behavioral, natural, and humanistic sciences. Approximately 750 to 1000 clinical hours. NPs choose a specialty training track in adult, acute care, pediatric, women's health, or gerontology
Certification/licensure	Separate accreditation and certification bodies require successful completion of an accredited program and NCCPA national certification exam	National certification is required in the majority of states
Recertification	Recertification requires 100 hours of CME every 2 years and an exam every 10 years. All PAs are licensed by their State Medical Board and the Medical Practice Act provisions	Recertification requires, on average, 75 CEUs every 5–6 years. NPs are licensed by their State Board of Nursing
Scope of practice	The supervising physician has relatively broad discretion in delegating medical tasks within his/her scope of practice to the PA in accordance with state regulations. Prescriptive privileges vary by sponsoring physician specialty and state regulations. On-site supervision is not required	NP scope of practice is based on licensure, accreditation, certification, and education. NPs have independent practice in the majority of states; some states have physician collaboration requirements. NPs may prescribe controlled substances. On-site supervision is not required
Third-party coverage and reimbursement	PAs are eligible for certification as Medicaid and Medicare providers. Commercial payer reimbursement is currently variable but is being promoted by the AAPA for improved payer consistency	NPs are eligible for certification as Medicaid and Medicare providers and generally receive favorable reimbursement from commercial payers

BSN, bachelor of science in nursing; *CEU*, continuing education unit; *CME*, continuing medical education; *NCCPA*, National Commission on Certification of Physician Assistants; *NP*, nurse practitioner; *PA*, physician assistant.
Adapted from Maryland Academy of Physician Assistants and American Academy of Physician Assistants. www.mdapa.org/maryland/differences.asp.

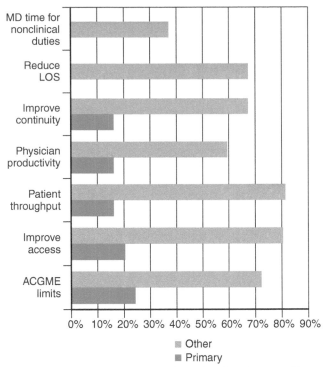

Fig. 86.1 Reasons for Hiring Nurse Practitioners and Physician Assistants as Reported by 25 Academic Medical Centers. *ACGME*, Accreditation Council for Graduate Medical Education; *LOS*, length of stay; *MD*, medical doctor. (Adapted from Moote et al.[11])

BOX 86.1 Roles of NPs and PAs in the ICU.

Patient care management
Rounding
Obtaining history and performing physical examinations
Diagnosing and treating illnesses
Ordering and interpreting tests
Initiating orders, often under protocols
Prescribing and performing diagnostic, pharmacologic, and therapeutic interventions consistent with education, practice, and state regulations
Performing procedures (as credentialed and privileged, such as arterial line insertion, suturing, and chest tube insertion)
Assessing and implementing nutrition
Collaborating and consulting with the interdisciplinary team, patient, and family
Surgical assisting in the operating room
Education of staff, patients, and families

Practice guideline implementation
Lead, monitor, and reinforce practice guidelines for ICU patients (e.g., central line insertion procedures, infection prevention measures, stress ulcer prophylaxis)
Clinical research
Data collection
Enrollment of subjects
Research study management
Quality assurance
Lead quality-assurance initiatives such as ventilator-associated pneumonia bundle, sepsis bundle, rapid response team
Communication
Promote and enhance communication with ICU staff, family members, and the multidisciplinary team
Discharge planning
Transfer and referral consultations
Patient and family education regarding anticipated plan of care

ICU, intensive care unit, *NP*, nurse practitioner, *PA*, physician assistant.
Adapted from Kleinpell RM, Ely EW, Grabenkort R. Nurse practitioners and physician assistants in the intensive care unit: an evidence-based review. *Crit Care Med.* 2008;36(10):2888-2897..

TABLE 86.2 Selected Studies on NP and PA Care in the ICU.

Study	Method/Focus	Main Results
Gershengorn et al., 2011[23]	Retrospective review of 590 daytime admissions to 2 MICUs with use of NPs and PA coverage	No significant difference in hospital mortality, ICU LOS, or hospital LOS. Discharge to a skilled care facility was similar for NP/PA care compared with medical resident care
Gershengorn et al., 2012[14]	Literature review of the use of NP and PA providers in the ICU	NPs and PAs have been used in ICUs as a replacement for physicians in training or to provide on-site semiclosed staffing to care for critically ill patients. Data suggest that use of NPs and PAs is safe and equally efficacious for patient care
Kapu et al., 2014[20]	Evaluation of impact of adding NP to the rapid response team	In 2011, the new teams responded to 898 calls, averaging 31.8 minutes per call. The most frequent diagnoses were respiratory distress (18%), postoperative pain (13%), hypotension (12%), and tachyarrhythmia (10%). The teams facilitated 360 transfers to intensive care and provided 3056 diagnostic and therapeutic interventions. Communication with the primary team was documented on 97% of the calls. After implementation, charge nurses were surveyed, with 96% expressing high satisfaction associated with enhanced service and quality
Kapu et al., 2014[20]	Retrospective, secondary analysis of return on investment after adding NPs to 5 teams	Gross collections compared with expenses for 4 NP-led teams for 2-year time periods were 62%, 36%, 47%, and 32%. Average risk-adjusted LOS for the 5 time periods after adding NPs decreased and charges decreased
Kawar and DiGiovine, 2011[22]	Comparison of clinical outcomes between patients admitted to a resident-run MICU and a PA-run MICU with retrospective analysis of prospectively collected data for 5346 patients admitted to an MICU from January 2004 through January 2007; 3971 patients were admitted to a resident-run MICU (resident group) and 1375 to a PA-run MICU (PA group)	There was no difference in hospital mortality or in ICU mortality between the two groups either in uncontrolled or controlled analyses. Survival analyses showed no difference in 28-day survival between the 2 groups
Landsperger et al., 2016[31]	MICU prospective cohort study of all admissions to an adult medical ICU in an academic, tertiary-care center during a single time period. The primary end point of 90-day survival was compared between patients cared for by ACNP and resident teams using Cox proportional hazards regression. Secondary end points included ICU and hospital mortality and ICU and hospital length of stay	Among 9066 admissions, there was no difference in 90-day survival for patients cared for by ACNP or resident teams (adjusted HR 0.94; 95% CI 0.85–1.04; $P = .21$). Although patients cared for by ACNPs had lower ICU mortality (6.3%) than resident team patients (11.6%; adjusted OR 0.77; 95% CI 0.63–0.94; $P = .01$), hospital mortality was not different (10.0% vs. 15.9%; adjusted OR 0.87; 95% CI 0.73–1.03; $P = .11$). ICU length of stay was similar between the ACNP and resident teams (3.4 ± 3.5 days vs. 3.7 ± 3.9 days [adjusted OR 1.01; 95% CI 0.93–1.1; $P = .81$]), but hospital length of stay was shorter for patients cared for by ACNPs (7.9 ± 11.2 days) than for resident patients (9.1 ± 11.2 days) (adjusted OR 0.87; 95% CI 0.80–0.95; $P = .001$)
McMillen et al., 2012[32]	Surgical ICU care for 13,020 patients by PA team in 12-bed stepdown unit	Annual surgical mortality decreased and surgical volume increased

Continued

TABLE 86.2   Selected Studies on NP and PA Care in the ICU.—cont'd

Study	Method/Focus	Main Results
Sirleaf et al., 2014[24]	Comparison of procedures by NPs, PAs, and MDs for 1404 patients	MDs performed 1020 procedures, with 21 complications (complication rate 2%). NP/PAs completed 555 procedures; with 11 complications (complication rate 2%). There was no difference in the mean ICU and hospital LOS. Mortality rates were also comparable between the 2 groups (MD 11% vs. NP/PA 9.7%)
Sise et al., 2011[33]	Prospective analysis of adding NPs to a level 1 trauma center. Analysis of demographics, injury severity scores, LOS, complications, total direct costs of care, and outcomes	After addition of NPs, a decrease in complications by 28.4%, LOS by 36.2, and costs of care by 30.4%

CI, confidence interval; *HR,* hazard ratio; *ICU,* intensive care unit; *LOS,* length of stay; *MD,* medical doctor; *MICU,* medical intensive care unit; *NP,* nurse practitioner; *OR,* odds ratio; *PA,* physician assistant; *UTI,* urinary tract infection.

BOX 86.2   NP- and PA-Performed Tasks That Enhance the Quality of Care.[15–26]

Reduced length of stay
Reduced rates of urinary tract infections
Reduced rates of skin breakdown
Reduced time to bladder catheter removal
Reduced time to mobilization
Reduced duration of mechanical ventilation
Increased compliance with clinical practice guidelines
Reduced rates of reintubation
Increased time in coordination of care activities and cost-effective care
Increased patient and family satisfaction

NP, nurse practitioner; *PA,* physician assistant.

CONCLUSIONS

NPs and PAs are increasingly being integrated into ICUs. Care provided by teams that include NPs and PAs has been demonstrated to be comparable to that provided in other staffing models.[29,30] Increasing patient acuity levels, burgeoning requirements for ICU care, and a need to have ICU-trained clinicians provide for critically ill patients presents an important opportunity to integrate NPs and PAs as ICU care providers. Continued dissemination of successful ICU staffing models integrating NPs and PAs as well as additional research on ICU staffing models that include NPs and PAs are needed to identify best strategies for promoting optimal care for critically ill patients.

AUTHORS' RECOMMENDATIONS

- ICU models of care that incorporate NPs and PAs should be disseminated through publications and presentations to promote replication and extension.
- Additional research that demonstrates the effect of NP and PA care for ICU patients is needed.
- Funding should be allocated for research that explores optimal ICU workforce and staffing models that include NPs and PAs.

REFERENCES

1. Society of Critical Care Medicine. Critical Care Statistics. 2018. Available at: http://www.sccm.org/Communications/Critical-Care-Statistics. Accessed November 5, 2018.
2. The Leapfrog Group. Hospital Survey. Factsheet: ICU Physician Staffing. April 2018. Available at: http://www.leapfrog-group.org/sites/default/files/Files/2018%20IPS%20Fact%20Sheet.pdf Accessed November 5, 2018.
3. Pastores SM, O'Connor MF, Kleinpell RM, et al. The Accreditation Council for Graduate Medical Education resident duty hour new standards: history, changes, and impact on staffing of intensive care units. *Crit Care Med.* 2011;39:2540-2549.
4. Ward NS, Afessa B, Kleinpell R, et al. Intensivist/patient ratios in closed ICUs: a statement from the Society of Critical Care Medicine Taskforce on ICU Staffing. *Crit Care Med.* 2013; 41:638-645.
5. American Association of Nurse Practitioners. *NP Fact Sheet.* August 2018. Available at: http://www.aanp.org/all-about-nps/np-fact-sheet. Accessed November 5, 2018.
6. American Academy of Physician Assistants. What is a PA? Available at: https://www.aapa.org/what-is-a-pa/. Accessed November 5, 2018.
7. Institute of Medicine. *The Future of Nursing: Leading Change, Advancing Health.* Washington, DC: National Academies Press; 2010:638-645.
8. National Council of State Boards of Nursing. *APRN Consensus Model.* Chicago, IL: NCSBN; 2008.
9. Kleinpell R, Cook ML, Padden DL. American Association of Nurse Practitioners National Nurse Practitioner sample survey: update on acute care nurse practitioner practice. *J Am Assoc Nurse Pract.* 2018;30(3):140-149.
10. Kleinpell RM, Boyle WA III, Buchman TG, eds. *Integrating Nurse Practitioners and Physician Assistants into the ICU: Strategies for Optimizing Contributions to Care.* Mount Prospect, IL: Society of Critical Care Medicine; 2012.
11. Moote M, Krsek C, Kleinpell R, Todd B. Physician assistant and nurse practitioner utilization in academic medical centers. *Am J Med Qual.* 2011;26(6):452-460.
12. Curren J. Nurse practitioners and physician assistants: do you know the difference? *Medsurg Nurs.* 2007;16(6):404-407.
13. Kleinpell RM, Ely EW, Grabenkort R. Nurse practitioners and physician assistants in the intensive care unit: an evidence-based review. *Crit Care Med.* 2008;36(10):2888-2897.

14. Gershengorn HB, Johnson MP, Factor P. The use of nonphysician providers in adult intensive care units. *Am J Respir Crit Care Med.* 2012;185(6):600-605.

15. Scherzer R, Dennis MP, Swan BA, Kavuru MS, Oxman DA. A comparison of usage and outcomes between nurse practitioner and resident-staffed medical ICUs. *Crit Care Med.* 2017;45(2): e132-e137.

16. Joffe AM, Pastores SM, Maerz LL, Mathur P, Lisco SJ. Utilization and impact on fellowship training of non-physician advanced practice providers in intensive care units of academic medical centers: a survey of critical care program directors. *J Crit Care.* 2014;29(1):112-115.

17. Gracias VH, Sicoutris CP, Stawicki SP, et al. Critical care nurse practitioners improve compliance with clinical practice guidelines in "semiclosed" surgical intensive care unit. *J Nurs Care Qual.* 2008;23(4):338-344.

18. Johal J, Dodd A. Physician extenders on surgical services: a systematic review. *Can J Surg.* 2017;60(3):172-178.

19. Woo BFY, Lee JXY, Tam WWS. The impact of the advanced practice nursing role on quality of care, clinical outcomes, patient satisfaction, and cost in the emergency and critical care settings: a systematic review. *Hum Resour Health.* 2017;15(1):63.

20. Kapu AN, Kleinpell R, Pilon B. Quality and financial impact of adding nurse practitioners to inpatient care teams. *J Nurs Adm.* 2014;44(2):87-96.

21. Paton A, Stein DE, D'Agostino R, Pastores SM, Halpern NA. Critical care medicine advanced practice provider model at a comprehensive cancer center: successes and challenges. *Am J Crit Care.* 2013;22(5):439-443.

22. Kawar E, DiGiovine B. MICU care delivered by PAs versus residents: do PAs measure up? *JAAPA.* 2011;24(1):36-41.

23. Gershengorn HB, Wunsch H, Wahab R, et al. Impact of nonphysician staffing on outcomes in a medical ICU. *Chest.* 2011;139(6):1347-1353.

24. Sirleaf M, Jefferson B, Christmas AB, Sing RF, Thomason MH, Huynh TT. Comparison of procedural complications between resident physicians and advanced clinical providers. *J Trauma Acute Care Surg.* 2014;77(1):143-147.

25. Barocas DA, Kulahalli CS, Ehrenfeld JM, et al. Benchmarking the use of a rapid response team by surgical services at a tertiary care hospital. *J Am Coll Surg.* 2014;218(1):66-72.

26. Kapu AN, Wheeler AP, Lee B. Addition of acute care nurse practitioners to medical and surgical rapid response teams: a pilot project. *Crit Care Nurse.* 2014;34(1):51-59.

27. Perlmutter L, Nataraja S. *Developing the Sustainable Critical Care Team.* Washington, DC: Advisory Board Company Physician Executive Council; 2012.

28. McCarthy C, O'Rourke NC, Madison JM. Integrating advanced practice providers into medical critical care teams. *Chest.* 2013;143(3):847-850.

29. Garland A, Gershengorn HB. Staffing in ICUs: physicians and alternative staffing models. *Chest.* 2013;143(1):214-221.

30. Adams EK, Markowitz S. Improving efficiency in the healthcare system: removing anticompetitive barriers for advanced practice registered nurses and physician assistants. Brookings Institute, Policy Proposal 2018-08. 2018.

31. Landsperger JS, Semler MW, Wang L, Byrne DW, Wheeler AP. Outcomes of Nurse Practitioner-Delivered Critical Care: A Prospective Cohort Study. *Chest.* 2016 May;149(5):1146-54.

32. McMillen MA, Boucher N, Keith D, Gould DS, Gave A, Hoffman D. Maintaining quality of care 24/7 in a nontrauma surgical intensive care unit. *J Trauma Acute Care Surg.* 2012 Jul;73(1):202-8.

33. Sise CB, Sise MJ, Kelley DM, Walker SB, Calvo RY, Shackford SR, Lome BR, Sack DI, Osler TM. Resource commitment to improve outcomes and increase value at a level I trauma center. *J Trauma.* 2011 Mar;70(3):560-8.

87

Do the Guidelines for Brain Death Determination Need to Be Revised?

Ariane Lewis and Sam D. Shemie

INTRODUCTION

Since the first description of death based on loss of function of the brain in 1959 by Mollaret and Goulon, guidelines for determination of death by neurologic criteria have been utilized around the world.[1-3] Recently, there have been a number of lawsuits in Canada, the United Kingdom, and the United States challenging the validity of these guidelines and contending that death should only be declared using the traditional cardiopulmonary criteria.[4-10] In light of this, we examine the question of whether current guidelines for brain death determination are sufficient, or if revisions are required. We argue that use of neurologic criteria to declare death is sound practice, but (1) guidelines are not universally accepted worldwide, (2) procedural and conceptual variability exists, and (3) in some cases, implementation is oversimplified. Therefore, to advance worldwide conformity in the determination of the death process, guideline revisions are necessary.

HISTORY OF GUIDELINES FOR DETERMINATION OF BRAIN DEATH AND PROFESSIONAL SOCIETY ENDORSEMENT

The first guidelines on brain death determination were written by an ad hoc committee at Harvard Medical School and published in 1968 in the *Journal of the American Medical Association*.[11] Multiple institutions around the United States, including the National Institutes of Health, University of Minnesota, United States Navy, University of Pennsylvania, and University of Pittsburgh, followed Harvard's example and created their own guidelines to declare brain death.[12] By 1978, there were over 30 different criteria for brain death determination.[13] In 1987, in the interest of providing guidance to their members about determination of brain death in children, the American Academy of Neurology (AAN), American Academy of Pediatrics (AAP), American Neurological Association (ANA), and Child Neurology Society (CNS) endorsed guidelines published by the Task Force for Determination of Brain Death in Children.[14] When these

guidelines were updated in 2011 by AAP, CNS, and the Society of Critical Care Medicine (SCCM), their value was affirmed by AAN and was endorsed by AAP, American Association of Critical Care Nurses, CNS, National Association of Pediatric Nurse Practitioners, SCCM, Society for Pediatric Anesthesia, Society for Pediatric Neuroradiology, and World Federation of Pediatric Intensive and Critical Care Societies.[15] Similarly, guidelines for determination of brain death in adults were published by AAN in 1995 and updated in 2010. These were endorsed by the American College of Radiology (ACR), CNS, Neurocritical Care Society (NCS), and the Radiological Society of North America.[16,17] In a 2018 publication on contemporary concerns about brain death determination in the United States, the aforementioned 2010 adult guidelines and 2011 pediatric guidelines were acknowledged as the accepted criteria for determination of brain death by AAN, AAP, American College of Chest Physicians, ACR, ANA, American Society of Neuroradiology, CNS, and NCS.[18]

While these guidelines for determination of brain death were being created and endorsed by multiple organizations in the United States, medical societies around the world were writing their own guidelines.[2] For example, the Academy of Medical Royal Colleges, Australian and New Zealand Intensive Care Society, Canadian Neurocritical Care Group, and the World Health Organization have all published their own guidelines for determination of brain death.[19-22] In fact, a 2002 review of 80 countries found that 88% had guidelines for brain death determination and a 2015 survey found that 77% of 91 countries had guidelines for determination of brain death.[2,3] Many of these guidelines are based on the 1995 AAN guidelines for brain death determination.[23]

CONTENTS OF GUIDELINES FOR DETERMINATION OF BRAIN DEATH

At a minimum, guidelines for determination of brain death provide information about prerequisites for determination of brain death, including exclusion of confounders, and procedures to conduct: (1) the clinical examination to confirm a person is in a coma and has brainstem areflexia, (2) apnea testing, and (3) nonclinical diagnostic testing. Some guidelines also include instructions on the observation time prior to a brain death evaluation, the number of examinations required, inter-examination observation time, qualifications for examiners, and documentation of brain death.[3,15,17,19–22]

RATIONALE BEHIND GUIDELINES FOR DETERMINATION OF BRAIN DEATH

Guidelines are necessary in order to ensure that brain death determinations are consistently performed in the same manner and that death is only declared in the setting of catastrophic irreversible loss of brain function. The process for determining brain death may be nuanced. Guidelines instruct examiners how to perform an accurate examination so as to avoid any risk of diagnostic errors and false-positive determinations of death.

PROBLEMS WITH GUIDELINES FOR DETERMINATION OF BRAIN DEATH

Guidelines for determination of brain death are imperfect: they are not universally present and, where they are in place, they may be overly simplistic and subject to both procedural and conceptual variability. Indeed, there is certainly no international consensus on the criteria for brain death determination, and variability exists even in individual countries. This is the result of inconsistencies between criteria published by different medical societies, in different hospital protocols, and in procedures used by different practitioners. Practice variability is most prone to lead to false-positive determinations of brain death in regions without guidelines, in hospitals with guidelines that differ from local medical society guidelines, and in situations in which practitioner procedure deviates from hospital and/or medical society guidelines.

Failure to Achieve Ubiquity

Although there are guidelines for determination of brain death in most countries, they do not exist everywhere.[2,3] A 2015 worldwide survey of international members of the NCS, country representatives from the World Federation of Neurology, corresponding authors from relevant clinical publications identified through a literature search and personal contacts of the authors found that many countries did not have brain death guidelines.[2] Some of these findings have been disputed.[2,3,23,24] Nonetheless, the 2015 survey highlights the fact that use of formal brain death criteria is far from universal, especially in low-income nations and in countries without organ transplant networks, perhaps reflecting insufficient expertise and/or lack of technology.[2] Conversely, Waweru-Siika et al.[25] noted that the lack of brain death policies in Sub-Saharan Africa also reflected a complex cultural, ethnic, religious, and political landscape that often precluded the creation of brain death guidelines. Despite these barriers, the authors noted that policy and legislative initiatives to develop brain death guidelines in the region are needed to (1) limit futile treatment,

(2) avoid prolonging family suffering, (3) standardize clinical practice, and (4) ensure appropriate resource allocation.

Procedural Variability

Brain death determination guidelines are universally rooted in the 1968 Harvard criteria. As such, they require an established etiology for brain injury, exclusion of confounding conditions, and demonstration that a person is comatose, has brainstem areflexia and is unable to breathe spontaneously.[11] However, comparisons of regional, national, and international brain death guidelines demonstrate that protocols are not universally consistent (Tables 87.1 and 87.2).[2,3,26–29]

Two studies, one in 2002 and one in 2015, assessed procedural variability worldwide.[2,3] In 2002, Wijdicks[3] reviewed protocols from 70 countries around the world and found variability that included (1) the length of the observation period before brain death evaluation (0–24 hours), (2) the number of physicians whose opinion was required (1–4), (3) the necessity to perform apnea testing (86% of 70 guidelines), (4) the inclusion of a $PaCO_2$ target to be used during apnea testing (59% of 70 guidelines), and (5) the requirement for ancillary testing (40% of 70 guidelines). Similarly, Wahlster et al.'s 2015 international survey reported multiple significant deviations from the AAN guidelines in 53% of respondents from 91 countries.[2] Only slightly more than half of respondents reported use of specific criteria for brain death determination in children. The observation time before brain death determination ranged from 0 to 26 hours. The number of physicians required to participate in a brain death determination ranged from 1 to 3. The components of the clinical evaluation were also dissimilar: 96% required absence of corneal reflexes and pupillary light responses; 92% required absence of oculovestibular reflexes; 90% required absence of oculocephalic reflexes; 87% required absence of gag and cough reflexes; 77% required absence of purposeful responses; 75% required pupils to be midposition or dilated; 74% required absence of grimace to stimulation; and 23% required absence of spinal reflexes. Although 93% of 70 guidelines required apnea testing, there was marked variation in the protocol to perform apnea testing. Lastly, the use of nonclinical diagnostic testing when determining brain death, i.e., ancillary testing (diagnostic testing used as an alternative test to one that cannot be conducted), supplemental testing (diagnostic testing used in addition to an already conducted test), or confirmatory testing (diagnostic testing to confirm a previously conducted test) and the testing modality (an assessment of brain activity vs. an assessment of brain blood flow) varied; 29% of the 70 guidelines required diagnostic testing (28% required an electroencephalogram, 6% required catheter-based angiography, 5% required transcranial Dopplers, 4% required a nuclear medicine scan; and 4% required computed tomographic angiography).

These findings are concordant with regional studies in Europe and Asia.[26–28] Citerio et al.[26,27] found that while 25/28 European countries have guidelines for brain death determination, the protocols vary based on the (1) requirement for established etiology for neurologic injury; (2) inclusion of prerequisites for normal temperature, acid–base status, blood pressure, electrolytes, and endocrine status; (3) number of

TABLE 87.1 Variability in Brain Death Guidelines.

Guideline Component	Region Variability was Identified
Examinations/Examiners	
Number of examinations	Asia, Europe, United States, worldwide[2,26–30]
Number of apnea tests	Worldwide[2]
Number of examiners	Asia, Europe, worldwide[2,3,26–28]
Observation time prior to examination	Worldwide[2,3,30]
Observation time between examinations	Asia, Europe, United States[26,28–30]
Prerequisites	
Establishment of etiology for neurologic injury	Europe, United States[26,29,30]
Confirmation of normal acid–base status	Europe, United States[26,29]
Confirmation of normal blood pressure	Europe, United States[26,29]
Confirmation of normal electrolytes	Europe, United States[26,29]
Confirmation of normal endocrine status	Europe, United States[26,29]
Confirmation of normal temperature	Europe, United States[26,29,30]
Confirmation of absence of sedatives	United States[29]
Confirmation of absence of paralytics	United States[29]
Clinical Examination	
Absence of grimace to stimulation on examination	United States, worldwide[2,29]
Absence of response to pain on the cranium on examination	United States[29]
Absence of purposeful response on examination	United States, worldwide[2,29]
Absence of pupillary response on examination	United States, worldwide[2,29]
Absence of oculocephalic reflex on examination	United States, worldwide[2,29]
Absence of vestibulo-ocular reflex on examination	United States, worldwide[2,29]
Absence of corneal reflex on examination	United States, worldwide[2,29]
Absence of gag reflex on examination	United States, worldwide[2,29]
Absence of cough reflex on examination	United States, worldwide[2,29]
Absence of spinal reflexes on examination	Worldwide[2]
Apnea Testing	
Apnea testing requirement	United States, worldwide[2,3,29,30]
Apnea testing technique	United States, worldwide[2,3,29]
Minimum duration for apnea testing	Worldwide[2]
Requirement for an arterial line during apnea testing	Worldwide[2]
Apnea testing threshold	Asia, United States, worldwide[2,3,28,29]
Ancillary Testing	
Ancillary testing requirement	Asia, Europe, United States, worldwide[2,3,26–29]
Electroencephalogram requirement	Worldwide[2]
Transcranial Doppler requirement	Worldwide[2]
Nuclear medicine scan requirement	Worldwide[2]
Catheter-based angiography requirement	Worldwide[2]
Computed tomographic angiography requirement	Worldwide[2]

examinations required (1–3); (4) number of doctors required (1–4); (5) minimum observation time between clinical examinations (0–12 hours); and (6) necessity to perform ancillary testing (11/25 countries). Similarly, Chua et al.[28] found that while 12/14 countries in Asia have guidelines for determination of brain death, the protocols vary based on the (1) need to perform serial examinations (11/12 countries); (2) time between examinations (0–48 hours); (3) number of personnel needed for certification (2–6); (4) apnea testing threshold (>50 mm Hg to >60 mm Hg); and (5) necessity to perform nonclinical diagnostic testing (4/12 countries).

In addition to these studies that demonstrate international variability in brain death guidelines, Greer et al.[29] and Hornby et al.[30] found that institutional guidelines within an

TABLE 87.2 Brain Death by the Numbers.

Requirement	Numbers
Number of age groups specified[29]	1–6 groups
Observation period before brain death determination[2,3,30]	0–26 hours
Number of practitioners[2,3,26,28]	1–6 physicians
Number of clinical examinations[3,26,29]	1–5 examinations
Time between clinical examinations[26,28–30]	0–48 hours
Number of apnea tests[2,3,17,19,20]	0–2 tests
Minimum systolic blood pressure[17,19,20]	90–100 mm Hg
Minimum temperature[15,17,19,20,29,73,74]	33–36°C
Minimum $PaCO_2$ target after apnea test[28]	50–60 mm Hg
Maximum pH after apnea test[20,32]	7.28–7.4
Number of ancillary tests[2]	0–1 tests

individual country (the United States and Canada, respectively) were inconsistent and did not routinely reflect local medical society guidelines.

After reviewing 492 institutional guidelines, Greer et al.[29] reported variability in (1) examiner qualifications, (2) number of examiners, (3) number of examinations, (4) time between examinations, (5) identification of a clear etiology for loss of neurologic function, (6) requirement of a minimum temperature of 36°C, (7) requirement of absence of sedatives and paralytics, (8) requirement of absence of confounding medical conditions (acid–base, endocrine, electrolyte disorders), (9) requirement of absence of hypotension, (10) clinical examination components, (11) apnea testing requirements and procedures including the need for preoxygenation, a baseline arterial blood gas, abortion of the test if the person is unstable, and a $PaCO_2$ target of ≥60 or 20 mm Hg above baseline, and (12) the need for nonclinical diagnostic testing (mandatory in 7% protocols).

Hornby et al.[30] reviewed brain death guidelines from 37 centers in Canada and found that they did not consistently: (1) indicate that there must be an established cause for loss of neurologic function (92% of protocols); (2) provide a minimum core temperature (81% of protocols); (3) include tests to assess all brainstem reflexes (73% of protocols); (4) require apnea testing (89% of protocols); and (5) stipulate an observation period before a brain death examination (14% of protocols).

Brevity

Although some guidelines are extensive and detailed (the Academy of Medical Royal Colleges guidelines are 42 pages long), others are relatively terse.[20] Key components of the process of excluding confounders, performing the neurologic evaluation, and completing apnea testing are ignored in some guidelines.[2,3,26,27,29] Basic information, such as notation of the number of physicians required to perform an evaluation, is not provided in all guidelines.[26] Some protocols address brain

death determination in complex situations, such as for a person who is missing an eye or an ear, while others do not.[17,19]

Two challenging situations that are often excluded from brain death guidelines are determination of brain death in persons on extracorporeal membrane oxygenation (ECMO) and determination of brain death in persons who were treated with therapeutic hypothermia.[17,19,20,31,32] Use of ECMO has expanded in recent years, but, unfortunately, 62–73% of people placed on ECMO die—and 18–28% are declared dead by neurologic criteria.[33–36] Apnea testing in patients on ECMO is more complex than apnea testing in other populations.[33,37] However, there are reports in the literature of effective and safe approaches to apnea testing on ECMO. While German guidelines do not allow brain death determination to be made for a patient on ECMO unless an apnea test is performed, formal recommendations for determination of brain death in persons on ECMO are not routinely included in all brain death guidelines.[37,38]

Just as the use of ECMO has become more common in the past decade, there has been an upsurge in the use of therapeutic hypothermia after two seminal trials in 2002 demonstrated improved morbidity and mortality in persons with cardiac arrest who were cooled.[39–41] However, despite use of therapeutic hypothermia, patients can progress to brain death.[42–44] Determination of brain death after therapeutic hypothermia can be challenging because hypothermia transiently leads to depression of central nervous system function. Additionally, hypothermia alters pharmacokinetics and pharmacodynamics; so the depression of function is prolonged in patients treated with consciousness-altering drugs prior to, or concomitant with, cooling.[45–49] The potential effects of therapeutic hypothermia on the neurologic examination are noted in some guidelines, but few provide clear instructions about the length of recovery time required following rewarming.[17,19,20] The importance of including the need to delay brain death determination after therapeutic hypothermia in brain death guidelines is illustrated by two cases advertised in the literature as being demonstrative of "reversible brain death;" both cases were ultimately discredited and serve as evidence that recent therapeutic hypothermia and sedative use can lead to premature brain death determination.[45–48,50] Research is required to establish evidence-based guidance on determination of brain death after hypothermia.

Conceptual Variability

In addition to procedural variability, there is international conceptual variability about the specific anatomical parts of the brain that must have absence of function for death by neurologic criteria to be declared. Most of the world embraces the "whole brain" perspective to define death using neurologic criteria. Based on this view, death by neurologic criteria requires complete loss of function of the entire brain, including the brainstem. However, in some countries such as India, Singapore, Taiwan, and the United Kingdom, the definition of death by neurologic criteria is based purely on loss of function of the brainstem.[51] The impact of this ideological variability is most notable when considering people who have primary brainstem pathology and appear to have loss of consciousness based on interruption of the ascending reticular activating system. In this situation, a clinical evaluation might suggest a person is dead based on both brainstem and whole brain criteria. However, determining whole brain criteria in the setting of primary brainstem pathology is not straightforward because supratentorial blood flow and cortical activity can persist despite catastrophic damage to the brainstem.[52–54] Varying philosophies about the definition of death by neurologic criteria could, therefore, result in a person being considered dead by neurologic criteria using brainstem criteria, but alive if the whole brain perspective is embraced.

Conceptual variability also exists because religious acceptance of the use of neurologic criteria to declare death is not pervasive. Although brain death is accepted in most religions, individual religious perspectives on death can vary even within a common religious faith.[55] Religious dissent played a role both in preventing the creation of brain death guidelines in Sub-Saharan Africa and in challenging the validity of the guidelines in Canada, the United Kingdom, and the United States.[4–10,25] Due to varying religious perspectives on the use of neurologic criteria to declare death, religious exemption legislation exists in some jurisdictions, including four states in the United States.[56–59] However, allowing individuals to legally accept or reject use of neurologic criteria to declare death based on religious beliefs can damage the credibility of the entire concept of brain death.

ATTACKS ON THE INTEGRITY OF GUIDELINES FOR DETERMINATION OF BRAIN DEATH

In addition to attacks on the integrity of brain death guidelines due to protocol variation, inconsistent practice, and religious/philosophical dissonance, attacks have been made in the general media, medical literature, and the legal system based on (1) reports of recovery after brain death, (2) the fact that there can be a lengthy delay between brain death determination and cardiopulmonary arrest if somatic support is provided, and (3) the contention that guidelines do not appropriately assess for complete loss of brain function because some hormonal function can persist despite determination of brain death[4–10,46,50,60–63]

When the 2010 AAN guidelines for determination of brain death in adults were written, a review of the literature from 1996 to 2009 failed to identify cases of neurologic recovery when the 1995 AAN guidelines were appropriately applied.[17] Since then, the integrity of guidelines for determination of brain death has been questioned in (1) general media headlines touting "recovery from brain death" due to inappropriate use of the term "brain death" when the term "coma" was more appropriate or when determination did not adhere to the guidelines, and in (2) the aforementioned case reports detailing brain death determination after therapeutic hypothermia that described the determination as being "reversible."[46,50,64–66]

Additionally, a 2015 lawsuit, the case of Jahi McMath, addressed the possibility of recovery of function after brain death.[7] In this case, two physicians argued that during the 4.5-year period between the time US criteria for brain death in children were originally met and the time she had a cardiac arrest, Jahi regained neurologic function.[67,68] Notably, neither of these neurologists based their conclusion on a clinical examination; one physician's findings were based on a review of an electroencephalogram that he believed was not isoelectric and a magnetic resonance angiogram that he believed demonstrated slow intracranial blood flow, while the other's findings were based on a review of videotapes that he reported to show movements in response to commands; interestingly, the second physician disagreed with the first's interpretation of both the electroencephalogram and the magnetic resonance angiogram.[67] While the opinions of these neurologists are provocative, in the absence of an unbiased evaluation to determine whether or not the patient regained function, this case does not suggest that brain death determination guidelines need to be altered.

The McMath case does, however, illustrate the uncertainty that may arise when provision of somatic support leads to the passage of a substantial period of time between brain death determination and cardiopulmonary arrest.[7] Similar findings have been reported in some meta-analyses.[69,70] The fact that the heart can continue beating with the provision of somatic support after brain death determination has caused some to question the integrity of brain death as death.[69,71]

Lastly, some philosophers and physicians have berated brain death guidelines for not requiring hormonal derangements (such as diabetes insipidus).[62,72] Diabetes insipidus may not exist due to the extradural blood supply of the posterior pituitary gland. Thus, while some protocols note that diabetes insipidus is common in brain death, they also indicate that absence of diabetes insipidus does not preclude such a determination.[17,19,20]

AUTHORS' RECOMMENDATIONS

- In the interest of maintaining public trust and ensuring that determinations of death are only made in the setting of irreversible catastrophic brain injury, it is the responsibility of the medical profession to respond to recent lawsuits about the use of neurologic criteria to declare death by critically reviewing brain death determination guidelines.
- Use of neurologic criteria to declare death is sound practice, but guidelines need to be homogenized worldwide.
- The distinction between death and life must be absolute, and the process for making this determination needs to be the same for every doctor, in every hospital, in every country, both within and across borders.
- Guidelines for the determination of brain death must be impervious and they must be adeptly utilized universally.
- Conceptual and procedural variability in the number of examinations/examiners, prerequisites, clinical examination, apnea testing, and ancillary testing for determination of brain death should be eliminated.
- Guidelines should address complex situations like brain death determination after therapeutic hypothermia or brain death determination on ECMO.

REFERENCES

1. Mollaret P, Goulon M. Le coma depasse. *Rev Neurol (Paris)*. 1959;101:3-15.

2. Wahlster S, Wijdicks E, Patel P, et al. Brain death declaration: practices and perceptions worldwide. *Neurology*. 2015;84(18):1870-1879.

3. Wijdicks EFM. Brain death worldwide: accepted fact but no global consensus in diagnostic criteria. *Neurology*. 2002;58: 20-25.

4. Re: A (A Child). 2015:EWHC 443 (Fam).

5. *In Re: Mirranda Grace Lawson.*, CL16-2358, City of Richmond Circuit Court (2016).

6. *In Re: Allen Callaway.*, DG-16-08 (2016).

7. *Jahi McMath and Nailah Winkfield vs. State of California, County of Alameda, Alameda County Department of Public Health, Muntu Davis, MD, MPH, Alameda County Coroner and Medical Examiner, Alameda County Counsel, David Nefouse, Scott Dickey, Alameda County.*, 3:15-CV-06042 (2015).

8. *In Re: Guardianship of Hailu.*, 361 P.3d 5 (2015).

9. *McKitty v. Hayani.*, CV-17-4125, Ontario Superior Court of Justice (2017).

10. *Shalom Ouanounou v. Humber River Hospital, Ali Ghafouri, Garret Pulle, Sanjay Manocha, Dr. David Giddons, Coroner, and Office of the Chief Coroner.*, CV-17-585553, Ontario Superior Court of Justice (2017).

11. A definition of irreversible coma. Report of the Ad Hoc Committee of the Harvard Medical School to Examine the Definition of Brain Death. *JAMA*. 1968;205(6):337-340.

12. Powner DJ, Snyder JV, Grenvik A. Brain death certification. A review. *Crit Care Med*. 1977;5(5):230-233.

13. Black PM. Brain death (second of two parts). *N Engl J Med*. 1978;299(8):393-401.

14. American Academy of Pediatrics Task Force on Brain Death in Children. Guidelines for the determination of brain death in children. *Pediatrics*. 1987;80(2):298-300.

15. Nakagawa TA, Ashwal S, Mathur M, Mysore M, Committee for Determination of Brain Death in Infants and Children. Guidelines for the determination of brain death in infants and children: an Update of the 1987 Task Force Recommendations—Executive Summary. *Ann Neurol*. 2012;71(4):573-585.

16. Wijdicks EFM. Determining brain death in adults. *Neurology*. 1995;45(5):1003-1011.

17. Wijdicks EFM, Varelas PN, Gronseth GS, Greer DM. Evidence-based guideline update: determining brain death in adults: report of the Quality Standards Subcommittee of the American Academy of Neurology. *Neurology*. 2010;74(23):1911-1918.

18. Lewis A, Bernat JL, Blosser S, et al. An interdisciplinary response to contemporary concerns about brain death determination. *Neurology*. 2018;90(9):423-426.

19. Australian and New Zealand Intensive Care Society. The Anzics Statement on Death and Organ Donation. 2013;3.2. Available at: https://www.anzics.com.au/wp-content/uploads/2018/08/ANZICS_Statement_on_Death_and_Organ_Donation_Edition_3.2.pdf.

20. Academy of Medical Royal Colleges. A code of practice for the diagnosis and confirmation of death. 2010. Available at: https://www.aomrc.org.uk/reports-guidance/ukdec-reports-and-guidance/code-practice-diagnosis-confirmation-death/.

21. Shemie SD, Hornby L, Baker A, et al. International guideline development for the determination of death. *Intensive Care Med*. 2014;40(6):788-797.

22. Guidelines for the diagnosis of brain death. Canadian Neuro-critical Care Group. *Can J Neurol Sci*. 1999;26(1):64-66.

23. Ding ZY, Zhang Q, Wu JW, Yang ZH, Zhao XQ. A comparison of brain death criteria between China and the United States. *Chin Med J (Engl)*. 2015;128(21):2896-2901.

24. Natori Y. Legal determination of brain death. *Japan Med Assoc J*. 2011;54(6):363-367.

25. Waweru-Siika W, Clement ME, Lukoko L, et al. Brain death determination: the imperative for policy and legal initiatives in Sub-Saharan Africa. *Glob Public Health*. 2017;12(5):589-600.

26. Citerio G, Crippa IA, Bronco A, Vargiolu A, Smith M. Variability in brain death determination in Europe: looking for a solution. *Neurocrit Care*. 2014;21(3):376-382.

27. Citerio G, Murphy PG. Brain death: the European perspective. *Semin Neurol*. 2015;35(2):139-144.

28. Chua HC, Kwek TK, Morihara H, Gao D. Brain death: the Asian perspective. *Semin Neurol*. 2015;35(2):152-161.

29. Greer DM, Wang HH, Robinson JD, Varelas PN, Henderson G V, Wijdicks EFM. Variability of brain death policies in the United States. *JAMA Neurol*. 2016;73(2):213-218.

30. Hornby K, Shemie SD, Teitelbaum J, Doig C. Variability in hospital-based brain death guidelines in Canada. *Can J Anaesth*. 2006;53(6):613-619.

31. Kreitler K, Cavarocchi N, Hirose H, et al. Declaring a patient brain dead on extracorporeal membrane oxygenation (ECMO): are there guidelines or misconceptions? *Am J Transpl*. 2015;15:A224.

32. Teitelbaum J, Shemi SD. Neurologic determination of death. *Neurol Clin*. 2011;29(4):787-799.

33. Saucha W, Solek-Pastuszka J, Bohatyrewicz R, Knapik P. Apnea test in the determination of brain death in patients treated with extracorporeal membrane oxygenation (ECMO). *Anaesthesiol Intensive Ther*. 2015;47(4):368-371.

34. Mao J, Paul S, Sedrakyan A. The evolving use of ECMO: the impact of the CESAR trial. *Int J Surg*. 2016;35:95-99.

35. Thiagarajan RR, Brogan TV, Scheurer MA, Laussen PC, Rycus PT, Bratton SL. Extracorporeal membrane oxygenation to support cardiopulmonary resuscitation in adults. *Ann Thorac Surg*. 2009;87(3):778-785.

36. Barrett CS, Bratton SL, Salvin JW, Laussen PC, Rycus PT, Thiagarajan RR. Neurological injury after extracorporeal membrane oxygenation use to aid pediatric cardiopulmonary resuscitation. *Pediatr Crit Care Med*. 2009;10(4):445-451.

37. Hoskote SS, Fugate JE, Wijdicks EFM. Performance of an apnea test for brain death determination in a patient receiving venoarterial extracorporeal membrane oxygenation. *J Cardiothorac Vasc Anesth*. 2014;28(4):1027-1029.

38. Winter S, Groesdonk HV, Beiderlinden M. [Apnea test for assessment of brain death under extracorporeal life support.] *Med Klin Intensivmed Notfmed*. 2019;114(1):15-20.

39. Hypothermia after Cardiac Arrest Study Group. Mild therapeutic hypothermia to improve the neurologic outcome after cardiac arrest. *N Engl J Med*. 2002;346(8):549-556.

40. Bernard SA, Gray TW, Buist MD, et al. Treatment of comatose survivors of out-of-hospital cardiac arrest with induced hypothermia. *N Engl J Med*. 2002;346(8):557-563.

41. Cariou A, Payen JF, Asehnoune K, et al. Targeted temperature management in the ICU: guidelines from a French expert panel. *Anaesth Crit Care Pain Med*. 2018;37(5):481-491.

42. Fugate JE, Wijdicks EFM, White RD, Rabinstein AA. Does therapeutic hypothermia affect time to awakening in cardiac arrest survivors? *Neurology*. 2011;77(14):1346-1350.

43. Moler FW, Hutchison JS, Nadkarni VM, et al. Targeted temperature management after pediatric cardiac arrest due to drowning: outcomes and complications. *Pediatr Crit Care Med.* 2016;17(8):712-720.

44. Mulder M, Gibbs HG, Smith SW, et al. Awakening and withdrawal of life-sustaining treatment in cardiac arrest survivors treated with therapeutic hypothermia. *Crit Care Med.* 2014;42(12):2493-2499.

45. Shemie SD, Langevin S, Farrell C. Therapeutic hypothermia after cardiac arrest: another confounding factor in brain-death testing. *Pediatr Neurol.* 2010;42(4):304.

46. Webb AC, Samuels OB. Reversible brain death after cardiopulmonary arrest and induced hypothermia. *Crit Care Med.* 2011;39(6):1538-1542.

47. Streat S. 'Reversible brain death'—Is it true, confounded, or 'not proven'? *Crit Care Med.* 2011;39(6):1601-1603.

48. Wijdicks EFM, Varelas PN, Gronseth GS, Greer DM. There is no reversible brain death. *Crit Care Med.* 2011;39(9):2204-2205.

49. Anderson KB, Poloyac SM, Kochanek PM, Empey PE. Effect of hypothermia and targeted temperature management on drug disposition and response following cardiac arrest: a comprehensive review of preclinical and clinical investigations. *Ther Hypothermia Temp Manag.* 2016;6(4):169-179.

50. Joffe AR, Kolski H, Duff J, deCaen AR. A 10-month-old infant with reversible findings of brain death. *Pediatr Neurol.* 2009;41(5):378-382.

51. Wijdicks EF. The transatlantic divide over brain death determination and the debate. *Brain.* 2012;135(Pt 4):1321-1331.

52. Ferbert A, Buchner H, Ringelstein EB, Hacke W. Isolated brain-stem death. Case report with demonstration of preserved visual evoked potentials (VEPs). *Electroencephalogr Clin Neurophysiol.* 1986;65(2):157-160.

53. De Groot Y, Bakker J, Epker J, Van Der Hoven B, Kompanje E. Brain death determination in patients with acute basilar artery occlusion; some pitfalls: a case series. *Intensive Care Med.* 2011;37:S72.

54. Varelas PN, Brady P, Rehman M, et al. Primary posterior fossa lesions and preserved supratentorial cerebral blood flow: implications for brain death determination. *Neurocrit Care.* 2017;27(3):407-414.

55. Setta SM, Shemie SD. An explanation and analysis of how world religions formulate their ethical decisions on withdrawing treatment and determining death. *Philos Ethics, Humanit Med.* 2015;10(1):1-22.

56. *Ca. Health & Saf. Code §1254.4.*

57. NJ Sharing Network. New Jersey Brain Death Statute. 2014. Available at: http://www.njsharingnetwork.org/file/Brain-Death-Guidelines-July-27-2014sq-2.pdf. Accessed March 23, 2015.

58. New York State Department of Health. New York State Guidelines for Determining Brain Death. 2011. Available at: http://www.health.ny.gov/professionals/hospital_administrator/letters/2011/brain_death_guidelines.htm. Accessed September 13, 2018.

59. *210 Ill. Comp. Stat. §85/6.24.*

60. Choong KA, Rady MY. Re A (A Child) and the United Kingdom Code of Practice for the Diagnosis and Confirmation of Death: Should a secular construct of death override religious values in a pluralistic society? *HEC Forum.* 2018;30(1):71-89.

61. Yanke G, Rady MY, Verheijde JL. When brain death belies belief. *J Relig Health.* 2016;55(6):2199-2213.

62. *McMath vs. California.*, No. 3:15-06042 N.D. Cal. (2015).

63. Shah SK, Truog RD, Miller FG. Death and legal fictions. *J Med Ethics.* 2011;37(12):719-722.

64. Chuck E. Taylor Hale, teen whose "brain had turned to mush," set to graduate high school. NBC News. Available at: https://www.nbcnews.com/news/us-news/teen-whose-brain-had-turned-mush-set-graduate-high-school-n359506. Published May 17, 2015. Accessed September 13, 2018.

65. Wang Y. A father's desperate—but dangerous—strategy to keep his 'brain dead' son on life support. The *Washington Post.* https://www.washingtonpost.com/news/morning-mix/wp/2015/12/23/texas-man-says-he-went-to-jail-for-swat-standoff-that-saved-sons-life/?noredirect=on&utm_term=.cc0f60b32e9a. Published December 23, 2015. Accessed September 13, 2018.

66. Morales N. "Dead" man recovering after ATV accident. NBC News. http://www.nbcnews.com/id/23768436/ns/dateline_nbc-newsmakers/t/dead-man-recovering-after-atv-accident/#.WUqxlJLytGF. Published March 23, 2008. Accessed September 13, 2018.

67. Lewis A. Reconciling the case of Jahi McMath. *Neurocrit Care.* 2018;29(1):20-22.

68. Goldschmidt D. Jahi McMath, California teen at center of brain-death controversy, has died. CNN.com. https://www.cnn.com/2018/06/29/health/jahi-mcmath-brain-dead-teen-death/index.html. Published June 29, 2018. Accessed September 13, 2018.

69. Shewmon DA. Chronic "brain death": meta-analysis and conceptual consequences. *Neurology.* 1998;51(6):1538-1545.

70. Powner DJ, Bernstein IM. Extended somatic support for pregnant women after brain death. *Crit Care Med.* 2003;31(4):1241-1249.

71. President's Council on Bioethics. *Controversies in the Determination of Death: A White Paper by the President's Council on Bioethics.* Washington D.C.; 2008.

72. Nair-Collins M, Northrup J, Olcese J. Hypothalamic–pituitary function in brain death. *J Intensive Care Med.* 2016;31(1):41-50.

73. Cronberg T, Brizzi M, Liedholm LJ, et al. Neurological prognostication after cardiac arrest-Recommendations from the Swedish Resuscitation Council. *Resuscitation.* 2013;84(7):867-872.

74. Sampson BG, Datson LD, Bihari S. Use of imaging studies for determination of brain death in South Australian intensive care units. *Crit Care Resusc.* 2017;19(1):57-63.

88

How Do I Diagnose, Treat, and Reduce Delirium in the Intensive Care Unit?

Christina Boncyk, E. Wesley Ely, and Pratik Pandharipande

Delirium is a ubiquitous problem that affects intensive care unit (ICU) patients. When properly assessed, the diagnosis can be made in up to 80% of adult ICU patients and in up to 50% of critically ill children. However, delirium is regularly underdiagnosed in practice.[1–5] Given the impact of delirium on longer durations of mechanical ventilation and ICU length of stay as well as an increased risk of death, disability, and long-term cognitive dysfunction, recognition and diagnosis remain crucial for both treatment and prognostication.[5–11] The impact of delirium on patients, families, healthcare providers, and society is likely to increase as the population ages, with elderly patients carrying an increased burden of diagnoses, and age remaining a strong independent risk factor for delirium, though it must be noted that critically ill preschool infants and children also carry a significant risk for delirium.[2,6]

This chapter aims to broadly define delirium, discuss the associated subtypes and risk factors, and provide the basis for clinicians to develop strategies aimed at preventing and treating delirium in their practice settings.

DEFINITION

The *Diagnostic and Statistical Manual of Mental Disorders* 5th edition (*DSM-5*)[12] defines delirium as (1) a disturbance of consciousness (i.e., reduced clarity of awareness of the environment) with reduced ability to focus, sustain, or shift attention. (2) A change in cognition (e.g., memory deficit, disorientation, language disturbance) or development of a perceptual disturbance that is not better accounted for by a preexisting, established, or evolving dementia. (3) The disturbance develops over a short period (usually hours to days) and tends to fluctuate during the course of the day. (4) There is evidence from the history, physical examination, or laboratory findings that the disturbance is caused by a direct physiologic consequence of a general medical condition, an intoxicating substance, medication use, or more than one cause.

Delirium has been further differentiated according to the level of alertness; the motoric subtypes consist of hyperactive, hypoactive, and mixed subtypes.[13] The hypoactive subtype is characterized by a flat affect, withdrawal, apathy, or lethargy.

The hyperactive delirious patient is described as agitated, restless, violent, or emotionally labile. Mixed delirium carries fluctuating components of both hypoactive and hyperactive delirium. Distribution of delirium in medical and surgical ICU patients suggests that the hypoactive subtype is by far the most prominent, accounting for over 60% of delirious patients, depending on ICU and study population analyzed.[6,13–16] This is followed by the mixed subtype, which accounts for approximately 30% of all delirious patients, whereas purely hyperactive patients consistently account for less than 10% of delirious patients. Although arguably the most challenging to manage clinically, the weight of evidence suggests that not only does the pure hyperactive subtype account for the vast minority of delirious patients, but that it might also carry a better overall prognosis when compared with purely hypoactive patients. The Delirium Motor Subtype Scale may aid in distinguishing these diagnoses. Identification may better facilitate both patient management and research efforts.[17]

Another commonly observed form of brain organ dysfunction is subsyndromal delirium. Subsyndromal delirium is essentially the intermediate state between normal mentation and DSM-5 delirium diagnosis.[18] It is most simply described as a less severe form of delirium that fulfills some, but not all, DSM-IV criteria. It does, however, carry more adverse outcomes than if a patient were to remain at normal baseline mentation (i.e., increased ICU and hospital length of stay, lower cognitive and functional outcomes), but has less severe long-term repercussions than a full delirium diagnosis.[19,20]

RISK FACTORS

The causes of delirium are multifactorial. The risk factors can be divided into predisposing factors (i.e., host factors) and precipitating factors (Table 88.1). Patients in the hospital at a higher risk for having delirium include those with dementia, chronic illness, advanced age, existing infection, and depression. Modifiable risk factors such as hypertension, poor nutrition, substance withdrawal, and tobacco use have also been shown to be associated with development of delirium in the hospital. Iatrogenic or

TABLE 88.1 Risk Factors for Delirium.

Host Factors	Acute Illness	Iatrogenic and Environmental Factors
Age 65 years or older	Acidosis	Immobilization
Male sex	Anemia	Medications (e.g., opioids, benzodiazepines)
Alcoholism	Fever, infection, sepsis	Anticholinergic drugs
Apolipoprotein E4 polymorphism	Hypotension	Alcohol or drug withdrawal
Cognitive impairment	Metabolic disturbances (e.g., sodium, calcium, blood urea nitrogen, bilirubin, albumin)	Sleep disturbances
Dementia	Respiratory disease	—
Chronic obstructive pulmonary disease	—	—
History of delirium	—	—
Depression	—	—
Hypertension	—	—
Smoking	—	—
Vision or hearing impairment	—	—

potentially modifiable factors include hypoxia, metabolic and electrolyte disturbances, infection, dehydration, hyperthermia, sepsis, psychoactive medications, and sleep deprivation.[5,6,21–23] The role of statins in delirium has also been explored, especially in those undergoing cardiopulmonary bypass, with a retrospective study showing a decreased incidence of delirium in patients pretreated with statins.[24] ICU statin use has been associated with reduced delirium, especially early during sepsis, whereas the discontinuation of a previously used statin was associated with increased delirium.[25–27] However, randomized controlled trials (RCTs) of statin vs. no statin have been unable to demonstrate any reduction in delirium outcomes with the use of statins.[28,29] Benzodiazepine use has also been associated with an increased incidence of delirium in adults and children.[6,30–32] Sedation-related delirium has recently been studied. A small subset of patients (about 10%) may experience rapidly reversible delirium on discontinuing sedation, and those patients do not experience worse outcomes.[33] However, the majority of sedation-related delirium persists and is associated with undesirable outcomes, including long-term cognitive impairment.[34]

Cardiac surgery without cardiopulmonary bypass appears to confer an advantage in decreasing delirium in some studies, suggesting that electrolyte or metabolic disturbances play a role in the development of delirium; however, these are not consistent findings.[35]

PATHOGENESIS

The pathogenesis of delirium is complex and still poorly understood. The different mechanisms proposed are "complementary, rather than mutually exclusive."[20] Imbalance or derangement of multiple neurotransmitter systems has been implicated in the pathophysiology of delirium.

Neuroinflammatory Hypothesis

Inflammatory mediators such as cytokines and chemokines are readily expressed in critical illness, trauma, sepsis, and after surgical interventions. Animal studies have demonstrated that the release of endogenous inflammatory mediators correlates with exaggerated cognitive and motor symptoms[36] and increased vascular permeability in the brain.[37] The neuroinflammatory hypothesis postulates that delirium is a central nervous system (CNS) manifestation of the body's proinflammatory state during illness. Peripheral inflammation can lead to neuronal inflammation, especially affecting the microglia, which might manifest as delirium.[38] Cholinergic inhibition may limit this, except in patients with neurodegenerative disease, older age, on anticholinergic medications. These individuals may have primed microglia and, as a result, overactive neuroinflammation that leads to severe delirium and cognitive impairment. Studies have shown that sepsis and septic shock are characterized by significantly elevated C-reactive protein (CRP), S-100β, and cortisol in those patients with delirium compared with those without delirium.[39–41] Cerebral autoregulation is disturbed and inflammation may impede endothelial function of the cerebral vasculature, thus making the blood–brain barrier more permeable to inflammatory insults. In support of this theory, a prospective study of 147 ICU patients revealed endothelial dysfunction to be associated with a greater duration of delirium.[42] In another study, higher levels of procalcitonin at ICU admission were associated with a prolonged duration of brain dysfunction, and higher levels of CRP showed trends toward an association.[43] This proinflammatory state at the time of delirium could further be an indicator of a baseline neuroregulatory dysfunction. Baseline decreases in antiinflammatory mediators are overwhelmed by proinflammatory cytokines following stress, resulting in increased risk for brain dysfunction or delirium presentation.[44] In addition, inflammation upregulates γ-aminobutyric acid $(GABA)_A$ receptors in the brain, contributing to the inhibitory tone within the brain and reducing brain synaptic connectivity.[45] Thus, the iatrogenic administration of GABA-ergic medications such as benzodiazepines probably further contributes to the inhibition of neural pathways and increases the risk of delirium.

Cholinergic Deficiency Hypothesis

Impaired oxidative metabolism in the brain results in a cholinergic deficiency. The finding that hypoxia impairs acetylcholine synthesis further supports this hypothesis. The reduction in cholinergic function results in an increase in the levels of glutamate, dopamine, and norepinephrine in the brain and possibly neuroinflammation, as described earlier. Serotonin and GABA are also reduced, possibly contributing to delirium.[46,47] Furthermore, increased serum levels of acetylcholinesterase enzyme have been shown to be associated with hypoactive delirium—the causality of which remains unclear.[48]

Monoamine Axis Hypothesis

Dopamine, norepinephrine, and serotonin have been implicated in acute brain dysfunction in the ICU. Dopamine is thought to increase the excitability of neurons, and acetylcholine and GABA decrease neuronal excitability.[49] Norepinephrine activity has been associated with hyperactive delirium, and the elevated norepinephrine levels seen after traumatic brain injury have been associated with poor neurologic status, decreased survival, and longer hospital length of stay.[50]

Serotonin

Elevated serotonin levels have been associated with impaired learning and memory and may be indirectly involved in the pathogenesis of acute brain dysfunction.[46] Higher levels of tryptophan, linked to increased formation of serotonin and melatonin in the brain, may lead to hypoactive delirium. Elevated levels of the serotonin metabolite 5-hydroxyindoleacetic acid (5-HIAA) in the cerebrospinal fluid (CSF) have also been associated with hyperactive delirium.[51] This finding supports the notion that increased serotoninergic neurotransmission plays a role in the pathophysiology.

Amino Acid Hypothesis

Amino acid entry into the brain is regulated by a sodium-independent large neutral amino acid transporter type-1. Increased cerebral uptake of tryptophan and phenylalanine, compared with that of other large neutral amino acids, can lead to elevated levels of dopamine and norepinephrine, two neurotransmitters that have been implicated in the pathogenesis of delirium.[52–54] Although tryptophan has been postulated to play a role in delirium, a major pathway for its metabolism also exists via the kynurenine pathway. Activation of this pathway in the presence of inflammation may produce neurotoxic metabolites, which may predispose patients to delirium.[55]

Impaired Oxidative Metabolism

Oxygen deprivation in the brain through either hypoxia or hypoperfusion has been implicated in delirium. Engel and Romano[56] described delirium as a state of "cerebral insufficiency" as early as 1959, when they showed that delirium was accompanied by diffuse slowing on electroencephalogram, suggesting a reduction in brain metabolism. This hypothesis may be further accentuated in the patient who already has compromised blood flow secondary to vascular dementia. Decreases in oxidative metabolism, as well as acetylcholine release, have been demonstrated in the aging brain,[57] and preexisting cognitive dysfunction in the elderly patient, suggestive of chronic changes from vascular insufficiency, has been shown to be the most significant predictor of the development of delirium in the postoperative period.[58] The mechanism involves insufficient oxidative metabolism required for adenosine triphosphatase pump systems to maintain ionic gradients, which leads to abnormal neurotransmitter release, free radial production, and decrease in cortical synaptic depolarization.[20]

RECOGNITION OF DELIRIUM

Early recognition of delirium is important, if only to avoid lengthening its course through iatrogenic exacerbation: therefore, clinicians must use assessment tools that allow for timely, accurate assessment by a broad range of practitioners in various settings. Recognition becomes additionally difficult in the ICU setting because patients may have altered sensorium secondary to sedation administered for procedures, pain, or mechanical ventilation. Therefore, assessment of a patient for delirium becomes a two-step process. It is important for the clinician to first establish the current level of arousal and sedation before assessing the patient for delirium. Examples of scales that can be used to assess sedation include the Ramsay Sedation Scale,[59] the Riker Sedation-Agitation Scale,[60] and the Richmond Agitation-Sedation Scale (RASS).[61,62]

Once the level of sedation has been established and the patient is responsive to verbal stimulus, it is then appropriate for the clinician to assess for the presence of delirium. Although there have been multiple instruments validated for use in non-ICU patients, only two are validated for diagnosing delirium in mechanically ventilated adults patients: the Intensive Care Delirium Screening Checklist (ICDSC)[63] and the Confusion Assessment Method for the ICU (CAM-ICU). The CAM-ICU is a scale that is based on the Confusion Assessment Method[64,65] but that has been amended to increase its applicability in the ICU setting. It takes a trained ICU nurse approximately 2 minutes to complete the CAM-ICU, and accuracy over a set of 471 paired observations in the ICU setting has resulted in an accuracy rate of 98.4% with excellent inter-rater reliability.[64] It has been validated in multiple ICU settings.[66] Recently, the CAM-ICU-7 Delirium Severity Scale has been shown to be reliable and valid in a multicenter study of over 500 ICU patients.[67]

A combination of the RASS for assessment of sedation (Fig. 88.1), followed by the CAM-ICU (Fig. 88.2) or the ICDSC (Table 88.2) can be used for the establishment of delirium in ICU patients. The diagnosis of delirium using the CAM-ICU (after establishing a RASS score of –3 or less) requires (1) acute

STEP 1: Assess sedation (RASS)

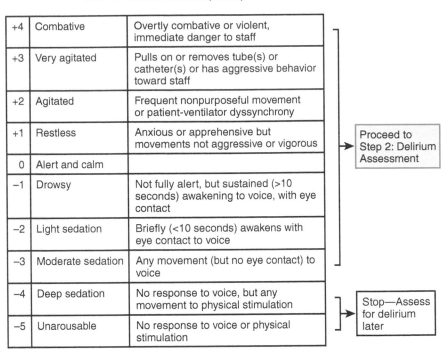

+4	Combative	Overtly combative or violent, immediate danger to staff
+3	Very agitated	Pulls on or removes tube(s) or catheter(s) or has aggressive behavior toward staff
+2	Agitated	Frequent nonpurposeful movement or patient-ventilator dyssynchrony
+1	Restless	Anxious or apprehensive but movements not aggressive or vigorous
0	Alert and calm	
−1	Drowsy	Not fully alert, but sustained (>10 seconds) awakening to voice, with eye contact
−2	Light sedation	Briefly (<10 seconds) awakens with eye contact to voice
−3	Moderate sedation	Any movement (but no eye contact) to voice
−4	Deep sedation	No response to voice, but any movement to physical stimulation
−5	Unarousable	No response to voice or physical stimulation

(+1 through −3 → Proceed to Step 2: Delirium Assessment)
(−4 and −5 → Stop—Assess for delirium later)

Fig. 88.1 Richmond Agitation-Sedation Scale (*RASS*),[61,62] which is used to determine the level of sedation.

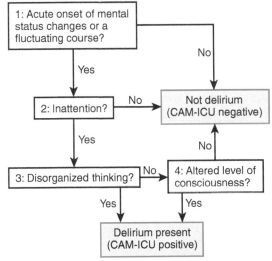

Fig. 88.2 Confusion Assessment Method for the Intensive Care Unit (*CAM-ICU*), which is used to determine the presence or absence of delirium after the level of sedation has been assessed. (From Ely E, Inouye S, Bernard G, et al. Delirium in mechanically ventilated patients: validity and reliability of the confusion assessment method for the intensive care unit (CAM-ICU). *JAMA*. 2001;286(21):2703-2710.

change or fluctuation in mental status (feature 1), *and* (2) inattention (feature 2), *and* (3) one of the following: (a) disorganized thinking (feature 3) *or* (b) altered level of consciousness (feature 4). Only those patients with a RASS score of −3 and higher are alert enough to respond to the test and thus can be assessed for delirium. For diagnosis of delirium with the ICDSC, patients who score at least 4 points are considered to have delirium. Subsyndromal delirium is diagnosed with

ICDSC scores ranging from 1 to 3.[19] While not the focus of this chapter, readers should be aware that there are delirium tools to monitor for delirium in critically ill children, which include the Pediatric CAM-ICU (pCAM-ICU),[68] the Preschool CAM-ICU (psCAM-ICU),[69] and the Cornell Assessment for Pediatric Delirium (CAP-D).[70]

Some studies have questioned whether delirium evaluations should be done while patients are receiving sedation.[33,71] As mentioned earlier, a small subset of patients (~10%) may have rapidly reversible sedation-related delirium.[33] Thus, when feasible, delirium evaluation should also be done after the interruption of sedation; however, delirium evaluations should not be forgone just because a patient is on sedation, as the omission would be far worse than overdiagnosing delirium in a handful of patients.

PRIMARY PREVENTION

The prevention of delirium in the ICU requires constant reassessment of patients' clinical courses and treatments. Several potential pathophysiologic contributors to delirium have been previously outlined. All have endpoints associated with cellular mechanisms, suggesting that avoiding metabolic derangements, including electrolyte abnormalities, hypoglycemia, hypoxia, dehydration, and hyperthermia, are paramount in the prevention of delirium. By far the easiest way to treat delirium is to prevent it from happening in the first place.

Medications, particularly benzodiazepines, have long been implicated in the development of delirium, either because of their side effects or their direct effects on the CNS. The number

TABLE 88.2 Intensive Care Delirium Screening Checklist.

Patient Evaluation

Altered level of consciousness (A–E)	Deep sedation/coma over entire shift [SAS = 1, 2; RASS = –4, –5] = Not assessable Agitation [SAS = 5, 6, or 7; RASS = 1–4] at any point = 1 point Normal wakefulness [SAS = 4; RASS = 0] over the entire shift = 0 points Light sedation [SAS = 3; RASS = –1, –2, –3]: = 1 point (if no recent sedatives) = 0 points (if recent sedatives)
Inattention	Difficulty in following a conversation or instructions. Easily distracted by external stimuli. Difficulty in shifting focuses. Any of these scores 1 point
Disorientation	Any obvious mistake in time, place, or person scores 1 point
Hallucinations–delusion–psychosis	The unequivocal clinical manifestation of hallucination or of behavior probably due to hallucination or delusion. Gross impairment in reality testing. Any of these scores 1 point
Psychomotor agitation or retardation	Hyperactivity requiring the use of additional sedative drugs or restraints to control potential danger to oneself or others. Hypoactivity or clinically noticeable psychomotor slowing
Inappropriate speech or mood	Inappropriate, disorganized, or incoherent speech. Inappropriate display of emotion related to events or situation. Any of these scores 1 point
Sleep/wake cycle disturbance	Sleeping less than 4 hours or waking frequently at night (do not consider wakefulness initiated by medical staff or loud environment). Sleeping during most of the day. Any of these scores 1 point
Symptom fluctuation	Fluctuation of the manifestation of any item or symptom over 24 hours scores 1 point
Total score (0–8)	

of medications administered[21] and their psychoactive effects[72] are suggestive of precipitating delirium.

Another major risk factor for delirium is alteration of the sleep cycle. Disruption of the sleep–wake cycle in the ICU may be necessary to continuously monitor and manage the critically ill patient. However, the toll on the patient may be high. Multiple studies have shown that sleep disruption has detrimental effects on cognition and memory even in the healthy, non-ICU patient.[73] Circadian rhythmicity is a key feature in multiple cellular processes responsible for wakefulness, hemodynamic or blood pressure variations, neurotransmitter systems, modulatory hormones, and cellular signal pathways that play significant roles in management, at the cellular level, to oxidative stressors.[20] Maintaining a sleep–wake cycle whenever possible through nonpharmacologic or pharmacologic means may help prevent delirium.[74]

There has been some debate about whether the "protocolization" of patient care may reduce the incidence of delirium. In a study that included 852 general medical patients older than 70 years, standardized geriatrician-led protocols were developed for six risk factors of delirium: cognitive impairment, sleep deprivation, immobility, visual impairment, hearing impairment, and dehydration. Using these protocols resulted in a 40% reduction in the initial development of delirium in the intervention patients (95 vs. 16%).[75] When these patients were assessed after 6 months for 10 outcomes, including items such as functional status, cognitive status, delirium, and rehospitalization, only incontinence was slightly less common in the intervention group.[76]

Patients in the ICU frequently receive continuous intravenous analgesics and sedatives. Accumulation in individual patients can predispose to a withdrawal syndrome on

discontinuation. Because substance-induced delirium is one of the etiologies recognized by the *DSM-5*, it is no surprise that analgesic and sedative polypharmacy contribute significantly; hence, strategies to reduce exposure to psychoactive medications need to be implemented.[77]

Benzodiazepines are known to increase the risk of delirium in a dose-dependent manner.[31,32] Many studies have shown that protocolized target-based sedation and daily spontaneous awakening trials reduce the number of days on mechanical ventilation. This also exposes the patient to lower cumulative doses of sedatives.[78,79]

For the improvement of patient outcome and recovery, a liberation and animation strategy focusing on the ABCDEFs (Assessing and treating pain, Both Awakening and Breathing Trials, Choice of appropriate sedation, Delirium monitoring and management, Early mobility and Exercise, and Family Engagement) has been proposed (http://www.sccm.org/ICULiberation/ABCDEF-Bundles) and compliance with this regimen has been shown to be associated with improved survival, decreased incidence of delirium and coma, and improvement in other patient outcomes.[80,81]

Studies have also shown that daily interruption of mechanical ventilation is superior to other varied approaches to ventilator weaning, and reduces the total time on mechanical ventilation.[82] The Awakening and Breathing controlled trial[83] combined the spontaneous awakening trial with the spontaneous breathing trial. This combination was associated with shorter duration of mechanical ventilation, a 4-day reduction in hospital length of stay, a remarkable 32% decrease in risk of dying at 1 year, with no long-term neuropsychological consequences of waking patients during critical illness.[84] Although delirium duration was not decreased, coma duration was reduced. Thus, more patients in the intervention group qualified for delirium evaluation as compared with the control group, where they were more likely to be in a state of coma: thus, ineligible for delirium evaluation.

Numerous studies have confirmed that benzodiazepines are associated with poor clinical outcomes.[1,32,85] Two studies comparing dexmedetomidine (alpha-2 agonist) with benzodiazepine infusions showed that the former reduced the burden of brain dysfunction.[86–88] Furthermore, there is a suggestion that the use of prophylactic dexmedetomidine following both cardiac and noncardiac surgery is preventive in the development of delirium in both intubated and nonintubated patients.[89,90] The mechanism is probably multifactorial, but it could include a decrease in administration of opioids due to analgesic and potentially opioid-sparing properties, improved pain scores, better quality of sleep, lack of anticholinergic effects, and/or association in decreased inflammatory biomarkers.[90,91] Studies comparing propofol with dexmedetomidine for ICU sedation have reported similar delirium rates,[92] although delirium was assessed days after patients were weaned off either sedative.

The need for larger safety and efficacy investigations into pharmacologic prevention studies is warranted. At this time, however, there are no recommendations for any prophylactic pharmacologic delirium protocol. This specifically includes the use of dexmedetomidine, cholinesterase inhibitors, and systemic corticosteroids. Cholinesterase inhibitors should not be used to prevent or treat delirium, as their use has been shown in a hypothesis-driven RCT to be associated with an increased duration of delirium as well as an elevated mortality risk.[93,94] The data on systemic corticosteroids have been mixed. Results in large patient cohorts show conflicting results—from an association between administration and transition from a nondelirious to a delirious state in medical and surgical patients[95–97] to a potential benefit in septic patients.[98] Further research into patient populations, potentially separating out glucocorticoid and mineralocorticoid activity, may clarify matters in the future. At the present time, the use of corticosteroids appears to offer no benefits, but also no major risks, pertaining to the development of delirium. The only prevention practice currently recommended is early mobility. Morris et al.[99] showed that early initiation of physical therapy in ICU patients was associated with decreased length of ICU and hospital polypharmacy. Schweickert et al.[100] looked at the efficacy of combining daily interruption of sedation with physical and occupational therapy on patient outcomes. Patients in the intervention arm had better functional outcomes at discharge, and early physical therapy was also associated with a 50% decrease in the duration of delirium in ICU and hospital stay. Needham et al.[101] conducted a quality improvement project with the use of a multidisciplinary team that focused on reducing sedation use. The authors reported that benzodiazepine use decreased and the patients had improved sedation and delirium status. A decrease in ICU and hospital length of stay was also noted.

We have included an empirical protocol (Fig. 88.3) that we use to treat delirium in ICU settings that is based on the current Society of Critical Care Medicine (SCCM) Clinical Practice Guidelines. It is merely an example of such a protocol, and the use of a similar protocol should be updated with current data and designed to be implemented specifically at an individual institution. The choice of particular antipsychotics is not described because there are limited data guiding such recommendations.

PHARMACOLOGIC INTERVENTION

Although antidelirium medications in either the preventive or treatment stage are appealing, there are currently none available that have the ability to alter the outcome of delirium. Before administering new psychotropic medications to the delirious patient, one must rule out all reversible causes that may either be the underlying etiology of the delirium or that may be exacerbating the current situation. Reversible causes that could precipitate or exacerbate delirium include hypoxia, hypercarbia, hypoglycemia, metabolic derangements, infection, or shock. Once a decision is made to use antipsychotic medications (typical or atypical), these medications should be individualized (and minimized) to avoid associated adverse events. Discontinuation plans should also be established, as antipsychotics initiated within the ICU are frequently inappropriately continued at hospital discharge and could pose long-term risks to patients continued on these medications.[102]

Recommendations for delirium treatment strategies suggest that dexmedetomidine may be a better treatment choice than a benzodiazepine. Specifically, for those patients with agitated delirium preventing liberation from mechanical ventilation, the addition of dexmedetomidine resulted in more ventilator-free hours compared with standard care or placebo, alone.[103]

Haloperidol is frequently used in the ICU for delirium. It may be given at an initial intravenous dose of 2–5 mg (0.5–2 mg in the elderly) and then repeated every 6 hours. The HOPE-ICU (HalOPeridol Effectiveness in ICU delirium) trial did not demonstrate that treatment with haloperidol was beneficial. The drug may still be considered for acute agitation (hyperactive delirium)[104] but haloperidol must be used with caution because it has a number of adverse side effects. These include dystonias, neuroleptic malignant syndrome, extrapyramidal effects, and, the most worrisome, torsades de pointes. Haloperidol should not be given to patients with electrocardiographic evidence of prolonged QT interval. Daily QT interval measurements are recommended when haloperidol is initiated.

Any of the atypical antipsychotic medications (olanzapine, risperidone, quetiapine, ziprasidone) may be considered for the treatment of delirium in the ICU, although data on their efficacy are sparse. In a small, 36-patient RCT, quetiapine was shown to be more efficacious in resolution of the first episode of delirium compared with placebo. Likewise, single-dose risperidone has been shown to reduce delirium in cardiac ICU patients.[105] These drugs also need to be used with caution and discontinued if high fever, QT prolongation, or

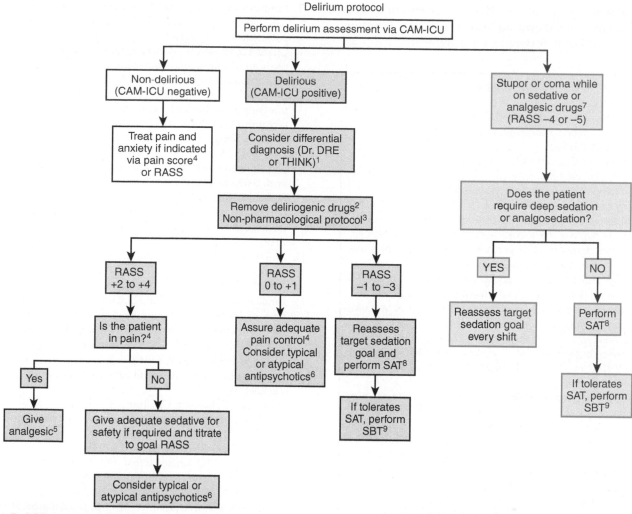

Delirium protocol

Perform delirium assessment via CAM-ICU

Non-delirious (CAM-ICU negative)

Treat pain and anxiety if indicated via pain score[4] or RASS

Delirious (CAM-ICU positive)

Consider differential diagnosis (Dr. DRE or THINK)[1]

Remove deliriogenic drugs[2] Non-pharmacological protocol[3]

RASS +2 to +4

Is the patient in pain?[4]

Yes — Give analgesic[5]

No — Give adequate sedative for safety if required and titrate to goal RASS

Consider typical or atypical antipsychotics[6]

RASS 0 to +1

Assure adequate pain control[4] Consider typical or atypical antipsychotics[6]

RASS −1 to −3

Reassess target sedation goal and perform SAT[8]

If tolerates SAT, perform SBT[9]

Stupor or coma while on sedative or analgesic drugs[7] (RASS −4 or −5)

Does the patient require deep sedation or analgosedation?

YES — Reassess target sedation goal every shift

NO — Perform SAT[8]

If tolerates SAT, perform SBT[9]

1. Dr. DRE:
   Diseases: Sepsis, CHF, COPD
   Drug Removal: SATs and stopping benzodiazepines/narcotics
   Environment: Immobilization, sleep and day/night orientation, hearing aids, eye glasses, noise
   THINK:
   Toxic Situations – CHF, shock, dehydration – Deliriogenic meds (tight titration) – New organ failure (liver, kidney, etc)
   Hypoxemia;
   Infection/sepsis (nosocomial), Immobilization
   Nonpharmacological interventions[3]
   K+ or Electrolyte problems
2. Consider stopping or substituting for deliriogenic medications such as benzodiazepines, anticholinergic medications (metoclopromide, H2 blockers, promethazine, diphenhydramine), steroids, etc.
3. See non pharmacological protocol – see below
4. If patient is non-verbal assess via CPOT or if patient is verbal assess via visual analog scale
5. Analgesia – Adequate pain control may decrease delirium. Consider opiates, non-steroidals, acetaminophen or gabapentin (neuropathic pain)
6. Typical or atypical antipsychotics. Thers is no evidence that haloperidol decreases the duratrion of delirium. Atypical antipsychotics may decrease the duration of delirium. Discontinue if high fever, QTc prolongation, or drug-induced rigidity.
7. Consider non-benzodiazepine sedation strategies (propofol or dexmedetomidine)
8. Spontaneous Awakening Trial (SAT) – If meets safety criteria (No active seizures, no alcohol withdrawal, no agitation, no myocardial ischemia, normal intracranial pressure, $FiO_2 \leq 70\%$)
9. Spontaneous Breathing Trial (SBT) – If meets safety criteria (No agitation, no myocardial ischemia, $FiO_2 \leq 50\%$, adequate inspiratory efforts, O_2 saturation $\geq 88\%$, no vasopressor use, PEEP ≤ 7.5 cm)

Non-pharmacological protocol[3]

Orientation
Provide visual and hearing aids
Encourage communication and reorient patient repetitively
Have familiar objects from patient's home in the room
Attempt consistency in nursing staff
Family engagement and empowerment

Environment
Sleep hygiene: Lights off at night, on during day.
Control excess noise (staff, equipment), earplugs
Early Mobilization and exercise
Music
Saturations >90%

Treat underlying metabolic derangements and infections

ABCDEF Bundle

http://www.icudelirium.org/medicalprofessionals.html

Fig. 88.3 An example of an empirical protocol used for the treatment of delirium in an intensive care unit setting. *CAM-ICU,* Confusion Assessment Method for the Intensive Care Unit; *CHF,* congestive heart failure; *COPD,* chronic obstructive pulmonary disease; *CPAP,* continuous positive airway pressure; *dx,* diagnosis; *PEEP,* positive end-expiratory pressure; *RASS,* Richmond Agitation-Sedation Scale. (From ICU Delirium and Cognitive Impairment Study Group (website). Resources: Delirium protocol. Vanderbilt University Medical Center. 2013. Courtesy Dr. E.W. Ely, http://www.icudelirium.org.)

drug-induced rigidity occurs. However, recent large, controlled studies have shown no benefit regarding decreasing duration of delirium or symptom management.

AUTHORS' RECOMMENDATIONS

- Delirium is a disturbance of consciousness and cognition occurring over a short period. It is associated with significantly increased morbidity and mortality in critically ill adults and children.
- Subtypes of delirium include hyperactive, hypoactive, and mixed. The subtype may carry a prognostic implication, with hyperactive having a better prognosis.
- Many risk factors are associated with delirium, and some of these are modifiable or preventable by the clinician, such as hypoxia, metabolic and electrolyte disturbances, infection, dehydration, hyperthermia, sepsis, psychoactive medications, and sleep deprivation.
- Various cellular and metabolic processes are proposed causes for delirium, all of which are probably interrelated.
- There are multiple validated assessment tools for delirium. Patients in the ICU must first be assessed for their level of sedation (with a scale such as the RASS) and then for the presence of delirium (with a scale such as the CAM-ICU or the ICDSC in adults and the pCAM-ICU, psCAM-ICU and CAP-D for children).
- Minimizing sedation by using tactics such as daily interruptions for sedation helps reduce the exposure to deliriogenic psychoactive medications.
- Benzodiazepines should be avoided in the ICU, except for the treatment of specific conditions. Alternatives for sedation include dexmedetomidine or propofol. Haloperidol and atypical antipsychotics may need to be utilized to control agitation but need to be discontinued as soon as possible, although additional studies are required to determine the role of these medications in preventing and treating delirium, given that they carry side effects.

REFERENCES

1. Dubois MJ, Bergeron N, Dumont M, Dial S, Skrobik Y. Delirium in an intensive care unit: a study of risk factors. *Intensive Care Med.* 2001;27(8):1297-1304.
2. Ely EW, Gautam S, Margolin R, et al. The impact of delirium in the intensive care unit on hospital length of stay. *Intensive Care Med.* 2001;27(12):1892-1900.
3. Pisani MA, Murphy TE, Van Ness PH, Araujo KL, Inouye SK. Characteristics associated with delirium in older patients in a medical intensive care unit. *Arch Intern Med.* 2007;167(15): 1629-1634.
4. Spronk PE, Riekerk B, Hofhuis J, Rommes JH. Occurrence of delirium is severely underestimated in the ICU during daily care. *Intensive Care Med.* 2009;35(7):1276-1280.
5. Traube C, Silver G, Reeder RW, et al. Delirium in critically ill children: an international point prevalence study. *Crit Care Med.* 2017;45(4):584-590.
6. Smith HAB, Gangopadhyay M, Goben CM, et al. Delirium and benzodiazepines associated with prolonged ICU stay in critically ill infants and young children. *Crit Care Med.* 2017;45(9): 1427-1435.
7. Pandharipande PP, Girard TD, Jackson JC, et al. Long-term cognitive impairment after critical illness. *N Engl J Med.* 2013;369(14):1306-1316.
8. Girard TD, Jackson JC, Pandharipande PP, et al. Delirium as a predictor of long-term cognitive impairment in survivors of critical illness. *Crit Care Med.* 2010;38(7):1513-1520.
9. Ely E, Shintani A, Truman B, et al. Delirium as a predictor of mortality in mechanically ventilated patients in the intensive care unit. *JAMA.* 2004;291:1753-1762.
10. Pisani M, Kong S, Kasl S, Murphy T, Araujo K, Van Ness P. Days of delirium are associated with 1-year mortality in an older intensive care unit population. *Am J Respir Crit Care Med.* 2009;180(11):1092-1097.
11. Shehabi Y, Riker R, Bokesch P, Wisemandle W. Delirium duration and mortality in lightly sedated, mechanically ventilated intensive care unit patients. *Crit Care Med.* 2010;38(12):2311-2318.
12. American Psychiatric Association. *Diagnostic and Statistical Manual of Mental Disorders.* 5th ed. DSM-5. Washington, DC: APA; 2013.
13. Pandharipande P, Cotton BA, Shintani A, et al. Motoric subtypes of delirium in mechanically ventilated surgical and trauma intensive care unit patients. *Intensive Care Med.* 2007;33(10):1726-1731.
14. Farina N, Smithburger P, Kane-Gill S. Screening and management of delirium in critically ill patients. *Hosp Pharm.* 2015;50(8):667-671.
15. Robinson TN, Raeburn CD, Tran ZV, Brenner LA, Moss M. The motor subtypes of post-operative delirium in the elderly. *Arch Surg.* 2011;146(3):295-300.
16. Kiely DK, Jones RN, Bergmann MA, Marcantonio ER. Association between psychomotor activity delirium subtypes and mortality among newly admitted postacute facility patients. *J Gerontol A Biol Sci Med Sci.* 2007;62(2):174-179.
17. Meagher D, Adamis D, Leonard M, et al. Development of an abbreviated version of the Delirium Motor Subtyping Scale (DMSS-4). *Int Psychogeriatr.* 2014;26(4):693-702.
18. Hughes CG, Brummel NE, Vasilevskis EE, Girard TD, Pandharipande PP. Future directions of delirium research and management. *Best Pract Res Clin Anaesthesiol.* 2012;26(3):395-405.
19. Ouimet S, Riker R, Bergeron N, Cossette M, Kavanagh B, Skrobik Y. Subsyndromal delirium in the ICU: evidence for a disease spectrum. *Intensive Care Med.* 2007;33(6):1007-1013.
20. Maldonado JR. Delirium pathophysiology: an updated hypothesis of the etiology of acute brain failure. *Int J Geriatr Psychiatry.* 2018;33(11):1428-1457.
21. Inouye SK, Charpentier PA. Precipitating factors for delirium in hospitalized elderly persons. Predictive model and interrelationship with baseline vulnerability. *JAMA.* 1996;275(11)852-857.
22. McNicoll L, Pisani MA, Zhang Y, Ely EW, Siegel MD, Inouye SK. Delirium in the intensive care unit: occurrence and clinical course in older patients. *J Am Geriatr Soc.* 2003;51(5):591-598.
23. Lin SM, Huang CD, Liu CY, et al. Risk factors for the development of early-onset delirium and the subsequent clinical outcome in mechanically ventilated patients. *J Crit Care.* 2008;23(3):372-379.
24. Katznelson R, Djaiani GN, Borger MA, et al. Preoperative use of statins is associated with reduced early delirium rates after cardiac surgery. *Anesthesiology.* 2009;110(1):67-73.
25. Pandharipande P, Shintani A, Hughes C, et al. Statin use and the daily risk of delirium in a prospective cohort of critically ill patients. *Am J Respir Crit Care Med.* 2012;185:A3646.

26. Morandi A, Hughes CG, Thompson JL, et al. Statins and delirium during critical illness: a multicenter, prospective cohort study. *Crit Care Med*. 2014;42(8):1899-1909.

27. Page VJ, David D, Zhao XB, et al. Statin use and risk of delirium in the critically ill. *Am J Respir Crit Care Med*. 2014;189(6):666-673.

28. Page VJ, Casarin A, Ely EW, et al. Evaluation of early administration of simvastatin in the prevention and treatment of delirium in critically ill patients undergoing mechanical ventilation (MoDUS): a randomised, double-blind, placebo-controlled trial. *Lancet Respir Med*. 2017;5(9):727-737.

29. Needham DM, Colantuoni E, Dinglas VD, et al. Rosuvastatin versus placebo for delirium in intensive care and subsequent cognitive impairment in patients with sepsis-associated acute respiratory distress syndrome: an ancillary study to a randomised controlled trial. *Lancet Respir Med*. 2016;4(3):203-212.

30. McPherson JA, Wagner CE, Boehm LM, et al. Delirium in the cardiovascular ICU: exploring modifiable risk factors. *Crit Care Med*. 2013;41(2):405-413.

31. Pandharipande P, Cotton BA, Shintani A, et al. Prevalence and risk factors for development of delirium in surgical and trauma intensive care unit patients. *J Trauma*. 2008;65(1):34-41.

32. Pandharipande P, Shintani A, Peterson J, et al. Lorazepam is an independent risk factor for transitioning to delirium in intensive care unit patients. *Anesthesiology*. 2006;104(1):21-26.

33. Patel SB, Poston JT, Pohlman A, Hall JB, Kress JP. Rapidly reversible, sedation-related delirium versus persistent delirium in the intensive care unit. *Am J Respir Crit Care Med*. 2014;189(6):658-665.

34. Girard TD, Thompson JL, Pandharipande PP, et al. Clinical phenotypes of delirium during critical illness and severity of subsequent long-term cognitive impairment: a prospective cohort study. *Lancet Respir Med*. 2018;6(3):213-222.

35. Bucerius J, Gummert JF, Borger MA, et al. Predictors of delirium after cardiac surgery delirium: effect of beating-heart (off-pump) surgery. *J Thoracic Cardiovasc Surg*. 2004;127(1):57-64.

36. Maldonado JR. Pathoetiological model of delirium: a comprehensive understanding of the neurobiology of delirium and an evidence-based approach to prevention and treatment. *Crit Care Clin*. 2008;24(4):789-856.

37. Cunningham C, Campion S, Lunnon K, et al. Systemic inflammation induces acute behavioral and cognitive changes and accelerates neurodegenerative disease. *Biol Psychiatry*. 2009;65(4):304-312.

38. van Gool WA, van de Beek D, Eikelenboom P. Systemic infection and delirium: when cytokines and acetylcholine collide. *Lancet*. 2010;375(9716):773-775.

39. van Munster BC, Bisschop PH, Zwinderman AH, et al. Cortisol, interleukins and S100B in delirium in the elderly. *Brain Cogn*. 2010;74(1):18-23.

40. Pfister D, Siegemund M, Dell-Kuster S, et al. Cerebral perfusion in sepsis-associated delirium. *Crit Care*. 2008;12(3):R63.

41. MacDonald A, Adamis D, Treloar A, Martin F. C-reactive protein levels predict the incidence of delirium and recovery from it. *Age Ageing*. 2007;36(2):222-225.

42. Hughes CG, Morandi A, Girard TD, et al. Association between endothelial dysfunction and acute brain dysfunction during critical illness. *Anesthesiology*. 2013;118(3):631-639.

43. McGrane S, Girard TD, Thompson JL, et al. Procalcitonin and C-reactive protein levels at admission as predictors of duration of acute brain dysfunction in critically ill patients. *Crit Care*. 2011;15(2):R78.

44. Westhoff D, Witlox J, Koenderman L, et al. Preoperative cerebrospinal fluid cytokine levels and the risk of postoperative delirium in elderly hip fracture patients. *J Neuroinflammation*. 2013;7(10):122.

45. Sanders RD. Hypothesis for the pathophysiology of delirium: role of baseline brain network connectivity and changes in inhibitory tone. *Med Hypotheses*. 2011;77(1):140-143.

46. Hshieh TT, Fong TG, Marcantonio ER, Inouye SK. Cholinergic deficiency hypothesis in delirium: a synthesis of current evidence. *J Gerontol A Biol Sci Med Sci*. 2008;63(7):764-772.

47. Plaschke K, Hill H, Engelhardt R, et al. EEG changes and serum anticholinergic activity measured in patients with delirium in the intensive care unit. *Anaesthesia*. 2007;62(12):1217-1223.

48. Jackson TA, Moorey HC, Sheehan B, Maclullich AM, Gladman JR, Lord JM. Acetylcholinesterase activity measurement and clinical features of delirium. *Dement Geriatr Cogn Disord*. 2017;43(1-2):29-37.

49. Trzepacz PT. Is there a final common neural pathway in delirium? Focus on acetylcholine and dopamine. *Semin Clin Neuropsychiatry*. 2000;5:132-148.

50. Tran TY, Dunne IE, German JW. Beta blockers exposure and traumatic brain injury: a literature review. *Neurosurg Focus*. 2008;25(4):E8.

51. Watne LO, Idland AV, Fekkes D, et al. Increased CSF levels of aromatic amino acids in hip fracture patients with delirium suggests higher monoaminergic activity. *BMC Geriatr*. 2016;16:149.

52. van der Mast RC, Fekkes D, Moleman P, Pepplinkhuizen L. Is postoperative delirium related to reduced plasma tryptophan? *Lancet*. 1991;338(8771):851-852.

53. Wurtman RJ, Hefti F, Melamed E. Precursor control of neurotransmitter synthesis. *Pharmacol Rev*. 1980;32(4):315-335.

54. Pandharipande P, Morandi A, Adams J, et al. Plasma tryptophan and tyrosine levels are independent risk factors for delirium in critically ill patients. *Intensive Care Med*. 2009;35(11):1886-1892.

55. Adams Wilson JR, Morandi A, Girard TD, et al. The association of the kynurenine pathway of tryptophan metabolism with acute brain dysfunction during critical illness. *Crit Care Med*. 2012;40(3):835-841.

56. Engel GL, Romano J. Delirium, a syndrome of cerebral insufficiency. *J Chronic Dis*. 1959;9(3):260-277.

57. Gibson GE, Peterson C. Aging decreases oxidative metabolism and the release and synthesis of acetylcholine. *J Neurochem*. 1981;37(4):978-984.

58. Robinson TN, Raeburn CD, Tran ZV, Angles EM, Brenner LA, Moss M. Postoperative delirium in the elderly: risk factors and outcomes. *Ann Surg*. 2009;249(1):173-178.

59. Keenan SP. Measuring level of sedation in the intensive care unit. *JAMA*. 2000;284(4):441-442.

60. Riker RR, Picard JT, Fraser GL. Prospective evaluation of the Sedation-Agitation Scale for adult critically ill patients. *Crit Care Med*. 1999;27(7):1325-1329.

61. Sessler CN, Gosnell MS, Grap M, et al. The Richmond Agitation-Sedation Scale: validity and reliability in adult intensive care unit patients. *Am J Respir Crit Care Med*. 2002;166(10):1338-1344.

62. Ely EW, Truman B, Shintani A, et al. Monitoring sedation status over time in ICU patients: reliability and validity of the Richmond Agitation-Sedation Scale (RASS). *JAMA*. 2003;289(22):2983-2991.

63. Bergeron N, Dubois MJ, Dumont M, Dial S, Skrobik Y. Intensive Care Delirium Screening Checklist: evaluation of a new screening tool. *Intensive Care Med.* 2001;27(5)859-864.

64. Ely E, Inouye S, Bernard G, et al. Delirium in mechanically ventilated patients: validity and reliability of the confusion assessment method for the intensive care unit (CAM-ICU). *JAMA.* 2001;286(21):2703-2710.

65. Inouye SK, van Dyck CH, Alessi C, Balkin S, Siegal AP, Horwitz RI. Clarifying confusion: the confusion assessment method. *Ann Intern Med.* 1990;113(12):941-948.

66. Pun BT, Gordon SM, Peterson JF, et al. Large-scale implementation of sedation and delirium monitoring in the intensive care unit: a report from two medical centers. *Crit Care Med.* 2005;33(6):1199-1205.

67. Khan BA, Perkins AJ, Gao S, et al. The Confusion Assessment Method for the ICU-7 Delirium Severity Scale: a novel delirium severity instrument for use in the ICU. *Crit Care Med.* 2017;45(5):851-857.

68. Smith HA, Boyd J, Fuchs DC, et al. Diagnosing delirium in critically ill children: validity and reliability of the Pediatric Confusion Assessment Method for the Intensive Care Unit. *Crit Care Med.* 2011;39(1):150-157.

69. Smith HA, Gangopadhyay M, Goben CM, et al. The Preschool Confusion Assessment Method for the ICU: valid and reliable delirium monitoring for critically ill infants and children. *Crit Care Med.* 2016;44(3):592-600.

70. Traube C, Silver G, Kearney J, et al. Cornell Assessment of Pediatric Delirium: a valid, rapid, observational tool for screening delirium in the PICU. *Crit Care Med.* 2014;42(3):656-663.

71. Haenggi M, Blum S, Brechbuehl R, Brunello A, Jakob SM, Takala J. Effect of sedation level on the prevalence of delirium when assessed with CAM-ICU and ICDSC. *Intensive Care Med.* 2013;39(12):2171-2179.

72. Marcantonio ER, Juarez G, Goldman L, et al. The relationship of postoperative delirium with psychoactive medications. *JAMA.* 1994;272(19):1518-1522.

73. Yoo SS, Hu PT, Gujar N, Jolesz FA, Walker MP. A deficit in the ability to form new human memories without sleep. *Nat Neurosci.* 2007;10(3):385-392.

74. Kamdar BB, King LM, Collop NA, et al. The effect of a quality improvement intervention on perceived sleep quality and cognition in a medical ICU. *Critical Care Med.* 2013;41(3):800-809.

75. Inouye SK, Bogardus Jr ST, Charpentier PA, et al. A multicomponent intervention to prevent delirium in hospitalized older patients. *N Engl J Med.* 1999;340(9):669-676.

76. Bogardus Jr ST, Desai MM, Williams CS, Leo-Summers L, Acampora D, Inouye SK. The effects of a targeted multicomponent delirium intervention on postdischarge outcomes for hospitalized older adults. *Am J Med.* 2003;114(5):383-390.

77. Devlin JW, Skrobik Y, Gélinas C, et al. Clinical practice guidelines for the prevention and management of pain, agitation/sedation, delirium, immobility, and sleep disruption in adult patients in the ICU. *Crit Care Med.* 2018;46(9):e825-e873.

78. Kollef MH, Levy NT, Ahrens TS, Schaiff R, Prentice D, Sherman G. The use of continuous i.v. sedation is associated with prolongation of mechanical ventilation. *Chest.* 1998;114(2):541-548.

79. Kress JP, Pohlman AS, O'Connor MF, Hall JB. Daily interruption of sedative infusions in critically ill patients undergoing mechanical ventilation. *N Engl J Med.* 2000;342(20):1471-1477.

80. Marra A, Ely EW, Pandharipande PP, Patel MB. The ABCDEF bundle in critical care. *Crit Care Clin.* 2017;33(2):225-243.

81. Barnes-Daly MA, Phillips G, Ely EW. Improving hospital survival and reducing brain dysfunction at seven California community hospitals: implementing PAD guidelines via the ABCDEF bundle in 6,064 patients. *Crit Care Med.* 2017;45(2):171-178.

82. Ely EW, Baker AM, Dunagan DP, et al. Effect on the duration of mechanical ventilation of identifying patients capable of breathing spontaneously. *N Engl J Med.* 1996;335(25):1864-1869.

83. Girard TD, Kress JP, Fuchs BD, et al. Efficacy and safety of a paired sedation and ventilator weaning protocol for mechanically ventilated patients in intensive care (Awakening and Breathing Controlled trial): a randomised controlled trial. *Lancet.* 2008;371(9607):126-134.

84. Jackson JC, Girard TD, Gordon SM, et al. Long-term cognitive and psychological outcomes in the Awakening and Breathing Controlled trial. *Am J Respir Crit Care Med.* 2010;182(2):183-191.

85. Marcantonio ER, Goldman L, Orav EJ, Cook EF, Lee TH. The association of intraoperative factors with the development of postoperative delirium. *Am J Med.* 1998;105(5):380-384.

86. Pandharipande PP, Pun BT, Herr DL, et al. Effect of sedation with dexmedetomidine vs. lorazepam on acute brain dysfunction in mechanically ventilated patients: the MENDS randomized controlled trial. *JAMA.* 2007;298(22):2644-2653.

87. Pandharipande PP, Sanders RD, Girard TD, et al. Effect of dexmedetomidine versus lorazepam on outcome in patients with sepsis: an a priori-designed analysis of the MENDS randomized controlled trial. *Crit Care.* 2010;14:R38.

88. Riker RR, Shehabi Y, Bokesch PM, et al. Dexmedetomidine vs. midazolam for sedation of critically ill patients: a randomized trial. *JAMA.* 2009;301(5):489-499.

89. Serafim RB, Bozza FA, Soares M, et al. Pharmacologic prevention and treatment of delirium in intensive care patients: a systematic review. *J Crit Care.* 2015;30(4):799-807.

90. Su X, Meng ZT, Wu XH, et al. Dexmedetomidine for prevention of delirium in elderly patients after non-cardiac surgery: a randomised double-blind, placebo-controlled trial. *Lancet.* 2016;388(10054):1893-1902.

91. Wu M, Liang Y, Dai Z, Wang S. Perioperative dexmedetomidine reduces delirium after cardiac surgery: a meta-analysis of randomized controlled trials. *J Clin Anesth.* 2018;27(50):33-42.

92. Jacob SM, Ruokonen E, Grounds RM. Dexmedetomidine vs. midazolam or propofol for sedation during prolonged mechanical ventilation: two randomized controlled trials. *JAMA.* 2012;307(11):1151-1160.

93. Devlin JW, Fraser GL, Ely EW, Kress JP, Skrobik Y, Dasta JF. Pharmacological management of sedation and delirium in mechanically ventilated ICU patients: remaining evidence gaps and controversies. *Semin Respir Crit Care Med.* 2013;34(2):201-215.

94. van Eijk MM, Roes KC, Honing ML, et al. Effect of rivastigmine as an adjunct to usual care with haloperidol on duration of delirium and mortality in critically ill patients: a multicentre, double-blind, placebo-controlled randomised trial. *Lancet.* 2010;376(9755):1829-1837.

95. Schreiber MP, Colantuoni E, Bienvenu OJ, et al. Corticosteroids and transition to delirium in patients with acute lung injury. *Crit Care Med.* 2014;42(6):1480-1486.

96. Sauër AM, Slooter AJ, Veldhuijzen DS, van Eijk MM, Devlin JW, van Dijk D. Intraoperative dexamethasone and delirium after cardiac surgery: a randomized clinical trial. *Anesth Analg.* 2014;119(5):1046-1052.

97. Wolters AE, Veldhuijzen DS, Zaal IJ, et al. Systemic corticosteroids and transition to delirium in critically ill patients. *Crit Care Med.* 2015;43(12):e585-e588.

98. Keh D, Trips E, Marx G, et al. Effect of hydrocortisone on development of shock among patients with severe sepsis: the HYPRESS randomized clinical trial. *JAMA.* 2016;316(17):1775-1785.

99. Morris PE, Goad A, Thompson C, et al. Early intensive care unit mobility therapy in the treatment of acute respiratory failure. *Crit Care Med.* 2008;36(8):2238-2243.

100. Schweickert WD, Pohlman MC, Pohlman AS, et al. Early physical and occupational therapy in mechanically ventilated, critically ill patients: a randomised controlled trial. *Lancet.* 2009;373(9678):1874-1882.

101. Needham DM, Korupolu R, Zanni JM, et al. Early physical medicine and rehabilitation for patients with acute respiratory failure: a quality improvement project. *Arch Phys Med Rehabil.* 2010;91(4):536-542.

102. Morandi A, Vasilevskis EE, Pandharipande PP, et al. Inappropriate medication prescriptions among elders surviving an intensive care unit (ICU) hospitalization. *J Am Geriatr Soc.* 2013;61(7):1128-1134.

103. Reade MC, Eastwood GM, Bellomo R, et al. Effect of dexmedetomidine added to standard care on ventilator-free time in patients with agitated delirium. *JAMA.* 2016;315(14):1460-1468.

104. Page VJ, Ely EW, Gates S, et al. Effect of intravenous haloperidol on the duration of delirium and coma in critically ill patients (HOPE-ICU): a randomised, double-blind, placebo-controlled trial. *Lancet Respir Med.* 2013;1(7):515-523.

105. Prakanrattana U, Prapaitrakool S. Efficacy of risperidone for prevention of postoperative delirium in cardiac surgery. *Anaesth Intensive Care.* 2007;35(5):714-719.